J. A. PETER PARÉ, M.D.

Director, Respiratory Division,
McGill University, Montreal, Quebec

ROBERT G. FRASER, M.D.

Professor, Diagnostic Radiology,
University of Alabama in Birmingham,
Birmingham, Alabama

SYNOPSIS OF DISEASES OF THE CHEST

W. B. SAUNDERS COMPANY

Philadelphia, London, Toronto, Mexico City, Rio de Janeiro, Sydney, Tokyo

W. B. Saunders Company: West Washington Square
                            Philadelphia, PA   19105

                            1 St. Anne's Road
                            Eastbourne, East Sussex BN21 3UN, England

                            1 Goldthorne Avenue
                            Toronto, Ontario M8Z 5T9, Canada

                            Apartado 26370—Cedro 512
                            Mexico 4, D.F., Mexico

                            Rua Coronel Cabrita, 8
                            Sao Cristovao Caixa Postal 21176
                            Rio de Janeiro, Brazil

                            9 Waltham Street
                            Artarmon, N.S.W. 2064, Australia

                            Ichibancho, Central Bldg., 22-1 Ichibancho
                            Chiyoda-Ku, Tokyo 102, Japan

Library of Congress Cataloging in Publication Data

Paré, J. A. Peter.

Synopsis of diseases of the chest.

1. Chest—Diseases.   I. Fraser, Robert G., 1921–
   II. Title.

RC941.P28 1983   617'.54   82–10616

ISBN 0–7216–7068–7

Synopsis of Diseases of the Chest   ISBN   0-7216-7068-7

Last digit is the print numnber: 9   8   7   6   5   4   3

This book is dedicated
to
OUR WIVES, ANNE and JOANNE

ACKNOWLEDGMENTS

The preparation of this book has required almost four years—a period of tedium and stoicism mixed with gratification. As might be expected in a task requiring the abridgment of a manuscript to approximately one-quarter its original size, the labor has been chiefly ours. However, the many steps necessary to the final product required the unselfish and enthusiastic contributions of several hands and minds, and the support and encouragement we received from many of our friends are duly acknowledged and greatly appreciated.

It is not possible to overstate our gratitude to our secretaries, who handled magnificently the tedious and necessarily exacting task of transcribing new manuscript and who cheerfully coped with all of the innumerable problems encountered. Mrs. Maria Karpowicz and Ms. Anna-Maria Messenzehl of the Montreal Chest Hospital Center and the Royal Victoria Hospital in Montreal and Miss Sheila Walker and Mrs. Carolyn Bryant of the University of Alabama Medical Center in Birmingham all exhibited exemplary patience and devotion in accomplishing this thorny chore. Miss Walker and Mrs. Bryant also carried out the tedious job of recording, filing, checking, and final validation of all references, a frustrating chore that they performed with meticulous accuracy.

Although the majority of illustrations were lifted from the second edition of *Diagnosis of Diseases of the Chest*, the few new figures required the superb photographic work of Susan Gray of the Department of Radiology, University of Alabama Medical Center in Birmingham. Joanne Fraser did much of the art work for the CT figures.

Throughout our labors, we have received tremendous support and cooperation from the publishers, notably Ms. Suzanne Boyd and Mr. Jack Hanley, who affectively and sympathetically minimized the many obstacles we encountered.

Finally, and with immense gratitude, we recall the patience and understanding displayed by our wives and children throughout our labors. Without their continuous encouragement, this book surely would not have been completed, and we acknowledge their many virtues with much love.

J. A. PETER PARÉ
ROBERT G. FRASER

PREFACE

In the preface to the second edition of our book *Diagnosis of Diseases of the Chest* published in 1977/78, we commented on the vast amount of new knowledge that had accumulated since the publication of the first edition in 1970 and on the resultant expansion of the book from two to four volumes. At the time, we recognized the risk that the book might become purely a reference work but remained hopeful that its organization would enable readers to be highly selective in the material they wished to read, thus preserving the textbook perspective. This has proven not to be the case: the more than 2300 pages of text have proven a formidable barrier to its acceptance as a tome to be read and digested from cover to cover. As a result, we recognized the need for a book that could be used as a text and yet would include information sufficient to a basic understanding of chest disease. Thus was born the idea of a synopsis, an abbreviated coverage of chest disease aimed at the resident in respiratory medicine or radiology, the senior medical student, or any physician or surgeon seeking a concise review of the subject.

The experience of writing the second edition taught us that the addition of new material to a book can be relatively straightforward; since there are few limitations placed on authors by the publisher, length is seldom a problem. By contrast, condensing manuscript can be a formidable task, as we soon discovered, and the abridgment of four volumes to one has proven to be a four-year undertaking. Not only has it been necessary to sacrifice much material—to "separate the wheat from the chaff"—but also to update virtually all sections of the book by adding new material that has appeared in the literature since 1978, compounding the effort to keep the book as short as possible. The 19 chapters in this book follow the same order as the major work, which we hope will make it easy to locate an expanded version of any subject in the four-volume set, if desired. The subdivision of virtually all descriptions of chest disease into etiology, pathogenesis, pathologic characteristics, roentgenographic manifestations, and clinical manifestations has been adhered to, permitting readers to cull the material appropriate to their discipline.

The last chapter is dedicated to tables of differential diagnosis and "decision trees." For purposes of brevity, only nine of 17 tables of differential diagnosis listed in the larger work have been included, comprising those patterns of disease that we have assumed offer the greatest challenge in differential diagnosis. Each table provides a nosologic approach to the differential diagnosis of disease of that pattern, including only minimal reference to clinical status. The decision trees that follow each table introduce into the diagnostic equation the clinical presentation of the patient, affording the reader an opportunity to correlate roentgenographic pattern with clinical signs and symptoms in order to reach the most likely diagnosis.

Since our intention has been to produce a textbook rather than a reference work, we have been very selective in our choice of referenced material, restricting the bibliography to those articles and books that we regarded as most essential for further reading on specific topics. Bibliographies have been placed at the end of each chapter. Illustrations have been reduced in both size and number to reveal only essential features of roentgenographic abnormality. Figures depicting normal and pathologic anatomy of the thorax by computed tomography were few in number in *Diagnosis of Diseases of the Chest,* an omission that has been corrected in *Synopsis.*

We have been concerned for many years with the wide range of terminology employed by physicians in the description of roentgenographic abnormalities in the thorax. In order to clarify the confusion, the Fleischner Society formed a Committee on Nomenclature several years ago that designed a glossary of roentgenologic words and terms. This task is nearing completion, and, with the permission of the Fleischner Society, we are including at the end of this book a glossary of selected words that we hope our readers will refer to and use.

Finally, we invite our readers to inform us of differences of opinion they may have with the contents of this book. It is only through such interchange of information and opinion that we can hope to establish on a firm basis the knowledge necessary for a full understanding of respiratory disease.

J. A. Peter Paré
Robert G. Fraser

CONTENTS

6

INFECTIOUS DISEASES OF THE LUNGS

10

PULMONARY HYPERTENSION AND EDEMA

11

DISEASES OF THE AIRWAYS

12

THE PNEUMOCONIOSES AND CHEMICALLY-INDUCED
LUNG DISEASES

13

DISEASES OF THE THORAX CAUSED BY EXTERNAL PHYSICAL AGENTS 616

14

DISEASES OF THE CHEST OF UNKNOWN ORIGIN 640

1

The Normal Chest

THE AIRWAYS AND PULMONARY VENTILATION

GENERAL CONSIDERATIONS

The function of the bronchial tree is to conduct air to the alveolar surface, where gas transfer takes place between respired air and gas dissolved in the blood of the alveolar capillaries. The inspired air should be evenly distributed to the alveolar capillary bed, with minimal resistance to flow. The greater part of the length and the smaller part of the volume of the respiratory tract are concerned only with the conduction of air; this part comprises the trachea and bronchi (whose walls contain cartilage) and nonalveolated bronchioles (no cartilage). The remainder of the respiratory tract, comprising the large bulk of the lungs, is concerned with both conduction and gas exchange, the terminal unit (the alveolus) being the only structure whose function is uniquely that of gas exchange. Thus the airway system can be subdivided into three zones, each with different structural and functional characteristics.

The conductive zone includes the trachea, bronchi, and nonalveolated bronchioles in which there is virtually no diffusion of gas through the well-developed wall. The nonparenchymatous pulmonary structures constitute this zone along with the pulmonary arteries and veins, lymphatic channels, nerves, connective tissues of the peribronchial and perivascular spaces, the interlobular septa, and the pleura.

The transitory zone, as its name implies, carries out both conductive and respiratory functions. It consists of the respiratory bronchioles, alveolar ducts, and alveolar sacs, all of which conduct air to the most peripheral alveoli. In addition, alveoli that arise from their walls are the site of gas exchange. This zone and the respiratory zone constitute the parenchyma, the spongy respiratory portion of the lung.

The respiratory zone consists of the alveoli, whose sole function is the exchange of gases between air and blood.

The descriptions that follow of the geometry, dimensions, and morphology of these zones are based on material gleaned largely from two sources—the publications of Horsfield, Cumming, and their associates,[1-3] and the 1963 monograph, "Morphometry of the Human Lung," by E. R. Weibel.[4]

THE CONDUCTIVE ZONE

GEOMETRY

Cumming and his associates[2] point out that usually, in nature, the distribution and collection of nutrients requires a branching system, and that biological branching systems show great similarity. For example, deciduous trees must provide large surface areas of leaves exposed to sunlight, so that photosynthesis can proceed with appropriate supplies transported from the ground. Observing a large oak in winter and in summer reveals how well the tree's branching system accomplishes this. Similar circumstances exist in the lung, in which a branching system of conducting airways is essential to transport the maximal amount of air, with minimal resistance, to the respiratory zone. Among the methods for comparative description of biological branching systems, the ones most conveniently applicable to the lung probably are those proposed by Strahler[5] and by Horsfield and Cumming.[6]

1

The basic branching pattern of the bronchial tree is dichotomous (*i.e.*, the parent branch divides into two parts). In any such system, the branching may be symmetric (two branches equal in all respects) or asymmetric (variation in the diameter or length of branches in a given generation, or in the number of divisions to the end branches, or a combination of these). In the bronchial tree, there is variation in both branch diameters and the number of divisions; thus, the system is one of *asymmetric dichotomy*.

DIMENSIONS

In their study of a cast of normal human lung, Horsfield and Cumming measured the length and diameter of every structure to an arbitrary anatomic site defined as the first point at which the measured diameter was ≤ 0.7 mm (700 μ); they measured the length of each branch between the two points of bifurcation, and the diameter at midpoint. Counting distally from the trachea, the number of generations to 0.7-mm airways ranged from 8 to 25; *i.e.*, the lobular branch with the shortest path length was reached after eight dichotomous branchings and the longest path length after 25. Analysis of the frequency distribution of divisions distally to lobular branches (Figure 1–1) showed a stepwise increase from division eight to a peak at 14, and a decrease from 15 to 25.[1]

A similar law is applicable to the *diameter* of the branching system, decreasing from the largest to the smallest in strict geometric progression so that the diameter in any given order is predictable. Similarly, the *length* of bronchial tree segments follows a fixed principle; the length of any branch can be found by dividing its parent's length by 1.49. The *volume* of airways from the carina to 0.7-mm branches was computed to be 71 ml. This volume, added to that of the upper airways from the mouth to the carina (80 ml), gives a total volume of

airways almost identical to the volume of anatomic dead space as determined by physiologic techniques.

In summary, two methods of counting (the Strahler and Horsfield-Cumming systems) permit accurate description of the tracheobronchial tree's dimensions (number, length, diameter, and volume of branches). Employing the Strahler system, counting proximally from branches 0.7 mm in diameter, the *number of orders* in the bronchial tree is 17. The branching ratio is 2.8 (*i.e.*, each branch gives rise to 2.8 daughter branches); this applies to all orders except the trachea (order 17), the main bronchi (order 16), and airways less than 0.7 mm in diameter (orders 1 through 5, respiratory bronchioles that have a regular dichotomous branching pattern). The *diameter* of the branching system decreases geometrically from the largest to the smallest, the diameter of an order being its parent's diameter divided by 1.4 (*i.e.*, half the value for the branching law). As with the branching law, this diameter law applies to order 6 and greater; below this, the airway diameter (0.7 mm, approximately) ceases to diminish. The *length* of the bronchial segments similarly is arranged according to a fixed relationship, the length of any branch being the length of its parent's divided by 1.49. Path lengths from the carina to the distal respiratory bronchiole range from 8 cm to 22 cm. The *volume* of airways from the carina to branches 0.7 mm in diameter is approximately 70 ml; the total volume (including mouth to carina) is 150 ml.

MORPHOLOGY

General Structure

The cartilages of the main-stem bronchi are horseshoe-shaped, as in the trachea (Figure 1–2). In lobar and segmental bronchi they consist of irregularly shaped plates and form much of the wall. As the pathway proceeds distally, the

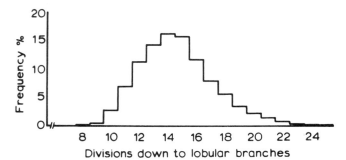

Figure 1–1. **Frequency Distribution of the Number of Divisions Down to the Lobular Branches.** (Reprinted from Horsfield, K., and Cumming, G.: J. Appl. Physiol., *24*:373, 1968, with permission of the authors, editor, and publisher.)

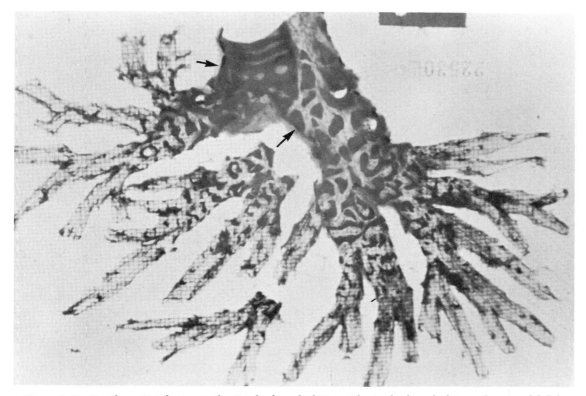

Figure 1–2. Cartilage Distribution in the Tracheobronchial Tree. The tracheobronchial tree of a normal left lung removed at necropsy has been dissected free, laid out on a wire mesh, and stained for cartilage. *Note* that the horseshoe-shaped cartilages in the trachea *(upper arrow)* extend for a short distance into the upper lobe bronchus but that the cartilage in the lower lobe bronchus *(lower arrow)* and peripheral bronchi forms discrete islands.

cartilages become progressively smaller and less complete until finally, in bronchi about 1 to 2 mm in diameter, they surround only the origins of the bronchioles arising from them. The bronchial muscle lies between the open ends of the horseshoe-shaped cartilages in the main bronchi, where it is attached to the inner perichondrium about 1 mm from their ends. As the cartilages become smaller and more irregular, the attachments extend further along the cartilages until, finally the bronchi are encircled by muscle. In the smaller bronchi and the bronchioles, the muscle bundles form a crisscrossed, spiral, geodesic network.

Bands of longitudinal elastic fibers form dense bundles in the membrana propria, causing a ridging of the bronchi that becomes less conspicuous distally. These fibers connect with circularly arranged elastic fibers that are in relation to the muscle layer, and, in the smaller bronchioles, through the circular elastic fibers to the surrounding alveolar and septal elastic tissues, thus forming a continuum through the lungs. It is believed that this radial tethering mechanism plays a major part in maintaining patency of the bronchioles. Connective tissue surrounds the bronchi to the point at which the bronchiolar walls become continuous with lung parenchyma; this peribronchial tissue is continuous with the periarterial connective tissue and, near the hilum, with the perivenous connective tissue. At the hilum and at the periphery of the lobules, the interlobular (septal) connective tissue is continuous with the subpleural connective tissue.

Ultrastructure

The bronchial mucosa contains four types of epithelial cells; ciliated pseudostratified columnar cells, goblet cells, "brush" cells (which bear microvilli at their free surfaces but no cilia), and "basal" cells. The last-named, which occupy the roughly triangular areas between the narrowed bases of the tall goblet and the ciliated cells, are thought to be multipotential, acting as stem cells from which the other types derive. The epithelial cells lie on a basement membrane that separates them from the lamina propria, which consists of a loose framework of collagen,

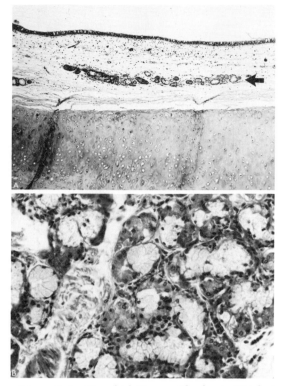

Figure 1–3. Bronchial Mucous Glands. *A,* Histologic section of a bronchial wall (low power magnification) showing from above downward the mucosa, submucosa containing mucous glands *(arrow)*, and cartilage. *B,* At higher power (× 250), a mucous gland is seen to contain two main types of cell, goblet or mucous cells (pale staining) and serous cells (deep staining). (Courtesy of Dr. James Hogg, University of British Columbia, and Dr. Nai-San Wang, McGill University, Montreal.)

elastic fibers, and reticular fibers, with an extensive plexus of nerves and blood vessels running through it. Within the lamina propria are various types of cells with specific physiologic functions: mast cells, which are a source of histamine, heparin, and serotonin; plasma cells, which are believed to be responsible for the production of IgA (an immunoglobulin which is in higher concentration in bronchial secretions than in the blood); and neutrophils, lymphocytes, and macrophages, which undoubtedly play an important role in host defense.

Extending into the lamina propria are the mucous glands, which develop from cells with an elaborate endoplasmic reticulum system and which produce most of the materials secreted into the bronchial lumen (Figure 1–3). Although the bronchial mucous glands belong chiefly to the lamina propria, many of them extend out to the cartilage or muscle wall. It has been estimated that an adult man has approximately 6000 tracheobronchial mucous glands, or about one gland per sq mm (Figure 1–4). Mucous glands extend to the small bronchi, roughly paralleling the distribution of cartilage. The goblet cells also are secretory, but they supply only a relatively small amount of mucus to the tracheobronchial tree. No differences have been demonstrated in the secretions from mucous glands and goblet cells,[6] and the teleological basis of these cells' coexistence is unknown. Goblet cells have basally located nuclei. Above the nuclei are prominent Golgi regions, in which secretory granules are formed; these

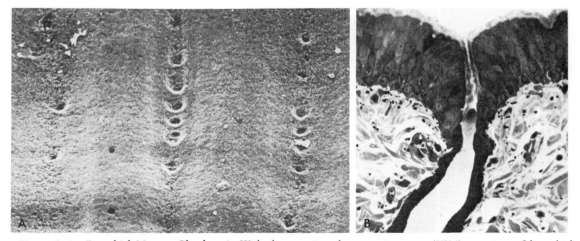

Figure 1–4. Bronchial Mucous Glands. *A,* With the scanning electron microscope (SEM), openings of bronchial glands appear as pits and form regular rows at the bottom of the longitudinal folds on the bronchial mucosa. (Swine SEM, × 250.) *B,* Cross section of a pitlike depression showing a normal opening of the bronchial gland; only a few ciliated cells extend into the duct. (Dog TBS, × 400.) *B* reprinted from Wang, Nai-San, et al.: Am. J. Pathol., 67:571, 1972, with permission of the authors and editor.)

granules are crowded into the upper parts of the cells until they are discharged. Goblet cells are more numerous proximally and commonly appear in clumps; there may be one goblet cell to four or five ciliated cells in the large airways in normal adults, compared with one to two for many hundreds of ciliated cells in the bronchioles. In the terminal bronchioles, the goblet cells have disappeared and the epithelium has become flattened. Here are found specialized low columnar cells (Clara cells), which bulge into the lumen of the bronchiole in the form of tongue- or flame-shaped cytoplasmic processes; it is probable that bronchiolar surfactant originates from these cells.

The periphery of the bronchial wall is composed of cartilage and muscle, the proportion of muscle increasing as the airway lumen decreases.

MUCUS RHEOLOGY

Biochemical Characteristics of Tracheobronchial Secretions

Secretions from the tracheobronchial tree are expectorated as sputum. Estimates of their volume in the normal human adult range from 10 to 100 ml per day.[6] Sputum consists of mucus (deriving from the mucous and serous cells of the bronchial glands and goblet cells), tissue fluid transudate, saliva, cellular material, enzymes, and immunoglobulins. Mucus is composed of about 95 per cent water and 1 per cent each of carbohydrate, protein, lipid, and inorganic material. Other than water, the main components are mucopolysaccharides—glycoproteins linked covalently to peptide by xylose-serine bonds to form mucopolysaccharide-protein complexes.

The mucous blanket plays a major role in protecting the lower respiratory tract from contamination with particles that are either inert or in the form of microorganisms. Antimicrobial activity also has been attributed to various enzymes and immunoglobulins in the tracheobronchial secretions.

Except under conditions of considerable irritation or infection, the principal immunoglobulin in tracheobronchial secretions is IgA. Immunofluorescent studies suggest that IgA in mucus is produced by plasma cells in the respiratory mucosa.

Expectorated bronchial secretions contain some cellular material, chiefly desquamated epithelial cells, alveolar macrophages, and polymorphonuclear leukocytes, whose numbers vary according to the nature of the irritant.

Physical Characteristics of Tracheobronchial Secretions

The chemical composition of tracheobronchial secretions and their content of corpuscular elements (blood cells, bacteria, and desquamated epithelium) make it incorrect to employ the term "viscosity" from a strict rheologic viewpoint. Both saliva and tracheobronchial secretions respond to applied forces not only by flowing, as do pure Newtonian liquids, but also by deforming, as do ideal elastic solids. The more suitable term to describe the physical properties of tracheobronchial secretions, therefore, is "viscoelastic."[7] The viscosity and elasticity of sputum vary considerably, not only from day to day but even during one day, and viscosity increases with decreasing humidity. Furthermore, purulent sputum is more viscous but less elastic than mucoid sputum, and the decrease in viscoelasticity with time at room temperature is considerably more rapid in purulent than in mucoid samples.

The Mucous Transport Mechanism

The mucociliary apparatus consists of innumerable cilia, which arise from the surface of pseudostratified columnar epithelial cells and lie in a fluid "sol layer" deep to less fluid mucous material, the "gel layer." Each ciliated cell has approximately 275 cilia (Figure 1–5), which beat at approximately 20 beats per second.[8] Ciliary motion consists of an effective stroke and a recovery stroke, both of which synchronize with the motions of cilia of neighboring cells.[9] As proposed by the Lucas-Douglas model of bronchial mucous transport,[8, 10] normally the cilia lie in a bath of clear serous fluid, supposedly of low viscosity; within this medium the cilia beat, propelling the mucus (gel layer), which floats like a blanket on the surface of the fluid in a manner analogous to a raft supported and propelled by many hands beneath it. Although the mucous blanket is separated from the surface of the epithelial cells by the less viscous sol layer, it is continuous with mucus projecting from the mouths of the mucous glands. Under normal conditions, the elastic component of mucous secretions does not impair the flow of the mucous blanket; in chronic bronchitis, however, the increased viscoelastic resistance of the mucus anchors the blanket into the mouths of the mucous glands, so that the rhythmic ciliary action can only stretch the extensions.

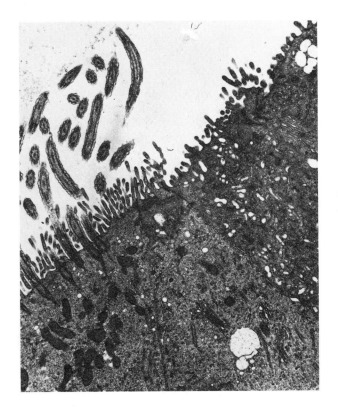

Figure 1–5. Epithelial Cells from a Major Bronchus. Note multiple cilia extending into the lumen. (Swine TEM, × 17,400.) (Reprinted from Wang, Nai-San, et al.: Am. J. Pathol., 67:571, 1972, with permission of the authors, editor, and publisher.)

Normal mucous transport is not synonymous with normal ciliary activity.[9] Changes in viscosity, pH, and perhaps even quantity of secretion can lead to a reduction in or complete cessation of transport despite normal ciliary motility. According to the Lucas-Douglas model,[10] mucostasis could result from reduced thickness of the sol layer (in which case the gel layer could clog the cilia) or from its increased thickness and the consequent removal of the gel layer from contact with the cilia. It is believed that the sol layer originates in the alveoli;[8] secretions from mucous glands, and goblet cells are added to form the gel layer when the sol layer reaches the terminal bronchioles, the most distal site of mucus production in the conducting system.

THE TRANSITORY ZONE

GEOMETRY

The bronchial cast studied by Horsfield and Cumming[1] permitted assessment of airways less than 0.7 mm in diameter under a dissecting microscope. These investigators made observations down to the last order of respiratory bronchioles—that is, the airway giving rise to an alveolar duct. They studied two lobules in each of 14 bronchopulmonary segments, measuring the length and diameter of every structure down to the terminal respiratory bronchioles (a total of 452 pathways).

In contrast to the asymmetric dichotomous branching system of the major airways, branching of structures distal to the terminal bronchioles was symmetrically dichotomous for three divisions. The walls of these airways bore the impressions of alveolar openings, whose number increased distally until, in the third generation, more than half the wall was occupied by openings. In many cases a side devoid of openings related to a contiguous branch of the pulmonary artery. Finally, there were several generations of alveolar ducts; their walls were distinctive, consisting entirely of rounded protuberances, the site of alveolar openings.

DIMENSIONS

Horsfield and Cumming[1] reported that each terminal bronchiole gave rise to an average of three generations of respiratory bronchioles (range, two to seven), and each distal respiratory bronchiole bore a structure that averaged six dichotomous divisions (range, three to nine). The alveolar ducts and sacs were computed to total 23×10^6. Each alveolar sac gave rise to 10 alveoli. The computed number of distal (last-order) respiratory bronchioles supplied by the trachea was 233,941.

Measurement of the diameter and length of each structure revealed a length-diameter ratio of approximately 1.5—that is, an airway whose length was 3 had a diameter of 2. Instead of continuous diminution with order, the diameter remained unaltered down to the alveolar sac.

MORPHOLOGY

As previously stated, the respiratory bronchioles, alveolar ducts, and alveolar sacs constituting the transitory zone carry out the dual function of conduction and gas exchange, the latter being performed by alveoli, which arise directly from the walls of these structures in increasing numbers distally; in fact, the walls of the alveolar ducts and sacs are formed entirely of alveoli.

THE RESPIRATORY ZONE

GEOMETRY

Weibel has greatly increased our knowledge of the geometry of the alveoli and their relationship to alveolar ducts,[4] and much of the following information is from his monograph on morphometry of the lung and reports of his earlier work with Gomez.[11]

Alveoli are small lateral outpouchings of respiratory bronchioles, alveolar ducts, and alveolar sacs. Malpighi, in 1697, likened the shape of the alveolus to the cell of a honeycomb. Weibel asserts that the honeycomb can serve as an acceptable alveolar model if one imagines it molded around the cylindrical surface of the alveolar duct, thereby transforming the hexagonal prism of the cell into a pyramidal wedge of the air sleeve surrounding the duct. The dome of an alveolus has a rather complex structure, usually consisting of more than three facets, formed by close packing of several alveoli belonging to adjacent alveolar ducts; therefore, each alveolus may have more than one vertex. The size and shape of the facets vary considerably, the arrangement more nearly resembling that of closely packed bubbles of soap foam (irregular polyhedral configuration). In general, three facets have a common line of junction at an average angle of 120 degrees, and it can be assumed that these facets are more or less flat if there is no pressure difference between contiguous alveoli.

DIMENSIONS

Until very recently it was generally accepted that the number of alveoli in the human lung remained fairly constant at about 300×10^6.[4, 12] However, in a study of 42 lungs free of chronic disease, from 32 subjects aged 19 to 85, Angus and Thurlbeck[13] recorded much greater variation in the number of alveoli; their computed totals ranged from 212×10^6 to 605×10^6 (mean, 375×10^6). Further, they found a highly significant relationship ($P < 0.001$) between alveolar number and body length. Since it is generally believed that new alveoli are added after birth, but that this multiplication ceases before somatic growth stops[12] (*i.e.*, alveolar number is determined before body length), it must be inferred that alveolar number is not governed solely by body length and lung volume. Angus and Thurlbeck[13] speculated that this might be genetically controlled and at least partly predetermined by future body height.

The lung contains only approximately 24×10^6 alveoli at birth, after which this number rapidly increases for some time.[12] It is currently held that alveolar multiplication ceases at the age of 8 years. Alveolar *dimensions* were obtained by Weibel[4] by direct measurement with an eyepiece micrometer from thin histologic sections. In adults, both maximal diameter and total depth (measured from the opening onto the alveolar duct or sac) averaged 250 to 300 μ. Total alveolar *surface area* determined by Weibel was approximately 70 to 80 sq m, which he considered consistent with an alveolar number of 300×10^6. In a study of nonemphysematous lungs, Thurlbeck estimated the total alveolar surface area to range from 40 to 100 sq m, depending upon body size.

MORPHOLOGY

The true lung parenchyma, composed of the alveoli and their capillaries, is set off sharply from surrounding connective tissue by a limiting membrane of dense elastic tissue and collagen that merges into the elastic fibers of alveolar walls.[14] The membrane forms a boundary separating the alveolar parenchyma from the loose connective tissue of the bronchovascular tree, interlobular septa, and pleura; at this last site the tissue constitutes the subpleural

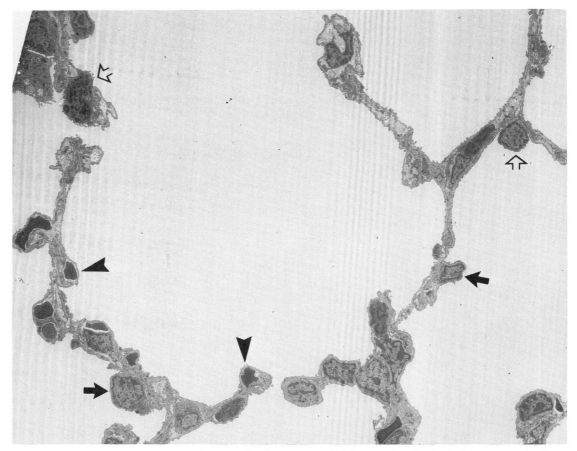

Figure 1–6. Single Pulmonary Alveolus. Visualized are type I *(solid arrows)* and type II *(open arrows)* cells, as well as alveolar capillaries *(arrowheads).* A pore of Kohn can be seen near the bottom of the figure. (Mouse lung, × 2300.) (Courtesy of Dr. Nai-San Wang, McGill University, Montreal.)

vascular layer. Blood vessels, nerves, and lymphatics lie in these compartments of loose connective tissue, which together form the interstitial space. Pressure may be more negative in this space than in the pleural cavity; air and fluid readily accumulate there.

In mammals, the alveolar wall is lined by a continuous layer of epithelial cells of two morphologically distinct types, type I and type II alveolar cells (Figure 1–6). Type II cells are responsible for the formation of the surface active agent, surfactant. A third cell type, the alveolar macrophage, is not truly a part of the alveolar wall, since it lies free within the alveolus, but it is convenient to describe its morphology and function here.

Type I Alveolar Epithelial Cell

This cell *(synonyms:* small alveolar cell, squamous lining cell, membranous pneumonocyte, and type A epithelial cell) lines most of the alveolar surface. It has a central nucleus surrounded by a rather thick cytoplasm, which stretches out in thin winglike processes to form part of the alveolar wall (Figure 1–7). These cells average 0.5 μ in thickness, the thinnest part of the cytoplasm measuring approximately 0.1 μ. This cytoplasmic process and the intracapillary erythrocytes are separated by a thin basement membrane composed of minute amounts of interalveolar substance and capillary endothelium. In some areas the basement membranes of the type I cells and the capillary endothelium appear to be fused, with little or no interalveolar substance: it is postulated that gas exchange takes place here.[15]

A feature of the alveolar septum that has been emphasized by Fishman[16] is its division into two functional zones when viewed on edge through the electron microscope—a "thin side" for gas exchange and a "thick side" for both support and water exchange (Figure 1–8). The difference between the two sides depends upon

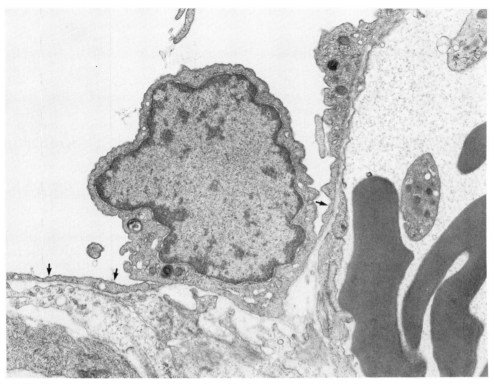

Figure 1–7. Type I Alveolar Epithelial Cell. Note the large nucleus and scanty cytoplasm that attenuates on both sides over the alveolar surface *(arrows)*. (Courtesy of Dr. Nai-San Wang, McGill University, Montreal.)

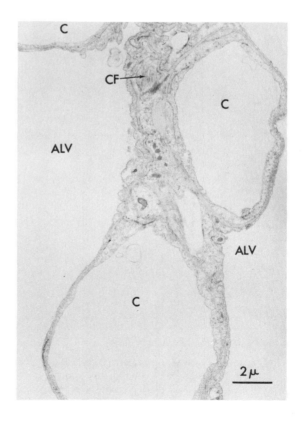

Figure 1–8. Edge-on View of the Alveolar-Capillary Membrane. Three capillaries *(C)* are present, suspended in the septum between alveoli *(ALV)*. On the right side of the middle capillary, the alveolar septum is thin; the opposite side is thick and contains supporting elements, including collagen fibers *(CF)*, in the interstitial space between the capillary and alveolar basement membranes. (TEM, × 10,000.) (Reprinted from Fishman, A. P.: Circulation, *46*:390, 1972, with permission of the author and editor and the American Heart Association, Inc.)

the amount of interstitial tissue separating the capillary endothelium from the alveolar epithelium. The thin side has very little interstitium, ranging from 300 to 500 Å in thickness, and thus consists basically of three anatomic layers: the alveolar epithelium, the capillary endothelium, and interposed fused basement membranes. In contrast, between the basement membranes of the thick side is an abundant interstitium consisting of collagen and elastic fibers, fibroblasts, macrophages, and ground substance. Thus, on this side, five layers separate alveolar air from capillary blood—alveolar epithelium, basement membrane, interstitial tissue, basement membrane, and capillary endothelium. This thick side not only provides support for the capillary network but constitutes an essential component of the water-exchanging apparatus of the lung, operating to expedite the movement of water and protein from the interstitial space of the alveolar septum toward the lymphatic capillaries.[16] It is clear that any one alveolus must consist of a multitude of thin and thick sides, creating what might be envisaged conceptually as an undulating contour of the alveolar surface. This concept of alveolar wall structure is of considerable importance in pulmonary edema.

In the type I cells, phagocytic ability is limited or absent.[17] Unlike type II cells, they have no microvilli protruding from their surfaces; they also appear to lack the capacity to regenerate, which is such a characteristic feature of type II cells, and, in fact, they may regenerate as transformed type II cells.

Intercellular clefts between type I alveolar epithelial cells are rather long and tortuous[18] in contrast to those between capillary endothelial cells (see page 37). In a study of the ultrastructural basis of alveolar-capillary membrane permeability, Schneeberger-Keeley and Karnovsky[18] described several areas along the course of the clefts in which the outer leaflets of the apposed membranes appeared fused, usually toward the luminal end of the cleft (Figure 1–9). These areas of fusion were observed consistently in all normal planes of section and were considered to be the "tight" junctions (zonulae occludentes) that represent the permeability barrier to the passage of low molecular weight proteins across the alveolar-capillary membrane. These tight junctions were in contrast to the "open" junctions (maculae occludentes) that characterized the intercellular clefts between capillary endothelial cells (Figure 1–10).

Type II Alveolar Epithelial Cell

The type II cell (*synonyms:* granular pneumonocyte, great or large alveolar cell, cuboidal secretory-type cell, corner alveolar cell, type B alveolar epithelial cell) is roughly cuboidal and often occupies corners in the alveolus[17] (Figure 1–11). It is 10 to 15 μ thick and usually contains

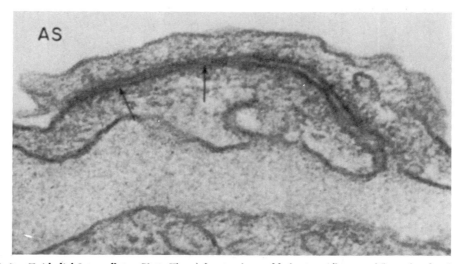

Figure 1–9. Epithelial Intercellular Cleft. The cleft extends roughly horizontally inward from the alveolar space *(AS)*. In several areas *(arrows)* the outer leaflets of the bounding unit membranes appear fused. This fusion usually occurs toward the alveolar end of the cleft. (Uninjected mouse lung; TEM, × 140,000). (Reprinted from Schneeberger-Keeley, E. E., and Karnovsky, M. J.: J. Cell Biol., 37:781, 1968, with permission of the authors and editor and by copyright permission of the Rockefeller University Press.)

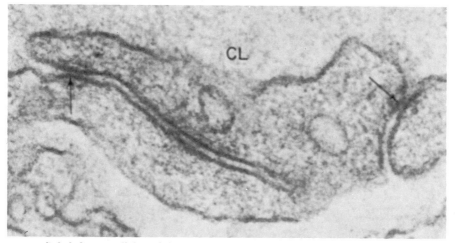

Figure 1–10. Endothelial Intercellular Cleft. A portion of a capillary lumen *(CL)* and two endothelial intercellular clefts can be seen. In the junction on the left *(arrow)* there is a distinct gap between the bounding unit membranes, whereas in the one on the right *(arrow)* details are obscured. (Uninjected mouse lung; TEM, × 140,000.) (Reprinted from Schneeberger-Keeley, E. E., and Karnovsky, M. J.: J. Cell Biol., 37:781, 1968, with permission of the authors and editor and by copyright permission of the Rockefeller University Press.)

numerous lamellar osmiophilic inclusion bodies.[17] Normally, the alveolus contains five to eight type II cells; in contrast to type I cells, however, they proliferate abundantly after diffuse alveolar injury caused by oxygen or various fumes.[15] Also in contrast to type I cells, type II cells have microvilli.

It is widely believed[15, 17, 19] that the osmiophilic inclusion bodies in type II alveolar epithelial cells are the precursors or storage form

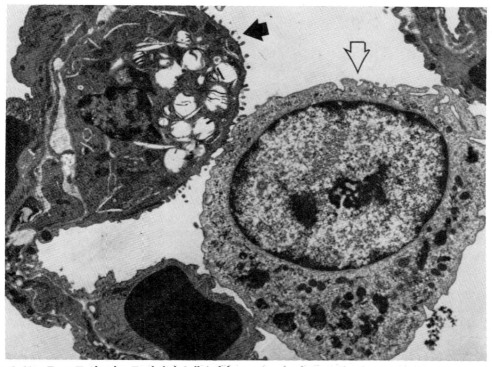

Figure 1–11. Type II Alveolar Epithelial Cell *(solid arrow)* **and Adjacent Alveolar Macrophage** *(open arrow)*. The contrasting ultrastructural features of each cell are well demonstrated. In this alveolus, the pneumonocyte lies on the flattened alveolar surface rather than in a corner location. (TEM, original magnification × 9900.) (Reprinted from Esterley, J. R., and Faulkner, C. S., II: Am. Rev. Resp. Dis., 101:869, 1970, with permission of the authors, editor, and publisher.)

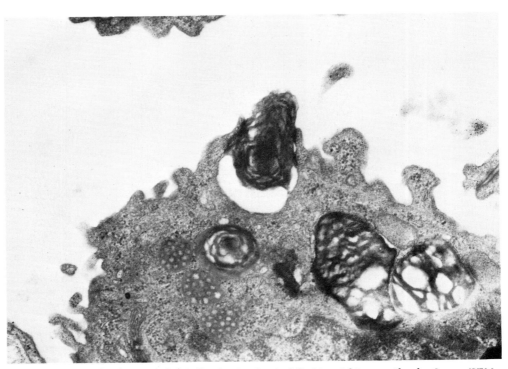

Figure 1–12. **Type II Alveolar Epithelial Cell Releasing Osmiophilic Material into an Alveolar Space.** (SEM, original magnification × 2800.) (Courtesy of Dr. Nai-San Wang, McGill University, Montreal.)

of pulmonary surfactant. Wang has shown by transmission electron microscopy the extrusion of osmiophilic material into an alveolar space (Figure 1–12).

The Alveolar Macrophage

This large cell, which may measure 12 μ in its longest diameter,[15] is known as the free cell of the lung because of its lack of attachment to a basement membrane and its presence in lung washings of the tracheobronchial tree. The primary role of the alveolar macrophage is that of host defense—the protection of the lung and the body from damage induced by microorganisms and inert particulate matter that reach the alveoli.

It has been estimated that 90 per cent of foreign material deposited on the mucosa of the tracheobronchial tree is cleared in less than 1 hour.[20] Most of this material is phagocytized by alveolar macrophages and disposed of via the tracheobronchial tree. The continual production of surfactant and its tendency to remain as a monolayer may provide a moving surface for macrophages and dust, thereby aiding their excretion via the airways. Similarly, respiratory excursion and, possibly, wavelike peristaltic patterns of alveolar fluid may help to transport macrophages that have ingested foreign material.

The very active complement of lysosomal enzymes in the alveolar macrophages plays a major role in the destruction of microorganisms. After an alveolar macrophage ingests a bacterium, its lysosomes attach themselves to the phagosomal membrane surrounding the bacterium; the lysosomal membrane becomes continuous with the phagosomal membrane; and the lytic enzymes kill and digest the bacterium. Foreign particles other than bacteria (*e.g.*, used surfactant)[19] are removed in a similar fashion from the alveoli by phagocytic activity of the alveolar macrophage (Figure 1–13).

SURFACTANT

On the basis of his observations that less pressure change was required to fully distend a fluid-filled than an air-filled lung, von Neergaard postulated a surface tension within the alveoli. Macklin recognized the need for a substance to regulate "surface tension" in the alveoli and surmised that it was secreted by a large alveolar epithelial cell, which he called a

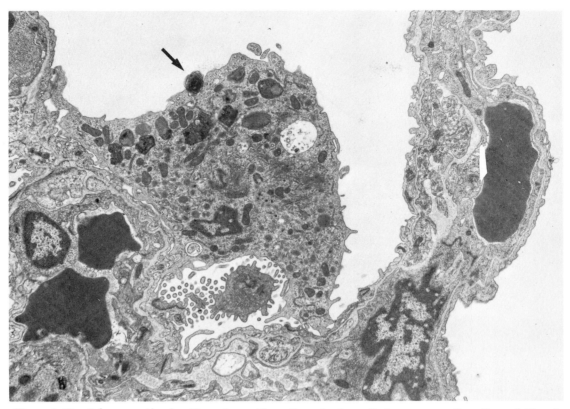

Figure 1–13. Pulmonary Alveolar Macrophage. View of an alveolar wall showing a capillary *(lower left)* and a macrophage on the alveolar surface engulfing osmiophilic material *(arrow)*. (TEM of mouse lung, × 9000.) (Courtesy of Dr. Nai-San Wang, McGill University, Montreal.)

"granular pneumocyte." Recent work employing tissue freezing, fixation of tissues through the vascular system, and technical improvements in electron microscopy has permitted definite identification of this acellular lining in all mammalian species studied, including man.[21, 22] In contrast to their polyhedral or pentagonal shape after conventional methods of tissue preparation, the alveoli appear spherical after rapid freezing, when fixed by vascular perfusion, or when viewed through the pleura of living animals. The common denominator of the three methods of inspection is the presence of air in the alveoli, which molds macrophages, epithelium, capillaries, and alveolar lining fluid into a continuous curved surface that probably represents the configuration consistent with the lowest surface energy. When the alveolar spaces are filled with fluid fixative, surface forces are eliminated and alveolar topography becomes dependent upon tissue and hemodynamic factors.

According to Gil and Weibel,[22] the acellular layer covering the alveolar surface consists of two functionally different components: (a) a film facing the alveolar air space, which is composed of densely spaced, highly surface-active phospholipids, and (b) deep to this film, a layer containing surface-active phospholipids in a different physicochemical configuration, possibly linked to proteins (Figure 1–14).

The composition of the pulmonary surface-active material was first identified in 1961 by Klaus and associates,[23] who concluded that the main component of the alveolar phospholipid was dipalmitoyl phosphatidylcholine (DPPC), also known as dipalmitoyl lecithin (DPL).

Electron microscopic and radioautographic studies have provided much circumstantial evidence linking osmiophilic inclusion bodies of the granular pneumocyte with surfactant.[19] Although the major clinical interest in surfactant relates to its underproduction and the resultant respiratory distress syndrome, the focus of attention has been extended by the finding that alveolar proteinosis *(see* Chapter 14) is related to overproduction of osmiophilic material by the type II alveolar cells or the formation of an

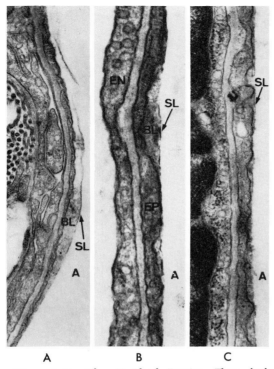

Figure 1–14. The Air-Blood Barrier. Three high-power magnifications show an extracellular duplex lining layer. Note the convexity of the surface in *A* and its flatness in *B* and *C*. These micrographs also demonstrate different appearances of the osmiophilic superficial layer *(SL)*. *BL* = base layer; *EN* = capillary endothelial cell; *EP* = alveolar epithelial cell; *A* = alveolus. (TEM, *A*, × 49,200; *B*, × 84,720; *C*, × 53,800.) (Reprinted from Gil, J., and Weibel, E. R.: Resp. Physiol., 8:13, 1969, with permission of the authors and editor.)

amount exceeding the capacity of the lungs to remove it.

Surfactant has a very rapid rate of turnover: in studies with dipalmitoyl lecithin labeled with radioactive palmitic acid, its half-life in normal adults has been reported as ranging from 14 hours[21] to somewhat less than 2 days.[19] It has been known for some time through chemical analysis of lipids that the concentration of surfactant is higher in the newborn than in the adult;[24] the rate of phospholipid synthesis reaches a peak at term and right after birth, declining rapidly to normal adult levels shortly thereafter. As pointed out by Avery,[25] pulmonary surfactant must be present at the moment of birth; otherwise every breath necessarily would resemble the first breath. Pulmonary surfactant allows for creation of a functional residual capacity.

An indicator of fetal lung development is the ratio of lecithin to sphingomyelin in amniotic fluid, a ratio that may prove to be a valuable guide as an index of the risk of neonatal respiratory distress. Warren and associates[26] found that the level of palmitic acid in amniotic fluid 24 hours or less before delivery clearly distinguishes those infants who are likely to develop respiratory distress syndrome from those who are mature. Palmitic acid measurement is rapid and simple and shows good agreement with the lecithin-sphingomyelin ratio. Thus, some methods of recognizing *in utero* the likelihood of respiratory distress syndrome (RDS) developing in the neonatal period obviously are of value.

THE LUNG UNIT

GENERAL ANATOMIC CONSIDERATIONS

The question of which portion of the lung parenchyma constitutes the "unit" of lung structure is still controversial, since each of the three basic units—the primary lobule, the secondary lobule, and the acinus—possesses characteristics that suit one set of circumstances better than another. As we shall attempt to show, however, the structure most uniformly acceptable for descriptive purposes, at least from the point of view of the roentgenologist and the physiologist, is the pulmonary acinus.

Of the many subdivisions of lung parenchyma that have been proposed as the lung unit (other than the acinus), those of William Snow Miller[27] have gained widest acceptance. He subdivided the parenchyma into two basic units, the primary and secondary lobules.

THE PRIMARY PULMONARY LOBULE OF MILLER

The primary lobule arises from the last respiratory bronchiole and consists of a series of alveolar ducts, atria, alveolar sacs, and alveoli, together with their accompanying blood vessels and nerves. Since there are approximately 23 million primary lobules in the human lung, it is clear that this unit is too small to be visualized roentgenographically when consolidated, and thus is of no practical roentgenologic significance.

THE SECONDARY PULMONARY LOBULE OF MILLER

The secondary lobule is defined as the smallest discrete portion of the lung that is surrounded by connective tissue septa.[27] Since the septa vary in size and extent, the size of the lobule varies; for example, it has been estimated that the number of primary lobules in a secondary lobule ranges from 30 to 50. The secondary lobule is irregularly polyhedral and is 1 to 2.5 cm in diameter. The septa dividing the lungs into lobules are most numerous in the lateral and anterior surfaces of the lower lobes, virtually nonexistent along the interlobar fissures and the posterior and mediastinal aspects of the lungs, and poorly developed in the central portion of the lungs. Although Heitzman and his colleagues[28, 29] regard the secondary pulmonary lobule as the basic unit of lung structure and function and hold that most pulmonary diseases are best considered in terms of this unit's pathology, we take exception to this view for two reasons: (1) the lobule varies greatly in size and distribution and exists in discrete form only on the lung surface; and (2) the secondary lobule seldom is recognizable roentgenographically as a structural unit (a fact, incidentally, with which Heitzman and his associates concur). Except for such uncommon events as the consolidation of a single secondary lobule—for example, by a pulmonary infarct—it is only when edematous fluid or other pathologic tissue occupies the interlobular septa and renders them visible as septal lines (B lines of Kerley) that the volume of lung between two lines can be recognized as a secondary lobule. We suggest that these two limitations negate the usefulness of Miller's definition for purposes of roentgenologic interpretation or for pathologic-roentgenologic correlation.

THE PULMONARY ACINUS

In the bronchial pathway to the lung periphery, the last purely conducting structure is the terminal bronchiole. The portion of lung distal to the terminal bronchiole is the acinus (Figure 1–15), which comprises respiratory bronchioles, alveolar ducts, alveolar sacs, and alveoli—the transitory and respiratory zones of the lung whose geometry, dimensions, and morphology were described earlier. Rindfleisch, who introduced the concept of the pulmonary acinus in 1872, likened it to a glandular structure possessing a round or oval body attached to an excretory duct like a berry on a stalk (Figure 1–16). According to Pump, the acinus measures approximately 7.5 × 8.5 mm on casts of lung inflated at a pressure equivalent to expiration.[30] This is somewhat larger than the 7.4-mm mean diameter reported by Gamsu and associates[31] in their roentgenographic study of the pulmonary acinus of lungs inflated and air-dried at a constant pressure of 30 cm of water, roughly equivalent to total lung capacity (*see* further on).

CHANNELS OF PERIPHERAL AIRWAY COMMUNICATION

Alveolar Pores

Pores of Kohn are present in the lungs of most mammals, in numbers varying with the species. In the human lung they are openings, or discontinuities, in the alveolar wall, about 3 to 13 μ in diameter; since the width of the

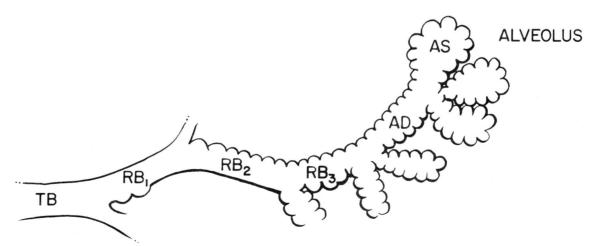

Figure 1–15. Component Parts of the Acinus. *TB* = terminal bronchiole. *RB* = respiratory bronchiole. *AD* = alveolar duct. *AS* = alveolar sac. (From Thurlbeck, W. M. *In* Sommers, S. C. (ed.): Pathology Annual: Nineteen Sixty-eight. New York, Appleton-Century-Crofts, 1968, p. 377.)

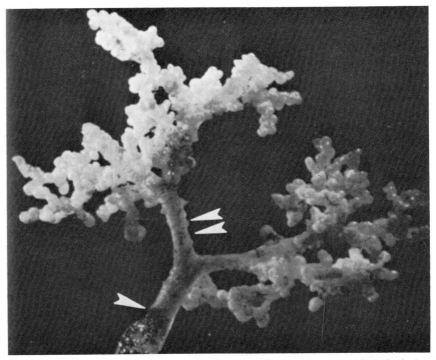

Figure 1–16. Cast of an Acinus Incompletely Filled with Resin. The smooth terminal bronchiole *(single arrowhead)* divides into two respiratory bronchioles, the upper one of which *(double arrowheads)* shows alveolar markings. After two or three generations the respiratory bronchioles divide to give rise to alveolar ducts, which are completely surrounded by alveoli. The rounded protuberances that are produced by partial filling of the alveoli with the resin are seen on the peripheral parts of the cast. (Reprinted from Horsfield, K., and Cumming, G.: J. Appl. Physiol., 24:373, 1968, with permission of the authors, editor, and publisher.)

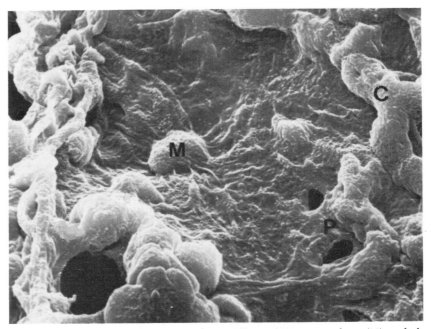

Figure 1–17. Surface of an Alveolus. Note surrounding capillaries *(C)*, a macrophage *(M)*, and alveolar pores *(P)*. (SEM, × 3650.) (Courtesy of Dr. Nai-San Wang, McGill University, Montreal.)

alveolar wall is dependent on lung volume and the degree of capillary engorgement, the width of the pores also varies with these factors. They are situated in intercapillary spaces and are lined with alveolar epithelium. Epithelial junctions are commonly if not invariably present on both sides of the pores, most of which are closely surrounded by capillary loops (Figure 1–17).[32] Pores are not present in the lungs of fetuses or newborn infants but increase rapidly in number with age. In the adult, a few alveoli have no pores; the majority contain one to six.

Canals of Lambert

Accessory bronchiolar-alveolar communications between alveoli and airways larger than the terminal bronchioles were first described by Lambert,[33] and their presence has been confirmed by others. These tubular structures are lined with epithelium; in lungs fixed in deflation they range in diameter from "practically closed" to 30 μ. The physiologic significance of these structures is not known, but obviously they provide an accessory route for the passage of air directly from bronchioles into alveoli.

Direct Airway Anastomoses

In both canine and human lungs, particles considerably larger than either pores of Kohn or canals of Lambert pass through collateral channels in lung parenchyma. Polystyrene spheres up to 64 μ have been passed through collateral channels in excised human lungs. Martin,[34] who observed the passage of insufflated India ink aerosols from one segment of a dog's lobe into an adjacent segment, reported that the particles were deposited only on collateral respiratory bronchioles that differed in several respects from Lambert's canals; however, his illustrations indicate that the collateral pathways were in fact first generation alveolar ducts.[32, 34] Although their precise anatomic nature is not clear, these channels are found relatively frequently and, because of their large size, may contribute significantly to collateral ventilation.

COLLATERAL VENTILATION

Even though we are still uncertain of the route by which air passes from one lung unit—acinus, lobule, segment, or lobe—to a contiguous unit, it has long been known that collateral ventilation occurs in the lungs of most mammalian species. In 1931, Van Allen and his colleagues[35] showed that air drift occurs readily between intralobar segments, but that interlobar drift occurs only when lobes are overdistended. More recently, a study of excised human lungs[36] demonstrated interlobar collateral air drift in three quarters of the normal lungs and in almost all the lungs with any degree of emphysema; the drift occurred throughout the whole range of lung volumes.

The anatomic site of the operative collateral channels is of major importance: if the obstructed unit is ventilated via a collateral respiratory bronchiole, the P_{O_2} would be higher than if collateral ventilation occurred from more distal parenchymal tissue, in which inspired air has been in contact with capillaries and thus has undergone gaseous exchange.

Resistance to air flow through collateral channels is much lower in emphysematous than in normal lungs; in fact, in excised emphysematous lungs, air flow resistance is much less through collateral channels than through regular conducting airways.[36]

THE ACINUS AS A ROENTGENOLOGIC UNIT

Since an acinus is visible macroscopically, it is reasonable to assume its visibility roentgenologically when completely or partially filled with contrast material or inflammatory exudate. In 1924, Aschoff suggested that consolidation of a single acinus by tuberculous inflammatory exudate or granulation tissue results in a rosette-like appearance, which he termed the "acino-nodose" lesion (Figure 1–18). However, it was not until recently that the precise roentgenologic nature of the acinus was established. Gamsu and his colleagues investigated the feasibility of roentgenographic visualization of individual acini in human lung.[31] Using a special tantalum suspension, they progressively opacified two or more segments of normal excised lungs distal to a wedged catheter, obtaining sequential roentgenograms on fine-grain film until almost total opacification was achieved. By correlating roentgenographic, microradiographic, and histologic appearances, they identified and differentiated terminal and respiratory bronchioles (Figure 1–19) and thus visualized individual acini. Progressive filling of a single acinus initially produced a rosette appearance and eventually a spherical lesion.

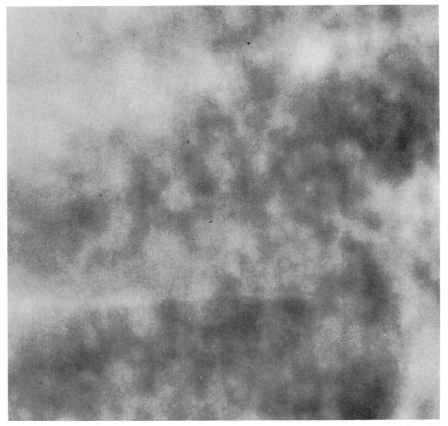

Figure 1–18. Acinar Shadows. Magnified view of a tomographic section of the right upper lobe of a patient with bronchogenic spread of tuberculosis from a cavity in the right lower lobe (not illustrated). On the original roentgenogram, individual acinar shadows measured 4 to 5 mm in diameter.

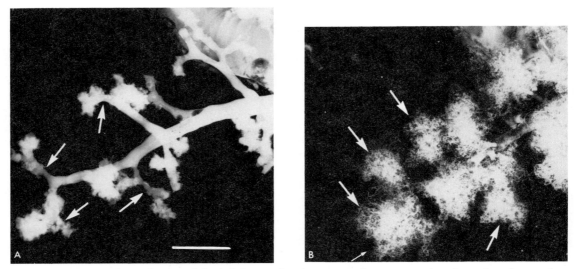

Figure 1–19. Bronchographic Morphology of the Peripheral Airways and Acinus. *A,* Selected area from the periphery of a bronchogram on a normal human lung removed at necropsy and opacified with a tantalum suspension. *Arrows* indicate terminal bronchioles, the majority of which are smooth-walled. *B,* Roentgenogram after air drying of the lung. There has now been further opacification of the intra-acinar airways. *Arrows* indicate partially opacified acini that can be related to the terminal bronchioles in *A*. The marker in *A* represents 5 mm. (Reprinted from Gamsu, G., et al.: Invest. Radiol., 6:171, 1971, with permission of the authors, editor, and publisher.)

Measurements of 25 acini revealed a mean diameter of 7.4 mm, in the range 6 to 10 mm. (These figures represent acinar caliber at a volume roughly equivalent to total lung capacity, since the lungs were fixed in inflation at a transpulmonary pressure of 30 cm of water.)

In the light of these facts and of previous discussions of the morphology and function of the lung parenchyma, we propose three reasons for accepting the acinus as a roentgenologic unit:

1. It is roentgenologically visible.

2. It is recognizable throughout the entire lung (in contrast to the secondary lobule, which is present in only the peripheral 2 to 3 cm or "cortex" of the lung).

3. It provides a useful correlation with function, since it constitutes the gas exchange (respiratory as well as conductive) portion of the lung.

THE ACINUS AS A FUNCTIONAL UNIT

As defined, the lung unit (analogous to the renal nephron) is that portion of the parenchyma distal to the terminal bronchiole. This definition is highly acceptable to both anatomists and roentgenologists, but is there evidence that this portion of the lung is also a functional unit? Most physiologists describe the alveolus as the unit of the lung. In so doing, however, they equate this not with the anatomic alveolus but with a hypothetical unit which, because of our lack of knowledge of correlation between physiology and anatomy, cannot be defined morphologically. In fact, it would be unrealistic to consider the structural alveolus as a physiologic unit. Each alveolus is one of a family of about ten[1] which arise from a common alveolar sac and which receive from a common arteriole capillaries that interconnect the alveoli.[37] It is unlikely that, in normal circumstances, the behavior of any one alveolus differs from that of its "siblings." Thus it seems likely that Miller's primary lobule, comprising the alveolar duct and its ramifications that arise from a last-order respiratory bronchiole, is the smallest portion that can be considered in the concept of a physiologic unit of lung function. Farther up the bronchial tree, at the level of the terminal bronchiole, a greater portion of the lung is included as a unit of function, since there are some 400 alveolar duct units distal to this point. Do all the alveoli that make up this acinus behave similarly? This question cannot

be answered yet, although accumulating evidence in the areas of both structure and physiology suggests that they do (as is discussed in relation to ventilation-perfusion ratios). For this reason, and in order to envisage a physiologic counterpart of the morphologic and roentgenologic unit, the basic functioning unit of the lung is taken to be the acinus—*i.e.*, all the lung parenchyma distal to the terminal bronchiole.

ROENTGENOLOGY OF THE AIRWAYS

It is of obvious importance for physicians interested in diseases of the chest to be familiar with the terminology and general spatial distribution of the bronchi and of the bronchopulmonary segments they supply. However, the number of variations from the norm of subdivision of the bronchial tree precludes detailed consideration of the subject in this book. In addition, we feel that a thorough understanding of pulmonary disease requires more familiarity with the anatomy of bronchopulmonary segments—the zones or regions of the lung supplied by the segmental bronchi—than with detailed knowledge of bronchial branching, since the former is only roughly dependent upon the latter.

In this section, therefore, we will present a standard nomenclature of bronchopulmonary anatomy and describe the prevailing pattern of segmental bronchial branching. Minor variations in the pattern that occur fairly frequently will be indicated.

In 1943 Jackson and Huber[38] published a nomenclature of the bronchial segments that was widely adopted and remains the generally accepted terminology in North America (Figures 1–20B and 1–22B).

Through common usage, the designation "main bronchi" is applied to the major bronchi arising from the bifurcation of the trachea down to the origin of the upper lobe bronchus on each side, and "intermediate bronchus" to the segment between the right upper lobe bronchus and the origins of the right middle and lower lobe bronchi.

THE TRACHEA AND MAIN BRONCHI

The trachea is, to all intents and purposes, a midline structure; a slight deviation to the right after entering the thorax is a normal finding and should not be misinterpreted as evidence of displacement (Figure 1–20). Its walls are parallel except on the left side just above the bifurcation, where the aorta commonly impresses a smooth indentation; rarely, the azygos vein causes a smaller indentation at the tracheobronchial angle on the right side. Bronchographically, the trachea, main bronchi, and intermediate bronchus have a smoothly serrated contour, created by the indentations of the horseshoe-shaped cartilage rings at regular intervals along these structures. A deficiency of the cartilage rings (the open end of the horseshoe) is closed by a pliable membranous sheath which produces a flat contour posteriorly.

In a recent computed tomographic study of the trachea, Kittredge[39] has shown considerable variability in the shape, position, and relationships of the trachea to other structures. Instead of the expected horseshoe configuration in cross section, the trachea may be round, oval, or concave posteriorly. Knowledge of these variations is of obvious importance in assessing the presence or absence of disease.

On a series of 350 roentgenograms of roughly equal numbers of male and female asymptomatic adults aged 30 to 80 years, we measured the anteroposterior and transverse dimensions of the tracheal air column 2 cm above the projected top of the aortic arch; the mean values were 19.5 mm (range, 11 to 30) and 17.5 mm (range, 11 to 26), respectively (unpublished data). Surprisingly, there were only negligible differences in transverse or anteroposterior dimensions on roentgenograms exposed at full inspiration and maximal expiration.

The trachea divides into the two major bronchi at the carina. The angle of bifurcation is varied and is most acute in asthenic subjects. In adults, the course of the right main bronchus distally is more direct than the left—a fact of considerable importance in relation to aspiration. By contrast, it has been shown[40] that in children the main bronchi arise from the trachea symmetrically up to the age of 15 years, following which the left bronchial angle increases; this symmetry explains the relatively equal incidence of right- and left-sided aspiration of foreign bodies in children compared with adults. In adults, the carinal angle ranges from 41 to 71 degrees in males (mean, 56.4) and from 41 to 74 degrees in females (mean, 57.7). The transverse diameter of the right main bronchus at total lung capacity is greater than that of the left (15.3 mm, compared with 13.0 mm[41]), although its length before the origin of the upper

lobe bronchus is shorter (average 2.2 cm, compared with 5 cm on the left).

The air column of the trachea, both major bronchi, and the intermediate bronchus should be plainly visible on well-exposed standard roentgenograms of the chest in frontal projection (see Figure 1–60, pages 90–91).

The combined thickness of the right tracheal wall and contiguous parietal and visceral pleura over the right upper lobe can almost always be identified on well-exposed posteroanterior roentgenograms as a vertically oriented linear opacity outlined by the air column of the trachea and contiguous lung parenchyma. Commonly referred to as the right paratracheal stripe, its width ranges from 1 to 4 mm but is usually approximately 2 mm;[42] a width greater than 4 mm constitutes reliable evidence of disease.

A thin vertical line shadow is usually well visualized on lateral chest roentgenograms, formed by the posterior boundary of the tracheal air column[43] (see Figure 1–61, pages 92–93). This thin band of uniform width consists chiefly of the posterior tracheal wall and is formed by two interfaces—anteriorly by the junction of the tracheal air column and the tracheal wall, and posteriorly by the junction of aerated lung in the right retrotracheal recess with the external aspect of the membranous tracheal sheath and a thin layer of mediastinal areolar tissue. Pathologic processes within the mediastinum (e.g., carcinoma of the mid-third of the esophagus) or in the medial portion of the right upper lobe can lead to deformity or obliteration of the posterior tracheal band, providing evidence for an abnormality which otherwise might not be readily apparent.[44, 115] There are also in lateral projection two roughly circular translucencies that are commonly visualized in a direct line with the tracheal air column (see Figure 1–61, pages 92–93); the upper translucency represents the right upper lobe bronchus viewed end-on, and the lower—approximately 2 to 3 cm distally—represents the left upper lobe bronchus viewed end-on. Occasionally, particularly in sthenic subjects, the lower of the two translucencies is produced by the left main-stem bronchus, owing to a more horizontal orientation of this bronchus in stocky individuals. Identification of these circular translucencies is important in diagnosis, since their displacement can be a subtle indicator of disease not evident on other roentgenographic projections.

Again in lateral projection, if one projects the shadow of the posterior tracheal stripe in a caudad direction beyond the circular shadow of the right upper lobe bronchus, one can identify a vertically oriented line shadow created by the posterior wall of the bronchus intermedius; this line shadow is formed by the air column of the bronchus itself anteriorly and by air-containing parenchyma of the right lower lobe posteriorly. The posterior wall of the left main bronchus does not form a similar line shadow, since it relates posteriorly to airless mediastinal tissue and the left pulmonary artery.

THE LOBAR BRONCHIAL SEGMENTS

On this and the following pages, the anatomic distribution of the bronchial segments is described and illustrated. Each segmental bronchus is considered separately, preceded by reproductions of a right bronchogram and corresponding drawings in posteroanterior and lateral projections (Figures 1–20 and 1–21), and of a left bronchogram similarly depicted (Figures 1–22 and 1–23).

Right Upper Lobe

The bronchus to the right upper lobe arises from the lateral aspect of the main-stem bronchus approximately 2.5 cm from the carina. The upper lobe bronchus divides at slightly more than 1 cm from its origin, most commonly into three branches. The pattern of branching in the right upper lobe varies, particularly in relation to the supply of the axillary portion of the lobe.

Right Middle Lobe

The intermediate bronchus continues distally for 3 to 4 cm from the takeoff of the right upper lobe bronchus and then bifurcates to become the bronchi to the middle and lower lobes. The middle lobe bronchus arises from the anterolateral wall of the intermediate bronchus, almost opposite the origin of the superior segmental bronchus of the lower lobe; 1 to 2 cm beyond its origin it bifurcates into lateral and medial segments.

Right Lower Lobe

The first branch originating in the lower lobe, the superior segmental bronchus arises from the posterior aspect of the lower lobe bronchus

immediately beyond its origin; thus, it is almost opposite the takeoff of the middle lobe bronchus. The four basal segments of the lower lobe can be readily identified roentgenologically by applying a few basic principles of anatomy. Reference to Figures 1–20 and 1–21 shows that in the frontal projection of a well-filled bronchogram, the order of the basal bronchi from the lateral to the medial aspect of the hemithorax is *anterior-lateral-posterior-medial*. As the patient is rotated into lateral projection, the relationship anterior-lateral-posterior is maintained; hence the acronym "ALP." The relationship of one basal bronchus to another is easily recognized by use of the ALP designation.

Left Upper Lobe

The left main bronchus is somewhat longer than the right, measuring approximately 5 cm in length. About 1 cm beyond its origin from the anterolateral aspect of the main bronchus, the bronchus to the left upper lobe either bifurcates or trifurcates, usually the former. In the bifurcation pattern, the upper division almost immediately divides again into two segmental branches, the apical posterior and anterior. The lower division is the lingular bronchus, which is roughly analogous to the middle lobe bronchus of the right lung. When trifurcation of the left upper lobe bronchus occurs, the apical posterior, anterior, and lingular bronchi originate simultaneously. As in the right upper lobe, the bronchial supply to regions of the left upper lobe is variable.

The lingular bronchus extends anteroinferiorly for 2 to 3 cm before bifurcating into superior and inferior divisions.

Left Lower Lobe

With one exception, the divisions of the left lower lobe bronchus are identical in name and anatomic distribution to those of the right lower lobe. The exception lies in the absence of a separate medial basal bronchus, the anterior and medial portions of the lobe being supplied by a single anteromedial bronchus. The mnemonic ALP applies as well to the left lower lobe as to the right for identification of the order of basilar bronchi and their relationship to one another in frontal, oblique, and lateral projections.

Text continued on page 30

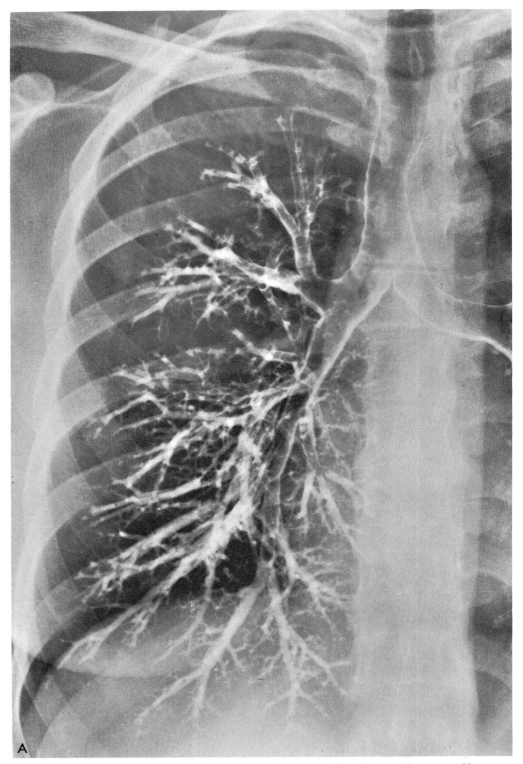

Figure 1–20. Right Bronchial Tree (Frontal Projection). *A,* Normal bronchogram of a 39-year-old woman.

Illustration continued on opposite page.

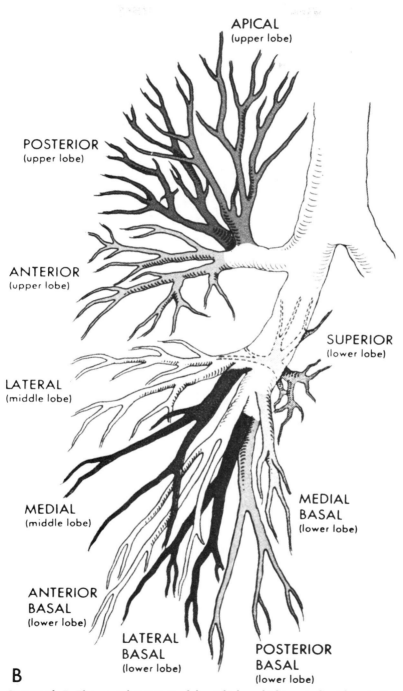

APICAL
(upper lobe)

POSTERIOR
(upper lobe)

ANTERIOR
(upper lobe)

SUPERIOR
(lower lobe)

LATERAL
(middle lobe)

MEDIAL
(middle lobe)

MEDIAL
BASAL
(lower lobe)

ANTERIOR
BASAL
(lower lobe)

LATERAL
BASAL
(lower lobe)

POSTERIOR
BASAL
(lower lobe)

B

Figure 1–20. *Continued. B,* The normal segments of the right bronchial tree in frontal projection. (Reproduced from Medical Radiography and Photography, Vol. 31, No. 2, 1955, with permission of the publisher, the Eastman Kodak Co.)

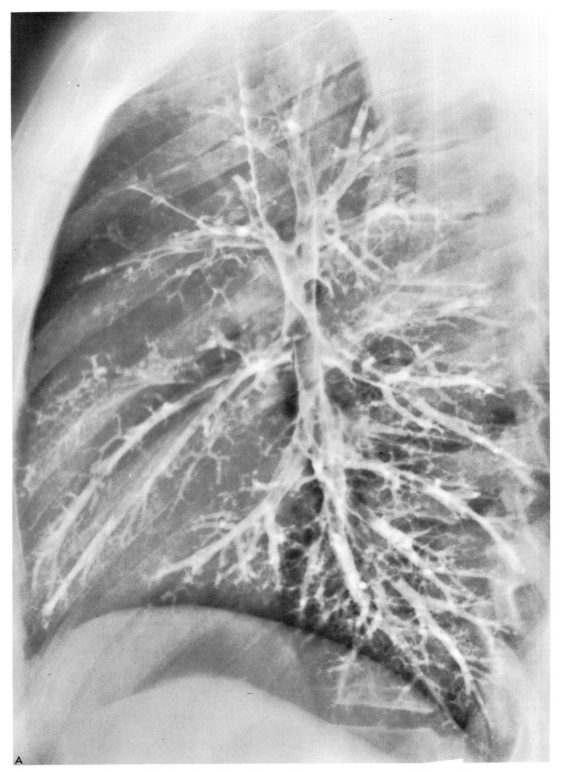

Figure 1–21. Right Bronchial Tree (Lateral Projection). *A,* Normal bronchogram of a 39-year-old woman.

Illustration continued on opposite page.

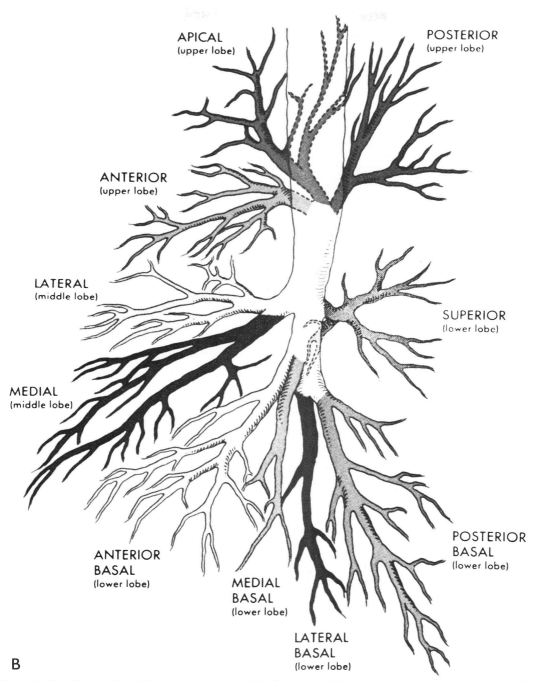

APICAL
(upper lobe)

POSTERIOR
(upper lobe)

ANTERIOR
(upper lobe)

LATERAL
(middle lobe)

SUPERIOR
(lower lobe)

MEDIAL
(middle lobe)

ANTERIOR
BASAL
(lower lobe)

MEDIAL
BASAL
(lower lobe)

LATERAL
BASAL
(lower lobe)

POSTERIOR
BASAL
(lower lobe)

B

Figure 1–21. *Continued. B,* The normal segments of the right bronchial tree in lateral projection. (Reproduced from Medical Radiography and Photography, Vol. 31, No. 2, 1955, with permission of the publisher, the Eastman Kodak Co.)

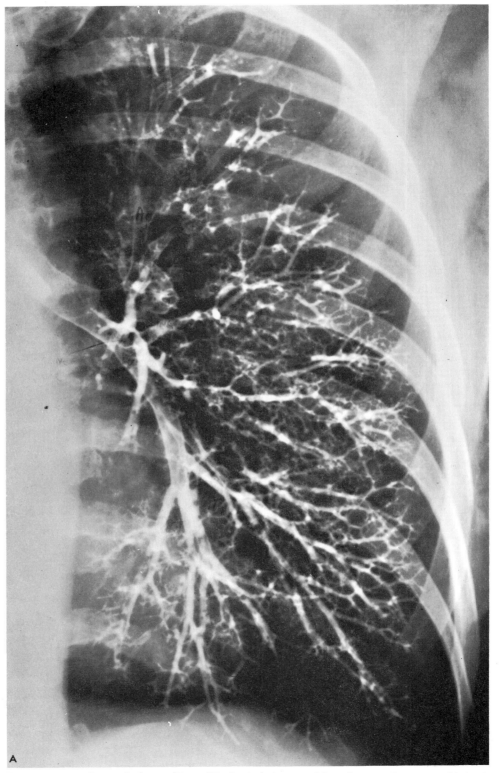

Figure 1–22. Left Bronchial Tree (Frontal Projection). *A*, Normal bronchogram of a 39-year-old woman.

Illustration continued on opposite page.

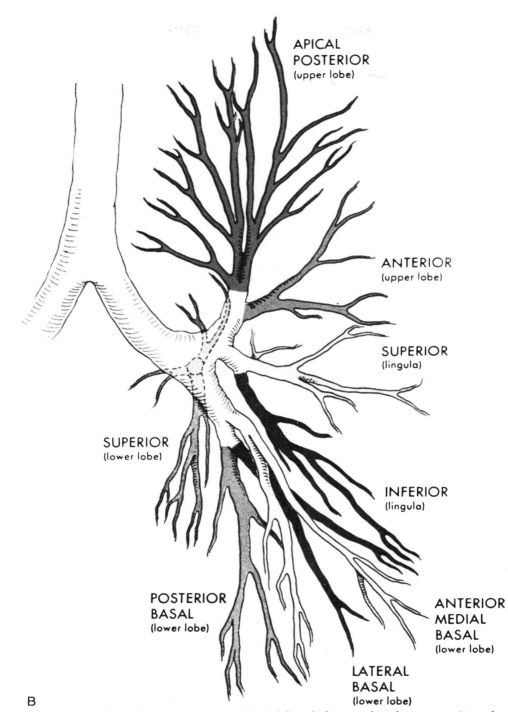

B

Figure 1–22. *Continued. B*, The normal segments of the left bronchial tree in frontal projection. (Reproduced from Medical Radiography and Photography, Vol. 31, No. 2, 1955, with permission of the publisher, the Eastman Kodak Co.)

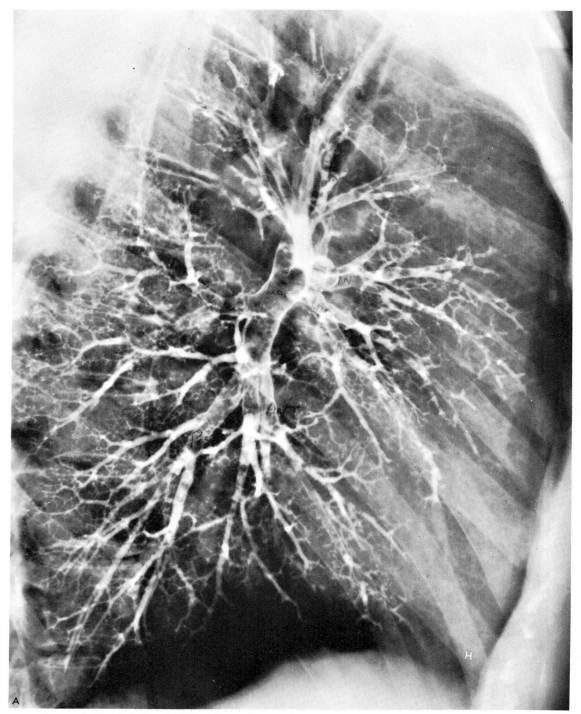

Figure 1–23. Left Bronchial Tree (Lateral Projection). *A*, Normal bronchogram of a 39-year-old woman.

Illustration continued on opposite page.

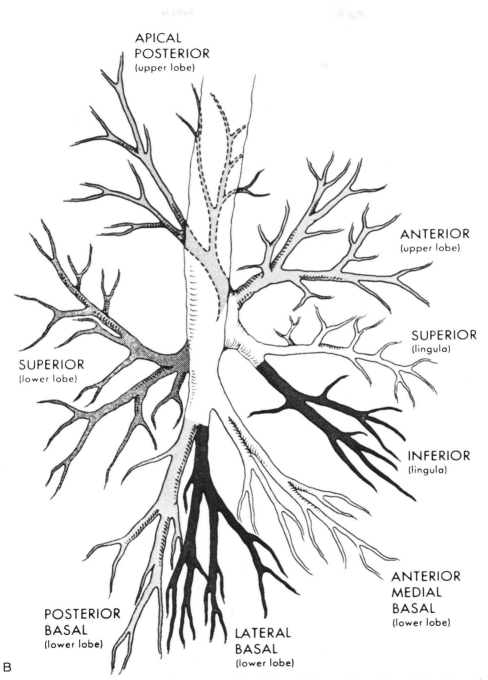

APICAL
POSTERIOR
(upper lobe)

ANTERIOR
(upper lobe)

SUPERIOR
(lingula)

SUPERIOR
(lower lobe)

INFERIOR
(lingula)

ANTERIOR
MEDIAL
BASAL
(lower lobe)

POSTERIOR
BASAL
(lower lobe)

LATERAL
BASAL
(lower lobe)

B

Figure 1–23. *Continued. B*, The normal segments of the left bronchial tree in lateral projection. (Reproduced from Medical Radiography and Photography, Vol. 31, No. 2, 1955, with permission of the publisher, the Eastman Kodak Co.)

FUNCTION OF THE AIRWAYS: PULMONARY VENTILATION

The purpose of respiration is to supply oxygen for the metabolic needs of cells and to remove carbon dioxide, one of the waste products of cellular metabolism. In the unicellular organism this is achieved simply by diffusion of these gases across the cell membrane; in man, although the basic purpose is the same, a complex mechanism is necessary. To bring oxygen from the atmosphere into contact with the cell membrane requires not only passage of the air down a long system of branching tubes, but also an additional means of transport to convey oxygen to even the most distant cells. This process utilizes two areas of diffusion, one in which oxygen is taken up by blood in pulmonary capillaries, and the other in which oxygen arrives at the tissue membrane. The elimination of carbon dioxide is accomplished by the same procedure in reverse: diffusion from tissues into blood, and then conveyance to lung capillaries, where the gas diffuses from liquid to gas phase and moves up the tubular conducting system and is exhaled.

Normal lung function requires the provision at the alveoli of sufficient oxygen to satisfy the demands of the tissues and sufficient movement of gas in the tracheobronchial tree to eliminate carbon dioxide brought to the alveoli. The needs of the tissues for oxygen—and consequently, the quantity of carbon dioxide eliminated—vary considerably, owing mainly to muscle activity. At rest, the oxygen requirement may be 200 to 250 ml per min, whereas during maximal exercise it may increase to 20 times this amount. To satisfy this variation in oxygen need under normal circumstances, a similar increase in volume of ventilation is necessary. This is accomplished by stimuli from various sources, the origin depending upon the circumstances of the need: oxygen lack, carbon dioxide excess in the blood, nervous reflexes from the lungs themselves, chemoreceptors in blood vessels, and other reflexes from somatic and visceral tissues, including the cerebral cortex, act directly or indirectly on the respiratory center to induce movement of the diaphragm and intercostal muscles and, thus, an appropriate increase in ventilation. It follows that this increase in ventilation to satisfy the need for oxygen will be to no avail if there is not a parallel increase in circulating blood through the lungs to carry oxygen to the tissues. Accordingly, rate and stroke volume increase and, during exercise, raise the cardiac output from,

for example, 5 liters per min to 25 to 30 liters per min.

Keeping in mind the chemical, nervous, and mechanical stimuli that act directly or indirectly on the respiratory center, cardiac muscle, airways, and pulmonary vessels and that vary the quantity of ventilation and perfusion of blood to the acinar unit, let us focus our attention on this unit, since it is here that the lung fulfills its role in respiration. To do this we shall consider (1) alveolar gas and its composition, (2) the mechanism by which this gas is moved in and out of the acinus, (3) perfusion of the acinus, (4) the process of diffusion of gas in the acinar unit and across the alveolocapillary membrane to red blood cells, (5) the matching of blood flow with ventilation in the acinar unit and the end result of these processes, and (6) blood gases and H ion concentration.

THE COMPOSITION OF GAS IN ALVEOLI

The composition of alveolar gas depends upon the rate and amount of oxygen removed and carbon dioxide added by capillary blood (which, in turn, depends upon aerobic metabolism of tissues) and the quantity and quality of the gas that reaches the acinus through the tracheobronchial tree.

Ventilation of the Acinus

At sea level, air contains approximately 21 per cent oxygen and 79 per cent nitrogen and has an atmospheric pressure of 760 mm Hg; the amount of carbon dioxide and other gases is negligible and can be disregarded. The partial pressures of these gases are approximately 159 mm Hg for oxygen ($P_{O_2} = 21/100 \times 760$) and 601 mm Hg for nitrogen ($P_{N_2} = 79/100 \times 760$). As air is inhaled into the tracheobronchial tree, the body temperature fully saturates it with water vapor at a partial pressure of 47 mm Hg, so that the partial pressure of oxygen drops to 149 mm Hg ($[760 - 47] \times 21/100$). At sea level, therefore, the ventilation of alveoli depends upon the quantity of gas containing oxygen, at a P_{O_2} of 149 mm Hg, that the thoracic "bellows" moves per minute into the acinus. Assuming that the conducting system is unobstructed, the quantity of gas reaching the alveoli depends upon the depth of respiration (tidal volume), the volume of the conducting system (dead space gas that does not reach the alveoli), and the number of breaths per minute. If a subject moves 450 ml with each breath, has a

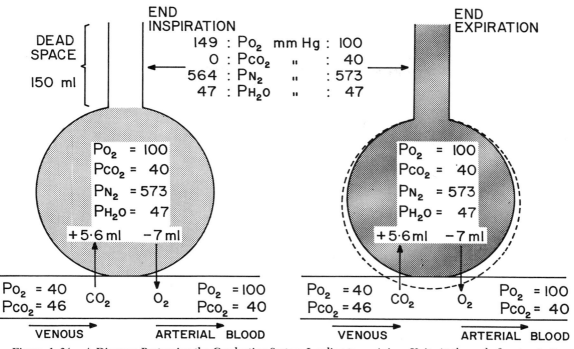

Figure 1–24. A Diagram Portraying the Conducting System Leading to an Acinar Unit. At the end of an inspiration of 450 ml of air, 150 ml of fresh air (saturated with water vapor) are situated within the conducting system and the remaining 300 ml have entered and mixed with alveolar gas. At end expiration the conducting system (dead space) is filled with alveolar air. Carbon dioxide moves from the capillary blood to the alveolus and oxygen from the alveolus to the capillary blood so that the gas composition of alveolar gas and blood are altered. *See* text.

respiratory dead space of 150 ml, and has a respiratory rate of 15 per minute, his total minute ventilation is 6750 ml (450 × 15); since each breath contributes 300 ml of fresh air to the alveolar spaces, total alveolar ventilation is 300 × 15, or 4.5 liters per min. However, it must be realized that at the end of the previous expiration the dead space was filled not with atmospheric air but with expired air having a composition equivalent to that in the acinus. This means, therefore, that with each inspiration the first 150 ml reaching the alveoli has the composition of alveolar gas and the next 300 ml is inspired air saturated with water vapor; these two differently composed gas volumes probably mix instantly in the acini. The remaining 150 ml of the tidal volume of 450 ml is in the conducting system at the end of the inspiration (Figure 1–24).

Alveolar-Capillary Gas Exchange

In addition to the contribution of ventilation to the composition of gas in the acinus, blood flow in the pulmonary capillaries varies the composition by the continuous removal of oxygen and addition of carbon dioxide. Obviously,

as a result of these two dynamic processes, the composition of alveolar gas fluctuates not only throughout the respiratory cycle but also from breath to breath and even from acinus to acinus (*see* page 46).

The quantity of oxygen removed from and carbon dioxide added to alveolar gas depends largely upon the metabolism of tissues. However, in a person at rest—assuming that perfusion of blood and ventilation of acinar units are well matched—every 100 ml of blood allows approximately 5.6 ml of carbon dioxide to diffuse into the alveolar spaces. At the same time, 7 ml of oxygen leaves the acinar units and is carried away by each 100 ml of blood going to the tissues. The partial pressure of carbon dioxide (PCO_2) in the acinus then is 40 mm Hg (713 × 5.6/100). The removal of oxygen, decreasing it from approximately 21 per cent to 14 per cent, gives a partial pressure of oxygen (PO_2) of 100 mm Hg (713 × 14/100) (Figure 1–24).

SUMMARY. **The composition of acinar gas varies with the metabolism of the tissues and the total alveolar ventilation. Increasing activity of tissues results in greater oxygen consumption and carbon dioxide production, which in turn lower the PO_2 and raise the PCO_2**

of the mixed venous blood returning to the lungs. The total alveolar ventilation depends upon tidal volume and respiratory rate.

MECHANICS OF ACINAR VENTILATION

Movement of atmospheric air down the conducting system to the acinar unit requires a certain force or pressure to overcome the "elastic" recoil of the lungs and the thoracic cage, the frictional resistance of pulmonary tissue and chest wall, and the resistance of the airways themselves. This pressure is produced by contraction of the muscles of inspiration, mainly the diaphragm, to a lesser extent the external intercostal muscles, and, in circumstances requiring greatly increased ventilation, the accessory respiratory muscles in the neck. At the end of inspiratory effort the inspiratory muscles relax; expiration usually occurs passively as the "elastic" parenchyma recoils to its resting state. If "elastic" recoil is defective, or if the conducting system is obstructed, expiratory muscles, particularly the abdominal muscles, come into play. This occurs also when large quantities of air are moved rapidly in and out of the chest.

Thus, air is brought to the acinus by the contraction of respiratory muscles, which exert a force or pressure to overcome the "elastic" recoil and frictional resistance of lung and thoracic cage, as well as the airway resistance of the tracheobronchial tree.

"Elastic" Recoil of Lung Parenchyma and the Thoracic Cage

The pressure in the pleural space normally is subatmospheric; i.e., 4 to 5 cm H_2O below that of the atmosphere. If air is introduced into this "space" and the visceral and parietal layers of pleura are allowed to separate, the lungs and the thoracic cage assume new positions, the former collapsing and the latter enlarging (Figures 1–25 and 1–26). This is the "elastic" recoil which is overcome by contraction of the respiratory muscles and expansion of the thoracic cage, and which represents the main mechanical impedance during quiet breathing.

On inspiration, the respiratory muscles act *initially* to overcome the "elastic" recoil of the lungs only; the thoracic cage, with an "elastic" recoil that allows a more expanded state, ac-

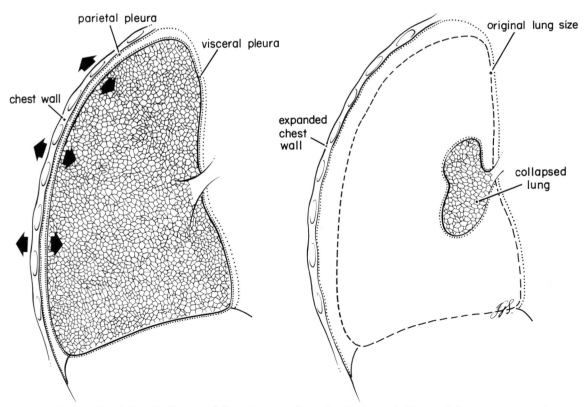

Figure 1–25. Elastic Recoil of Lung and Cage. Arrows indicate the elastic recoil of lung and thoracic cage. Introduction of air into the pleural cavity causes lung and thoracic cage to assume "resting" positions.

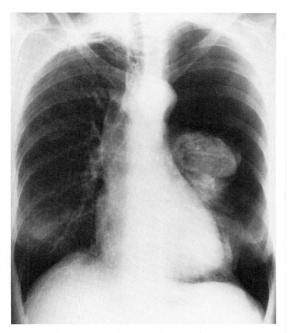

Figure 1–26. Spontaneous Pneumothorax. A poster-oanterior roentgenogram of a 28-year-old man shortly after the development of spontaneous pneumothorax. The volume of the left hemithorax is considerably larger than that of the right, due not to "tension" in the pleural space but to loss of the influence of the inward pull of the elastic recoil of the lung on the chest wall.

tually aids pulmonary inflation. As inspiration continues, the chest wall goes beyond its resting position and the force of muscular contraction then is exerted against the recoil of both lung and thoracic cage. As the cage expands, the intrapleural pressure becomes more subatmospheric, the acini and conducting tubes enlarge, gaseous pressure in the alveoli decreases in relation to atmospheric pressure at the mouth, and air moves down the conducting system. The force or pressure exerted on the lungs by muscle contraction overcomes both "elastic" recoil and flow resistance; this pressure is measurable, since it is reflected in the degree of change in intrapleural pressure. Measurement is made directly or, more conveniently, by use of an intraesophageal balloon that reflects changes in intrapleural pressure. **The relationship of the change in intrapleural pressure to the volume of gas that moves into the lungs is expressed as liters/cm H_2O and is known as lung compliance.** To distinguish the force or pressure needed to overcome "elastic" recoil from that required to overcome resistance in the airways and lung tissue, measurement is made with breathing suspended, when flow in the bronchi ceases and flow resistance is elimi-

nated. Under these conditions, only the pressure required to overcome elasticity is measured. The resulting volume change affected by the pressure change is the **static compliance** (Figure 1–27). As the normal lung becomes more inflated it becomes less compliant; for this reason it is more informative to express compliance as the change in intrapleural pressure required to produce a volume change at a specific degree of lung inflation, usually functional residual capacity (FRC). Edema and fibrotic or granulomatous infiltration render the lungs stiffer and less compliant, so that more pressure is required to move a given volume of gas; or, to put it differently, a given pressure moves a smaller volume. When the elastic architecture of the lung is faulty, as in emphysema, a given pressure may actually produce a greater volume change than in the normal lung; in such a case, compliance is increased.

"Elastic" recoil of the lung has been attributed in part to the peculiar arrangement of collagenous and elastic fibers. The helical structure of this fibrous network gives the lungs an elastic behavior similar to that of a coil spring. However, tissue elasticity is not the only component of the "elastic recoil" of the lungs, as indicated by the fact that less pressure change is required to fully distend a fluid-filled than an air-filled lung. This is due to surface tension, a force that tends to contract alveolar spaces and to resist expansion, existing in each alveolus between its lining and its gas content. Surface tension accounts for most of the lung's "elastic" recoil and is eliminated when gas is replaced by liquid.

Surface Tension and Surfactant

Surface tension at the air-liquid interface of the alveolar wall varies, depending upon whether the lungs are inflating or deflating. The layer lining the alveoli contains a substance that can lower surface tension as alveolar spaces decrease in size during expiration. Perhaps surface tension is best exemplified by a child's bubble pipe: the bubble on the mouth of the bowl tends to retract into the pipe and a distending force is necessary to counteract this effect.[45] A soap bubble, however, has a constant surface tension. An analogous but somewhat different situation exists in relation to the acinus on the end of the terminal bronchiole or the alveoli on the end of the alveolar sac. As distending pressure decreases and alveoli become smaller during expiration, the collapse that occurs in the child's bubble pipe is prevented by

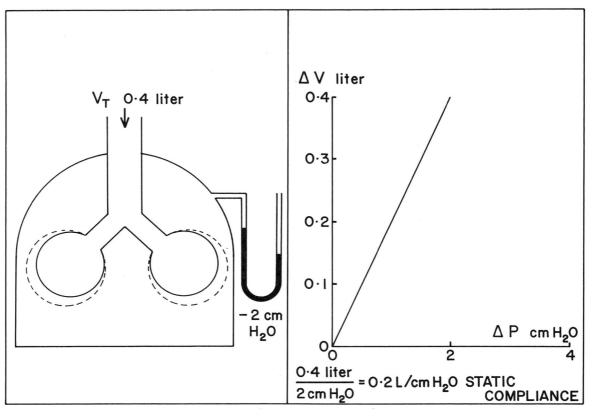

Figure 1–27. Pressure-Volume Relationships. A change of 2 cm H_2O in pleural pressure (ΔP) results in a volume change (ΔV) of 0.4 liters of tidal air (V_T) in two hypothetical acini. The diagram on the right depicts the change in volume of 0.4 liters and the change in pressure of 2 cm H_2O. The static compliance in this example is 0.2 liters/cm H_2O.

the presence in the lining membrane of a surface-active substance, surfactant, that can reduce surface tension almost to zero.

It is believed that deep breaths or perhaps even normal ventilation are required to replenish the surface-active substance and that continued shallow breathing eventually may lead to collapse. The implications of the effect of surface tension and surfactant on the capillary circulation are considerable; they are discussed in a subsequent section.

Resistance of the Airways

During quiet breathing, most of the work of the respiratory muscles is required to overcome "elastic" recoil; when ventilation becomes more rapid, flow increases and increased work is necessary to overcome resistance in the conducting airways. Resistance increases in direct proportion to the length of a tubular conducting system, so that twice as much pressure is required to maintain the same flow in a tube doubled in length. However, reduction in the radius of a tube by one-half requires a sixteen-fold increase in pressure to maintain the same flow. These principles of laminar flow pertain to rigid, smooth tubes. Bronchial flow and airway resistance are more complicated: not only are the bronchial tubes irregular but they also branch frequently and vary in caliber throughout the respiratory cycle. These additional features create turbulence, which adds to resistance. Resistance is different during inspiration and expiration and varies with both lung volume and flow rate. Because of the nature of the branching of the bronchial tree, the total cross-sectional area becomes markedly increased with each new generation beyond the segmental bronchi, so that resistance is much lower in the bronchioles than in the bronchi.

Anatomic differences between the larger cartilaginous bronchi and the smaller membranous bronchioles suggest different functions for these two portions of the conducting system, and this has been supported by physiological studies. Bronchi that contain cartilage remain patent after removal from the body; bronchioles, however, because of their content of elastic and muscle tissue, collapse under similar circumstances. During life, these cartilages not only maintain patency of the larger airways during expiration, but also prevent overdistention during maximal inspiration. These two portions of the conducting system differ not only in the construction of their walls but also in the fact that they occupy different thoracic cage "compartments," which are separated by a strong elastic limiting membrane.[14] The cartilage-containing airways appear to have a potential space around them[37] and are affected more by changes in transpulmonary pressure (the difference between pressure at the mouth and intrapleural pressure) than by changes in lung volume. The bronchioles, on the other hand, lie on the other side of a limiting membrane that fuses with the bronchial walls at the point at which the cartilage disappears.[14] They lie within the lobule, tightly connected to the pulmonary parenchyma, and the patency of their lumina is influenced by changes in lung volume.

During expiration, as lung volume becomes smaller and intrapleural pressure becomes less subatmospheric, resistance in both bronchi and bronchioles increases. Most of the increase in resistance, however, is in the bronchi and is due to their bronchomotor tone. In the absence of bronchomotor tone, there is very little increase in resistance as lung volume decreases until lung volume becomes very small.

In addition to these passive forces acting on the conducting system and causing increase or decrease in resistance, there are active stimuli to both bronchodilatation and bronchoconstriction. These are mediated through nervous pathways or by the action of chemicals, either on the receptor sites for postganglionic fibers or through direct action on smooth muscle.

Reflex local bronchoconstriction occurs when adjacent major pulmonary arteries are obstructed, constituting what appears to be a compensatory mechanism to divert ventilation to perfused areas. The operation of this mechanism can be prevented by the inhalation of 3 to 5 per cent carbon dioxide, in which circumstances it is thought that bronchoconstriction is due to the reduced P_{CO_2}.

A sudden increase in resistance, as occurs during attacks of asthma, prolongs expiration and thereby prevents complete emptying of the acinar unit; the next inspiration enlarges the unit and thus increases the functional residual capacity. This increase in lung volume augments "elastic" recoil to supply greater expiratory force. However, in prolonged asthmatic attacks, increasing overinflation may be associated with a decrease in "elastic" recoil.

Obstruction in the airways is not always the result of constriction of smooth muscle; it may be due to mucus in the bronchi or bronchioles or, as in emphysema, to "weak" walls. In this condition airway resistance is increased both because of loss of elastic tissue to hold open the smaller bronchi or bronchioles, and because of the development of a high intrapleural pressure in an attempt to force air out of the alveolar spaces.

Tissue Resistance

During movement of the chest, in addition to airway resistance tissue resistance also is present; this is caused by displacement of lung tissue itself, the rib cage, the diaphragm, and the abdominal contents. It is generally thought that in a healthy person, tissue resistance accounts for about 20 per cent and airway resistance for 80 per cent of total pulmonary resistance. This, however, may be an overestimate.[46] Tissue resistance is increased when the lung is infiltrated by granulomatous, fibrotic, or malignant tissue. During expiration some of the elastic force is used to overcome this additional frictional resistance, and, since there is less force available to overcome resistance in the conducting system, expiration is slowed.

SUMMARY. **The force required to overcome the "elastic" recoil and the resistance of lungs, bronchial tubes, and thoracic cage is measured as a pressure in centimeters of water. The relationship of pressure to volume of gas moved in and out of the lungs is known as compliance and is expressed as liters/cm H_2O. Compliance is decreased when the lung is made stiffer by fibrotic or granulomatous infiltration; it is increased when pulmonary elastic recoil is reduced, as in emphysema. "Elastic" recoil is only partially due to the elasticity of lung parenchyma. A major component is dependent upon alveolar surface tension, which increases with inspiration and decreases with expiration. This tension is modified by a substance known as surfactant, which is present in the alveoli.**

During quiet breathing most of the work of the respiratory muscles is required to overcome "elastic" recoil. During rapid respirations the increase in flow, the irregularity of the bronchi (which produces turbulence), and the bronchomotor tone add a significant impedance to ventilation. Bronchospasm or mucus in the airways adds to this resistance.

Loss of elastic support to the smaller bronchi and bronchioles and development of a high intrapleural pressure during expiration are responsible for the severe degree of airway resistance that develops in emphysema. Parenchymal and thoracic wall tissues also create a resistance to respiration, and this may be considerable when diseased lungs are infiltrated diffusely.

THE PULMONARY VASCULAR SYSTEM

MORPHOLOGY OF THE VASCULAR SYSTEM

The pulmonary arterial system accompanies the bronchial tree and divides with it, a branch always accompanying the appropriate bronchial division; these have been termed "conventional" branches. However, many accessory branches of the pulmonary artery arise at points other than corresponding bronchial divisions. These accessory branches outnumber the conventional ones; they originate throughout the length of the arterial tree and are most frequent peripherally.

The pulmonary arterial system may be conveniently divided into three types—elastic, transitional, and muscular. The arteries that accompany bronchi are elastic, and those that run with nonrespiratory bronchioles are muscular: the former vessels have a well-defined internal and external elastic lamina, with seven or more elastic laminae between, and the latter have an internal and an external elastic lamina with less than four elastic laminae between. Vessels that have intermediate amounts of elastic tissue are termed "transitional" arteries. The number of generations of the types of artery differs in various pathways. In the anterior basal segment artery (Figure 1–28) elastic arteries stop at about the sixth order, followed by two orders of transitional arteries coinciding with the end of the cartilage in the bronchi. Beyond this the vessels are muscular in type. Many muscular vessels arise proximally from elastic vessels that correspond to side branches along lateral pathways of the bronchial tree. The muscular arteries measure about 2000 μ in diameter at their point of origin and diminish to about 100 μ at the level of the terminal bronchiole. The walls become progressively thinner, with loss of elastic lamina and muscle. Beyond the level of the terminal bronchioles the arteries lose their continuous muscle coat

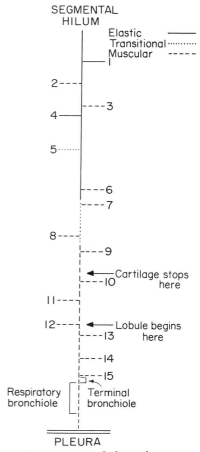

Figure 1–28. Structure of the Pulmonary Arteries. Diagrammatic representation (drawn to scale) of the full length of an anterior basal segmental artery. The structure of the artery is related to bronchial generations, and only conventional branches are included—those which accompany airways. (Reproduced with the permission of the Editor of *Clinical Radiology* and of the authors—Elliott, F. M., and Reid, I.: Clin. Radiol., *16*:193, 1965.)

and become arterioles, with a single elastic lamina. Within the acinus, arterioles continue to divide and accompany their respective branches of the respiratory tree to the level of the alveolar sacs. Many accessory branches are given off to supply the walls of the acinar pathways and the alveoli. These branches, as well as those that terminate around the alveolar sacs, are sometimes called precapillary arterioles; they break up to form the capillary network of the alveoli themselves. The capillary network of the alveoli is the densest in the body; its geometry and dimensions are discussed in the following section.

The *bronchial arteries*, usually three in number but sometimes more, vary in origin. The usual pattern consists of one bronchial artery on the right, originating from the third intercostal artery (the first right intercostal artery that arises directly from the aorta), and two on the left (arising directly from the aorta on its ventral aspect, usually opposite the fifth and sixth thoracic vertebrae). The bronchial arteries supply the bronchial wall as far as the terminal bronchioles, forming one arterial plexus in the peribronchium and another in the tunica propria. They also supply the loose peribronchial and perivascular connective tissue, the tracheal wall, the middle third of the esophagus, the visceral pleura over the mediastinal and diaphragmatic surfaces of the lungs (the visceral pleura over the lung convexities is supplied by pulmonary arteries), the paratracheal, carinal, hilar, and intrapulmonary lymph nodes and lymphoid tissue, the vagus and bronchopulmonary nerves, and sometimes the parietal layer of pericardium and the thymus. In addition the vasa vasorum of the aortic arch, the pulmonary arteries, and the pulmonary veins are fed by branches of the bronchial arteries. Distal branches anastomose with one another. In some forms of bronchiectasis the bronchial arterial system is greatly hypertrophied and blood flow through the arteries may be greatly increased.

The *pulmonary venous radicles* arise from capillaries distal to the alveolar meshwork and from the capillary network of the pleura. Except for their position, venules are histologically indistinguishable from arterioles. The venous system drains by way of the interlobular septa, and thus does not accompany the corresponding arterial tree. A bronchial vein plexus, which corresponds to the bronchial artery plexus, extends proximally from the level of respiratory bronchioles and connects at intervals with the pulmonary veins; most of the veins of the intrapulmonary bronchi drain into the pulmonary veins. The venous drainage of the large bronchi and the tracheal bifurcation form a few small trunks (bronchial veins) that drain into the azygos system and receive branches from the mediastinum; these veins connect with the intrabronchial venous plexus. Approximately two thirds of the blood carried by bronchial arteries returns to the left atrium via the pulmonary veins, and the remaining one third flows through other bronchial veins via the azygos or hemiazygos veins into the right atrium.

GEOMETRY AND DIMENSIONS OF THE ALVEOLAR CAPILLARY NETWORK

Reports from Weibel's laboratory[4, 11] point out that the basic element of the *systemic*

capillaries is a rather long, thin tube that may be connected at either end with other capillaries, thus forming a capillary network of fairly loose mesh. By contrast, the *pulmonary* capillaries form a dense network, enclosed in the alveolar wall. The basic elements of this network, the capillary segments, fundamentally are shaped like short cylindric tubes, modified at their bases in the form of wedges in order to allow each segment to join at either end with two adjacent segments. In the vast majority of instances three of these segments join, but junctures of four may easily occur. This results in an average angle of juncture of about 120 degrees. Thus, the basic geometric structures of the capillary network is hexagonal, each mesh being surrounded, on average, by six segments. This two-dimensional network on the alveolar facets becomes three-dimensional when three septal facets join, achieved by the rotation of the plane of juncture of three segments by approximately 90 degrees.

Weibel found that the external diameter of capillary segments in fresh lung averaged 8.6 μ; allowing 0.3 μ for the average thickness of the capillary endothelium, the average internal capillary diameter was estimated to be 8 μ. The axial *length* of capillary segments ranged from 9 to 13 μ (average, 10.3). Weibel deduced that each alveolus is surrounded by about 1800 to 2000 capillary segments and that the total number of capillary segments in the entire lung shows a group average of about 280 billion. He estimated total capillary blood volume to be 140 ml; total capillary surface of the lung was 70 sq m, only slightly less than that of the alveolar surface. The volume of blood per alveolus was estimated at 4.7×10^{-7} ml and the capillary surface per alveolus at 23.4×10^{-4} sq cm.

MORPHOLOGY OF THE ALVEOLAR CAPILLARY

The endothelium of the pulmonary capillaries is continuous and nonfenestrated,[18] the cells lying on a continuous basement membrane. The endothelial cells are separated by clefts approximately 200 Å wide, which are narrowed at irregular intervals from the capillary ostea to form "pores" or "junctions" 40 to 50 Å wide (Figure 1–29). These "open" junctions (maculae occludentes) permit the passage of low molecular weight proteins (such as horseradish peroxidase[18]) across the endothelial wall and contrast with the "tight" junctions between alveolar cells (zonulae occludentes—*see* Figure

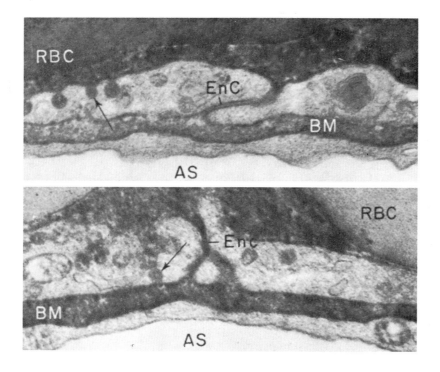

Figure 1-29. Endothelial Intercellular Cleft. Section of alveolar wall from the lung of a mouse sacrificed 90 sec after horseradish peroxidase injection. Reaction product in the capillary lumen (indicated by *RBC*) extends through the endothelial intercellular cleft *(EnC)* into the adjacent basement membrane (BM). In *A*, the staining of horseradish peroxidase is quite light, whereas in *B* the basement membrane is deeply stained. Reaction product is present in endothelial invaginations on both the capillary side *(arrow in A)* and the alveolar side *(arrow in B)* of the cell. (TEM, × 46,000.) (Reprinted from Schneeberger-Keeley, E. E., and Karnovsky, M. J.: J. Cell. Biol., 37:781, 1968, with permission of the authors, editor, and publisher and by copyright permission of the Rockefeller University Press.)

1–9, page 10) which act as a permeability barrier to such proteins.

ROENTGENOLOGY OF THE VASCULAR SYSTEM

The *main pulmonary artery* curves upward from the pulmonic valve to form a segment of the left border of the heart. At the level of the carina and slightly to the left of the midline it bifurcates into right and left branches (Figure 1–30). The right branch is almost horizontal and divides into two main branches while still within the mediastinum and before reaching the hilum; the left curves sharply *upward* and backward as it passes into the left hilum, which, therefore, is situated slightly higher and more posterior than the right. In one series of 500 normal subjects, the left hilum was higher than the right in 97 per cent.[47] In 3 per cent the hila were at the same level, and in none was the right hilum higher than the left.

The *right pulmonary artery* lies posterior to the aorta and the superior vena cava and anterior to the right main bronchus (Figures 1–30 and 1–31). Its superior branch, the truncus anterior, supplies most of the upper lobe. It curves superiorly and anteriorly over the upper lobe bronchus and then divides into three branches which follow the anterior, apical, and posterior segmental bronchi.

The inferior of the two pulmonary arteries in the right hilum (the interlobar artery) is much larger than the truncus anterior (Figure 1–31); it passes in front of the intermediate bronchus, and on the lateral aspect of this bronchus descends abruptly into the major fissure. It supplies one branch to the middle lobe, one to the superior segment of the lower lobe, and, in random order, four branches that accompany the basal bronchi of the lower lobe.

The *left pulmonary artery* splits into two branches within the left hilum after passing immediately anterior and lateral to the lower portion of the left main bronchus. The left pulmonary artery is on a more posterior plane than the right, a difference that usually allows for distinction between the two vessels on lateral roentgenograms. The upper (and smaller) of the two divisions of the left pulmonary artery sends two or more branches to the apical posterior segments and one to the anterior segment of the upper lobe, following closely the anatomic distribution of the segmental bronchi. Thus, no major vessel to the left upper lobe is analogous to the truncus anterior to the right. The lower of the two main vessels in the hilum (the interlobar artery) curves sharply over the top of the upper lobe bronchus and descends abruptly, along the lateral aspect of the lower lobe bronchus, into the major fissure (*see* Figure 1–61, pages 92–93). The lingular artery, with its two branches, arises from the anterior aspect

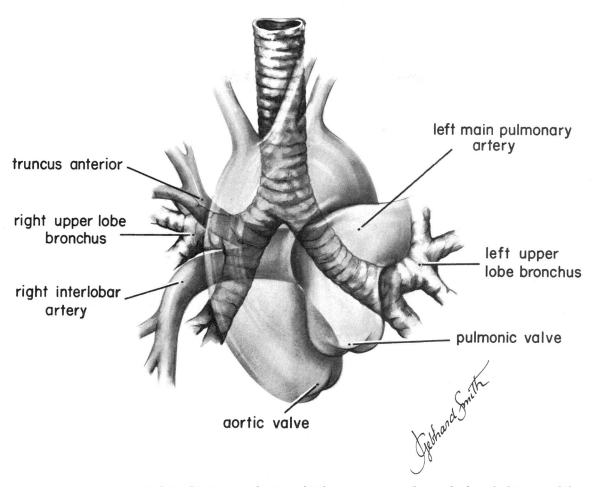

truncus anterior

right upper lobe
bronchus

right interlobar
artery

left main pulmonary
artery

left upper
lobe bronchus

pulmonic valve

aortic valve

Figure 1–30. Anatomic Relationship Between the Central Pulmonary Arteries, the Tracheobronchial Tree, and the Aorta. The *right pulmonary artery* lies posterior to the ascending aorta and anterior to the right main bronchus. Its superior branch (the truncus anterior) curves superiorly and anteriorly over the upper lobe bronchus; its inferior branch (the interlobar artery) passes in front of the intermediate bronchus and curves abruptly downward along the lateral aspect of this bronchus. The *left pulmonary artery* passes immediately anterior and lateral to the lower portion of the left main bronchus; the lower of its two main branches in the hilum (the interlobar artery) curves slightly posteriorly over the top of the upper lobe bronchus and descends abruptly along the lateral aspect of the lower lobe bronchus (*see* Figure 1–33, page 42).

of this vessel. The superior segmental artery of the lower lobe arises from the posterior aspect of the descending artery, just proximal to the origin of the lingular artery. The arterial ramifications to the remainder of the lower lobe are similar in name and number to the basal bronchi they accompany.

The spatial distribution of pulmonary veins is even more variable than that of the arteries (Figures 1–31B and 1–32). The commonest pattern consists of two large veins on each side that enter the mediastinum slightly below the pulmonary arteries and anterior to them. On the right side, the superior pulmonary vein drains the upper lobe and usually the middle lobe, although in some cases a separate vein

from the middle lobe drains directly into the left atrium or joins with the inferior pulmonary vein; the inferior vein drains the whole of the lower lobe. On the left side, the superior and inferior pulmonary veins drain the upper and lower lobes, respectively, although lingular drainage is into the inferior vein in some cases.

Arterial and venous trunks within the lungs are usually distinguished without difficulty if certain anatomic relationships are kept in mind (Figure 1–32). The course of the veins is remote from the bronchoarterial bundles, a remoteness that begins in the lung periphery, where the arterial system is in the center of the lobules and the venous system is within the interlobular septa. This relationship persists, so that in all

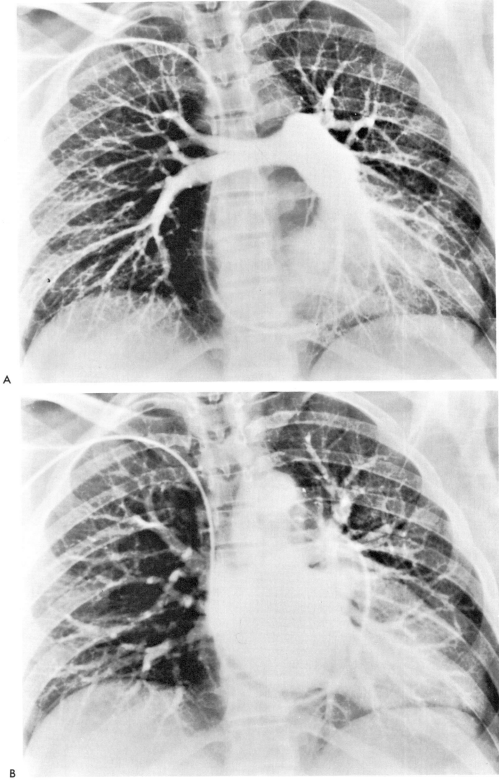

Figure 1–31. Pulmonary Angiogram. *A*, Arterial phase. *B*, Venous phase. *See* text for description.

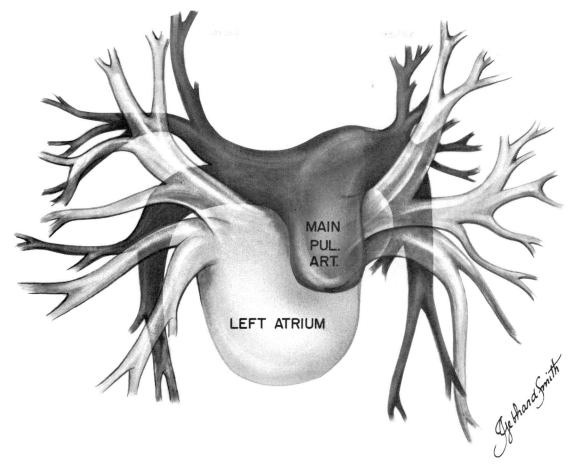

Figure 1–32. Anatomic Relationship Between Pulmonary Arteries and Veins. In the upper portions of the lungs, the veins *(light shading)* run lateral to their respective arteries *(dark shading)*; in the mid• and lower lung zones, the veins lie inferior to the arteries.

areas the arteries and their corresponding veins are separated by air-containing lung parenchyma and thus should be distinguishable. When not superimposed, the veins run either lateral or inferior to their respective arteries. Arteries and veins usually are distinguished more easily in the lower lobes because of the general vascular topography: the relatively horizontal position of the venous channels contrasts with the almost vertical course of the arteries, a relationship that usually can be seen clearly in the right lower lobe on a frontal roentgenogram. In the lateral projection, confluence of the pulmonary veins is on a plane slightly anterior to the course of the pulmonary arteries.

The anatomy of the major arteries, veins, and airways, particularly in the region of the hila, frequently can be seen with great clarity on lateral projections of the thorax, both on standard roentgenograms and on tomograms (Figure 1–33). The superb treatise by Proto and Speckman[48] dealing with the anatomy of the thorax on left lateral roentgenograms is highly recommended to readers desiring more complete knowledge of this important subject.

The caliber of the hilar pulmonary arteries is of considerable importance in roentgenologic diagnosis and should be assessed carefully. The most significant sign is a change in caliber from one examination to another, particularly in relation to the diagnosis of pulmonary embolism; when comparison is not possible or when evidence of pulmonary arterial hypertension is sought, roentgenographic measurement of segments of the pulmonary vascular tree may provide useful information. The figures supplied by Chang,[49] who measured the right descending pulmonary artery in more than 1000 normal adult subjects, appear to be the most accurate available. Measuring the transverse diameter of the interlobar artery from its lateral aspect to the air column of the intermediate bronchus,

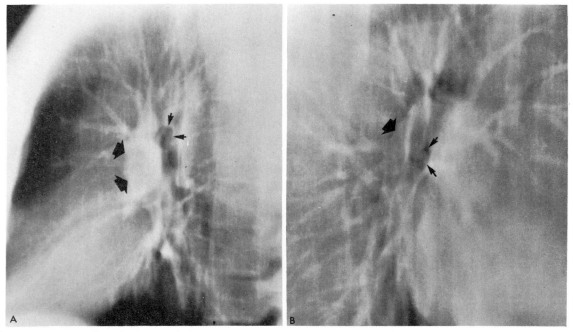

Figure 1–33.   The Hila in Lateral Projection. *A,* In a lateral tomographic section through the *right* hilum, the tracheal air column is well seen. The oval shadow of the right interlobar pulmonary artery *(thick arrows)* lies immediately anterior to the air column of the main-stem and intermediate bronchi; immediately above and slightly posterior to this vessel is the circular air column of the right upper lobe bronchus cut across *(thin arrows)*; the lower lobe vessels can be seen descending in a slightly posterior direction. *B,* A tomographic section of the *left* hilum reveals certain differences from the right that permit their distinction; the left pulmonary artery is superimposed on the air column of the left main bronchus and immediately above the circular air column of the left upper lobe bronchus *(thin arrows)*; the interlobar artery *(thick arrow)* curves posteriorly and inferiorly across the aortic window, giving origin from its posterior surface to the branch of the superior segment of the left lower lobe. The lower lobe veins can be seen to cross the arteries at a sharp angle.

he found the upper limit during inspiration to be 16 mm in males and 15 mm in females, 1 to 3 mm greater than during expiration.

FUNCTION OF THE VASCULAR SYSTEM

PERFUSION OF THE ACINAR UNIT

Pulmonary blood volume (PBV) is defined as the volume of blood within the pulmonary arteries, pulmonary capillaries, pulmonary veins, and an indeterminate portion of the left atrium. When measured with a dye technique in 15 normal subjects it ranged from 204 to 314 ml per sq m body surface area (mean, 271 ml/m²),[50] indicating that the amount of blood in the lungs at any one time is about 10 per cent of total blood volume. The capillary blood volume (Vc), which represents about 20 to 25 per cent of the PBV, is estimated to be 60 to 140 ml in the resting subject, increasing to 150 to 250 ml during exercise.[37, 50] These figures, largely calculated by measuring CO uptake by intracapillary erythrocytes, closely agree with

estimates made by anatomic techniques.[51, 52] This may be interpreted as indicating that the capillary vascular bed, whose surface area measures 70 to 100 sq m, is maximally distended during peak exercise.

Various pressures modify the flow of blood through the capillaries. (1) *The mean intravascular pressure* is only 14 mm Hg in the pulmonary artery, despite the fact that it handles the same cardiac output as the systemic circulation. (2) *The transmural vascular pressure* is the intravascular pressure minus intrapleural pressure in larger vessels outside the lobular limiting membrane. In smaller vessels and capillaries within the membrane it is best expressed as the difference between intravascular hydrostatic pressure and alveolar pressure. (3) *The driving pressure* in the pulmonary circulation is the difference between arterial and pulmonary venous or left atrial pressures in the lower part of the lung and the difference between arterial and alveolar pressures in the upper part of the lung, in upright subjects at rest (Figure 1–34). The pressure in capillaries cannot be measured directly; it must average more than

5 mm Hg (left atrial pressure) for blood to move, and is estimated to be about 9 mm Hg at the arterial end and 6 mm Hg at the venous end. It is influenced by gravity. Since the colloidal osmotic pressure is thought to be 25 to 30 mm Hg, under normal resting conditions a considerable force keeps the alveoli dry; and even during maximal exercise, when cardiac output increases to 25 to 30 liters per min in healthy individuals, the hydrostatic pressure does not exceed the osmotic pressure.

The hemodynamics of the pulmonary circulation cannot be deduced on the basis of laws that relate to a rigid tubular system. Like the conducting system, the circulatory system is distensible; it branches and bends; it is subject to changing pressure on its walls and has a pressure at each end, either or both of which may vary in degree in certain circumstances. Flow is pulsatile but probably always laminar in small vessels and sometimes turbulent in

larger ones. Viscosity is greater in the main vessels, but overall resistance to flow is mainly from arterioles and capillaries. When the left atrial pressure and transpleural (alveolar minus intrapleural) pressure are constant, an increase in pulmonary artery pressure causes vessels to distend (transmural pressure increase). As with the conducting system, doubling or halving the radius causes a sixteenfold change in resistance; in this case, as cardiac output increases, vessels widen, and closed capillaries open, leading to a fall in resistance.

SUMMARY. **Both physiologic and anatomic measurements indicate that the amount of blood in the capillaries in a resting subject is 60 to 140 ml, increasing to 150 to 250 ml during exercise.**

Various pressures influence the flow of blood through pulmonary capillaries. The mean hydrostatic intravascular pressure in the pulmonary artery is only 14 mm Hg. The transmural vascular pressure is the intravascular pressure minus the intrapleural pressure in the larger vessels, and in smaller vessels and capillaries it is thought to be the difference between the intravascular hydrostatic and alveolar pressures. The driving pressure in the pulmonary circulation is greatly influenced by gravity. In erect subjects the driving pressure in the upper lung (in which alveolar pressure is greater than pulmonary venous pressure) is the difference between arterial and alveolar pressures. In the lower lung the driving pressure is the difference between arterial and venous pressures.

The intravascular pressure in the capillaries is considered to be in the range of 6 to 9 mm Hg, and the great distensibility of these vessels prevents a significant rise even during severe exertion. The colloidal osmotic pressure, which is 25 to 30 mm Hg, serves to keep the alveoli dry (or ideally moist) even with a fivefold increase in cardiac output.

FACTORS INFLUENCING PULMONARY CIRCULATION

Gravity

The lung measures approximately 30 cm from apex to base, and the hilum is positioned at about the midline. The pulmonary artery enters the lung at the hilum. Since a column of blood 15 cm high is equivalent to a column of mercury 11 mm high, in the erect subject gravity affects the intravascular pressure to the extent that systolic, diastolic, and mean pressures are reduced by 11 mm Hg at the apex and are

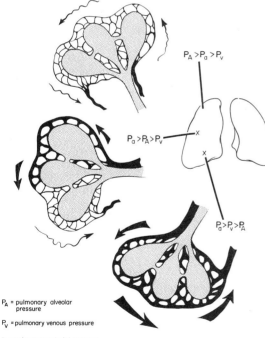

$P_A > P_a > P_v$

$P_a > P_A > P_v$

$P_a > P_v > P_A$

P_A = pulmonary alveolar pressure

P_v = pulmonary venous pressure

P_a = pulmonary arterial pressure

Figure 1–34. Diagram Depicting the Influence of Gravity on Perfusion of Acinar Units in Upright Man. *In the upper unit,* alveolar pressure (P_A) may in certain circumstances become higher than pulmonary artery pressure (P_a) so that the capillaries are virtually empty. *In the midlung,* alveolar pressure (P_A) is lower than arterial pressure (P_a) but higher than venous pressure (P_v), so that blood flow occurs through the arterial end of the capillaries but is impeded on the venous end. *The unit at the base of the lung* shows dilated capillaries throughout since both arterial (P_a) and venous (P_v) pressures are greater than alveolar pressure (P_A).

increased by 11 mm Hg at the base. If pulmonary arterial pressure in the hilar vessels is taken as 20/9 mm Hg, it follows that pressure at the extreme apex will be 9/−2 and that no perfusion will occur in the apical zone during diastole; at the base, the pressure will be 31/20, which will increase the capillary pressure in this area and will render the lung base more susceptible to transudation of fluid into the alveoli. Since the pulmonary veins enter the left atrium at approximately the same level, there also will be a similar and proportional variation in venous pressure (Figure 1–34).

Gravity largely governs the distribution of blood flow in the lungs. At the extreme apex in the upright person at rest there is just enough pressure under normal conditions to overcome the effect of gravity. However, when the hydrostatic pressure falls, as in states of shock, or the alveolar pressure rises, as a consequence of positive pressure breathing, the unperfused but ventilated apices become alveolar dead space. Farther down the lung, pressure on the arterial side rises but is opposed by alveolar pressure, which readily compresses the thin-walled capillaries. Therefore, the driving pressure in the upper part of the lung is the difference between arterial and alveolar pressures. Since alveolar pressure is not influenced by gravity, and arterial pressure gradually increases down the lung, the driving pressure and, therefore, blood flow also increase. However, because intravascular pressure decreases in the passage of blood from arteriole to venule, alveolar pressure is greater than venous pressure in the upper lung, and the venous end of the capillary is constricted. The degree of constriction decreases gradually as the increasing effect of gravity causes a rise in venous pressure and allows a greater flow of blood as the lung base is approached (Figure 1–34). At one point, venous pressure rises above alveolar pressure; below that point the driving pressure of blood through the lung is the difference between arterial and venous pressures. Because arterial and venous pressures are influenced equally by gravity, despite the lack of increase in driving pressure blood flow continues to increase as the base of the lung is approached. This is due to the increasing intravascular pressure or transmural pressure on both arterial and venous ends, which dilates the vessels and thereby reduces pulmonary vascular resistance to flow. At the base of the lung, at low lung volumes, the regional blood flow decreases where the parenchyma is least expanded. This is due to increased resistance of the extra-alveolar vessels, which narrow when surrounding lung tissue is poorly inflated.

SUMMARY. **Gravity reduces the circulation in the upper lobes and increases it in the lower lobes. Circulation at the extreme apex, which depends on the gradient between pulmonary intravascular and alveolar pressures, is barely maintained in erect resting subjects. The pulmonary artery pressure increases from apex to base, and the driving pressure of blood through the lungs becomes the difference between arterial and venous pressures as soon as the effect of gravity causes pulmonary venous pressure to exceed alveolar pressure. As the base of the lung is approached pulmonary circulation continues to increase, not because of an increase in driving pressure (this cannot occur because arterial and venous pressures are equally affected by gravity) but through the increased transmural pressure which dilates the pulmonary vasculature and reduces resistance. At low lung volumes extra-alveolar vessels at the base of the lung are narrowed, so that local pulmonary resistance increases and pulmonary capillary circulation decreases.**

Intrapleural Pressure and Lung Volume

We have seen that the conducting system to the acinar unit runs in two separate "lung compartments." Similarly, larger arteries and veins are outside the lobular limiting membrane and are influenced by their own transmural pressures, the vessels dilating during inspiration as the pressure difference between the lumen and intrapleural "spaces" increases and constricting during expiration as the pressure difference decreases. Vessels within the limiting membrane, like the membranous airways, are affected by changes in lung volume. The small muscular arteries and arterioles lie beside the airways, whereas the veins are between the lobules at the periphery. During inspiration, the increased lung volume dilates the vessels, which are closely interconnected with alveolar tissue within the compartment. During expiration, as the lung assumes a position of rest, the vessels narrow and their blood volume decreases.

It is not known what effect changes in lung volume exert on the pulmonary capillaries. Some believe that dilatation of the capillaries reduces pulmonary vascular resistance during lung inflation. The majority, however, consider that these thin-walled vessels are compressed during inspiration, thereby increasing vascular resistance.[53] During inspiration the compression of the pulmonary capillary bed and the consequent decrease in blood volume are probably offset by the rise in volume in the larger vessels. Still an unknown quantity in this regard is the part played by surface tension, which is thought to increase as alveoli distend (see page 12) and, consequently, would be expected to counteract the effect of compression by pulling away from capillary walls. This concept is strongly supported by studies of the pulmonary ultrastructure, using the vascular system for perfusion of fixatives.[22] In contrast to previous work, these studies showed smooth intra-alveolar lining with a gradually curved alveolus.

SUMMARY. **The larger pulmonary arteries and veins dilate during inspiration as the difference between intravascular and intrapleural pressures (transmural pressure) increases, and constrict during expiration as the pressure difference decreases. The smaller arteries and arterioles, closely interconnected with alveolar tissue, dilate as lung volume increases during inspiration and narrow during expiration. The capillaries probably are compressed during inspiration, leading to an increase in resistance. Intra-alveolar surface tension, which increases during inspiration, may counteract the compressing effect of alveolar distention.**

Neurogenic and Chemical Effects

In addition to the pressure and volume changes that passively influence the pulmonary vasculature, some active stimuli can modify capillary circulation to acinar units. Hypoxemia and acidosis appear to be the most potent. Such stimuli not only have a vasomotor effect but also a direct action on the myocardium (and, hence, on cardiac output) as well as an indirect effect on both myocardium and vessels via the sympathicoadrenal system; thus, their influence on the hemodynamics of the pulmonary circulation is complex. Systemic hypoxemia acts on the carotid body, triggering a reflex mechanism that gives rise to arteriolar vasoconstriction. Local hypoxia is reported to produce vasoconstriction locally,[54] probably by acting on the arteriole that accompanies the terminal bronchiole, i.e., in the circulation that supplies the acinar unit. This is an ideal area in which to reduce circulation when ventilation is inadequate. Acidosis, whether metabolic (e.g., diabetic ketosis, lactic acidosis, or due to renal failure) or resulting from an increase in the P_{CO_2}, also causes local vasoconstriction and in poorly ventilated acini acts synergistically with the hypoxemic effect. Increased left atrial or

pulmonary venous pressure is thought to be the stimulus for arteriolar constriction, which protects capillaries from excessive hydrostatic pressure in conditions such as mitral stenosis.

The existence of precapillary anastomotic channels between bronchial and pulmonary vessels in the normal lung is controversial, but it is known that they are present in certain disease states. Several types have been found in association with congenital pulmonary artery stenosis, bronchiectasis, and pulmonary diseases that give rise to interstitial fibrosis, and their functioning has been demonstrated with angiographic techniques and by analysis of oxygen saturation during catheterization of lobar arteries. Since systemic arterial pressure is six to eight times greater than pulmonary artery pressure, flow is from bronchial to pulmonary vessels.

SUMMARY. **Hypoxemia and acidosis appear to be potent vasomotor stimuli to the pulmonary vasculature. A local vasoconstrictive effect, possibly at the level of the arteriole accompanying the terminal bronchiole, is considered responsible for limiting circulation of poorly ventilated acinar units. In certain disease states, bronchial-pulmonary artery anastomoses may increase the vascular resistance in damaged and underventilated areas, thereby diverting pulmonary blood flow to functioning units.**

DIFFUSION OF GAS FROM ACINAR UNITS TO RED BLOOD CELLS

Diffusion in the Acinar Unit

Diffusion of a gas occurs passively from an area of higher partial pressure of the gas to one of lower partial pressure. In a gaseous medium, a light gas diffuses faster than a heavier one. In a liquid or in tissue the rate of diffusion is largely dependent upon the solubility of the particular gas in that medium. Oxygen is slightly lighter than carbon dioxide and, therefore, diffuses more rapidly in acinar gas. In water and tissue, carbon dioxide is more soluble than oxygen, and diffuses through these media 20 times faster than does oxygen. Since both are able to diffuse many thousands of times more rapidly in a gaseous medium than in water or tissue, diffusion out of acini consists largely of getting through the alveolocapillary membrane and plasma and in and out of the red cell. Because diffusion through these structures is accomplished much more readily by carbon dioxide than by oxygen, outward diffusion of carbon dioxide is never a clinical problem, and further discussion need concern only the diffusion of oxygen.

Assuming a tidal volume of 450 ml and a dead space of 150 ml, 300 ml of fresh air and 150 ml of dead space alveolar air from the previous expiration enter the acinar units during each inspiration (Figure 1–24, page 31). Since the units already contain seven or eight times this volume (functional residual capacity), the "fresh" air that enters last may fill only the respiratory bronchioles and main ducts. In the normal lung, however, because of the rapid diffusion of oxygen in a gaseous medium, complete mixing of this fresh air with intra-acinar gas is probably instantaneous. In obstructive emphysema, with the breakdown of alveolar septa and the creation of much larger air spaces, mixing may be delayed, and in these circumstances gaseous diffusion may limit the diffusing capacity.

Diffusion Across the Alveolocapillary Membrane

The membrane through which oxygen diffuses to reach plasma in capillaries comprises (1) a surface-active liquid that lines the intra-alveolar membrane, (2) alveolar epithelial cells with attenuated cytoplasm, (3) basement membrane to the epithelial layer, (4) loose connective tissue, (5) basement membrane to the capillary endothelium, and (6) capillary endothelium. It is thought that diffusion takes place only through the lateral cytoplasmic extensions of the type I alveolar epithelial cells, and that the "blood-air pathway" in a normal lung is 0.36 to 2.5 μ thick.[15] Through this thin membrane, with a driving pressure of approximately 60 mm Hg (P_{O_2} of alveolar gas minus P_{O_2} of mixed venous blood [$100 - 40 = 60$ mm Hg]), under resting conditions oxygen almost fully saturates the blood in one third of the time taken by blood to traverse the pulmonary capillaries. During exercise, with increased cardiac output and pulmonary capillary blood volume, the transit time is reduced. Nevertheless, aided by the slightly higher P_{O_2} due to increased ventilation, the blood is virtually saturated by oxygen by the time it reaches the end of the capillary. With decreased alveolar P_{O_2} (e.g., due to atmospheric conditions at high altitude, respiratory center depression, or neuromuscular disease), the driving pressure of oxygen is reduced; exercise under these conditions results in a shortened transit time which, together with the reduced driving pressure, may limit diffusion, so that the end capillary blood may be only partly oxygenated. Although the transit time is thought of in relation to capillaries only, it is probable that the process of diffusion starts in the arterioles which are the origin of capillaries, since their walls are in direct contact with alveolar air.[37, 55]

In addition to the aforementioned factors that affect diffusion, the total area in which flowing blood comes in contact with ventilated acinar units influences the capacity for diffusion. This is exemplified by the decrease in diffusion that occurs after pneumonectomy, and may be responsible in part for the decrease in diffusing capacity that occurs in emphysema, in which a considerable amount of the alveolocapillary membrane often is destroyed. The amount of *effective* alveolocapillary membrane usually is reduced because of mismatching of capillary circulation with acinar ventilation (see further on). Since this may be an inevitable accompaniment of diseases that thicken the alveolocapillary membrane, assessment of responsibility for diffusion impairment may be difficult.[56]

Many diseases may involve the acinar unit in such a way as to interfere with diffusion (Figure 1–35). In such cases the arterial oxygen saturation may be normal in patients at rest, despite significant reduction in diffusing capacity; however, exercise elicits hypoxemia because the transit time through capillaries is decreased.

Intravascular Diffusion

The crossing of the alveolocapillary membrane by oxygen does not complete the process of diffusion, and it is probable that resistance to gas movement into red cells is often greater than that to gas movement from the alveoli into the blood.[57] This is due not to the distance to be traversed through plasma to the red cell but to the rate of reaction of oxygen molecules with red cell contents. Differences in the rate of gas exchange in the red cell, the final phase of diffusion, are not important in relation to normal lungs breathing air, but they play a significant role in diffusion impairment in states of low alveolar oxygen tension and in anemia.

SUMMARY. **The diffusion of oxygen from alveolus to red blood cell is influenced by the difference between alveolar and mixed venous P_{O_2}, the total area and thickness of alveolocapillary membrane, and the number of red blood cells and their transit time in the pulmonary capillaries.**

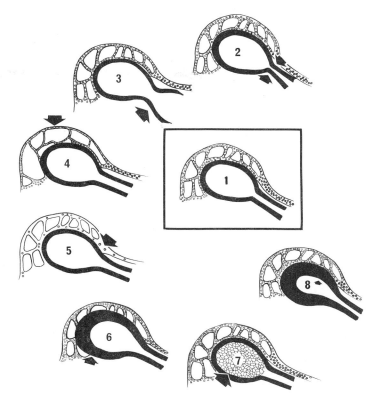

Figure 1–35. Pathophysiology of Diffusion Defect. The structure in the center of the diagram (1) is a normal air-containing acinar unit in which are depicted a conducting system, an alveolar cell lining, a normal amount of tissue between air space and capillary endothelium, and a capillary network containing a normal number of red blood cells. The acinar units around the periphery depict various mechanisms of diffusion defect: (2) obstruction to air entry; (3) dilatation and confluence of respiratory bronchioles (resulting in an increased pathway for diffusion, as in centrilobular emphysema); (4) loss of capillaries; (5) anemia; (6) increase in tissue between air space and capillary endothelium; (7) replacement of air in air space by edema, exudate, or blood; and (8) increase in alveolar lining cells.

MATCHING CAPILLARY BLOOD FLOW WITH VENTILATION IN THE ACINUS

Ideally, alveolar ventilation and alveolar perfusion should be uniform; *i.e.,* each acinus should receive just the right amount of air to oxygenate the hemoglobin completely and to remove the carbon dioxide given off during gas exchange. This would mean that each of the 33,000 acini, with its 400 alveolar ducts and 8,000 alveoli, would receive equal portions of the alveolar ventilation ($\dot{V}A$), which is estimated to average 4.5 liters per min, and of the alveolar perfusion ($\dot{Q}$), which averages 5 liters per min. In other words, not only would the ratio of ventilation to perfusion ($\dot{V}A/\dot{Q}$) be 4.5:5.0 liters or 0.9 for each lung, but each acinar unit would have an identical ratio. Despite the fact that this is not true even for the normal lung, the concept of an "ideal" $\dot{V}A/\dot{Q}$ ratio is useful as a point of reference in judging relationships between ventilation and perfusion within the acini.

When the $\dot{V}A/\dot{Q}$ ratio is not ideal (*i.e.,* other than 0.9), it is either because perfusion is reduced relative to ventilation or because ventilation is decreased relative to blood flow.

The effect of gravity is to increase blood flow to the most dependent portion of lung. In an upright person this is the lung base. The increase in blood flow in the middle part of the lung is due to rising hydrostatic pressure in the arteries and arterioles; since intra-alveolar pressure does not change, the rise in hydrostatic pressure increases driving pressure. In the lower lung, in which pulmonary venous pressure exceeds alveolar, the driving pressure of blood through the lung is the difference between pressure on the arterial end and that on the venous end of the capillary. Since gravity affects the intravascular pressure on the venous and arterial ends equally, the driving pressure does not change as the base of the lung is approached. However, vessel distention caused by the increased intramural pressure reduces resistance in this part of the pulmonary circulation and thus permits ever-increasing blood flow down to the lung base.

Ventilation of the lung also is modified by gravity.[58] The effect of gravity is to increase intrapleural pressure down the lung (*i.e.,* make it less subatmospheric) and thus decrease transpulmonary pressure. Therefore, at the end of a quiet expiration, the acinar units are less distended and their volume is smaller in the lower than in the upper lung regions. In experiments on dogs frozen intact in the erect (head up) position, Glazier and associates[59] showed that in expiration the volume of an alveolus 25 cm from the lung's apex was half that of an alveolus at 5 cm. During the next inspiration any change in transpulmonary pressure results in relatively more regional ventilation of lower than of upper lung zones. In other words, since functional residual capacity is proportionally less in lower than in upper lung regions, the lower regions receive a larger percentage of inspired air. If this increase in ventilation from apex to base were directly proportional to the increase in blood flow, the $\dot{V}A/\dot{Q}$ ratio would not vary throughout the lung. This is not the case, however, and since the effect of gravity is greater on perfusion than on ventilation, blood and gas are slightly mismatched; i.e., $\dot{V}A/\dot{Q}$ ratio changes down the lung.

Areas with reduced or absent perfusion contribute little or no carbon dioxide to the expired air; if their ventilation volume is large enough they cause significant dilution of the carbon dioxide to the total expired gas, since inspired gas going to unperfused areas contains insignificant amounts of carbon dioxide and the gas is expired virtually unchanged. In such circumstances, comparison of the PCO_2 of arterial blood and that of expired gas coming from the alveoli shows that the normal gradient of 2 mm Hg is increased to 6 mm Hg, or more.

More recently, radioactive gases have been used to determine regional ventilation and perfusion. These techniques detect inequality of perfusion and ventilation at various levels in the lungs of normal subjects. The counters, which measure the radioactivity, "look" at many hundreds of acinar units at one time and obviously reflect the sum total of their $\dot{V}A/\dot{Q}$ ratios. In contrast to other methods of assessing ventilation and perfusion distribution, they record the regional ratios. These methods are useful in studies of the normal lung and are proving their worth in measurement of lung function in various diseases.

Many investigators using radioactive gases have shown beyond question that gravity changes the $\dot{V}A/\dot{Q}$ ratio from "ideal" values in the normal subject. The $\dot{V}A/\dot{Q}$ ratio varies between 2 and 3 at the apex of the lung and between 0.5 and 1.0 at the base. The top-to-bottom gravity effect becomes anterior-to-posterior when the subject is supine and is reversed in the head down position; it is exaggerated at the apices when pulmonary arterial pressure falls and at both top and bottom during acceleration of the body. This last maneuver not only deprives the upper lung of blood but also diverts flow to the lower lung, which may be unventilated because of closure of the conducting system due to the increase in intrapleural pressure.[60]

Increased Ventilation-Perfusion Ratios

Increase in the $\dot{V}A/\dot{Q}$ ratio indicates too much ventilation in relation to the amount of blood flowing through that area. Under normal conditions the highest ratios are at the extreme apices of the lungs, where some acini may not be perfused in a subject standing at rest. Therefore, the ratio in such an acinus that is still ventilated can be expressed as infinity. The existence of such units is predicted from knowledge of the effect of gravity on intravascular pressure, which indicates that alveolar pressure may be higher than capillary pressure in this region. But some perfusion of the lung may occur even when capillary pressure is slightly less than alveolar pressure; intra-alveolar surface tension, pulling away from the capillary wall and thus keeping the capillary open, has been given responsibility for this phenomenon.

Ventilation of totally underperfused acinar units serves no purpose, nor does a portion of that to units that are better ventilated than perfused. The disproportion in ventilation in relation to blood flow, which can be determined, is referred to as "wasted ventilation" or "alveolar dead space." When it is added to the volume of the conducting system (i.e., the anatomic dead space), the total is expressed as the "physiologic" dead space. This may be greatly increased in certain disease states, such as embolism to large pulmonary arteries, in which ventilation persists despite little or no circulation, or when large bullous or cystic areas communicate with the conducting system. In such conditions the number of acinar units available for gas exchange is decreased; thus, if cardiac output remains unchanged, ventilation has to increase to expel the usual amount of carbon dioxide and to maintain the usual level of oxygenation. The PCO_2 of arterial blood can be kept within normal limits by this adjustment (see page 49), but the PCO_2 of the end tidal gas (the expired gas, after subtracting the volume from the anatomic dead space) is reduced by the contribution from the alveolar dead space. This alveolar-arterial gradient for PCO_2 can result only from overventilation relative to perfusion; i.e., a predominance of acinar units with high $\dot{V}A/\dot{Q}$ ratios.

Decreased Ventilation-Perfusion Ratios

Conversely—and this applies to the base of the lung in the normal, upright human subject—there may be too little ventilation in relation to the amount of pulmonary blood flow. In such circumstances, an acinar unit, which is totally unventilated but is perfused, has a $\dot{V}A/\dot{Q}$ ratio of zero. An underventilated unit does not raise the PO_2 or lower the PCO_2 of the end capillary blood to the same degree as does a unit with uniform ventilation and perfusion. Therefore blood leaving acinar units with low $\dot{V}A/\dot{Q}$ ratios and going to the left side of the heart and to the systemic circulation decreases the PO_2 of arterial blood and increases the PCO_2. This is equivalent to saying that there is some "wasted blood flow" from these units, analogous to the wasted ventilation that contributes to the expired gas from units that are overventilated relative to their blood flow. This blood adds to the venous admixture caused by "absolute shunts," which exist even in normal lungs. Absolute shunting (*i.e.*, the passage of venous blood through the lungs, without any contact with alveolar gas) occurs in the normal state because bronchial blood flow is partially taken up in the pulmonary venules. In diseased lungs, absolute shunts may develop between pulmonary arterioles and venules, by-passing acinar units, and may contribute significant amounts of blood to the venous admixture. The relative amounts of blood contributed to the venous admixture by absolute shunts and by acini with low $\dot{V}A/\dot{Q}$ ratios can be calculated while the subject breathes 100 per cent oxygen. Poorly ventilated acini may result from a loss of distensibility (compliance) of the lung units, from obstruction to flow (resistance) in the conducting system which prevents satisfactory ventilation in the time taken for a respiratory cycle, or from an abnormally long distance for gas diffusion to the alveolar wall. Regardless of cause, inhalation of 100 per cent oxygen gradually replaces nitrogen by oxygen even in the most poorly ventilated unit, fully saturating blood leaving the unit. On the other hand, this inspired gas with a high PO_2 (670 mm Hg) does not come in contact with blood flowing through absolute shunts; thus, any hypoxemia of arterial blood that remains during the inspiration of 100 per cent oxygen is due to absolute shunting. However, because 100 per cent oxygen not only saturates hemoglobin completely but also dissolves 2 ml oxygen per 100 ml blood, as against 0.3 ml when room air is breathed, an absolute shunt of 20 per cent or less may be undetected if only oxygen saturation of arterial blood is measured and not PO_2. This is because oxygen dissolved in plasma attaches to and fully saturates hemoglobin when blood coming from the lungs, which are exposed to a partial pressure of 100 per cent oxygen, mixes with shunted blood on the left side of the heart. The venous admixture from a shunt of 20 per cent or less can be detected, however, by determining the PO_2 of arterial blood; in the absence of an absolute shunt, this should be approximately 600 mm Hg.

Since both a lowered PO_2 (indirectly) and a raised PCO_2 (directly) stimulate the respiratory center and augment ventilation, if some acinar units are underventilated and thus create hypoxemia and hypercarbia, total alveolar ventilation is increased. This affects well-ventilated acinar units in that carbon dioxide is washed out and their alveolar PCO_2 is reduced, allowing a higher PCO_2 gradient and, therefore, a greater driving pressure for diffusion between blood and gas. Consequently, excess carbon dioxide retained by blood circulating through poorly ventilated units is balanced by a supranormal output from units that are perfused and well ventilated. Comparison of the dissociation curves for carbon dioxide and oxygen (Figure 1–36) shows that, although this compensation can be accomplished readily for carbon dioxide, the shape of the oxygen curve prevents further significant oxygenation at high levels of PO_2. Even if the ventilation of an acinar unit is doubled, raising the PO_2 from 100 to 125 mm Hg, the curve is so nearly horizontal in this range that arterial oxygen saturation increases from 97.5 per cent to only 98.5 per cent. In other words, ventilation-perfusion inequality leading to hypoxemia is not associated with carbon dioxide retention so long as sufficient numbers of acinar units are well ventilated.

Significance of Ventilation/Perfusion Inequality

Although gravity effects considerable changes in perfusion and in $\dot{V}A/\dot{Q}$ ratios from top to bottom of the lung, the overall effect on gas exchange in the normal upright individual is small. It has been estimated that the PO_2 of arterial blood would be only 3 mm Hg higher if perfusion matched ventilation exactly.[60] Increased flow to the lungs, as occurs during exercise or in the presence of left-to-right cardiac shunts, produces a more even distribution of blood, as does pulmonary arterial or venous hypertension.

Unevenness of ventilation and perfusion is

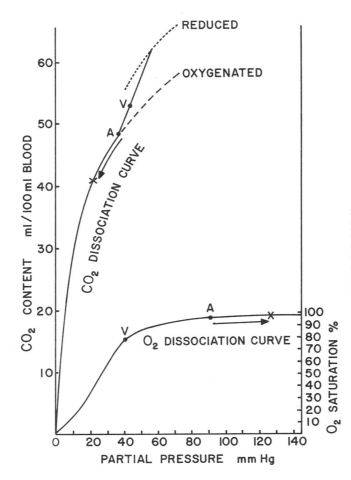

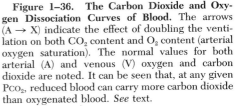

Figure 1–36. The Carbon Dioxide and Oxygen Dissociation Curves of Blood. The arrows (A → X) indicate the effect of doubling the ventilation on both CO_2 content and O_2 content (arterial oxygen saturation). The normal values for both arterial (A) and venous (V) oxygen and carbon dioxide are noted. It can be seen that, at any given P_{CO_2}, reduced blood can carry more carbon dioxide than oxygenated blood. *See* text.

the major cause of cyanosis in patients with respiratory disease. However, it is remarkable how severely the lung may be diseased without deviation of the arterial oxygen saturation from the normal range of 95 to 100 per cent, even when a lobe or an entire lung has been destroyed by bronchiectasis or emphysema. In many cases this may be explained by the simultaneous destruction by disease of vessels and airways. In such circumstances, the unevenness of ventilation and perfusion are so matched that the $\dot{V}_A/\dot{Q}$ ratios approach "ideal." In addition to these fortuitous "pathologic occurrences," compensatory physiologic mechanisms tend to maintain $\dot{V}_A/\dot{Q}$ ratios and arterial oxygen saturation within normal limits. Since the pulmonary microcirculation lacks sphincters and innervation,[37] it appears that blood distribution in capillaries is purely random and is influenced by such minor factors as blocked capillaries (by microembolism and leukocytes) and, perhaps, even the angle of a capillary as it comes off the arteriole. If this is so, some regional control is required to match ventilation and perfusion at entry to the lung unit. Thus it seems logical to assume that the very close association of terminal bronchiole and arteriole in the same connective tissue sheath is more than a chance occurrence: this would be an ideal site to shut off perfusion when ventilation was inadequate or to reduce ventilation when blood flow was lacking. A low P_{O_2} in the gas approaching the acinus may act at this site; by constricting the pulmonary arteriole it may divert blood to better ventilated areas. Studies with an electrode inserted into pulmonary arteries 2 mm in diameter clearly show that inspired gas diffuses into the lumen of such vessels. There is also a mechanism for reducing ventilation in areas with little or no perfusion. The stimulus to this bronchiolar or bronchial constriction is a low P_{CO_2}, but the exact site of action has not been determined.[61]

SUMMARY. **Even in the normal lung there is mismatching of ventilation and perfusion. Both are affected by gravity, perfusion to a greater extent than ventilation; therefore, the upper lung is overventilated and the lower underven-**

tilated relative to circulation. The distribution of inspired gas can be detected, using an inert gas. Blood distribution can be measured by comparing the P_{CO_2} of arterial blood with the P_{CO_2} of mixed alveolar expired gas. These methods of determining distribution indicate the likelihood of gross mismatching of blood and gas but do not indicate which lung areas are responsible. Regional ventilation and perfusion can be estimated by use of scintillation counters over the chest wall after inhalation of a radioactive gas or its injection into a systemic vein. Each counter measures the sum total of $\dot{V}_A/\dot{Q}$ ratios of large numbers of acini.

An *increased* ventilation-perfusion ratio (greater than 0.9) indicates more ventilation than perfusion, as is normal in the upper lung zones. The surplus of ventilation can be calculated and is known as "wasted ventilation." This, together with the anatomic dead space, represents the "physiologic" dead space. In certain disease states, such as pulmonary embolism or large bullae that communicate with the bronchial tree, the physiologic dead space may be considerable and is reflected in increased arterial-alveolar P_{CO_2} gradient.

A *decreased* ventilation-perfusion ratio (less than 0.9) indicates less ventilation than perfusion, as is normal in the lower lung zones. The surplus of perfusion ("waste blood flow") is indicated by the degree of reduction in arterial blood P_{O_2}.

The inhalation of 100 per cent oxygen distinguishes hypoxemia due to underventilated alveoli from that due to absolute shunts in the lung: it raises P_{O_2} to the normal level of 600 mm Hg or more, in cases of hypoventilation resulting from any cause. Some degree of absolute shunt is present if this level is not reached.

Pulmonary capillary blood leaving underventilated areas is not fully saturated with oxygen and has a raised P_{CO_2}. When there is sufficient healthy lung, increased ventilation allows maintenance of the P_{CO_2} at a normal level in the arterial blood, but, because of the shape of the oxygen dissociation curve, usually does not correct hypoxemia.

The effect of gravity in the normal upright subject is to decrease the P_{O_2} to 3 mm Hg less than it would be under "ideal" circumstances. Even when the pulmonary parenchyma is largely destroyed there may be very little mismatching of perfusion and ventilation. Simultaneous destruction of blood vessels and air spaces partly accounts for this, but there are physiologic mechanisms as well that pre-vent circulation to poorly ventilated areas and ventilation to poorly perfused areas.

BLOOD GASES AND ACID-BASE BALANCE

Blood Gases

The ability of the lung to perform its prime function—the exchange of oxygen and carbon dioxide—is readily determined from analysis of a sample of arterial blood. The oxygen carried can be measured as arterial oxygen saturation or as P_{O_2}. Arterial oxygen saturation = O_2 content/O_2 capacity (per cent). Since each 1.0 g of hemoglobin can combine with 1.37 ml O_2, the oxygen capacity of a subject with 15 g hemoglobin per 100 ml blood is approximately 20 ml/100 ml blood. The content is the amount of oxygen that the blood actually contains; this can be determined in a sample by extraction under anaerobic conditions. In a subject with normal lungs breathing air at sea level this amounts to 19 ml (or slightly more) and, therefore, oxygen saturation is 19/20 × 100, or 95 per cent.

The P_{O_2} is best measured directly by use of an electrode. The oxygen dissociation curve provides an indirect measurement that is unreliable because values vary with the pH and temperature of the blood and because of the horizontal slope of the upper part of the curve (Figure 1–36).

In contrast to oxygen, which is carried almost entirely by hemoglobin, approximately 75 per cent of carbon dioxide is contained in plasma. In the resting subject, while mixed venous blood holds about 15 ml O_2/100 ml blood at a P_{O_2} of 40 mm Hg and an oxygen saturation of 75 per cent, its carbon dioxide content is about 52 ml/100 ml blood at a P_{CO_2} of 45 mm Hg. Although the red blood cell carries only 25 per cent of the carbon dioxide, it plays an essential role in the transport of this gas to the lungs; it contains the enzyme carbonic anhydrase, which rapidly hydrates the carbon dioxide passing through the erythrocyte membrane and converts it into carbonic acid, H ions, and bicarbonate ions. The bicarbonate ions (HCO_3) quickly permeate the cell membrane and enter the plasma in exchange for chloride ions; in this manner, as bicarbonate, most of the carbon dioxide from the tissues is carried by the blood. Since blood that contains reduced hemoglobin can carry more carbon dioxide than can fully oxygenated blood at the same P_{CO_2}, the circumstances are ideal for the uptake of carbon dioxide in the tissues and for its unloading in the pulmonary capillaries when the hemoglobin has been reoxygenated (Figure 1–36).

In anemia, no matter how severe, PO_2 is normal and hemoglobin is fully saturated, oxygen content and capacity being reduced. However, the small amount of oxygen taken up by the blood indicates the anemia and the resultant reduction in total oxygen transport to the tissues. When normal hemoglobin is replaced by methemoglobin, sulfhemoglobin, or carboxyhemoglobin, the PO_2 remains normal, although spectrophotometric analysis of the sample reveals reduced oxygen saturation.

Arterial hypoxemia may be due to one or more of four mechanisms—diffusion defect, true shunt, ventilation-perfusion inequality, or hypoventilation.

Reduced diffusing capacity is commonest in emphysema, in which it is due to ventilation-perfusion inequality and loss of alveolocapillary membrane, and in diseases that thicken the alveolocapillary membrane by granulomatous, fibrotic, or neoplastic infiltration. This latter group may have $\dot{V}A/\dot{Q}$ inequality also, which in some patients undoubtedly plays a major role in reducing the capacity for diffusion. Hypoxemia may be absent at rest, but during exercise, when intracapillary transit time is reduced, arterial oxygen saturation and PO_2 are decreased. The PCO_2 is normal or may even be reduced, because carbon dioxide diffuses through a tissue membrane 20 times as readily as oxygen; also, these subjects tend to hyperventilate and thereby have decreased carbon dioxide and secondarily decreased bicarbonate, to compensate for the respiratory alkalosis.

A true shunt of venous blood to systemic circulation may be due to congenital cardiac disease, arteriovenous aneurysm of the lung, or, in some diseases that affect the parenchyma, precapillary anastomosis of the pulmonary arteriole and venule. The shunted blood never comes in contact with acinar units, whether or not these are ventilated, and for this reason the PO_2 of the arterial blood cannot be raised to a normal value (approximately 600 mm Hg) during inhalation of 100 per cent oxygen. In fact, when the shunt handles 10 per cent or more of the cardiac output, the arterial PO_2 cannot rise above 500 mm Hg. All other mechanisms that produce hypoxemia can be fully corrected by the inspiration of 100 per cent oxygen, which replaces nitrogen in even the most poorly ventilated acini. In true shunt, no matter how large, the PCO_2 is always normal or low, since additional ventilation removes more carbon dioxide

from acini that are perfused and ventilated. The inability of this compensatory hyperventilation to improve uptake of oxygen significantly is apparent on study of the oxygen and carbon dioxide dissociation curves (Figure 1–36). Doubling the ventilation decreases PCO_2 from 40 to 20 mm Hg and eliminates considerable amounts of carbon dioxide, whereas the increase in PO_2 that results from increase in ventilation insignificantly increases arterial-blood oxygen content and saturation.

In most cases the hypoxemia and cyanosis that accompany pulmonary disease are due to $\dot{V}A/\dot{Q}$ inequality. Chronic bronchitis and emphysema are the clinical conditions most commonly associated with this physiologic disturbance. The capillary blood that flows by underventilated acinar units is not fully saturated and does not release normal amounts of carbon dioxide, since the gradient between the PCO_2 of blood and of the acinus is reduced. However, again because of the difference in the dissociation curves, hyperventilation of well-ventilated acini, with consequent reduction in PCO_2 in such areas, increases the blood-to-acinus gradient and eliminates more carbon dioxide from these areas. Consequently, in patients with $\dot{V}A/\dot{Q}$ inequality the PCO_2 may be low, normal, or increased. The PCO_2 increases as the disease advances, the harder work of breathing causing the respiratory muscles to produce more carbon dioxide than can be eliminated by the fewer normally functioning acini; or, perhaps more correctly, the PCO_2 rises when the patient, exposed to the discomfort of excessive respiratory effort, settles subconsciously for a higher arterial blood PCO_2. Incidentally, this is a compensatory mechanism, since it increases the PCO_2 gradient between blood and acinus. Patients with diseases that give rise to $\dot{V}A/\dot{Q}$ inequality can correct their hypoxemia and cyanosis by breathing 100 per cent oxygen, since oxygen replaces nitrogen in even the most poorly ventilated areas. When carbon dioxide retention also is present, prolonged inhalation of oxygen increases the concentration of carbon dioxide in arterial blood, and confusion and coma may result. This further retention of carbon dioxide during oxygen breathing is due to removal of the carotid body's hypoxemic stimulus to ventilation.

In diseases of the respiratory center itself and in neuromuscular disease affecting the thoracic cage, the overall decrease in ventilation may be generalized, resulting in underventilation despite normal perfusion; i.e., the $\dot{V}A/\dot{Q}$ ratio may be reduced in every acinus in both lungs.

When obesity is associated with hypoventilation, with resultant polycythemia, hypoxemia, and carbon dioxide retention, the $\dot{V}A/\dot{Q}$ inequality may be localized to the lung bases. This form of hypoxemia can be corrected readily by a few deep breaths of even room air; this finding, together with good function test values of bronchial flow, differentiates this condition from obstructive lung disease. The inhalation of 100 per cent oxygen by patients with general hypoventilation causes them to respond with further decrease in ventilation and its consequences, as occurs in other diseases that cause $\dot{V}A/\dot{Q}$ inequality.

Acid-Base Balance

Together with the analysis of arterial blood to determine P_{O_2} (or oxygen saturation)—which detects physiologic abnormality and when combined with clinical information aids in diagnosis—determination of the H^+ (pH) concentration is of utmost importance. The highly complex acid-base state and its regulation have been reviewed in detail, and the interested reader desiring more comprehensive coverage is referred to these treatises.[62] The section that follows is a simplified account of disturbances in H^+ concentration [H^+] with particular reference to the commoner clinical states likely to be encountered by physicians interested in respiratory diseases.

Under normal conditions, values for H^+ concentration [H^+], pH, bicarbonate concentration [HCO_3^-], and P_{CO_2} remain within a relatively narrow range. In arterial blood, the [H^+] may vary from 35 to 45 nM/L, pH from 7.35 to 7.45, [HCO_3^-] from 22 to 28 nM/L, and P_{CO_2} from 35 to 45 mm Hg. Interpretation of disturbances of acid-base balance requires knowledge not only of the various biochemical components but also of the clinical picture. For descriptive purposes it is simplest to consider disturbances of acid-base balance as physiologic derangements, defining acidosis as an abnormal condition or process that would *decrease* the pH or *increase* the [H^+] of the blood if there were no secondary changes. Similarly, alkalosis can be defined as a process that tends to *increase* the pH or *decrease* [H^+] of the blood if there are no secondary changes. The terms acidemia and alkalemia are best restricted to situations in which arterial pH falls or rises, respectively.

Disturbances of acid-base balance can be further divided into those that are respiratory in origin and those that are primarily nonrespiratory (metabolic). Respiratory changes in the balance are due to overventilation or underventilation, with excess removal or retention of carbon dioxide, which decreases or increases the total "carbonic acid pool" of the extracellular fluid. Nonrespiratory disturbances are the result of increase or decrease in noncarbonic acid or a loss or gain of bicarbonate by the extracellular fluid. Acidosis or alkalosis may be "simple," *i.e.*, purely respiratory or metabolic, or "mixed," reflecting physiologic disturbances that are both respiratory and nonrespiratory in nature, such as derangements of tissue perfusion and renal function, and the assimilation or loss of excessive acid or base through the gastrointestinal tract. The commonest type of "mixed" acidosis seen by the chest physician is that due to severe acute pulmonary edema, in which CO_2 retention occurs and tissue hypoxia permits anaerobic glycolysis and the formation of lactic acid.

COMPENSATORY MECHANISMS. The range of blood [H^+] compatible with life is about 20 to 160 nM/L (pH 6.8 to 7.7). When the [H^+] moves from the accepted normal range (38 to 42 nM/L) the body's homeostatic mechanisms react to restore the balance. The type and magnitude of the mechanisms evoked depend on the degree of disturbance, its duration, and the type of imbalance (carbonic or noncarbonic). For adequate body function, it is more important to maintain near normality of [H^+] than to maintain CO_2 or bicarbonate in the range found in health. In fact, regulation of acid-base balance is often reflected in abnormally high or low levels of carbon dioxide and bicarbonate in the extracellular fluid. Homeostatic mechanisms that operate in acid-base derangement include (1) buffering of the excess H^+ or HCO_3^- in intracellular and extracellular fluids, (2) compensatory increase or decrease in alveolar ventilation, and (3) renal response.

The buffer components in extracellular fluids are hemoglobin, plasma proteins, bicarbonate, and phosphate. In the blood itself, buffering is complete within a few minutes and is largely dependent on the bicarbonate and hemoglobin system. The bicarbonate also moves from the interstitial fluid spaces into the blood in situations of H^+ excess; this may take 25 minutes to 2 hours. Within the cells, buffering depends upon the presence of protein and phosphate radicals.

The respiratory compensatory mechanism is a result of [H^+]-induced stimulation of receptors in the central nervous system and the aortic and carotid bodies. Elimination or retention of carbon dioxide has been reported to take minutes to hours.

Shifts of H^+, K^+, and Na^+ from various tissues, particularly muscle, and carbonate from bone are somewhat slower in compensating for disturbances in acid-base balance, but quantitatively they are of great importance. The movement of H^+ into the cells is reflected in increased $[K^+]$ in the extracellular fluid.

The renal response to disturbances in acid-base balance may take up to 1 week for completion; in respiratory acidosis it is well developed in 48 hours and usually maximal within 5 days.[63] Renal compensation for alkalosis depends upon the rapidity of development of the alkalosis and, in chronic states, on the depletion of sodium, chloride, and potassium.

RESPIRATORY ACIDOSIS. Respiratory acidosis results from alveolar hypoventilation. CO_2 retention develops as a result of $\dot{V}Q$ inequality (i.e., regional hypoventilation of well-perfused areas in the lung) or generalized hypoventilation; in the latter, the lung parenchyma may be entirely normal but a neuromuscular defect limits movement of the thoracic cage. $\dot{V}Q$ abnormality is usually due to obstructive lung disease. Generalized alveolar underventilation results from malfunction of the respiratory center or from injury or disease of the efferent neural pathway in the spinal cord, anterior horn cells, or peripheral nerves innervating the diaphragm and intercostal muscles. Myopathy or myositis, and extreme deformity of the thoracic cage, as in kyphoscoliosis, also may restrict alveolar ventilation.

Respiratory acidosis may be acute or chronic. The acute form occurs in severe status asthmaticus, acute respiratory center depression caused by drug intoxication, and rarely from neuromuscular disorders. Hypoventilation leading to chronic respiratory acidosis occurs in chronic bronchitis, emphysema, diseases in which the anterior horn cells are destroyed, and the muscular dystrophies. A rare cause of chronic respiratory failure is upper airway obstruction; this may be due to endotracheal cicatricial stenosis, functional obstruction associated with obesity, or tracheal tumor. Perhaps the commonest examples of respiratory acidosis are those due to acute infection or drug-precipitated acute respiratory center depression complicating chronic obstructive pulmonary disease in patients with compensated chronic respiratory acidosis. For further discussion, see Chapter 18.

COMPENSATORY MECHANISMS IN RESPIRATORY ACIDOSIS. Sudden alveolar hypoventilation increases the PA_{CO_2} (partial pressure of alveolar CO_2) and hence the Pa_{CO_2} (partial pressure of arterial CO_2), forming carbonic acid and shifting the Henderson equation to the right ($H_2O + CO_2 \rightleftarrows H_2CO_3 \rightleftarrows H^+ + HCO_3^-$), thereby increasing both $[H^+]$ and HCO_3^-. The increased carbonic acid is buffered within a few minutes, chiefly by hemoglobin and plasma proteins. The degree of acid-base disturbance depends upon the extent of CO_2 retention and subsequent compensation. Ion shifts, lasting hours to days, occur between extracellular and intracellular fluids, especially in muscle and bone. H^+ ions penetrate cell membrane, allowing K^+ to escape and increasing extracellular potassium.

When CO_2 retention is prolonged there is a renal response, which also helps to keep $[H^+]$ within normal range. This mechanism is well developed by 48 hours and usually maximal within 5 days.[63] The kidney reacts to the acidosis by increasing its ability to reabsorb and generate HCO_3^-. The raised arterial P_{CO_2} apparently stimulates bicarbonate conservation; the raised P_{CO_2} in the renal tubule cells increases the formation of carbonic acid (H_2CO_3) and enhances renal intracellular $[H^+]$ and H^+ secretion; and the augmented renal tubule H^+ secretion—resulting from carbonic acid dissociation—gives rise to de novo generation of HCO_3^- by the renal tubules. The end result of the compensatory HCO_3^- reabsorption and generation is increased excretion of Cl^- ions, with consequent hypochloremia.

RESPIRATORY ALKALOSIS. Respiratory alkalosis results from hyperventilation. It is commonest in tension or anxiety states, in which circumstances it is usually acute and rarely prolonged. Some drugs (e.g., salicylic acid, paraldehyde, epinephrine, and progesterone) may cause hyperventilation by stimulating the respiratory center. Traumatic, infectious, or vascular lesions of the central nervous system may produce respiratory alkalosis. Fever and gram-negative bacteremia can induce hyperventilation, but if shock develops this is often rapidly balanced by lactic acidosis—the result of tissue hypoperfusion. Several pulmonary diseases are associated with mild respiratory alkalosis. In these circumstances the stimuli to hyperventilation are probably a combination of hypoxemia and reflexes initiated in the lung parenchyma. Some of these pulmonary diseases are acute (e.g., asthma and pulmonary emboli) and others are chronic (e.g., granulomatous and fibrotic interstitial disorders that cause compensated respiratory alkalosis). Excessive artificial ventilation also may give rise to acute or chronic respiratory alkalosis.

COMPENSATORY MECHANISMS IN RESPIRATORY ALKALOSIS. Hyperventilation decreases $PACO_2$ and hence $PaCO_2$: the decrease in arterial PCO_2 shifts the Henderson equation to the left ($H_2O + CO_2 \rightleftarrows H_2CO_3 \rightleftarrows H^+ + HCO_3^-$ and decreases both $[H^+]$ and $[HCO_3^-]$. H^+ moves from the intracellular fluid, where it is replaced by sodium and potassium, and increased amounts of lactic acid are produced in the tissues. This increase in lactic acid formation has been attributed to several factors, including intracellular alkalosis, hypocapnia (perhaps due to pyruvate carboxylase inhibition and subsequent increase in pyruvate and lactate), and tissue hypoxia. The resultant decreased efficiency of oxygen delivery reflects both peripheral vasoconstriction and the reduced ability of hemoglobin to release oxygen. Buffering in the extracellular fluid and extracellular-intracellular ion shifts occur within minutes to hours.

Persistence of the alkalotic state evokes a renal response: the urinary excretion of H^+ decreases and that of HCO_3^- and K^+ increases.

METABOLIC ACIDOSIS. Metabolic or nonrespiratory acidosis results from increased $[H^+]$ from noncarbonic acid or decreased $[HCO_3^-]$ in the extracellular fluid. The H^+ excess can result from ingestion or infusion of noncarbonic acid, excess acid metabolic products within the body, or decreased renal excretion of H^+.

Extraneous sources of noncarbonic acid include various drugs and toxic substances, including salicylates, paraldehyde, phenformin, methyl alcohol, ethylene glycol, ammonium chloride (NH_4Cl), and arginine and lysine hydrochloride. The acid-citrate-dextrose added to stored bank blood may cause metabolic acidosis, through anaerobic conversion of dextrose to lactic acid.

Endogenous H^+ formation may result from the accumulation of large quantities of the keto acids—beta-hydroxybutyric acid and acetoacetic acid—in uncontrolled diabetes, starvation, and occasionally alcoholism. Lactic acid is the other major source of noncarbonic acid within the body: it is produced in tissue hypoxia and diffuses out of the cells in the un-ionized acid form, producing a temporary excess of noncarbonic acid in the extracellular fluid. Clinical situations in which lactic acid is produced include heavy muscular exercise and acute severe tissue hypoxemia or hypoperfusion secondary to arterial hypotension or high levels of circulating catecholamines. Lactic acid is formed also when oxygen supplies at the tissue level are reduced, as in severe hypocapnia, reflecting both the inability of hemoglobin to release oxygen in these circumstances and the vasoconstriction induced by low PCO_2. Lactic acid may play a major role in increasing the $[H^+]$ in acute pulmonary edema due to left ventricular failure, although in some instances there is a superimposed respiratory acidosis. In acute left ventricular failure with metabolic acidosis, lactic acid may be produced even in the absence of hypotension or clinical evidence of shock.

Hydration can cause acidosis by diluting the extracellular $[HCO_3^-]$ and thereby increasing $[H^+]$, but this minor degree of acidosis is rapidly corrected by compensatory hypocapnia.

In renal failure the deficiency in H^+ excretion is largely due to impaired ammonia secretion. In renal tubular acidosis, and sometimes in chronic pyelonephritis, major difficulty appears to be inability to maintain the maximal H^+ gradient between renal tubule cells and the luminal fluid. The loss of HCO_3^- or other conjugate base from the extracellular fluid, through the kidneys or gastrointestinal tract, increases the H^+ concentration; in the kidneys this occurs with the use of the carbonic anhydrase inhibitor acetazolamide (Diamox) and in the gastrointestinal tract it follows severe diarrhea or fistula.

COMPENSATORY MECHANISMS IN METABOLIC ACIDOSIS. A rise in $[H^+]$ resulting from noncarbonic acid in the extracellular fluid elicits immediate buffering from hemoglobin, plasma proteins, bicarbonate, and phosphate. The Henderson equation shifts to the left, almost immediately decreasing $[HCO_3^-]$ and increasing carbonic acid (which is dissipated in the lungs as carbon dioxide). The action of the increased $[H^+]$, particularly on brain stem receptors but also on the peripheral aortic and carotid chemoreceptors, augments alveolar ventilation and rapidly eliminates carbon dioxide produced by the buffering of the excess H^+. Hyperventilation, which develops within minutes, depends upon normality of the respiratory center and adequacy of ventilatory mechanics. The degree of compensatory hyperventilation reflects the severity of the metabolic acidosis, but it appears to be maximal when the PCO_2 reaches 12 mm Hg and $[H^+]$ is 80 nM/L (pH 7.10). In these circumstances the limiting factor may be the muscular effort required over a prolonged period.[63]

Intracellular buffering, with the replacement by H^+ of K^+, Na^+, and Ca^{++} in tissues, including bone, is slower than extracellular buffering, but eventually more noncarbonic acid is buffered intracellularly than in the extracellular fluid; carbonate [CO_3^-] is released from bone and combines with some of the extra H^+ to form HCO_3^-.

As long as renal function is satisfactory there is a considerable adaptive increase in H^+ excretion, which may reach ten times normal; simultaneously, virtually all HCO_3^- filtered by the kidney is reabsorbed through the renal tubules. This compensatory mechanism, which operates for from hours to days, obviously cannot develop when the noncarbonic acid excess is due to renal failure.

METABOLIC ALKALOSIS. Metabolic alkalosis results when the [H^+] in extracellular fluid is decreased by loss of noncarbonic acid or increase in alkali.

A common cause of metabolic alkalosis is the excessive loss of noncarbonic acid during severe, prolonged vomiting; the hydrochloric acid eliminated in this way depletes not only the H^+ in extracellular fluid but also chloride ions and fluid volume, both of which contribute to the alkalosis. The acute metabolic alkalosis that may result from excessive ingestion or infusion of alkali such as $NaHCO_3$ or $CaCo_3$ or trishydroxymethylamine methane (THAM) is readily reversed by increased urinary HCO_3^- excretion.

Patients who produce or are treated with large amounts of corticosteroid hormones retain Na^+ and HCO_3^-. The mechanism of the alkalosis that develops has not been clearly established, but is known to depend on enhanced excretion of potassium.

Undoubtedly, the most common cause of metabolic alkalosis is the treatment of chronic carbon dioxide retention. In such patients the [HCO_3^-] increases to compensate for the increased [H^+]. In most cases a decrease in chloride ions occurs in association with the increased renal acid excretion that compensates for the chronic respiratory acidosis. In such cases there may be cardiac as well as respiratory failure, and treatment will be directed toward correcting both decompensated states. If artificial ventilation is used to reduce the P_{CO_2} quickly, the patient is left with excess HCO_3^- and, therefore, with metabolic alkalosis. This will worsen if corticosteroids also are given. The diuretics and low sodium diet used in the treatment of heart failure deplete the body not only of Na^+ and Cl^- but also of extracellular fluid. As a result, the patient—originally in respiratory acidosis and perhaps still having CO_2 retention—now has an excess of HCO_3^- and a lack of Cl^- in a decreased extracellular fluid space, all factors that prolong the alkalosis.

The renal attempt to regulate acid-base balance in the face of these difficult conditions is discussed further on.

COMPENSATORY MECHANISMS IN ALKALOSIS. An increased concentration of HCO_3^- is buffered in both extracellular and intracellular compartments. Lactic acid moves from the cells into the extracellular fluid, so that HCO_3^- and other conjugate bases are converted to the conjugate acids.

It is to be expected that the respiratory apparatus compensates for H^+ depletion or HCO_3^- excess by underventilation. This certainly occurs with alkalosis induced by sodium bicarbonate infusion, by THAM, and by ethacrynic acid. Hypoventilation compensating for metabolic alkalosis also occurs following excessive and prolonged vomiting.

The renal response to acute metabolic alkalosis, which is prompt, is increased HCO_3^- excretion. If the cause of the alkalosis is not quickly corrected, however, compensation at the kidney level is complicated by such factors as the demand for renal Na^+ reabsorption and the Cl^- concentration in the extracellular fluid. As described earlier, some patients with chronic respiratory acidosis become depleted of Cl^- during therapy; in addition, the extracellular fluid volume decreases, requiring increased Na^+ reabsorption. What is called for in these circumstances is bicarbonate diuresis, but this is impossible because the unavailability of Cl^- and the strong stimulus for Na^+ reabsorption demand reabsorption of bicarbonate. To maintain electroneutrality, Na^+ reabsorption must be accompanied by reabsorption of an anion or excretion of the equivalent amount of cation. The cations available for excretion to enhance Na^+ reabsorption are H^+ and K^+. Under these circumstances of chronic metabolic alkalosis the urine is already rich in K^+ and H^+; should K^+ depletion supervene, even more H^+ will have to be excreted, further aggravating the metabolic state. The result of this complicated interaction of multiple factors is the production of acid urine free of HCO_3^-; thus the kidney not only fails to excrete the excess alkali but reabsorbs it as it acidifies the urine. This situation can be corrected only by restoring the extracellular fluid volume and by providing Cl^-, K^+, and Na^+; this is readily accomplished by infusion of NaCl supplemented with K.

ACID-BASE NOMOGRAMS. Clinical information is indispensable for the correct interpretation of acid-base disturbances. Nevertheless, nomograms based on in vivo studies in humans and animals, delineating 95 per cent significance bands, may be very useful in determining

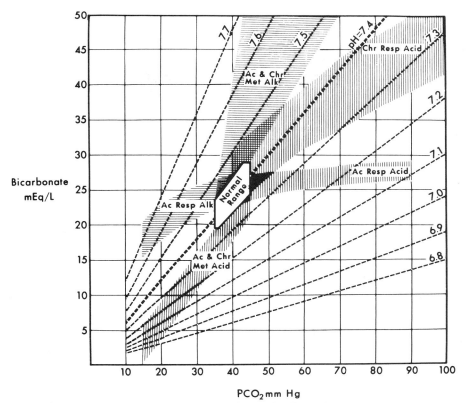

Figure 1–37. Acid-Base Nomogram. *In vitro* nomogram showing bands for defining a single respiratory or metabolic acid-base disturbance. (Reprinted from Arbus, G. S.: Can. Med. Assoc. J., *109*:291, 1973, with permission of the author, editor, and publisher.)

whether the disturbance is "pure" or "mixed": significance bands in acid-base balance[64] define the range of acid-base values expected in 95 per cent of cases of a specific acid-base disorder. Values for P_{CO_2}, H^+, and HCO_3^- in response to acute[65] and chronic[66] hypoventilation and hyperventilation have been established. Unlike respiratory disorders, however, acute and chronic metabolic acid-base disturbances do not have clearly, delineated significance bands. Arbus[67] recently reviewed the data of metabolic acidosis and alkalosis.

The great variety of acid-base diagrams or nomograms suggested for clinical use[67] plot either P_{CO_2} against H^+ (pH) or P_{CO_2} against HCO_3^-, with linear isopleths of the third component radiating from the origin. Figure 1–37, which depicts such a nomogram, shows 95 per cent significance bands for defining a single respiratory or metabolic acid-base disturbance. *Although values outside the bands almost certainly represent "mixed" disturbances, those within the bands do not necessarily represent a single disturbance.*

SUMMARY. **The amount of oxygen carried by the arterial blood can be measured by determining its content per 100 ml blood and dividing this by the total amount of oxygen the same blood can carry when exposed to oxygen (oxygen capacity); this ratio is known as the arterial oxygen saturation. A more reliable method is to measure the P_{O_2} of arterial blood with an electrode.**

Most of the carbon dioxide is carried in the plasma as bicarbonate. The red blood cell, however, contains carbonic anhydrase, an enzyme that converts carbon dioxide into carbonic acid, H ions, and bicarbonate, the last of which crosses the cell membrane in exchange for chloride ions. Blood that contains reduced hemoglobin can carry more carbon dioxide, an ideal circumstance for assimilating carbon dioxide in the tissues and releasing it in the lungs.

In diffuse infiltrative disease of the alveolar septa, arterial hypoxemia is due partly to $\dot{V}_A/\dot{Q}$ inequality and partly to diffusion defect and may be manifest only during exercise. Since carbon dioxide diffuses 20 times as readily as oxygen, in these diseases the diffusion defect is for oxygen only and the P_{CO_2} is normal or low.

A true or absolute shunt results in hypoxemia without carbon dioxide retention: patients with this condition hyperventilate and maintain low or normal levels of carbon dioxide. In chronic bronchitis and emphysema, hypoxemia is due mainly to $\dot{V}A/\dot{Q}$ abnormality; the PCO_2 is low, normal, or high, depending upon the patient's ability to hyperventilate and the amount of remaining functioning lung to compensate. Disease of the neuromuscular system or the respiratory center causes general hypoventilation and, therefore, hypoxemia and carbon dioxide retention. In the hypoventilation associated with obesity the $\dot{V}Q$ ratio at the lung bases appears to be grossly decreased; the unsaturation and carbon dioxide retention are corrected easily by the patients' taking a few deep breaths of even room air.

Measurement of the H^+ concentration of the arterial blood is an essential part of blood-gas analysis. Acute carbon dioxide retention is manifested by a rise in PCO_2 and a normal level of bicarbonate and, therefore, increase in H^+ concentration. Chronic carbon dioxide retention is accompanied by raised bicarbonate and normal H^+ concentrations. Similarly, a low PCO_2 with decreased H^+ indicates acute hyperventilation and, with normal H^+ concentration, chronic hyperventilation. Secondary hyperventilation and hypoventilation may be initiated by nonrespiratory acidosis or alkalosis. Respiratory and nonrespiratory acid/base disturbances may occur simultaneously and can be interpreted only with full knowledge of the clinical situation.

NONRESPIRATORY FUNCTIONS OF THE LUNG

It is obvious that the prime function of the lung is respiratory, involving gas exchange. The nonrespiratory functions of the lung encompass three general areas—metabolism, host defense mechanisms, and certain physical and related functions.

PHYSICAL AND RELATED FUNCTIONS

Since the entire cardiac output flows through their huge capillary network, the lungs are in an advantageous position to carry out certain physical functions. These relate chiefly to their capacity to act as a sieve. For example, they filter various types of emboli; in this regard, studies in animals in which glass beads up to 120 μ in diameter passed through the pulmonary circulation confirm the clinical suspicion of passage of emboli exceeding the diameter of pulmonary capillaries (averaging 8 to 9 μ) and indicate precapillary arteriovenous communications. The lung probably serves as a physiologic sieve for blood cells also, including leukocytes, platelets, and megakaryocytes; the megakaryocytes from the bone marrow may permit the production of platelets *in situ*.

The lungs also play a role in the excretion of volatile substances other than CO_2. For example, they help in the regulation of water balance; the estimated average loss of water through the lungs per 24 hours is 250 ml in health,[68] increasing with fever or hyperpnea. The main solute excreted at the alveolar-capillary interface is CO_2. Other nonrespiratory metabolites in the blood that are volatile at 37° C and that diffuse into alveolar gas include acetone in diabetes and fasting; methylmercaptan and ammonia in liver cell failure; methanol of unknown source; allicin following garlic ingestion; a breakdown product of dimethyl sulfoxide (DMSO) which, when applied to the skin, smells like garlic; paraldehyde; and ethanol, used for determining the blood level of alcohol in automobile drivers.

Collections of neural tissue have been identified in the vascular system of the lung, suggesting a possible role as baroreceptors or chemoreceptors. These include (1) the "glomus pulmonale," which is situated in the adventitia of the pulmonary artery of several mammals, including man, and resembles the carotid body, and (2) various baroreceptors believed to have sensory endings that are situated in the large pulmonary arteries, pulmonary veins, and left atrium. Despite the anatomic identification of these collections of neural tissue, their precise function is not known.

FUNCTIONS INVOLVED IN HOST DEFENSE

The contents of the pulmonary airways and air spaces are a direct extension of our environment, and the lungs possess a remarkable array of mechanisms to prevent damage from natural and man-made pollution.[20] It is important to realize that the phagocytic alveolar macrophages, whose capacity to engulf microorganisms and particles that penetrate to the respiratory portion of the lungs was described earlier, constitute the last line of defense, virtually all potentially pathogenic material being removed at a higher level in the tracheobronchial tree. Large particles impact on the surface of the lining membrane and are excreted on the mucociliary blanket. Very small particles (0.2 to 0.3 μ) remain suspended in air and are exhaled, rarely being deposited. Particles measuring 0.5 to 3 μ in diameter may penetrate to the respiratory portion of the lung, in which 90 per cent are deposited by gravity and are engulfed by alveolar macrophages that are excreted largely via the tracheobronchial tree.

The reaction to irritating or noxious gases is different. The first line of defense is cessation of ventilation; gases that do enter the conducting system are absorbed on the moist surface of the upper airways or are detoxified by chemical combination with a substance within the mucous blanket or elaborated by the lung as an antagonist or inhibitor.

There are several noncellular enzymes and circulating chemical substances that have a protective function, including lysozymes, lactoferrin, interferon, and, of course, surfactant. In addition, there are natural defense mechanisms against allergens entering the respiratory tract as particles or gases: IgG is produced by plasma cells and lymphocytes in the lamina propria of the tracheobronchial tree, and IgE by mast cells; similarly, epithelial cells of the respiratory tract give rise to a secretory piece that combines with plasma IgA to form a specific immunoglobulin in airway secretions. All these host defense mechanisms are adversely affected by hypoxia and hyperoxia, and by acidosis, cigarette smoke, corticosteroids, and various gases such as ozone.

METABOLIC FUNCTIONS

The lungs are involved in the storage, transformation, degradation, and synthesis of a large variety of substances.[68] The presence in the lung of enzymes known to play a part in metabolic synthesis indicates their origin from lung tissue, but in most instances the specific site of synthesis within the lung is unknown. Studies of metabolic activity, including oxygen consumption, have identified intrapulmonary cells that contain the elements commonly associated with high metabolic activity[68, 69]—large alveolar epithelial cells, Clara cells, alveolar macrophages, mast cells, and endothelial cells of the pulmonary vasculature. The first three were described previously, and it remains to discuss the activities of mast cells and vascular endothelial cells.

Mast cells are pleomorphic tissue elements of mesodermal origin which, in mammals, tend to be concentrated in the subpleural area. They contain histologically visible cytoplasmic granules of fine reticular or vacuolar structure, in addition to numerous other elements commonly associated with active metabolic cells. They are rich in heparin, histamine, slow-reacting substance (SRS), and several proteolytic and other enzymes. The number of mast cells in the lung appears to relate to the content of histamine, heparin, and SRS, but it is not known whether the mast cell synthesizes these chemical substances or simply stores them for release on demand.

The precise action and interaction of these substances in the human lung is not known, but it seems probable that they have specific activities. For example, histamine may play a role in anaphylactic shock. Since heparin, an antithromboplastin and antithrombin agent, inhibits fibrin formation, probably one of its main roles within the lung is to promote hemofluidity. In addition, heparin inhibits hyaluronidase and has an antihistaminic effect. Its therapeutic efficacy in preventing bronchoconstriction in pulmonary thromboembolism has led to the suggestion that its role in the lung is to inhibit histamine released coincidentally from mast cells. The vast endothelial network of the pulmonary capillaries appears to serve not only as a barrier between blood and gas but also as a source of materials for fibrinolysis.[68] The lungs contain large amounts of plasmin activator and thrombokinase, the former converting plasminogen to plasmin and the latter converting the circulating precursor prothrombin to thrombin. Thrombin plays a key role in the conversion of fibrinogen to fibrin. Plasmin, which is an active proteolytic enzyme, dissolves fibrin.

It is apparent that this protective mechanism for preventing occlusion of the pulmonary vessels has limitations, in view of the development of pulmonary hypertension resulting from multiple small pulmonary emboli (*see* Chapter 9). Sometimes, following pulmonary manipulation in cardiac resuscitation or during pulmonary or open heart surgery, fibrinolysis becomes excessive, probably as a result of the release of large amounts of plasmin activator into the circulation.

Reference has already been made to phospholipid synthesis by large alveolar epithelial cells, and there is no question that the lungs are engaged in lipid metabolism. The presence of lipoprotein lipases within or on the surface of capillary endothelial cells indicates that the lungs have an enormous capacity for lipolysis. Lipids, especially long-chain fatty acids absorbed by the intestinal tract, enter the blood-stream as chylomicra (glycerides in stable emulsion), which pass up the thoracic duct and thence through the right side of the heart to the pulmonary vascular bed. The fatty acids released by hydrolysis of lipid ester bonds may be used by tissues, including the lung, both as a substrate for oxidative metabolism and for the formation of complex lipids. In addition, both *in vivo* and *in vitro* studies in animals have shown the lung's ability to synthesize protein and glycoprotein.

Other biologically active substances, about which even less is known, are stored, transformed, or synthesized in the lungs. Serotonin is metabolized to 5-hydroxyindoleacetic acid and may be taken up by platelets within the lung. In cases of malignant carcinoid neoplasms (*see* Chapter 8), the excessive serotonin scleroses the valves of the right side of the heart and may cause bronchoconstriction. The presence in lung tissue of enzymes known to be active in catecholamine synthesis and degradation suggests that the norepinephrine and epinephrine in the walls of bronchi and blood vessels may be produced and rendered inactive at these sites. Both E and F prostaglandins have been identified in lipid extracts of lungs from several mammalian species, including man. They appear to act directly on the muscle of bronchi and pulmonary vessels, prostaglandin E causing relaxation and F causing constriction; their physiologic effects may be altered by the enzyme prostaglandin dehydrogenase in lung tissue. Prostaglandins are not only synthesized and apparently extracted by the lung, but also are released from pulmonary tissue.

Vasoactive polypeptides also may be released from or inactivated by the lung;[68, 69] these include components of the bradykininogen-kallikrein system and the conversion of the decapeptide angiotensin I to the more vasoactive angiotensin II.

DEVELOPMENT OF THE LUNG

The whole subject of the growth and remodeling of the lung in health and disease has been reviewed by Reid,[70] and both this article and its exhaustive bibliography are recommended as sources of detailed information about a topic considered only superficially in the following paragraphs.

Intrauterine development can be conveniently, if somewhat arbitrarily, divided into four periods: embryonic, pseudoglandular, canalicular, and terminal sac.[71]

Embryonic Period

The lung begins to develop as a ventral outpouching or diverticulum of the foregut at 24 days of embryonic life (embryos of about 17 to 20 somites; Figure 1–38A). This first indication of the lungs occurs high up, near the junction of the occipital and cervical segments.[71] The outpouching is lined by endodermal epithelium and is invested by splanchnic mesenchyme. During the next 2 to 3 days (26 to 28 days of intrauterine life, the embryo measuring 4 to 5 mm), it gives rise to right and left lung buds which, even at this early stage, show a characteristic direction of growth, the one on the right being more downward and the one on the left more transverse (Figure 1–38B and C). As the lung buds elongate, the respiratory portion of the gut becomes separated from the esophageal portion by lateral ingrowths of surrounding mesoderm that progressively meet to form the tracheoesophageal septum (Figure 1–38D). By the end of another two days (28 to 30 days, embryos of 6 to 7 mm) the lung buds have elongated into primary lung sacs or primary bronchi. By days 30 to 32, the five lobar bronchi appear as monopodial outgrowths of the primary bronchi (Figure 1–38D). Thus, by the end of the fifth week, the airways destined to become the five lobar bronchi have begun their development, marking the end of the embryonic period[72] (Figure 1–38E).

Pseudoglandular Period

This extends from the end of the fifth to the sixteenth week of gestation. Following the appearance of the five lobar bronchi as outgrowths of primary bronchi, branching occurs quite quickly, more or less dichotomously. All segmental bronchi are present by 34 to 36 days (embryos of 11.0 to 13.6 mm), and all subsegmental bronchi are represented, with many undergoing further subdivision by days 38 to 40 (Figure 1–38F). Preacinar airway branching is complete by the seventeenth week. During this period, the airways are blind tubules lined by columnar or cuboidal epithelium. Cartilage and bronchial glands continue to develop until the twenty-fourth week.

Canalicular Period

From the sixteenth to the twenty-fourth week of intrauterine development, the peripheral portion of the bronchial tree produces airways destined to be the future respiratory bronchioles, and lung tissue adjacent to the res-

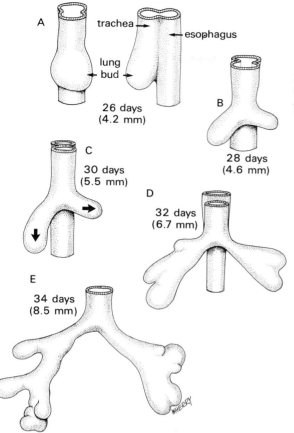

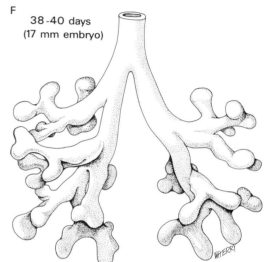

Figure 1–38. Development of the Human Lung. Diagrammatic representation of the development of human lung in the embryonic and pseudoglandular periods. A is depicted from the front and the side, all others from the front only. *See* text for description.

piratory bronchioles becomes vascularized through ingrowth of capillaries.

Terminal Sac Period

Further branching and remodeling of intra-acinar airways follows. By the twenty-fourth week the lung has developed terminal clusters of airways termed "saccules," a stage of development that marks the beginning of the terminal sac period; this lasts until birth. By the twenty-eighth week of gestation there are usually three generations of respiratory bronchioles opening into transitional ducts (destined to become alveolar ducts in the adult), with several generations of saccules arising from them. The entire acinar pathway is lined by flattened epithelium. At this stage a blood-gas barrier exists which is capable of permitting gas exchange. Eventually, the saccules become the alveolar ducts, alveolar sacs, and alveoli, but properly speaking this stage of development does not occur until after birth.

It has been shown that, at birth, there are three generations of respiratory bronchioles, one of transitional ducts, and three of saccules that end in a terminal saccule, all of which are the usual components of an acinar unit. True alveoli are not visible at birth, being represented by shallow depressions in the saccule walls. During early postnatal development, not only do the alveoli multiply in number but each part of the acinus increases in length; also, terminal bronchioles are transformed into respiratory bronchioles and distal respiratory bronchioles into alveolar ducts.[72] Alveolar sacs are believed to form from terminal saccules after birth, each sac giving rise to many alveoli. The proximal part of the terminal saccule becomes an alveolar duct, and the distal part an atrium.

The "alveoli" number approximately 24,000,000 at birth, and probably multiply until about eight years, at which time the adult complement is reached. This is generally accepted to be approximately 300 million,[12] although a more recent study of adult lungs by Angus and Thurlbeck[13] showed an estimated range of 212 to 605 million (mean, 375 million), with a highly significant statistical relationship between alveolar number and body length. Although estimates of the time at which alveolar multiplication stops are controversial, there is

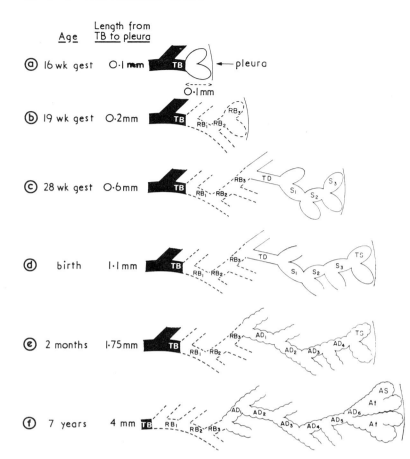

Figure 1–39. Development of the Acinus. Diagrammatic representation of the acinus at six stages of development. At all ages airway generations are drawn the same length so that increase in length represents an increase in generations. A given generation may be traced down the same vertical line, permitting remodeling in its structure to be followed. Actual increase in size is shown by the length from the terminal bronchiole *(TB)* to the pleura. *RB* = Respiratory bronchiole; *TD* = transitional duct; *S* = saccule; *TS* = terminal saccule; *AD* = alveolar duct; *At* = atrium; *AS* = alveolar sac. (Reprinted from Hislop, A., and Reid, L.: Thorax, 29:90, 1974, with permission of the authors, editor, and publisher.)

no question that alveoli enlarge from childhood to adulthood. The area of the air-tissue interface increases from 2.8 m² at birth, to 32 m² at eight years, to 75 m² in the adult, an increase that also is related linearly to body surface area.[12]

The length of the acinus increases from early gestation to the age of seven years (Figure 1–39). By seven years the lung's respiratory zone appears adult, but it further lengthens and the alveoli enlarge with increase in body size, until the adult acinus measures 5 to 10 mm long.[72]

Structural changes also occur in the intra-acinar arteries after birth: in the fetus, the pulmonary artery walls are relatively thick, as a result of their high muscle content; immediately after birth the wall thickness of vessels less than 200 μ in diameter diminishes, due to dilatation of the intra-acinar pulmonary arterial bed. This relative lack of musculature in vessels accompanying alveolar ducts and respiratory bronchioles permits ready diffusion of gases through airway walls. During the first four months after birth the wall thickness of larger pulmonary vessels decreases to adult levels, suggesting a growth rate change in the muscle cells.

In their study of fetal and infant lungs, Hislop and Reid[73] injected the pulmonary veins with a radiopaque medium and described their drainage pattern and structure. As in the arterial system, the preacinar drainage pattern was complete halfway through fetal life and the intra-acinar pattern developed during childhood. The pattern of growth in the size and number of veins and in their branching is similar to that of the arteries, although muscle development in the veins is slower.

The earlier discussion on surfactant outlined the changes in the fatty acid pattern of pulmonary phospholipids, particularly dipalmitoyl lecithin; the rate of synthesis of this substance increases from about 34 weeks to maximum at term, and shortly after birth and thereafter it rapidly declines to normal adult levels.

THE NERVOUS SYSTEM

Sensory fibers from the lung run in the vagus. They are derived from various sources. The bronchial epithelium contains nerve endings sensitive to tactile stimulation that continue as far as respiratory bronchioles. Stretch receptors are present in the lamina propria, muscle, and cartilage of the bronchi. The pulmonary veins are particularly well supplied, and the terminals of the subendothelial nerves probably are chemoreceptors. Branches associated with venules lie in septa in the periphery of lobules, and it is likely that these are sensitive to stretch. Pressor receptors are present in the muscle of pulmonary arteries and veins.

The motor supply is derived from both sympathetic and parasympathetic systems. The sympathetic supply is from the second, third, and fourth thoracic sympathetic ganglia, and the parasympathetic, through the vagus, forms peribronchial and perivenous ganglia. Motor supply in the bronchial tree extends as far as the terminal bronchioles, and in the pulmonary artery and vein to the limit of muscle. The bronchial arteries also have a rich nerve supply.

A recent "state of the art" review by Richardson[74] summarizes current knowledge on the nerve supply of the lung in humans and is highly recommended.

THE PLEURA

MORPHOLOGY

The lung is encased in the visceral pleura, a stable membrane separated from the limiting membrane of the lung by a layer of loose connective tissue. The pleura is only loosely attached to the limiting membrane—the two are readily separated in the plane of the subpleural connective tissue, and fluid or air may collect in this layer. Lung expansion is somewhat restricted by the limiting membrane and the pleura, as evidenced by the close correlation between total lung volume at full inspiration during life and lung volume after death, even with high transpulmonary pressures. Further, impressions caused by the heart and great vessels remain after death, despite inflation to high transpulmonary pressure.

The pleura consists of a thin superficial layer or endopleura and a denser, deeper layer known as the chief layer. The superficial layer is composed of a delicate sheet of elastic and collagenous fibers, in no particular pattern, underlying a sheet of mesothelial cells. These cells are thin and flattened, a few microns thick, and about 30 μ in diameter; they may swell to become cuboidal and can multiply rapidly. Cilia up to 2 μ long have been observed by electron microscopy on the free border of large mesothelial cells of human visceral pleura. The chief

layer of the pleura, which is responsible for its mechanical stability, consists of dense collagenous and elastic tissue.

The subpleural connective tissue is made up of loose connective tissue which is a continuation of the pulmonary interstitial tissue. Lymphatic channels, veins, arteries, and a rich capillary network are present in this layer, which is also referred to as the vascular layer of the pleura. In the parietal pleura, the lymphatic vessels are mainly subjacent to the intercostal muscles and the muscular part of the diaphragm, whereas the blood vessels relate mainly to the ribs.[14]

ROENTGENOLOGY

The combined thickness of the parietal and visceral pleural layers over the convexity of the lungs and over the diaphragmatic and mediastinal surfaces is insufficient to render these layers roentgenographically visible in the normal human subject. The diaphragmatic and mediastinal pleura, even if moderately and uniformly thickened, is never visible, its water density precluding roentgenographic separation from contiguous diaphragm and mediastinum. Over the convexity of the lungs, however, even slight thickening (1 to 2 mm, for example) can be appreciated because of the greater density of contiguous ribs. Such an appearance is evidence of current pleural disease or residual thickening from past disease.

In the interlobar regions, contiguous layers of visceral pleura are roentgenographically visible because of the presence of air-containing lung on both sides. Interlobar fissures become visible when the x-ray beam passes tangentially along their surfaces; when visualized, these are of value in the assessment of disease of the pulmonary lobes that form them.

FISSURES

Normal Interlobar Fissures

Fissures form the contact surfaces between pulmonary lobes. Their depth varies from complete lobar separation to a superficial slit not more than 1 to 2 cm deep in the lung surface. The depth of interlobar fissures is important: the less complete a fissure line, the larger the bridge of lung parenchyma connecting two contiguous lobes. Schall and Hoffman[75] are said to have found failure of the main fissure to reach the mediastinal surface above or below the hilum in 50 per cent of lungs. Kent and Blades[76] found incompleteness of the major fissure in approximately 30 per cent of their cases, an incidence identical to that of Medlar[77] but considerably lower than the 70 per cent of 50 right lungs studied by Raasch and his colleagues.[78] Such parenchymal bridges provide a ready pathway for collateral air drift or for the spread of disease to another lobe, creating roentgenographic signs that may give rise to erroneous conclusions. Therefore, the assessment of certain diseases should include consideration of interlobar fissure depth.

Interlobar surfaces seldom appear flat anatomically. For example, in their study of 100 fixed, inflated lungs (50 right, 50 left), Raasch and his associates[78] found certain differences of potential importance in the orientation of the two major fissures: on the right side, the upper portion of the major fissure almost always faced laterally and was usually concave; in over 80 per cent of cases, the lower portion of the fissure also faced laterally but was convex. By contrast, on the left side, although the upper portion of the fissure almost always faced laterally and was usually concave (as on the right), the lower portion faced medially and was usually convex, similar to an airplane propeller. Similarly, the minor fissure, although in a generally horizontal plane, may make a double curve, the medial portion being convex upward and the lateral half convex downward, creating a shallow **S** configuration.

Oblique (Major) Fissure

The oblique (major) fissure (Figure 1–40), which separates the upper (and middle) lobe from the lower lobe, begins at or about the level of the fifth thoracic vertebra and extends obliquely downward and forward, roughly paralleling the sixth rib, ending at the diaphragm a few centimeters behind the anterior pleural gutter.

Horizontal (Minor) Fissure

The horizontal (minor) fissure (Figure 1–40), which separates the anterior segment of the right upper lobe from the right middle lobe, lies roughly horizontal at about the level of the fourth rib anteriorly. Anatomically the minor fissure rarely reaches the mediastinum, and then only in its anterior portion; despite this, one of the more constant relationships is the fissure's medial termination at the lateral margin of the interlobar pulmonary artery.

Accessory (Supernumerary) Fissures

Any segment of lung may be partly or completely separated from adjacent segments by an accessory pleural fissure. The anatomic incidence is much higher than is generally appreciated, amounting to about 50 per cent of lungs. These fissures vary in their degree of develop-

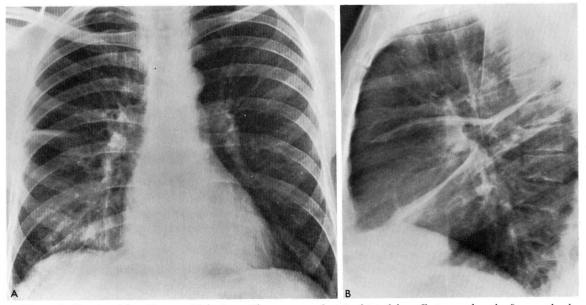

Figure 1–40. Interlobar Fissures, Right Lung. The presence of minimal interlobar effusion renders the fissures clearly visible in posteroanterior (A) and lateral (B) roentgenograms.

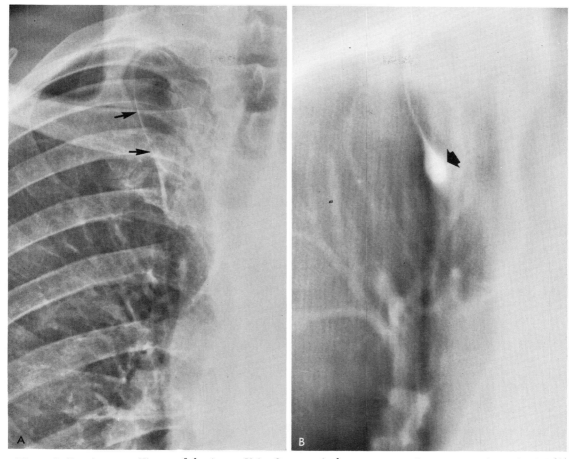

Figure 1–41. Accessory Fissure of the Azygos Vein. On a standard roentgenogram in posteroanterior projection *(A)*, the fissure can be identified as a curvilinear shadow *(arrows)* extending obliquely across the upper portion of the right lung, its lower end some distance above the right hilum. A tomographic section with the patient in the supine position *(B)* permits better visualization of the tear-drop shadow of the vein *(arrow)* because of distention.

ment, from superficial slits in the lung surface not more than 1 or 2 cm deep to complete fissures that extend all the way to the hilum. Most of these accessory fissures are of little more than academic interest roentgenologically.

Perhaps the best known of the accessory fissures, although of no known pathologic significance, is the *azygos fissure* (the meso-azygos), which is created by downward invagination of the azygos vein through the apical portion of the right upper lobe (Figure 1–41). The familiar curvilinear shadow that extends obliquely across the upper portion of the right lung is formed by four pleural layers (two parietal and two visceral), since the azygos vein runs outside the parietal pleura and thus invaginates four layers in its downward course. The fissure terminates in the "tear-drop" shadow caused by the vein itself at a variable distance above the right hilum.

PHYSIOLOGY

The visceral and parietal pleura form smooth membranes that facilitate the movement of the lungs within the pleural space. The membranes secrete and absorb pleural fluid, which facilitates movement. The following material on pressures within the pleural cavity and the formation and absorption of pleural fluid is only a brief summary of these complex subjects, and the reader interested in acquiring additional information is directed to the excellent reviews by Agostoni[79] and Black.[80]

PRESSURES

Pressure within the pleural cavity represents the difference between the elastic forces of the chest wall and of the lungs. Lung tissue has a natural tendency to recoil and continues to do so even after the lungs have been removed from the body. Thus, even at the end of a maximal expiration (residual volume), the lungs tend to collapse. By contrast, the chest wall rests at about 55 per cent of vital capacity; below this volume it has a natural tendency to expand, and above this it tends to recoil inward toward the resting position. At resting lung volume (at the end of a quiet expiration, or functional residual capacity) the chest wall is still below its resting position of 55 per cent of the vital capacity. Thus, the chest wall's expansion outward is opposed by an equal opposite force from the lungs (*see* Figure 1–25). At this point pleural pressure is about −5 cm H_2O. However, pleural pressure is not uniform through the pleural cavity, although its precise variation and its cause and effects are not certain.[58] Pleural pressure is more negative at the apex of the pleural cavity than at the base, and the gradient probably is about 0.2 cm H_2O per centimeter vertical height—although a steeper pressure gradient has been suggested.[81] The gradient is not uniform; it is greater over the upper than the lower zones of the lung. It is gravity-dependent, being reversed in subjects in the head-down position.

The effects of this gradient have been demonstrated by Milic-Emili and others,[58] who have shown that the upper lung zones are more expanded than the lower in subjects in the upright position at all lung volumes other than total lung capacity. The lower lung zones expand more than the upper during inspiration, and this is reflected by the greater ventilation of the lower zones in healthy, young, erect subjects. Regional volume behavior of the lung has been compared to that of an easily extensible coiled spring.[58] If the spring is held at its upper end so that it is acted upon only by the force of gravity, the coils will be further apart at the upper than at the lower end: this is analogous to the greater alveolar volume in the upper than in the lower lung zones. If the spring is lengthened by applying a weight at the bottom, the distances between coils will increase until they are equal: the change in distance between the coils is greater at the lower end, corresponding to the greater change in volume at the bottom of the lung.

FLUID FORMATION AND ABSORPTION

The volume of liquid in a single pleural space in man is approximately 2 ml. Human pleural fluid is reported to have an average protein concentration of 1.77 g per 100 ml (range, 1.38

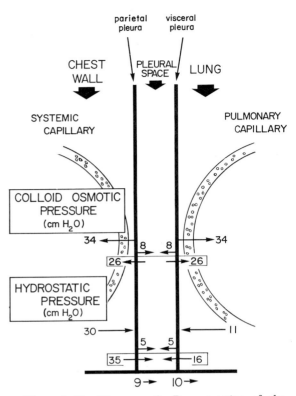

Figure 1–42. Diagrammatic Representation of the Pressures Involved in the Formation and Absorption of Pleural Fluid. *See* text for description.

to 3.35), and to contain sodium, potassium, and calcium concentrations similar to those of interstitial fluid.

In normal man, transudation and absorption of fluid within the pleural cavity follow the Starling equation and depend upon a combination of hydrostatic, colloid osmotic, and tissue pressures. The tissue pressures are not known, but knowledge of the first two suggests that, in health, fluid is formed at the parietal pleura and absorbed at the visceral pleura (Figure 1–42). The net hydrostatic pressure which forces fluid out of the parietal pleura results from the hydrostatic pressure in systemic capillaries that supply the parietal pleura (30 cm H_2O) and the pleural pressure (−5 cm H_2O at functional residual capacity). Thus, the net hydrostatic drive is 35 cm H_2O pressure. The colloid osmotic pressure in the systemic capillaries is 34 cm H_2O, and that of the pleura[82] approximately 8 cm H_2O, yielding a net drive of 26 cm colloid osmotic pressure from the pleural space to the capillaries of the parietal pleura. The balance of these forces (35 − 26 cm = 9 cm H_2O) is directed from the parietal pleura to the pleural cavity. The visceral pleura, other than over the mediastinal surfaces, is supplied by pulmonary artery capillaries, whose hydrostatic pressure is approximately 11 cm H_2O. Other pressures remain roughly constant. Thus, the net hydrostatic pressure from visceral pleura toward pleural cavity is 16 cm H_2O (11 + 5 cm). The osmotic colloid pressures remain constant, with a pressure of 26 cm away from the pleural cavity. The net effect of these forces is a drive of 10 cm H_2O (26 − 16 cm) toward the visceral pleural capillaries.

As has been noted, in health the pleural fluid has a low protein content,[83] permitting fluid formation by the parietal pleural capillaries and its absorption by the visceral pleural capillaries according to Starling's principles. When the protein concentration of pleural fluid rises sufficiently, the effect of colloid osmotic pressure in visceral pleural capillaries is reduced to negligible proportions, and the only route of absorption of pleural fluid is by bulk flow via the lymphatics.[84] Nearly all lymphatic absorption takes place in the parietal pleura. Communication between lymphatics and the pleural cavity appears to be through temporary dehiscence of adjoining mesothelial cells, which occurs when the pleura is stretched. Since parietal pleural lymphatic vessels pass through the diaphragm and intercostal muscles, movement of the chest wall might increase lymphatic flow and the speed of absorption from the pleural space. Stewart[83] found that in humans the rate of absorption of fluid high in protein falls significantly during the night, and he postulated that the decreased rate and depth of respiration during sleep might account for this.

It is apparent that abnormal amounts of fluid may accumulate when hydrostatic pressure or capillary permeability is increased or colloid osmotic pressure is decreased. Increased hydrostatic pressure causes the pleural effusion that occurs in heart failure, and increased capillary permeability is responsible in inflammatory and neoplastic disease of the pleura.

THE LYMPHATIC SYSTEM

LYMPHATICS OF THE LUNGS AND PLEURA

Although the entire cardiac output passes through the lungs, which have a rich lymphatic supply, lymphatic flow from them is small compared with that which drains the systemic circulation. The pleural lymphatics vary in size and number and are much more numerous over the lower than the upper lobes (Figure 1–43A). Lymph flows in them for a variable distance on the surface of the lung and then passes centrally to the hilum, via the septal, perivenous, and peribronchial lymphatics. Lymphatic ducts start in the region of the alveolar ducts and the respiratory bronchioles, lymph flowing centripetally in the bronchovascular sheath toward the hilum (Figure 1–43B). Although lymphatic capillaries are not found at the level of the air–blood barrier or the interalveolar septa, some have been described adjacent to alveolar walls related to small "juxta-alveolar" blood vessels.[85, 86] Lymphatic channels also drain the periphery of the lung lobules, where they run in the lobular septa along with the pulmonary veins (the site of Kerley B lines). Lymph flow in these also is toward the hilum. Anastomotic channels connect the perivenous lymphatics and those in the bronchovascular sheath; they are up to 4 cm long and usually lie approximately midway between the hilum and periphery of the lung. (Distention of these communicating lymphatics and edema of their surrounding connective tissues results in Kerley A lines.) Numerous valves, 1 to 2 mm apart, direct lymph flow in both pleural and intrapulmonary lymphatics.

The pulmonary lymphatic vessels help to clear interstitial fluid from the lungs and to remove foreign particles and antigens that have reached the alveoli.[114] The flow of lymph through pulmonary lymphatic channels may depend on a "pumping" action of ventilation, and Fleischner[87] postulated that the "butterfly" pattern of pulmonary edema may be caused by the greater ventilatory excursion of the periphery (cortex) than of the central portion (medulla) of the lung, thereby facilitating clearance of edema fluid from peripheral zones.

In many mammals the lung periphery contains abundant lymphoid tissue. Lymph nodules—collections of lymphoid tissue lacking obvious capsules or trabeculae—are frequent along the large bronchi; their structure is similar to that of a primary nodule in the lymph node.[15] In other areas of the lung, nonencapsulated, poorly demarcated lymphoid aggregates occur more peripherally.

THE THORACIC DUCT AND RIGHT LYMPHATIC DUCT

The radiologic anatomy of the *thoracic duct* has been described in detail by Rosenberger and Abrams[88] on the basis of 390 sequential lymphangiograms. The duct originates at the junction of two lumbar lymphatic trunks, the initial prominent confluence being the cisterna

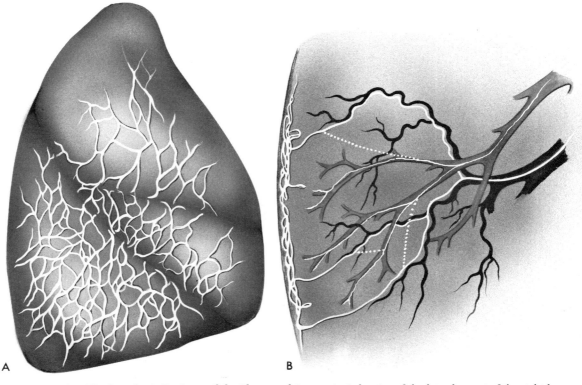

Figure 1–43. The Lymphatic Drainage of the Pleura and Lungs. *A*, A drawing of the lateral aspect of the right lung shows the pleural lymphatics to be much more numerous over the lower half of the lung than over the upper. *B*, In a coronal section through the midportion of the lung, lymphatic channels from the pleura enter the lung at the interlobular septa and extend medially to the hilum along venous radicals *(dark shaded vessels)*; lymphatic channels originating in the peripheral parenchyma extend medially in the bronchovascular bundles *(light shaded vessels)*. Communicating lymphatics *(dotted lines)* extend between the peribronchial and perivenous lymphatics.

chyli on the anterior aspect of the vertebral column from T12 to L2. The thoracic duct, which is a continuation of the cisterna chyli, enters the thorax through the aortic hiatus of the diaphragm. In the majority of subjects it lies to the right of the aorta and follows its course cephalad; thus, in the lower portion of the thorax it lies roughly in the midline of the vertebral column or slightly to one side. In patients with a markedly tortuous aorta the duct lies to the left of the spine. At roughly the level of the carina, the duct crosses the left main-stem bronchus and runs cephalad in a plane parallel to the left lateral wall of the trachea and slightly posterior to it. The duct leaves the thorax between the esophagus and left subclavian artery and runs posterior to the left innominate vein; much of the cephalic one-third (the cervical portion) is supraclavicular. It joins the venous system most commonly by emptying into the internal jugular vein and sometimes into the subclavian, innominate, and external jugular veins.

The roentgenologic anatomy of the *right lymphatic duct* has not been described, since this vessel cannot be suitably opacified. This duct is an inconstant channel: the three trunks—the right jugular, right subclavian, and right mediastinal—often open separately into the jugular, subclavian, and innominate veins, respectively.

LYMPHATICS OF THE MEDIASTINUM

Although our major concern is with lymphatic drainage of the lungs and pleura, involvement of the mediastinal lymph nodes is fairly common in diseases arising in the breast, chest wall, diaphragm, or intra-abdominal or retroperitoneal structures. Therefore, a thorough understanding of all afferent and efferent drainage pathways and of nodal anatomy is imperative. Individual patterns of lymph node enlargement may supply an important clue to the origin or nature of a disease process arising inside or outside the thorax.

Intrathoracic lymph nodes are usually divided into two main anatomic groups, the parietal and visceral mediastinal nodes. The former drain the thoracic wall and certain extrathoracic tissues, and the latter are concerned almost entirely with intrathoracic structures. For purposes of roentgenographic description, however, a more useful classification is based on subdivision of groups of nodes in relation to the three mediastinal compartments. Since extensive communications exist not only between the parietal and visceral groups of nodes but also within the visceral group itself, an anatomic description based on mediastinal zones possesses considerable merit.

THE ANTERIOR MEDIASTINAL COMPARTMENT

Two chains of lymph nodes are present in the anterior compartment—the sternal (parietal) and the anterior mediastinal (visceral) groups (Figure 1–44).

Sternal (Anterior Parietal or Internal Mammary) Group

This group is situated extrapleurally. The nodes are scattered along the internal mammary arteries and behind the anterior intercostal spaces and costal cartilages bilaterally. Two or three may be directly retrosternal. These nodes vary in number but occur more consistently superiorly. Their afferent channels drain the upper anterior abdominal wall, the anterior thoracic wall, the anterior portion of the diaphragm, and the medial portions of the breast. They communicate with the visceral group of anterior mediastinal nodes and the cervical nodes, and their main efferent channels are the right lymphatic duct or bronchomediastinal duct on the right and the thoracic duct on the left.

Anterior Mediastinal (Prevascular) Group

This comprises the second group of nodes in the anterior mediastinal compartment; they belong to the visceral collection. A few nodes are posterior to the sternum in the lower thorax, but the majority are grouped in the prevascular areas bilaterally, along the superior vena cava and innominate vein on the right and in front of the aorta and carotid artery on the left side. A few lie anterior to the thymus behind the manubrium. These nodes drain most of the structures in the anterior mediastinum, including the pericardium, part of the heart, the thymus, thyroid, diaphragmatic and mediastinal pleura, and the anterior portions of the hila bilaterally. Their efferent channels drain via the bronchomediastinal trunk or thoracic duct.

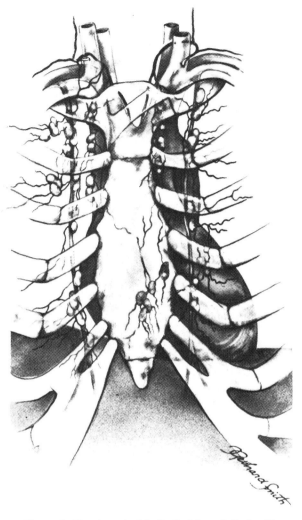

Figure 1–44.   Anterior Mediastinal Lymph Nodes. The nodes illustrated are chiefly those of the anterior parietal group scattered along the internal mammary arteries and behind the anterior intercostal spaces and costal cartilages bilaterally. The prevascular (visceral) group relates to the superior vena cava and innominate vein on the right and to the aorta and carotid artery on the left.

THE POSTERIOR MEDIASTINAL COMPARTMENT

Groups of nodes belonging to both the parietal and the visceral chains lie in the posterior mediastinum (Figure 1–45).

Intercostal (Posterior Parietal) Group

This group lies laterally, in the intercostal spaces, and medially, in the paravertebral areas adjacent to the heads of the ribs. Both groups drain the intercostal spaces, parietal pleura, and vertebral column. They communicate with the posterior mediastinal group of visceral nodes and have efferent channels that drain to the

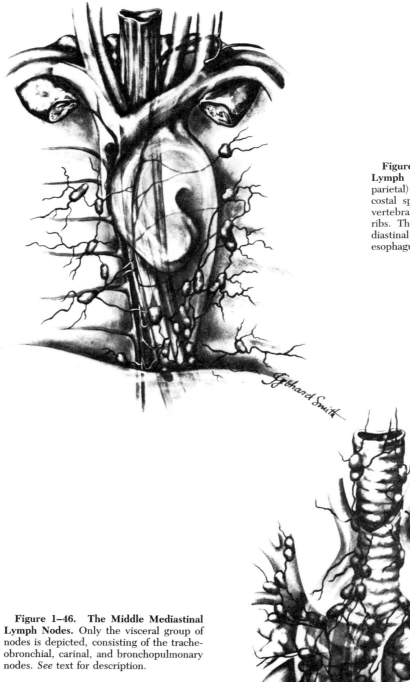

Figure 1–45. Posterior Mediastinal Lymph Nodes. The intercostal (posterior parietal) group lies laterally, in the intercostal spaces, and medially, in the paravertebral areas adjacent to the heads of the ribs. The visceral group of posterior mediastinal nodes is situated along the lower esophagus and descending aorta.

Figure 1–46. The Middle Mediastinal Lymph Nodes. Only the visceral group of nodes is depicted, consisting of the tracheobronchial, carinal, and bronchopulmonary nodes. *See* text for description.

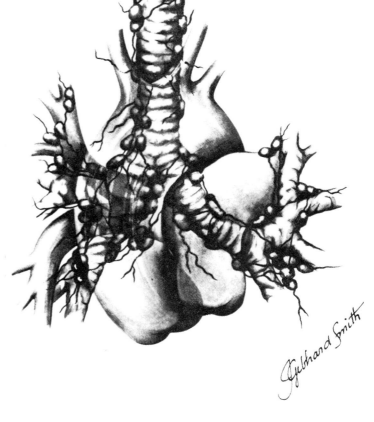

thoracic duct from the upper portions of the thorax and to the cisterna chyli from the lower thoracic area.

Posterior Mediastinal Group

This group of visceral nodes is situated along the lower esophagus and descending aorta. The nodes possess afferent channels from the posterior portion of the diaphragm, the pericardium, esophagus, and directly from the lower lobes of the lungs. They communicate with the bifurcation group of tracheobronchial nodes and drain mainly via the thoracic duct.

THE MIDDLE MEDIASTINAL COMPARTMENT

This compartment also includes parietal and visceral components.

Parietal Group

These nodes are situated mainly around the pericardial attachment to the diaphragm; they drain the diaphragm and portions of the liver via efferent pathways that pass anteriorly to the sternal or anterior mediastinal nodes and posteriorly to the posterior mediastinal nodes. Formerly thought to be of little importance roentgenologically, these nodes are now known to be involved in some cases of lymphoma.[89] Enlargement of the nodes in the cardiophrenic angles particularly may hinder differentiation from other masses arising locally and may be mistaken for pleuropericardial fat pads.

From a roentgenologic point of view the other lymph nodes in the middle mediastinal compartment constitute the most important group in the thorax: the *tracheobronchial, carinal,* and *bronchopulmonary* nodes (Figure 1–46). Although these groups freely communicate with one another, involvement often is predominantly in one group.

Tracheobronchial Nodes

These nodes are scattered along the lateral aspects of the trachea and in the tracheobronchial angles and are more numerous on the right than on the left. One node which is fairly constant in position is situated in the right tracheobronchial angle contiguous with the azygos vein; this is commonly referred to as the azygos node. Afferent channels arise from the bronchopulmonary and bifurcation nodes, from the trachea and esophagus, and from the right or left lung directly without diversion via

the bronchopulmonary or bifurcation nodes. Direct communication exists with the anterior and posterior groups of visceral mediastinal nodes. The efferent channels are the bronchomediastinal trunk on the right and the thoracic duct on the left.

Bifurcation (Carinal) Nodes

These are situated along the anterior and inferior aspects of the carina and extend downward along the medial aspects of the main bronchi to the origin of the lower lobe bronchi bilaterally. They receive afferent drainage from the bronchopulmonary nodes, the anterior and posterior mediastinal nodes, the heart, pericardium, and esophagus, and directly from both lungs. Efferent drainage is to the right tracheobronchial group.

Bronchopulmonary Nodes

These nodes, which are numerous bilaterally, vary in number. They lie in the angles between the bronchial bifurcations in the hilar regions and are closely related to the arteries and veins. Their afferent supply is from all pulmonary lobes, and efferent drainage is to the bifurcation and tracheobronchial nodes.

PATTERNS OF LYMPHATIC DRAINAGE OF THE LUNGS

The location of enlarged lymph nodes within the mediastinum may be important in determining the intrapulmonary site of origin of infections or neoplasms. Much of our knowledge of patterns of regional lymph node drainage from the lung derives from Rouvière's treatise[90] on the anatomy of the human lymphatic system, published in 1938, which was based on necropsy studies of 200 fetuses, neonates, amd children. Many of his observations have since been confirmed. Rouvière subdivided the lungs into three main drainage areas—the superior, middle, and inferior—without correspondence to pulmonary lobes.

On the right side, in the superior area, lymph drains directly into the paratracheal and upper bronchopulmonary nodes. The middle zone drains directly into the paratracheal nodes, the bifurcation nodes, and the central group of bronchopulmonary nodes. The inferior zone drains into the inferior bronchopulmonary and bifurcation nodes and the posterior mediastinal chain. Thus, on the right side, all the lymph drains eventually via the right lymphatic duct.

Rouvière[90] stated that, *on the left side*, in the superior area, lymph drains both into the prevascular group of anterior mediastinal nodes and directly into the left paratracheal nodes. The middle zone drains mainly via the bifurcation and central group of bronchopulmonary nodes and partly directly into the left paratracheal group. The inferior zone drains into the bifurcation and inferior bronchopulmonary nodes and into the posterior mediastinal chain. Thus, according to Rouvière,[90] the superior portion and part of the middle zone drain via the left paratracheal nodes into the thoracic duct, and lymph drainage from the remainder of the left lung empties eventually into the right lymphatic duct.

This "crossover" phenomenon was long thought to be of diagnostic and therapeutic importance in diseases originating in the middle or lower portion of the left lung, but more recent investigations have cast some doubt on the validity of the phenomenon in adults. For example, Baird[91] performed bilateral prescalene node biopsies in 218 patients, 110 of whom had bronchogenic carcinoma; the direction of lymphatic spread within the mediastinum was cephalad and usually ipsilateral, irrespective of the location of the primary growth. Contralateral spread was uncommon and about equally frequent from either lung.

THE MEDIASTINUM

Our knowledge of the roentgenographic anatomy of the mediastinum has accumulated over the years by the studies of many investigators and was consolidated into a superb treatise on the subject by Heitzman in 1977.[92] A great deal of useful information about the anatomy of the mediastinum can be gleaned from standard roentgenograms and conventional tomograms of the thorax in posteroanterior, lateral, and oblique projections, but with the introduction of computed tomography (CT) in 1973 we were provided with a technique of examining mediastinal structures with much greater precision than with conventional roentgenography. In the vast majority of clinical settings, however, conventional roentgenography is all that is necessary for adequate evaluation of the mediastinal compartments, and CT should be reserved for the selective investigation of particular problems. In this book, we have chosen to describe mediastinal anatomy by both standard roentgenographic and CT techniques, the former following hereafter and the latter beginning on page 78.

The mediastinum constitutes a compartmented septum or partition that divides the thorax vertically (Figures 1–47 and 1–48). Traditionally, it is divided into two major compartments, the superior and the inferior, the latter being subdivided into anterior, middle, and posterior compartments. Since each compartment contains anatomic structures almost unique to it, many of the affections to which the mediastinum is subject tend to occur *predominantly* in one or the other compartment; thus, we feel that this anatomic subdivision has considerable merit. For a number of reasons, however, Heitzman[92] has taken issue with this anatomic classification and has devised an alternate scheme based on a division of the right and left sides of the mediastinum into areas of somewhat similar size separated by a major vascular channel. In his classification, the traditional middle and posterior mediastinal compartments are subdivided into four areas based on the aortic and azygos arches: the regions above and below the aortic arch on the left side and above and below the azygos arch on the right side. We have examined this approach to mediastinal anatomy in considerable detail and have concluded that it possesses both advantages and disadvantages over the traditional method: both are to some extent arbitrary, yet each can be employed satisfactorily in the majority of clinical situations. During the many years we have attempted to analyze mediastinal abnormalities using the traditional subdivision into three compartments, we have found the system to work reasonably well and have decided to stick with this classification in this book. However, for those who wish to seek the other point of view, we strongly recommend study of the excellent treatise on the subject by Heitzman.[92]

Two further points deserve emphasis. First, the superior mediastinal compartment is defined as that region extending from the thoracic inlet to a line drawn from the angle of Louis to the lower edge of the body of the fourth thoracic vertebra; we feel that this compartment possesses little practical importance as a separate division and have excluded it from the classification. Secondly, since the posterior limit of the mediastinum has been precisely defined anatomically as the anterior surface of the vertebral column, the paravertebral zones and posterior gutters are not technically included in the definition. However, because these areas contain structures of importance in the etiology of posterior mediastinal masses, for purposes of roentgenologic differential diagnosis they are considered part of the posterior mediastinum.

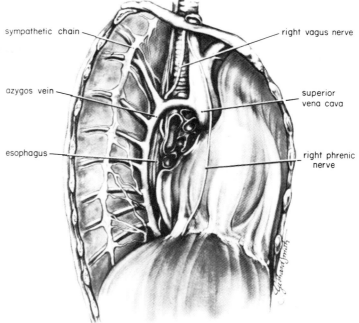

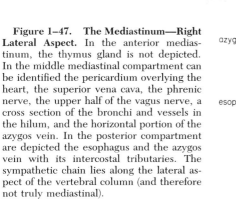

Figure 1–47. The Mediastinum—Right Lateral Aspect. In the anterior mediastinum, the thymus gland is not depicted. In the middle mediastinal compartment can be identified the pericardium overlying the heart, the superior vena cava, the phrenic nerve, the upper half of the vagus nerve, a cross section of the bronchi and vessels in the hilum, and the horizontal portion of the azygos vein. In the posterior compartment are depicted the esophagus and the azygos vein with its intercostal tributaries. The sympathetic chain lies along the lateral aspect of the vertebral column (and therefore not truly mediastinal).

MEDIASTINAL COMPARTMENTS

ANTERIOR MEDIASTINAL COMPARTMENT

The anterior mediastinal compartment (Figures 1–47 and 1–48) is bounded anteriorly by the sternum and posteriorly by the pericardium, aorta, and brachiocephalic vessels. It contains the thymus gland, the anterior mediastinal lymph nodes, including both parietal and visceral groups, and the internal mammary

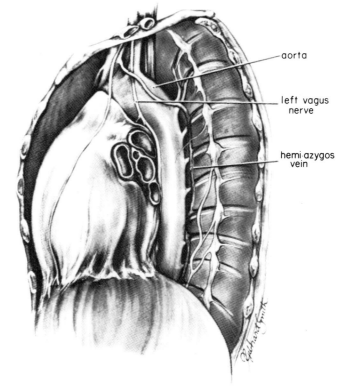

Figure 1–48. The Mediastinum—Left Lateral Aspect. No anatomic structures are depicted in the anterior mediastinum. In the middle mediastinal compartment, in addition to the structures already described in Figure 1–47 are the ascending and transverse arch of the aorta and the brachiocephalic arteries. Most of the vagus nerve can be identified. In the posterior mediastinal compartment the descending thoracic aorta and hemiazygos veins can be seen.

arteries and veins in the parasternal areas bilaterally. It is relatively narrow, particularly inferiorly, where the pericardium overlying the right ventricle touches the lower portion of the sternum.

MIDDLE MEDIASTINAL COMPARTMENT

The middle mediastinal compartment (Figures 1–47 and 1–48) contains the pericardium and heart, the ascending and transverse arch of the aorta, the superior and inferior vena cavae, the brachiocephalic arteries and veins, the phrenic nerves and upper portion of the vagus nerves, the trachea and main bronchi and their contiguous lymph nodes, and the pulmonary arteries and veins.

POSTERIOR MEDIASTINAL COMPARTMENT

The posterior mediastinal compartment (Figures 1–47 and 1–48) lies between the pericardium and the spinal column. It contains the descending thoracic aorta, esophagus, thoracic duct, azygos and hemiazygos veins, sympathetic chains and the lower portion of the vagus nerves, and the posterior group of mediastinal lymph nodes; as previously mentioned, for practical purposes the paravertebral zones and posterior gutters are included in this compartment.

MEDIASTINAL PLEURAL REFLECTIONS

It is important to recognize certain lines within the mediastinal contour on well-exposed frontal or lateral chest roentgenograms, since deviations in their pattern may supply important clues in diagnosis. These lines, caused by the reflection of pleura over certain structures, are conveniently considered according to their anatomic location—in the anterior, posterior, and middle mediastinal compartments.

ANTERIOR MEDIASTINAL PLEURAL REFLECTIONS

Anterior Junction Line

Because the heart and major vessels deviate from the sternum superiorly, the anterior mediastinum deepens and the right and left lungs come into apposition, creating the anterior mediastinal septum. This thin hairline shadow, the *anterior junction line* (synonym: anterior mediastinal line) represents the thickness of the

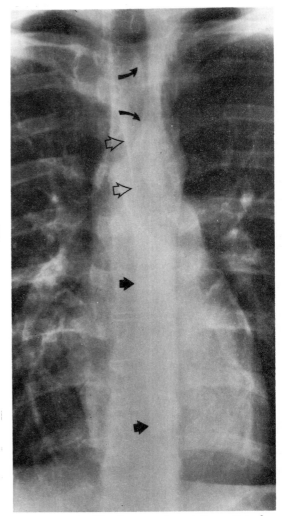

Figure 1–49. The Azygoesophageal Recess Interface, Posterior Junction Line, and Anterior Junction Line. A detail view of the mediastinum from a PA roentgenogram reveals a slightly curved shadow convex to the right *(solid arrows)* projected in front of the thoracic spine; this represents the azygoesophageal recess interface. Superiorly a second curved line shadow convex to the left *(curved arrows)* and projected over the air column of the trachea represents the posterior junction line. Between the two is the thin hairline shadow of the anterior junction line *(open arrows)*.

visceral and parietal pleura of the two contiguous upper lobes, possibly with a small amount of areolar tissue interposed. Measuring no more than 1 to 2 mm in diameter, it is commonly identified on posteroanterior roentgenograms projected over the air column of the trachea for several centimeters distal to the plane of the junction of the manubrium and the body of the sternum (Figure 1–49). It thus projects considerably lower than the supra-aortic posterior junction line *(see further on)*, a similar linear shadow with which it is sometimes confused. The anterior mediastinal line usually deviates slightly from right to left from above downward.

POSTERIOR MEDIASTINAL PLEURAL REFLECTIONS

Four lines or interfaces are visible within the mediastinal contour on many well-exposed frontal chest roentgenograms —the supra-aortic posterior junction line, the azygoesophageal recess interface, the descending aortic interface, and the paraspinal interface.

Supra-aortic Posterior Junction Line

This line (synonym: the esophageal-pleural stripe) is formed by contact of the parietal and visceral layers of pleura of the right and left lungs, which come into contact above the aortic and azygos arches, behind the trachea and esophagus, and in front of the upper thoracic spine. As the arch of the azygos vein curves anteriorly at the level of the aortic arch and right main bronchus (see further on), it causes a superior reflection of the posterior mediastinal pleura that creates the right side of the supra-aortic posterior junction line. This cephalad sweep of the mediastinal pleura from the azygos arch usually comes in contact with the left lung behind the esophagus and trachea, so that the pleural surfaces of the two lungs come together in the supra-aortic triangle of the posterior mediastinal compartment (Figure 1–49). This line of apposition projects over the air column of the trachea; since its center is at the plane of the upper surface of the manubrium, it is invariably projected at a level higher than the anterior junction line. Its right side is usually gently concave. Since the esophagus is close to the posterior aspect of the trachea in the supra-aortic triangle and slightly to the left of midline, the left-sided lung may sometimes outline the left lateral esophageal wall, especially if the esophagus is distended with gas. Cimmino[93] has shown by computed tomography that there is some variability in the relationship of the esophagus to the trachea, the two sometimes being side by side with the esophagus to the left.

Azygos Vein and Azygoesophageal Recess Interface

The importance of the azygos vein and its pleural reflections in assessing normality and pathologic processes affecting the mediastinum was first detailed by Heitzman and colleagues

in 1971,[94a, 94b] and more recently has been described in detail by Kieffer and Heitzman in terms of cross-sectional anatomy and computerized tomography.[95] In their superb anatomic-roentgenologic studies, these authors pointed out that the course of the azygos vein within the mediastinum determines the anatomic arrangement of the right posterior mediastinal pleura and contiguous lung, and that the interfaces thus produced provide useful landmarks for roentgen evaluation of the mediastinum.

The azygos vein, the cephalad continuation of the right ascending lumbar vein, passes through the aortic hiatus of the diaphragm and ascends within the thorax on the anterior aspect of the thoracic spine. In many cases it deviates slightly to the right in its ascent. It receives the hemiazygos vein at the level of T8 or T9, becoming 1 cm or more in diameter in its ascent to the level of T4 or T5; there it angulates sharply anteriorly and slightly to the right to terminate in the posterior wall of the superior vena cava just above the entry of that vessel into the right atrium. As the azygos vein passes anteriorly across the right side of the mediastinum, it relates to the superior aspect of the right upper lobe bronchus and the truncus anterior branch of the right pulmonary artery.

Along most of its ascent up the vertebral column, the azygos vein is intimately related to the pleura of the right lower lobe and to the esophagus that lies just anterior to it. Between the esophagus and the vein is a space into which lung inserts. Termed by anatomists the crista pulmonis, this intrusion has been designated the azygoesophageal recess by Heitzman and his colleagues; the interface that is created on a frontal roentgenogram represents the medial extent of the azygoesophageal recess (Figure 1–49). Sometimes the lung in the azygoesophageal recess contacts the right side of the descending aorta.

The azygoesophageal recess interface extends from above the diaphragm, in front of the thoracic vertebrae, to the level of the aortic arch and right main bronchus. Its right side is sharply delineated by air-containing lung. Its left side is usually of unit density because of contiguity of the azygos vein, esophagus, and aorta; however, if gas is present in the esophagus, the combined thickness of the right esophageal wall and contiguous visceral and parietal pleura creates a linear opacity or stripe.

The main portion of the vein may be visible in its retrotracheal course as it curves anteriorly contiguous to the arch of the aorta.[96] It is seen through the air column of the trachea as an indistinct soft tissue shadow, analogous to the aortic knob created by the transverse arch of

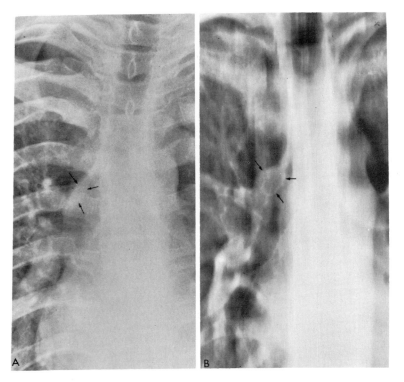

Figure 1–50. Effect of Body Position on Azygos Vein Diameter. *A*, A roentgenogram in the erect position shows the azygos vein as an elliptic shadow projected in the right tracheobronchial angle *(arrows).* *B*, In the same subject, a tomographic section of the mid-mediastinum in the supine position demonstrates a much larger vein shadow *(arrows)* owing to distention brought about by the supine body position.

the aorta, and has been termed by Heitzman and associates the "azygos knob." It is of obvious importance not to mistake this opacity for an enlarged mediastinal node or tracheal mass.

Mensuration of the azygos vein is important in some diseases, notably portal hypertension, obstruction of the superior vena cava, and right atrial hypertension (as in decompensation of the right side of the heart). The only segment that can be measured accurately on standard roentgenograms is the point at which it is visualized roughly tangentially in the right tracheobronchial angle just before entering the superior vena cava. In this location the vein often is visible on frontal chest roentgenograms as an elliptical opacity (Figure 1–50). Felson[97] states that on teleroentgenograms of erect normal subjects the transverse diameter of the vein measured from its outer border to the contiguous air column of the right main bronchus may be up to 10 mm, and we have observed the same diameter in many normal subjects. It is reasonable to adopt the following general rules regarding the diameter of this vein. In the majority of normal subjects in the erect position the azygos vein diameter is 7 mm or less; a diameter of 7 to 10 mm is seen sometimes and is almost always within the normal range; a diameter exceeding 10 mm should be regarded as pathologic except in pregnant women. In the latter group, the maximum diameter can

be as large as 15 mm, a normal effect of pregnancy which should be borne in mind when considering the differential diagnosis of azygos vein enlargement.

Vascular distention due to change in body position from erect to recumbent increases the vein's diameter (Figure 1–50). Doyle and his associates,[98] using a tomographic technique with a shortened focus-film distance, measured the maximal diameter in 48 healthy subjects in a supine position and found a mean azygos vein diameter of 14.2 mm; the diameter exceeded 16 mm in only eight subjects.

Descending Aortic Interface

This is an interface formed by contact of the left lower lobe with the lateral aspect of the descending thoracic aorta. In young asthenic subjects it may be barely visible as a vertically oriented interface projecting just to the left of the spine, but in sthenic subjects it is generally clearly visible. In the presence of aortic elongation from whatever cause, the interface assumes a gentle convex configuration laterally.

Paraspinal Interface

The reflection of pleura from the posterior thoracic wall onto the *right* side of the mediastinum is smooth and normally is uninterrupted by protruding structures. Thus it is invisible on frontal roentgenograms of the chest unless thoracic spine osteophytes displace it laterally and permit its visualization. By contrast, on the *left* side the descending thoracic aorta protrudes slightly laterally in the posterior mediastinal compartment, causing lateral displacement of the mediastinal pleura posterior to it. This creates the paraspinal interface (*synonyms:* left paraspinal reflection, paraspinal line). This longitudinal shadow is projected about midway between the outer border of the descending thoracic aorta and the vertebral column (Figure 1–51); it extends from the aortic arch down to the diaphragm. As might be expected, elongation of the thoracic aorta displaces the paraspinal interface laterally, the relationship of the interface to the lateral border of the aorta and the spine being maintained at roughly mid-position; both conventional and computerized tomography have shown that in such circumstances the space between the paraspinal interface and the spine is occupied by fat.

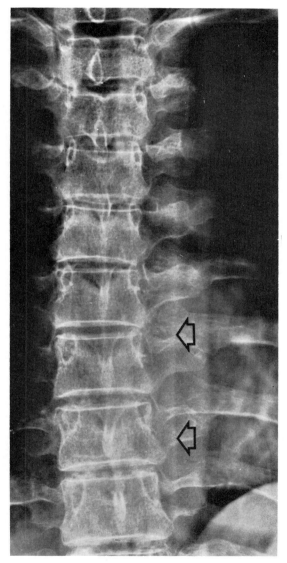

Figure 1–51. The Paraspinal Interface. A roentgenogram of the mediastinum in anteroposterior projection, supine position; normal 42-year-old male. A longitudinal shadow *(arrows)* extending from the arch of the aorta to the diaphragm is projected about midway between the lateral border of the descending aorta and the vertebral column; this shadow is caused by the paravertebral mediastinal pleura being displaced laterally by the descending aorta.

MIDDLE MEDIASTINAL PLEURAL REFLECTIONS

Right Cardiovascular Contour

In a posteroanterior roentgenogram of the chest (*see* Figure 1–60, pages 90–91), the right mediastinal border from the right atrium to the lung apex is formed by the superior vena cava and right brachiocephalic vein. In healthy subjects, provided that the chest is correctly centered, the ascending aorta contributes nothing to the mediastinal contour. The extreme cephalad portion of the mediastinum in the plane of the second and third posterior interspaces may be formed by the right subclavian artery. In some cases the shadow of the inferior vena cava is visible running downward and laterally from the median, across the right cardiophrenic angle. This represents the intrathoracic portion of the vein as it ascends to the right atrium.

Physiologic accumulations of fatty tissue are common in the cardiophrenic recesses bilaterally, producing an obtuse angular configuration of the inferior mediastinum at its junction with the diaphragm. Their density may be slightly less than that of the heart, allowing identification through them of the approximate position of the cardiac borders. These pleuropericardial fat shadows should not be misinterpreted as cardiac enlargement or as mediastinal or diaphragmatic masses of possible importance. However, the bilateral cardiophrenic regions contain parietal lymph nodes of the middle mediastinal chain, whose enlargement in patients with lymphoma may simulate pleuropericardial fat pads.[89]

Left Cardiovascular Contour

On the left side, the contour of the mediastinum cephalad from the diaphragm includes the left ventricle, left atrial appendage (seldom, if ever, visualized as a separate shadow on static teleroentgenograms of normal subjects), the left border of the undivided pulmonary artery, the pleural reflection from the aorta downward on to the main pulmonary artery, and the aortic knob. The silhouette of the superior mediastinum above the arch of the aorta is formed mostly by the left subclavian artery.

An interface of considerable importance in the left mediastinal contour, particularly from the point of view of mediastinal lymph node enlargement, is a "window" formed by the arch of the aorta and the left pulmonary artery—thus, the *aortopulmonary window interface.* The boundaries of this space are the posterior surface of the ascending aorta, the anterior surface of the descending aorta, the inferior surface of the aortic arch, and the upper surface of the left pulmonary artery. The trachea, left main bronchus, and esophagus form its medial boundary and the left lung its lateral boundary. Within this space are situated fat, the ligament of the ductus arteriosus, the left recurrent laryngeal nerve, and ductal lymph nodes. On a frontal chest roentgenogram, the interface is normally flat or concave; enlargement of ductal lymph nodes displaces the interface laterally, thus creating a convex configuration that is a subtle but important sign of disease.

The Heart Generally

It is beyond the scope of this book to discuss the heart in detail. However, it is important to recognize that certain deviations in the normal roentgen anatomy of the cardiovascular silhouette may give rise to confusion.

In a frontal roentgenogram of the normal chest (*see* Figure 1–60, pages 90–91), the position of the heart in relation to the midline of the thorax depends largely upon the patient's build. Assuming roentgenographic exposure with lungs fully inflated, in asthenic patients the heart shadow is almost exactly midline in position, projecting only slightly more to the left; in those of stockier build it lies a little more to the left of midline (in the range of three-quarters to one-quarter).[99]

In normal subjects, the transverse diameter of the heart measured on standard teleroentgenograms is mostly in the range of 11.5 to 15.5 cm;[99] it is less than 11.5 cm in approximately 5 per cent, and only rarely exceeds 15.5 cm (in very heavy subjects of stocky build, often

manual laborers). The custom of trying to assess cardiac size by relating it to the transverse diameter of the chest, *i.e.*, cardiothoracic ratio, is inaccurate. Although 50 per cent is widely accepted as the upper limit of normal for this ratio, in fact it exceeds 50 per cent in at least 10 per cent of normal subjects.[99] This ratio is especially fallacious in patients who have a small heart. As pointed out by Simon,[99] in a person with an 8-cm transverse cardiac diameter in a 24-cm thorax, the heart would have to enlarge 4 cm before the cardiothoracic ratio reached the mythic 50 per cent. In our view, it is preferable to evaluate cardiac size subjectively on the basis of experience; alternatively, it is reasonable to assume that a heart whose transverse diameter exceeds 15.5 to 16 cm is enlarged until proved otherwise.

Chiefly as a result of the influence of systole and diastole, both the size and contour of the heart may vary from one examination to another, even when all examinations are made with an identical degree of lung inflation. In a series of 200 normal subjects,[99] the difference in transverse cardiac diameter on successive examinations showed a group average of 0.5 cm. A rough guide in this assessment is that a heart whose transverse diameter has increased by 1.5 cm or more on sequential examinations has very likely increased in size.

COMPUTED TOMOGRAPHY OF THE NORMAL MEDIASTINUM

On the following pages is depicted the anatomy of the normal mediastinum as seen on computed tomographic (CT) scans (Figures 1–52 to 1–56). Only five levels have been selected to illustrate the most important anatomic relationships; thus, the subject has not been dealt with exhaustively and the interested reader is directed to more complete works on the subject, particularly the monograph by Kieffer and Heitzman.[95] In each figure, the precise level of the CT scan is indicated on a scout view; this is followed by the scan and a diagrammatic representation of the scan. All scans were performed on a young asymptomatic male volunteer, using a General Electric CT/T Model 8800 total body scanner with a scanning time of 4.8 sec/slice. There was no contrast enhancement. For further details of the technique of and indications for CT scanning of the thorax, see page 107.

Text continued on page 85

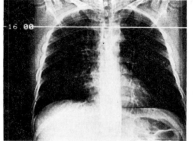

A

**List of Anatomic Structures
for Figure 1–52**
1. Manubrium
2. Left brachiocephalic vein
3. Right brachiocephalic vein
4. Calcified lymph node
5. Innominate artery
6. Left carotid artery
7. Trachea
8. Lymph node
9. Thoracic duct
10. Left subclavian artery
11. Esophagus
12. Spinal cord

Figure 1–52. Normal Cross-Sectional Anatomy of the Mediastinum at a Level Immediately Cephalad to the Arch of the Aorta. *A*, Scout view indicating level of cut. *B*, CT scan. *C*, Drawing of anatomic structures. Immediately behind the manubrium sterni (1) is the longitudinal shadow of the left brachiocephalic (innominate) vein (2), as it passes from left to right to join the right brachiocephalic vein (3) to form the superior vena cava. Situated in the angle formed by the junction of these two vessels is a tiny densely calcified lymph node (4). Immediately posterior to and contiguous with the left brachiocephalic vein is the innominate artery to the right (5) and left carotid artery to the left (6). The tracheal air column (7) can be clearly seen immediately posterior to the innominate artery. To the left of the trachea is a collection of mediastinal fat in which are situated a small lymph node (8) and the thoracic duct (9). Also within this fatty tissue posteriorly is the circular image of the left subclavian artery (10). Posterior to the trachea and slightly to the left is the shadow of the esophagus containing a small amount of gas (11). The spinal cord (12) can be readily identified within the spinal canal.

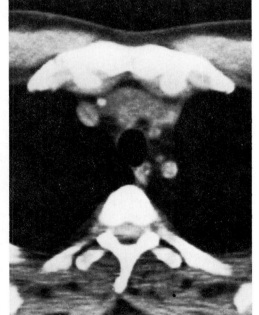

B

C

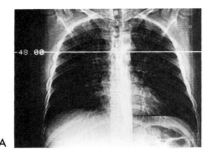

A

**List of Anatomic Structures
for Figure 1–53**

1. Anterior mediastinal fat
2. Ascending aorta
3. Superior vena cava
4. Trachea
5. Fat in aortopulmonary window
6. Lymph nodes
7. Descending aorta
8. Esophagus
9. Azygos vein

Figure 1–53. Normal Cross-Sectional Anatomy of the Mediastinum at a Level Immediately Caudad to the Arch of the Aorta. *A,* Scout view indicating level of cut. *B,* CT scan. *C,* Drawing of anatomic structures. Immediately posterior to the sternum is a roughly triangular opacity of low attenuation (1) representing an accumulation of fat in the anterior mediastinal septum between the right and left lungs. Posterior to this fatty accumulation is the circular shadow of the ascending aorta (2), to the right of which is the superior vena cava (3). The tracheal air column (4) is readily identified in the midline posterior to the ascending aorta. To the left of the trachea is a rather indistinct zone of relatively low attenuation which represents the upper level of the aortopulmonary window (5); two small lymph nodes (6) can be seen in the lateral portion of the window. The descending aorta (7) relates to the window posteriorly. The shadow of the esophagus (8) is situated directly behind the trachea and close to the right lateral wall of the descending aorta. On the right posterolateral aspect of the trachea is the shadow of the posterior portion of the azygos vein (9) as it begins its horizontal course from the spine toward the superior vena cava.

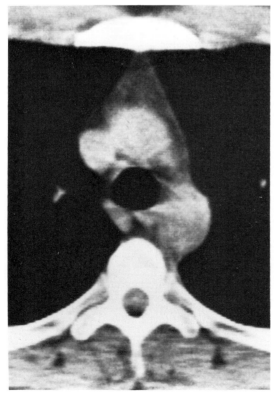

B

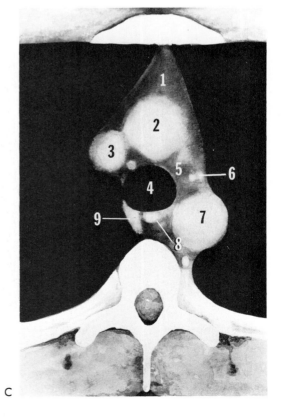

C

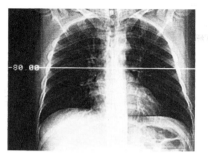

A

**List of Anatomic Structures
for Figure 1–54**

1. Anterior junction line
2. Ascending aorta
3. Main pulmonary artery
4. Right pulmonary artery
5. Left pulmonary artery
6. Left main bronchus
7. Superior vena cava
8. Right main bronchus
9. Descending aorta
10. Esophagus
11. Azygos vein
12. Inferior accessory azygos vein

Figure 1–54. Normal Cross-Sectional Anatomy of the Mediastinum at a Level Immediately Caudad to the Carina. *A,* Scout view indicating level of cut. *B,* CT scan. *C,* Drawing of anatomic structures. Immediately posterior to the sternum is the very thin linear opacity (1) representing the anterior junction line which blends rather abruptly into a triangular opacity of low attenuation representing anterior mediastinal fat. Immediately posterior to this fatty accumulation are two readily separable opacities, the ascending aorta on the right (2) and the main pulmonary artery on the left (3). Immediately posteriorly, the latter vessel bifurcates into right (4) and left (5) branches. Behind the left branch is the left main bronchus (6). Posterior and slightly to the right of the ascending aorta is the rather poorly defined shadow of the superior vena cava (7), behind which is the right main bronchus (8). The shadow of the descending aorta (9) is readily identifiable on the anterolateral aspect of the vertebral body; anterior to the aorta and slightly to the right is the gas-containing esophagus (10). Immediately anterior to the vertebral body is the small shadow of the azygos vein (11); situated within the V created by the azygos vein and descending aorta is a very small opacity which probably represents the thoracic duct. Identifiable as only a very thin shadow immediately to the left of the vertebral body is the inferior accessory azygos vein (12). Because of the relatively high level setting of this CT scan, the anterior junction line and azygoesophageal recess are poorly visualized, but these can be seen to better advantage in Figure 1–55 at lung window settings.

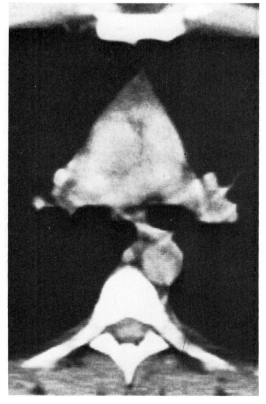

B

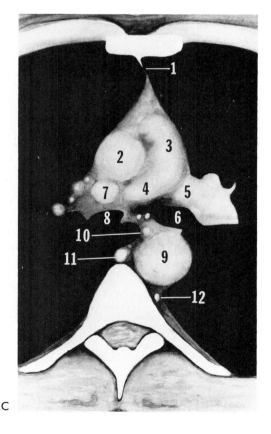

C

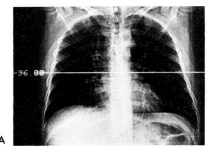

A

**List of Anatomic Structures
for Figure 1–55**

1. Anterior junction line
2. Right intermediate bronchus
3. Azygos vein
4. Aorta
5. Left upper lobe bronchus
6. Right interlobar artery
7. Left interlobar artery

Figure 1–55. **Two Representative CT Scans of the Thorax at Lung Window Settings to Illustrate the Anterior Junction Line, the Azygoesophageal Recess, the Major Hilar Pulmonary Structures, and the Pulmonary Veins.** In *A*, *B*, and *C*, the scan is at a level 16 mm caudad to the cut in Figure 1–54 and thus through the midportion of both hila. Note the slight inclination of the anterior junction line (1) from right to left. The azygoesophageal recess is clearly depicted *(arrows in C)*, its anterior boundary being formed by the thin posterior wall of the right intermediate bronchus (2). The small bump on the medial aspect of the azygoesophageal recess represents the azygos vein (3). Seen only in profile is the shadow of the descending thoracic aorta (4). The longitudinal air column in the left hilum is the left upper lobe bronchus (5). The right interlobar artery (6) is directly lateral to the right intermediate bronchus, whereas the left interlobar artery (7) relates to the posterolateral aspect of the left upper lobe bronchus.

Illustration continued on opposite page.

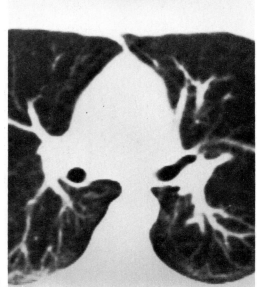

B

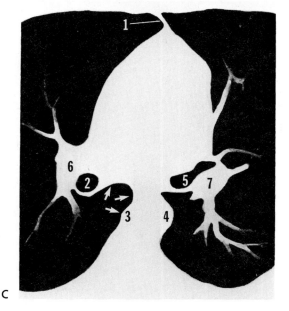

C

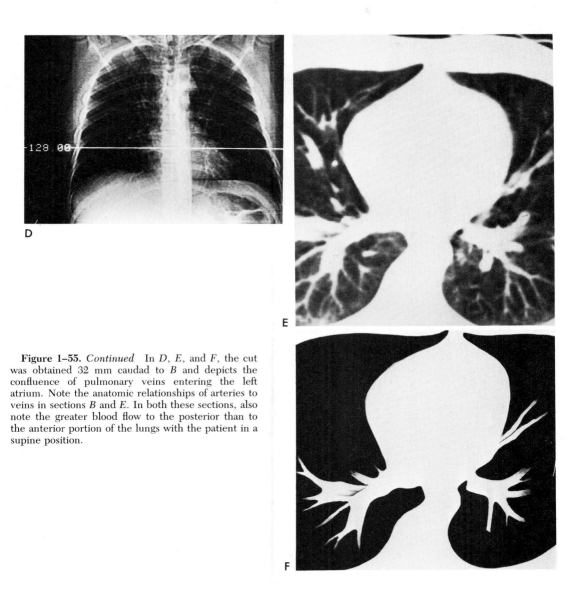

Figure 1–55. *Continued* In *D, E,* and *F,* the cut was obtained 32 mm caudad to *B* and depicts the confluence of pulmonary veins entering the left atrium. Note the anatomic relationships of arteries to veins in sections *B* and *E.* In both these sections, also note the greater blood flow to the posterior than to the anterior portion of the lungs with the patient in a supine position.

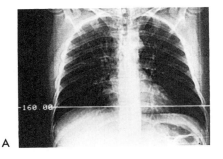

A

**List of Anatomic Structures
for Figure 1–56**

1. Liver
2. left hemidiaphragm
3. Pericardial fat
4. Pericardium
5. Epicardial fat
6. Left ventricle
7. Right ventricle
8. Right atrium
9. Descending aorta
10. Esophagus
11. Azygos vein
12. Hemiazygos vein

Figure 1–56. Normal Cross-Sectional Anatomy of the Mediastinum at the Level of the Dome of the Right Hemidiaphragm. *A,* Scout view indicating level of cut. *B,* CT scan. *C,* Drawing of anatomic structures. The large central opacity in the right hemithorax is the liver (1), and the smaller opacity in the left hemithorax is a small portion of the dome of the left hemidiaphragm (2). Situated immediately posterior to the xiphoid process of the sternum is an irregular accumulation of tissue of low attenuation (3) which represents pericardial fat on the anterior aspect of the pericardium. The pericardial membrane itself can be identified as a very thin linear structure (4) extending around the front and right lateral aspect of the heart. Deep to the pericardium, particularly anteriorly, is a thin layer of epicardial fat (5). Various components of the heart can be vaguely identified, including the left ventricle (6), the right ventricle (7) and the right atrium (8). In the posterior mediastinum can be identified the descending thoracic aorta (9), the gas-containing esophagus lying immediately anterior to the aorta (10), the azygos vein (11), and the hemiazygos vein (12).

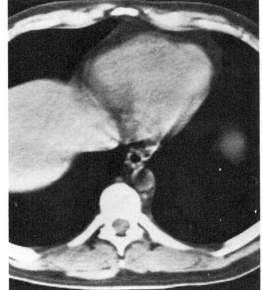

B

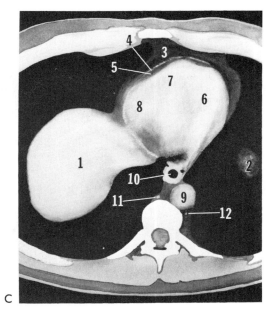

C

THE DIAPHRAGM

The diaphragm is a musculotendinous sheet separating the thoracic and abdominal cavities (Figure 1–57). The central tendon is a broad sheet of decussating tendon fibers, in shape similar to a broad-bladed Australian boomerang; the point of the "boomerang" is directed toward the sternum and the concavity toward the spine. The muscle fibers arise anteriorly from the xiphoid process, around the convexity of the thorax from ribs 7 to 12, posteriorly from the lateral margins of the first, second, and third lumbar vertebrae on the right side, and from the first and second lumbar vertebrae on the left. These fibers converge toward the central

tendon and are inserted into it nearly perpendicular to its margin. The muscle fibers are of varied length, from 5 cm anteriorly at the sternal origin to 14 cm posterolaterally where they originate from the ninth, tenth, and eleventh ribs.[14] Von Hayek[14] points out that it is the posterolateral portion of the hemidiaphragms, in which the muscle fibers are longest, that undergoes the greatest excursion on respiration. The muscle fibers that compose the sternal attachment and those that arise from the seventh rib are separated bilaterally by triangular spaces poor in muscular and tendinous tissue. These triangular spaces (the foramina of Morgagni) constitute weak areas in the diaphragm. Deficiencies in the origins of the mus-

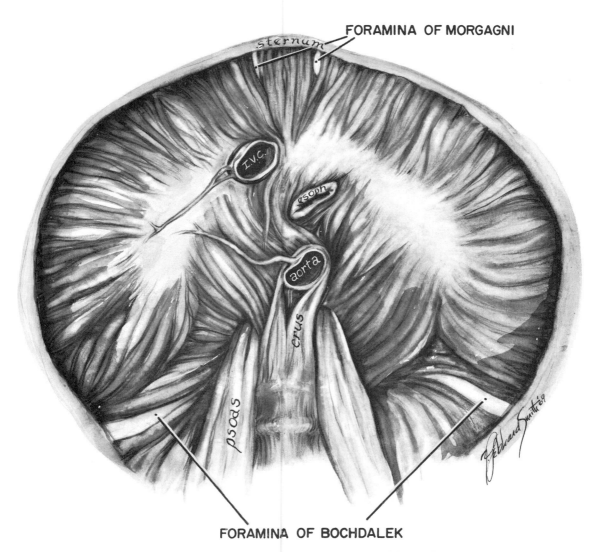

FORAMINA OF MORGAGNI

FORAMINA OF BOCHDALEK

Figure 1–57. **Anatomy of the Normal Diaphragm Viewed from Below.** *See* text.

cle bundles from the posterolateral rib cage (the foramina of Bochdalek) similarly create areas of potential weakness.

RELATIONSHIP BETWEEN THE HEIGHT OF THE RIGHT AND LEFT HEMIDIAPHRAGMS

The tendency for the plane of the right diaphragmatic dome to be about half an interspace higher than the left is well recognized, but in 9 per cent of 500 normal subjects examined by Felson[97] both were at the same height or the left was higher than the right.

It is a common error for students to ascribe the higher position of the right hemidiaphragm to the mass of the liver beneath it. In fact, the lower position of the left hemidiaphragmatic dome relates to the contiguous mass of the left side of the heart.

RANGE OF DIAPHRAGMATIC EXCURSION ON RESPIRATION

In their study of 114 healthy young males, Young and Simon[100] found a range of diaphragmatic excursion from 0.8 to 8.1 cm; it was 5 to 7 cm in 57 persons (50 per cent) and less than 3 cm in 16 (14 per cent). These authors emphasized that diaphragmatic excursion less than 3 cm is not necessarily abnormal, which has been our experience also. In fact, they found no relationship between diaphragmatic movement and vital capacity, some patients with mean diaphragmatic excursions of less than 3 cm having a vital capacity of over 5 liters.

THE CHEST WALL

The structures of the thoracic wall, both soft tissue and osseous, form a complex of shadows on roentgenograms of the chest that may be important to roentgenographic analysis, and a working knowledge of their normal anatomy and variations is indispensable.

SOFT TISSUES

On frontal roentgenograms of the thorax (*see* Figure 1–60, pages 90–91) the soft tissues, consisting of the skin, subcutaneous fat, and muscles, usually are distinguishable over the shoulders and along the thoracic wall. The pectoral muscles form the anterior axillary fold,

a structure that normally is visible in both male and female patients, curving smoothly downward and medially from the axilla to the rib cage. In men, particularly those with heavy muscular development, the inferior border of the pectoralis major muscle may be seen as a downward extension of the anterior axillary fold, passing obliquely across the middle portion of both lungs. In women, this shadow is obscured by the breasts, whose presence and size must be taken into consideration in assessing the density of the lower lung zones.

BONES

In the absence of pulmonary or pleural disease, deformity of the spine, or congenital anomalies of the ribs themselves, the rib cage should be perfectly symmetric on both sides. Both the upper and lower borders of the ribs should be sharply defined except in the middle and lower thoracic regions; here, the thin flanges created by the vascular sulci on the inferior aspects of the ribs posteriorly are visualized *en face*, creating a less distinct inferior margin.

Calcification of the rib cartilages is common, and probably never of pathologic significance. The first rib cartilage usually is the first to calcify, often shortly after the age of 20.

Thin, smooth shadows of water density that parallel the ribs and measure 1 to 2 mm in diameter project adjacent to the inferior and inferolateral margins of the first and second ribs and to the axillary portions of the lower ribs. These "companion shadows" (Figure 1–58) are caused by a combination of muscle tissue, fascia, and adipose tissue between the rib and parietal pleura. The bulk of these "companion shadows" is probably caused by fat. Vix[101] has shown by pathologic-roentgenologic correlation that extrapleural fat is most abundant over the fourth to eighth ribs posterolaterally and that it relates chiefly to the ribs rather than to the interspaces.

Congenital anomalies of the ribs are relatively uncommon; supernumerary ribs arising from the seventh cervical vertebra were identified in 1.5 per cent of 350 normal subjects examined by Felson;[97] nearly all were bilateral but many had developed asymmetrically.

Sometimes the inferior aspect of the clavicles has an irregular notch or indentation 2 to 3 cm from the sternal articulation; its size and shape are varied, from a superficial saucer-shaped defect to a deep notch 2 cm wide by 1.0 to 1.5 cm deep. These *rhomboid fossae* (Figure 1–59) give rise to the costoclavicular or rhomboid

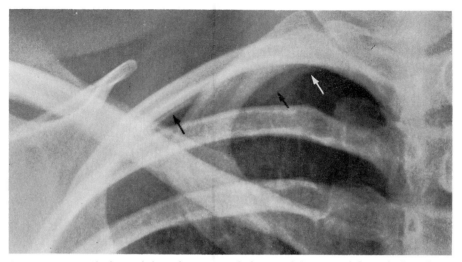

Figure 1–58. Companion Shadows of the Ribs. A magnified view of the apex of the right hemithorax reveals thin smooth shadows of water density lying roughly parallel to the inferior surfaces of the first and second ribs *(arrows)*. These companion shadows are caused by visualization in tangential projection of a combination of parietal pleura and the soft tissues immediately external to the pleura.

ligaments that radiate downward to bind the clavicles to the first rib.

The normal *thoracic spine* is straight in frontal projection and gently concave anteriorly in lateral projection. Its roentgenographic density in lateral projection decreases uniformly from above downward, and any deviation from this should arouse suspicion of intrathoracic disease.

THE NORMAL CHEST ROENTGENOGRAM

As the preceding sections have shown, the lungs are composed of an almost incredible complex of tissues, each of which separately has a unique function but all of which together perform the act of respiration. The morphologist can examine each tissue and pronounce on its normal or abnormal characteristics. In many ways, through the application of special techniques such as bronchography and angiography, the roentgenologist similarly can assess individual components of the lungs, although his or her methods are necessarily more gross. However, the bulk of the chest roentgenograms that the diagnostician must interpret are plain films, taken without contrast media, and therefore he or she is dealing with a summation of relatively low contrast objects forming a complex group of roentgenographic shadows of varied definition and density. The composition of the lungs in relation to their "density" and to their roentgenographic pattern has received insufficient attention in the literature, and in this section an attempt is made to clarify some of these issues.

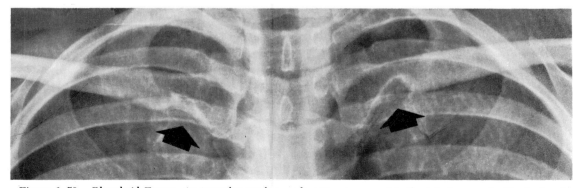

Figure 1–59. Rhomboid Fossae. An irregular notch or indentation is present in the inferior aspect of both clavicles approximately 2 cm from their sternal end *(arrows)*. These fossae give origin to the costoclavicular or rhomboid ligaments.

TABLE 1–1. PULMONARY TISSUE AND BLOOD
VOLUMES IN ML

	EXTRAVASCULAR PULMONARY TISSUE VOLUME	BLOOD VOLUME	TOTAL MAXIMAL TISSUE VOLUME
Staub,[37] 1963*	275	350	625
Loyd et al., 1966†	420	430	850
Average	350	390	740

*Estimate of the lungs of a 70-kg man, based on anatomic studies of five healthy men.

†Estimate of the lungs of a 70-kg man, 70 in in height, derived from a nomogram constructed by Loyd and his associates;[102] from physiologic data (based on the determination of pulmonary tissue volume described by Sackner and his coworkers[103] and of pulmonary blood volume described by McGaff and his associates[104]).

NORMAL LUNG DENSITY

It is readily apparent that the "roentgenographic density" of the lungs is the result of the absorptive powers of each of its component parts—gas, blood, and tissue. Although precise figures for the contributions of blood and tissue vary somewhat depending upon whether results are obtained by anatomic or physiologic methods, data have been compiled which allow a reasonable approximation (*see* Table 1–1).

Weibel[51] estimated that the lung parenchyma comprises 90 per cent of total lung volume. Using a point counting technique, he measured the volumetric proportion of the three components of lung parenchyma: *air* accounted for 92 per cent, and *tissue and capillary blood* for 8.0 per cent (including interstitium, endothelial and epithelial cells, vessel walls, and blood). On the basis of Weibel's figures and assuming a total lung volume of 7240 ml, the parenchymal component is approximately 6500 ml (90 per cent of 7240 ml), 500 ml of which consist of tissue and blood (8 per cent of 6500 ml). Thus, *the density of lung parenchyma at total lung capacity is 0.08 (500 g: 6500 ml). It follows that in a chest roentgenogram all the tissue visible in the peripheral 2 cm of the lung or between vascular shadows has a density of 0.08 g per ml.*

ALTERATION IN LUNG DENSITY

In any clinical situation, alteration in roentgenographic lung density may be due to one of three mechanisms or a combination thereof.

Physiologic Mechanisms

A frequently observed physiologic variation in lung density is the change that may occur from one examination to another on the same subject, depending upon depth of inspiration. Such variation is readily explained by comparing the contributions of the three components of the lung to its density. For example, consider a 20-year-old man, 170 cm in height, and assume that pulmonary blood volume and tissue volume are reasonably constant at different degrees of lung inflation. According to the tables of normal values constructed by Goldman and Becklake,[105] predicted lung volumes for such a subject will be: total lung capacity, 6.5 liters; functional residual capacity, 3.4 liters; and residual volume, 1.5 liters. Assuming a total maximal tissue volume of 740 ml, average lung density at total lung capacity is 0.10; at functional residual capacity, density is almost double (0.18); and at residual volume it is more than treble (0.33). Thus it is clear that, assuming total pulmonary blood volume to be constant at different degrees of lung inflation, *lung density is inversely proportional to the amount of contained gas.*

Physical (or Technical) Mechanisms

Symmetry of roentgenographic density of the two lungs in a normal subject depends upon proper positioning for roentgenography. If the patient is rotated as little as 2 to 3 degrees, the density of the lung closer to the film will be uniformly *greater* than that of the other lung. This effect is produced by the greater thickness of thoracic-wall musculature through which the x-ray beam must pass when a patient is rotated to one side. A similar effect is produced by scoliosis. Since comparison of the density of the two lungs plays such an important part in the assessment of chest roentgenograms, correct positioning of the patient and centering of the x-ray beam are crucial.

Pathologic Mechanisms

Excluding from consideration the contribution to roentgenographic density from the soft tissues of the thoracic wall, and provided that physiologic and physical causes can be excluded, variation in lung density is always due to increase or decrease in one or more of the three elements—air, blood, and tissue. In the majority of clinical situations, change in density, whether increased or decreased, local or diffuse, is the result of change in all three components.

THE PULMONARY MARKINGS

Physicians should have a thorough knowledge of the pattern of linear markings throughout the normal lung. Unfortunately, such knowledge cannot be gained through didactic teaching; it requires exposure to thousands of normal chest roentgenograms to acquire the experience—perhaps, more, the art—to be able to distinguish normal from abnormal. It requires not only familiarity with the distribution and pattern of branching of these markings (described in the section on roentgen anatomy), but also an awareness of normal caliber, extent of normal roentgenologic visibility, and changes that may occur in different phases of respiration and in various body positions. There are two main reasons for needing such knowledge: (1) a change in the caliber of arteries and veins constitutes one of the most valuable roentgenologic signs of pulmonary venous and pulmonary arterial hypertension, and (2) a redistribution of vessels, with consequent modification of the number of roentgenologically visible markings, may constitute the major evidence for pulmonary collapse or previous pulmonary resection.

The linear markings are created by a complex bundle of structures that are intimately related to one another in their passage through the lungs (Figures 1–60 and 1–61). These structures are the pulmonary arteries, bronchial arteries, bronchi, nerves, and the lymphatic channels and lymphoid collections. All of these structures are connected, at least proximal to the arterioles, by a cuff of loose areolar tissue. The arterial bundles fan outward from both hila, tapering gradually as they proceed distally. In the normal state they are visible up to about 1 to 2 cm from the visceral pleural surface over the convexity of the lung, at which point lung structure becomes totally acinar and the lung markings invisible (the lung parenchyma).

As indicated in the section dealing with the pulmonary vascular tree, the anatomic remoteness of the pulmonary veins from the arteries often renders their distinction possible roentgenographically. In the region of the pulmonary ligaments, especially, these vessels should be readily distinguishable, since the pulmonary

veins in the lower lung zones lie almost horizontally and on a lower plane than the arteries (*see* Figure 1–32, page 41, and Figure 1–55, page 82). A horizontal line drawn across a posteroanterior roentgenogram of the chest at a midpoint between the apex and diaphragm separates the pulmonary artery complex in the hila (at or above this line) and the veins (below the line). It is probable that in roughly half of all patients the upper lobe arteries and veins cannot be distinguished on plain roentgenograms of the chest in posteroanterior projection. When the vessels can be visualized separately, the veins that drain the upper lobes always project lateral to their respective arteries—a relationship particularly valuable in the right hilar region, in which the superior pulmonary vein forms the lateral aspect of the hilum superiorly and thus produces the upper limb of its concave configuration (Figure 1–60).

The posteroanterior chest roentgenogram of a normal erect subject invariably shows some discrepancy in size of the linear markings in the upper lung zones compared to the lower, owing to less perfusion of the former. In erect subjects, hydrostatic pressure increases pulmonary blood flow progressively from apex to base, a unit volume of lung at the base of the thorax having approximately four times the blood flow of a similar volume at the apex. In recumbent subjects, absence of the influence of gravity renders this discrepancy in vascular size minimal. The caliber of the upper lobe vessels in supine patients is influenced also by the recumbency-induced increase in pulmonary blood volume, which is said to amount to about 30 per cent.[106] Thus the gravitational advantage enjoyed by the upper lobes in the supine position may make the upper lobe vasculature look quite different in such films than it does in films made in the erect position, a discrepancy that must not be misinterpreted as evidence of disease.

Complex interrelationships between transthoracic pressure and pulmonary blood flow occur during inspiration and expiration and during the Valsalva or Mueller maneuver.* Use of the Valsalva and Mueller maneuvers to pro-

Text continued on page 95

---

*The Valsalva maneuver consists of forced expiration against a closed glottis, and the Mueller maneuver consists of inspiration against a closed glottis. For proper hemodynamic effect, pressures of plus and minus 40 to 50 cm H_2O, respectively, should be maintained for 7 to 10 seconds. For roentgenograms to be comparable, both maneuvers should be performed at the same degree of lung inflation, preferably at the end of a quiet inspiration.

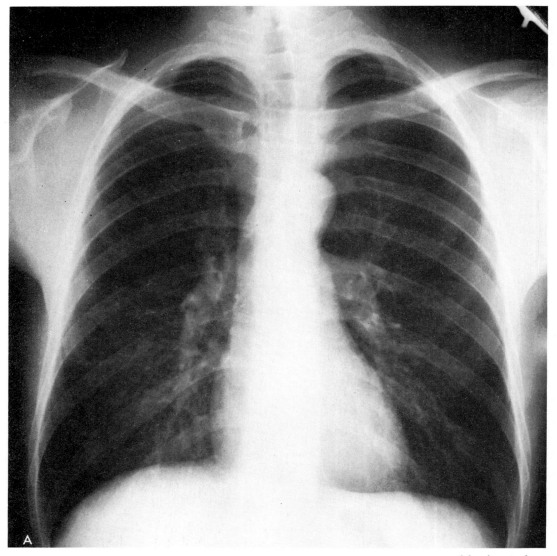

Figure 1–60. Normal Chest Roentgenogram, Posteroanterior Projection. A, A roentgenogram of the chest in the erect position of an asymptomatic 26-year-old man.

Illustration continued on opposite page.

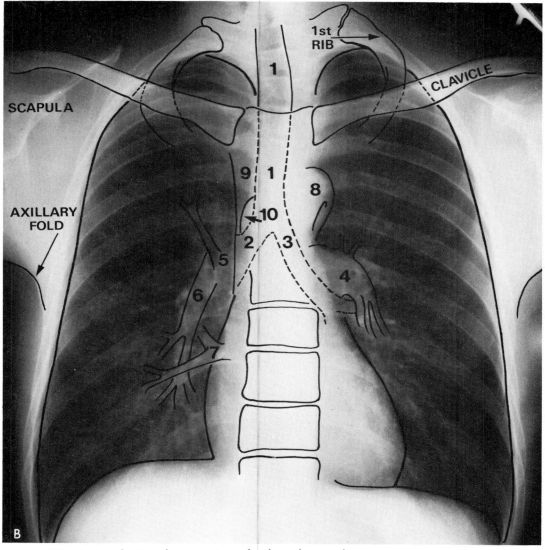

Figure 1–60. *Continued.* *B*, A diagrammatic overlay shows the normal anatomic structures numbered or labeled: (1) trachea; (2) right main bronchus; (3) left main bronchus; (4) left pulmonary artery; (5) right upper lobe pulmonary vein; (6) right interlobar artery; (7) right lower and middle lobe vein; (8) aortic knob; (9) superior vena cava; (10) azygos vein.

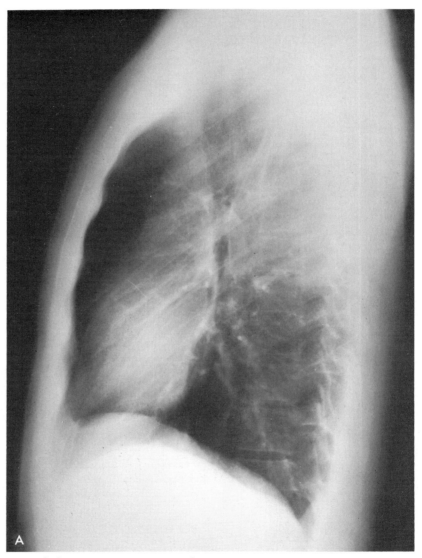

Figure 1–61.   Normal Chest Roentgenogram, Lateral Projection. *A*, A roentgenogram of the chest in the erect position of an asymptomatic 26-year-old man.

Illustration continued on opposite page.

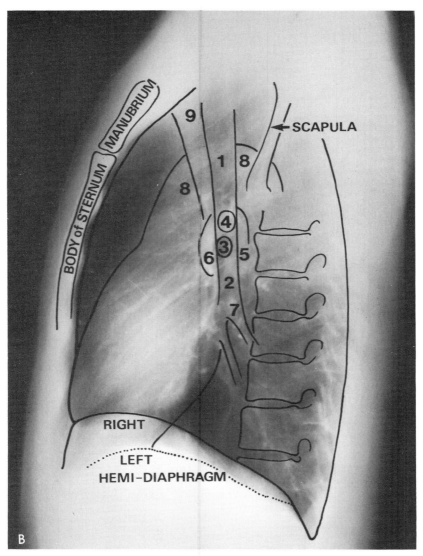

Figure 1–61. *Continued.* *B,* A diagrammatic overlay shows the normal anatomic structures numbered or labeled: (1) tracheal air column; (2) right intermediate bronchus; (3) left upper lobe bronchus; (4) right upper lobe bronchus; (5) left interlobar artery; (6) right interlobar artery; (7) confluence of pulmonary veins; (8) aortic arch; (9) brachiocephalic vessels.

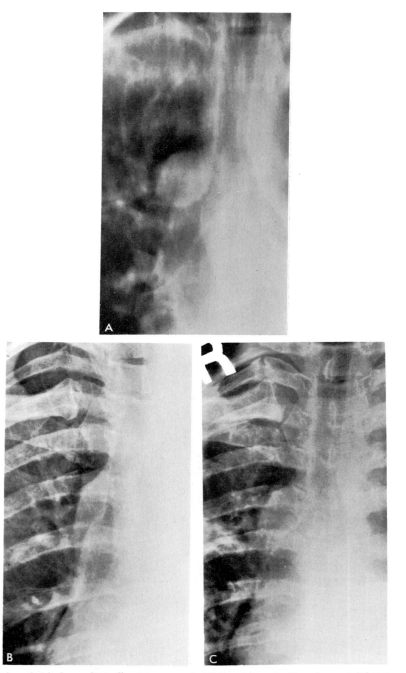

Figure 1–62. Value of Valsalva and Mueller Maneuvers in Distinguishing the Vascular or Solid Nature of Intrathoracic Lesions. *A*, A tomographic section of the midmediastinum reveals a well-defined circular shadow situated in the right tracheobronchial angle; differential diagnosis includes an enlarged azygos lymph node or a markedly dilated azygos vein. *B*, A roentgenogram of the same area in the erect position during the Valsalva maneuver reveals a marked reduction in the size of the shadow. *C*, A similar projection during the Mueller maneuver shows a considerable increase in the size of the shadow compared to *B*. Subsequent angiographic studies proved the shadow to be a markedly dilated azygos vein associated with azygos continuation of the inferior vena cava.

duce increase and decrease, respectively, in intra-alveolar pressure has important but limited application in roentgen diagnosis. The Valsalva maneuver may be used to advantage in the differentiation of vascular and solid lesions within the thorax.[107] Vascular structures are reduced in size when intra-alveolar pressure is increased, whereas solid lesions remain unchanged. The method is of particular value in the differentiation of an azygos vein from an enlarged azygos lymph node (Figure 1–62), or a pulmonary arteriovenous fistula from a solid mass. Tomography may be used to advantage during these maneuvers.

These examples of the use of the Valsalva and Mueller maneuvers indicate a trend increasingly emphasized in recent years—the application of physiologic principles to roentgen diagnosis. Knowledge of pathophysiology has played a major role in the roentgenologic study of the cardiovascular system for many years, but probably has not received the attention it deserves in pulmonary diseases.

PERCEPTION IN CHEST ROENTGENOLOGY

OBSERVER ERROR

The roentgenologic diagnosis of chest disease begins with *identification* of an abnormality on a roentgenogram: that which is not *seen* cannot be appreciated. These statements may appear self-evident, but they express an observation that deserves constant re-emphasis. The gain in confidence in one's ability to *interpret* changes apparent roentgenographically must not be mistaken by the roentgenologist for an improvement in the accuracy with which one sees them in the first place. Many studies of the accuracy of diagnostic procedures have revealed an astonishingly high incidence of both intraobserver* and interobserver† error among experienced roentgenologists. For example, in one series based only on positive roentgenograms interobserver error ranged from 9 to 24 per cent and intraobserver error from 3 to 31 per cent. Since these figures are derived from studies by competent, experienced observers, it is clear that no roentgenologist should be lulled

---

*Inconsistent observations made by one roentgenologist on two separate readings of the same roentgenograms.

†Inconsistent observations made by two or more roentgenologists on the same roentgenograms.

into a false sense of security concerning his or her competence to "see" a lesion: confidence should be continually modified by studied scientific reserve.

The reasons for observer error are both subjective and objective and are highly complex, every physician concerned with the interpretation of chest roentgenograms must become thoroughly familiar with the physical and physiologic principles of perception, so that errors are kept to a minimum. Some of the more important of these principles are outlined here.

A roentgenogram can be inspected in two ways, each of which may be usefully employed in different situations. *Directed search* is a method whereby a specific pattern of inspection is carried out, commonly along such lines as thoracic and extrathoracic soft tissues, bony thorax, mediastinum, diaphragm, pleura, and, finally, the lungs themselves, the latter usually by individual inspection and comparison of the zones of the two lungs from apex to base. Such a method should probably be employed by trainees, for it is only through the exercise of this routine during thousands of examinations that the *pattern* of the normal chest can be recognized. The alternative method of inspection is *free search*, in which the roentgenogram is scanned without a preconceived orderly pattern. This technique is the scanning method employed by the majority of expert roentgenologists; our experience supports this. However, we consider that discovery of an abnormality during free-search scanning must be followed by an orderly pattern of inspection so that other, less obvious, abnormalities are not overlooked.

It is important to view every chest roentgenogram from a distance of at least 6 to 8 ft, or through diminishing lenses. The reasons are twofold: (1) the slight nuances of density variation between similar zones of the two lungs can be better appreciated at a distance than from the traditional viewing position, and (2) the visibility of shadows with ill-defined margins is significantly improved by minification. The physiologic mechanisms underlying this improved visibility have been explained by Tuddenham.[108] The perception of a roentgenologic shadow in the lungs depends largely upon the gradation of density at the border of the lesion or its sharpness of definition. At standard viewing distance the retina more readily appreciates a lesion whose borders are sharply defined than one whose borders are indistinct. Since such appreciation is dependent upon the visual angle which the border of the lesion subtends at the observer's retina, increased viewing distance (or the use of a diminishing lens), by reducing this visual angle, enhances appreciation of a lesion with indistinct borders.

THRESHOLD VISIBILITY

In a study reported by Newell and Garneau[109] in 1951 in which Lucite disks were employed as test objects, it was found that a structure of unit density must be at least 3 mm in thickness to be roentgenographically visible. Further, it was observed that this *threshold visibility* applied only if the margins of the Lucite disks were parallel to the plane of the roentgen beam—visibility diminished progressively as the margins were increasingly beveled. In 1963, Spratt and his associates[110] found that roentgenologists could locate the shadows of Lucite balls regularly only if the balls were at least 1 to 2 cm in diameter; balls 0.6 cm in diameter could be located only when projected over intercostal spaces, and those as small as 0.3 cm could be identified only in retrospect. The difference between the 3 mm measurement of Newell and Garneau[109] and the larger figures reported by Spratt and his colleagues[110] lies in the character of the *border* of the shadow: the 3-mm measurement applies only to lesions whose borders are sharply defined, and lesions with indistinctly defined or beveled margins (such as a sphere) must be greater than 3 mm in diameter to be roentgenographically visible. Some support is lent to these observations by roentgenologic-pathologic studies which have shown that most solitary tumors are not visualized roentgenologically until their diameter exceeds 6 mm,[110] and that a cancer less than 1.0 cm in diameter is seldom identified by standard roentgenographic methods.[111]

These limits of visibility apply, of course, to individual shadows within the lung rather than to multiple diffuse nodular opacities produced, for example, by miliary tuberculosis. In the latter instance, the question of summation of images is raised, and, although we are not able to enter into a discussion of the pros and cons of summation as a roentgenographic effect, we consider that the proposals put forward by Resink[112] possess considerable merit. This author suggests that wide distribution of a large number of small lesions throughout the lungs allows visibility of individual deposits only when they are *not* summated and that when sum-

mation does occur the appreciation of individual deposits is lost through blurring. (It should be noted that concepts of the effects of summation are conflicting; for example, Newell and Garneau[109] state that objects of subliminal absorption may be brought above threshold by summation of their shadows.)

Certain objective reasons for missing lesions during roentgenologic interpretation have been clarified by studies in which postmortem roentgenography of the chest has been correlated with subsequent morphologic study of the lungs. In one such study[113] of more than 300 cadavers, the lesions most often missed roentgenologically were small calcified or uncalcified nodules 3 mm or slightly more in diameter in the region of the pleura or subpleural parenchyma. Many metastatic nodules measuring up to 1 cm in diameter were not visualized. In four of the 300 cases, lesions measuring 2 to 5 cm in diameter which were discovered on roentgenography of the removed lungs were not visible even in retrospect in films taken with the lungs *in situ*. These authors describe two areas within the thorax in which it is difficult to project a lesion so that it is related to air-containing parenchyma without a superimposed confusion of overlying bones and major blood vessels: over the convexity of the lungs in close proximity to the pleura and rib cage, and in the paramediastinal regions, where the shadows of the aorta, heart, and spine are quite dense. Lesions in close proximity to the diaphragm probably come within the same category. Clearly, it is important to be aware of these relatively "blind" areas in the thorax and to pay particular attention to them in the development of a scanning routine.

Another area of particular importance in the interpretation of chest roentgenograms comprises all the structures outside the limits of the thorax. The importance to diagnosis of such abnormalities as hepatomegaly or splenomegaly, calcification in these organs, displacement or alteration in the contour of the gastric air bubble, and calcification within the thoracic soft tissues cannot be overstressed. Finally, we have been repeatedly impressed by the information to be gained from thorough inspection of the "corners and borders" of roentgenograms. In most departments the name and age of the patient is inscribed thereon by photographic imprinting, particulars which should be noted for definite identification; similarly, an appreciation of dextrocardia or transposition of the thoracic and abdominal viscera may depend upon the position of the "right" or "left" marker.

PSYCHOLOGIC ASPECTS OF ROENTGENOLOGIC INTERPRETATION

This subject is all too often neglected. Three aspects will be considered briefly.

Reader Fatigue

The recent enormous increase in the use of roentgenologic services has resulted in a significant increase in the number of examinations each roentgenologist may be required to report. The inevitable result is "reader fatigue." No experienced roentgenologist denies the diminution in visual and mental acuity that develops during the day when the workload necessitates a heavy reporting schedule. The degree of susceptibility varies, but fatigue eventually affects all to a point at which lack of efficiency accrues to the detriment of the patient. Each individual must set his or her own standards, but two mechanisms can be employed to reduce reader fatigue to a minimum: frequent "rest periods" away from the viewbox and the establishment of a reasonable maximal number of examinations to be reported each day.

Physical Aspects

The atmosphere in which reporting is carried out deserves more attention than it is usually given. Quiet surroundings, away from distracting influences, are most desirable for necessary thought and reflection. Viewing facilities should be optimal. The illuminator probably is the least expensive and yet one of the most important pieces of apparatus in any department of roentgenology; yet, all too often, insufficient attention is paid to such aspects as light intensity and background illumination. The necessity for comfort and convenience of viewing and dictation requires no comment.

Intangible Factors

Intimately linked with the complex causes of observer error are several abstract phenomena that inevitably confront all roentgenologists but that defy adequate explanation. A typical example is the variation with which the same examination may be reported from one day to another: a roentgenogram of the chest (often in the troublesome borderland between normal and abnormal) may be pronounced normal on Monday morning and be interpreted by the same observer as showing "diffuse interstitial disease" on Friday afternoon! It is a moot point whether fatigue is the dominant influence in these intraobserver disagreements; rather, they may be more realistically ascribed to a "state of mind" which is continually fluctuating and which represents an intangible influence on one's approach to a problem. Intraobserver disagreements are bound to occur but every physician must constantly strive to reduce their incidence by effecting the most efficient system of roentgenographic perception of which he or she is capable.

REFERENCES

1. Horsfield, K., and Cumming, G.: Morphology of the bronchial tree in man. J. Appl. Physiol., 24:373, 1968.
2. Cumming, G., Horsfield, K., Harding, L. K., and Prowse, K.: Biological branching systems with special reference to the lung airways. Bull. Physiopathol. Resp., 7:31, 1971.
3. Cumming, G.: Airway morphology and its consequences. Bull. Physiopathol. Resp., 8:527, 1972.
4. Weibel, E. R.: Morphometry of the Human Lung. New York, Academic Press, Inc., 1963.
5. Strahler, A. N.: Equilibrium theory of erosional slopes approached by frequency distribution analysis. Am. J. Sci., 248:673, 1950.
6. Yeager, H., Jr.: Tracheobronchial secretions. Am. J. Med., 50:493, 1971.
7. Denton, R., Forsman, W., Hwang, S. H., Litt, M., and Miller, C. E.: Viscoelasticity of mucus. Its role in ciliary transport of pulmonary secretions. Am. Rev. Resp. Dis., 98:380, 1968.
8. Litt, M.: Mucus rheology. Relevance to mucociliary clearance. Arch. Intern. Med., 126:417, 1970.
9. Dalhamn, T.: Ciliary motility studies. Arch. Intern. Med., 126:424, 1970.
10. Lucas, A. M., and Douglas, L. C.: Direction of flow of nasal mucus. Proc. Soc. Exp. Biol. Med., 31:320, 1934.
11. Weibel, E. R., and Gomez, D. M.: Architecture of the human lung. Science, 137:577, 1962.
12. Dunnill, M. S.: Postnatal growth of the lung. Thorax, 17:329, 1962.
13. Angus, G. E., and Thurlbeck, W. M.: Number of alveoli in the human lung. J. Appl Physiol., 32:483, 1972.
14. von Hayek, H.: The Human Lung. New York, Hafner Publishing Co., 1960.
15. Nagaishi, C.: Functional Anatomy and Histology of the Lung. Baltimore and London, University Park Press, 1972.
16. Fishman, A. P.: Pulmonary edema: The water-exchanging function of the lung. Circulation, 46:390, 1972.
17. Esterly, J. R., and Faulkner, C. S., II: The granular pneumonocyte. Absence of phagocytic activity. Am. Rev. Resp. Dis., 101:869, 1970.
18. Schneeberger-Keeley, E. E., and Karnovsky, M. J.: The ultrastructural basis of alveolar-capillary membrane permeability to peroxidase used as a tracer. J. Cell Biol., 37:781, 1968.

19. Clements, J. A.: Pulmonary surfactant. Am. Rev. Resp. Dis., *101*:984, 1970.

20. Green, G. M.: The J. Burns Amberson Lecture. In defense of the lung. Am. Rev. Resp. Dis., *102*:691, 1970.

21. Morgan, T. E.: Pulmonary surfactant. N. Engl. J. Med., *284*:1185, 1971.

22. Gil, J., and Weibel, E. R.: Improvements in demonstration of lining layer of lung alveoli by electron microscopy. Resp. Physiol., *8*:13, 1969.

23. Klaus, M. H., Clements, J. A., and Havel, R. J.: Composition of surface-active material isolated from beef lung. Proc. Natl. Acad. Sci. USA, *47*:1858, 1961.

24. Scarpelli, E. M.: The Surfactant System of the Lung. Philadelphia, Lea & Febiger, 1968.

25. Avery, M. E.: The J. Burns Amberson Lecture. In pursuit of understanding the first breath. Am. Rev. Resp. Dis., *100*:295, 1969.

26. Warren, C., Holton, J. B., and Allen, J. T.: Assessment of fetal lung maturity by estimation of amniotic fluid palmitic acid. Br. Med. J., *1*:94, 1974.

27. Miller, W. S.: The Lung. Springfield, Ill., Charles C Thomas, Publisher, 1937.

28. Heitzman, E. R., Markarian, B., Berger, I., and Dailey, E.: The secondary pulmonary lobule: A practical concept for interpretation of chest radiographs. I. Roentgen anatomy of the normal secondary pulmonary lobule. Radiology, *93*:507, 1969.

29. Heitzman, E. R., Markarian, B., Berger, I., and Dailey, E.: The secondary pulmonary lobule: A practical concept for interpretation of chest radiographs. II. Application of the anatomic concept to an understanding of roentgen pattern in disease states. Radiology, *93*:513, 1969.

30. Pump, K. K.: Morphology of the acinus of the human lung. Dis. Chest, *56*:126, 1969.

31. Gamsu, G., Thurlbeck, W. M., Macklem, P. T., and Fraser, R. G.: Roentgenographic appearance of the human pulmonary acinus. Invest. Radiol., *6*:171, 1971.

32. Macklem, P. T.: Airway obstruction and collateral ventilation. Physiol. Rev., *51*:368, 1971.

33. Lambert, M. W.: Accessory bronchiole-alveolar communications. J. Pathol. Bacteriol., *70*:311, 1955.

34. Martin, H. B.: Respiratory bronchioles as the pathway for collateral ventilation. J. Appl. Physiol., *21*:1443, 1966.

35. Van Allen, C. M., Lindskog, G. E., and Richter, H. G.: Collateral respiration. Transfer of air collaterally between pulmonary lobules. J. Clin. Invest., *10*:559, 1931.

36. Hogg, J. C., Macklem, P. T., and Thurlbeck, W. M.: The resistance of collateral channels in excised human lungs. J. Clin. Invest., *48*:42, 1969.

37. Staub, N. C.: The interdependence of pulmonary structure and function. Anesthesiology, *24*:831, 1963.

38. Jackson, C. L., and Huber, J. F.: Correlated applied anatomy of the bronchial tree and lungs with a system of nomenclature. Dis. Chest, *9*:319, 1943.

39. Kittredge, R. D.: Computed tomography of the trachea: A review. CT, *5*:44, 1981.

40. Cleveland, R. H.: Symmetry of bronchial angles in children. Radiology, *133*:89, 1979.

41. Fraser, R. G.: Measurements of the calibre of human bronchi in three phases of respiration by cinebronchography. J. Can. Assoc. Radiol., *12*:102, 1961.

42. Savoca, C. J., Austin, J. H. M., and Goldberg, H. I.: The right paratracheal stripe. Radiology, *122*:295, 1977.

43. Palayew, M. J.: The tracheo-esophageal stripe and the posterior tracheal band. Radiology, *132*:11, 1979.

44. Daffner, R. H., Postlethwait, R. W., and Putman, C. E.: Retrotracheal abnormalities in esophageal carcinoma: Prognostic implications. Am. J. Roentgenol., *130*:719, 1978.

45. Tierney, D. F.: Pulmonary surfactant in health and disease. Dis. Chest, *47*:247, 1965.

46. Macklem, P. T., and Mead, J.: Resistance of central and peripheral airways measured by a retrograde catheter. J. Appl. Physiol., *22*:395, 1967.

47. Felson, B.: Chest Roentgenology. Philadelphia, W. B. Saunders Co., 1973.

48. Proto, A. V., and Speckman, J. M.: The left lateral radiograph of the chest. Med. Radiogr. Photogr., *55*:30, 1979.

49. Chang, C. H. (Joseph): The normal roentgenographic measurement of the right descending pulmonary artery in 1,085 cases. Am. J. Roentgenol., *87*:929, 1962.

50. Yu, P. N.: Pulmonary Blood Volume in Health and Disease. Philadelphia, Lea & Febiger, 1969.

51. Weibel, E. R.: Morphometrische Analyse von Zahl, Volumen und Oberfläche der Alveolen und Kapillären der menschlichen Lunge. Z. Zellforsch. Mikrosk. Anat., *57*:648, 1962.

52. Cander, L., and Forster, R. E.: Determination of pulmonary parenchymal tissue volume and pulmonary capillary blood flow in man. J. Appl. Physiol., *14*:541, 1959.

53. Permutt, S., Howell, J. B. L., Proctor, D. F., and Riley, R. L.: Effect of lung inflation on static pressure-volume characteristics of pulmonary vessels. J. Appl. Physiol., *16*:64, 1961.

54. Fishman, A. P.: Respiratory gases in the regulation of the pulmonary circulation. Physiol. Rev., *41*:214, 1961.

55. Jameson, A. G.: Diffusion of gases from alveolus to precapillary arteries. Science, *139*:826, 1963.

56. Finley, T. N., Swenson, E. W., and Comroe, J. H., Jr.: The cause of arterial hypoxemia at rest in patients with "alveolar-capillary block syndrome." J. Clin. Invest., *41*:618, 1962.

57. Forster, R. E., Craw, M. R., Constantine, H. P., and Morello, J. A.: Gas exchange processes in the pulmonary capillaries. *In* de Reuck, A. V. S., and O'Connor, M. (eds.), Ciba Foundation: Symposium on Pulmonary Structure and Function. London, J. & A. Churchill, 1962, pp. 215–231.

58. Milic-Emili, J., Henderson, J. A. M., Dolovich, M. B., Trop, D., and Kaneko, K.: Regional distribution of inspired gas in the lung. J. Appl. Physiol., *21*:749, 1966.

59. Glazier, J. B., Hughes, J. M. B., Maloney, J. E., and West, J. B.: Vertical gradient of alveolar size in lungs of dogs frozen intact. J. Appl. Physiol., *23*:694, 1967.

60. West, J. B.: Ventilation: Blood Flow and Gas Exchange. Oxford, Blackwell, 1965.

61. Newhouse, M. T., Becklake, M. R., Macklem, P. T., and McGregor, M.: Effect of alterations in end-tidal CO_2 tension on flow resistance. J. Appl. Physiol., *19*:745, 1964.

62. Davenport, H. W.: The ABC of Acid-Base Chemistry; The Elements of Physiological Blood-Gas Chemistry for Medical Students and Physicians, 5th ed. Chicago, University of Chicago Press, 1969.

63. Siegel, P. D.: The physiologic approach to acid-base balance. Med. Clin. North Am., 57:863, 1973.
64. Schwartz, W. B., Brackett, N. C., Jr., and Cohen, J. J.: The response of extracellular hydrogen ion concentration to graded degrees of chronic hypercapnia: The physiologic limits of the defense of pH. J. Clin. Invest., 44:291, 1965.
65. Brackett, N. C., Jr., Cohen, J. J., and Schwartz, W. B.: Carbon dioxide titration curve of normal man. Effect of increasing degrees of acute hypercapnia on acid-base equilibrium. N. Engl. J. Med., 272:6, 1965.
66. Gennari, F. J., Goldstein, M. B., and Schwartz, W. B.: The nature of the renal adaptation to chronic hypocapnia. J. Clin. Invest., 51:1722, 1972.
67. Arbus, G. S.: An *in vitro* acid-base nomogram for clinical use. Can. Med. Assoc. J., 109:291, 1973.
68. Heinemann, H. O., and Fishman, A. P.: Nonrespiratory functions of mammalian lung. Physiol. Rev., 49:1, 1969.
69. Said, S. I.: The lung as a metabolic organ. N. Engl. J. Med., 279:1330, 1968.
70. Reid, L.: The lung: Its growth and remodeling in health and disease. 1976 Edward B. D. Neuhauser lecture. Am. J. Roentgenol., 129:777, 1977.
71. Boyden, E. A.: Developmental anomalies of the lungs. Am. J. Surg., 89:79, 1955.
72. Hislop, A., and Reid, L.: Development of the acinus in the human lung. Thorax, 29:90, 1974.
73. Hislop, A., and Reid, L: Fetal and childhood development of the intrapulmonary veins in man Branching pattern and structure. Thorax, 28:313, 1973.
74. Richardson, J. B.: Nerve supply to the lungs. Am. Rev. Resp. Dis., 119:785, 1979.
75. Kerley, P.: In Shanks, S. C., and Kerley, P. (eds.): A Textbook of X-ray Diagnosis. Vol. II, 3rd ed. Philadelphia, W. B. Saunders Co., 1962, p. 403.
76. Kent, E. M., and Blades, B.: The surgical anatomy of the pulmonary lobes. J. Thorac. Surg., 12:18, 1942.
77. Medlar, E. M.: Variations in interlobar fissures. Am. J. Roentgenol., 57:723, 1947.
78. Raasch, B. N., Carsky, E. W., Lane, E. J., O'Callaghan, J. P., and Heitzman, E. R.: Correlated radiographic anatomy of the interlobar fissures, in press.
79. Agostoni, E.: Mechanics of the pleural space. Physiol Rev., 52:57, 1972.
80. Black, L. F.: The pleural space and pleural fluid Mayo Clin. Proc., 47:493, 1972.
81. Rutishauser, W. J., Banchero, N., Tsakiris, A. G., Edmundowicz, A. C., and Wood, E. H.: Pleural pressures at dorsal and ventral sites in supine and prone body positions. J. Appl. Physiol., 21:1500, 1966.
82. Agostoni, E., and Mead, J.: Statics of the respiratory system. *In* Fenn, W. O., and Rahn, H. (eds.): Handbook of Physiology, Section 3, Respiration. Vol. 1. Washington, D.C., American Physiological Society, 1964, pp. 387–409.
83. Stewart, P. B.: The rate of formation and lymphatic removal of fluid in pleural effusions. J. Clin. Invest., 42:258, 1963.
84. Burgen, A. S. V., and Stewart, P. B.: A method for measuring the turnover of fluid in the pleural and other serous cavities. J. Lab. Clin. Med., 52:118, 1958.
85. Lauweryns, J. M.: The juxta-alveolar lymphatics in the human adult lung. Histologic studies in 15 cases of drowning. Am. Rev. Resp. Dis., 102:877, 1970.
86. Tobin, C. E.: Lymphatics of the pulmonary alveoli. Anat. Rec., 120:625, 1954.
87. Fleischner, F. G.: The butterfly pattern of acute pulmonary edema. Am. J. Cardiol., 20:39, 1967.
88. Rosenberger, A., and Abrams, H. L.: Radiology of the thoracic duct. Am. J. Roentgenol., 111:807, 1971.
89. Castellino, R. A., and Blank, N.: Adenopathy of the cardiophrenic angle (diaphragmatic) lymph nodes. Am. J. Roentgenol., 114:509, 1972.
90. Rouvière, H.: Anatomy of the Human Lymphatic System. (Translated by Tobias, M. J.) Ann Arbor, Mich., Edwards, 1938.
91. Baird, J. A.: The pathways of lymphatic spread of carcinoma of the lung. Br. J. Surg., 52:868, 1965.
92. Heitzman, E. R.: The Mediastinum: Radiologic Correlations with Anatomy and Pathology. St. Louis, The C. V. Mosby Co., 1977.
93. Cimmino, C. V.: The esophageal-pleural stripe: An update. Radiology, 140:609, 1981.
94a. Heitzman, E. R., Scrivani, J. V., Martino, J., and Moro, J.: The azygos vein and its pleural reflections. I. Normal roentgen anatomy. Radiology, 101:249, 1971.
94b. Heitzman, E. R., Scrivani, J. V., Martino, J., and Moro, J.: The azygos vein and its pleural reflections. II. Applications in the radiological diagnosis of mediastinal abnormality. Radiology, 101:259, 1971.
95. Kieffer, S. A., and Heitzman, E. R.: An Atlas of Cross-Sectional Anatomy: Computed Tomography, Ultrasound, Radiography, Gross Anatomy. Hagerstown, Md., Harper and Row, 1979.
96. Austin, J. H. M., and Thorsen, M. K.: Normal azygos arch: Retrotracheal visualization on frontal chest tomograms. Am. J. Roentgenol., 137:1205, 1981.
97. Felson, B.: Chest Roentgenology. Philadelphia, W. B. Saunders Co., 1973.
98. Doyle, F. H., Read, R. E., and Evans, K. T.: The mediastinum in portal hypertension. Clin. Radiol., 12:114, 1961.
99. Simon, G.: Principles of Chest X-Ray Diagnosis 3rd ed. London, Butterworth, 1971.
100. Young, D. A., and Simon, G.: Certain movements measured on inspiration-expiration chest radiographs correlated with pulmonary function studies. Clin. Radiol., 23:37, 1972.
101. Vix, V. A.: Extrapleural costal fat. Radiology, 112:563, 1974.
102. Loyd, H. M., String, S. T., and DuBois, A. B.: Radiographic and plethysmographic determination of total lung capacity. Radiology, 86:7, 1966.
103. Sackner, M. A., Feisal, K. A., and DuBois, A. B.: Determination of tissue volume and carbon dioxide dissociation slope of the lungs in man. J. Appl. Physiol., 19:374, 1964.
104. McGaff, C. J., Roveti, G. C., Glassman, E., and Milnor, W. R.: The pulmonary blood volume in rheumatic heart disease and its alteration by isoproterenol. Circulation, 27:77, 1963.
105. Goldman, H. I., and Becklake, M. R.: Respiratory function tests: Normal values at median altitudes and the prediction of normal results. Am. Rev. Tuberc., 79:457, 1959.
106. Daley, R., Goodwin, J. F., and Steiner, R. E. (eds.): Clinical Disorders of the Pulmonary Circulation. London, J. & A. Churchill, 1960.

107. Rigler, L. G.: Functional roentgen diagnosis: Anatomical image—physiological interpretation. Am. J. Roentgenol., 82:1, 1959.
108. Tuddenham, W. J.: Problems of perception in chest roentgenology: Facts and fallacies. Radiol. Clin. North Am., 1:277, 1963.
109. Newell, R. R., and Garneau, R.: The threshold visibility of pulmonary shadows. Radiology, 56:409, 1951.
110. Spratt, J. S., Jr., Ter-Pogossian, M., and Long, R. T. L.: The detection and growth of intrathoracic neoplasms: The lower limits of radiographic distinction, the antemortum size, the duration, and the pattern of growth as determined by direct mensuration of tumor diameters from random thoracic roentgenograms. Arch. Surg., 86:283, 1963.

111. Goldmeier, E.: Limits of visibility of bronchiogenic carcinoma. Am. Rev. Resp. Dis., 91:232, 1965.
112. Resink, J. E. J.: Is a roentgenogram of fine structures a summation image or a real picture? Acta Radiol., 32:391, 1949.
113. Greening, R. R., and Pendergrass, E. P.: Postmortem roentgenography with particular emphasis upon the lung. Radiology, 62:720, 1954.
114. Yoffey, J. M., and Courtice, F. C.: Lymphatics, Lymph and the Lymphomyeloid Complex. New York, Academic Press, Inc., 1970, p. 294.
115. Lindell, M. M., Jr., Hill, C. A., and Libshitz, H. I.: Esophageal cancer: Radiographic chest findings and their prognostic significance. Am. J. Roentgenol., 133:461, 1979.

2

Methods of Roentgenologic and Pathologic Investigation

ROENTGENOLOGIC EXAMINATION

In this book the approach to the diagnosis of chest disease involves two basic steps in a logical sequence of events: first, *identification* of a pathologic process roentgenologically; and second, through *correlation* of these preliminary roentgenographic findings *with the clinical picture*, arrival at a diagnosis that takes into account the results of special roentgenographic procedures, laboratory tests, pulmonary function tests, scintillation scanning, and surgical procedures (such as bronchoscopy and biopsy). In this chapter the roentgenographic and pathologic methods we employ are described. Emphasis is placed on the techniques that have proved most valuable in our experience. Procedures that others have employed to advantage but we have found unrewarding are described briefly, together with our reasons for regarding them as unprofitable.

The cornerstone of roentgen diagnosis is the plain roentgenogram. This statement cannot be overemphasized. All other roentgen procedures, such as fluoroscopy, tomography, and special contrast studies, are strictly ancillary. With a few exceptions, to which we refer later on, establishing the *presence* of a disease process by plain roentgenography of the chest should constitute the first step; if this first examination does not show clearly the nature and extent of the lesion, additional studies can be carried out to *complement* the plain roentgenogram.

STANDARD ROENTGENOGRAPHY

ROUTINE PROJECTIONS

Roentgenologists vary in their appreciation of which projections of the thorax constitute the most satisfactory basic or "routine" views for preliminary evaluation. The great majority, including the authors, prefer posteroanterior and lateral projections. As basic projections of the thorax, these provide the essential requirement of a three-dimensional view of the chest. Variations on this routine are numerous, depending upon economic circumstances and the whims of the roentgenologist. For example, roentgenography of the chest as a screening procedure (as used in mass surveys) is carried out on such a colossal scale that it has become economically unsound to take more than a single posteroanterior view. One cannot be overly critical of this practice, since the subjects are ostensibly asymptomatic.

In these days of burgeoning health costs, it is vital that all physicians give due consideration to the benefit—or perhaps more importantly the lack of benefit—to be derived from examinations performed in specific clinical settings that have customarily been regarded as "routine." For example, from an analysis of over 10,000 chest roentgenographic examinations of a hospital-based population, Sagel and his colleagues[1] concluded that routine screening examinations, obtained solely because of hospital admission regulations or scheduled surgery, are not warranted in patients under 20, and that the lateral projection can be safely eliminated from routine screening examinations in patients 20 to 39 years of age but should be included whenever chest disease is suspected and in screening examinations of patients 40 years of age or older. In a similar analysis of the charts and routine preoperative chest roentgenograms of 350 children admitted for elective pediatric surgery,[2] it was found that for the most part such roentgenograms revealed no useful information and that they were not indicated in the absence of clinical suspicion of pulmonary or cardiovascular disease. Similar conclusions were drawn from a retrospective study of routine prenatal chest roentgenograms of 12,109 pregnant women delivered consecutively at the Mayo Clinic:[3] of the 48 patients who showed appreciable roentgenographic abnormalities, *all* had a positive history or abnormal physical findings that would have suggested the presence of disease and the requirement for chest roentgenography.

ROENTGENOGRAPHIC TECHNIQUE

The basic principles of roentgenographic technique are as follows: (1) Positioning must be such that the x-ray beam is properly centered, the patient's body is not rotated, and the scapulae are rotated sufficiently anteriorly as to be projected free of the lungs. (2) Respiration must be fully suspended, preferably at TLC. In this regard, the studies of Crapo and his associates are important:[4] these authors showed that in erect chest roentgenography, normal subjects routinely inhale to approximately 95 per cent TLC *without coaxing*; thus, such roentgenograms can be of value in estimating lung volume and, by comparison with subsequent roentgenograms, in appreciating increase or decrease in volume as a result of disease. (3) Exposure factors should be such that the resultant roentgenogram permits faint visualization of the thoracic spine *and* the intervertebral disks so that lung markings behind the heart are clearly visible; exposure should be as short as possible, consistent with the production of adequate contrast. Unfortunately, all too frequently technical factors are such that optimal roentgenographic density is achieved over the lungs generally but without adequate penetration of the mediastinum or the left side of the heart, a tendency that seriously limits roentgen interpretation. With perseverance, it is always possible to develop roentgenographic techniques that obviate problems of underexposure.

To achieve consistently high quality chest roentgenograms we recommend a high kilovoltage technique (in the range of 110 to 150). To obtain adequate exposure of the mediastinum while maintaining a proper level of exposure of the lungs, we use a tunnel-wedge filter, developed in the Royal Victoria Hospital by G. A. Wilkinson.[5] In addition to reducing exposure to the apices, wedge filtration provides increased exposure over the width of the mediastinum and because of its beam "hardening" effect tends to reduce scatter from the mediastinum. As well as providing better penetration of the mediastinum, these films yield a clearer visualization of the pulmonary vasculature than can be obtained with more standard techniques. The only possible drawback is the diminished visibility of calcium, resulting from the lower coefficient of x-ray absorption, but this has not proved troublesome in practice.

The *lordotic projection* can be made in the anteroposterior projection or in a modified posteroanterior projection. We are not particularly impressed by the value of this projection. Much time and money are wasted by performing examinations in lordotic projection when a direct approach by tomography would yield more information.

At the time of writing, *digital radiography* has just appeared on the horizon, and the impact that this exciting new technique will have on chest radiology—in fact all of radiology—is yet to be felt. Some liberal thinkers feel that within the foreseeable future—and certainly by the last decade of the century—the majority of x-ray images of the thorax will be interpreted from a CRT monitor.

INSPIRATORY-EXPIRATORY ROENTGENOGRAPHY

Roentgenograms exposed in full inspiration (total lung capacity) and maximal expiration (residual volume) may supply useful information in two specific situations.

1. The main indication for such studies is the investigation of air trapping, either general or local. When air trapping is widespread, as in spasmodic asthma or emphysema, diaphragmatic excursion is reduced symmetrically and lung density changes little; when air trapping is local, as results from a check valve bronchial obstruction or from lobar emphysema, the expiratory roentgenogram reveals restricted ipsilateral diaphragmatic elevation, a shift of the mediastinum toward the contralateral hemithorax, and relative absence of density change

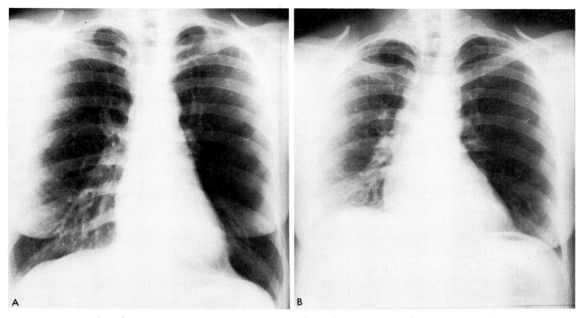

Figure 2–1. Value of Inspiratory-Expiratory Roentgenography in the Assessment of Air Trapping. *A*, A roentgenogram in full inspiration (TLC) of a 31-year-old woman with unilateral obliterative bronchiolitis (Swyer-James' syndrome). *B*, In full expiration (RV), the presence of left-sided air trapping is evidenced by a shift of the mediastinum to the right, reduction in left hemidiaphragmatic excursion, and a marked discrepancy in overall density of the two lungs.

in involved bronchopulmonary segments (Figure 2–1).

2. When pneumothorax is suspected, and the visceral-pleural line is not visible on the standard inspiratory roentgenogram or the findings are equivocal, a film taken in full expiration may show the line more clearly. This is because at full expiration (a) the volume of air in the pleural space is relatively greater in relation to the volume of lung, providing better separation of the pleural surfaces, and (b) the relationship of the pleural line to overlying ribs changes.

VALSALVA AND MUELLER MANEUVERS

As discussed in Chapter 1, these may aid in determining the vascular or solid nature of intrathoracic masses. Pressures should be sustained for a minimum of 10 sec before exposure. Either the erect or recumbent position can be employed, depending upon the information sought.

ROENTGENOGRAPHY IN THE SUPINE POSITION

The majority of chest roentgenography is performed with the patient erect, but occasionally circumstances demand that the patient be supine, usually postoperatively or in cases of severe illness. Because of the shorter focal film

distance usually required and the anteroposterior direction of the x-ray beam, magnification of the heart and superior mediastinum often amounts to 15 to 20 per cent, compared with 5 per cent in conventional posteroanterior teleroentgenography. Roentgenography in supine patients is liable to result in diagnostic error in relation to the pulmonary vascular shadows also. As discussed in Chapter 1, pulmonary blood flow is approximately 30 per cent greater in supine than in erect subjects, and, therefore, the pulmonary vascular shadows, may appear larger. In the upper lungs, this dilatation is enhanced by removal of the effects of gravity and consequent increased flow to upper lung zones. This must not be misinterpreted as evidence of pulmonary venous hypertension.

The number of requests for roentgenographic examination of the chest with mobile apparatus at a patient's bedside has increased enormously in recent years, owing partly to a remarkable growth of intensive care units and partly to the introduction of complex cardiovascular surgical procedures that require close postoperative surveillance. Unfortunately such roentgenograms are almost invariably technically inferior to those obtained in the standard manner in a radiology department. This inferior quality derives from multiple factors, some of which are uncontrollable (*e.g.*, the patient's supine position, a short focal film distance, and the restricted ability of many such patients to suspend respiration). Other factors, including the technical ones employed in the exposure, are subject to control. All too frequently these roentgenograms are over- or underexposed, often to a degree that limits or even precludes recognition of the subtle changes that are so important in the postoperative period. To obviate these problems, we and others[6] strongly recommend the use of high kVp techniques with mobile apparatus now available. As an alternative, a technique employing a double screen–double film combination in a single cassette[7] has been found useful.

ROENTGENOGRAPHY IN THE LATERAL DECUBITUS POSITION

In this technique, the patient lies on one side and the x-ray beam is oriented horizontally. Since in the majority of instances the dependent hemithorax is the side being specifically examined, it is desirable to elevate the thorax on a nonabsorbing support such as a foam cushion or mattress. The technique is invaluable for the identification of small pleural effusions and for confirming the presence of subpulmonic effusions (Figure 2–2). Less than 100 ml of fluid may be identified on well-exposed roentgeno-

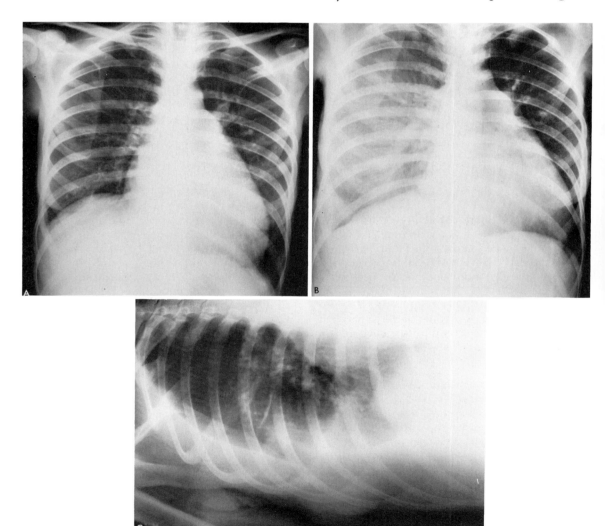

Figure 2–2. Value of Lateral Decubitus Roentgenography in the Assessment of Pleural Effusion. A posteroanterior roentgenogram in the erect position (A) reveals what appears to be marked elevation of the right hemidiaphragm, although slight thickening of the axillary pleura in the region of the costophrenic sulcus suggests the possibility of infrapulmonary effusion. Roentgenography in the supine position (B) reveals a marked increase in the opacity of the right hemithorax, owing to the presence of fluid in the posterior pleural space; the right hemidiaphragm is now viewed in proper perspective, whereas in A it was obscured by subpulmonic effusion. A lateral decubitus roentgenogram (C) shows the fluid to much better advantage along the costal margin and reveals how much fluid can be accommodated in the subpulmonic space.

grams in this position, whereas those taken with the patient erect seldom reveal pleural effusions of less than 300 ml.[8] Roentgenography in the lateral decubitus position is useful also to demonstrate a small pneumothorax in the superior hemithorax when evidence in other positions, particularly the supine, is equivocal. Occasionally, it may be of value to reveal a change in position of an air-fluid level in a cavity or to ascertain whether a structure that forms part of a cavity represents a freely moving intracavitary foreign body (*e.g.*, a fungus ball or mycetoma).

ROENTGENOGRAPHY IN THE OBLIQUE POSITION

Oblique studies are sometimes useful in locating a disease process or showing it to better advantage (*e.g.*, pleural plaques in asbestosis), but in most situations we prefer to employ more searching techniques, such as tomography.

ROENTGENOLOGIC PROCEDURES FOR THE EVALUATION OF INTRATHORACIC DYNAMICS

FLUOROSCOPY

The fluoroscopic screen registers a constant image of the object being examined and thus allows appreciation of the dynamic activity of roentgenographically visible intrathoracic structures. *With few exceptions, fluoroscopy should be restricted to this purpose.*

Fluoroscopy may supply information concerning movement of the diaphragm and thoracic wall during respiration. Particularly in acute subphrenic disease restricted excursion of one hemidiaphragm may constitute an important clue to its presence. Similarly, when local air trapping is present, as in lobar or unilateral emphysema or soon after impaction of a foreign body, restricted diaphragmatic excursion and rib approximation on the affected side during forced expiration may be the sole evidence of an abnormality that may give rise to only very subtle changes on roentgenograms exposed in full inspiration. Mediastinal swing during deep breathing is sometimes better appreciated by observing dynamic movement than by studying roentgenograms made during inspiration and expiration.

Fluoroscopy may indicate the presence or absence of pulsation in an intrapulmonary mass, allowing differentiation between its vascular and solid nature (provided the mass is not contiguous to the heart or a vigorously pulsating vessel). Similarly, the amplitude and regularity of pulsation of the cardiac chambers, aorta, and pulmonary arteries can be readily appreciated fluoroscopically, as can calcifications in a cardiac valve, the pericardium, and the major vessels. Such findings may be of major importance in assessment of pulmonary diseases of cardiovascular origin.

Identification of abnormalities of esophageal position or contour can be important in roentgenologic diagnosis. Deformity caused by enlarged mediastinal lymph nodes may constitute a cardinal sign in the diagnosis of bronchogenic cancer or in the assessment of operability once the diagnosis has been established. Disturbed esophageal dynamics, as in achalasia or scleroderma, may be the chief indication of the origin of the patchy consolidation seen in aspiration pneumonitis or the diffuse reticular pattern of interstitial fibrosis. Fluoroscopy should always precede roentgenography in the investigation of esophageal disease: not only is it the only method for revealing abnormalities of dynamics (*e.g.*, aperistalsis), but it also allows appreciation of minimal but persistent irregularities of contour that might appear insignificant on roentgenograms of the barium-filled esophagus.

STANDARD TOMOGRAPHY

TECHNIQUES

Tomography (*synonyms:* body section roentgenography, planigraphy, laminagraphy, stratigraphy, and sectional roentgenography) allows selective visualization of a particular layer of tissue to the exclusion of structures lying superficial or deep to it. Regardless of the type of motion employed, the technique involves reciprocal movement of the x-ray tube and film at proportional velocity. The reciprocal motion causes blurring of all structures not continuously "in focus" during excursions of the tube and film, so that the image of only a thin "slice" is recorded in detail on the roentgenogram. The level of tomographic "cut" is controlled by the ratio of the tube-object distance to the object-film distance, so that this level can be altered by varying the ratio. The thickness of the "cut" is governed by the length of tube-film travel— the shorter the excursion, the thicker the layer recorded (zonography). Various reciprocal movements of tube and film have been developed, including rectilinear, circular, elliptical, and hypocycloidal. Although rectilinear tomography is probably the simplest to perform and most widely available, Littleton and his colleagues[9] have concluded from a recent tomographic study of a fresh frozen human cadaver that a rectilinear tomogram is not a true sectional image and that it does not truthfully represent the planar anatomy of the intended layer; by contrast, pluridirectional tomograms, particularly trispiral, accurately depict the anatomic section in fine detail. These authors strongly recommend the use of pluridirectional techniques in chest tomography. However, in a more recent study in which full lung linear and pluridirectional tomography were compared in the detection of pulmonary nodules, Bein and Stone[10] found no superiority of the latter method, ostensibly because small nodules could remain undetected on slices at 1-cm intervals with the extremely thin (1 mm) focal plane characteristic of the pluridirectional technique.

The value of computerized axial tomography in the study of thoracic disease is now in little doubt, and it is clear that this revolutionary technique will prove a great boon in the assessment of pulmonary and mediastinal abnormalities. This subject is dealt with in some detail in the following pages.

INDICATIONS

There are two main indications for standard tomography of the thorax.

1. The need for precise knowledge of the morphologic characteristics of lesions visible on plain roentgenograms whose nature is obscured by superimposed images lying superficial and deep to them. Perhaps the best example of this indication is the detection of pulmonary cavitation. In a study of 271 tomograms of 172 patients with pulmonary tuberculosis,[11] in 10.7 per cent tomography revealed cavitation unsuspected on conventional roentgenograms; conversely, in 18.8 per cent tomography failed to show cavities suspected on plain roentgenograms. Other examples of this indication include identification of calcium in pulmonary nodules and the separation of potentially confusing hilar shadows.

2. Clearer visualization of shadows that on plain roentgenograms are indistinct because of image summation: the prime example of this indication is study of the bronchi and the pulmonary vasculature. Visualization of the trachea and proximal large bronchi is very clear tomographically. Posterior oblique tomography at an angle of 55 degrees has been recommended for displaying a clearer outline of the anatomic components of the hila.[12]

For some years, the place of full lung tomography in the investigation of metastatic disease has been disputed, but certain general principles now appear to be fairly well accepted. It is well known that if a primary malignant lesion has been eradicated, removal of a single metastasis from the lungs may be curative; therefore, when a single metastatic lesion is visualized in a lung on standard roentgenograms, therapeutic and prognostic implications demand thorough tomographic search of both lungs for other metastatic foci. In patients in whom no metastases are identified on plain roentgenograms, the situation is not quite so simple. There is now no doubt that in some patients, metastatic lesions will be discovered on full lung tomograms that are not seen on plain roentgenograms: of 410 patients with a variety of malignant neoplasms studied retrospectively by Sindelar and his colleagues,[13] 54 had confirmed metastatic disease; of these, metastases were identified by full lung tomography in 51 patients (94.4 per cent) but in only 36 patients (66.7 per cent) on standard chest roentgenograms. Thus, in this series 15 of the patients with normal chest roentgenograms had metastatic lesions demonstrated on tomograms. This suggests that full lung tomography is indicated in all patients with primary malignant neoplasms arising outside the thorax in whom surgical resection (rather than cytotoxic therapy) is the treatment of choice. However, we suspect that cost-benefit analysis of *all* patients with extrathoracic cancer would show that tomography is of real value only in those with neoplasms that show propensity for spread to the lungs, notably malignant melanoma and primaries arising in the urogenital and skeletal systems. This attitude is lent some support by a recent study by Curtis and her colleagues[14] of 144 patients with proven breast carcinoma and a negative chest roentgenogram in which it was shown convincingly that full lung tomography is not warranted as a screening procedure in these patients, chiefly because of the low propensity for carcinoma of the breast to metastasize to the lungs. Incidentally, if full lung tomography is to be performed for the detection of metastatic pulmonary nodules, a recent study comparing full lung tomograms obtained at 1- and 2-cm intervals showed that the detection rate was significantly improved with 1-cm sections.[15]

Still open to question is the issue of whole lung tomography versus computed tomography (CT) in the investigation of metastatic disease. At the time of writing the most thorough study that has been performed in this regard is that of Muhm and his colleagues[16] in which 91 patients with known malignancy were studied by both whole lung tomography and computed tomography of the lungs. In 32 (35 per cent) of the 91 patients, more pulmonary nodules were detected by CT than by whole lung tomography. In five of the 32 patients, whole lung tomography showed no pulmonary nodules but CT showed one or more; in 13 patients, one nodule was seen on whole lung tomography but two or more were detected by CT; in an additional 13 patients, bilateral pulmonary nodules were detected by CT after whole lung tomography had demonstrated nodules in only one lung. Of considerable interest was the observation that in four of the 91 patients in this series fewer nodules were detected by CT than by whole lung tomography. It seems to us that the final answer is not yet in on this controversy.

In summary, there is now little doubt that in patients with primary malignancies that show a propensity for metastasizing to lungs and for whom surgical rather than cytotoxic therapy is planned, full lung tomography should be carried out before attacking the primary lesion. Whether CT should replace full lung tomography in this regard is still open to question.

COMPUTERIZED TOMOGRAPHY (CT)

TECHNIQUES

Since the introduction of this revolutionary British invention into North America in 1973, clinical evaluation of the technique has burgeoned and it has demonstrated beyond question its enormous value in the investigation and diagnosis of disease. Although its use in the diagnosis of intracranial disease has undoubtedly been of greatest value, the development of the body scanner has enabled us to look into the thorax and abdomen and see things heretofore beyond the scope of diagnostic techniques. At the time of writing, CT of the thorax has rather limited application; nevertheless, it serves as a noninvasive technique capable of demonstrating soft tissue structures and of detecting small differences in their densities.

A computerized tomographic scan consists of a group of pictures of the body in a series of transverse slices. It replaces the standard transmission roentgenographic image with a system that measures the quantity of x-ray photons that are absorbed by the different elements within the body. As in most roentgenographic procedures, the variable forming the CT image is the difference in x-ray attenuation properties of various tissues; for example, the attenuation coefficient of fat is less than that of muscle, which is less than that of bone, thus permitting their distinction. In CT, a series of profiles of x-ray attenuations is obtained at different angles to the object examined. By the use of a computer-applied algorithm, these profiles yield cross-sectional images of the x-ray attenuation coefficients. These images depict anatomic structures and pathologic alterations heretofore invisible by conventional radiologic techniques. As pointed out by Ter-Pogossian,[17] the success of CT stems from three factors: (1) utilization of a narrow beam of x-rays and highly collimated detectors to provide a signal that is nearly free of scattered radiation; (2) the properties of CT detectors to be significantly more free of noise than conventional screen-film combinations; and (3) reconstruction of a cross-sectional image unencumbered by superimposed activity. Anatomic structures often can be identified by CT although the difference in their attentuation coefficients is negligible, provided these structures are separated by interfaces of different attenuation properties; for instance, in the abdomen the liver and pancreas can be distinguished from each other and from other structures because of the presence of fat-containing interfaces of low attenuation. In addition, the attenuation coefficient of one tissue compared with another can be established in relative terms by determining their "CT numbers." This simple procedure can be greatly aided by the IV injection of a contrast medium, which brings about a rise in CT numbers in proportion to the blood content of the tissue being measured; for example, contrast enhancement will usually permit distinction of a mediastinal cyst from an aortic aneurysm or a highly vascular solid neoplasm.

Briefly, the technique involves the rotation of a single beam of x-rays 360 degrees around the body in 1 degree steps, taking measurements of the transmitted radiation at each interval during rotation. The x-ray beam is collimated to a width ranging from 5 to 12 mm so that each scan represents a slice of body of that thickness. Obviously, multiple slices are required to cover the whole thorax.

INDICATIONS

In July, 1979, the Society for Computed Body Tomography published a new series of indications for body CT,[18] and the following, with some modification, represent the recommendations of that organization. Indications for CT in chest diseases have been reviewed more recently by Raval and associates.[19] These indications can conveniently be divided into abnormalities affecting the mediastinum, lungs, pleura, and chest wall.

Mediastinum

EVALUATION OF PROBLEMS IDENTIFIED ON STANDARD CHEST ROENTGENOGRAMS. The differentiation of the cystic, fatty, or solid nature of mediastinal masses, and the localization of such masses relative to other mediastinal structures; the assessment of whether mediastinal widening is pathologic or is simply an anatomic variation or caused by physiologic fat deposition; the distinction of a solid mass from a vascular anomaly or aneurysm (generally by contrast enhancement); the differentiation of a dilated pulmonary artery from a solid mass in a hilum (*e.g.*, enlarged lymph nodes) when conventional tomography fails or is not capable of making this distinction (however, *see* further on); the differentiation of lymph node enlargement, vascular cause, or anatomic variant in the presence of deformity of the paraspinal line; and finally, determination of the extent of mediastinal spread in patients with bronchogenic carcinoma.

SEARCH FOR OCCULT THYMIC LESION. The detection of thymoma or hyperplasia in selected patients with myasthenia gravis when standard chest roentgenograms are negative or suspicious.

Lungs

SEARCH FOR PULMONARY LESIONS. The detection of occult pulmonary metastases when either extensive surgery is planned for a known primary neoplasm with a high propensity for lung metastases or a solitary lung metastasis is identified on a chest roentgenogram; the detection of a primary neoplasm in a patient with positive sputum cytology and negative chest roentgenography and fiberoptic bronchoscopy.

SEARCH FOR DIFFUSE OR CENTRAL CALCIFICATION. This search is made in a pulmonary nodule when conventional tomography is indeterminate. In this regard, the exciting results obtained by Siegelman and his colleagues in the differentiation of benign and malignant solitary pulmonary nodules are worthy of note[20] by assessing CT numbers from thin sections of 91 apparently noncalcified pulmonary nodules in 88 patients, these authors showed that benign lesions had relatively high CT numbers, presumably because of diffuse calcification, and that malignant lesions had comparatively lower numbers.

Pleura

DETECTION OF PLEURAL EFFUSION. When its presence may be obscured by a pulmonary opacity and when simpler roentgenographic techniques fail to clarify; assessment of the postpneumonectomy fibrothorax for recurrent disease.

DETERMINATION OF THE EXTENT OF PLEURAL INVOLVEMENT. In the investigation of selected patients with bronchogenic carcinoma.

Chest Wall

DETERMINATION OF THE EXTENT OF NEOPLASTIC DISEASE. Assessment of bone, muscle, and subcutaneous tissue involvement and the detection of intrusion into the thoracic cavity or spinal canal.

Additional indications might include assisting in the percutaneous biopsy of lesions such as mediastinal masses when fluoroscopic guidance is inadequate; the localization of loculated collections of fluid within the pleural space when standard roentgenographic, fluoroscopic, or ultrasonic techniques prove inadequate; and (possibly) the early detection of pulmonary emphysema and characterization of its severity.[21]

In a prospective study, Mintzer and his colleagues[22] compared the value of conventional chest tomography and CT in the evaluation of 100 patients with proven chest malignancies. Generally, the mediastinum was better assessed by CT, particularly in identifying neoplastic invasion. By contrast, conventional tomograms were found to be more useful in evaluating the hila. In the study as a whole, either full lung tomography or CT (or both) directly affected therapy in 18 patients. In a more recent study in which plain roentgenography, conventional tomography, and computed tomography were compared in the detection of intrathoracic lymph node metastases from lung carcinoma,[23] it was shown that all modalities demonstrated about the same accuracy; however, in patients with hilar or mediastinal lymph node enlargement (or both), CT was more sensitive but not more specific than the other two, and conventional tomography was no more accurate than CT for hilar evaluation.

BRONCHOGRAPHY

Physicians in general and radiologists in particular are becoming increasingly concerned about the efficacy of certain roentgenologic procedures in clarifying the nature of an illness. This concern derives partly from a desire to reduce the burgeoning costs of medical care (by restricting diagnostic procedures to their most productive minimum) and partly from a growing awareness that the discovery rate of some procedures is low in relation to patient benefit. In our opinion, bronchography is one of these procedures. Avery joins in this opinion by suggesting that bronchography may be an "outmoded procedure."[24]

Perhaps more than any other roentgenologic procedure, bronchography has been the subject of controversy as to its value in the diagnosis of pulmonary disease. Supporters of the procedure (who, we suspect, are in the minority) speak enthusiastically of its ability to demonstrate differentiation between infectious and neoplastic pulmonary lesions by revealing characteristic deformity of the airways.[25] Although bronchography probably can provide this differentiation in some situations, the question remains: "If efficacious treatment depends on identification of the offending microorganisms or neoplastic cells, why employ bronchography to make a *general* distinction between the two processes in the first place?" With few exceptions, to which reference is made further on, the *diagnosis* of pulmonary disease depends on microbiologic or morphologic examination, and the many recently developed procedures to obtain adequate material for study permit precise diagnosis in most cases without recourse to bronchography. Biopsies of most lesions affecting the major airways can be performed bronchoscopically, and prior roentgenographic location of the lesion is usually as accurate by tomography as by bronchography—and with considerably less hazard. With few exceptions, biopsies of lesions in the lung periphery beyond the reach of the bronchoscope can be done by transthoracic needle or bronchial brush—or the diagnosis may have been confirmed already by cytologic examination of sputum or bronchial washings.

As with most special diagnostic procedures, the indications for bronchography vary widely in different institutions. Our own experience has led us to adopt a conservative approach, not only because more direct diagnostic procedures are more informative and less hazardous, but also because with some conditions (*e.g.*, hemoptysis in association with a normal chest roentgenogram) bronchography has a low discovery rate.

In our view, there is only one indication for bronchography—the investigation of the presence and extent of bronchiectasis, and then only when the clinical state of the patient is such that surgical resection of local disease could be performed with benefit. Although the plain roentgenogram reveals bronchiectasis in approximately 93 per cent of patients with the disease,[26] only bronchography shows its severity and distribution. Whenever bronchiectasis is suspected or proved and surgery is contemplated, all 19 bronchopulmonary segments must be visualized bronchographically to exclude abnormality in areas in which no changes are apparent on the plain roentgenogram. One cautionary note: simple dilatation of segmental bronchi without destruction—reversible bronchiectasis—is a frequent concomitant of acute pneumonia and, although temporary, may persist as long as 3 to 4 months. During this period, bronchography may reveal bronchial deformity indistinguishable from irreversible cylindrical bronchiectasis; despite clinical suspicion of chronic disease, therefore, definitive investigation should be postponed for at least 4 months after acute pneumonia.

It is to be emphasized that in a patient with hemoptysis and a normal chest roentgenogram, bronchography rarely reveals abnormality and seldom is indicated, an opinion with which Forrest and his associates are in complete agreement.[27] A similar but more vexing problem develops when sputum cytology findings are repeatedly positive for malignant cells but the plain roentgenographic and bronchoscopic appearances are normal. In such cases, we find bronchography just as unrevealing as in cases of hemoptysis from an unidentified site; we feel that the most logical next step in the investigation of these patients is a CT scan. If the scan is normal, watchful waiting is recommended, with plain roentgenograms taken at 3-month intervals or less until either a lesion is demonstrated or the length of the follow-up has excluded a reasonable possibility of neoplasm (false positive cytologic findings).

The bronchographic techniques most widely used include supraglottic injection, the transglottic catheter method (the catheter is inserted through the glottis via the nose or mouth), and the percutaneous cricothyroid technique (administration directly through a needle or by a modified Seldinger technique). We prefer the transglottic technique, in which a soft rubber urethral catheter is inserted through the larynx via a naris and into a selected site in the bronchial tree. A complete description of the technique we employ can be found in the text Diagnosis of Diseases of the Chest (page 214).

ANGIOGRAPHY

This includes all procedures in which contrast media are injected into the vascular structures of the thorax for investigating thoracic disease. These methods include pulmonary angiography, aortography, bronchial arteriography, superior vena cava angiography, and azygography. Only the general indications for their use are considered here; detailed discussion in relation to specific diseases is presented in relevant chapters.

Our attitude toward thoracic angiography is clearly more conservative than that of many others. In several situations in which others successfully employ angiography, such as assessing the operability of lung cancer, we rely more heavily on traditional noninvasive methods of roentgenologic investigation, including CT scanning. It is inevitable that the contents of this book reflect this attitude. However, to disregard the experience of others would be negligent; therefore, wherever these procedures are mentioned, our discussion of angiographic techniques and findings is based largely on the observations of others.

PULMONARY ANGIOGRAPHY

Generally speaking, direct injection into the main pulmonary artery or one of its branches invariably produces clearer opacification of the pulmonary vascular tree than does venous or intracardiac injection; the superior visualization usually outweighs any disadvantage inherent in the catheterization procedure.

There are four major indications for pulmonary angiography.

(a) Detection of congenital anomalies of the pulmonary vascular tree, including agenesis or hypoplasia of a pulmonary artery, coarctation of one or more pulmonary arteries (peripheral pulmonic stenosis), idiopathic dilatation of a pulmonary artery, arteriovenous malformation of the lung, anomalous pulmonary venous drainage, and pulmonary venous varix.

(b) Investigation of acquired disease of the pulmonary arterial and venous circulation: primary pulmonary arterial hypertension, secondary pulmonary arterial and venous hyperten-

sion, and conditions of obscure origin leading to pulmonary venous obstruction (e.g., mediastinitis).

(c) Investigation of the resectability of bronchogenic cancer.

(d) Investigation of thromboembolic disease of the lungs. The important role that pulmonary angiography can play in the investigation of thromboembolic disease is no longer in dispute; in selected cases it may be of great diagnostic importance. No significant side effects of pulmonary angiography have been observed except in cases of primary pulmonary arterial hypertension, in which the risk of morbidity or mortality is increased.

At the time of writing, the role to be played by digital subtraction angiography in the study of the pulmonary circulation has not been clarified.

AORTOGRAPHY

The preferred technique is direct catheterization of the thoracic aorta percutaneously, with either flooding of the aorta or selective catheterization of a particular vessel. Indications are threefold.

(a) In the differential diagnosis of space-occupying lesions in the mediastinum; e.g., to distinguish aneurysms of the aorta from other mediastinal masses contiguous with the aorta. Selective angiography of the subclavian and internal mammary arteries can be used for investigating and differentiating anterior mediastinal masses. Aortography is imperative in patients in whom mediastinal widening is observed following severe deceleration injuries. When the widening is recognized, emergency aortography is indicated (1) to distinguish purely venous hematoma from major arterial injury, and (2) to show the number and sites of arterial lesions.

(b) Precise identification of aortic anomalies, such as patent ductus arteriosus or aortic coarctation.

(c) Identification of anomalous vessels, such as an artery supplying a sequestered lobe.

BRONCHIAL ARTERIOGRAPHY

Optimal opacification can be achieved only by selective catheterization, usually via a percutaneous transfemoral approach;[28] the tip of the catheter is wedged into a bronchial artery at the level of the fifth or sixth thoracic vertebra.

Bronchial arteriography has been recommended for investigating severe hemoptysis, particularly when a possible source of bleeding is not apparent from the plain roentgenogram. In patients with cataclysmic, life-threatening hemoptysis in whom resectional surgery is contraindicated for one reason or another, the technique of therapeutic embolization of bronchial arteries has been gaining increasing attention.[29, 30] A number of substances can be employed for occlusion, including Gianturco coils, Ivalon, Gelfoam, or inflatable balloons. A similar technique has been employed in controlling severe hemorrhage from pulmonary arteries, such as from a Rasmussen aneurysm[29] and from multiple pulmonary artery fistulas.[31]

SUPERIOR VENA CAVA ANGIOGRAPHY

This procedure can be carried out by unilateral or simultaneous bilateral arm-vein injection or via a catheter inserted into the superior vena cava or one of its large tributary veins. There are two main indications.

(a) To investigate obstruction of the superior vena cava (the superior vena cava syndrome).

(b) To investigate space-occupying lesions, either within the mediastinum or within the lung contiguous to the superior mediastinum, in which involvement of the great vein may indicate inoperability.

AZYGOGRAPHY

Although other techniques (*e.g.*, intraosseous injection into a rib) can result in satisfactory opacification of the azygos system, a more precise method involves the introduction of a catheter directly into the azygos via the femoral vein, right atrium, and superior vena cava; in addition to the superior opacification it provides, the technique permits recording of intravascular pressures. In our view, there is only one real indication for this procedure, the investigation of an enlarged azygos vein. Severe cirrhosis of the liver, obstruction of the superior vena cava, congestive heart failure, or anomalous pulmonary venous drainage may cause enlargement of the azygos vein in the right tracheobronchial angle. When the inferior vena cava is congenitally absent (infrahepatic interruption with azygos continuation), the azygos system becomes the main route for the return of systemic blood from beneath the diaphragm. Azygography may aid in the investigation, but the true nature of the anomaly is better elucidated by injection of contrast medium into the

femoral vein below. Although this anomaly is harmless *per se*, its common association with other congenital cardiovascular anomalies must be borne in mind.

CONTRAST STUDIES BY GAS INSUFFLATION

Insufflation of gas into pleural, mediastinal, or abdominal compartments has been used for diagnostic purposes with various degrees of success. It has not received the enthusiastic endorsement of most diagnosticians, probably because other simpler and less time-consuming techniques accurately yield the information required in most situations. In some cases, however, gas insufflation may provide information not available from other techniques. These techniques and their indications are described in considerable detail in Diagnosis of Diseases of the Chest (page 225), and the interested reader is directed there for more information.

ROENTGENOLOGIC METHODS IN THE ASSESSMENT OF LUNG FUNCTION

It is inevitable that over the years roentgenographic techniques have been devised to estimate parameters of lung function. Some, notably the determination of lung volume, are very accurate compared with physiologic methods of measurement; the majority, however, either lack sufficient precision or necessitate the use of highly complex apparatus not generally available. Whereas the refined techniques of pulmonary function testing described in Chapter 3 serve as the sheet anchor of physiologic investigation in most cases, certain roentgenologic procedures are useful as rough screening methods or when physiologic techniques are not available.

DETERMINATION OF LUNG VOLUMES

Of the many roentgenographic methods that have been devised for determining lung volume, that described by Harris and his colleagues[32] in 1971 is perhaps the most widely used and the easiest to perform. The outlines of the lungs on posteroanterior and lateral roentgenograms are traced, their areas measured with a planimeter, and a regression equation applied to these measurements. Measurements of TLC thus obtained approximate those achieved in the body plethysmograph both in healthy subjects and in patients with obstructive or restrictive diseases. Of potential promise is the technique described by Herman and his coworkers[33] which employs computerized graphic-to-digital conversion of tracings directly from posteroanterior and lateral roentgenograms. The procedure can be performed in less than 60 sec, and in a test on 53 subjects it showed good correlation with physiologic measurements ($r = 0.85$). Lung volumes can also be measured with reasonable accuracy by CT scanning.

STUDIES OF VENTILATION

Fluoroscopy and roentgenography may be useful as rough screening measures in the in vestigation of pulmonary ventilation. Estimates of diaphragmatic and costal excursion during quiet and forced respiration may indicate restricted ventilation, either bilaterally symmetric, as in diffuse bronchospasm or emphysema, or asymmetric, as may occur in association with a partly obstructing bronchial neoplasm or foreign body.

STUDIES OF PERFUSION

Since the volume of extravascular interstitial tissue presumably is constant, the roentgenographic density of lung is dependent upon the ratio of the amount of blood in the vascular tree to the amount of gas in the airways. At any one time, therefore, at a given degree of lung inflation, lung density should reflect the absolute amount of blood within the vascular tree, including capillaries. Oligemia or pleonemia, if of sufficient degree, can be appreciated on standard roentgenograms of the chest through assessment of decrease or increase, respectively, in the size of pulmonary vascular markings and sometimes by subjective evaluation of background lung density; the latter evaluation can be considerably facilitated by full lung tomography.

The most widely used method of assessing regional pulmonary ventilation and perfusion is lung scintiscanning. Techniques most commonly used are described in the following section.

LUNG SCANNING

Although the number of indications for lung scanning has increased, the major clinical application is in two relatively narrow fields of interest—thromboembolic disease and ventilation-perfusion studies of lung function.

INSTRUMENTATION

Generally speaking, the use of radioactive isotopes in lung studies involves the recording on sensitive devices of the gamma radiation produced by radionuclides injected intravenously into the bloodstream or inhaled into the air spaces. The imaging devices are basically of two types—the rectilinear scanner, which covers the field of interest in "strips," and the scintillation or gamma camera, which records in a single exposure the flux of gamma radiation from the lungs. The latter is much more versatile, permitting viewing of a large area at one time; in addition, the gamma camera permits isotopic angiography and angiocardiography.

RADIOPHARMACEUTICALS

These substances may be particulate or gaseous. The former has the advantage of allowing more time for scanning. For this, an intravenous injection is given of a standard quantity of tagged MAA (macroaggregates of human serum albumin) containing radioactive particles largely in the range of 10 to 50 μ in diameter. Being larger than the capillaries, they lodge in the first capillary bed encountered. Since the particles remain lodged for a considerable time before they disintegrate, they can be scanned with either the relatively slow, widely available rectilinear scanner or the gamma camera. Imaging with gaseous radionuclides—^{133}Xe, for example—requires performance of the scan over a relatively brief period, necessitating use of the scintillation camera. The properties of commonly used radiopharmaceuticals in lung scanning are summarized in Table 2–1.

The gaseous radiopharmaceutical most widely used for studying the pulmonary circulation is ^{133}Xe. The ^{133}Xe (10 mCi dissolved in saline) is injected intravenously; while the patient holds his or her breath, a gamma camera picture records perfusion. Since the xenon passes almost instantly into the alveoli, during subsequent respiration the distribution of xenon throughout all areas of ventilated lung, including those poorly perfused, can be recorded. Xenon is cleared from the lungs in 3 to 4 min in normally ventilated regions but is delayed in poorly ventilated regions (that is, those with air trapping).

Techniques for assessing pulmonary ventilation involve the inhalation of a radioactive gas (such as ^{133}Xe) or a nebulized aerosol of a radioactive material (such as albumin labeled with ^{131}I or ^{99m}Tc) (Figure 2–3). For the latter, the particles must be sufficiently small—less than 1 μ in diameter—to reach the alveoli.

TABLE 2–1. PROPERTIES OF COMMONLY USED LUNG SCANNING AGENTS

RADIONUCLIDE	PHYSICAL T½	PRINCIPAL GAMMA KEV	BETA	PARTICLE	BIOLOGIC LUNG T½	SCANNING DOSE ROUTE	RADIATION TO LUNGS
^{131}I	8 days	364	Yes	Macroaggregated albumin	8 hr	300 μCi IV	1.2–1.8 rad
^{113m}In	100 min	390	No	Ferric hydroxide	4–12 hr	2 mCi IV	1.5 rad
^{99m}Tc	6 hr	140	No	Macroaggregated albumin		2 mCi IV	0.8 rad
^{99m}Tc	6 hr	140	No	Ferric hydroxide	6–20 hr	2 mCi IV	1.2 rad
^{99m}Tc	6 hr	140	No	Albumin microsphere	4.5 hr	2 mCi IV	0.8 rad
^{113m}In	100 min	390	No	Albumin microsphere		2 mCi IV	1.5 rad
^{133}Xe	5.27 days	81 31	Yes	Aqueous solution	0.5 min	10 mCi IV	28–50 mrad

(Reprinted from Mishkin, F. S., and Brashear, R. E.: Use and Interpretation of the Lung Scan. Springfield, Ill., Charles C Thomas, Publisher, 1971, by permission of the authors and publisher.)

PERFUSION

AEROSOL

XENON

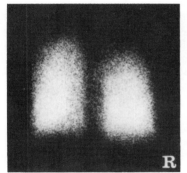
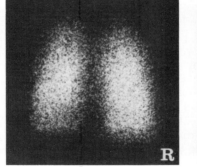
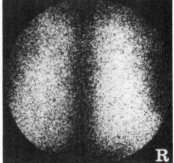

Initial

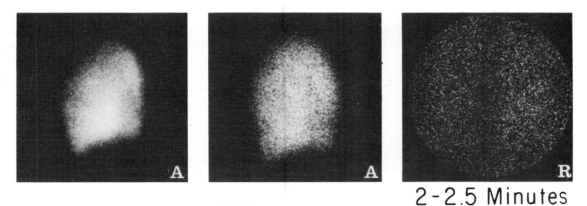

2-2.5 Minutes

Figure 2–3. Normal Perfusion, Airway Patency, and Ventilation Lung Scans. The two perfusion lung images on the left (posterior and lateral) were obtained following injection of ^{99m}Tc MAA, the airway patency images in the middle following inhalation of ^{99m}Tc sulfur colloid, and the inhalation images on the right following injection of ^{133}Xe. In all three procedures, the radiopharmaceutical was delivered and the images recorded in the erect position with a gamma camera. Note that the upper lung zones are better ventilated than perfused. The initial xenon image was made during breath-holding; washout is nearly complete in 2.0 to 2.5 minutes. (Courtesy of the late Dr. George Taplin, University of California, Los Angeles.)

INDICATIONS

Of the several indications for lung scanning summarized by DeLand and Wagner,[34] the following five seem to be most clinically useful.

(a) Detection of pulmonary thromboembolism.

(b) Monitoring the natural history or treatment of thromboembolism.

(c) Quantitative evaluation of the distribution of infectious, obstructive, and other pulmonary diseases.

(d) Preoperative evaluation of patients with emphysema, neoplasms, and bronchiectasis.

(e) Early detection of carcinoma of the lung (e.g., in patients with positive cytologic findings and a normal chest roentgenogram).

Of the several other indications for lung scan that have been reported, perhaps the most frequent are those relating to the use of [67]Gallium-citrate. In a review of the use of ^{67}Ga in pulmonary disorders, Siemsen and colleagues[35] pointed out that this isotope possesses limited value in the differential diagnosis of pulmonary diseases because of its nonspecific affinity for both neoplastic and inflammatory processes. However, based on personal observations of over 1100 patients with a variety of pulmonary diseases, they concluded that the judicious use of ^{67}Ga in selected patients can be of value in a number of clinical situations, specifically in the preoperative evaluation of hilar and mediastinal involvement in pulmonary neoplasms, in the differential diagnosis of pulmonary infarction and bacterial pneumonia, in the assessment of activity in patients with sarcoidosis, including evaluation of the effects of corticosteroid therapy, in the early detection of neoplastic and infectious diseases before roentgenographic abnormality becomes apparent, particularly in diffuse carcinomatosis and *Pneumocystis carinii* pneumonia, and in the interstitial pulmonary disease caused by bleomycin therapy.[36] Because of its affinity for active inflammatory tissue, ^{67}Ga can be of value in estimating the degree of activity in patients with cryptogenic fibrosing alveolitis and in following the response to therapy, a feature emphasized by Line and his colleagues.[37] It has also been reported to be useful in following the response to therapy in patients with lymphoma.[38]

In summarizing their experience in over 1000 cases, Siemsen and his colleagues[35] concluded that "it remains to be seen whether gallium imaging statistically provides essential additional information in these indications when compared to cheaper conventional techniques."

The major indication for lung scanning is the investigation of thromboembolic diseases. Briefly, studies with tagged MAA are of diagnostic value only when the scan image is compared with the chest roentgenogram. Many physiologic and pathologic conditions (such as the patient's posture during tracer injection, obesity, cardiomegaly, and cardiac decompensation) alter lung images, and must be taken into account for correct interpretation.[39] Since any disease characterized by consolidation or atelectasis or both can diminish pulmonary artery perfusion, and since the airless lung can absorb radiation, reduced or absent radioactivity on scanning does not necessarily indicate embolism. When the clinical picture suggests embolism, however, and the chest roentgenogram shows no opacity, scintillation studies may be diagnostic. This is especially true when the perfusion scan shows one or more defects and the ventilation scan is normal (just as a normal lung scan virtually excludes a major pulmonary embolism). Since pulmonary embolism may be medically or surgically curable, the diagnosis must be made by whatever tools are at the physician's disposal. In many cases the diagnosis can be established by isotopic studies, but *the majority of pulmonary emboli can be identified only by integrating information gained from all methods of investigation.*

DIAGNOSTIC ULTRASOUND

This technique has limited but potentially important applications within the thorax. The limitations are imposed by the physical composition of the intrathoracic structures in that neither air nor bone transmits sound, instead absorbing or reflecting incoming sonic energy and preventing the collection of information about acoustic interfaces behind ribs or lung tissue. But there are "windows" in the thorax through which ultrasonography can garner information useful in the investigation of thoracic disease. Undoubtedly the most important of these are the intercostal spaces, through which ultrasonic beams can be directed toward the heart and pericardium. It is in this field of echocardiography that ultrasonography has made its greatest impact in the assessment of thoracic disease, particularly in establishing the nature of valvular deformity, the volume of cardiac chambers, and the thickness of their walls. It is also valuable for detecting pericardial effusion, assessing its size, and differentiating it from cardiomegaly.

The second most useful application of ultrasonography in the thorax is in assessing local pleural thickening, usually loculated empyema. Differentiation of liquid from solid pleural collections, which may be exceedingly difficult with standard roentgenographic techniques, is achieved easily with ultrasonography (Figure 2–4). Furthermore, it provides an assessment of the amount of fluid loculated in a pleural pocket, indicates the anatomic point for thoracentesis, and simplifies fluid aspiration by permitting insertion of a needle directly through a special transducer.

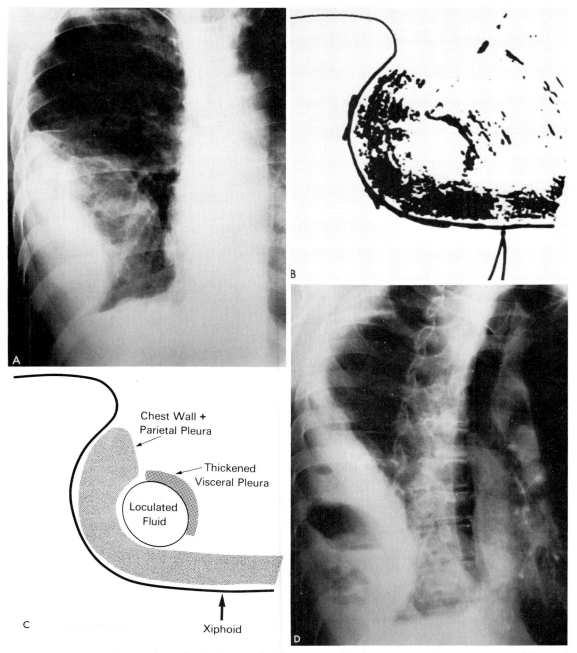

Chest Wall +
Parietal Pleura

Thickened
Visceral Pleura

Loculated
Fluid

Xiphoid

Figure 2–4. Identification of Loculated Empyema by Ultrasonography. An anteroposterior roentgenogram (A) reveals a large, homogeneous opacity in the right lower hemithorax laterally whose configuration strongly suggests fluid loculation. An ultrasonic B-scan of the lower chest (B) shows a roughly elliptical, sharply demarcated sonolucent space posterolaterally, possessing the typical characteristics of a fluid-filled space. A drawing (C) indicates important landmarks. Thoracentesis was carried out, pus withdrawn, and air introduced; an oblique roentgenogram (D) reveals the space corresponding to the sonolucent zone in the ultrasound recording. (Courtesy of Dr. Reggie Greene, Massachusetts General Hospital, Boston.)

MASS CHEST ROENTGENOGRAPHY AS A SCREENING PROCEDURE

The vastly increasing use of ionizing radiation in the diagnosis of chest disease, particularly in mass chest roentgenography, has caused many to ponder the efficacy of such programs, especially in relation to the potentially harmful effect of such vast quantities of radiation on populations as a whole. A most useful, succinct policy statement stemming from these deliberations was prepared by the Bureau of Radiological Health of the U.S. Department of Health, Education, and Welfare, in collaboration with the American Colleges of Radiology and Chest Physicians.[40] We reproduce here verbatim the recommendations contained in this policy statement, which has been endorsed by the U.S. National Tuberculosis and Respiratory Disease Association and the Centers for Disease Control. We enthusiastically endorse these recommendations.

1. Community chest x-ray surveys among the general population are not productive as a screening procedure for the detection of tuberculosis and should not be done. In a high tuberculosis incidence area where fixed x-ray facilities are limited or not available, it may be necessary to screen selected groups of the population by x-ray in conjunction with the tuberculin skin test. In such circumstances, full follow-up treatment facilities must be available as an essential component of the community tuberculosis control program. Tuberculin skin tests should be performed for those under age 21 *in lieu* of chest x-ray examinations, even if periodic physical examinations are required for food handlers or school employees. Those jurisdictions requiring chest x-ray examinations should re-evaluate this procedure. The primary screening of grade and high school children for tuberculosis should not be by x-ray examination. The chest x-ray examination would thus be restricted to the positive reactors to the tuberculin test in the younger age groups. In low prevalence groups, consideration should also be given to the tuberculin skin test as the initial screening examination for case finding. X-ray examination should be restricted to the positive reactors.

2. Community chest x-ray surveys among the general population for detection of other pulmonary disease or heart disease have not proved sufficiently rewarding and should not be done.

3. When radiologic screening of selected groups of the general population may be productive, the full size film is preferred. The use of the photofluorographic unit as a screening device is justified only under the following conditions:

    a. A definitive interpretation must be made by qualified physicians such as certified radiologists or other physicians with demonstrated competence in the interpretation of chest radiographs.

    b. The radiographs and the reports should be made available upon request to the private physician, public health, and hospital agencies for a period of at least 5 years.

    c. The equipment used must meet the requirements of the NCRP Report No. 33, or appropriate State and Federal regulations.

4. While community chest x-ray surveys among the general population are not recommended, x-ray facilities for individuals should be available. These may be located in a public health department, private office or health centre.

PATHOLOGIC EXAMINATION

The proper management of pulmonary, pleural, or mediastinal disease depends upon accurate diagnosis. By "proper management" is meant not only the initiation of appropriate therapy but also the requirement, with a few exceptions, of informing the patient of the nature of the disease and the prognosis. In some cases the clinical findings or roentgenographic manifestations, either alone or in combination, are sufficiently characteristic to indicate the diagnosis without further investigation. In many others the diagnosis can be established by noninvasive methods; for example, identification of a causative microorganism on smear or culture; or of specific cells by cytologic examination of expectorated material, bronchial washings, or pleural fluid; or of specific antibodies in serum, increased numbers of eosinophils in the blood, or abnormalities of pulmonary function. Despite these and other investigative procedures available to the physician, however, there are inevitably a few cases in which thorough study does not reveal the diagnosis. Therefore one must decide whether an invasive diagnostic procedure is justified in the face of the accompanying potential morbidity or even mortality.

Techniques of pathologic examination are considered under three headings: cytology, biopsy, and necropsy.

METHODS OF PATHOLOGIC EXAMINATION (CYTOLOGY)

CYTOLOGY OF PULMONARY SECRETIONS

Exfoliative cytologic examination of pulmonary secretions with the Papanicolaou technique, although time-consuming, is a simple and relatively reliable method for diagnosing bronchogenic carcinoma. For the experienced it may represent the most accurate method of reaching a confident diagnosis; in fact, its accuracy and reliability are superior to both bronchoscopy and biopsy of prescalene lymph nodes, although these procedures are frequently complementary. Positive diagnosis by this technique in large series of patients with confirmed lung cancer ranges from 71 per cent[41] to 90 per cent.[42]

At least two studies have shown that sputum specimens are at least equal to bronchial washings as a source of material for cytologic examination. However, it may be necessary to resort to bronchial washings for positive diagnosis, particularly when sputum specimens are not readily obtainable.

Positive findings in exfoliative cytologic studies in cases of lung cancer are commoner with central than peripheral neoplasms or metastases.[41]

False positive results—single or repeated identification of class V cells by the Papanicolaou technique—are rare, being reported in only 1 to 3 per cent in most series. False negative results—ranging in incidence from 10 to 30 per cent of histologically proved cases—may be caused by lack of communication between the neoplasm and the bronchial lumen, by bronchial stenosis, or by misinterpretation of the smears.

Fluorescence microscopy combined with exfoliative cytology in screening for lung cancer roughly halves the time needed for the Papanicolaou method but reduces the discovery rate to only 83 per cent.

CYTOLOGY OF PLEURAL FLUID

Nonmalignant Cells

The relative numbers of erythrocytes, polymorphonuclear leukocytes, eosinophils, and lymphocytes in pleural fluid may indicate the etiology of an effusion.

ERYTHROCYTES. Light and associates[43] found RBC counts greater than 10,000 per cu mm common to all types of effusions and therefore of no discriminatory value. Counts exceeding 100,000 per cu mm most often were associated with malignant neoplasm, pulmonary infarction, or traumatic hemorrhage.

NEUTROPHILS. A large number of neutrophils in pleural fluid usually indicates bacterial pneumonia but may also be found in pancreatitis and pulmonary infarction and occasionally in malignant neoplasm and tuberculosis.[43] However, an effusion containing more than 50 per cent neutrophils is almost certainly not due to tuberculosis.

LYMPHOCYTES. In contrast to the "50 per cent rule" for neutrophils and tuberculosis, an effusion containing 50 per cent or more lymphocytes is almost certainly tuberculous or neoplastic.[43] Although the predominance of lymphocytes does not help to differentiate between tuberculosis and metastatic cancer, a grossly bloody effusion or one containing 100,000 RBC per cu mm is much more likely to be of neoplastic than of tuberculous origin.

EOSINOPHILS. Tuberculosis or neoplastic effusions rarely contain eosinophils,[43] which is perhaps the most important observation in regard to eosinophilia in pleural fluid. Eosinophilic pleural effusion, not necessarily associated with blood eosinophilia, may be present in a wide variety of diseases. Pulmonary infarction is said to be a relatively frequent cause and histoplasmosis, coccidioidomycosis, and actinomycosis occasional causes of eosinophilic effusion.

Malignant Cells

Positive findings in exfoliative cytologic examination of pleural effusions of malignant origin range from 33 to 66 per cent. This comparatively small yield probably results, at least in part, from the fact that some of these effusions are secondary to pneumonitis distal to an obstructing bronchogenic carcinoma or to lymphatic obstruction. False positive findings are common because of the difficulty of distinguishing malignant from mesothelial cells.

METHODS OF PATHOLOGIC EXAMINATION (BIOPSY)

In the textbook *Diagnosis of Diseases of the Chest*, we described in considerable detail the techniques currently available for biopsy of the lung. Further, we discussed indications and contraindications, summarized the results obtained by various investigators, and proposed approaches to specific problems. The interested reader is directed to this book (page 244) for detailed information. In the following pages we have attempted to summarize the current status of lung biopsy and to consider how individual situations should be approached. Although we have taken the extensive experience of other investigators into due consideration, our recommendations reflect the approaches we have adopted on the basis of personal experience. It is emphasized at the outset that in formulating indications for lung biopsy there are no rules that apply to every situation; each patient must be considered individually, and the merits of all the variables must be weighed before making a decision.

Clinical and roentgenologic variables will influence the decision as to whether to perform biopsy and which procedure to use. The first four of the following variables must be taken into account in *all* situations when biopsy is being considered.

1. No invasive procedure is indicated if the diagnosis can be established by simpler, noninvasive techniques (for example, sputum culture and cytologic study and tracheobronchial aspiration).

2. Biopsy is not indicated if the possibility of malignancy has been excluded by certain roentgenographic signs; for example, calcification within a solitary pulmonary nodule or confirmation of lack of change in the size of a solitary nodule when compared with previous roentgenograms obtained at least two years previously.

3. The patient's general condition must be such that it does not contraindicate an invasive procedure; for example, biopsy of a small peripheral nodule for purposes of diagnosis alone might be justified in a patient with severe COPD in whom thoracotomy and surgical resection would not be feasible, but the patient should have enough breathing reserve to withstand the almost inevitable pneumothorax.

4. The expertise of the operator must be an important consideration in the choice of technique for biopsy. If the operator has had a very low incidence of false negative results in needle aspiration biopsy of peripheral nodules, this procedure should be preferred over alternative methods.

5. The patient's age is very important in some situations; for example, solitary peripheral nodules in a 25-year-old woman and a 50-year-old man require different approaches.

6. A history of exposure to carcinogens can be of major significance. The commonest example is a long history of cigarette smoking; patient exposure to such substances as asbestos, arsenic, or radioactive materials also will influence judgment.

7. The presence or absence of symptoms is a vital factor in establishing the requirement for biopsy in many cases; for example, entirely different approaches are needed for multiple pulmonary nodules in a patient with polyarthritis and in an asymptomatic person.

8. Evidence of disease elsewhere in the body constitutes a major factor in the decision as to whether to do a biopsy; for example, multiple pulmonary nodules in a patient with a large renal mass would lead to a reasonably confident diagnosis of metastases, but when associated with nasal ulceration and hematuria would strongly suggest Wegener's granulomatosis.

9. Finally, timing is an important consideration in all cases. While drawing up these recommendations, we thought of patients we have seen whose roentgenograms revealed lesions of unknown etiology, and while biopsy was being considered for definitive diagnosis the lesions either diminished or were no longer apparent on films obtained a few days later—spontaneously or as a result of nonspecific therapy. In many instances, therefore, it is advisable to watch a lesion for several days before carrying out an invasive procedure, particularly when infection is a distinct possibility.

There are six basic roentgenographic patterns of disease for which the indications for and techniques of biopsy are different. In the recommendations to follow, these patterns are discussed in relation to variables of major importance to each, leading to a decision as to whether to recommend an invasive procedure, and which procedure, for each lesion.

1. *Solitary pulmonary nodule 2 cm or less in diameter in the lung periphery* (Figure 2–5): such a lesion in a patient under 30 years of age is almost certainly benign; biopsy is not warranted even if no previous roentgenograms are available for comparison or an earlier film showed no similar shadow. In such cases, however, chest roentgenograms are desirable every 3 months or so for about a year to confirm the benign nature of the lesion. (Occasionally, a solitary nodule will simply disappear.) Calcium within the lesion (not eccentrically situated) establishes its benign nature beyond reasonable doubt and indicates no further follow-up. (Eccentric calcification should raise the possibility of so-called scar carcinoma and such a lesion either should be investigated promptly or watched closely.)

In patients over 30 years of age, particularly those in the 40 to 60 age group, a solitary uncalcified lesion must be regarded as a bronchogenic carcinoma until proved otherwise. If previous roentgenograms are not available for comparison, or such roentgenograms reveal no lesion or a smaller lesion than is now apparent, in most cases we recommend surgical resection. This approach is governed largely by the incidence of false negative results of needle aspiration biopsy reported by most investigators and the very low incidence of morbidity and mortality following thoracotomy and wedge resection.

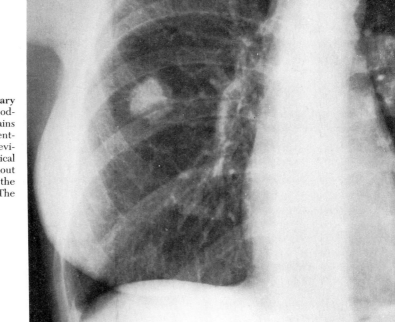

Figure 2–5. Solitary Pulmonary Nodule 2 cm in Diameter. This nodule is of uniform density and contains no demonstrable calcium. A roentgenogram from several years previously revealed no lesion. Surgical resection was carried out without biopsy study of the nature of the lesion. Anaplastic carcinoma. The patient is a 51-year-old woman.

If such a patient refuses surgery, or surgery is contraindicated by severe impairment of lung function or concomitant disease elsewhere, there is reasonable justification for biopsy—either by needle aspiration or by the transbronchial approach with a brush or biting forceps. In the same category are patients with a solitary peripheral nodule and clinical or roentgenologic evidence of metastatic disease elsewhere. The rationale for an invasive procedure in each of these circumstances is difficult to define but is chiefly the establishment of a diagnosis for prognostic purposes.

2. *A pulmonary mass larger than 2 cm in diameter, with or without cavitation* (Figure 2–6): the clinical presentation may broadly suggest the etiology of such a mass. In an asymptomatic patient who is not a compromised host, the possibility of primary bronchogenic carcinoma ranks high on the list of differential diagnoses and investigation must be aggressive. If repeated cytologic examinations of sputum and bronchial washings have proved negative, we recommend transbronchial biopsy, first with brushing and then followed if necessary by one of the cutting techniques to obtain tissue. In a patient who presents with fever and constitutional symptoms, an infectious etiology is obviously much more likely (note, however, that a compromised host may have such a lesion without concomitant fever or constitutional

symptoms). Again, provided that the etiologic agent has not been identified on sputum smear or culture, a more direct approach may be necessary. If the lesion has cavitated, percutaneous needle aspiration biopsy or transbronchial brushing will yield diagnostic material in most cases; if the mass is solid, a transbronchial approach probably is preferable, beginning with brushing and followed if necessary by tissue biopsy.

3. *Consolidation of lung parenchyma, usually but not always segmentally distributed and associated with loss of volume* (Figure 2–7): in most patients with this pattern an endobronchial lesion is producing obstructive pneumonitis, and bronchoscopy and direct tissue biopsy usually reveal the diagnosis. Despite the potential hazard of serious hemorrhage from vascular lesions, it is usually desirable if not essential for the surgeon to know the precise nature of the lesion before thoracotomy so that he or she can design an appropriate operative procedure. If biopsy proves that the lesion is malignant, thoracotomy should always be preceded by mediastinoscopy and node biopsy. The roentgenographic pattern may not suggest an endobronchial obstructing lesion (*e.g.*, if the process is nonsegmental or an air bronchogram is identified) or whether the lesion is neoplastic (*e.g.*, bronchioloalveolar carcinoma) or infectious (*e.g.*, pneumonia), and biopsy

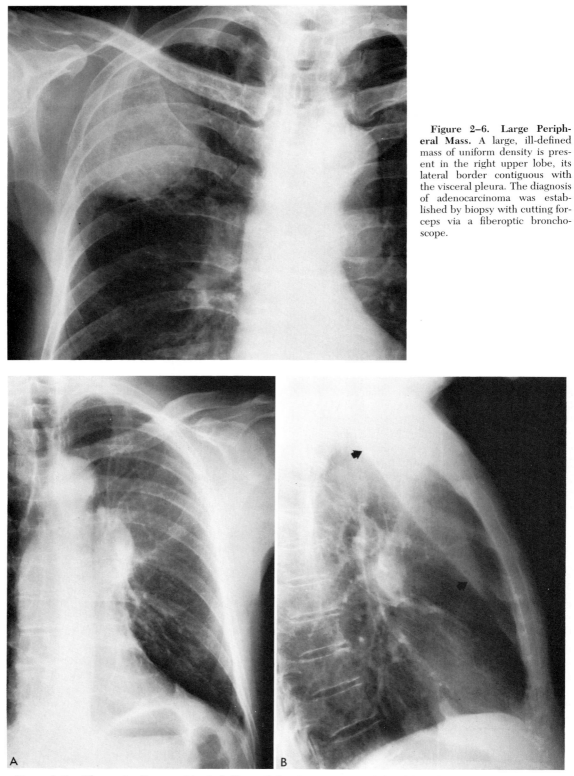

Figure 2–6. Large Peripheral Mass. A large, ill-defined mass of uniform density is present in the right upper lobe, its lateral border contiguous with the visceral pleura. The diagnosis of adenocarcinoma was established by biopsy with cutting forceps via a fiberoptic bronchoscope.

Figure 2–7. Obstructive Pneumonitis, Left Upper Lobe. Posteroanterior *(A)* and lateral *(B)* roentgenograms reveal moderate loss of volume of the left upper lobe *(arrows* in *B* point to anteriorly displaced major fissure). The collapsed lobe is uniformly opaque and shows no air bronchogram. Bronchoscopic biopsy results revealed squamous-cell carcinoma. The patient is a 63-year-old man.

may be required to obtain tissue or cells for diagnosis. Although percutaneous needle aspiration biopsy may suffice in such circumstances, we prefer the transbronchial approach, which gives a higher yield of positive diagnoses.

4. *Multiple pulmonary nodules, with or without cavitation:* in many patients with this roentgenographic pattern the diagnosis is evident and there is no need to obtain tissue for cytologic or histologic examination. Such patients include those with an established primary neoplasm elsewhere (metastases); those who have upper respiratory tract disease and hematuria (Wegener's granulomatosis); those with a long history of polyarthritis (rheumatoid necrobiotic nodules); and those with multiple pulmonary cavitary lesions and suppurative infection elsewhere (pyemic abscesses). If these diagnoses have been excluded, the remaining possibilities are rather limited: (a) multiple infectious granulomas, particularly as caused by histoplasmosis or coccidioidomycosis (skin tests may be helpful, or knowledge that the patient lives in or has traveled through an endemic zone); and (b) multiple hamartomas (there is no way of establishing a positive diagnosis short of obtaining tissue).

Many patients with multiple metastatic nodules are asymptomatic, despite the roentgenographic pattern. In the majority, tissue is required only to establish the diagnosis for prognosis, but in rare cases a specific vaccine can be made from metastatic nodules (*e.g.*, in melanosarcoma, in which case thoracotomy must be performed to obtain an adequate tissue sample). We believe that roentgenographic investigation of multiple organ systems, in search of a primary lesion, is so often unrewarding that it is seldom indicated. A direct approach to the pulmonary nodules themselves is less time-consuming, less expensive, and more informative: biopsy by percutaneous needle aspiration or by a transbronchial technique usually suffices. Open lung or cutting needle biopsy should be reserved for cases in which less traumatic procedures have yielded negative results and the metastatic nature of the lesions is reasonably certain.

5. *Acute diffuse lung disease* (Figure 2–8): the great majority of these patients are compromised hosts. Although the symptomatology may be unimpressive despite rapidly progressive pulmonary disease, in many cases dyspnea and cough indicate a rapidly disseminating infec-

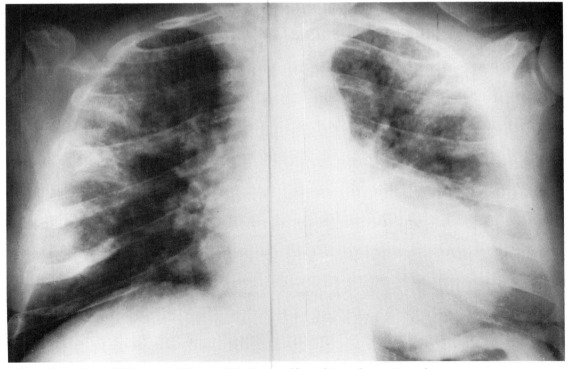

Figure 2–8. Acute Diffuse Lung Disease. This 32-year-old renal transplant patient who was on immunosuppressive therapy presented with low-grade fever, increasing dyspnea, and cough. Sputum and transtracheal aspirates failed to reveal an etiologic agent but transbronchial brushing showed *Pneumocystis carinii* organisms.

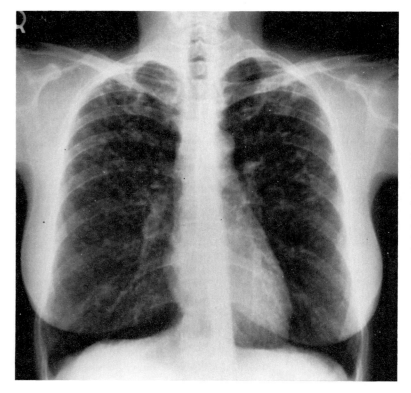

Figure 2–9. Chronic Diffuse Lung Disease. This 46-year-old woman presented with a 6-months' history of increasing shortness of breath on exertion and mild nonproductive cough. A rather coarse reticulonodular pattern is present, with moderate upper zone predominance. Open lung biopsy revealed histiocytosis X.

tious disease. Prompt etiologic diagnosis is of the utmost importance, since appropriate antimicrobial therapy may be life-saving. Unfortunately, more often than not the precise diagnosis cannot be made by study of the sputum or tracheobronchial aspirates, and biopsy must be performed without delay. Since these patients are usually seriously ill, thrombocytopenic, and with decreased respiratory reserve, every attempt must be made to avoid the more traumatic procedures such as percutaneous cutting needle biopsy or thoracotomy. A transbronchial technique usually will suffice, beginning with brushing and followed by a cutting technique if necessary. Percutaneous needle aspiration biopsy may be equally productive, particularly in cases of *Pneumocystis carinii* pneumonia. Should these fail to yield diagnostic material, one may have to resort to open lung biopsy.

Although most compromised hosts presenting with this pattern are found to harbor opportunistic infections (most commonly *Pneumocystis carinii* or cytomegalovirus), it is vital that iatrogenic pulmonary disease be excluded. This is usually achieved by abrupt withdrawal of most therapeutic agents, including corticosteroids and chemotherapeutic and immunosuppressive drugs. Careful appraisal of the antibiotic regi-

men is imperative. In a significant number of compromised hosts, these steps alone bring about a prompt remission of the infectious process, and, if the disease is drug-induced, may even banish the roentgenographic abnormality.

6. *Chronic diffuse pulmonary disease* (Figure 2–9): the pattern of the disease is predominantly interstitial in most cases but in some primarily involves air spaces. Onset is usually insidious. Many of these patients are asymptomatic, and it is debatable whether an invasive diagnostic procedure is justified despite the low risk. For example, the patient with a diffuse reticular pattern, hilar lymph node enlargement, and anergy almost certainly has sarcoidosis and requires no further investigation, not even scalene node biopsy. However, there are large numbers of patients in whom diffuse progressive disease has produced symptoms and in whom the roentgenographic pattern and clinical picture reveal nothing specific to suggest the diagnosis. In this situation, unless the patient is too old or too ill to warrant the slight risk, biopsy is mandatory. In some of our patients biopsy has resulted in diagnosis of a treatable condition. Also, we have faced the dilemma of seeing patients become so disabled by dyspnea that we hesitated to recommend biopsy; in such circumstances we think it wise to restrict inva-

sive procedures to those least likely to provoke complications, since therapy other than with corticosteroids is unlikely to be indicated by biopsy regardless of the result. As the first step we recommend a transbronchial approach for biopsy of the peripheral parenchyma with a cutting instrument; should this prove unrewarding, open lung biopsy should be performed. In our opinion, the low yield of needle biopsy contraindicates this procedure.

METHODS FOR PATHOLOGIC EXAMINATION (NECROPSY)

The lungs collapse after removal from the body and must be reinflated postmortem if emphysema is to be recognized. Further, reinflation is useful in diagnosing many other disorders. The lung is a large organ of complex arrangement and few diseases affect it uniformly throughout, making a random section technique of examination inadequate. There are some special techniques that may be extremely valuable in assessment of the general patterns of the bronchi and pulmonary vasculature and these may be reviewed if desired in the text *Diagnosis of Diseases of the Chest* (page 270). Subjects discussed in that section include postmortem inflation of the lung, pathologic examination of the lung, recording and storage, lung morphometry, and handling of surgical specimens.

REFERENCES

1. Sagel, S. S., Evens, R. G., Forrest, J. V., and Bramson, R. T.: Efficacy of routine screening and lateral chest radiographs in a hospital-based population. N. Engl. J. Med., *291*:1001, 1974.
2. Farnsworth, P. B., Steiner, E., Klein, R. M., and SanFilippo, J. A.: The value of routine preoperative chest roentgenograms in infants and children. J.A.M.A., *244*:582, 1980.
3. Bonebrake, C. R., Noller, K. L., Loehnen, C. P., Muhm, J. R., and Fish, C. R.: Routine chest roentgenography in pregnancy. J.A.M.A., *240*:2747, 1978.
4. Crapo, R. O., Montague, T., and Armstrong, J.: Inspiratory lung volume achieved on routine chest films. Invest. Radiol., *14*:137, 1979.
5. Wilkinson, G. A., and Fraser, R. G.: Roentgenography of the chest. Appl. Radiol., *4*:41, 1975.
6. Tabrisky, J., Herman, M. W., Torrance, D. J., and Hieshima, G. B.: Mobile 240 kVp phototimed chest radiography. Am. J. Roentgenol., *135*:295, 1980.
7. Wilkinson, G. A., and Fraser, R. G.: Use of a double screen-film combination in bedside chest roentgenography. Radiology, *117*:222, 1975.
8. Rigler, L. G.: Roentgen diagnosis of small pleural effusion: A new roentgenographic position. J.A.M.A., *96*:104, 1931.
9. Littleton, J. T., Durizch, M. L., and Callahan, W. P.: Linear vs. pluridirectional tomography of the chest. Correlative radiographic anatomic study. Am. J. Roentgenol., *134*:241, 1980.
10. Bein, M. E., and Stone, D. N.: Full lung linear and pluridirectional tomography: A preliminary evaluation of nodule detection. Am. J. Roentgenol., *136*:1013, 1981.
11. Favis, E. A.: Planigraphy (body section radiography) in detecting tuberculous pulmonary cavitation. Dis. Chest, *27*:668, 1955.
12. Janower, M. L.: 55° posterior oblique tomography of the pulmonary hilum. J. Can. Assoc. Radiol., *29*:158, 1978.
13. Sindelar, W. F., Bagley, D. H., Felix, E. L., Doppman, J. L., and Ketcham, A. S.: Lung tomography in cancer patients. Full-lung tomograms in screening for pulmonary metastases. J.A.M.A., *240*:2060, 1978.
14. Curtis, A. M., Ravin, C. E., Collier, P. E., Putman, C. E., McLoud, T., and Greenspan, R. H.: Detection of metastatic disease from carcinoma of the breast: Limited value of full lung tomography. Am. J. Roentgenol., *134*:253, 1980.
15. Bein, M. E., Greenberg, M., Liu, P.-Y., Ohara, J., Bassett, L. W., Schaefer, C. J., and Steckel, R. J.: Pulmonary nodules: Detection in 1 and 2 cm full lung linear tomography. Am. J. Roentgenol., *135*:513, 1980.
16. Muhm, J. R., Brown, L. R., Crowe, J. K., Sheedy, P. F., II, Hattery, R. R., and Stephens, D. H.: Comparison of whole lung tomography and computed tomography for detecting pulmonary nodules. Am. J. Roentgenol., *131*:981, 1978.
17. Ter-Pogossian, M. M.: The challenge of computed tomography. Am. J. Roentgenol., *127*:1, 1976.
18. Society for Computed Body Tomography: Special report. New indications for computed body tomography. Am. J. Roentgenol., *133*:115, 1979.
19. Raval, B., Lamki, N., and Carey, L. S.: Computed tomography in chest diseases. CT, *5*:91, 1981.
20. Siegelman, S. S., Zerhouni, E. A., Leo, F. P., Khouri, N. F., and Stitik, F. P.: CT of the solitary pulmonary nodule. Am. J. Roentgenol., *135*:1, 1980.
21. Rosenblum, L. J., Mauceri, R. A., Wellenstein, D. E., Bassano, D. A., Cohen, W. N., and Heitzman, E. R.: Computed tomography of the lung. Radiology, *129*:521, 1978.
22. Mintzer, R. A., Malave, S. R., Neiman, H. L., Michaelis, L. L., Vanecko, R. M., and Sanders, J. H.: Computed vs. conventional tomography in evaluation of primary and secondary pulmonary neoplasms. Radiology, *132*:653, 1979.
23. Osborne, D. R., Korobkin, M., Ravin, C. E., Putman, C. E., Wolfe, W. G., Sealy, W. C., Young, W. G., Breiman, R., Heaston, D., Ram, P., and Halber, M.: Comparison of plain radiography, conventional tomography, and computed tomography in detecting intrathoracic lymph node metastases from lung carcinoma. Radiology, *142*:157, 1982.
24. Avery, M. E.: Bronchography: Outmoded procedure? Pediatrics, *46*:333, 1970.
25. Molnar, W., and Riebel, F. A.: Bronchography: An aid in the diagnosis of peripheral pulmonary carcinoma. Radiol. Clin. North Am., *1*:303, 1963.
26. Gudbjerg, C. E.: Bronchiectasis; radiological diagnosis and prognosis after operative treatment. Acta Radiol. (Suppl.), *143*, 1957.

27. Forrest, J. V., Sagel, S. S., and Omell, G. H.: Bronchography in patients with hemoptysis. Am. J. Roentgenol., *126*:597, 1976.

28. Nordenström, B.: Selective catheterization and angiography of bronchial and mediastinal arteries in man. Acta. Radiol., *6*:13, 1967.

29. Remy, J., Smith, M., Lemaitre, L., Marache, P., and Fournier, E.: Treatment of massive hemoptysis by occlusion of a Rasmussen aneurysm. Am. J. Roentgenol., *135*:605, 1980.

30. Remy, J., Arnaud, A., Fardou, H., Giraud, R., and Voisin, C.: Treatment of hemoptysis by embolization of bronchial arteries. Radiology, *122*:33, 1977.

31. Castaneda-Zuniga, W., Epstein, M., Zollikofer, C., Nath, P. H., Formanek, A., Ben-Shachar, G., and Amplatz, K.: Embolization of multiple pulmonary artery fistulas. Radiology, *134*:309, 1980.

32. Harris, T. R., Pratt, P. C., and Kilburn, K. H.: Total lung capacity measured by roentgenograms. Am. J. Med., *50*:756, 1971.

33. Herman, P. G., Sandor, T., Mann, B. E., McFadden, E. R., Korngold, E., Murphy, M. A., and Mellins, H. Z.: Rapid computerized lung volume determination from chest roentgenograms. Am. J. Roentgenol., *124*:477, 1975.

34. Deland, F. H., and Wagner, H. N., Jr.: Atlas of Nuclear Medicine. Vol. II: Lung and Heart. Philadelphia, W. B. Saunders Co., 1970.

35. Siemsen, J. K., Grebe, S. F., and Waxman, A. D.: The use of gallium-67 in pulmonary disorders. Semin. Nucl. Med., *8*:235, 1978.

36. Richman, S. D., Levenson, S. M., Bunn, P. A., Flinn, G. S., Johnston, G. S., and DeVita, V. T.: ^{67}Ga accumulation in pulmonary lesions associated with bleomycin toxicity. Cancer, *36*:1966, 1975.

37. Line, B. R., Fulmer, J. D., Reynolds, H. Y., Roberts, W. C., Jones, A. E., Harris, E. K., and Crystal, R. G.: Gallium-67 citrate scanning in the staging of idiopathic pulmonary fibrosis: Correlation with physiologic and morphologic features and bronchoalveolar lavage. Am. Rev. Resp. Dis., *118*:355, 1978.

38. Turner, D. A., Fordham, E. W., Ali, A., and Slayton, R. E.: Gallium-67 imaging in the management of Hodgkin's disease and other malignant lymphomas. Semin. Nucl. Med., *8*:205, 1978.

39. Poe, N. D., Swanson, L. A., and Taplin, G. V.: Physiological factors affecting lung scan interpretations. Radiology, *89*:661, 1967.

40. U.S. Department of Health, Education and Welfare, in collaboration with the American College of Radiology and the American College of Chest Physicians: The Chest X-Ray as a Screening Procedure for Cardiopulmonary Disease. A Policy Statement. Washington, D.C., Publication No. (FDA) 73–8036, April, 1973.

41. Rosa, U. W., Prolla, J. C., and da Silva Gastal, E.: Cytology in diagnosis of cancer affecting the lung. Results in 1,000 consecutive patients. Chest, *63*:203, 1973.

42. Oswald, N. C., Hinson, K. F. W., Canti, G., and Miller, A. B.: The diagnosis of primary lung cancer with special reference to sputum cytology. Thorax, *26*:623, 1971.

43. Light, R. W., Erozan, Y. S., and Ball, W. C., Jr.: Cells in pleural fluid. Their value in differential diagnosis. Arch. Intern. Med., *132*:854, 1973.

3

Methods in Clinical, Laboratory, and Functional Investigation

CLINICAL HISTORY

In pulmonary disease the key to solution of abnormal roentgenographic shadows most often lies in thorough awareness of the patient's complaints. In some cases, despite symptoms indicating advanced and disabling disease, the chest roentgenogram may be normal, a finding which, in itself, limits the diagnostic possibilities and excludes diseases invariably associated with an abnormal roentgenogram. The symptoms of respiratory disease are cough and expectoration, shortness of breath, chest pain, and hemoptysis. These will be considered individually, after which further consideration will be given to the pertinence of personal, occupational, and residential history and to disease of other organ systems commonly associated with respiratory disorders.

SYMPTOMS OF RESPIRATORY DISEASE

COUGH AND EXPECTORATION

Cough is a defensive mechanism designed to rid the conducting passages of mucus and foreign material. It is generally accepted that the acinar units do not contain nerve endings for the initiation of coughing. The cough reflex is stimulated when material originating from disease in the alveoli arrives in the larger airways. The efferent pathways of the cough reflex are lie in the recurrent laryngeal nerve, which causes closure of the glottis, and in the phrenic and spinal nerves, which effect contraction of the diaphragm and other respiratory muscles against a closed glottis. The most sensitive areas of the conducting system are in the larynx and epicarina and at the bifurcation of the major bronchi.

A cough may be dry or productive. An acute dry cough often develops in the early stages of virus infections involving both upper and lower respiratory tracts. A dry cough may occur in association with bronchogenic carcinoma, although the majority of these patients smoke cigarettes and therefore have bronchitis and produce some mucoid expectoration. A dry, very irritating cough, often occurring in spasms, may be an early symptom of left-sided heart failure. A short, dry cough may be a nervous habit. Most dry coughs, if sufficiently prolonged, eventually become productive.

The time of occurrence of the cough may be useful in determining its origin. Most people with a chronic cough complain that it is worse when they lie down at night; this is particularly true of those who have bronchiectasis or a postnasal drip from chronic sinusitis. The patient with chronic bronchitis or bronchiectasis also expectorates when he or she gets up in the morning. Spasms of coughing due to bronchial asthma or left-sided heart failure frequently occur at night and may awaken the patient. A cough in association with or shortly after ingestion of food may indicate aspiration into the tracheobronchial tree.

The character and quantity of expectorated material may suggest the diagnosis. The patient with chronic bronchitis expectorates daily in small quantities, usually mucoid material, but with "colds" this may become yellow or green and sometimes slightly blood-streaked. Saccular bronchiectasis gives rise to copious, purulent, and often blood-streaked expectoration every day. Bacterial pneumonia is associated with thick yellow or greenish sputum. A foul or fetid

125

odor indicates infection from anaerobic organisms. Bronchial tree casts, consisting of inspissated mucus, are seen in cases of bronchitis, spasmodic asthma, or mucoid impaction, the last often in association with hypersensitivity aspergillosis.

Although a cough itself may not indicate the underlying disease process, its combination with other symptoms may be highly suggestive. If it occurs suddenly during an acute febrile episode and is associated with hoarseness, viral laryngotracheobronchitis is very likely the cause. When it is accompanied by stridor, some intrinsic or extrinsic obstruction to the upper respiratory passages is present. An associated generalized wheeze usually indicates acute bronchospasm, although rarely an endotracheal or mediastinal lesion in the region of the carina may be responsible. A persistent local wheeze during expiration often indicates an intrinsic bronchogenic lesion, such as carcinoma.

An alarming, although rare, symptom following a spasm of coughing is syncope; the patients usually are of stocky build and smoke and drink heavily.

Cough and mucoid expectoration are very common symptoms in patients with chronic bronchitis; any change in the character of a cough may indicate bronchogenic malignancy, just as a change in bowel habit may be indicative of carcinoma of the lower bowel.

HOARSENESS

When this symptom is acute and associated with symptoms of infection of the upper respiratory tract, it indicates viral laryngitis. Patients who from habit or in their occupation talk a lot may regain their normal voice only with difficulty. If the symptom persists for more than a month, the vocal cords should be examined for evidence of an intrinsic neoplasm or granulomatous process or unilateral abductor palsy. The common pulmonary cause of persistent hoarseness is a mediastinal lesion, usually bronchogenic carcinoma involving the recurrent laryngeal nerve. Secondary laryngeal lesions may develop in cases of pulmonary tuberculosis with cavitation.

SHORTNESS OF BREATH

The symptom of dyspnea or awareness of breathing is caused by an increase in stiffness of the lung, in airway resistance, in exercise ventilation, or, most commonly, by a combination of these.

A detailed description is most useful in differentiating organic causes of shortness of breath from functional or psychoneurotic dyspnea. The latter variety, which is related to tension or anxiety, is the commonest cause of shortness of breath; it is said to occur in 10 per cent of patients of specialists in internal medicine.[2] It often is associated with various other symptoms but can occur independently. Usually it is described as an inability to take a deep breath or to get air "down to the bottom of the lungs," and patients often spontaneously demonstrate by taking a deep breath. Patients who are short of breath at rest and not during exercise almost invariably have functional dyspnea. An exception to this rule is the patient with spasmodic asthma.

Inability to lie flat because of a feeling of suffocation or waking during the night with shortness of breath strongly suggests organic disease. Since attacks of asthma often occur during the night, this symptom does not necessarily indicate left ventricular failure, but it should arouse suspicion and a careful physical examination should be directed toward exclusion of this possibility. Although the desire for three or four pillows under one's head while in bed commonly relates to mitral stenosis or left ventricular failure, many patients with chronic bronchitis and emphysema are more comfortable in this position, particularly when the disease is advanced or when coughing and expectoration are severe.

Shortness of breath only during exertion is strong evidence for organic disease and renders functional dyspnea unlikely. Some patients do not complain of undue dyspnea during exertion but state that it develops afterward, while they are at rest. Often this indicates some form of left-sided heart failure, but it may be due to a variant of chronic bronchitis or asthma in which bronchospasm or increase in bronchial secretions is precipitated by exercise.

Of equal importance to the event that precipitates it is the relationship of dyspnea to other symptoms. In bronchitis or emphysema, dyspnea that develops during exertion is almost invariably preceded by a long history of cough and expectoration. In angina pectoris, shortness of breath may be so closely linked to "tightness" in the chest that patients with coronary insufficiency may have difficulty in determining which symptom limits their activity and even may be unable to differentiate one sensation from the other. Patients with heart disease who cannot increase their cardiac output to meet the tissues' demand for extra oxygen during exercise may experience not only shortness of breath but also weakness. Dyspnea of functional or psychoneurotic origin may be associated with a great variety of symptoms. The dyspnea may be confused with weakness and fatigue, and many of these patients describe these sensations as if they were identical.

CHEST PAIN

Pleural Pain

Disease of the lung itself may progress to an advanced stage and result in death without producing even minor chest pain; this is because the lung tissue and visceral pleura lack a sensory apparatus to detect pain. The parietal pleura, on the other hand, is richly supplied with sensory nerves deriving from the intercostal nerves and the nerves to the diaphragm. The nerve endings are stimulated by inflammation and stretching of the membrane, and not, as was thought in the past, by the friction of visceral pleura against parietal pleura. Pleural pain may vary in degree, from lancinating discomfort during slight inspiratory effort to a less severe but still sharp pain that may "catch" the patient at the end of a maximal inspiration. Pleural pain often disappears or is reduced to a dull ache during expiration or breath-holding. Pressure over the intercostal muscles in the area of pain may not elicit discomfort, and when it does, the pain is mild compared to the subjective sensation. This is in contrast to chest wall pain, which is associated with a palpable zone of extreme tenderness, often localized to a very small area of muscle. Except when it involves the diaphragm, the diseased area of pleura, which often is secondary to a pulmonary parenchymal lesion, typically underlies the area in which pain is perceived. The central part of the diaphragm is innervated by the phrenic nerve, and the sensory afferent fibers enter the cervical cord mainly in the third and fourth cervical posterior nerve roots; hence, irritation of the central portion of the diaphragmatic pleura is referred to the neck and the upper part of the shoulder. The outer parts of the diaphragmatic pleura are supplied by lower intercostal nerves, which enter the thoracic cord in the seventh to twelfth dorsal posterior nerve roots; irritation of this portion of the pleura causes referred pain in the lower thorax, lumbar area, and upper abdominal region. Pleural pain usually signifies inflammatory or malignant disease but also may accompany pneumothorax.

Mediastinal Pain

The trachea, esophagus, pericardium, aorta, thymus gland, and many lymph nodes are situated in the mediastinum, and disease involving any of these may cause pain in that region. Inflammation or neoplastic infiltration of the mediastinal compartment itself may cause discomfort locally. The pain may be felt in the retrosternal or precordial area and may radiate to the neck or arms or through to the back. The most common retrosternal pain is that due to myocardial ischemia; this is described as "squeezing," "pressing," or "choking" and may extend to the neck or down the left arm or both arms; onset is abrupt and the pain may be associated with circulatory collapse. The severe pain due to myocardial infarction may be closely simulated in other entities; these include massive pulmonary embolism and severe chronic pulmonary hypertension due to mitral stenosis or multiple small pulmonary emboli. Acute pericarditis may cause pain confusingly similar to that produced by myocardial disease; the pain often has a precordial distribution and may be made worse by breathing or swallowing and be relieved by bending forward.[3] Dissecting aneurysm of the aorta also may give rise to similar pain and should be suspected when pain is severe from the outset, instead of gradually increasing, and when it radiates to the back and down the abdomen into the lower limbs. A local aneurysm of the aorta may cause "boring" retrosternal or back pain when it erodes sternum, ribs, or vertebrae. Esophageal disease may give rise to "burning" pain and usually is clearly associated with the ingestion of food or assumption of the recumbent position.

Chest Wall Pain

Pain originating in or referred to the chest wall, not due to parietal pleural irritation, is common. When this pain appears to originate in intercostal muscle fibers there may be a history of trauma which produced strain or even tearing, but more often there is no obvious precipitating cause and the condition is labeled as myositis or fibrositis. In such cases tenderness may be elicited by pressure over the painful area. This pain can be differentiated from true "pleural pain" by its limited or lack of increase during deep inspiration and its aggravation by coughing or trunk movement.

Another chest wall pain is that due to pressure or inflammation irritating the posterior nerve root. Called radicular pain, this follows the specific intercostal nerve distribution and radiates around the chest from behind or, in some cases, is localized to one area. Usually it is described as dull and aching and is made worse by movement, particularly coughing. It may be due to a protruded intervertebral disk, rheumatoid spondylitis, or inflammatory or malignant disease involving the vertebrae or spinal canal. A variety of intercostal nerve root pain whose origin may be difficult to identify in the early stages, before the appearance of the typical rash, is that due to herpes zoster. The pain is usually described as "burning," most often over a wide area unilaterally along the pathway of one or more intercostal nerves.

Pain confined to vertebral and paravertebral areas may originate in inflammatory or neoplastic disease of the vertebrae, and percussion over the vertebral spines may elicit local tenderness due to disease in the underlying vertebral body. An unusual form of pain, usually in bone, is that experienced by patients with Hodgkin's disease or other neoplasms; this lasts for an hour or more after the ingestion of even small amounts of alcohol.

Pain in the chest wall may be due to disease of the ribs. In addition to those of known traumatic origin, rib fractures may result from prolonged episodes of severe coughing. The costochondral junctions of the ribs may be the site of perichondritis, often associated with tenderness and swelling (Tietze's syndrome). The ribs may be involved in a metastatic process or multiple myeloma and rarely by a primary tumor such as a fibrosarcoma; the pain usually is appreciated before the mass develops, at first poorly localized but later as a dull, boring ache over the area of invasion.

"Precordial Catch"

This is a benign transitory pain of undetermined origin characterized by a severe, sharp pain, occurring at rest or during mild activity over the left side of the chest, usually at the cardiac apex, and lasting from 30 sec to 5 min.[3] The mechanism is unknown, the condition is very common, and its importance lies solely in its differentiation from other chest pain of more serious consequence.

HEMOPTYSIS

Every patient who complains of an initial episode of hemoptysis should have at least a chest roentgenogram and many require extensive investigation. Bleeding may be from the upper respiratory tract and usually can be distinguished clinically from hemoptysis originating in the lower respiratory tract. When there is doubt as to the source of bleeding, the patient should be assumed to have lung disease and should be examined accordingly. Patients with a history of acute or chronic bronchitis sometimes expectorate blood-streaked sputum. Bleeding is a common complaint of patients with bronchial adenoma or carcinoma. In bronchiectasis, bloody expectoration may be the only symptom; usually it is abundant and originates in granulation tissue. Less frequent causes of bleeding from the bronchial tree are the erosion of broncholiths through the wall of the bronchus, erosion of a bronchus by an aortic aneurysm, and dilatation of bronchial veins in association with mitral stenosis. Unlike hematemesis, hemoptysis is rarely exsanguinating. The major causes of such massive hemoptysis are tuberculosis, lung abscess, bronchiectasis, and carcinoma. A mortality rate of 37 per cent occurred among patients who lost 600 ml of blood within 48 hours, a rate that rose to 75 per cent with greater losses within 16 hours.[4]

Bleeding from the lung itself may be due to a local lesion, such as pulmonary infarction, pneumonia, lung abscesses and cysts, and various granulomata, including tuberculosis, mycotic infections, and Wegener's granuloma. Although systemic disorders with a bleeding tendency are rarely if ever manifested by isolated bleeding from the lower respiratory tract, they may give rise to severe hemoptysis accompanied by bleeding into other viscera and the skin. The possibility of pulmonary or bronchial lesions as a source of bleeding should be investigated when patients on anticoagulant therapy cough up blood. A few patients who complain of blood "welling up" in the throat have hematemesis from esophageal varices, a possibility that should not be overlooked, particularly when bleeding is brisk and the blood is dark.

When the sputum is frankly bloody and does not contain mucoid or purulent material it is more likely due to pulmonary infarction than to pneumonia, particularly if it persists unchanged for several days. Bloody material mixed with pus should suggest pneumonia or lung abscess in acute illness and bronchiectasis in chronic disease.

In Western countries, in which the diagnosis is established in approximately 50 per cent of patients with hemoptysis, bronchitis and bronchiectasis are the commonest causes when a specific diagnosis can be made. In Western Europe and North America, bronchogenic carcinoma is said to be responsible for hemoptysis in 5 to 10 per cent of cases. Bronchiectasis associated with inactive tuberculosis of the upper lobes has been reported to be a commoner cause than active tuberculosis, and this has been our experience. The percentage of patients with hemoptysis but normal roentgenograms in whom no definite diagnosis can be made ranges from 15 to 58 per cent.

PAST ILLNESSES AND PERSONAL HISTORY

Establishing the correct diagnosis may depend upon a knowledge of the patient's medical history or personal habits: the respiratory symptoms or abnormal chest roentgenogram simply may represent previous active lung disease that has left its imprint on the pulmonary parenchyma, or a lung lesion may be a belated metastasis from a primary malignancy elsewhere that was removed many years earlier. Previous chest roentgenograms should be obtained for comparison with the present one. Patients should be questioned about medication: for example, lipoid pneumonia may follow the use of nose drops or laxatives containing mineral oil. Respiratory failure may be wholly or partly attributable to recent sedation. A patient's cigarette consumption may be of significance in suspected cases of bronchogenic carcinoma or bronchitis and emphysema. Corticosteroid therapy, poor diet, and heavy alcohol intake may play a major part in lowering resistance to infection. The personal history is not complete without inquiry about contact with animals, domestic and wild. This pertains not only to the patient with allergies, whose bronchospasm may be due to a household pet, but also, for example, to the patient with an acute pneumonic lesion who may have contracted ornithosis from a sick bird, tularemia from skinning a wild rabbit, or Q fever from inhalation of dust contaminated by sheep or cattle.

FAMILY HISTORY

In pulmonary disease, this aspect is most important in relation to a potential source of infection. Tuberculosis remains the most serious of the pulmonary diseases that spread in the home, but many acute virus infections may be disseminated throughout a household.

Some pulmonary diseases have a familial incidence, presumably on a genetic basis. They include mucoviscidosis, some cases of pulmonary emphysema, a hereditary form of Hamman-Rich syndrome (familial fibrocystic pulmonary dysplasia), hereditary telangiectasia, Kartagener's syndrome, pulmonary myomatosis, and alveolar microlithiasis. These diseases are rare and may be recognized only when a familial incidence is revealed.

OCCUPATIONAL AND RESIDENTIAL HISTORY

A complete occupational history from the time of first employment is essential when the chest roentgenogram reveals diffuse pulmonary disease. In addition to the pneumoconioses that cause diffuse granulomatous and fibrotic parenchymal disease, exposure to various chemical fumes and dusts may result in bronchial damage or may elicit severe, although in most cases reversible, bronchitis and bronchospasm. Farmers appear to be particularly liable to occupational lung diseases such as extrinsic allergic alveolitis (farmer's lung), histoplasmosis, and silo-filler's disease. Pollution from industry or even residence in an area of heavy atmospheric pollution may not only have a nonspecific irritating effect on patients with chronic obstructive disease, but also may contain more specific hazards, such as asbestos and beryllium, which are known to cause granuloma and fibrosis.

A history of residence in, and even travel through, an area where coccidioidomycosis or histoplasmosis is endemic may be pertinent, and parasitic diseases should be suspected in emigrants from areas in which they are endemic.

SYSTEMIC INQUIRY

Since lung involvement may be only one manifestation of a general disease process, inquiry concerning all body systems may prove revealing. For example, systemic inquiry may reveal symptoms indicating a primary site for multiple discrete nodules in the lung which had been suspected of being metastatic deposits. Bronchogenic oat-cell carcinoma may be associated with abnormality in almost any organ or tissue (*see* Chapter 8), and symptoms of the extrapulmonary manifestations of this unusual neoplasm can be elicited by systemic inquiry.

PHYSICAL EXAMINATION

The roentgenogram has not replaced the physician's eyes, ears, and hands; rather, it is an additional, valuable diagnostic method, complementary to the technique of physical examination, providing information the latter cannot give. The present-day student is fortunate in having roentgenography and pulmonary function tests as indispensable aids in perfecting his technique in physical examination.

It is to be emphasized that the chest roentgenogram may be interpreted as being normal when there is serious and advanced pulmonary disease detectable only by physical examination; conversely, roentgenography may reveal severe abnormality when physical findings are normal.

METHOD OF EXAMINATION AND SIGNIFICANT CHEST SIGNS

Examination of the front of the thorax is best performed with the patient supine and the back with the patient sitting or standing; patients who are too weak to sit upright unaided should be supported by someone standing at the foot of the bed and holding their hands. When this is impossible because of extreme weakness or serious illness, the patient should lie on the right side and then roll over onto the left side, the uppermost hemithorax being examined in turn. It is important to keep in mind always that examination of the chest is a comparative exercise. Each region of one side is compared with the same area on the other side; this rule applies equally for inspection, palpation, percussion, and auscultation.

INSPECTION

Inspection of the patient is well under way by the time the physical examination has begun. Throughout history-taking the physician has had ample opportunity to note the character of a cough, the presence or absence of hyperpnea, sighing respirations, or grimaces of pain accompanying cough or respiration. In the examining room the thoracic cage is inspected for evidence of deformity and the skin for its color and evidence of collateral venous circulation. Chest

movement is observed and the rate of respiration is noted.

A lag during inspiration or an area of diminished movement seen or felt and involving all or part of a hemithorax may be the only physical sign indicating disease of the lung or pleura. It indicates loss of elasticity of the underlying tissues, or compensatory spasm of intercostal and diaphragmatic musculature to avoid pain on movement. This sign is present in acute disease such as atelectasis, pneumonia, or pleurisy; or it may indicate a long-standing chronic or inactive fibrotic process of the lung or pleura, and then often is associated with scoliosis of the dorsal spine, with the concavity to the disease side. When the loss of volume is considerable, whether due to an acute or a chronic lesion, there may be a shift of the mediastinum; this is detectable as displacement of the apical cardiac impulse and the trachea toward the involved side.

PALPATION

The apical cardiac impulse and the trachea should be palpated, a shift from normal position indicating loss of volume or a relative increase in volume of one hemithorax in comparison with the other. The left parasternal region should be palpated to determine whether a heave is present, denoting right ventricular hypertrophy. The intercostal spaces and ribs should be palpated for tumor masses and to elicit any tenderness to pressure. The axillae and the cervical region should be explored carefully to detect enlarged lymph nodes.

PERCUSSION

The percussion note is produced by vibration of the percussed finger and sympathetic vibrations of the chest wall and underlying tissues and organs. The quality of the note is composed of its loudness, pitch, and timbre. The amplitude of vibrations (loudness) is much less over solid organs, such as the heart and liver, than over healthy lung, which, because of its elasticity, vibrates more. The loudness also depends upon the force of the stroke and the thickness of the chest wall. An accumulation of fluid between the percussed finger and underlying lung reduces intensity or loudness. Resonance elicited by percussion over healthy aerated lung is distinguishable from the dull note obtained over a solid organ by the rapidity of vibrations (pitch) and by overtones superimposed on the basic note (timbre); the resonant note has a lower pitch and more overtones. The difference between the normal, resonant note and the tympanitic note—as is heard on percussion over gas in the stomach—is due largely to difference in timbre. In the presence of lung disease the percussion note varies from the impaired resonance heard over an area of pneumonia that is partially consolidated to the extreme dullness or flatness that indicates a large accumulation of pleural fluid. At the other end of the scale, the note is hyper-resonant in cases of emphysema and pneumothorax and sometimes is tympanitic over large superficial cavities or pneumothorax. An unusual form, known as "skodaic resonance," is heard sometimes over a partly compressed upper lung region when the lower portion is collapsed by pleural effusion. It should be stressed that the lung tissue assessed by the percussing finger is only the superficial 5 cm. No matter how much force is used in this method of examination, the central portion of the lung remains "silent."

AUSCULTATION

The quality and intensity of the breath sounds, as well as the presence or absence of adventitious noises, are ascertained by listening while the patient breathes quietly and then deeply, with the bell or diaphragm held firmly against the chest. The quality of breath sounds varies from region to region, even in normal subjects, depending upon the proximity of larger bronchi to the chest wall. In the axillae or at the lung bases a vesicular sound is heard during inspiration and often early in expiration that has been likened to the rustle of wind in the trees. The sound of air flow has a somewhat different quality over the trachea and upper retrosternal area; the pitch is higher, and expiration is clearly audible and lasts longer than the inspiratory phase. Between the scapulae and anteriorly under the clavicles, particularly on the right side, the breath sounds assume characteristics of both vesicular and bronchial air flow and are described as bronchovesicular.

The intensity of "air entry" of breath sounds should be appraised. Again, this depends upon the thickness of the chest wall and the region of the lung examined, as well as upon the depth of respiration.

The mechanism of production of breath sounds is not thoroughly understood. Forgacs and colleagues,[5] who measured the intensity of breath sounds at the mouth while eliminating such adventitious sounds as wheezing and stridor, found that the sound of breathing is generated by turbulent flow in the upper respiratory tract; when turbulent flow was reduced by the inspiration of helium, breath sounds were eradicated. Auscultation over the glottis normally reveals a high-pitched noise during inspiration, followed by a pause and then by a higher-pitched, louder, longer expiration. This sound, which is heard very well over the trachea, is modified slightly in the bronchial tubes, in which expiration becomes even more high-pitched. However, at the periphery of the lung the character of the sound is radically changed: inspiration is louder than expiration, which is short and may not even be heard. There is no pause between inspiration and expiration, and the sound has a soft, rustling quality known as "vesicular breathing." This alteration in the original "glottic" noise is believed to be due to a dampening effect of the spongy lung tissue and also to the entry of air from thousands of narrow terminal bronchioles into acinar units.

Many factors may contribute to reduction or complete abolition of vesicular breathing. It may be difficult to hear breath sounds during shallow breathing due to weakness or neuromuscular disease. Diminished air entry, due to complete obstruction of a lobar or segmental bronchus or reduction in compliance resulting from edema or fibrosis of interstitial tissue, respectively, may eliminate or diminish the vesicular murmur. Complete destruction of acinar units, as in chronic obstructive emphysema, may result in very faint air entry. The transmission of breath sounds may be interrupted by an excess of subcutaneous fat or may be completely suppressed by fluid or air in the pleural cavity.

The quality of breath sounds changes from vesicular to bronchovesicular or bronchial when underlying parenchyma partly or completely loses its air content; this occurs in pneumonia and in "nonobstructive" (adhesive) atelectasis. Consolidated or airless lung tissue is an excellent conductor of high-pitched, prolonged expiratory sounds that emanate from adjacent bronchi.

The voice sounds may provide clues to pathologic changes. Normally, a soft, confused, barely audible sound is heard over lung distant from large bronchi. In the presence of consolidation or nonobstructive atelectasis, voice sounds become more distinct and produce a noise known as "bronchophony"; in many cases of consolidation the words are distinctly audible

TABLE 3–1. A Classification of Adventitious Sounds that Is Simple and Widely Used

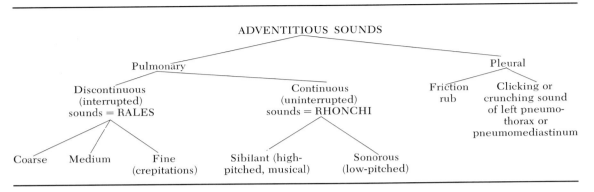

over the involved area when the patient whispers "ninety-nine"; this "whispering pectoriloquy" is a useful confirmatory sign of pneumonic consolidation.

Adventitious sounds are divided into those having their origin in the bronchopulmonary tree and those indicating disease of the pleura. We use a terminology that is descriptive and simple and probably is the most widely accepted by present-day physicians (*see* Table 3–1). *Rales* are discontinuous noises which may be fine (usually at the end of inspiration, as air enters the acinar unit), medium (often during both inspiration and expiration, as air flows by an excess of fluid in the smaller bronchi), and coarse (the low-pitched, bubbling sounds that result from the accumulation of secretions in larger bronchi and the trachea). Rales are present more often during inspiration, when air flow is faster. They may be elicited during a rapid, deep breath, or—particularly when they are fine—during a deep breath after maximal expiration ended by a cough (post-tussive rales). Fine rales sometimes are detected at the end of a deep inspiration, and usually at the lung bases, even in normal subjects; they are thought to represent the opening of atelectatic acinar units after shallow breathing, a consequence of insufficiently deep inspirations to replenish the alveolar surface-active substance. Fine rales, however, are usually persistent and multiple and often occur in showers; they indicate pulmonary edema or the alveolar exudate of pneumonia. They may be modified in the proximity of a cavity or pneumothorax; these act as resonating chambers and alter the timbre. They have a high-pitched superficial quality in cases of diffuse interstitial disease associated with general loss of lung volume.

Other adventitious sounds that originate in the bronchopulmonary tree are the high-pitched (sibilant) and low-pitched (sonorous) continuous noises that should be called *rhonchi*. These indicate partial obstruction by thick mucus in the bronchial lumen, edema, spasm, or a local lesion of the bronchial wall. A wheeze is the sound of a rhonchus heard at a distance without the aid of a stethoscope or which the patient himself can detect. The term *wheezing respirations* is used sometimes to denote the persistent inspiratory and expiratory rhonchi, usually of the musical, sibilant variety, heard all over the chest during bronchospasm. Rhonchi not appreciated during quiet breathing may become audible when the rate of air flow is increased during fast, deep breathing or when the bronchial tubes are narrowed during maximal expiration.

The other group of adventitious sounds represents manifestations of pleural disease, in which inflammation of the pleura roughens these membranes and covers them with sticky, fibrinous exudate. During both inspiration and expiration, and particularly in areas in which excursion of the thoracic cage is greatest, a rubbing, rasping, or leathery sound may be heard as the visceral lining moves against the parietal lining. The noise usually is associated with pain. Its disappearance during breath-holding, but not during coughing, renders it unlike rhonchi due to partial bronchial obstruction by mucus, which can closely resemble pleural friction rub.

Hamman[6] described a crunching or clicking sound over the lower retrosternal area, synchronous with the heart beat, which he thought was pathognomonic of air in the mediastinum. Scadding and Wood[7] found it more commonly associated with a small left pneumothorax, an opinion now held by most. In a series of 24 patients in whom this sound was heard, 22 had left-sided pneumothorax and only two had pneumomediastinum.[8]

A continuous murmur heard on auscultation

over the lung may indicate pulmonary arteriovenous fistula or severe bronchiectasis, especially if the murmur corresponds with a nodule or an inhomogeneous opacity observed on a chest roentgenogram.

Clinical examination of the heart is essential in every suspected case of pulmonary disease, since certain abnormalities may provide important clues to the etiology. For example, disease affecting either the parenchyma or the pulmonary vasculature may cause pulmonary arterial hypertension; this is evidenced by right ventricular heave, accentuated second pulmonic sound, or pulmonic or tricuspid regurgitant murmurs. In a minority of cases of diffuse pulmonary edema secondary to mitral stenosis or acute left ventricular decompensation, convincing roentgenographic evidence of cardiac enlargement is absent; in such cases, a mitral valve murmur, severe arterial hypertension, or clinical signs of left ventricular strain suggest the cause of the edema. Pulsus paradoxus, an abnormality usually associated with cardiac tamponade, may be observed in patients with obstructive pulmonary disease, particularly severe asthma. Normally the systolic arterial pressure falls 5 mm Hg or less during inspiration.

EXTRATHORACIC MANIFESTATIONS OF PULMONARY DISEASE

Complete physical examination is essential in every case of lung disease. The diagnosis may be suggested by discovery of a mass or an enlarged abdominal organ. The skin and the endocrine and central nervous systems are most commonly involved and these manifestations are discussed in appropriate chapters. The section that follows is concerned with clubbing and cyanosis, one or both of which are found in many and must be sought in all cases of pulmonary or pleural disease.

CLUBBING AND HYPERTROPHIC PULMONARY OSTEOARTHROPATHY

These are not synonymous: clubbing frequently occurs in the absence of full-blown osteoarthropathy, and "pulmonary osteoarthropathy" occasionally occurs without clubbing. Confusion of simple clubbing with pulmonary osteoarthropathy is probably responsible for the great variation in reported incidence of these two conditions in patients with bronchogenic carcinoma, ranging from 2 to 48 per cent.

There are four generally accepted criteria for clubbing: (1) increased bulk of the terminal pulp; (2) change in the angle between the nail and the proximal skin to greater than 180 degrees; (3) sponginess of the nail bed when pressure is applied to the nail; and (4) increased nail curvature.

The diagnosis of pulmonary osteoarthropathy requires joint symptoms, namely, arthralgia with swelling and stiffness affecting mainly the fingers, wrists, ankles, and knees, or deep-seated bone pain. The roentgenogram usually shows subperiosteal new bone formation in the long bones of the lower limbs, and some consider this finding essential to diagnosis. Malignant chest tumors account for 90 per cent of typical pulmonary osteoarthropathy; the majority of these are primary but a few are metastatic. The pathogenetic mechanism of this unusual picture is not fully understood, but it is agreed that the earliest anatomic change in the limbs is an overgrowth of highly vascular connective tissue, followed by subperiosteal new bone formation.

In patients with acquired symmetric *clubbing* of the fingers and toes blood flow to the digits is increased, whereas in those with acquired hypertrophic pulmonary osteoarthropathy, although blood flow to the extremities is increased, most of this appears to be shunted through arteriovenous communications in the areas of osteoarthropathy. In most cases the increase in blood flow to the extremities appears to be secondary to a reflex mechanism, the vagus nerve serving as the afferent pathway; the stimulus presumably comes indirectly, from abnormal intrathoracic "masses" or ischemic tissue distal to them. Procedures such as the removal of a primary lung lesion, exploratory thoracotomy, or unilateral vagotomy often are followed by a prompt reduction in blood flow, then by resolution of soft tissue overgrowth, and some weeks later by regression of the bony changes; however, the clubbing itself may not disappear completely.

CYANOSIS

Many patients with lung disease have blue or bluish-gray skin and mucous membranes; this is most obvious in the nail beds or buccal mucosa and usually reflects severe hypoxemia of arterial blood due to ventilation-perfusion inequality. Cyanosis is best appreciated in adequate daylight and is virtually unrecognizable under a fluorescent lamp.[9] It is estimated that 5 g hemoglobin/100 ml blood has to be reduced before cyanosis is visible, and, therefore, this sign is never present in patients with severe anemia. It may be due to inadequate saturation of arterial blood leaving the left side of the heart, excessive slowing in the peripheral capillaries, or both.

The central or hypoxemic variety associated with lung disease is commonest in patients with chronic obstructive emphysema in whom a large volume of underventilated lung is still being perfused with venous blood. In other lung diseases, such as severe acute alveolar pneumonia with circulatory collapse, both central and peripheral factors undoubtedly play a part: the venous blood in pulmonary capillaries encounters airless acini, and the same blood stagnates in systemic capillaries and allows excessive removal of oxygen by the tissues.

Peripheral cyanosis either is paroxysmal and precipitated by cold, as in Raynaud's disease, or general and prolonged, in the latter case often with systemic hypotension and indications of circulatory collapse. The former type occurs in scleroderma, which commonly involves the lung; the latter is commoner in primary heart disease, such as myocardial infarction, than in lung conditions, but may occur in association with cor pulmonale and hypoxemia and then indicates a very poor prognosis.

When cyanosis is central in origin the nail beds usually are deep blue or blue-gray and the skin is warm, whereas peripheral cyanosis is usually associated with cold, clammy skin and dusky, livid nail beds. Frequently it is not possible on appearance alone to differentiate with certainty between central and peripheral cyanosis. However, the degree of oxygen saturation of arterial blood will give the answer.

When the pathogenesis of cyanosis appears obscure, methemoglobinemia or sulfhemoglobinemia should be considered.

SPECIAL DIAGNOSTIC PROCEDURES

ENDOSCOPIC EXAMINATION

LARYNGOSCOPY

The larynx can be examined indirectly, by use of a mirror, or directly; the latter may be combined with bronchoscopy.

Laryngoscopy should be performed in any patient who complains of a persistent, dry, hacking or brassy cough, particularly when this is associated with hoarseness. The vocal cords should be well visualized, not only to exclude a local lesion but also to detect paralysis that would account for the hoarseness. In the latter instance, roentgenography may reveal a mediastinal lesion involving a recurrent laryngeal nerve.

BRONCHOSCOPY

This procedure, which formerly was the prerogative of the otolaryngologist, is now more widely adopted by internists and surgeons specializing in lung disease. This is right, for in most cases the results must be considered in the light of other findings and a general knowledge of lung disease. Since the commonest indication for this procedure is suspicion of endobronchial neoplasm, the obvious person to look down the bronchoscope is the surgeon, who requires a clear picture of the extent of the lesion and its position in the bronchial tree in order to assess resectability and to determine how much lung should be removed.

If at all possible, bronchoscopy should be done under local anesthesia: the patient's cooperation is required to obtain a satisfactory specimen of bronchial lavage, and the loss of cough reflex while under general anesthesia usually results in an inadequate specimen. With reassurance and premedication with sedatives the patient is able to relax and need not be restrained. The local anesthetic is applied first with a nebulizer and subsequently by spraying the vocal cords and trachea under direct view by the bronchoscopist. Since an essential feature of most bronchoscopies is bronchial lavage to obtain secretions from the bronchial tree, it should be kept in mind that some local anesthetics have antibacterial action. Bronchoscopy can be performed with either a rigid or a fiberoptic bronchoscope, the latter possessing several advantages over the former. In experienced hands, this instrument makes the examination considerably less traumatic; it permits thorough examination of the entire tracheobronchial tree, including the upper lobes, down to subsegmental levels; and it can be introduced through the nose, a rigid metal bronchoscope, or an endotracheal tube. The fiberscope also can be used in artificially ventilated patients, a special adaptor being fitted to prevent air leak.

The major indication for bronchoscopy is roentgenographic evidence of bronchial obstruction, either partial or complete. Approximately 50 per cent of lung cancers are visible through the rigid bronchoscope, compared with approximately 60 per cent through the bronchofiberscope.[10] A positive diagnosis of lesions not seen endoscopically because of their peripheral location can be made in a high percentage of cases by biopsy with minute forceps inserted down the bronchoscope, by bronchial brushing, or by cytologic examination of aspirated material (see page 116).

Another indication for bronchoscopy is hemoptysis. Despite the danger inherent in the procedure during active bleeding, sometimes it is necessary when bleeding is copious and the roentgenogram does not indicate the source. Knowledge of the site of bleeding aids resectional surgery if exsanguination appears imminent.

The risk inherent in bronchoscopic examination appears slight, although the associated occurrence of cardiac arrhythmias is not unusual. Tachycardia appears to be mainly reflex in origin, since it occurs when the bronchoscope touches the trachea. The commonest complication of bronchoscopy per se is laryngospasm, which probably can be avoided if sufficient local anesthetic is used. The mortality in one series was 0.01 per cent, the deaths resulting from extreme hypoxemia in patients who were already hypoxic.

Bronchoscopic examination without biopsy is unlikely to cause severe bleeding, although extreme care should be exercised when an aortic aneurysm is suspected.

A promising procedure employed in conjunction with bronchoscopy is the use of a fluorescent hematoporphyrin derivative that accumulates preferentially in neoplastic tissue. The value of this diagnostic procedure has recently been greatly enhanced by a technique wherein a small quantity of hematoporphyrin is injected and a fluorescence-detection system is employed simultaneously with conventional illumination during flexible bronchoscopy.[11]

MEDIASTINOSCOPY

This endoscopic examination is used diagnostically to obtain tissue within the mediastinum. The procedure is carried out through an incision in the suprasternal notch; the soft areolar tissues are dissected along the whole trachea, and biopsy material is removed under direct vision through an instrument similar to that used for esophagoscopy in children. The space explored is roughly the upper half of the mediastinum, including tissues around the intrathoracic portion of the trachea, the tracheal bifurcation, and the proximal part of the major bronchi. In some cases it may be impossible to carry out more than finger palpation.

Complications of mediastinoscopy are uncommon and usually not serious; one review of the literature[12] estimated their incidence as 3 to 4 per cent. The most serious complication is hemorrhage, usually venous.

ESOPHAGOSCOPY

Pulmonary disease such as aspiration pneumonia and scleroderma may occur in association with esophageal disease, and diagnosis may be facilitated by direct endoscopic examination of the esophagus. The procedure should be preceded by fluoroscopic examination with barium.

BACTERIOLOGY IN PULMONARY DISEASE

COLLECTION OF MATERIAL

Sputum

A most important aid to the definitive diagnosis of lung disease lies in the proper collection of sputum and the diagnostic methods used in its examination. Almost every clinical situation in chest disease requires that the bacteriology laboratory receive a fresh specimen of sputum, preferably from well down in the lungs.

Fresh specimens are required in bacterial, mycotic, and viral diseases. The only indications for collecting expectorated material over a prolonged period are to determine its quantity and quality and to obtain material for acid-fast culture, which is positive most often when sputum is collected for 24 to 72 hours. However, since acid-fast bacilli are often detectable on film smears of freshly expectorated material, longer collection may not be necessary in many cases of cavitary disease or lobar consolidation suspected to be due to tuberculosis.

When a patient fails to respond to antibiotic therapy appropriate to the pathogen originally detected, further cultures should be made, since another pathogenic agent, perhaps acquired in the hospital, may be responsible for the lack of clinical improvement.

In patients whose expectoration is negligible, a well-established method of inducing sputum production is the use of an aerosol solution of propylene glycol or sulfur dioxide mixed with 10 per cent normal saline. Sputum induction has been shown to be superior to gastric lavage in establishing a diagnosis of pulmonary tuberculosis although the two methods are complementary.

Gastric Lavage

A plastic tube is passed down into the patient's stomach upon awakening in the morning and swallowed pulmonary secretions are siphoned out; the material should be cultured immediately for acid-fast organisms.

Tracheal Aspiration and Lavage

A technique for bypassing the upper respiratory passages and obtaining material directly from the trachea originally described by Pecora[13] is now widely used. This procedure, known as transtracheal aspiration (TTA), is performed by introducing a 14-gauge needle through the cricothyroid membrane and anterior tracheal wall followed by the insertion of a polyethylene catheter through the needle; suction is applied to the catheter to obtain material for smear and culture.

The main value of TTA is in determining the etiology of severe pneumonia in obtunded patients who are unable to expectorate. It is also the only reliable method for definitive diagnosis of anaerobic infections because it avoids contamination of sputum specimens with mouth organisms.

Although complications from TTA are uncommon and usually mild, some fatalities have been reported. Copious intratracheal hemorrhage and aspiration pneumonitis do occur occasionally and may be serious complications in patients with a poor cough reflex; for this reason, this procedure should not be carried out on patients with a bleeding tendency. Hypoxemia with cardiac arrhythmias and arrest can be avoided by 100 per cent oxygen breathing, which should be mandatory in all patients undergoing TTA. As with the majority of invasive diagnostic procedures, risk is significantly decreased with experience. Transtracheal aspiration should be performed only by trained experts and not inexperienced house staff.

Swabs of Upper Respiratory Tract

Laryngeal swabs for screening for tuberculosis activity are simple to obtain and often yield organisms. Swabs of the pharynx or nasopharynx, which frequently are taken in suspected virus disease, should be placed immediately in a liquid solution containing salt and either gelatin or bovine serum albumin, with or without antibiotics. This material should be delivered immediately to the laboratory for inoculation; when preparation is delayed for a few hours the specimen should be kept at $-40°C$ or, if for longer, at $-70°C$.

Examination of Stool

As can be appreciated from Table 3–2, microscopic examination of slides (with coverslip) of fecal material is indicated in many parasitic diseases of the lungs; also, viruses can often be isolated in stools. Centrifugation filtration methods can be used to concentrate parasites or eggs.

Blood

A culture should be made at the height of fever, using an aseptic technique, in every case of acute fulminating pneumonia. In cases of lung disease thought to be viral, the blood should be drawn early in the disease, part of the aliquot being used for culture and part for identifying antibodies to pathogens (*see* later discussion).

Pleural Effusion

The presence of pleural effusion is determined by the roentgenographic appearance and physical signs. The area of maximal accumulation is judged from posteroanterior and lateral roentgenograms; it is confirmed by percussion of the chest wall or, when available, by reflected ultrasound. In most cases thoracentesis is performed through the interspace at the site of maximal dullness, usually posteriorly or posterolaterally. However, in many cases of pleural effusion apparent roentgenographically, the history or physical examination or both may arouse suspicion of an underlying parenchymal lesion. In such cases as much fluid as possible should be removed to give a clearer view of underlying lung parenchyma that may be hidden by the opacification of a large accumulation of effusion. In these circumstances the needle should be inserted low in the thoracic cage. It is unwise to remove fluid too rapidly from patients who are in heart failure or who have severe anemia, since acute pulmonary edema is likely to develop. Only a limited amount should be removed at any one time, and the use of a vacuum bottle is contraindicated.

TABLE 3–2. PARASITIC PULMONARY INFESTATIONS

| | ISOLATION AND IDENTIFICATION | | | |
ORGANISM	MICROSCOPIC AND CULTURAL CHARACTERISTICS	SEROLOGIC TESTS	SKIN TESTS	LEUKOCYTE COUNT°
Endamoeba histolytica	Amebae in sputum or stool; cysts in stool	Precipitation and indirect hemagglutination	Nil	Moderate, sometimes with eosinophilia
Toxoplasma gondii	Inoculation of mice with suspected material and demonstration of intracellular crescent-shaped protozoan	Sabin-Feldman dye, indirect hemagglutination, and fluorescent antibody	Yes	Normal with some lymphocytosis
Pneumocystis carinii	1 to 3 μ irregular organism may be found in sputum or in lung biopsy	Complement fixation	Nil	Mild to considerable with neutrophilia
Ascaris lumbricoides	Adult worms or typical mammilated outer shell ova in stools	Nil	Nil	Mild to moderate with eosinophilia
Strongyloides stercoralis	Larvae in stools and rarely in sputum	Nil	Nil	Mild to considerable with eosinophilia
Ancylostoma duodenale, Necator americanus	Ova or mature worms in stools	Nil	Nil	Eosinophilia; leukopenia to moderate leukocytosis; usually normal
Trichinella spiralis	Larvae seen in muscle biopsy specimens 10 days postinfection	Precipitation, complement fixation, and flocculation	Yes	Mild to considerable with eosinophilia
Filaria species (tropical eosinophilia)	Lung biopsy or microfilariae in nocturnal blood rarely	Complement fixation of limited value	Yes	Considerable with extreme degree of eosinophilia
Toxocara species (visceral larva migrans)	Larvae seen in eosinophilic granuloma in liver biopsy	Indirect hemagglutination	Nil	Considerable with extreme eosinophilia
Echinococcus granulosus	Scolices found in sputum	Complement fixation, indirect hemagglutination	Yes	Normal to moderate in 20 to 25%; slight eosinophilia
Cysticercus cellulosae	Ova or mature worms in stools; biopsy of subcutaneous lesions	Complement fixation of limited value	Yes	Normal to mild, no eosinophilia
Paragonimus westermani	Typical operculated eggs in sputum or stool	Complement fixation	Yes	Usually normal without eosinophilia
Schistosoma mansoni S. japonicum S. haematobium	Typical ova of each variety in stool, urine, and rarely in sputum; lung biopsy	Specific complement fixation and precipitation	Yes	Moderate leukocytosis and eosinophilia

*Leukocyte count: <5,000 = Leukopenia
5,000–10,000 = Normal
10,000–12,000 = Mild leukocytosis
12,000–15,000 = Moderate
>15,000 = Considerable

The techniques of thoracentesis and pleural biopsy are described in detail in the text *Diagnosis of Diseases of the Chest* (page 301).

It is our opinion that in the majority of cases initial thoracentesis should be combined with biopsy of the parietal pleura. When the diagnosis is "certain" and the effusion is considered to be secondary to pneumonia, heart failure, or kidney disease, pleural biopsy may not be required; nevertheless, even in these cases the etiology of an effusion is often doubtful, and pleural biopsy does not result in serious complications and often provides information of diagnostic importance.

SMEARS AND CULTURES

All patients acutely ill with pneumonia when admitted to the hospital should be encouraged to cough and spit into a sputum box as soon as possible; if they are seriously ill and unable to expectorate, transtracheal aspiration is indicated. The fresh sputum or aspirate should be smeared on a slide, gram-stained, and inoculated on a culture medium. The choice of antibiotic should be made on the basis of the Gram stain, before obtaining culture and sensitivity results from the bacteriology laboratory. This does not mean that one can diagnose the etiologic agent of pneumonia by the smear alone; subsequent culture may reveal a pathogen different from that suspected from the preliminary smear. However, since patients with severe acute pneumonia may die before the results of culture are forthcoming, this smear represents the most dependable method of making a tentative diagnosis and instituting appropriate therapy. Although the normal person without bronchopulmonary disease has sterile bronchi,[14] his or her upper respiratory tract contains nonpathogenic cocci and bacilli which are apparent on routine smears. For this reason, in cases of fulminating pneumonia it is important to get a specimen that originates in the lower respiratory tract.

Furthermore, even positive sputum cultures of a pathogenic bacterium do not necessarily signify that a pneumonic process is due to the cultured organism. When the growth is heavy or pure, more reliance can be placed on this finding, but decisions concerning therapy and management must be based on clinical features as well. It has been suggested that the results of culture are more reliable if expectorated sputum is repeatedly washed beforehand.[15]

Mycobacterium tuberculosis and other mycobacteria may be apparent in sputum smears stained by the Ziehl-Neelsen method. A presumptive diagnosis of tuberculosis can be made on this evidence, but definitive diagnosis can be made only when culture reports are received.

Table 3–3 summarizes the bacteriologic features of the many bacterial and viral diseases that may affect the lungs, and Table 3–4 those of the mycoses.

Isolation of the organism, whether it be bacterium, virus, rickettsia, or fungus, is the only conclusive means of diagnosing infectious disease, but the culture of some pathogens is fraught with danger and may lead to laboratory-acquired disease. The etiologic agents of tularemia and Q fever fall into this category, and great care should be taken in handling material in cases of suspected or known disease of this type. It may even be wise to settle for a presumptive diagnosis based on the results of serologic and skin tests. Fungus disease also has been reported to originate in the laboratory due to *Coccidioides immitis* and *Histoplasma capsulatum*.

TABLE 3–3. BACTERIAL, RICKETTSIAL, AND VIRAL PULMONARY INFECTIONS

	ISOLATION AND IDENTIFICATION			
ORGANISM	MICROSCOPIC AND CULTURAL CHARACTERISTICS	SEROLOGIC TESTS	SKIN TESTS	LEUKOCYTE COUNT°
Streptococcus pneumoniae	Tentative identification on smear; culture on blood agar; mouse inoculation	Specific antiserum to identify type	Nil	Considerable with neutrophilia
Staphylococcus aureus	Tentative on smear; colonies hemolyze blood agar; organism is coagulase-positive	Nil	Nil	Considerable with neutrophilia
Streptococcus pyogenes	Tentative on smear; Lancefield group A on culture; beta hemolysis on blood agar	Antibodies to streptolysin O	Nil	Considerable with neutrophilia
Bacillus anthracis	Tentative on smear, culture on peptone agar	Indirect fluorescent antibody, agar gel diffusion, complement fixation, and hemagglutination	Nil	Normal to considerable with neutrophilia
Listeria monocytogenes	Motile organism showing hemolysis on blood agar; conjunctival inoculation in rabbit or guinea pig	Agglutination (IgG)	Nil	Moderate with lymphocytosis
Pseudomonas aeruginosa	Tentative on smear; heavy growth on artificial medium required for pathogenicity	Nil	Nil	Leukopenia to moderate
Pseudomonas pseudomallei (Malleomyces pseudomallei)	Aerobic or anaerobic standard culture media; motile pleomorphic with one or two flagellae at one pole	Hemagglutination and complement fixation	Nil	Normal to moderate

TABLE 3–3. BACTERIAL, RICKETTSIAL, AND VIRAL PULMONARY INFECTIONS *(Continued)*

| ORGANISM | ISOLATION AND IDENTIFICATION | | | |
	MICROSCOPIC AND CULTURAL CHARACTERISTICS	SEROLOGIC TESTS	SKIN TESTS	LEUKOCYTE COUNT°
Klebsiella aerogenes	Tentative on smear; mucoid gelatinous colonies on agar; biochemical tests and type specific capsule	Specific antiserum to identify type	Nil	Leukopenia to moderate
Escherichia coli	Tentative on smear; heavy growth on artificial medium required for pathogenicity	Nil	Nil	Normal to moderate
Proteus species	Tentative on smear; heavy growth on artificial medium required for pathogenicity	Nil	Nil	Normal to considerable
Salmonella species	Tentative on smear; *S. typhi* or *S. choleraesuis,* usually; differentiation on basis of biochemical and agglutination	Agglutination	Nil	Leukopenia to moderate
Legionnella pneumophila	Direct immunofluorescent staining of respiratory tract secretions or tissue; culture of blood, pleural fluid, or TTA on charcoal yeast extract medium.	Indirect immunofluorescent antibody, a micro hemagglutination technique, is promising	Nil	Moderate leukocytosis with lymphopenia
Haemophilus influenzae	Encapsulated organism with capsular swelling in appropriate biologic fluid; nasopharyngeal swab culture on blood agar in children	Specific antiserum to identify type	Nil	Normal to moderate
Bordetella pertussis	Smear nasopharyngeal swab on Bordet-Gengou agar	Fluorescent antibody, complement fixation, and agglutination	Nil	Moderate to considerable with lymphocytosis
Francisella tularensis (Pasteurella tularensis), Brucella tularensis)	Tentative on smear; body fluids cultured on blood agar directly or after passage through mouse or guinea pig	Agglutination	Yes	Normal to considerable
Yersinia pestis (Pasteurella pestis)	Tentative on smear; body fluids cultured on blood agar directly or after passage through mouse or guinea pig	Fluorescent antibody, agglutination, and complement fixation	Nil	Mild to moderate
Bacteria anitratum	Large white or mucoid colony on agar; inability to reduce nitrates	Nil	Nil	Mild to moderate
Brucella species	10% CO_2 needed for *B. abortus* culture on tryptose phosphate; differentiate species on basis of biochemical and serologic tests	Agglutination and complement fixation	Yes	Leukopenia to normal
Pseudomonas mallei (Malleomyces mallei)	Species differentiated antigenically; culture on enriched agar; guinea pig inoculation	Agglutination and complement fixation	Yes	Leukopenia to normal
Bacteroides species	Anaerobic culture required of transtracheal or needle aspirated material; frequently combined with anaerobic streptococci and fusospirochetal organisms.	Nil	Nil	Normal to moderate
Mycobacterium tuberculosis and unclassified	Tentative identification on smear; colony appearance identifies strain; animal inoculation	Agar double diffusion and hemagglutination of limited value	Yes	Normal to mild with monocytosis
Mycoplasma pneumoniae	Growth of pleuropneumonia like organism on enriched agar or beef broth; cultivation in simian cell tissue culture and chorioallantoic membrane	Cold agglutination, complement fixation, and fluorescent antibody	Nil	Usually normal, rarely from mild to considerable

Table continued on next page

TABLE 3–3. BACTERIAL, RICKETTSIAL, AND VIRAL PULMONARY INFECTIONS *(Continued)*

	ISOLATION AND IDENTIFICATION			
ORGANISM	MICROSCOPIC AND CULTURAL CHARACTERISTICS	SEROLOGIC TESTS	SKIN TESTS	LEUKOCYTE COUNT°
Influenza virus	Human and simian cell tissue culture; inoculation of chick embryo	Complement fixation, hemagglutination, and neutralization, fluorescent antibody	Nil	In primary virus pneumonia mild to severe with neutrophilia
Parainfluenza virus	Human and simian cell tissue culture	Neutralization, complement fixation, and hemabsorption with guinea pig erythrocytes	Nil	Usually normal, rarely mild to moderate leukocytosis
Respiratory syncytial virus	Human, simian, and bovine cell tissue culture from nasal or pharyngeal secretions	Neutralization, complement fixation, and hemagglutination-inhibition	Nil	Usually normal
Rubeola virus	Human and simian cell tissue culture; inoculation of chick embryos; giant cells in urine or throat washings	Hemagglutination-inhibition, neutralization, and complement fixation	Nil	Normal to moderate
Coxsackie virus	Culture in human amnion or Rhesus monkey kidney	Neutralization	Nil	Leukopenia to moderate
ECHO viruses	Human and simian cell tissue culture	Neutralization and complement fixation	Nil	Normal to moderate
Adenoviruses	Human and simian cell tissue culture	Complement fixation	Nil	Normal to mild
Herpes zoster (varicella)	Human cell tissue culture; intranuclear inclusion bodies in sputum cells of patients with pneumonia	Complement fixation, neutralization, and fluorescent antibody	Nil	Normal to considerable
Cytomegalovirus	Human cell tissue culture	Complement fixation and agglutination	Nil	Normal or perhaps abnormal due to underlying primary disease
Lymphocytic choriomeningitis	Simian cell tissue culture; inoculation of chick embryos	Complement fixation	Nil	Leukopenia to moderate
Infectious mononucleosis	Causative agent not isolated; Epstein-Barr virus (?)	Heterophile antibody agglutination, EBV antibodies by fluorescent antibody, complement fixation, and immunodiffusion	Nil	Leukocytosis early; leukopenia with mononucleosis later
Cat scratch fever	Causative agent not isolated	Nil	Intradermal test with cat scratch antigen	Normal
Chlamydia species (psittacosis, ornithosis)	Inoculation of mice or chick embryos with sputum or blood	Complement fixation	Nil	Usually normal; rarely leukopenia or mild to moderate leukocytosis
Chlamydia species (lymphogranuloma venereum)	Tissue culture; inoculation of chick embryos	Complement fixation	Frei	Mild to moderate
Coxiella burnetti (Q fever)	Culture of body fluids in chick embryos; guinea pig	Complement fixation	Nil	Normal in 60%, mild to moderate
Rickettsia tsutsugamushi (scrub typhus)	Peritoneal inoculation of mice with blood	Agglutination to *Proteus* OX-K antigen and fluorescent antibody	Nil	Leukopenia to normal

°Leukocyte count: <5,000 = Leukopenia
　　　　　　　5,000–10,000 = Normal
　　　　　　　10,000–12,000 = Mild leukocytosis
　　　　　　　12,000–15,000 = Moderate
　　　　　　　>15,000 = Considerable

SEROLOGIC AND SKIN TESTS

These methods are particularly useful in the diagnosis of pulmonary viral or mycotic infections. They portray the antigen-antibody reactions that take place in the skin and the test tube, usually as a result of the development of antibodies in the patient. These tests are widely used to diagnose a number of chronic pulmonary disorders and epidemiologically to establish the prevalence of diseases of infectious origin in specific geographic areas. Since the patient has usually recovered by the time the antibody titer rises, indicating the diagnosis, these tests are seldom of direct diagnostic value in acute disease.

SEROLOGIC TESTING

This technique is most often used to determine the causative pathogens in various bacterial, viral, mycotic, and parasitic diseases (see Tables 3–2, 3–3, and 3–4). In the great majority of instances the test is dependent upon the development in the patient's serum of antibodies that cause agglutination, precipitation, or complement fixation, when exposed to specific antigens. Although very high titers on one occasion may strongly suggest the specific etiologic agent, rising or falling titers in serial or paired serologic tests some time apart constitute much stronger evidence.

Serologic testing is of most practical value in relation to chronic pulmonary disease, and this is well exemplified in fungal infections. The two major pathogenic mycoses in which serologic tests play a distinct role in diagnosis are coccidioidomycosis and histoplasmosis. The most useful serologic test in histoplasmosis is the complement-fixation (CF) test, using both histoplasmin and a saline suspension of yeast form as antigens. Using these two antigens, positive results will be obtained in approximately 95 per cent of culturally proved cases of progressive pulmonary disease.[16] The yeast form gives a positive result earlier. In disseminated infections the CF reaction is less reliable, giving positive results in 56 to 80 per cent of cases.[16] Other serologic tests of value in detecting histoplasmosis are indicated in Table 3–4.

In coccidioidomycosis, screening is recommended with agar gel–double diffusion as well as a latex particle agglutination test, and positive reactors should be tested by complement fixation and tubular precipitin. The CF test is used primarily to determine whether the disease is disseminated: a titer rising above 1:16 should arouse suspicion of dissemination. Precipitins may be detected within 1 to 3 weeks after the onset of primary infections; the CF test, however, is not usually positive until 4 to 6 weeks after infection, by which time the precipitin test usually has reverted to negative. Spherulin (antigen prepared from the sporangium [spherule] of C. immitis) is more sensitive than coccidioidin (antigen derived from the mycelial form).

Less common mycotic infections caused by pathogenic (in contrast to opportunistic) fungi in which serologic testing may prove useful are sporotrichosis and paracoccidioidomycosis (South American blastomycosis). Results of serologic tests are negative in cutaneous sporotrichosis, but the complement-fixation test is highly specific and usually positive in the active pulmonary form.

The detection of antibodies as a reflection of host tissue invasion may be extremely useful in opportunistic fungal infections, whereas the culture of fungi from sputum or transtracheal aspirates is of limited value, since these organisms are common commensals. However, since opportunistic fungi infect compromised hosts, antibody production is often not forthcoming because of defective immune response.

Serologic tests may also assist in the diagnosis of several parasitic diseases; for example, invasive amebiasis can be detected by both gel diffusion precipitin and indirect hemagglutination tests. Obviously the results of such tests are more reliable in North Americans than in patients from areas in which these diseases are highly endemic, on whom they must be interpreted with caution. The three most reliable serologic tests for diagnosing toxoplasmosis are the indirect fluorescent antibody, indirect hemagglutination, and Sabin-Feldman dye tests. Hydatid disease is almost always associated with the production of antibodies, and rupture of a cyst often results in a rise in titer. Serologic testing is also used in trichinosis, although here its value is limited by the short clinical course of the infestation and by delay in the development of antibodies.

In addition to the more or less specific antibodies, nonspecific cold agglutination antibodies and antibodies to Streptococcus MG are found in approximately 50 per cent of patients with Mycoplasma pneumoniae infections and constitute strong evidence of this disease. However, cold agglutinins sometimes develop in other infectious diseases involving the lungs.

The mixing of specific serum with an antigen

TABLE 3–4. MYCOTIC PULMONARY INFECTIONS

| ORGANISM | ISOLATION AND IDENTIFICATION | | SKIN TESTS | LEUKOCYTE COUNT° |
	MICROSCOPIC AND CULTURAL CHARACTERISTICS	SEROLOGIC TESTS		
Histoplasma capsulatum	On glucose agar at 30°C mycelial growth with tuberculate spores; on cysteine blood agar at 37°C or in tissues stained with silver nitrate 2 $\mu \times 4\ \mu$ yeast cells occur; mice inoculation useful	Complement fixation with mycelial and yeast antigens, latex agglutination, agar gel double diffusion, and indirect fluorescent antibody	Yes	Normal to mild; rarely considerable in cavitary disease; leukopenia in disseminated cases
Coccidioides immitis	On glucose agar at 30°C mycelial growth with arthrospores; in human body fluids or tissues or after inoculation into mice or guinea pigs 20 to 80 μ spherules are seen	Agar gel double diffusion agglutination, tubular precipitation, and complement fixation	Yes	Normal to moderate; eosinophilia usually with erythema nodosum
Blastomyces dermatitidis	On glucose agar grows slowly as mycelia with conidia; on blood agar grows as single budding–doubly refractile walled yeast organisms	Agar gel double diffusion and indirect fluorescent antibody for yeast form only	Yes	Normal to moderate; rarely considerable
Cryptococcus neoformans	On glucose agar and on blood agar at 37°C 4 to 20 μ yeast cells; these spherical organisms with a thick capsule may be identified in body fluids with India ink stain	Indirect fluorescent antibody, agglutination for both antibody and antigens	Nil	Normal to moderate
Actinomyces israelii	On enriched agar under anaerobic conditions delicate gram-positive hyphae; in tissues or body fluids mycelial clumps (sulfur granules) may be identified	Indirect fluorescent antibody	Nil	Normal to moderate
Nocardia species	On glucose agar and on blood agar under aerobic conditions delicate branching filamentous hyphae; organism is gram-positive and some strains are acid fast	Nil	Yes	Moderate, usually neutrophilia; occasionally lymphocytosis or leukopenia
Aspergillus species	On glucose agar broad septate hyphae with characteristic conidiophores expanding into large vesicle form	Precipitation	Yes	Normal to moderate, sometimes eosinophilia

from the patient comprises a different form of antigen-antibody reaction which is not strictly a serologic test; this technique has thrown new light on the early immunologic diagnosis of infectious diseases. Antigen and specific antibody, one of which is labeled with fluorescent dye, are mixed and processed; the histologic sections are washed thoroughly to remove unbound reagent, and antigen-antibody reactions become apparent as fluorescent areas. In most instances antiserum to the suspected organism is mixed with tracheobronchial secretions or cultures of this material. This is the direct method, which requires labeling of the specific antibody to the suspected antigen. An indirect method which does not require fluorescent dye tagging of specific antibody is of even greater practical value: this consists of an anti-immunoglobulin to one species of animal prepared in another species. This antiglobulin fluorescent conjugate can then be overlaid on the histologic preparation and in this way a number of specific antibodies to suspected antigenic organisms can be looked for at the same time. This procedure

TABLE 3–4.   MYCOTIC PULMONARY INFECTIONS (*Continued*)

	ISOLATION AND IDENTIFICATION			
ORGANISM	MICROSCOPIC AND CULTURAL CHARACTERISTICS	SEROLOGIC TESTS	SKIN TESTS	LEUKOCYTE COUNT*
Candida species	On cornmeal agar thick-walled chlamydospores; in body fluids and tissues 2 to 4 μ thin-walled oval budding yeasts are seen	Agglutination and precipitation	Nil	Normal to moderate
Phycomycetes (mucormycosis)	On glucose agar wide nonseptate hyphae bearing large (100 μ) globular sporangia develop	Nil	Nil	
Geotrichum species	On glucose agar oval or spherical arthrospores separated from hyphae; in sputum there may be large rectangular arthrospores with rounded ends	Agglutination	Yes	Eosinophilia in bronchial form
Sporotrix schenckii	On glucose agar at 30°C delicate hyphae supporting conidiophores; on enriched media at 37°C cigar-shaped gram-positive yeasts are found	Agglutination, complement fixation, agar gel diffusion, and indirect fluorescent antibody	Yes	Normal to moderate
Blastomyces brasiliensis	On glucose agar mycelial growth with branching hyphae and conidia; in tissues or on culture at 37°C multiple budding yeast organisms are seen	Complement fixation and agar gel double diffusion	Yes	
Allescheria boydii	On glucose agar thin hyphae with stalks bearing single conidium; large (50 to 200 μ) flask-shaped ascospores are also seen	Nil	Nil	
Torulopsis glabrata	On glucose agar reproduces by budding but fails to produce septate hyphae	Nil	Nil	Normal

*Leukocyte count: < 5,000 = Leukopenia
5.000–10,000 = Normal
10,000–12,000 = Mild leukocytosis
12,000–15,000 = Moderate
>15,000 = Considerable

permits diagnosis in the acute phase of various infections, and its use in *Mycoplasma pneumoniae*, *H. capsulatum*, respiratory syncytial virus, *Legionella pneumophila*, and many other infections has been reported (*see* Tables 3–2, 3–3, and 3–4).

SKIN TESTS

These tests can be divided into those used to detect hypersensitivity to allergens that produce immediate reactions and those used to diagnose bacterial, fungal, and parasitic diseases that usually give rise to delayed reactions.

Immediate Reactivity

Scratch or intradermal tests are used to detect atopy, seasonal and perennial rhinitis, and asthma, using common inhalants such as pollens, molds, dusts, and danders; foods and drugs are used when the patient's history indicates specific sensitivity. Application of the allergens provokes more or less specific reactions, although some have a nonspecific irritating quality. Pollen extracts are almost always specific and usually of clinical significance. This is true also for mold spore extracts and for many danders and some foods, but not for house dust, feathers, wool, kapok, and silk. Skin tests are particularly useful when they confirm a history indicating specific allergy and form the basis of a desensitization program.

Skin Tests for Bacteria, Fungi, and Parasites

Tables 3–2, 3–3, and 3–4 summarize the uses of these reactions for diagnostic purposes. Skin tests of value for diagnosing bacterial infections are those used in suspected mycobacterial disease and tularemia.

Intermediate-strength purified protein derivative (PPD) 0.0001 mg or 5 tuberculin units (TU) is usually employed for diagnostic skin testing for tuberculosis. If a patient fails to react to intermediate strength PPD, a second strength (PPD-S 250 TU) can be used, although a positive reaction at this strength is less significant.

The skin test is carried out as follows. The solution (0.1 ml) is injected intradermally through disposable 26- or 27-gauge short-beveled needles on the volar aspect of the forearm, with the needle bevel pointing upward. Tests should be read on the second or third day after injection, the diameter of induration being measured transversely to the long axis of the forearm and recorded in millimeters. The degree of erythema is of no significance and need not be estimated. A Mantoux reaction of 10 mm or larger is positive, 5 to 9 mm is doubtful, and less than 5 mm is negative.

A positive tuberculin reaction is strong evidence that a patient has or has had tuberculosis, particularly if the induration is 10 mm or more in diameter. False positive reactions are rare and represent cross-reactions due to infection from atypical mycobacteria. The larger the size of the tuberculin reaction, the greater the risk of clinical tuberculosis in the future.[18]

The major drawback to the tuberculin test lies in the considerable incidence of false negative reactions. (For practical diagnostic purposes, a false negative reaction is one in which the intracutaneous injection of 0.1 ml of 5 TU PPD-S results in induration less than 10 mm diameter.) False negative reactions may be due to (1) faulty technique of administration, (2) faulty interpretation of the reaction, (3) lack of

potency of the injected material or (4) diminished immunologic response to tuberculin.[19]

Patients infected with *M. tuberculosis* show negative reactions during the 3 to 9 weeks of incubation while the cell-mediated delayed hypersensitivity is developing. Various acute exanthemata, particularly measles, transiently depress the tuberculin reaction; a more permanent diminution or loss of delayed skin hypersensitivity may occur in sarcoidosis, lymphoma, chronic leukemia, amyloidosis, syphilis, hypothyroidism, and advanced carcinoma.[17] In addition, corticosteroids may render previously positive reactors negative.

In contrast to the waning sensitivity to tuberculin that may occur with aging or with treatment of early disease, an occasional patient may show enhanced reaction associated with repeated Mantoux testing. The potential error in calling a test negative when the induration measures 5 mm or less is revealed by this phenomenon, since the booster effect of subsequent tuberculin testing may produce a positive reaction of 10 mm or more and lead to the assumption that tuberculosis has developed.[18]

Negative reactions to 5 TU of stable PPD (treated with Tween 80 to prevent adsorption) may occur in cases of relatively mild infection with positive sputum culture.[19-21] An incidence of 10 to 17 per cent of this phenomenon has been reported in unselected series; unfortunately, serial tuberculin testing, which would reveal whether true sensitivity was developing or the patients were basically anergic, was not carried out. True anergy associated with a negative response to PPD is seen in patients with overwhelming tuberculous infections.

The skin test for tularemia is a delayed hypersensitivity reaction; following intradermal injection of antibody, it is read after 48 hours.

Skin tests for fungus infections aid in the diagnosis of histoplasmosis and coccidioidomycosis but not blastomycosis. A strong argument can be made for avoiding histoplasmin intradermal skin testing in adults suspected of having active histoplasmosis. Intradermal injection of histoplasmin can increase circulating antibodies, although complement-fixing antibody titers seldom rise above one-sixteenth. If blood is drawn at the same time as or within 4 days of skin testing, a spurious rise in antibody titer will not have had time to develop. On the other hand, the first serologic tests frequently show equivocal values and repeat tests are required to ascertain activity; skin testing may thus interfere with the interpretation of serial rises in antibody titers.

In patients suspected of having coccidioidomycosis, sensitivity is determined by intradermal injection of antigen from lysates of the mycelial (coccidioidin) or spherule form (spherulin); both are highly specific but neither appears useful in disseminated disease. A skin test with coccidioidin has the same significance as the tuberculin reaction, becoming positive 3 to 4 weeks after infection and 12 to 20 days after the onset of clinical illness. Spherulin appears to be just as specific but more sensitive than coccidioidin.

PLEURAL FLUID

Pleural fluid should be examined for cellular content, and aliquots should be sent to bacteriology, pathology, and biochemistry laboratories.

Protein Content

The terms "transudate" and "exudate" are still used in relation to pleural effusion, but the present tendency is to group effusions according to protein content rather than specific gravity. Protein concentration almost always differentiates transudates of congestive heart failure from exudates due to cancer or tuberculosis, levels in the former being less than 3.0 g per 100 ml of fluid and in the latter more than 3.0 g per 100 ml.

In a prospective study of 150 pleural effusions, Light and associates[22] described a more elaborate attempt to separate transudates from exudates. Employing diagnostic criteria based on clinical presentation, they classified 47 effusions as transudates and 103 as exudates. Biochemically, there were three differentiating characteristics: (1) a fluid-to-serum protein ratio greater than 0.5; (2) pleural fluid LDH greater than 200 IU; and (3) a fluid-to-serum LDH ratio greater than 0.6. All but one of the clinically diagnosed exudates had at least one of these characteristics, whereas only one transudate had any.

Glucose Content

Several authors have reported very low glucose concentrations in pleural effusion secondary to tuberculosis and rheumatoid arthritis, and it is probable that values below 26 mg per 100 ml usually indicate one of these diseases. However, very low glucose content in neoplastic pleural effusions also has been reported.

pH of Pleural Fluid

Light and associates[22] found that a pH below 7.30 was highly suggestive of tuberculosis, whereas values greater than 7.40 usually indicated malignancy. These authors also found that pH levels of pleural effusions associated with pneumonia but not grossly purulent can help in deciding the mode of therapy, particularly the need for tube drainage: complete resolution of the effusions was achieved with antibiotic therapy alone in all 19 patients with pneumonic effusions with a pH greater than 7.20, whereas no improvement resulted from antibiotics and thoracentesis in the 5 patients with effusions with a pH of less than 7.20.

Fat Content

Chylothorax should be suspected when the gross appearance of the effusion is cloudy or milky. The fat content exceeds 400 mg per 100 ml, and the protein content is almost invariably greater than 3 g per 100 ml.[23] In some cases effusions due to tuberculosis and rheumatoid disease contain cholesterol and may resemble chylothorax.

Other Biochemicals in Pleural Effusion

Pleural effusion, usually left-sided and sometimes hemorrhagic, is present in 5 to 15 per cent of patients with acute pancreatitis.[24] A high amylase content in the fluid is highly suggestive of this diagnosis but may also be found in patients with esophageal perforation, presumably as a result of the presence of saliva which contains considerable amylase.

Reduced pleural fluid complement has been reported in lupus erythematosus and rheumatoid arthritis. Hyaluronic acid may be present in pleural effusions caused by pleural mesothelioma. A high level of alkaline phosphatase in the pleural fluid was reported in one case of alveolar cell carcinoma, possibly indicating production of this enzyme by the tumor.

The etiologic characteristics of pleural effusions were reviewed by an American Thoracic Society committee on therapy of pleural effusions, and the conclusions of their 1968 report[25] are summarized in Table 3–5.

TABLE 3–5. ETIOLOGIC CHARACTERISTICS OF PLEURAL EFFUSIONS

	TUBERCULOSIS	MALIGNANCY	CONGESTIVE FAILURE	PNEUMONIA AND OTHER NONTUBERCULOUS INFECTIONS	RHEUMATOID ARTHRITIS AND COLLAGEN DISEASES	PULMONARY EMBOLISM	FUNGAL INFECTION	TRAUMA	CHYLOTHORAX
Clinical	Younger patient, exposure to tuberculosis, good health prior to effusion	Older patient, poor health prior to effusion	Signs and symptoms of congestive failure	Signs and symptoms of respiratory tract infection	History of joint involvement may or may not be present, subcutaneous nodules	Postoperative patient, immobilized patient, venous disease	Exposure in endemic area	History of trauma	History of trauma, known malignancy
Gross appearance	Usually serous, may be sanguineous	Often sanguineous	Serous	Serous	Turbid or yellow-green	Often sanguineous	Serous	Sanguineous	Chylous
Microscopic examination	Positive for acid-fast bacilli 30 to 70 per cent of cases, cholesterol crystals	Cytology positive in 40 per cent	0	May or may not be positive for bacilli	0	0	May or may not be positive for fungi	0	Fat droplets
Cell count	5 per cent over 10,000 erythrocytes; 75 per cent over 1,000 leukocytes, mainly lymphocytes	65 per cent bloody, 40 per cent over 1,000 leukocytes, mainly lymphocytes	10 per cent over 10,000 erythrocytes; 10 per cent over 1,000 leukocytes	Polymorphonuclears predominate	Lymphocytes predominate	Erythrocytes predominate	0	Erythrocytes	0

Culture	10 to 70 per cent pleural effusion culture positive; 10 to 15 per cent sputum or gastric culture positive	0	May or may not be positive	0	May or may not be positive	0	0
Specific gravity	75 per cent over 1.016	90 per cent under 1.016 (unless pulmonary embolism)	Over 1.016	Over 1.016	Over 1.016	Over 1.016	Over 1.016
Protein	90 per cent 3 g or more	75 per cent less than 3 g	3.0 g or more	3.0 g or more	3.0 g or more	3.0 g or more	3.0 g or more
Sugar	60 per cent less than 60 mg per 100 ml	0	Occasionally less than 60 mg per 100 ml	5–17 mg per 100 ml (only in rheumatoid arthritis)	0	0	0
Other	No mesothelial cells on cytology; the cause in 75 per cent of males under 25 years of age, 50 per cent of males 25 or over; tuberculin test usually positive	Right-sided in 55 to 70 per cent	If hemorrhagic fluid 65 per cent due to tumor; tends to continue to form after removed	Rapid clotting time; lupus erythematosus cell or rheumatoid factor may be present	Associated with opacity on roentgenogram	Source of emboli may or may not be noted	Skin and serologic tests may be helpful

HEMATOLOGIC PROCEDURES IN LUNG DISEASE

Polycythemia frequently but not invariably occurs in association with chronic hypoxemia in pulmonary disease. By contrast, anemia is uncommon. It may develop with a chronic infectious process or widespread malignancy, and in some cases of idiopathic pulmonary hemorrhage or Goodpasture's syndrome anemia may be noted even before the patient expectorates blood.

The kidneys, and to a lesser extent other organs (particularly the liver and spleen), produce erythropoietin in response to hypoxia; the intraerythrocytic level of 2,3-diphosphoglycerate (DPG) increases and the oxygen dissociation curve shifts to the right.

Variations in the total and differential leukocyte count may play a major role in the differential diagnosis of lung disease (*see* Tables 3–2, 3–3, and 3–4). A leukocytosis of over 15,000 white cells per cu mm, with a predominance of polymorphonuclear cells, is strong evidence for bacterial rather than viral pneumonia. It must be remembered, however, that fulminating bacterial pneumonia may be associated with normal or even low white cell counts.

ELECTROCARDIOGRAPHY

An electrocardiogram is of fundamental importance in differentiating myocardial infarction from acute massive pulmonary embolism. It is also useful in indicating lung disease as a cause of heart failure in patients who might otherwise be considered to be suffering from coronary artery insufficiency or myocardial disease.

PULMONARY FUNCTION TESTS

INTRODUCTION

Pulmonary function tests can play a useful role in detecting respiratory disease, in leading to a definitive diagnosis when correlated with clinical and roentgenologic findings, and in managing various pulmonary disorders through sequential objective assessment of the degree of dysfunction. To screen a patient with respiratory disease adequately, a *variety* of function tests is usually required. This section deals only with procedures that the authors have found most successful; it does not attempt to review the entire subject of pulmonary function analysis, which has been done so well by others.[1]

Measurements of lung volumes and capacities, flow rates, and arterial blood gases remain the basic means of assessing disturbed pulmonary physiology. A Collins 13.5-liter water-sealed spirometer is the least expensive and most dependable method of determining vital capacity, timed vital capacity, functional residual capacity, and mixing; the last two measurements require integration of a closed-circuit helium apparatus. Maximal breathing capacity and expiratory flow rates are usually recorded on a spirometer with low-flow resistance, using a high-speed kymograph. Bedside measurements can be made with a simplified instrument such as a McKesson Vitalor.[26] Because these methods are time-consuming, many investigators in recent years have worked to develop electronic spirometers providing rapid on-line reports of function.

Measurements of blood gases and pH using appropriate electrodes and determinations of diffusing capacity by the single-breath or steady-state carbon monoxide method should be possible in a well-equipped screening laboratory.

Direct measurements of resistance and of static and dynamic compliances, which require more expensive equipment, may give valuable information not revealed by the usual screening tests. The determination of regional ventilation and perfusion, using radioactive gases, can be applied clinically and, although time-consuming and expensive, can provide important diagnostic information.

Since dyspnea on exertion is a major complaint of patients with respiratory disease, it is appropriate to study the physiology of such patients while they are exercising; circuits have been constructed for this purpose that measure workload, ventilation, O_2 uptake, CO_2 production, diffusing capacity, and resistance.

Procedures to evaluate the sensitivity of the respiratory center and respiratory muscle strength are required less often but can be carried out without expensive equipment in any laboratory. Chemoreceptors in the brain stem are exposed to increasing concentrations of CO_2 by the rebreathing or steady-state technique, and the degree of ventilatory response is recorded. Diaphragmatic paralysis or fatigue may be a cause of dyspnea or respiratory failure and may be suspected when paradoxical movement of the abdominal muscles is associated with a decrease in lung volumes and expiratory flow rates and abnormal gas exchange. Respiratory muscle function can be determined by measuring maximal inspiratory pressure or transdiaphragmatic pressure or from electromyograms of the diaphragm (*see* Chapter 18).

Predicted Normal Values of Pulmonary Function

Interpretation of the results of pulmonary function tests is based on the degree of deviation from predicted normal values calculated from regression equations that usually take into account variations attributable to age, sex, and height. There is a wide range of scatter among "normals," and it has been recommended that on average a 20 per cent loss of function must occur before an individual result can be considered of pathologic significance. It is always wise to interpret the test results in the light of clinical and roentgenographic manifestations. A more dependable assessment of impaired function can be obtained from repeating the pulmonary function tests at intervals, the patient serving as his or her own control.

Prediction formulas for spirometric measurements in healthy persons show negative correlations with age and positive correlations with height. In addition to age, sex, and height, other factors such as ethnic origin, physical activity, environmental conditions, and tobacco smoking can affect normal values of ventilatory function.

Lung Volumes

Lung volumes and capacities can be appreciated from a study of the diagram in Figure 3–1. There are four volumes: (1) tidal volume (TV), which is the amount of gas moving in and out of the lung with each respiratory cycle; (2) residual volume (RV), which is the amount remaining in the lung after a maximal expiration and is the only lung volume that cannot be measured directly by spirometry; (3) inspiratory reserve volume (IRV), the additional gas that can be inspired from the end of a quiet inspiration; and (4) expiratory reserve volume (ERV), the additional amount of gas that can be expired from the resting or end expiratory level.

There are also four capacities, each of which contains two or more volumes: (a) total lung capacity (TLC), the gas contained in the lung at the end of a maximal inspiration; (b) vital capacity (VC), the amount that can be expired after a maximal inspiration; (c) inspiratory capacity (IC), the amount of gas that can be inspired from the end of a quiet expiration; and (d) functional residual capacity (FRC), the volume of gas remaining in the lungs at the end of a quiet expiration.

Vital Capacity (VC) and Its Subdivisions

Although this volume of gas can be measured from the end of a maximal expiration to full inspiration, it is usually expressed as the amount of air expelled from the lungs after a maximal inspiration. In obstructive lung disease, because air is trapped in the lungs, the VC is less when maximal inspiration is followed by maximal expiration and when expressed as forced vital capacity (FVC) than when it is determined from the end of maximal expiration to maximal inspiration. VC usually is measured with a spirometer; predicted normal values have been calculated based on age, sex, and height. The

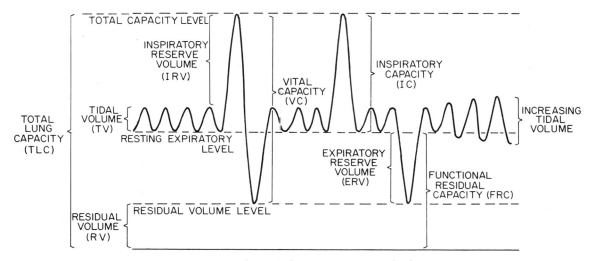

Figure 3–1. Lung Volumes and Capacities. *See* text for description.

VC also varies with the position of the patient, the volume being less in the supine than in the erect position.

The VC serves little purpose as an independent measurement of pulmonary function, but can be of much value when considered in conjunction with the results of other tests of pulmonary function. It is a useful index of day-to-day changes in the clinical state of patients with neuromuscular disease. The subdivisions of VC, particularly inspiratory capacity and inspiratory reserve volume, rarely are useful in assessing pulmonary function. ERV is greatly reduced in patients with obesity and hypoventilation syndrome, in which state the $\dot{V}_A/\dot{Q}$ ratios are low at the lung bases. TV varies greatly in normal subjects, and this measurement by itself usually is not informative; however, multiplication of TV by the respiratory rate per minute yields the minute volume, and in some cases alveolar hypoventilation can be assessed on these two indices alone.

The ratio of forced expiratory volume in one second (FEV_1) to forced vital capacity (FVC) indicates whether insufficiency is "restrictive" or "obstructive." In obstructive disease the VC is relatively well maintained in comparison to FEV_1, whereas in restrictive disease the FEV_1 may be close to normal and the VC very definitely decreased.

Functional Residual Capacity (FRC) and Residual Volume (RV)

These compartments are measured by a closed circuit method using helium or by placing the patient in a body plethysmograph. With the closed-circuit method the patient breathes from a spirometer containing a known concentration of helium. At the beginning of the experiment the helium concentration in the lungs is zero; as the patient breathes in and out of the spirometer, the gas mixes between spirometer and lungs until the concentration of helium is the same in both. FRC is calculated from the concentration of helium before and at the end of the experiment and the volume in the spirometer. When the lung contains poorly ventilated areas it may be necessary to continue the test for upward of 20 min before equilibrium is attained. The RV is readily obtained by subtracting from FRC the ERV as measured on the spirometer.

When the thorax contains volumes of gas that barely communicate with the conducting tubes, equilibrium between patient and spirometer may appear to be reached while gas is still entering these areas so slowly as to go undetected. To measure the true thoracic gas volume in these circumstances, it is necessary to place the patient in a body box (plethysmograph). With this apparatus the thoracic volume can be calculated by applying Boyle's law, which states the relationship between changes in pressure and volume of a gas at constant temperature.

In common with VC values, measurements of lung volumes by themselves are of little use in the assessment of lung function, but they may be most informative when considered with the results of other pulmonary function tests.

Total Lung Capacity (TLC)

The TLC is calculated simply by the addition of RV and VC. This measurement in itself can be misleading, since TLC may be normal in the presence of serious disease—and, in fact, may be much greater than normal in patients with emphysema, because of increase in the FRC. In "restrictive" disease of the lungs or thoracic cage, the TLC is decreased because of decrease in VC or RV or both.

As with RV and FRC, the TLC may be falsely low when measured by the helium method. Volumetric determination based on posteroanterior and lateral roentgenograms of the chest has been shown to correlate better with values obtained by body plethysmography in emphysematous patients and with the planimetric method may be accomplished by experienced workers in less than a minute.[27]

MEASUREMENT OF ALVEOLAR GAS COMPOSITION

As stated in Chapter 1, the composition of gas in the acinar unit is dependent upon alveolar ventilation and mixed venous P_{O_2} and P_{CO_2} of the blood in the pulmonary capillaries. The mixed venous blood gases can be determined by analysis of samples obtained through a catheter in the right side of the heart. This procedure is not suitable for routine use, but in intensive care units these gases can be monitored easily by sampling through catheters inserted for measurement of central venous pressure. Mixed venous P_{CO_2} can be measured accurately by a rebreathing method,[28] and arterial P_{CO_2} can be calculated from these results by assuming a constant arterial-venous P_{CO_2} difference of 6 mm.

Ventilation of the acinar unit can be estimated accurately in normal subjects. Alveolar ventilation can be calculated from an end tidal sample of carbon dioxide or oxygen, the volume of expired gas, and the volume and gas content inspired. When the lungs are diseased, however, the situation is not so simple, since there may be many acinar units not uniformly ventilated that empty late in expiration. In such circumstances it is difficult, if not impossible, to obtain a true alveolar (or acinar) sample, and a reliable estimate of alveolar ventilation requires measurement of the total minute ventilation and subtraction from this of an assumed volume of anatomic dead space. The volume of alveolar ventilation per minute of a patient with diseased lungs may equal that of a subject with healthy lungs of the same age, sex, and build. Despite the fact that the patient has some units that are barely ventilated, he or she has others that are overventilated, and therefore total ventilation may be normal.

There is no doubt, however, that the most accurate index of alveolar ventilation is analysis of an arterial blood sample, which gives values for P_{CO_2} and P_{O_2}; a P_{CO_2} value above the normal range indicates that many acinar units are poorly ventilated.

MEASUREMENT OF MECHANICS OF ACINAR VENTILATION

Measurement of Compliance

Compliance is the relationship between the pressure required to overcome "elastic recoil"

and the volume of air that moves into the lung as a result of this pressure change. To avoid the effect of resistance and to measure compliance alone, the test is done in a "static" position; that is, while the breath is held with the glottis open. As the normal lung becomes more inflated it becomes less compliant and the pressure-volume curve becomes more horizontal (Figure 3–2). Compliance is expressed in liters/cm H_2O. Pressure is measured by a manometer attached to a tube leading to a thin-walled balloon which is swallowed to the mid-esophagus. The volume is measured either by use of a pneumotachograph at the mouth, with integration of the pneumotachogram signal, or while the patient breathes from a spirometer. This pressure-volume curve includes measurement of the "elastic" properties of the elastic and collagen tissues of the lungs and those of the thoracic cage, and the force required to overcome the surface tension effect of the alveoli.

Measurement of Total Pulmonary Resistance

SPIROMETRY. This is an indirect method for determining the resistance of the airways and lung tissue. A single forced inspiratory or expiratory curve is measured on a revolving drum or a bellows-type apparatus and is expressed as liters per min moved in or out of the lung. The "timed vital capacity" may be used to quantify expiration; after an inspiration, the patient exhales as rapidly as possible all of the air in the

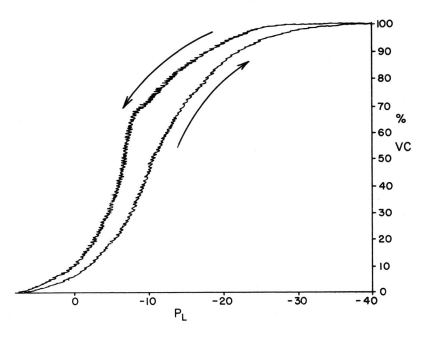

Figure 3–2. Pressure-Volume Curve. A pressure-volume tracing of a young male adult measured in both inspiration and expiration from residual volume to total lung capacity and back to residual volume. The upper curve represents the expiratory tracing. Notice the more horizontal appearance (decrease in compliance) as total lung capacity is reached.

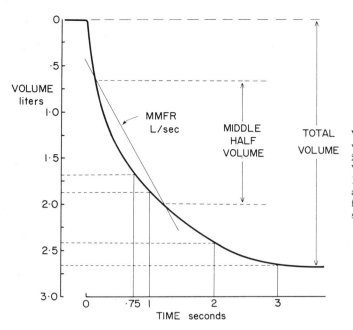

Figure 3–3. Measurement of Ventilatory Volumes. This graph depicts the curve of a forced vital capacity (FVC) in which a total volume of 2.6 liters has been expired in 3 seconds ($FEV_{3.0}$). Volumes expired during the 3/4 second ($FEV_{0.75}$), 1 second ($FEV_{1.0}$), and 2 second ($FEV_{2.0}$) intervals are also indicated. The maximal midexpiratory flow rate (MMFR) can be calculated at 1.3 liters/sec.

lungs. This is the forced expiratory volume (FEV); the amounts expired during the first 1.0 sec and the first 3.0 sec are expressed as $FEV_{1.0}$ and $FEV_{3.0}$. Normal persons exhale approximately 83 per cent of VC in 1.0 sec and approximately 97 per cent in 3.0 sec, whereas expiratory flow curves of patients with obstructive lung disease are prolonged. On the other hand, although patients with a restrictive lung condition such as fibrosis may have a substantially reduced VC, they can have almost normal $FEV_{1.0}$ and $FEV_{3.0}$ values, since there is no bronchial obstruction.

Many ways of expressing the forced expiration curve have been devised. In our laboratory we measure FEV on a rapidly revolving drum and from this curve determine FEV_1 (the volume expired in the first second). In addition, we measure the middle half of the FEV curve (MMFR or MMF) and express this volume in liters per sec (Figure 3–3).

FLOW-VOLUME CURVE. Another way of depicting airway resistance is by the flow-volume curve or loop. In contrast to the forced vital capacity curve (FVC), for which flow is plotted against time, in this technique flow is plotted against the actual volume of lung at which flow is occurring. The flow-volume loop actually measures inspiration *and* expiration and is particularly useful in identifying obstruction in the larger airways. The configuration of the flow-volume loop in normal subjects and in patients with tracheal obstruction is considered in greater detail in Chapter 11.

Although these indirect methods for assessing resistance in the lungs are simple to perform and are widely used, they must be interpreted with caution. (1) Maximum expiratory flow (MEF) is largely effort-dependent near TLC; this must be kept in mind in assessing the significance of FEV_1, since falsely low values may be recorded in patients unable or unwilling to cooperate. On the other hand, MEF is relatively independent of effort over the major portion of VC, including the midexpiratory portion of the curve (MMF). (2) The flow-volume curve does not indicate specific mechanical abnormalities, since patients with decreased compliance have reduced flow rates; direct measurements of resistance are therefore preferable.

USE OF BODY PLETHYSMOGRAPH. Since resistance equals the pressure difference divided by the volume flow, resistance in the airways can be determined only with knowledge of the instantaneous air flow and the difference between atmospheric and alveolar pressures. Air flow can be determined with a pneumotachograph, but the measurement of alveolar pressure requires a more elaborate procedure. The patient breathes in and out in an airtight box, and the pressure in the box is measured and recorded by a very sensitive manometer. Alveolar pressure can be calculated from the pressure change in the box during the respiratory cycle.

Normal values of respiratory resistance as determined by the body plethysmograph during rapid, shallow breathing range from 0.6 to 2.4

cm H$_2$O/liter/sec, with flow rates of 0.5 liter/sec in adults.

USE OF MOUTH PRESSURE FOR DETERMINING AIRWAY RESISTANCE. Alveolar pressure can be determined indirectly by using an electrically controlled shutter; while this device momentarily shuts off flow during inspiration, the mouth pressure (which, presumably, is equal to the alveolar pressure immediately before interruption) is recorded. The apparatus is cheaper but yields less accurate values than the body plethysmograph.

Measurement of Resistance in Small Airways

Measurements of lung volumes and the indirect and direct methods of determining airway resistance described previously may yield normal values in patients with chronic obstructive lung disease, since chronic bronchitis is primarily a disease of the distal conducting system. It has been shown experimentally that the main site of resistance to air flow in the tracheobronchial tree is the central airways, particularly those with an internal diameter of 4 to 8 mm, and that peripheral airways less than 2 mm internal diameter contribute only 10 to 20 per cent of total pulmonary resistance (Figure 3–4). Because peripheral resistance is such a minor component of total resistance, even a fairly large obstruction in the small airways of the lungs may not be detected in measurements of total airway resistance. The hypothetical situation described by Macklem[30] illustrates this point very nicely (Fig. 3–5). In this two-compartment lung model, obstructing half the peripheral airways doubled the resistance contributed by these airways; since central resistance remained unchanged, total pulmonary resistance increased by only 10 per cent—an amount virtually impossible to detect clinically using present-day tests designed to measure resistance. In this hypothetical situation, peripheral airways to half the total lung parenchyma are obstructed; since these parenchymal units can be ventilated only by collateral air flow, ventilation distribution and gas exchange will be

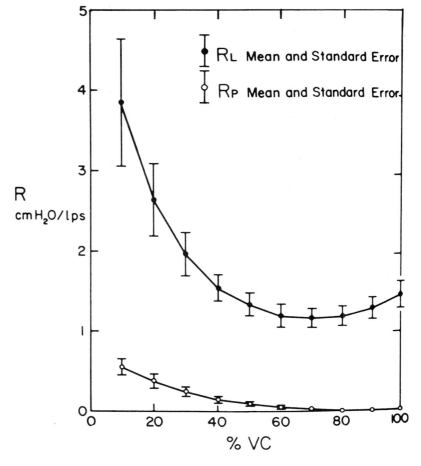

Figure 3–4. **Contribution of Peripheral Airway Resistance to Total Resistance in Dogs.** Mean values $\pm$ SE for total resistance (R_L) and peripheral resistance (R_P) at different lung volumes in eight living dogs. At 10 per cent VC, data were obtainable in only six dogs because the catheter tended to become obstructed at these low lung volumes. *See* text. (Reprinted from Macklem, P. T., and Mead, J.: J. Appl. Physiol., 22:395, 1967, with permission of the authors, editor, and publisher.)

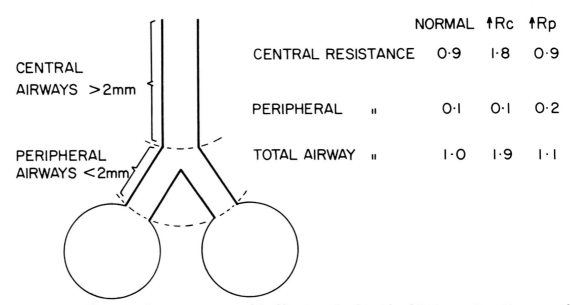

	NORMAL	↑Rc	↑Rp
CENTRAL RESISTANCE	0·9	1·8	0·9
PERIPHERAL "	0·1	0·1	0·2
TOTAL AIRWAY "	1·0	1·9	1·1

CENTRAL AIRWAYS >2mm

PERIPHERAL AIRWAYS <2mm

Figure 3–5. Effect on Total Airway Resistance of Doubling Central and Peripheral Resistance. Since 90 per cent of airway resistance is in airways larger than 2 mm and only 10 per cent in peripheral airways, nine units are allotted to central and one unit to peripheral airways. When central airway resistance is doubled a highly significant change takes place in total airway resistance, whereas if peripheral airway resistance is doubled the change in total resistance is insignificant. (Slightly modified from Macklem, P. T.: Med. Clin. North Am., 57:669, 1973, with permission of the author, editor, and publisher.)

seriously affected. Thus, as previously noted, the peripheral airways may be regarded as a "quiet zone"[31] within the lungs.

The realization that extensive disease could be present in small airways despite normal results with conventional tests of pulmonary function led to the assumption that there could be many individuals with "early" obstructive pulmonary disease, with or without symptoms, in whom the presence of disease could be detected only with more sensitive tests of respiratory function. Three of these tests will be described in some detail, along with data attesting to their relative value. They are (1) dynamic compliance of small airways; (2) flow-volume rates and curves at low lung volumes (including the effect on the flow-volume curve of helium and oxygen breathing in contrast to air breathing); and (3) closing volumes and closing capacity.

DYNAMIC COMPLIANCE. We have already seen that compliance — the relationship between pressure changes and the volume of air that moves in and out of the lungs—is measured in a "static" position to determine elastic recoil; similar measurements can be made when the subject is breathing. In most normal lungs, dynamic compliance does not vary with respiratory frequencies up to 100 breaths per minute.[1] This maintenance of the relationship be-

tween pressure and volume changes in different circumstances reflects the remarkably synchronous action of acinar units throughout the lungs. A falling compliance—a decrease in volume change for a given change in pressure—with increasing respiratory frequency indicates asynchrony that may be due to decreased elastic recoil or airway obstruction. When results of standard pulmonary function tests are normal (including resistance and static compliance), it is very likely that some acinar units are inadequately ventilated because of obstruction in smaller airways.[32] In such circumstances, if the respiratory rate is slow enough, air enters and leaves the unit whose airway is obstructed via collateral channels, so that ventilation is not impaired. With increasing rates of respiration, however, there is insufficient time for air to enter and leave during the shorter respiratory cycle; the consequence is impaired ventilation (Figure 3–6).

FLOW-TIME AND FLOW-VOLUME CURVES. Flow-time curves (see Figure 3–3) are recordings of expiratory flow during maximal effort from TLC, plotted against time. Flow-volume curves also measure the forced vital capacity from TLC, but instantaneous expiratory air flow is plotted against lung volume instead of time (Figure 3–7). Since flow rates measured close to RV are believed to reflect the state of the

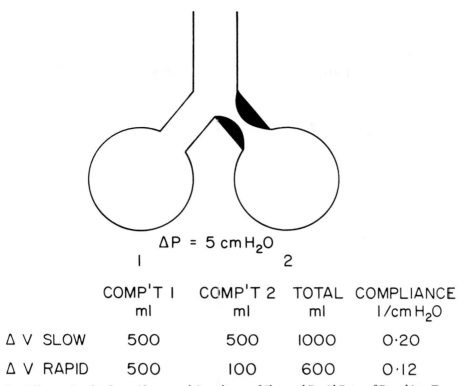

	COMP'T I ml	COMP'T 2 ml	TOTAL ml	COMPLIANCE l/cm H_2O
Δ V SLOW	500	500	1000	0·20
Δ V RAPID	500	100	600	0·12

Figure 3–6. Effect on Total Volume Change and Compliance of Slow and Rapid Rates of Breathing. Two-compartment lung model showing that at slow rates of breathing 500 ml can enter the obstructed compartment just as readily as the unobstructed one, giving a total volume change of 1 liter. However, with rapid breathing insufficient time is available for ventilation of the obstructed compartment and the total change in volume—and hence compliance—falls. ΔP = change in pressure; ΔV = change in volume. (Reprinted from Macklem, P. T.: Med. Clin. North Am., 57:669, 1973, with permission of the author, editor, and publisher.)

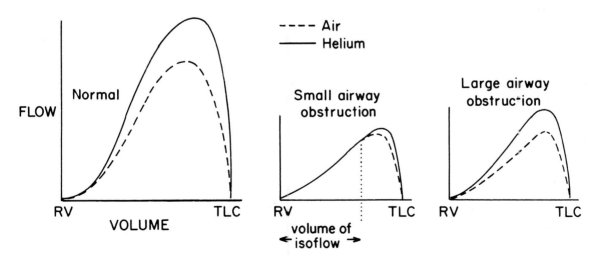

Figure 3–7. Effect on Flow-Volume Curve of Helium Breathing in Patients with Small and Large Airway Obstruction. Expiratory flow-volume curves from a normal subject and from patients with small and large airway obstruction are compared. The improvement in flow that occurs in the normal subject and in the patient with large airway obstruction while breathing helium is not seen in the patient with small airway obstruction; the volume of isoflow is greatly increased in the latter patient. *RV* = residual volume; *TLC* = total lung capacity.

smaller airways, the MMFR obtained from the flow-time curve and flow rates calculated from the flow-volume curve at 75 per cent or less of VC help to detect abnormalities in small airways when other function parameters are normal or near normal.

Comparison of the maximal expiratory flow-volume curves while breathing air and while breathing a mixture of 80 per cent helium and 20 per cent oxygen also is useful in determining the site of airway obstruction.[33] Since gas flow in large airways is chiefly turbulent, and helium reduces turbulence, maximal expiratory flow in both normal subjects and patients with obstructed large airways improves when they breathe this gas. However, since gas flow in small airways is laminar rather than turbulent, patients with obstruction largely confined to these airways show no improvement in the flow-volume curve when breathing helium (Figure 3–7). Using this technique to study age-matched groups of asymptomatic light smokers and non-smokers, Hutcheon and associates[34] found that the volume of isoflow—the point at which flow-volume curves while breathing air and while breathing 80 per cent helium with 20 per cent oxygen come together (Figure 3–7)—most clearly separated the two groups.

CLOSING VOLUME. This has been defined as the lung volume at which dependent lung zones cease to ventilate, presumably because of airway closure. Airway closure occurs at low lung volumes in the dependent lung zones (lung bases) as a result of the gravity-dependent gradient in pleural pressure:[35] pleural pressure is least negative at the lung bases and may even become positive near the end of expiration, allowing dependent portions of the lung to assume minimal volume. Elastic recoil of these deflated regions then may be insufficient to maintain patency of local airways, permitting closure. In disease, premature airway closure and therefore increased closing volume may result from intrinsic small airway disease or loss of lung elastic recoil; the latter may be due to elastic tissue destruction or diminished surfactant or a combination of both.

Two techniques have been proposed for measuring closing volume, both entailing exhalation from TLC to RV and measurement of inert marker gases at the mouth. The bolus technique requires the inhalation from RV of a small amount of helium.[36] Since airways in dependent lung zones are closed at low lung volumes, the inert gas is preferentially distributed to upper lung zones as the patient inspires to TLC;[37] this results in a much higher concen-

tration of gas in upper lung zones, the lower zones being filled with room air or oxygen, whichever is used to complete the inspiration. During the next expiration from TLC, helium is monitored at the mouthpiece and its concentration is plotted against lung volume on an XY recorder.

The other technique commonly used for measuring closing volume is the nitrogen method devised by Anthonisen and his colleagues[38] and based on a modification of Fowler's single-breath nitrogen test[39] (Figures 3–8). As with the other techniques this test begins at RV, at which point the dependent lung parenchyma has a relatively lower volume than the upper lung zones and hence contains less nitrogen. From RV, a single breath of 100 per cent oxygen is inspired to TLC; since all alveoli in the lungs are equally and fully expanded at TLC, more oxygen flows to lower lung zones, diluting the nitrogen already present and creating a concentration gradient for nitrogen between the top and bottom of the lung of approximately 2:1. The patient then expires at a flow rate of about 0.5 liter per sec, the expired gas being sampled close to the mouth with a nitrogen analyzer; the nitrogen concentration is plotted against lung volume on an XY recorder. Phase I of this curve represents the anatomic dead space, which contained 100 per cent oxygen, and phase II is the rapidly increasing nitrogen concentration from mixed alveolar and dead space gas; phase III—the alveolar "plateau"—reflects the nitrogen content of acinar units, with a gradually increasing contribution from upper lung zones. Phase IV, the closing volume, is the curve's final steep slope due to emptying of upper lung zone units; it begins with airway closure in dependent lung zones. Closing volume (CV) can be expressed as the amount of gas from the point of airway closure to RV or as the amount remaining within the lungs from the beginning of phase IV (which would therefore include RV). Alternatively, CV added to RV is known as closing capacity (CC). These measurements usually are represented as percentages of VC and TLC. CC-TLC is more accurate than CV-VC, presumably due to the influence of RV in CC-TLC and the fact that RV increases early with airway obstruction.

SIGNIFICANCE OF ABNORMAL TESTS. These techniques are considered indicators of small airway abnormalities at an "early" stage and are used extensively to screen population groups. The most widely used is the nitrogen single-breath method, mainly because it is less time-consuming and requires less expensive equip-

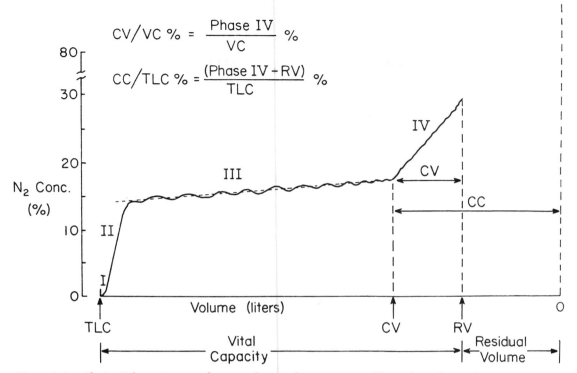

$$CV/VC \% = \frac{Phase\ IV}{VC} \%$$

$$CC/TLC \% = \frac{(Phase\ IV - RV)}{TLC} \%$$

Figure 3–8. Closing Volume. Diagram depicting closing volume as measured by analysis of expired nitrogen concentration after inhalation of a single breath of 100 per cent oxygen from RV to TLC. The presumed point of bronchial closure in dependent lung zones occurs at the point indicated by CV. For further explanation, *see* text.

ment. In all studies to date, predicted normal values for closing volumes show an increase with age, presumably reflecting loss of elastic recoil. Abnormal values have been obtained by a variety of techniques in cigarette smokers and in patients with viral infections or interstitial pulmonary edema. Follow-up studies after correction of the cause has shown a return of values to normal.

When closing volume exceeds FRC, patients manifest impaired gas exchange even at rest and when breathing at TV; this result of VQ inequality is most obvious in the supine position. Grossly obese patients are particularly susceptible to abnormal gas exchange from increased closing volume because of their reduced ERV.

MEASUREMENT OF PERFUSION OF ACINAR UNITS

Measurement of Volume, Flow, and Pressure

Although volume, pressure, and flow of blood in individual acinar units cannot be determined, their values in the lungs as a whole can be measured during catheterization of the right side of the heart. Cardiac output can be measured during catheterization of the right side of the heart. Cardiac output can be measured while the patient is resting or exercising, using the Fick method or dye dilution curves. Instantaneous pulmonary capillary volume (Vc) can be measured by two methods. In the first, the patient inhales a mixture of 80 per cent nitrous oxide and 20 per cent oxygen while seated in a body plethysmograph; the sensitive manometer that records the pressure around the patient shows an abrupt fall as nitrous oxide leaves the acini to dissolve in the blood. Carbon monoxide is used in the second method to measure diffusion; the membrane component can be separated from that due to the blood, and the Vc can be estimated.[40]

Measurement of the Distribution of Capillary Blood Flow

Methods for determining the distribution of pulmonary capillary blood make use of a radioactive gas, such as xenon; this is injected and its regional distribution throughout the lungs is measured by scintillation counters placed over the chest wall. Radioactive carbon dioxide, which is inhaled, can be used similarly.

MEASUREMENT OF THE DIFFUSION OF GAS IN ACINAR UNITS

The diffusing capacity for carbon monoxide (DL_{CO}) is computed as follows:

$$DL_{CO} = \frac{\text{ml of CO taken up by capillary blood}}{\text{mean alveolar } P_{CO} - \text{mean capillary } P_{CO}}$$

The amount of carbon monoxide taken up by capillary blood is calculated by subtracting volume × CO concentration of expired gas from volume × CO concentration of inspired gas. Determination of the denominator of this equation is more subject to error in cases of lung diseases. In normal subjects, a sample of gas expired at the end of tidal volume reflects accurately the mean alveolar P_{CO}, and, since the normal mean capillary P_{CO} is so small that it can be ignored, the diffusing capacity can be calculated reliably. However, in diseased lungs which have relatively underventilated areas that empty late, the normal sharp division between dead space gas and alveolar gas is lost and the end tidal sample does not necessarily represent the mean alveolar P_{CO}.

Several techniques for use with carbon monoxide have been devised for measuring diffusing capacity. The main differences between these techniques are the length of time the carbon monoxide is kept in the lungs and the methods of determining mean alveolar P_{CO}. The single-breath method entails the inhalation of a gas that contains minute quantities of carbon monoxide followed by breath-holding for 10 seconds. It is useful for screening, particularly in patients with unimpaired distribution of inhaled gas. The steady-state technique requires inhalation of the carbon monoxide gas mixture for several breaths, until alveolar P_{CO} remains constant. In addition to diffusing capacity, fractional removal of carbon monoxide is calculated from the end tidal sample; this confirms the accuracy of the diffusing capacity value, since both decrease simultaneously in most cases.

The fractional uptake of carbon monoxide is the amount removed divided by the amount inspired. Thus:

$$\text{CO uptake (\%)} = \frac{\text{CO inspired} - \text{CO expired}}{\text{CO inspired}}$$

During hyperventilation, fractional carbon dioxide uptake may decrease, but the diffusing capacity is unchanged. During hypoventilation, however, the diffusing capacity may be reduced due to a very low tidal volume, whereas fractional carbon monoxide uptake decreases to a lesser extent. Although this measurement has proved of some use in validating steady-state diffusing capacity, it is worthless as a screening test for chronic respiratory disease. Diffusing capacity during exercise can be determined by the steady-state method. However, an end tidal sample obtained in these circumstances is not reliable; and since the numerator of the equation for calculating the diffusing capacity for carbon monoxide becomes the chief determinant, in such instances it is valid to calculate alveolar P_{CO} from the inspired and expired carbon monoxide concentrations, assuming a value for the respiratory dead space.

The diffusing capacity reflects not only the thickness of the alveolocapillary membrane but also the total area of this membrane and the hemoglobin content of the pulmonary capillary blood. Removal of a lobe or an entire lung reduces the overall diffusing area. Inequality in the ventilation-perfusion ratio results in decreased diffusing capacity, because less carbon monoxide is taken up by poorly ventilated or poorly perfused areas than by areas with normal perfusion and ventilation. Since the uptake of carbon monoxide by capillary blood is due mainly to its great affinity for hemoglobin, in cases of anemia the diffusing capacity is reduced because of lack of hemoglobin.

Thus, despite the relative simplicity of the measurement of diffusion with carbon monoxide, it does not differentiate "true diffusion defects" from shunts or ventilation-perfusion inequalities.

MEASUREMENT OF MATCHING OF BLOOD FLOW AND VENTILATION

Measurement of Distribution of Inspired Air

Poorly ventilated acinar units receive less oxygen from a single deep breath of 100 per cent oxygen and empty later during the next expiration than well-ventilated acini. This is the rationale of the single-breath 100 per cent oxygen test with continuous analysis by nitrogen meter of expired air.[41] After a single inspiration of 100 per cent oxygen, the first part of the expiration contains 100 per cent oxygen, which comes from the dead space. Next, the expired gas comes from the acini; if these empty synchronously and are equally ventilated the nitrogen meter curve shows a horizontal line throughout the rest of the expiration. Poorly ventilated acini receive smaller amounts of oxygen and empty late so that during the next complete expiration the nitrogen curve slopes upward as it records their contribution. A modification of this method is used to determine closing volume (*see* Figure 3–8).

Another method for determining the distribution of inspired gas uses a helium closed-circuit apparatus; the result is expressed as mixing efficiency (ME). This apparatus also can be used to calculate lung volumes, including RV. The patient is connected to the circuit and breathes from a spirometer containing helium;[42] the concentration of expired gas is measured by a katharometer, and the distribution is determined by recording the number of breaths taken before the helium concentration remains steady.

Measurement of Distribution of Pulmonary Capillary Blood

Uneven distribution of pulmonary capillary blood despite relatively uniform ventilation can be detected when large areas of lung are unperfused. The alveolar PCO_2, determined by analysis of a sample of expired gas taken at the end of tidal volume (end tidal) or at the end of maximal expiration (end expiratory), is compared with the arterial PCO_2. A difference of greater than 6 mm Hg indicates large numbers of unperfused acini; the expired gas from these areas contains no carbon dioxide and, therefore, decreases the PCO_2 of the total sample of gas. This measurement becomes less accurate with the development of compensatory mechanisms that decrease ventilation to unperfused areas and divert inspired air to areas that are well perfused.

Measurement of Inequality of Ventilation-Perfusion Ratios

Unlike the single-breath method, which utilizes an inert gas that measures the distribution of inspired air only, continuous analysis of a single expiration with a carbon dioxide analyzer gives information pertaining to both ventilation and perfusion and their uniformity. A rise in the carbon dioxide concentration throughout expiration indicates perfusion of poorly ventilated areas that empty late in the expiratory phase.

Radionuclides are being used increasingly in the study of lung function. Regional ventilation-perfusion inequality in the lungs can be measured with radioactive oxygen and carbon dioxide and with ^{133}Xe. Xenon is particularly useful for demonstrating relatively normal ventilation in unperfused areas secondary to pulmonary embolism and for measuring closing volume. The clinical application of radioactive gas in the study of pulmonary function is somewhat limited by the highly complex and expensive equipment required, the time involved, and the need for technical expertise.

MEASUREMENT OF BLOOD GASES AND H$^+$ ION CONCENTRATION

Arterial blood can be obtained almost as easily as venous blood. Brachial or radial arteries are preferred to femoral arteries, which should be punctured only as a last resort. Since arteries are deeper than veins they are more evasive; therefore, the area should be infiltrated with local anesthetic, which serves the double purpose of reducing pain and vasospasm. Significant morbidity as a result of arterial puncture is rare; in our laboratories we have never encountered a serious complication after many thousands of percutaneous punctures, mainly of the radial artery, although clinical sequelae of puncture of other arteries appear to be commoner.[43]

The Van Slyke method of measuring oxygen content and oxygen capacity of arterial blood is still used in modern pulmonary function laboratories as a yardstick of the accuracy of newer methods. In our routine laboratory we use a spectrophotometric method to determine arterial oxygen saturation and simultaneously measure arterial blood PO_2 with an electrode. This assessment of arterial blood oxygen by two methods is useful for detecting technical errors, the accuracy of values being ascertained by reference to the oxygen dissociation curve. The results of blood gas analysis can be interpreted with tables and graphs that quantify shuntlike effects. In 1973 Mays[44] published normal values for arterial blood gas tension during rest, voluntary breath-holding, and maximal voluntary hyperventilation; reference to a diagram provides a simple, rapid, clinical method of estimating the severity of blood gas disturbances that reflect $\dot{V}/\dot{Q}$ mismatching at any physiologic level of alveolar ventilation (Figure 3–9).

PCO_2 and H$^+$ ion concentration also can be measured with electrodes. It is essential that the accuracy of these delicate instruments be checked periodically by duplicate measurement with an Astrup apparatus.

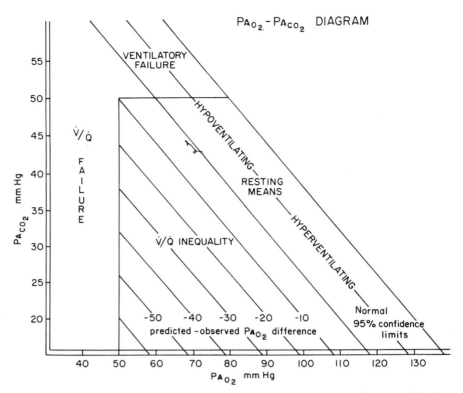

Figure 3–9. $P_{A_{O_2}}$-$P_{A_{CO_2}}$ Diagram. To use, plot patient value (resting, exercising or hyperventilating) on appropriate intercept. Values which indicate $\dot{V}/\dot{Q}$ disturbance are quantitated by reference to the slanting isopleths to left of, and paralleling, the normal regression slope. Degree of $\dot{V}/\dot{Q}$ disturbance is expressed in millimeters of mercury predicted-observed $P_{A_{O_2}}$ difference, at the level of alveolar ventilation reflected by the observed $P_{A_{CO_2}}$. Normal and failure zones are self-explanatory. (Reprinted from Mays, E. E.: Chest, 63:793, 1973, with permission of the author and editor.)

VENTILATORY RESPONSE

Interest in the sensitivity of the respiratory center has largely centered on its response to CO_2, and particularly on the great individual variation. Response usually is represented as change in ventilation with increments of arterial P_{CO_2} (or end tidal P_{CO_2}) as the patient breathes increasing concentrations of carbon dioxide. Rebuck and Read,[45] who explored the limits of normality by performing studies of ventilatory response to CO_2 in 17 outstanding athletes, found a fourteen-fold range, from 0.57 to 8.17 liters per min per mm Hg P_{CO_2}. Rebuck and Campbell[46] found a similar intersubject range in response to hypoxia; further, subjects who failed to respond to hypoxia also showed no response to hypercapnia.

Methods

Ventilatory response to CO_2 can be measured with a steady-state method by adding various concentrations of the gas to the inspired mixture, and minute ventilation is measured when the arterial or end tidal P_{CO_2} has reached a plateau. In a simpler but equally effective method, the patient rebreathes from a 4- or 5-liter bag that contains 50 per cent oxygen and enough carbon dioxide to make the Pa_{CO_2} equivalent to the P_{CO_2} of mixed venous blood. With this technique, P_{CO_2} equilibrium is rapidly established between mixed venous blood, arterial blood, and end expiratory gas. Response curves relating ventilation to end expiratory P_{CO_2} or arterial P_{CO_2}, which are linear, are reproducible by this method.

The ventilatory response to hypoxia can be assessed by a similar method in which end tidal P_{CO_2} is kept constant in the rebreathing bag at "mixed venous" level.[46] Studies with this method in normal subjects show that the ventilatory response to decreasing P_{O_2} in inspired gas is linear and is reproducible.

Another method of measuring respiratory center drive is to determine phrenic nerve activity. Lourenço and Miranda[47] determined electromyographic activity of the diaphragm in normal subjects and those with bronchitis while rebreathing, using a bipolar lead introduced via the esophagus to the level of the diaphragm. They found decreased diaphragmatic activity in some patients with chronic obstructive lung disease. The increase in neuronal discharge produced by a given rise of $PaCO_2$ was reduced at least tenfold in those with hypercapnia compared with normal subjects, suggesting markedly decreased respiratory center sensitivity.

Because of its simplicity and reliability, perhaps the most promising procedure for evaluating respiratory center output is the measurement of inspiratory pressure at the time of sudden airway occlusion. This index of ventilatory drive (change in pressure/change in PCO_2) correlates significantly with ventilatory response to carbon dioxide and degree of airway obstruction.

Significance of Variation in Ventilatory Drive

Rarely, a primary defect in sensitivity of the respiratory center causes hypoxemia and carbon dioxide retention. This appears to be the mechanism involved in chronic hypoventilation in some obese patients and particularly in cases of CO_2 retention in nonobese polycythemic and hypoxemic patients. However, the classic example of a chronic hypoventilator who fails to respond adequately to increasing concentrations of inspired carbon dioxide is the patient with obstructive pulmonary disease. Many studies have shown that added airway resistance in normal subjects or in patients with chronic obstructive pulmonary disease reduces the ventilatory response to CO_2. However, correlation between degree of air flow obstruction and ventilatory response is poor, and some patients with severe air flow obstruction have a relatively good ventilatory response and normal PCO_2. This lack of relationship between ventilatory drive and FEV_1 has led to the conclusion that constitutional variation in respiratory center sensitivity may be the major determinant of CO_2 retention when there is airway obstruction. Certainly the wide range of response to CO_2 in normal subjects supports this hypothesis. Nevertheless, obstructive lung disease reduces the ventilatory results of a given amount of respiratory muscle work and modifies the ventilatory response to CO_2.

EXERCISE TESTING

Although most patients with cardiac and respiratory disease have no symptoms until stressed by exertion, they seldom are assessed physiologically in the laboratory by exercise testing. This is understandable, since clinical findings or pulmonary function measurements at rest usually provide sufficient information for diagnosis. A thorough evaluation of pathophysiology during exercise is usually time-consuming and requires exceptional technical expertise and intricate, expensive equipment that needs careful maintenance. Nevertheless, the clinician is faced with a significant number of patients whose problems cannot be properly understood without exercise testing.

There are two situations in which physiologic data while exercising are essential: (1) when the patient complains of dyspnea on exertion, has normal pulmonary function values, and the clinical data do not indicate the pathogenesis of this symptom; and (2) to assess physiologic disability objectively in order to determine the value of a planned training program.

A few patients with bronchospastic disease fail to show abnormal physical findings and pulmonary dysfunction at rest. In such instances, resistance measurements immediately after specific exercise provide valuable information. An even more perplexing problem is the patient with absent or equivocal evidence of cardiac and pulmonary disability whose dyspnea on effort is not clearly attributable to malfunction of the heart or lungs. Management of such patients requires knowledge of the mechanism of dyspnea, and Campbell has aptly questioned the ethics of prescribing or proscribing the physical activity of such patients without first determining their capabilities under exercise conditions.

Physical training programs for disabled patients with chronic obstructive pulmonary disease are being carried out in many centers. Although undoubtedly some of the benefit is psychological, careful studies have indicated physiologic improvement as well; each case must be assessed objectively to determine whether continuation of the program is warranted.

Direct measurement of maximal oxygen uptake is the classic test of physical fitness. In untrained, unhealthy, and older subjects, it is preferable to carry out submaximal testing, the patient being studied during two or more workloads on a cycle ergometer. The maximal oxygen uptake can be obtained by extrapolating the relationship to the predicted maximal heart rate. Most clinical physiologists in this field advocate a simple screening test first, followed by more complicated procedures if the results of screening indicate the need.[48] The stage 1 exercise testing proposed by Jones[48] consists of gradually increasing workload while heart rate and minute ventilation are measured and the electrocardiograph is monitored; the degree of tachycardia and minute ventilation are compared with normal values for each workload. If the results of stage 1 testing indicate a need for further information, more complicated studies can be carried out. Stage 2 is performed in a steady state at one or more workloads. Tidal volume CO_2 output, oxygen intake, respiratory exchange ratio, mixed expired PCO_2, end tidal PCO_2, and mixed venous PCO_2 are determined, in addition to heart rate, ventilation, and respiratory rate. These data not only define the state of respiratory function while under stress but also reflect cardiac function and the degree of anaerobic muscle metabolism. Stage 3 exercise testing is identical to stage 2 with the addition of direct arterial blood sampling.

Exercise testing in asthmatics is best carried out on a treadmill or, even more simply, after running or walking rapidly through corridors or up stairs; flow rates are measured at the height of dyspnea and during the next 15 to 20 minutes.

Some patients who complain of dyspnea perform normally on exercise testing, with appropriate increase in heart rate and ventilation. In these circumstances symptoms may be psychological or due to obesity or poor physical condition. Such patients can be reassured and encouraged to lose weight and follow a specific physical conditioning program. When heart rate and ventilation are inappropriate to the workload, additional pertinent information can be obtained from measurement of cardiac output and the behavior of blood gases under exercise conditions. As a general rule, an inappropriate degree of tachycardia is an index of primary cardiac disease, whereas excessive minute ventilation correlates more closely with impaired lung function.

REFERENCES

1. Bates, D. V., Macklem, P. T., and Christie, R. V.: Respiratory Function in Disease; An Introduction to the Integrated Study of the Lung, 2nd ed. Philadelphia, W. B. Saunders Co., 1971.
2. Rice, R. L.: Symptom patterns of the hyperventilation syndrome. Am. J. Med., 8:691, 1950.
3. Lichstein, E., and Seckler, S. G.: Evaluation of acute chest pain. Med. Clin. North Am., 57:1481, 1973.
4. Crocco, J. A., Rooney, J. J., Fankushen, D. S., Di-Benedetto, R. J., and Lyons, H. A.: Massive hemoptysis. Arch. Intern. Med., 121:495, 1968.
5. Forgacs, P., Nathoo, A. R., and Richardson, H. D.: Breath sounds. Thorax, 26:288, 1971.
6. Hamman, L.: Spontaneous mediastinal emphysema. Bull. Johns Hopkins Hosp., 64:1, 1939.
7. Scadding, J. G., and Wood, P.: Systolic clicks due to left-sided pneumothorax. Lancet, 2:1208, 1939.
8. Semple, T., and Lancaster, W. M.: Noisy pneumothorax: Observations based on 24 cases. Br. Med. J., 1:1342, 1961.
9. Kelman, G. R., and Nunn, J. F.: Clinical recognition of hypoxaemia under fluorescent lamps. Lancet, 1:1400, 1966.
10. Martiny, O., Berson, S. D., Solomon, A., Collins, T. F. B., and Webster, I.: An evaluation of needle punch biopsy specimens in the diagnosis of diffuse lung disease. Am. Rev. Resp. Dis., 107:209, 1973.
11. Kinsey, J. H., Cortese, D. A., and Sanderson, D. R.: Detection of hematoporphyrin fluorescence during fiberoptic bronchoscopy to localized early bronchogenic carcinoma. Mayo Clin. Proc., 53:594, 1978.
12. Hájek, M., and Homan van der Heide, J. N.: Early detection of mediastinal spread of pulmonary carcinoma by mediastinoscopy. Thorax, 25:720, 1970.
13. Pecora, D. V.: A comparison of transtracheal aspiration with other methods of determining the bacterial flora of the lower respiratory tract. N. Engl. J. Med., 269:664, 1963.
14. Laurenzi, G. A., Potter, R. T., and Kass, E. H.: Bacteriologic flora of the lower respiratory tract. N. Engl. J. Med., 265:1273, 1961.
15. Lapinski, E. M., Flakas, E. D., and Taylor, B. C.: An evaluation of some methods for culturing sputum from patients with bronchitis and emphysema. Am. Rev. Resp. Dis., 89:760, 1964.
16. Buechner, H. A., Seabury, J. H., Campbell, C. C., Georg, L. K., Kaufman, L., and Kaplan, W.: The current status of serologic, immunologic and skin tests in the diagnosis of pulmonary mycoses. Report of the committee on fungus diseases and subcommittee on criteria for clinical diagnosis—American College of Chest Physicians. Chest, 63:259, 1973.
17. Leading article: Tuberculin anergy. Br. Med. J., 4:573, 1970.
18. Comstock, G. W., Furcolow, M. L., Greenberg, R. A., Grzybowski, S., MacLean, R. A., Baer, H., and Edwards, P. Q.: The tuberculin skin test: A statement by the Committee on Diagnostic Skin Testing, American Thoracic Society. Am. Rev. Resp. Dis., 104:769, 1971.
19. Schachter, E. N.: Tuberculin negative tuberculosis. Am. Rev. Resp. Dis., 106:587, 1972.
20. Hyde, L.: Clinical significance of the tuberculin skin test. Am. Rev. Resp. Dis., 105:453, 1972.
21. Holden, M., Dubin, M. R., and Diamond, P. H.: Frequency of negative intermediate-strength tuberculin sensitivity in patients with active tuberculosis. N. Engl. J. Med., 285:1506, 1971.
22. Light, R. W., MacGregor, M. I., Luchsinger, P. C., and Ball, W. C., Jr.: Pleural effusions: The diagnostic separation of transudates and exudates. Ann. Intern. Med., 77:507, 1972.
23. Leuallen, E. C., and Carr, D. J.: Pleural effusion. A statistical study of 436 patients. N. Engl. J. Med., 252:79, 1955.
24. Light, R. W., and Ball, W. C., Jr.: Glucose and amylase in pleural effusions. J.A.M.A., 225:257, 1973.
25. Busey, J. F., Fenger, E. P. K., Hepper, N. G., Kent, D. C., Kilburn, K. H., Matthews, L. W., Simpson, D. G., and Grzybowski, S.: Therapy of pleural effusion. A statement by the Committee on Therapy.

American Thoracic Society. Medical Section of the National Tuberculosis Association. Am. Rev. Resp Dis., 97:479, 1968.

26. McKerrow, C. B.: The McKesson Vitalor. J.A.M.A. 177:865, 1961.

27. Harris, T. R., Pratt, P. C., and Kilburn, K. H.: Total lung capacity measured by roentgenograms. Am. J. Med., 50:756, 1971.

28. Collier, C. R.: Determination of mixed venous CO_2 tensions by rebreathing. J. Appl. Physiol., 9:25, 1956.

29. Macklem, P. T., and Mead, J.: Resistance of central and peripheral airways measured by a retrograde catheter. J. Appl. Physiol., 22:395, 1967.

30. Macklem, P. T.: The pathophysiology of chronic bronchitis and emphysema. Med. Clin. North Am., 57:669, 1973.

31. Mead, J.: The lung's "quiet zone." (Editorial). N. Engl. J. Med., 282:1318, 1970.

32. Woolcock, A. J., Vincent, N. J., and Macklem, P. T.: Frequency dependence of compliance as a test for obstruction in the small airways. J. Clin. Invest., 48:1097, 1969.

33. Despas, P. J., Leroux, M., and Macklem, P. T.: Site of airway obstruction in asthma as determined by measuring maximal expiratory flow breathing air and a helium-oxygen mixture. J. Clin. Invest., 51:3235, 1972.

34. Hutcheon, M., Griffin, P., Levison, H., and Zamel, N.: Volume of isoflow. A new test in detection of mild abnormalities of lung mechanics. Am. Rev. Resp. Dis., 110:458, 1974.

35. Anthonisen, N. R., Robertson, P. C., and Ross, W. R. D.: Gravity-dependent sequential emptying of lung regions. J. Appl. Physiol., 28:589, 1970.

36. Green, M., Travis, D. M., and Mead, J.: A simple measurement of phase IV ("closing volume") using a critical orifice helium analyzer. J. Appl. Physiol., 33:827, 1972.

37. Milic-Emili, J., Henderson, J. A. M., Dolovich, M. B., Trop, D., and Kaneko, K.: Regional distribution of inspired gas in the lung. J. Appl. Physiol., 21:749, 1966.

38. Anthonisen, N. R., Danson, J., Robertson, P. C., and Ross, W. R. D.: Airway closure as a function of age. Resp. Physiol., 8:58, 1969–70.

39. Fowler, W. S.: Lung function studies. III. Uneven pulmonary ventilation in normal subjects and in patients with pulmonary disease. J. Appl. Physiol., 2:283, 1949.

40. Roughton, F. J. W., and Forster, R. E.: Relative importance of diffusion and chemical reaction rates in determining rate of exchange of gases in the human lung, with special reference to true diffusing capacity of pulmonary membrane and volume of blood in the lung capillaries. J. Appl. Physiol., 11:290, 1957.

41. Comroe, J. H., Jr., and Fowler, W. S.: Lung function studies. VI. Detection of uneven alveolar ventilation during a single breath of oxygen. Am. J. Med., 10:408, 1951.

42. Bates, D. V., Woolf, C. R., and Paul, G. I.: Chronic bronchitis: A report on the first two stages of the coordinated study of chronic bronchitis in the Department of Veterans Affairs, Canada. Med. Ser. J. Can., 18:211, 1962.

43. Mortensen, J. D.: Clinical sequelae from arterial needle puncture, cannulation, and incision. Circulation. 35:1118, 1967.

44. Mays, E. E.: An arterial blood gas diagram for clinical use. Chest, 63:793, 1973.

45. Rebuck, A. S., and Read, J.: Patterns of ventilatory response to carbon dioxide during recovery from severe asthma. Clin. Sci., 41:13, 1971.

46. Rebuck, A. S., and Campbell, E. J. M.: A clinical method for assessing the ventilatory response to hypoxia. Am. Rev. Resp. Dis., 109:345, 1974.

47. Lourenço, R. V., and Miranda, J. M.: Drive and performance of the ventilatory apparatus in chronic obstructive lung disease. N. Engl. J. Med., 279:53, 1968.

48. Jones, N. L.: Exercise testing. Br. J. Dis. Chest, 61:169, 1967.

4

Roentgenologic Signs in the Diagnosis of Chest Disease

The integration of information obtained from systematic interpretation of the chest roentgenogram and careful analysis of the clinical status of the patient yields a high degree of diagnostic accuracy in most chest diseases. However, although the final assessment must take into account the patient's history, physical examination, laboratory tests, and pulmonary function studies, the physician should glean as much information as possible from an objective assessment of the roentgenogram *before* attempting clinical correlation. A roentgenographic pattern of disease may be sufficiently distinctive that an etiologic diagnosis can be made with reasonable certainty on that evidence alone; confirmation will depend upon whether the roentgenologic conclusions and the clinical picture can be reconciled.

The roentgenographic characteristics of specific disease entities are given in the relevant chapters. This chapter describes *basic roentgen signs* as they indicate the *fundamental nature* of disease. It is subdivided into three major sections: increased roentgenographic density, decreased roentgenographic density, and diseases of the pleura.

LUNG DISEASES THAT INCREASE ROENTGENOGRAPHIC DENSITY

In essence, the lung consists of two main functioning tissues: that for *conduction* (bronchi, blood vessels, and lymphatics) and that for *gaseous exchange* (acini, or lung parenchyma, made up of peripheral air spaces, extravascular interstitial tissue, and capillaries) (Figure 4–1). Excluding the vascular system, it is obvious that all pulmonary disease that increases density in the lung periphery involves change in one or both of two components, the air spaces and extravascular interstitial tissue. Although most diseases that affect the acinus so as to produce an increase in roentgenographic density involve *both* the air spaces and interstitial tissue to a variable extent, it is helpful to divide these diseases into three general groups, *depending upon which component is predominantly affected:*

1. *Air spaces.* The air may be replaced either by tissue or by fluid (consolidation) or absorbed and not replaced (atelectasis).
2. *Interstitial tissues.*
3. *Total acinus* (combined air spaces and interstitial tissues).

PREDOMINANTLY AIR-SPACE DISEASE

PARENCHYMAL CONSOLIDATION

In this situation the air within the acinus is *replaced* by liquid or tissue, the result being *consolidation* of the parenchyma (Figure 4–2). Typically, many contiguous acini are involved, producing uniform shadows of increased density varying in size from a few centimeters to a whole lobe. Sometimes, however, *individual shadows* approximately 7 mm in diameter can be identified that coincide roughly with the size and configuration of single acini and are a distinctive feature of air-space consolidation.

The Acinar Shadow

Since the acinus is a unit of parenchymal structure approximately 7 mm in diameter (*see* page 15, Chapter 1), it can be assumed that replacing its air with liquid or tissue of unit density would result in a roentgenographic shadow approximately 7 mm in diameter, fairly

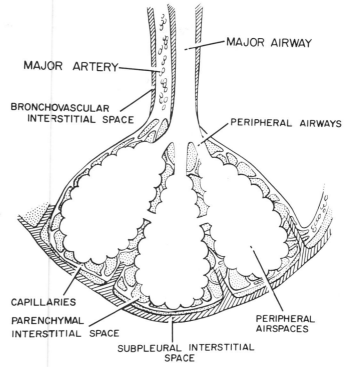

Figure 4–1.   Diagrammatic Representation of the Lung. This diagram depicts the components of the lung that are involved in the majority of pulmonary diseases—the large and small airways, the peripheral air spaces (including communicating channels), the arteries, veins, and capillaries, and the bronchovascular, subpleural, and parenchymal interstitial space. Throughout the chapter this diagrammatic representation of the normal lung is reproduced alongside diagrams depicting disturbances in morphology.

well circumscribed, and with a slightly irregular contour. In diffuse diseases of the lung characterized by air-space consolidation (*e.g.*, acute pulmonary edema and idiopathic pulmonary hemorrhage [Figure 4–3]), in many cases one or more discrete acinar shadows can be seen,

although confluence precludes visualization of individual acini in most areas of the lungs. Groups of confluent acinar shadows are often separated by normal air-containing parenchyma, creating a pattern of numerous "fluffy," rather poorly defined shadows throughout the

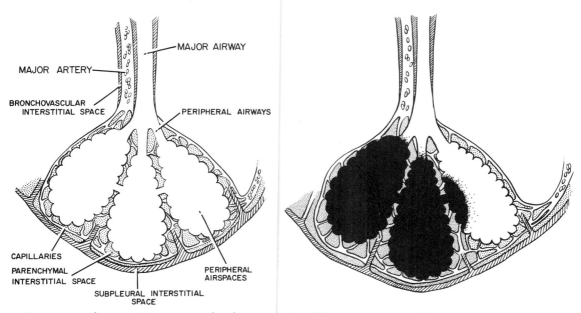

Figure 4–2.   The Lung Diagram: Peripheral Air-space Consolidation. Exudate has filled two of the air spaces and is flowing into the third via pores of Kohn. Volume is unaffected, and the airways are patent. The parenchymal interstitial tissue is increased in amount around the consolidated air spaces.

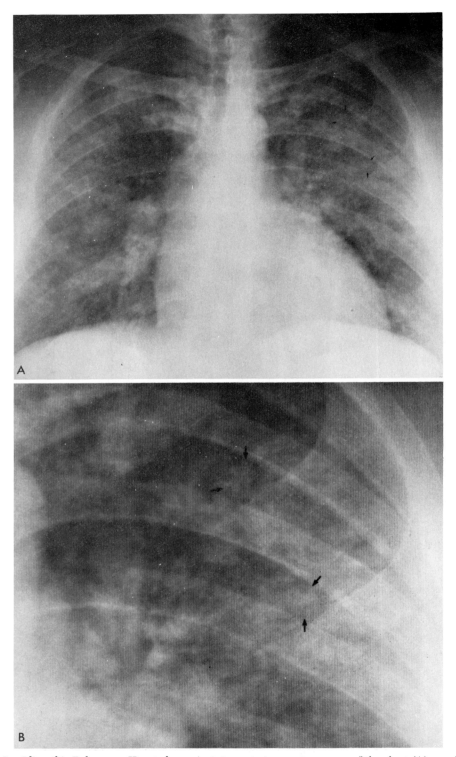

Figure 4–3. Idiopathic Pulmonary Hemorrhage. A posteroanterior roentgenogram of the chest (A) reveals extensive air-space consolidation throughout both lungs, confluent in many areas but patchy in others, permitting identification of individual acinar shadows (B, arrows).

lung. The overall picture may suggest an inhomogeneous consolidation, and it is important to recognize that *each individual group* of acinar lesions is homogeneous—an observation that establishes the true nature of the underlying pathology. In localized diseases, such as acute diplococcal pneumonia or exudative tuberculosis, acinar shadows are confluent, so that the density is more or less homogeneous throughout but may have, at its borders, occasional acinar shadows whose margins are either completely surrounded by air-containing lung or only partly obscured by the consolidation.

Obviously, identification of an acinar shadow establishes the *anatomic location* of a disease process, *not* its mechanism of production, and extends the differential diagnosis to a multitude of diseases of varying pathogenesis that characteristically produce acinar consolidation, such as acute alveolar edema, bleeding into the acini, aspiration of blood or lipid, certain primary lung neoplasms, and idiopathic conditions such as alveolar proteinosis.

Each of these is capable of producing acinar

shadows; once the anatomic location has been established, analysis of the pattern and distribution of roentgenographic changes should reduce the number of differential diagnostic possibilities to relatively few entities and occasionally will permit confident diagnosis; when this is not possible from objective evidence alone, correlation with clinical information usually leads to a positive diagnosis.

Nonsegmental Distribution

A characteristic feature of diseases associated with air-space consolidation is failure to respect segmental boundaries. In widely disseminated disease, such as acute pulmonary edema, lack of segmental distribution is not unexpected. Even in localized disease, however, intersegmental spread occurs; for example, in acute diplococcal pneumonia, infection is propagated centrifugally via the pores of Kohn or other channels of collateral drift (Figure 4–4).[1] Since segment boundaries do not impede the passage of air or fluid via these pores, the exudate of

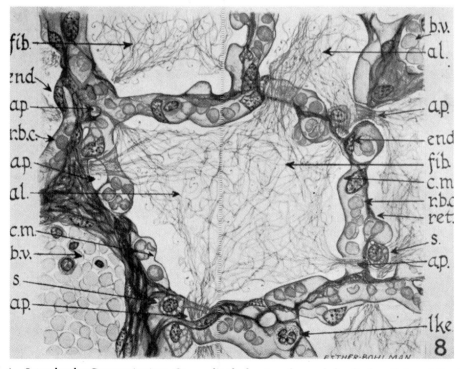

Figure 4–4. Interalveolar Communications. Camera lucida drawing of several alveoli of a rat's lung following injection of sterile heparinized plasma into the bronchial tree. Fibrin threads can be seen to be passing through several pores of Kohn. Key to labels: *al.*, alveolar space; *a.p.*, alveolar pore; *a.ph.*, alveolar phagocyte; *b.v.*, blood vessel; *cap.*, blood capillary; *c.m.*, capillary membrane; *end.*, endothelial cell of capillary; *fib.*, fibrin network; *L.*, lymphocyte; *lke.*, granular leukocyte; *r.b.c.*, red blood cell; *ret.*, reticulum; *s.*, septal cell. (From Loosli, C. G.: A.M.A. Arch. Pathol., 24:743, 1937.)

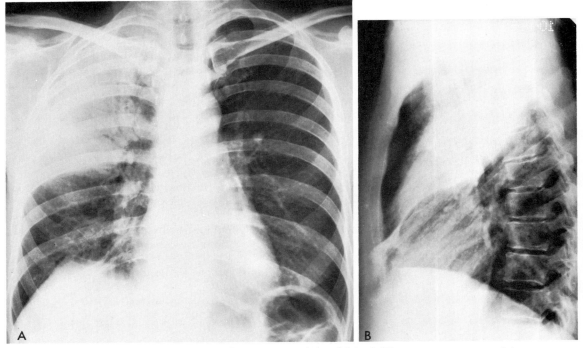

Figure 4–5. Acute Air-space Pneumonia. Posteroanterior *(A)* and lateral *(B)* roentgenograms reveal homogeneous consolidation of the right upper lobe (heavy growth of *S. pneumoniae* from the sputum); a well-defined air bronchogram is present. There is no loss of volume and, in fact, the upper half of the chief fissure is bulged slightly posteriorly. The anterior (retrosternal) portion of the lobe is unaffected, in keeping with the nonsegmental character of acute air-space pneumonia. (From Fraser, R. G., and Wortzman, G.: J. Can. Assoc. Radiol., *10:*37, 1959.)

acute alveolar pneumonia can spread throughout the lung periphery (Figure 4–5). Consequently, such diseases do not conform precisely to bronchopulmonary segments, an observation of major importance in establishing the pathogenesis of the disease process and thereby in arriving at an etiologic diagnosis.[2, 3]

The Air Bronchogram

Consolidation of the lung parenchyma, with little or no involvement of conducting airways, creates another important roentgenographic sign. In acute alveolar pneumonia, for example, consolidation usually begins in subpleural parenchyma (Figure 4–6), the exudate rapidly spreading centrifugally to surround bronchi and bronchioles as it advances toward the hilum. Since the consolidation is entirely parenchymal, air in the bronchi is not displaced. This produces contrast between the air within the bronchial tree and the surrounding airless parenchyma, so that the normally invisible bronchial air column becomes roentgenographically visible (Figure 4–5). Two situations must exist for an air bronchogram to be visualized: the airways

must be air-containing (the bronchus cannot be completely occluded at its origin), and surrounding lung parenchyma must be of markedly reduced air content or *airless*. Since the parenchyma may be airless when its air has been *replaced* by fluid or tissue (consolidation) or when it has been *absorbed* and *not replaced* (atelectasis), an air bronchogram may be seen in either circumstance *but only when the supplying bronchus is not occluded.* As discussed in the next section, there are four mechanisms that may cause atelectasis, the commonest being obstruction of a supplying bronchus; in such circumstances an air bronchogram cannot exist, since the distal parenchyma no longer communicates with the mouth. In the other three types of atelectasis—relaxation, cicatrization, and adhesive—no bronchus is occluded, and since the parenchyma surrounding air-containing bronchi is of reduced air content or airless, an air bronchogram is anticipated. In fact, "pure" interstitial lung disease of sufficient severity can be associated with a prominent air bronchogram.

When only a small volume of lung parenchyma is consolidated, in some cases one may

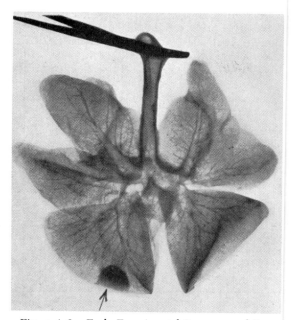

Figure 4–6. Early Experimental Pneumococcal Pneumonia. Roentgenogram of the excised lungs of a dog removed 1 hour after intrabronchial injection of 0.5 ml type 1 *S. pneumoniae* culture. The consolidation is subpleural in location *(arrow)* and is still situated within the confines of the segment into which the culture was injected. Its rounded margin indicates centrifugal spread, however, and suggests that the inflammatory exudate soon will extend beyond the segmental boundary. (From Robertson, O. H., Coggeshall, L. T., and Terrell, E. E.: J. Clin. Invest., *12*:467, 1933.)

visualize small branching airways whose diameter identifies them as bronchioles rather than bronchi; in such circumstances, the term "air bronchiologram" is appropriate. Like the air bronchogram, it signifies airlessness of surrounding parenchyma; it may be apparent in both consolidative processes and diseases in which atelectasis predominates (*e.g.*, hyaline membrane disease of the newborn).

In summary, regardless of its etiology, any pathologic process associated with an air bronchogram or air bronchiologram must fulfill three critiera: (1) it must be anatomically situated within the lung parenchyma; (2) the parenchyma must be completely or almost airless as a result of consolidation or atelectasis or both; and (3) the lumen of the bronchus leading to the affected parenchyma must not be totally occluded.

Absence of Collapse

In acinar consolidation, absence of volume loss is understandable when one considers the pathogenesis of these processes. In the first place, air in the acini is replaced by an equal or almost equal quantity of liquid or tissue. Second, since the process is predominantly parenchymal, airways leading to affected portions of lung remain patent; thus there is no reason for collapse before exudate fills the air spaces. Again there are occasional exceptions to this rule; for example, pulmonary infarction, in which volume may be decreased by causes other than airway obstruction.

In summary, therefore, the roentgenologic signs associated with air-space (acinar) consolidation are as follows.

1. The acinar shadow.

2. Relatively homogeneous density when acinar consolidation is confluent.

3. The air bronchogram (or air bronchiologram).

4. Nonsegmental distribution.

5. Negligible collapse.

PARENCHYMAL ATELECTASIS

In its pure form atelectasis may be regarded conceptually as the antithesis of consolidation: in the former, air is absorbed and not replaced, and in the latter, air is replaced by fluid or tissue of approximately equal volume. Thus, from a roentgenologic point of view, the major difference is one of volume: in consolidation, volume is normal; in atelectasis, it is reduced.

The terminology of pulmonary atelectasis is controversial. We prefer to use the word in its broad sense—to denote *diminished air within the lung associated with reduced lung volume.* This definition simply implies loss of volume, not increase in roentgenographic density. Perhaps one of the commonest forms of atelectasis occurs in a lobe where blood supply has been interrupted by thromboembolism. This may be accompanied by considerable volume loss of the affected lobe or segment, and manifested by diaphragmatic elevation and fissure displacement but no increase in roentgenographic density; in fact, density may be reduced because of the oligemia resulting from arterial obstruction. This example indicates the importance of *regarding atelectasis as a process in which the only direct roentgenographic sign is loss of lung volume, and it is in this context that "atelectasis" is used throughout this book.*

Since we have described atelectasis essentially in terms of lung volume, it is important to consider the mechanisms that keep the lung expanded. Alterations in these mechanisms provide a suitable basis for classifying atelectasis.

Varieties of Atelectasis

PASSIVE (RELAXATION) ATELECTASIS. The lung has a natural tendency to collapse and does so when removed from the chest. While the lungs are in the thoracic cavity, this tendency is opposed by the chest wall, and at the resting respiratory position (FRC) the tendency of the lung to collapse and for the chest wall to expand are equal and opposite. When the thorax contains a space-occupying process (*e.g.*, pneumothorax), the lung retracts and its volume decreases; this is *passive or relaxation atelectasis*.

CICATRIZATION ATELECTASIS. In a static system, the volume attained by the lung depends upon the applied force and the opposing elastic forces, the sum of which is generally termed compliance or change in volume per unit change in pressure. It follows that when the lung is stiffer than normal, *i.e.*, when compliance is decreased, lung volume is decreased. This classically occurs with pulmonary fibrosis and is called *cicatrization atelectasis*.

ADHESIVE ATELECTASIS. The pressure-volume behavior also depends upon the forces acting at the air–tissue interface of the alveolar wall. As alveoli diminish in volume, the surface tension of the interface is diminished by the "alveolar lining fluid," or surfactant. When the action of surfactant is interfered with, as may occur in the respiratory distress syndrome, there may be widespread collapse of alveoli.

This type of atelectasis has been referred to as microatelectasis or nonobstructive atelectasis, but we shall refer to it as *adhesive atelectasis*.

RESORPTION ATELECTASIS. The most common form of atelectasis, and the most complex, is caused by the resorption of gas from the alveoli, as may occur in acute bronchial obstruction. Since we have classified other forms of atelectasis on the basis of mechanism rather than etiology, this type of atelectasis is best termed *resorption atelectasis*.

Resorption Atelectasis

This occurs when communications between alveoli and trachea are obstructed (Figure 4–7). The mechanism of resorption is simple: the partial pressure of gases is lower in mixed venous blood than in alveolar air; as blood passes through the alveolar capillaries, the partial pressures of its gases equilibrate with alveolar pressure. The alveoli diminish in volume corresponding to the quantity of oxygen absorbed, their pressure remaining atmospheric; consequently, the partial pressures of carbon dioxide and nitrogen in the alveoli rise relative to capillary blood, and both gases diffuse into blood to maintain equilibrium. Thus alveolar volume is further reduced, with a consequent rise in the alveolar-capillary blood P_{O_2} gradient; oxygen diffuses into capillary blood, and this cycle is repeated until all alveolar gas is absorbed. In a previously healthy lobe, all air will

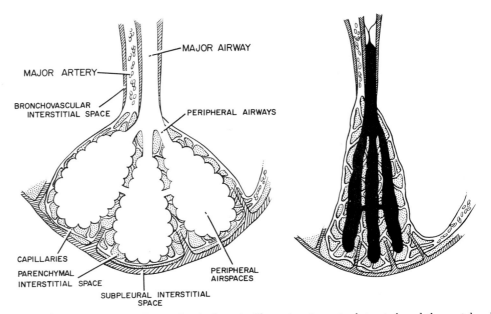

Figure 4–7. The Lung Diagram: Resorption Atelectasis. The major airway is obstructed, and the peripheral airways and air spaces are airless and collapsed.

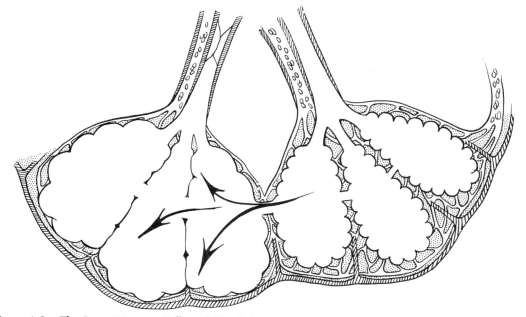

Figure 4–8. The Lung Diagram: Collateral Ventilation Associated with Air Trapping. The airway on the left is obstructed, that on the right patent; the parenchyma distal to the obstructed airway is being ventilated by collateral air drift. The diagram depicts a situation in which air enters the obstructed segment more easily than it leaves, thus resulting in air trapping.

have disappeared after 18 to 24 hours. Since oxygen is absorbed selectively much more rapidly than nitrogen, when a lobe is filled with oxygen at the moment of occlusion (a situation that might pertain during anesthesia), collapse occurs much more rapidly and should be roentgenographically apparent within minutes. This effect may be observed in both infants and adults in whom malposition of endotracheal tubes has caused bronchial occlusion, and it is vital that the physician be aware of the exceptional rapidity with which an obstructed lung or lobe can collapse in such circumstances.

It is important to realize that *resorption atelectasis is not the inevitable or only accompaniment of bronchial obstruction, nor is obstruction of a major bronchus the only cause of resorption atelectasis.* The effect of obstruction of the airways depends upon the site and extent of bronchial or bronchiolar obstruction, the pre-existing condition of the lung tissue, and collateral air drift. This last feature is so important that it deserves special mention.

Collateral Air Drift

Collateral ventilation or collateral air drift are the terms used to describe ventilation of alveoli other than by direct airway connections. There are three routes of collateral ventilation: (1) *The pores of Kohn,* which are circular or oval discontinuities in alveolar walls. (2) *The canals of Lambert,* which are epithelium-lined tubules between preterminal bronchioles and surrounding alveoli. (3) *Direct airway anastomoses,* about 120 μ in diameter. It is not known which of these routes is the most important in man, but it is clear that considerable collateral ventilation can occur, even from upper to lower lobes. Of particular importance is the possibility of air trapping in collaterally ventilated lung (Figure 4–8). The observation[4] that overinflation occurs distal to congenital bronchial atresia suggests that collateral ventilation is a potent force in causing chronic air trapping and resultant alveolar overdistention.

Customarily collateral air drift has been regarded as occurring readily between lobar segments but not between pulmonary lobes; such a conclusion seems obvious in view of the fissures separating the lobes and the impossibility of air passing across the pleural space. However, in a study at necropsy of eight normal and eight emphysematous excised human lungs in which the resistance of collateral channels was measured, Hogg and his associates[5] found the fissures between upper and lower lobes complete in only three normal lungs and one emphysematous lung. Thus collateral drift occurred between these two lobes in five of the eight normal lungs and in seven of the eight emphysematous lungs. This observation is of obvious importance in the assessment of roentgenographic signs when an endobronchial mass in a lobar bronchus appears to occlude its lumen completely; in one of our patients a bronchial adenoma at the origin of the left lower lobe bronchus prevented passage of bronchographic contrast material, but the lower lobe was air-containing although slightly reduced in volume.

If collateral air drift is such a potent force in preventing parenchymal collapse, under what circumstances does collapse occur? This depends chiefly upon the site of bronchial obstruction. If the obstruction is in a lobar bronchus, the development of atelectasis is readily explained by the absence of a parenchymal bridge from the involved lobe to a contiguous lobe; if the obstruction is in a segmental or subsegmental bronchus, collapse must be caused by some influence *preventing* collateral air drift[4]—probably inflammatory exudate. In personal communication, Fleischner confirmed the existence of alveolar exudate in cases of "platelike" atelectasis.

Even excluding the effect of collateral air drift, the end result of bronchial obstruction is not necessarily a collapsed, airless lobe. For example, intralobar infection may lead to pneumonic consolidation severe enough to limit loss of volume (Figure 4–9). Infection is frequent with slowly progressive, obstructive processes such as bronchogenic carcinoma or bronchial adenoma, so that loss of volume may be only slight or moderate (Figure 4–10). Pneumonitis,

bronchiectasis, and abscesses that develop behind the obstruction are usually of sufficient degree to counteract, at least partly, collapse induced by air absorption. The characteristic roentgenographic picture of "obstructive pneumonitis" should immediately alert the physician to the presence of an obstructing endobronchial lesion.

Even in the absence of infection fluid exudation occurs to some extent in all cases of acute obstructive atelectasis. Although assessment of volumetric reduction necessarily is rough, it might reasonably be estimated that 24 to 48 hours after complete bronchial occlusion in a patient breathing room air the volume of a pulmonary lobe seldom is reduced more than 50 per cent. Since a completely collapsed lung (as in total pneumothorax, for example) occupies a volume no larger than a man's fist, obviously a very large amount of fluid must exude into the substance of a lobe before its volume is reduced by only 50 per cent. This accumulation of sterile edema fluid and blood behind a bronchial obstruction is euphemistically termed "drowned lung," although the bulk of the accumulated liquid probably is blood rather than water (edema). If the obstruction persists and the obstructed lobe remains sterile, volumetric readjustment occurs within the hemithorax whereby other compensatory processes try to restore normal volume. As these other mechanisms play an increasingly important role in restoring pleural pressure to normal levels,

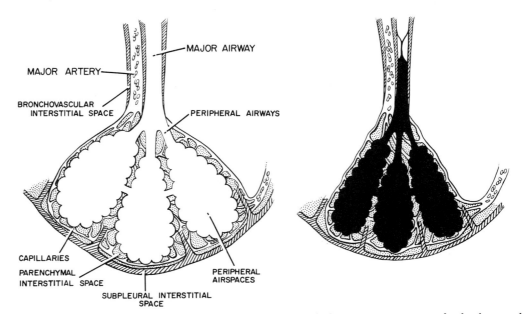

Figure 4–9. The Lung Diagram: Obstructive Pneumonitis. Although the major airway is completely obstructed, loss of volume of the peripheral air spaces is only moderate; outpouring of edematous fluid (or inflammatory exudate) has prevented the complete collapse depicted in Figure 4–7.

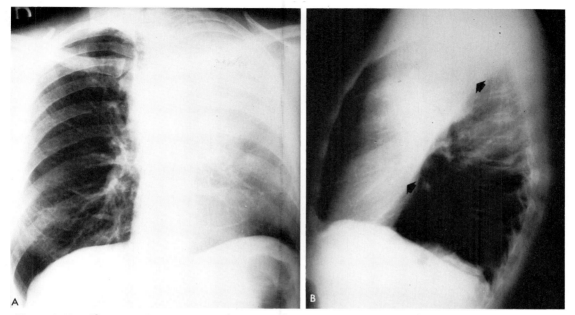

Figure 4–10. Obstructive Pneumonitis—Left Upper Lobe. Posteroanterior *(A)* and lateral *(B)* roentgenograms reveal homogeneous opacification of the left upper lobe; there is no air bronchogram. The chief fissure *(arrows)* is not displaced forward, and the only signs indicating loss of volume are slight mediastinal shift and hemidiaphragmatic elevation. Collapse was prevented by the development of severe pneumonia distal to a completely obstructed left upper lobe bronchus—the "drowned lung." Proved bronchogenic carcinoma.

excess edema fluid and blood within the "drowned lobe" gradually are reabsorbed, and eventually the lobe occupies the smallest possible volume. The result is chronic uncomplicated atelectasis. The collapsed lobe may be so small that it is almost invisible roentgenographically, and then the diagnostician must rely heavily on evidence of compensatory phenomena.

Resorption atelectasis may occur in the absence of occlusion of a major bronchus but cannot develop unless there is interruption of communication between alveoli and a major airway. Perhaps the best example is lower lobe bronchiectasis consequent upon childhood bronchopulmonary infection. In this situation permanent atelectasis ensues and, together with bronchial infection, results in bronchiectasis. This, of course, is an oversimplification; since the chain of events leading to irreversible bronchiectasis doubtless also would result in fibrosis, the mechanisms underlying the development of bronchiectasis relate to both resorption and cicatrization.

Passive Atelectasis

This term *(synonym; relaxation atelectasis)* denotes pulmonary collapse in the presence of pneumothorax or hydrothorax (Figure 4–11).

Provided the pleural space is free (*i.e.*, without adhesions), collapse of any portion of lung is proportional to the amount of gas or liquid in the adjacent pleural space. In upright man, the tendency for gas to pass to the upper portion of the pleural space results in a relatively greater degree of collapse of upper lobe parenchyma than of lower. For this reason, identification of a very small pneumothorax, particularly in infants, is easier with the patient in the lateral decubitus position, using a horizontal roentgen beam.

It might be thought logical that shrinkage of a lung to half its normal projected area would double roentgenologic density. That this is not so is illustrated by the difficulty commonly experienced in visualizing the lung edge in any case of spontaneous pneumothorax, even of moderate degree (Fig. 4–12A). As a lung shrinks under pneumothorax, its density does not increase notably until its projected area is reduced to about one tenth its normal area at total lung capacity.[2] The probable explanation for this anomalous situation is twofold: first, the reduction in lung volume is approximately balanced by reduction in blood content, net roentgenographic density being altered only slightly; and second, air in the pleural space both anteriorly and posteriorly serves as a nonabsorbing medium, contributing to the overall radiolucency of the roentgenographic image.

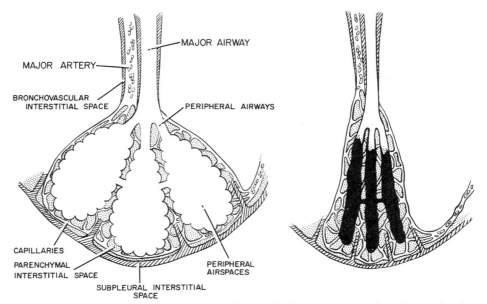

Figure 4–11. The Lung Diagram: Passive Atelectasis. The peripheral air spaces are collapsed and airless but in contrast to the situation in resorption atelectasis (*see* Figure 4–7), the airways are patent.

Even when pneumothorax-induced collapse is total, the lung mass is not completely airless—the lobar and larger segmental bronchi are sufficiently stable structurally to resist collapse; therefore, they remain air-filled and, although reduced in caliber, should be apparent as an air bronchogram (Figure 4–12*B*). For obvious reasons it is essential that this sign be sought carefully in any case of total or almost total pneumothorax; absence of an air bronchogram should immediately arouse suspicion of an endobronchial obstruction. It is clear that, in such circumstances, the lung will not reexpand no matter how rigorous the therapeutic maneuvers to reduce the pneumothorax.

So-called "compression" or "mantle" atelec-

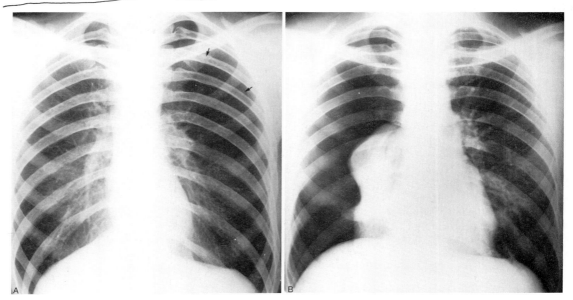

Figure 4–12. Spontaneous Pneumothorax. The posteroanterior roentgenograms of two patients are illustrated. In *A*, the left-sided pneumothorax is small (*arrows* point to the visceral pleural line). Note that the left hemithorax is more radiolucent than the right and of greater volume than the right because of the removal of the influence of elastic recoil of the lung on the chest wall. In *B*, the right pneumothorax is total. Note the small volume occupied by the whole lung when totally collapsed. The well-defined air bronchogram indicates airway patency.

tasis, formerly classified separately, differs so little from passive atelectasis that it does not warrant a separate category. The term has been used to designate parenchymal collapse contiguous to a space-occupying mass within the thorax and therefore local rather than general atelectasis as in pneumothorax. Any intrathoracic space-occupying process—for example, a bronchogenic cyst or pneumatocele—induces airlessness of a thin layer of contiguous lung parenchyma; although this could reasonably be regarded as "compression," the lung's elastic recoil properties render a concept of "relaxation" more logical. Thus we prefer to regard this process as a form of passive atelectasis.

An unusual and undoubtedly very uncommon form of atelectasis has recently been described under the name "rounded atelectasis."[6] Presenting as a fairly homogeneous, rather ill-defined opacity up to 5 cm in greatest diameter, these lesions are invariably pleural-based and are most commonly situated along the posterior surface of a lower lobe. The bronchovascular bundles in the vicinity of the mass appear to be gathered together in a sheaf as they curve posteriorly toward the mass, simulating the tail of a comet. The mass is always in contact with chronically thickened pleura, which is alleged to be the basic pathogenesis of the process. In fact, an association has been observed with asbestos-related pleural disease. In a number of patients on whom thoracotomy has been performed for a mistaken diagnosis of cancer, the collapsed pulmonary parenchyma has reexpanded following decortication of the thickened pleura; as a consequence, it is reasonable to regard this form of atelectasis as the passive or relaxation type.

Adhesive Atelectasis

This term describes alveolar collapse in the presence of patent airway connections and, thus, is true "nonobstructive" atelectasis. The condition is controversial and poorly understood. The best examples are the respiratory distress syndrome of newborn infants and acute radiation pneumonitis (Figure 4–13). In both conditions atelectasis may be a prominent feature and may be related, at least in part, to an inactivation of surfactant. Clements[7] showed that surfactants reduce the surface tension of an alveolus as its surface area or volume decreases. In other words, they protect against collapse in that the critical closing pressure of alveoli occurs at a lower volume and distending pressure. Absence of surfactant has been reported in studies of purely atelectatic human lung.[8]

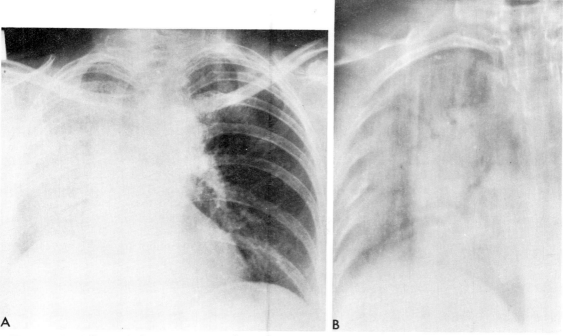

A   **B**

Figure 4–13. Adhesive Atelectasis in Acute Radiation Pneumonitis. A posteroanterior roentgenogram (*A*) reveals severe loss of volume of the right lung associated with marked mediastinal shift and hemidiaphragmatic elevation; the density is rather granular (the oblique shadow across the left upper lung is an artifact). A well-defined air bronchogram (seen to better advantage on the anteroposterior tomogram—*B*) indicates major airway patency.

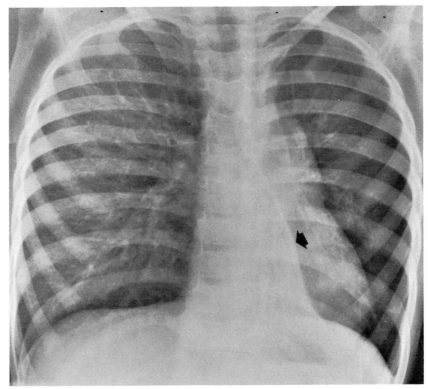

Figure 4–14. Adhesive Atelectasis Caused by Surfactant Deficit or Peripheral Airway Obstruction. The left lower lobe is almost completely collapsed (*arrow* points to the interface between the displaced major fissure and the overinflated upper lobe). Despite the severe atelectasis, a well-defined air bronchogram can be clearly identified out to the periphery. Bronchoscopy showed no evidence of bronchial obstruction. Three-and-one-half year old girl approximately 2 years following acute adenoviral pneumonia of the left lung; the lobe eventually re-expanded spontaneously. (Reprinted from MacPherson, R. I., Cumming, G. R., and Chernick, V.: J. Canad. Assoc. Radiol., *20*:225, 1969, with permission of the authors and editor.)

In all forms of adhesive atelectasis in which there is increased roentgenographic density, since the process is peripheral, an air bronchogram will be present (Figure 4–14).

Cicatrization Atelectasis

Some may object to the inclusion of loss of lung volume casued by fibrosis as a type of atelectasis, but we believe this entity is best described here. The pathologic process is one of fibrosis with resultant cicatrization; the former may or may not be associated with parenchymal destruction, but in either event it results in loss of volume of the affected portion of lung. Not only is air per unit lung volume decreased, but, also, tissue per unit lung volume is increased, thus increasing roentgenographic density. The roentgenologic signs depend upon whether the process is local or general.

Localized disease is best exemplified by chronic infection, often granulomatous in nature, and epitomized by long-standing produc-

tive pulmonary tuberculosis. In essence, it is a chronic "nonobstructive" atelectasis in which the destruction of lung parenchyma is followed by fibrosis and progressive loss of volume through cicatrization. The more proximal bronchi become dilated, so that the morphologic picture is one of chronic bronchiectasis and parenchymal scarring. The roentgenologic signs are as might be expected (Figure 4–15): a segment or lobe occupying a volume smaller than normal, with a density rendered inhomogeneous by dilated air-containing bronchi, and with irregular thickened strands extending from the collapsed segment to the hilum. The compensatory signs of chronic loss of volume are usually evident.

Generalized fibrotic disease of the lungs also may be associated with loss of volume. In chronic interstitial pulmonary fibrosis, for example, involvement of the parenchymal interstitial space results in widespread reduction in the volume of air-containing parenchyma; this may be evidenced roentgenologically by eleva-

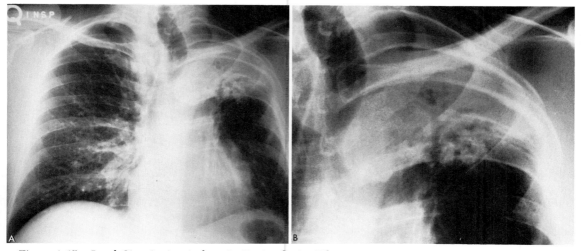

Figure 4–15.   Local Cicatrization Atelectasis: Postirradiation Fibrosis. A posteroanterior roentgenogram *(A)* reveals considerable loss of volume of the left upper lung, with displacement of the trachea to the left, approximation of the left upper ribs, and elevation of the left hilum. A magnified view *(B)* shows a prominent air bronchogram in an otherwise homogeneous opacity. One and one-half years previously, this 48-year-old man was found to have inoperable squamous-cell carcinoma of the left upper lobe, for which he had received an intensive course of cobalt therapy.

tion of the diaphragm and overall reduction in lung size (Figure 4–16).

In summary, atelectasis may occur by means of four mechanisms which, in any given situation, may operate independently or in combination.

1. *Resorption atelectasis* occurs when communications between the trachea and alveoli are obstructed.

2. *Passive (relaxation) atelectasis* denotes loss of volume accompanying an intrathoracic space-occupying process, particularly pneumothorax or hydrothorax.

3. *Adhesive atelectasis* is related to a complex group of forces, of which abnormality of surfactant is probably the most common. As with passive and cicatrization atelectasis, this form of collapse is associated with patent large airway communications.

4. *Cicatrization atelectasis* designates volume loss resulting from local or general pulmonary fibrosis.

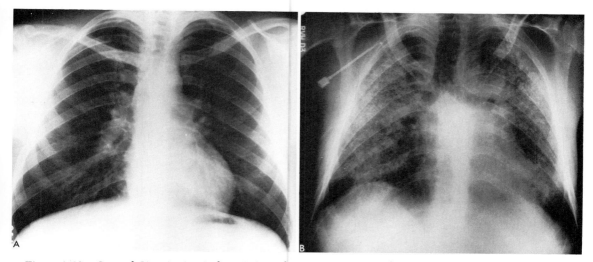

Figure 4–16.   General Cicatrization Atelectasis Secondary to Intravenous Talcosis in a Heroin Addict. At the time of the normal chest roentgenogram illustrated in *A*, this 19-year-old white man had been taking drugs (both heroin and methadone) intravenously for over 2 years. Six years later, a roentgenogram *(B)* reveals diffuse interstitial disease throughout both lungs associated with severe loss of lung volume as evidenced by elevation of the diaphragm and smallness of the thoracic cage. This represents diffuse interstitial fibrosis caused by intravenously injected talc.

ROENTGENOLOGIC SIGNS OF ATELECTASIS

The roentgenologic signs of atelectasis may be both *direct* and *indirect*, the latter consisting chiefly of compensatory phenomena.

Direct Signs

DISPLACEMENT OF INTERLOBAR FISSURES. We define atelectasis simply as loss of lung volume. Accordingly, the only *direct* sign is *displacement of interlobar fissures*. Although local increase in density is a common manifestation of pulmonary atelectasis, it is not essential to the definition and therefore cannot be construed as a direct sign. In addition, displacement of the fissures that form the boundary of a collapsed lobe is one of the most dependable and easily recognized signs of atelectasis (Figure 4–17). The only exception to this general rule occurs when a main bronchus is obstructed, resulting in atelectasis of a whole lung; in such circumstances, since major fissures are not truly displaced, *direct* signs consist of those described later, notably diaphragmatic elevation and mediastinal displacement.

Indirect Signs

LOCAL INCREASE IN DENSITY. This is the most important indirect sign of atelectasis and is caused by airless lung. The volume of an airless lobe or segment depends not only upon which order of bronchus is obstructed, but also upon the amount of sequestered blood and edema fluid, either sterile or infected, within the obstructed parenchyma.

The chief indirect roentgenologic signs of atelectasis, other than local opacity, are those processes that compensate for the reduction in intrapleural pressure—diaphragmatic elevation, mediastinal shift, approximation of ribs, and overinflation of the remainder of the lung (Figures 4–17 and 4–18). The part played by each compensatory mechanism in any given situation is somewhat unpredictable, although predominance is dictated largely by the anatomic position of the collapsed lobe; all four mechanisms may operate fairly equally, or one or two may predominate to the exclusion of others. Two general rules deserve emphasis. (1) Displacement of the diaphragm and mediastinum is maximal contiguous to the major collapse; for example, lower lobe collapse tends to elevate the posterior more than the anterior portion of the hemidiaphragm and to displace

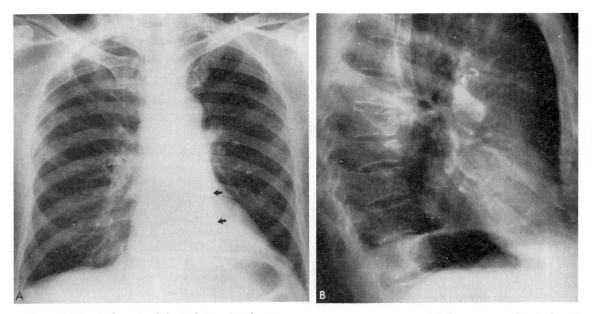

Figure 4–17.   Atelectasis of the Left Lower Lobe. A posteroanterior roentgenogram *(A)* shows a triangular shadow of homogeneous density in the inferomedial portion of the left hemithorax. Its lateral margin *(arrows)* represents the interface between the collapsed left lower lobe and overinflated left upper lobe. Indirect signs of atelectasis include increased radiolucency of the left upper compared with the right upper lobe, redistribution of vascular markings, and elevation of the left hemidiaphragm. The mediastinum shows little or no shift. In lateral projection *(B)*, the shadow is barely visible as an area of increased density situated in the posterior costophrenic sulcus, but its presence is indicated by the loss of visibility of the posterior portion of the left hemidiaphragm (the silhouette sign).

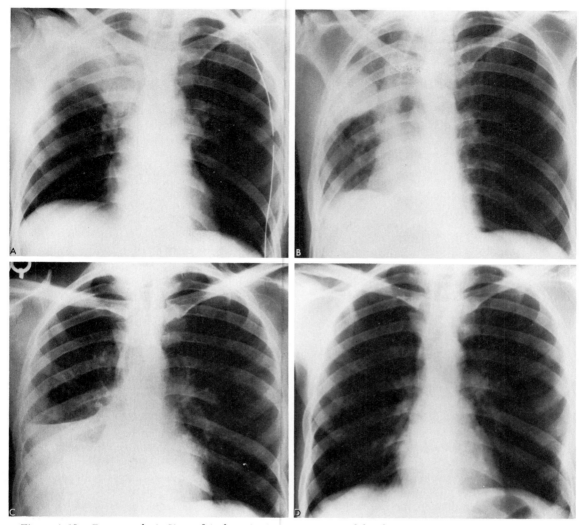

Figure 4–18. **Roentgenologic Signs of Atelectasis.** A roentgenogram of the chest in anteroposterior projection, supine position (A), reveals a homogeneous shadow in the upper portion of the right hemithorax; its concave lower margin is formed by the upwardly displaced horizontal fissure; the right hemidiaphragm is slightly elevated. Atelectasis of the right upper lobe (24 hours postoperative for thoracoabdominal repair of hiatus hernia). Twenty-four hours later (B), the right upper lobe collapse is clearing, but the diaphragmatic elevation has increased and the mediastinum has shifted markedly to the right; note the approximation of ribs. These signs indicate acute obstruction of the right intermediate bronchus with progressing collapse of the middle and lower lobes, undoubtedly caused by a mucous plug displaced from the upper lobe bronchus. Twenty-four hours later (C), the middle and lower lobes are virtually airless; the right upper lobe has completely re-expanded. Twenty-four hours later (D), following bronchoscopic removal of a mucous plug from the intermediate bronchus, all signs have disappeared and the lungs are now roentgenologically normal.

the inferior more than the superior mediastinum. Conversely, upper lobe collapse is associated with upper mediastinal displacement, often with little hemidiaphragmatic elevation. (2) The briefer the atelectasis, the greater the predominance of diaphragmatic and mediastinal displacement (Figure 4–18); the more chronic the collapse, the more will compensatory overinflation predominate (Figure 4–17).

ELEVATION OF THE HEMIDIAPHRAGM. As already stated, hemidiaphragmatic elevation is

always a more prominent feature of lower than of upper lobe collapse (compare Figure 4–18A and C). In the lower lung zones, elevation tends to occur in the area contiguous to the lobe involved—posterior elevation in lower lobe collapse and anterior elevation in middle lobe or lingular collapse (although, in the latter situation, diaphragmatic displacement is seldom severe).

MEDIASTINAL DISPLACEMENT. The normal mediastinum is a surprisingly mobile structure and reacts promptly to differences in pressure between the two halves of the thorax (Figure 4–18). The anterior and middle mediastinal compartments are less stable than the posterior and, therefore, shift to a greater extent. The degree of shift is usually greatest in the region of major pulmonary collapse; thus tracheal and upper mediastinal displacement is a feature of upper lobe collapse and may be negligible when the lower lobes are involved; in the latter instance, the inferior mediastinum undergoes the greatest displacement.

COMPENSATORY OVERINFLATION. Overinflation of the remainder of the ipsilateral lung is one of the most important and reliable indirect signs of atelectasis (Figure 4–17). It seldom occurs rapidly and, in the early stages of lobar collapse, usually is of less diagnostic help than the other compensatory phenomena, such as diaphragmatic elevation and mediastinal displacement. As the period of collapse lengthens, however, overinflation becomes more prominent and the diaphragmatic and mediastinal changes regress.

Roentgenologic evidence of compensatory overinflation may be extremely subtle. It may be difficult to estimate the increase in lung translucency resulting from the greater air-blood ratio, but appreciation may be enhanced by viewing the roentgenogram from a distance of several feet or through minification lenses. Clearly, more reliable evidence for overinflation is supplied by the *alteration in vascular markings* resultant upon the increased lung volume (Figure 4–17); the vessels are more widely spaced and sparser than in the normal contralateral lung. When a considerable volume of one lung becomes atelectatic, there is a tendency for overinflation to involve the contralateral lung; this may progress to a stage in which the opposite lung displaces the mediastinal septum locally. This displacement occurs chiefly in the anterior mediastinal compartment, at the level of the first three or four costal cartilages, limited anteriorly by the sternum and posteriorly by the great vessels. Roentgenologic appreciation of anterior mediastinal displacement is usually easy, through visualization of the displaced anterior mediastinal line; the curvilinear opacity of the apposed pleural surfaces usually visible on a posteroanterior roentgenogram, protruding into the involved hemithorax; in lateral projection the anterior mediastinum appears exceptionally radiolucent and increased in depth.

DISPLACEMENT OF THE HILA. The hila are often involved in the redistribution of anatomic structures within the thorax in the presence of atelectasis, and such displacement constitutes an invaluable sign of collapse (Figure 4–19). It occurs more predictably in collapse of the upper than of the lower lobes and usually is more marked the more chronic the atelectasis.

A cardinal sign of lower lobe collapse is loss of visibility of the interlobar artery; since the lung parenchyma adjacent to the artery is airless, the air-tissue interface is lost and the vessel becomes invisible. This sign is particularly valuable on the left side, where pleural effusion sometimes creates a triangular shadow in the posterior paravertebral zone that simulates total left lower lobe collapse. Preservation of the shadow of the interlobar artery establishes the pleural origin of the opacity, whereas its obliteration indicates lobar collapse.

CHANGES IN THE CHEST WALL. Approximation of the ribs is, in our experience, the least dependable of all compensatory signs of atelectasis. The difficulty may be compounded by alterations in rib angulation, produced by even minor degrees of scoliosis. While approximation of ribs as a sign of smallness of a hemithorax may be of some value in cases of chronic loss of volume, as from cicatrization, we feel that it should not be relied upon too heavily as an accurate indicator of reduction in hemithoracic volume in cases of acute lobar collapse.

ABSENCE OF AN AIR BRONCHOGRAM. For the most part, *resorption atelectasis* cannot be present if air is visible in the bronchial tree. If bronchial obstruction is severe enough to cause absorption of air from the parenchyma of the affected lobe or segment, it also must cause absorption of gas from the bronchial tree. Particularly when pneumonitis behind the obstruction is so severe that consolidation exceeds atelectasis, absence of an air bronchogram is a roentgenologic sign of vital importance, since it may be the only aid to differentiating an obstruction by a bronchogenic carcinoma from a consolidative process such as simple bacterial pneumonia.

The preceding statements apply only to atelectasis produced by resorption and not by the other three mechanisms (passive, adhesive, and cicatrization). In the first two particularly, an air bronchogram is virtually always present.

In summary, the roentgenologic signs of atelectasis are:

A. *Direct:*
1. **Displacement of interlobar fissures.**
B. *Indirect:*
1. **Local increase in density.**
2. **Elevation of the hemidiaphragm.**
3. **Displacement of the mediastinum.**
4. **Compensatory overinflation.**

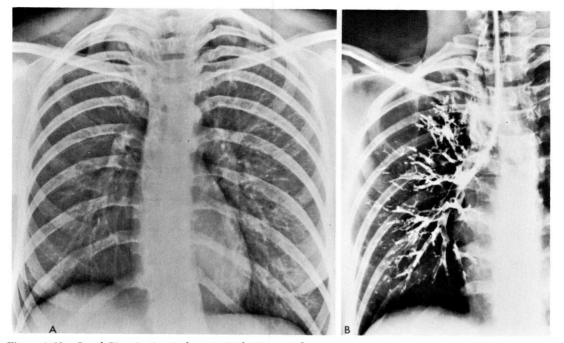

Figure 4–19.   Local Cicatrization Atelectasis, Right Upper Lobe. A posteroanterior roentgenogram *(A)* shows a poorly defined shadow lying in the right superior paramediastinal zone. Marked loss of volume of the right upper lobe is indicated by elevation of the right hilum and displacement of the trachea to the right. In a right bronchogram *(B)*, displacement of the trachea is well shown as is dilatation and distortion of the upper lobe segmental bronchi, particularly the apical segment. Chronic fibroproductive tuberculosis with tuberculous bronchiectasis.

5. **Displacement of hila.**
6. **Approximation of ribs.**
7. **Absence of an air bronchogram (in cases of resorption atelectasis only).**

PATTERNS OF LOBAR AND SEGMENTAL ATELECTASIS

Since the degree of collapse of a lobe is governed largely by the amount of exudation into it, the resultant roentgenographic image varies from a consolidated lobe in which there is only minimal loss of volume to a state of total lobar collapse; therefore, the anatomicospatial relationships in each lobe are described from a state of normal volume through all stages to total atelectasis.

Provided that the pleural space is intact (*i.e.*, no pneumothorax or hydrothorax), certain basic characteristics are common to all forms of pulmonary collapse, regardless of the lobe involved or whether the collapse is of a whole lung or a subsegment. It is important to realize that, regardless of the severity of collapse, the *visceral pleural surface of the affected lobe or segment continues to relate intimately to the*

parietal pleura; in other words, the visceral pleural surface never retracts inward so as to lose contact with the parietal pleura over the convex or mediastinal surfaces of the hemithorax. Since movement thus is restricted hilarward, and the medial aspect of the lobe is relatively fixed at the hilum, the form the collapsed lobe eventually must adopt is limited. The resultant shape also is partly affected by the semi-rigid components of the lung (the bronchi, arteries, and veins), which can be crowded together in very close apposition in one plane but have a limited capacity for shortening. Thus, any pulmonary lobe in its fully inflated state may be likened to a pyramid with its apex at the hilum and its base contiguous to the parietal pleura; as the lobe loses volume, two surfaces of the pyramid approximate, the end result of total collapse being a flattened triangle or triangular "pancake" whose apex and base maintain contiguity with the hilum and parietal pleura, respectively.

Total Pulmonary Atelectasis

When an entire lung collapses because of obstruction of a main bronchus, the compensa-

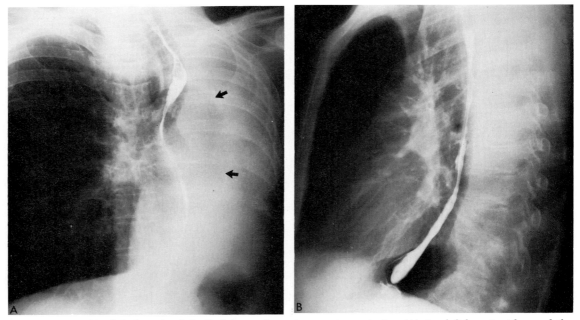

Figure 4–20. Total Atelectasis of the Left Lung. In posteroanterior projection *(A)*, the left lung is airless and the mediastinum shifted markedly to the left. The interface between the overinflated right lung and collapsed left lung is indicated by *arrows*. The left hemidiaphragm (indicated by the position of the gastric fundus) is only slightly elevated. In lateral projection *(B)*, roughly the anterior half of the left hemithorax is occupied by overinflated right lung that has extended in front of the heart and major vessels into the left hemithorax.

tory phenomena are identical in character to those that develop with less severe pulmonary collapse but obviously are greater in degree and in some respects less readily apparent (Figure 4–20). Elevation of the ipsilateral hemidiaphragm is recognizable only on the left side, the stomach bubble indicating its position. The hemithorax usually evidences retraction. It is on the mediastinum, however, that the most important effect is exerted by the net difference in pressure between the two halves of the thorax. As the normal contralateral lung overinflates, the whole mediastinum moves to the affected side, the greatest shift occurring anteriorly, where the mediastinum is weakest. As the overinflated lung moves across the midline, it displaces the heart, aorta, and collapsed lung posteriorly. The resultant roentgenologic signs are virtually diagnostic: in lateral projection, depth and radiolucency of the retrosternal air space are increased, with a general increase in roentgenographic density in the posterior portion of the thorax (Figure 4–20). In posteroanterior projection, the uniform opacity caused by the superimposed cardiovascular structures and collapsed lung is interrupted by the radiolucency of overinflated contralateral lung that has passed across the midline of the thorax. The margin of the overinflated lung is usually visible extending into the involved hemithorax.

Lobar Atelectasis

The patterns created by atelectasis of the right and left upper lobes differ and, therefore, are described separately; the lower lobes have almost identical patterns and are considered together.

RIGHT UPPER LOBE. The minor fissure and the upper half of the major fissure approximate by shifting upward (Figure 4–21). Both fissures become gently curved, with their convexity upward in lateral projection; the minor fissure shows roughly the same curvature in posteroanterior projection (Figure 4–22). As volume loss increases, the visceral pleural surface sweeps upward over the apex of the hemithorax, so that the lobe comes to occupy a flattened position contiguous with the superior mediastinum. In lateral projection, the collapsed lobe may appear as an indistinctly defined triangular shadow with its apex at the hilum and its base contiguous with the parietal pleura just posterior to the extreme apex of the hemithorax (the "mediastinal wedge").

LEFT UPPER LOBE. The major difference between collapse of the left and right upper lobes is the absence of a minor fissure on the left, on which side all lung tissue anterior to the major fissure is involved (Figure 4–23). This fissure, which is slightly more vertical than the chief

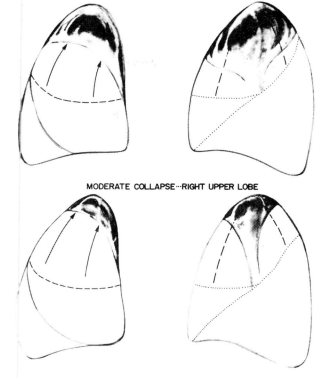

Figure 4–21. Patterns of Lobar Collapse: Right Upper Lobe. *See* text for description.

MODERATE COLLAPSE···RIGHT UPPER LOBE

SEVERE COLLAPSE···RIGHT UPPER LOBE

fissure on the right, is displaced forward in a plane roughly parallel to the anterior chest wall, a relationship depicted particularly well on lateral roentgenograms (Figure 4–24). As volume loss increases, the fissure moves further anteriorly and slightly medially, until on lateral projection the shadow of the lobe is no more than a broad linear opacity contiguous with and parallel to the anterior chest wall. The contiguity of the collapsed lobe with the anterior mediastinum obliterates the left cardiac border in frontal projection (the "silhouette sign"). The

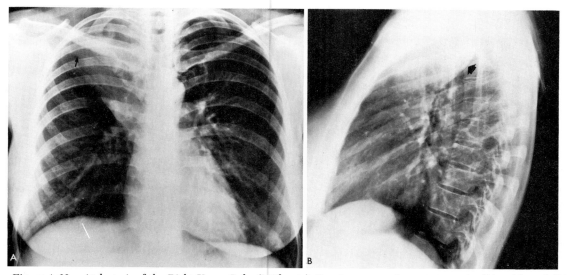

Figure 4–22. Atelectasis of the Right Upper Lobe (Moderate). Roentgenograms in posteroanterior *(A)* and lateral *(B)* projection show a homogeneous opacity in the upper portion of the right hemithorax. In posteroanterior projection the lower border of the shadow is formed by the upward displaced minor fissure *(arrow)*. The upward displaced major fissure is seen clearly in lateral projection *(arrow)*. Bronchial adenoma totally obstructing the right upper lobe bronchus.

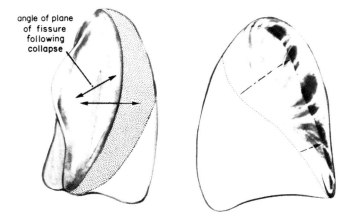

angle of plane
of fissure
following
collapse

MODERATE COLLAPSE···LEFT UPPER LOBE

Figure 4–23. **Patterns of Lobar Collapse: Left Upper Lobe.** *See* text for description.

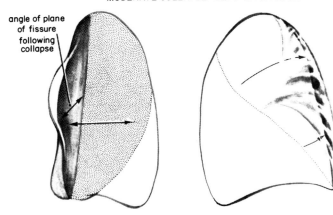

angle of plane
of fissure
following
collapse

SEVERE COLLAPSE···LEFT UPPER LOBE

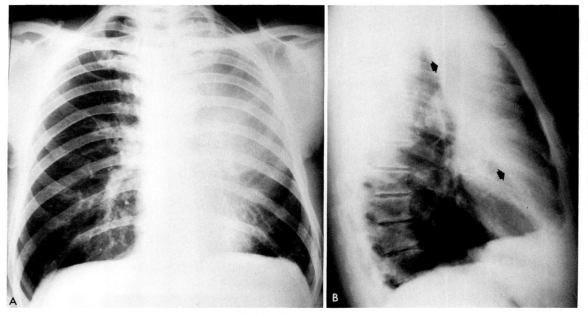

Figure 4–24. **Atelectasis of the Left Upper Lobe (Moderate).** In posteroanterior projection *(A)*, the entire left border of the heart is obscured by a homogeneous opacity projected over the upper two thirds of the left hemithorax. In lateral projection *(B)*, the chief fissure is displaced anteriorly *(arrows)*. Note the absence of an air bronchogram, indicating bronchial obstruction. The left hemidiaphragm is moderately elevated. Bronchogenic carcinoma left upper lobe bronchus, with obstructive pneumonitis.

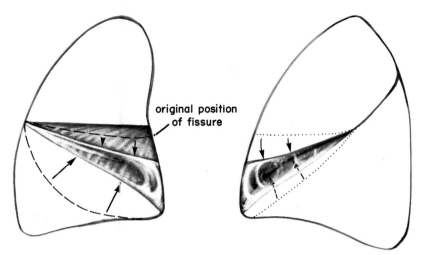

original position of fissure

Figure 4–25. Patterns of Lobar Collapse: Right Middle Lobe. *See* text for description.

apical segment tends to retract downward, the space it vacates being occupied by the overinflated superior bronchopulmonary segment of the lower lobe; the apex of the hemithorax thus contains aerated lung.

RIGHT MIDDLE LOBE. Atelectasis of the right middle lobe is one of the easiest diagnoses to make on lateral roentgenography and one of the most difficult on posteroanterior projection. With progressive loss of volume, the minor fissure and the lower half of the major fissure approximate; they are almost in contact when collapse is complete (Figure 4–25). The resultant triangular "pancake" of tissue has its apex at the hilum and its base contiguous to the parietal pleura over the anterolateral convexity of the thorax. In lateral projection it appears as a linear shadow of increased density, sometimes no more than 2 or 3 mm wide; in posteroanterior projection there may be no discernible increase in density—the only evidence of disease may be obliteration of part of the right cardiac border (the "silhouette sign") owing to contiguity of the right atrium and the collapsed lobe. This lack of density on posteroanterior projection is caused by the obliquity of the collapsed lobe in a superoinferior plane. At any point its thickness is insufficient to cast a discernible roentgenographic shadow. When the patient assumes a lordotic position, the downward displaced minor fissure becomes oriented in a plane parallel to the roentgen beam, so that the collapsed lobe is visualized as a thin "sail-like" shadow extending from the lateral chest wall medially and slightly inferiorly along the right cardiac border (Figure 4–26).

LOWER LOBES. The fissures approximate in such a manner that the upper half of the chief fissure swings downward and the lower half backward (Figure 4–27). This displacement is

best appreciated in lateral projection, but during its downward displacement the upper half of the fissure may become clearly evident in posteroanterior projection as an opacity with a sharply defined upper surface extending obliquely downward and laterally from the region of the hilum (Figure 4–28). As collapse progresses, the lobe moves posteromedially to occupy a position in the posterior costophrenic gutter and medial costovertebral angle. Since the flat surface of the triangular "pancake" lies against the mediastinum, the thickness of tissue traversed by the roentgen beam in lateral projection may be insufficient to cast a shadow in this projection. In frontal projection, provided that exposure factors ensure adequate penetration of the heart, the collapsed lobe should be plainly visible as a diminutive triangular opacity in the costovertebral angle.

"Segmental Atelectasis"

These words have been placed in quotation marks to emphasize the fact that the term is probably a misnomer, at least in a pure sense. The reasons for the semantic inaccuracy are relatively simple. We have already seen that collateral channels can exert a potent force in ventilating alveoli other than by direct airway connections. Since collateral channels exist in profusion within segments, obstruction of a segmental or subsegmental bronchus cannot result in collapse unless some influence is present that prevents collateral air drift. In fact, provided that there is no infection, the presence of a complete obstruction in a segmental bronchus over a long period of time often results in overinflation of distal parenchyma rather than collapse. When an opacity is present distal to an obstructed segmental bronchus, the influ-

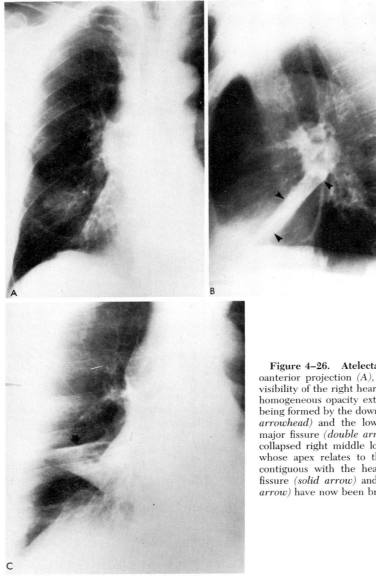

Figure 4–26. Atelectasis of the Right Middle Lobe. In posteroanterior projection *(A)*, the major evidence of disease is loss of visibility of the right heart border. In lateral projection *(B)*, a broad homogeneous opacity extends anteroinferiorly, the upper interface being formed by the downwardly displaced horizontal fissure *(single arrowhead)* and the lower interface by the anteriorly displaced major fissure *(double arrowheads)*. In lordotic projection *(C)*, the collapsed right middle lobe is clearly seen as a triangular opacity whose apex relates to the lateral chest wall and whose base is contiguous with the heart; the downwardly displaced horizontal fissure *(solid arrow)* and upwardly displaced major fissure *(open arrow)* have now been brought into profile.

ence that prevents collateral air drift in the majority of cases is inflammatory exudate so that in effect the pathologic process is one of pneumonia (Figure 4–29). Since the pneumonia has developed as a consequence of obstruction of a segmental bronchus, the correct appellation is "obstructive pneumonitis." Thus, a homogeneous opacity that conforms to the anatomic distribution of a bronchopulmonary segment and in which no air bronchogram is identifiable should immediately alert the physician to the presence of an obstructing endobronchial lesion. Obviously the caveat regarding the use of the term "segmental atelectasis" applies equally to subsegments although, as will be discussed

later (*see* page 211), it is conceivable that linear opacities commonly observed in the lung bases could be caused by subsegmental atelectasis in which collapse of alveoli resulted from surfactant deficit.

As might be anticipated, the opacity resulting from segmental or subsegmental obstructive pneumonitis depends not only upon the original volume of lung parenchyma affected but also upon the amount of exudation into it. Thus, the shadow can vary from a large conical opacity in which there is very little loss of volume to little more than a broad linear opacity in which atelectasis has predominated over inflammatory exudation. Regardless of the severity of the loss

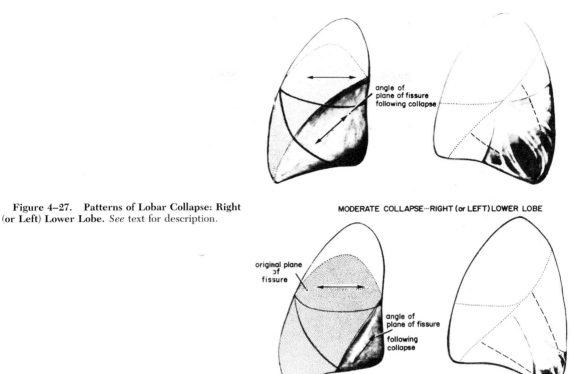

Figure 4–27. Patterns of Lobar Collapse: Right (or Left) Lower Lobe. *See* text for description.

MODERATE COLLAPSE···RIGHT (or LEFT) LOWER LOBE

SEVERE COLLAPSE···RIGHT (or LEFT) LOWER LOBE

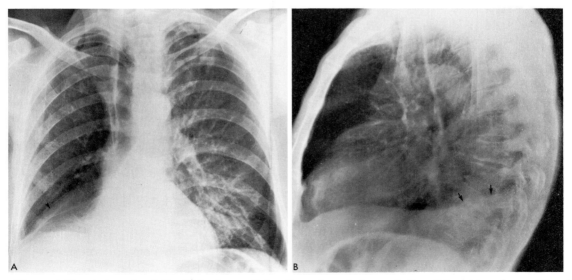

Figure 4–28. Atelectasis of the Right Lower Lobe. In posteroanterior projection *(A)*, a triangular opacity of homogeneous density is projected in the plane of the right cardiophrenic angle. Its upper border, produced by the interface between the downward displaced chief fissure and contiguous aerated lung, is sharply circumscribed *(solid arrows)*. Compensatory overinflation has occurred in the right upper and middle lobes and in the whole of the left lung (indicated by displacement of the anterior mediastinal septum to the right—*open arrows*). In lateral projection *(B)*, a poorly defined opacity can be identified posteroinferiorly, obscuring the costophrenic gutter and the posterior portion of the right hemidiaphragm *(arrows)*. A mediastinal wedge cannot be seen.

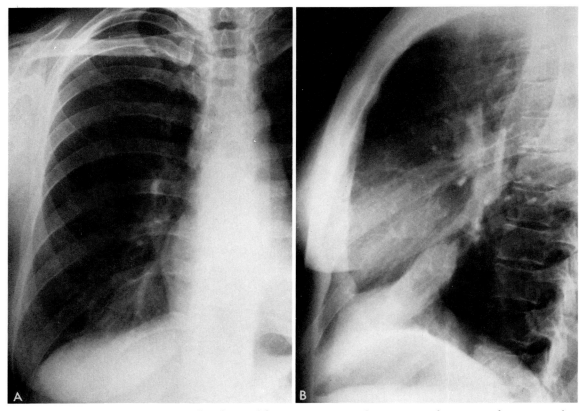

Figure 4–29. "Segmental Atelectasis" and Consolidation, Anterior Basal Segment, Right Lower Lobe. A triangular opacity of homogeneous density is situated in the inferior portion of the right lower lobe, conforming to the anatomic distribution of the anterior basal bronchopulmonary segment; there is moderate loss of volume; the absence of an air bronchogram indicates bronchial obstruction. The shadow is rather indistinctly defined in posteroanterior projection *(A)*, but well-circumscribed in lateral projection *(B)*. Bronchostenosis secondary to endobronchial tuberculosis in a 29-year-old woman.

of volume, however, it is recommended that the term "segmental atelectasis" be struck from our descriptive vocabulary and that we employ terminology that more accurately reflects the true nature of an important pathologic process.

PREDOMINANTLY INTERSTITIAL DISEASE

This heading covers the multitude of pulmonary diseases characterized by predominant involvement of the interstitial tissues of the lung. Conceptually, these diseases are the antithesis of the alveolar consolidative processes, in that *alveolar air is largely preserved and it is the tissues surrounding the air spaces and airways that are increased in volume.* An enormous number of diseases can produce predominantly interstitial involvement of the lungs. The roentgenographic pattern may be so dis-

tinctive that in some cases a confident diagnosis can be made based on these appearances alone. In others, the diagnosis may be strongly suggested when roentgenographic changes are considered in relation to the history or to evidence supplied by special roentgenographic procedures, laboratory findings, or pulmonary function values. In the majority, however, architectural disturbance is so similar that a definitive diagnosis cannot be made without recourse to histologic examination of tissue removed at biopsy.

CONCEPTS OF ROENTGENOLOGIC ANATOMY

It will be recalled that the lung parenchyma is sharply demarcated from the connective tissues of the bronchovascular tree, the interlobular septa, and the pleura by a limiting membrane. This membrane is composed of dense elastic tissue and collagen that merges into the elastic fibers of alveolar walls. The blood vessels, nerves, and lymphatics lie in this compartment of loose connective tissue, called the *perivascular (or axial) interstitial space*. In addition, there is a small interstitial space in the walls of the alveoli themselves; this is referred to as the *parenchymal (or acinar) interstitial space*, in keeping with our use of the term "parenchyma" to denote the gas-exchanging part of the lung.

The *perivascular interstitial space* consists of the sheath of loose connective tissue around the bronchovascular bundles that form the visible lung markings. This interstitial sheath extends out to the peripheral bronchioles, beyond which the airways are intimately related to the parenchyma. A similar sheath exists around the venous radicals within the lung, and this interstitial space is continuous with the peripheral interlobular septa that contain the veins and lymphatics that drain the peripheral parenchyma; it is also continuous with the subpleural interstitial space. The *parenchymal (acinar) interstitial space* lies between the alveolar and capillary basement membranes. This small space is made up of elastic and collagen fibers

Since interstitial diseases of the lung usually, if not always, affect both "compartments" to some degree, it might be argued that their subdivision is arbitrary and of little practical importance. From a roentgenologic point of view, however, we have found their distinction to be of some value, chiefly because their individual involvement usually produces distinguishable roentgenographic patterns. For example, one of the common abnormalities affecting the interstitial tissues of the lung is pulmonary edema. In studies of rapidly frozen dog lungs in which pulmonary venous pressures were raised by graded levels, Staub and his colleagues[9] showed a definite sequence of fluid accumulation in various compartments of the lung (Figure 4–30). Fluid appeared first in the interstitial connective tissue compartment around the large blood vessels and airways; thickening of the alveolar wall followed, but it was not until the interstitial compartment was well filled that alveolar edema appeared; alveolar filling occurred independently and rapidly in individual alveoli. It is this anatomic localization in the perivascular and lobular interstitium that produces the typical roentgenographic pattern of loss of the normal sharp definition of the pulmonary vascular markings and thickening of the interlobular septa (B lines of Kerley) (Figure 4–31). Edema fluid that accumulates in the *parenchymal* interstitial tissues in these cir-

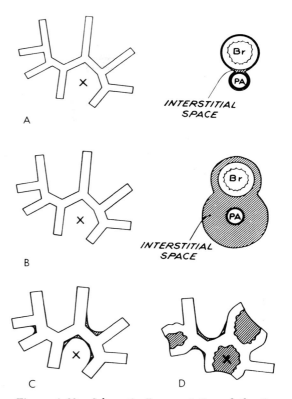

Figure 4–30. Schematic Representation of the Sequence of Fluid Accumulation in Acute Pulmonary Edema. *A*, Normal lung (alveolar wall and alveoli on the left, bronchovascular bundle on the right). *B*, Interstitial edema in which fluid accumulated preferentially in the loose interstitial space around the conducting blood vessels and airways without affecting the alveolar walls. *C*, Early alveolar edema showing loose interstitial spaces filled and fluid overflowing into alveoli, preferentially at the corners at which the curvature is greatest. *D*, Alveolar flooding. (Slightly modified from Staub, N. E., Nagano, H., and Pearce, M. L.: J. Appl. Physiol., 22:227, 1967, with permission of the authors and editor.)

cumstances usually produces little or no discernible roentgenographic change. The pattern of roentgenologic abnormality in such instances shows predominantly perivascular interstitial tissue involvement.

It is probable that the same statement can be made about other types of interstitial disease in which the alveolar wall is widened without much associated distortion of lung architecture. Since the number of alveoli in the human lung ranges from 300 to 600 million,[10] it is most unlikely that an increase in the wall thickness of these tiny structures could produce individually identifiable roentgenographic opacities. As with interstitial pulmonary edema that widens the alveolar wall, it is possible that such an abnormality could result in a haze over the lungs or in a ground-glass opacity, but it is

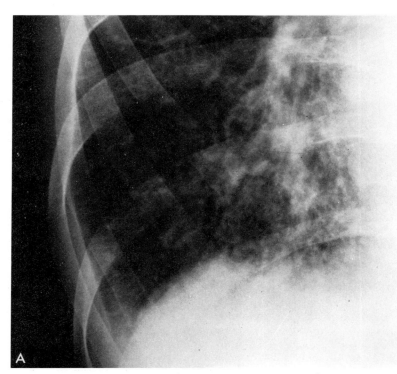

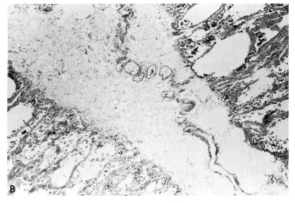

Figure 4–31. Pulmonary Interstitial Edema. A magnified view of the lower half of the right lung *(A)* shows the vascular markings to be hazy and indistinct because of the accumulation of fluid in the perivascular interstitial space. Thin horizontal lines of increased density measuring approximately 1 cm in length can be identified along the axillary lung margin inferiorly; these are due to accumulation of edema fluid in the interlobular septa (Kerley B lines). A photomicrograph *(B)* of an identical shadow of another patient studied at necropsy reveals a markedly thickened edematous interlobular septum extending across the field, the parenchyma above and below showing congestion and hemosiderosis; a slightly distended lymphatic channel can be seen passing through the center of the edematous septum. The line shadow observed roentgenographically is caused by edema of the septum rather than by distention of the lymphatic.

probably more often associated with a normal chest roentgenogram. We suspect that the reticulonodular pattern that characterizes the majority of diffuse interstitial lung diseases results from predominant involvement of the bronchovascular interstitium (Figure 4–32).

Generalized interstitial diseases may affect all parenchymal elements to varying degrees, although involvement of the interstitium is predominant. For example, in desquamative interstitial pneumonitis (fibrosing alveolitis), the morphologic picture is not one of simple thickening of alveolar walls with maintenance of pulmonary architecture but of an abundance of macrophages and desquamated alveolar lining cells within the alveoli; thus, the disease affects

both interstitium and air spaces. In its advanced stages the disease obliterates alveoli and dilates bronchioles proximal to obliterated acini, resulting in severe disorganization of lung architecture characteristic of the so-called honeycomb pattern and end-stage lung (*see* later on).

The concept of predominance is important. Those who criticize the logic of dividing diffuse lung disease into interstitial and air space patterns state that histologically the majority of diseases affect both anatomic compartments to some degree and that their distinction is therefore arbitrary. This is perhaps true, but we submit that the division is nevertheless valid if one accepts the concept of *predominant* involvement: an acinar pattern indicates *predominant*

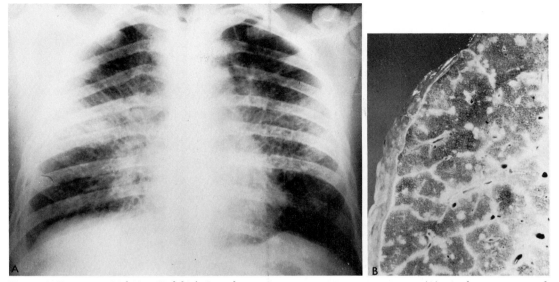

Figure 4–32. Interstitial Non-Hodgkin's Lymphoma. A posteroanterior roentgenogram *(A)* reveals extensive involvement of both lungs by a rather coarse reticular pattern. A photograph of the anterior portion of the lung removed at necropsy and sliced in a sagittal plane *(B)* reveals extensive thickening of the interlobular septa and perivascular interstitial tissues. The patient was an 18-year-old male with non-Hodgkin's lymphoma.

involvement of the parenchymal air spaces and a nodular or reticular pattern indicates *predominant* involvement of the interstitium. Bearing this in mind, pattern recognition becomes a logical and useful technique in roentgenologic interpretation.

ROENTGENOGRAPHIC PATTERNS OF DIFFUSE INTERSTITIAL DISEASE

Confusion in the interpretation of diffuse interstitial lung disease is not surprising—not only are the patterns numerous and extremely varied, but also our knowledge of their precise nature suffers from a lack of accurate roentgenologic-pathologic correlation. We still cannot accurately predict the pathologic anatomy in a number of these diseases. However, in most situations abnormal interstitial patterns can be described and classified precisely enough to allow reasonable conclusions to be drawn concerning their morphologic characteristics.

Before discussing specific roentgenographic manifestations of diffuse interstitial lung diseases, we shall indicate the roentgenologic changes common to all and without which the predominantly interstitial site of involvement should be doubted. Since the disease is anatomically interstitial, the acini remain air-containing, although their volume may be reduced by such effects as cicatrization. Therefore, diffuse

interstitial disease must be of inhomogeneous roentgenographic density; in most cases this feature alone distinguishes interstitial from air-space disease. Secondly, and for the same reason, the airways seldom are involved to any major extent, so that, by and large, there is nothing to prevent air from reaching the lung parenchyma. Therefore, *volume reduction due to airway obstruction is not a feature of interstitial disease* (although volume may decrease when interstitial fibrosis leads to cicatrization).

Five basic roentgenographic patterns of interstitial disease may be recognized: (1) ground glass, or granular, (2) nodular, (3) reticular, (4) reticulonodular, and (5) honeycomb.

Ground-Glass Pattern

This pattern *(synonyms:* granular stippling, reticulogranular, granular) is produced when interstitial tissue has increased to such an extent that density is increased, but the deposits are individually invisible. The roentgenographic appearance is of relatively homogeneous "clouding" or haze over the lungs. When the roentgenographic technique allows visibility of extremely fine detail, it is sometimes possible with a magnifying glass to identify tiny nodular opacities (as in early miliary tuberculosis) or extremely fine reticulation (as in early asbestosis).

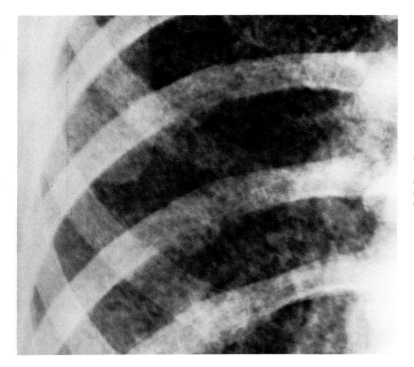

Figure 4–33. Patterns of Interstitial Disease: Nodular. A magnified view of the right lower zone of a posteroanterior roentgenogram of a patient with proved miliary tuberculosis; the pattern is purely nodular. (Courtesy of Dr. Romeo Ethier, Montreal Neurological Hospital.)

The ground-glass appearance has been described as typical of the early stages of asbestosis and berylliosis, in both of which it may be reasonably attributed to minimal fibrosis or granulomatous inflammation in the parenchymal interstitial space. It is logical to assume that this ground-glass opacification or granular stippling might be roentgenologically apparent in the early stages of the majority of interstitial lung diseases.

Nodular Pattern

Purely nodular interstitial diseases of the lungs are perhaps best epitomized by hematogenous infections such as miliary tuberculosis (Figure 4–33). Since the infecting organism reaches the lungs via the circulation and is trapped in the capillary sieve, it *must* be purely interstitial in location (at least early in its course; as the infection spreads, it may involve acinar air spaces). As the tubercles grow, they create a ground-glass pattern and eventually become large enough to be roentgenographically visible as tiny, discrete, punctate opacities. Early disseminated hematogenous carcinomatosis may have an identical appearance.

Reticular Pattern

This consists of a network of linear opacities, conceptually a series of rings surrounding spaces of air density (Figure 4–34). The precise pattern of the reticulation depends upon several variables, the two most important being the degree of thickening of the interstitial space and the effects the interstitial involvement exerts on parenchymal air spaces. It is useful to describe a reticular pattern according to the size of the "net"; the terms fine, medium, and coarse, although arbitrary, are in wide use and appear to be generally acceptable.

The observation that different roentgenographic patterns of reticulation merely indicate different degrees of severity of interstitial replacement is lent some support by numerous reports describing transition from a fine reticular pattern (even beginning with a ground-glass pattern), through all stages of fine, medium, and coarse reticulation, to honeycombing. This progression of changes has been described in many varied disease processes, including idiopathic interstitial fibrosis, rheumatoid lung, asbestosis, and lymphangiomyomatosis. The majority of diffuse interstitial diseases of the lung probably would be found to follow the same pattern of progression if they could be observed throughout their course.

Reticulonodular Pattern

Although a linear network throughout the interstitial tissue may present roentgenographically as a purely reticular pattern, orientation

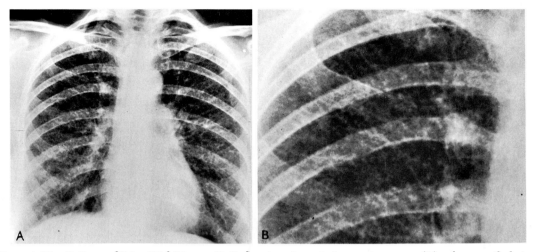

Figure 4–34. Patterns of Interstitial Disease: Reticular. A posteroanterior roentgenogram *(A)* and a magnified view of the right upper lung *(B)* reveal a fine network pattern characteristic of reticulation. Sarcoidosis.

of some linear opacities parallel to the x-ray beam frequently suggests a nodular component in addition to the reticular. Although in any given situation a reticulonodular pattern may be produced by this mechanism, it also may be produced by *admixture* of nodular deposits and diffuse linear thickening throughout the interstitial space, as, for example, in lymphangitic carcinomatosis.

Honeycomb Pattern

As mentioned earlier, the term "honeycombing" probably is overused. In our view, it should be restricted to a roentgenographic pattern that roughly resembles a true honeycomb—*air-containing cystic spaces 5 to 10 mm in diameter surrounded by thick walls* (Figure 4–35).

The morphologic counterpart of honeycomb

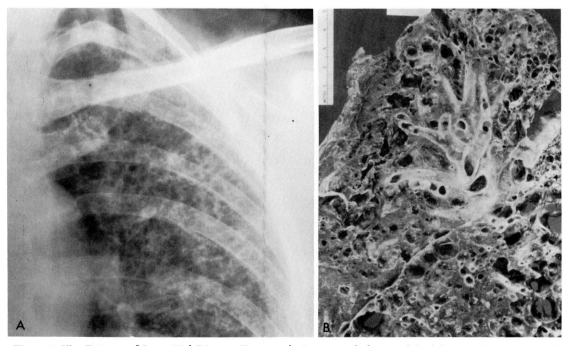

Figure 4–35. Patterns of Interstitial Disease: Honeycomb. In a magnified view of the left upper lung *(A)*, irregular cystic spaces can be identified ranging in size from 3 to 10 mm and possessing fairly thick walls. This is the characteristic appearance of the honeycomb pattern. A photograph of a cross section of the whole lung removed at necropsy *(B)* shows gross disorganization of lung architecture with small and large cystic spaces scattered widely throughout the lung.

lung, as defined above, has three characteristic features (Figure 4–35B): (1) the formation of cysts, 5 mm or more in diameter, commonly lined by bronchiolar epithelium; (2) the presence of thickened fibrous walls around the cysts; and (3) gross distortion and often obliteration of intervening lung parenchyma. It is to be emphasized that since the pathogenesis of honeycombing involves both the interstitium and air spaces, it is incorrect to label this pattern of disease "interstitial." In fact, the pathologic process cuts a swath across the lung parenchyma, affecting all elements and resulting in a morphologic and roentgenologic picture of the end-stage lung.

The roentgenographic pattern of honeycombing may be produced by a number of diseases, including histiocytosis X, idiopathic pulmonary fibrosis (cryptogenic fibrosing alveolitis), rheumatoid lung, lymphangiomyomatosis or tuberous sclerosis, scleroderma, asbestosis, chronic interstitial fungal infections, and occasionally end-stage sarcoidosis. Anatomic predominance of the pattern aids considerably in differential diagnosis; for example, histiocytosis X and sarcoidosis show a predilection for upper lung zones, whereas the remainder of the diseases listed above tend to lower zonal predominance. It is clear from this short list that restriction of the term "honeycomb lung" to the pattern described here reduces the diagnostic possibilities to relatively few diseases, especially if one takes into account anatomic predilection. We submit that this is the only way to bring some order to the confusion that surrounds diffuse interstitial lung disease.

Modifying Influences

Certain secondary effects sometimes produced by diffuse interstitial disease may considerably modify the basic roentgenographic pattern. For example, emphysema, either secondary to bronchiolar obstruction or compensatory to pulmonary fibrosis, may distort the pulmonary architecture and render the original disease pattern unrecognizable: the combination of conglomerate shadows and compensatory emphysema in advanced silicosis exemplifies this situation. Similarly, cicatrization produced by diffuse interstitial fibrosis may reduce lung volume severely, with resultant crowding of the reticular markings. Such modifying influences usually occur in relation to fairly definite etiologic and pathogenetic circumstances and, therefore, may help one to differentiate the many diseases in which the interstitial space of the lungs is diffusely affected.

COMBINED AIR-SPACE CONSOLIDATION AND INTERSTITIAL DISEASE

The pattern created by this combination is best exemplified by pulmonary edema secondary to pulmonary venous hypertension. The roentgenographic manifestations of *interstitial involvement* are largely those of a change in the perivascular interstitial sheath: edema fluid within the sheath increases the size and reduces the definition of lung markings in a distinctive pattern. The roentgenographic manifestations of *parenchymal air-space consolidation*, produced by edema fluid within the acini, consist of a few discrete and several confluent "fluffy" opacities characteristic of acinar-filling processes. This combination of interstitial and acinar patterns is highly suggestive of pulmonary edema of cardiac origin.

Another example of combined involvement of this type is acute pneumonitis of *Mycoplasma* or viral etiology. This infection characteristically causes acute interstitial inflammation, creating a pattern early in its course of fine to medium reticulation in segmental distribution. This "pure" interstitial involvement is often of short duration, the inflammatory reaction soon extending into the parenchymal air spaces and resulting in consolidation.

COMBINED CONSOLIDATION, ATELECTASIS, AND INTERSTITIAL DISEASE

This type of involvement perhaps is best exemplified by acute bronchopneumonia. The inflammation involves bronchial and bronchiolar walls and produces acute bronchitis and bronchiolitis; the bronchovascular interstitial sheath is inflamed and edematous; dissemination of the infection peripherally leads to patchy air-space consolidation; and the bronchitis and bronchiolitis lead to irregular airway obstruction, resulting in focal areas of air-space collapse (Figure 4–36). Patchy areas of lung parenchyma may show no abnormality or may overinflate to compensate for the focal atelectasis. Because of the mechanism of spread, the involvement is necessarily segmental. The resultant roentgenographic pattern of changes depicts the interstitial involvement, irregular zones of peripheral air-space consolidation, peripheral air-space collapse, and normal or overinflated parenchyma. Because of this admixture, individual acinar shadows are seldom recognizable. Depending upon the degree of consolidation, volume loss in the segment may be slight or

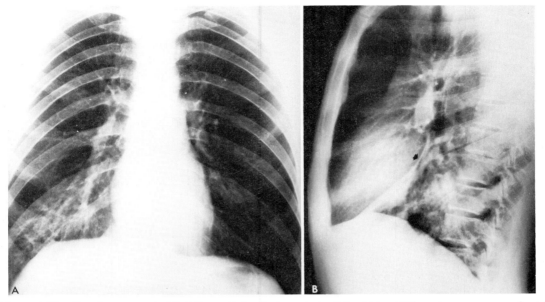

Figure 4–36. Bronchopneumonia, Right Lower Lobe. Posteroanterior *(A)* and lateral *(B)* roentgenograms reveal patchy consolidation of the anterior and lateral basal segments of the right lower lobe. Posterior bowing of the chief fissure *(arrow)* indicates some degree of loss of volume. The inhomogeneous nature of the disease suggests combined air-space consolidation, focal atelectasis, and focal compensatory overinflation.

moderate; overall density is inhomogeneous as a result of the foci of normal or overinflated parenchyma.

GENERAL SIGNS IN DISEASE THAT INCREASE ROENTGENOGRAPHIC DENSITY

In addition to the basic signs already described, there are several others that may aid in determining the nature of a pathologic process within the lungs.

a. Characteristics of the border of a pulmonary lesion.

b. Bulging of interlobar fissures.

c. Cavitation.

d. Calcification.

e. Distribution of disease within the lungs (anatomic bias).

f. Roentgenologic localization of pulmonary disease (the "silhouette sign").

g. Time factor in roentgenologic diagnosis.

CHARACTERISTICS OF THE BORDER OF A PULMONARY LESION

SHARPNESS OF DEFINITION. Roentgenographic assessment of the margin of a pulmo-

nary lesion coincides reasonably accurately with the morphologic appearance of the junction of consolidated tissue and normal lung parenchyma. Unfortunately, what is seen is an anatomic border, not the nature of the cells forming the border. In an analysis of 155 solitary lung lesions, Bateson[11] found that 58 of 80 primary carcinomas (73.5 per cent) had indistinctly defined margins and the remaining 22 were well defined; of 20 inflammatory lesions, 15 had ill-defined margins and five were well defined; only the 40 mixed tumors and other benign lesions had sharply defined margins in all cases. It may be concluded, therefore, that although the sharpness of definition of a pulmonary opacity gives *some* indication of its nature, it cannot be a sign of *absolute* value in establishing a diagnosis (Figure 4–37).

LOBULATION. Lobulation (as distinct from smoothness of contour) has a significance in many respects similar to that of sharpness of definition. *In general,* smoothness of contour suggests benignity, and lobulation indicates malignancy (Figure 4–37). Of 100 solitary circumscribed bronchogenic carcinomas studied by Bateson,[12] 29 had well-defined margins and *all* of these were lobulated. Probably the "umbilication" or notching of the border of a solitary pulmonary nodule described by Rigler[13] as a sign of malignancy is merely a manifestation of lobulation. Unfortunately, umbilication is not

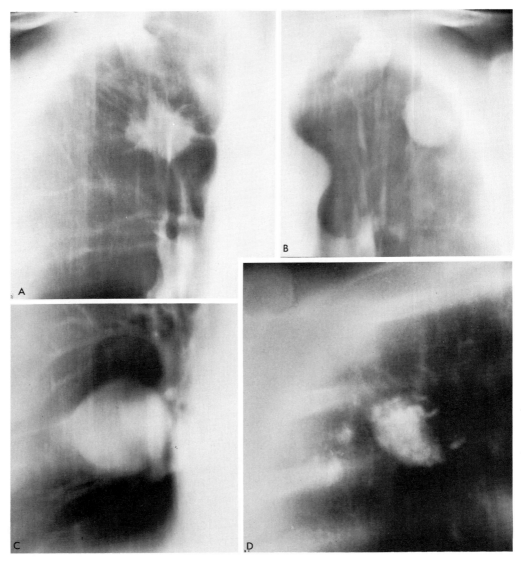

Figure 4–37.   Characteristics of the Border of Four Different Pulmonary Nodules Observed Tomographically. *A*, Shaggy, lobulated border of a primary adenocarcinoma; *B*, a smooth, nonlobulated contour of a primary adenocarcinoma; *C*, a smooth, nonlobulated border of a solitary metastasis from embryonal carcinoma of the testis; *D*, a sharply defined, somewhat lobulated contour of a histoplasmoma, with several satellite lesions situated laterally; both the larger nodule and the satellite lesions are calcified.

an infallible sign of malignancy, since in our experience it is present in a significant number of inflammatory nodules.

SATELLITE LESIONS. These are small punctate opacities in close proximity to a larger lesion, usually a solitary peripheral nodule, and in the great majority of cases suggest an infectious nature of a parenchymal lesion, particularly of tuberculous etiology (Figure 4–37).

RELATIONSHIP OF A LESION TO THE PLEURA. The contour of an opacity that relates to the pleura, either over the convexity of the thorax or contiguous with the mediastinum or diaphragm, can provide a useful clue to whether the process is intra- or extrapulmonary in origin. A mass that originates within the pleural space or extrapleurally displaces the pleura and underlying lung inward such that the angle formed by the margins of the mass and the chest wall is obtuse; by contrast, an intrapulmonary mass tends to relate to contiguous pleura with an acute angle. It should be obvious that these general rules apply only when such lesions are viewed tangentially.

BULGING OF INTERLOBAR FISSURES

Displacement of fissures toward a zone of increased density constitutes the only direct sign of lobar atelectasis. An equally valuable but less frequent sign is displacement of interlobar fissures in the opposite direction from the involved lobe—in other words, bulging of the fissures. This occurs most commonly in acute exudative infections of the lung in which the virulence of the organism produces an abundant exudate; the commonest of these is pneumonia caused by *Klebsiella pneumoniae* (Friedländer's pneumonia). Acute lung abscess often expands a lobe, particularly when air trapping by a check-valve mechanism in the communicating airway distends the abscess cavity (Figure 4–38).

In addition to the acute pneumonias, any space-occupying mass within a lobe may displace a fissure if the lesion occupies significant volume or if it is contiguous with the fissure; peripheral bronchogenic carcinoma is perhaps the most common of these masses.

The fissures are ordinarily an efficient barrier to the interlobar spread of parenchymal disease. A few diseases, however, have a propensity for crossing pleural boundaries, undoubtedly the commonest of these being mycotic infection of the lungs, particularly actinomycosis; these organisms not only pass across interlobar fissures but also across the visceral and parietal pleural layers over the convexity of the lung, and they may incite abscesses and osteomyelitis in the chest wall. Pulmonary tuberculosis, particularly in children, may transgress pleural boundaries; bronchogenic carcinoma rarely does so.

CAVITATION

The word "cavity" implies a focus of increased density whose central portion has been replaced by air. The presence of an air-fluid level is not necessary to the definition, nor is size of the cavity or thickness of its wall. The terms "cavity" and "abscess" are not synonymous; an intrapulmonary abscess without communication with the bronchial tree is roentgenographically opaque; only when the abscess communicates with the bronchial tree, allowing air to replace necrotic material, should "cavity" be applied.

The great majority of pulmonary cavities are caused by tissue necrosis and the expulsion of necrotic material into the bronchial tree. The mechanism by which necrosis occurs varies according to the underlying disease. In infectious processes such as acute staphylococcal pneumonia, the virulence of the infection leads to tissue death; the necrosis of neoplasms probably is related at least partly to deficient blood supply, although the very small size (not exceeding 1 cm in diameter) of some neoplasms that undergo cavitation suggests another mechanism, perhaps delayed hypersensitivity reaction.

The roentgenographic demonstration of pul-

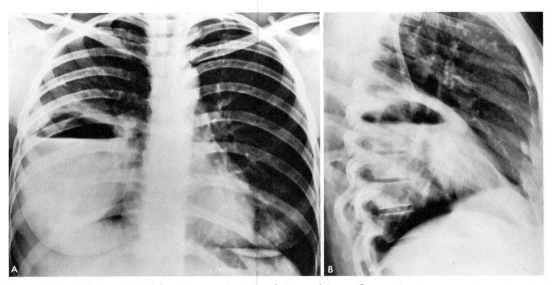

Figure 4–38. Bulging of Interlobar Fissures: Acute Staphylococcal Lung Abscess. Roentgenograms in posteroanterior *(A)* and lateral *(B)* projection reveal a large abscess in the right lower lobe producing upward bulging of the major fissure.

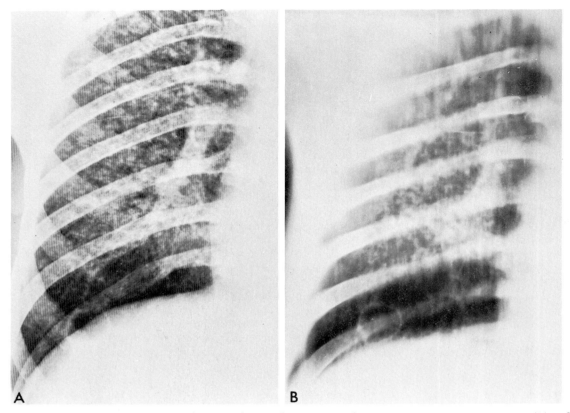

Figure 4–39. Tuberculous Lung Abscess with Bronchogenic Spread. A posteroanterior roentgenogram *(A)* and anteroposterior tomogram *(B)* of the right lung reveal a well-defined thin-walled cavity in the base of the right lower lobe. Multiple poorly defined shadows possessing the typical characteristics of acinar lesions can be identified throughout much of the right lung, representing bronchogenic spread from the tuberculous cavity. This combination of changes comprises almost certain evidence of a tuberculous etiology. (Courtesy of Dr. Richard Lesperance, formerly of the Montreal Chest Hospital Center.)

monary cavitation may be simple or exceedingly difficult. If the cavity contains fluid, as is frequently the case, the identification of an air-fluid level is clearly pathognomonic. In the absence of an air-fluid level, tomography may be essential to confirm the diagnosis or, perhaps more commonly, to identify cavitary disease that was not even remotely suspected on plain roentgenography.

Although the nature of cavity formation within specific disease groups varies considerably, in most cases the general patterns give some indication of the underlying etiology (Figure 4–39). The following examples indicate prevailing patterns; in each category there are occasional exceptions to the general rule.

CAVITY WALL. This is usually thick in acute lung abscess (Figure 4–38), primary (Figure 4–40) and metastatic carcinoma, and Wegener's granulomatosis and usually is thin in infected bullae and post-traumatic cysts. From a study of 65 solitary cavities in the lung designed to evaluate diagnostic implications of cavity wall

thickness, Woodring and his colleagues[14] found that all lesions in which the thickest part of the cavity wall was 1 mm were benign; of the lesions whose thickest measurement was 4 mm or less, 92 per cent were benign; of cavities that were 5 to 15 mm in their thickest part, benign and malignant lesions were equally divided; when the cavity wall was over 15 mm in thickness, 95 per cent of lesions were malignant. These authors concluded that measurement of the thickest part of a cavity wall provides a more reliable indication of benignancy or malignancy than measurement of the thinnest part.

CHARACTER OF INNER LINING. This is usually irregular and nodular in carcinoma (Figure 4–40), shaggy in acute lung abscess (Figure 4–38), and smooth in most other cavitary lesions.

NATURE OF CONTENTS. In the majority of cases the contents are fluid, with no distinctive characteristics. In contrast to the usually flat, smooth character of air-fluid levels, in certain diseases the contents may be so typical as to be diagnostic; for example, the intracavitary fungus

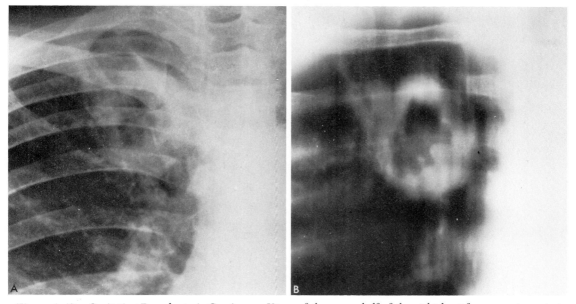

Figure 4–40.   Cavitating Bronchogenic Carcinoma. Views of the upper half of the right lung from a posteroanterior roentgenogram *(A)* and an anteroposterior tomogram *(B)* reveal a rather poorly defined cavitating mass. The thickness of the wall and irregular nodular character of the inner lining are highly suggestive of bronchogenic carcinoma. Proved highly differentiated squamous-cell cancer.

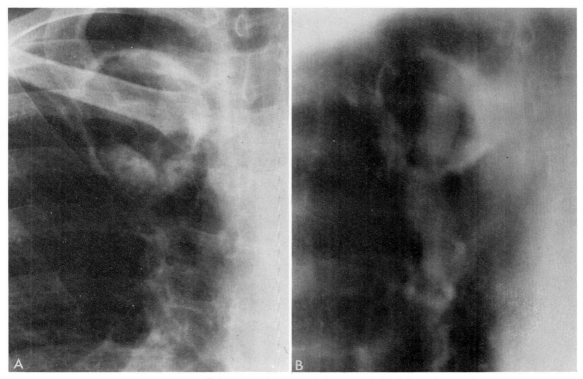

Figure 4–41.   Intracavitary Fungus Ball (Mycetoma). Views of the upper half of the right lung from a posteroanterior roentgenogram *(A)* and an anteroposterior tomogram *(B)* reveal a rather thin-walled but irregular cavity in the paramediastinal zone. Situated within it is a smooth oblong shadow of homogeneous density whose relationships to the wall of the cavity change from the erect *(A)* to the supine *(B)* positions. Histologically, the intracavitary mass was composed of multiple mycelial threads characteristic of *Aspergillus*. The cavity was of tuberculous etiology.

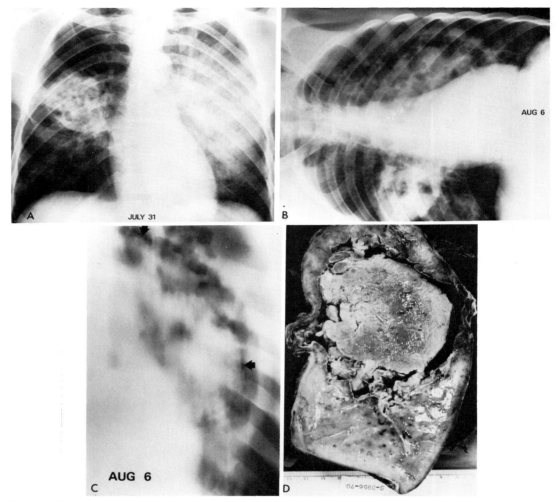

Figure 4–42. Acute Lung Gangrene in Klebsiella Pneumonia. On admission to hospital, a chest roentgenogram (not illustrated) of this 37-year-old man revealed massive air-space consolidation throughout much of the left lung and midportion of the right lung. He was exceedingly ill and required assisted ventilation. *K. pneumoniae* was grown from the sputum; blood cultures were negative. Although 11 days later his clinical condition had improved somewhat, a roentgenogram (*A*) revealed a change in the texture of the consolidation in that its homogeneity was disturbed by multiple poorly defined air-containing spaces, seen to better advantage in the right than the left lung. This represents the earliest roentgenologic sign of acute lung gangrene. One week later, a lateral decubitus roentgenogram (*B*) revealed a large, irregular, shaggy mass within a huge cavity in the left lung indicated to better advantage in an anteroposterior tomogram (*arrows* in *C*). The left lower lobe was resected and the specimen (*D*) showed a large necrotic mass lying within a huge cavity and completely separated from the cavity walls. (Reprinted from Knight, L., Fraser, R. G., and Robson, H. G.: Can. Med. Assoc. J., *112*:196, 1975, with permission of the authors and editor.)

ball (mycetoma; aspergilloma—Figure 4–41) or intracavitary blood clot or fibrin ball, which form freely mobile intracavitary masses; or the collapsed membranes of a ruptured echinococcus cyst, which float on top of the fluid within the cyst and create the characteristic "water-lily" sign or the "sign of the camalote" (a water plant found in South American rivers).

A rare but characteristic intracavitary mass is that associated with massive pulmonary gangrene, in which extensive necrosis of lung tissue occurs in cases of acute Friedländer's or pneu-mococcal pneumonia; irregular pieces of sloughed lung parenchyma float like icebergs in the cavity fluid (Figure 4–42).

MULTIPLICITY OF LESIONS. Some cavitary disease is characteristically solitary—for example, primary bronchogenic carcinoma, acute lung abscess, and post-traumatic lung cyst; other diseases are characteristically multiple—for example, metastatic neoplasm, Wegener's granulomatosis, acute coccidioidomycosis, and acute pyemic abscesses.

We will mention briefly simulation of cavities—an uncommon occurrence. At necropsy some "cavitary" lesions visible on premortem roentgenograms are found to contain no air and to have no communication with the bronchial tree. Histologically, the center of such lesions is necrotic, and it is assumed that some histochemical change has occurred in this necrotic material whereby its lipid content is sufficiently high to cause a relatively radiolucent shadow roentgenographically, thus simulating cavitation.[15]

CALCIFICATION

Intrathoracic calcification is an important parameter of pulmonary disease. In the majority of cases it is dystrophic, usually in tissue that has degenerated and become necrotic. Although metastatic calcification occurs, presumably because of the low pH of lung tissue, it is seldom roentgenographically visible.

Both the distribution and character of calcification should be noted, since each has diagnostic significance. It is convenient to consider intrathoracic calcification under five headings, depending on its anatomic location and distribution: local parenchymal, widespread parenchymal, lymph nodal, pleural, and other.

LOCAL PARENCHYMAL CALCIFICATION. The commonest form of pulmonary calcification is the single, often densely calcified focus, situated anywhere in the lungs and representing calcification of a healed primary granulomatous lesion. It is most frequently caused by histoplasmosis, and less often by tuberculosis. This Ghon lesion is usually part of a duo (the Ranke complex), the other component being calcification of a hilar or mediastinal drainage lymph node. Although calcification nearly always is associated with healing of the infectious process, it does not necessarily indicate that the lesion is inactive.

Calcification within *solitary pulmonary nodules* is a useful indicator of the nature of these perplexing lesions. Most importantly, it is the most reliable single piece of evidence that a lesion is benign.[16] The major exception to this general rule is the isolated instance of a peripheral primary carcinoma engulfing an existing granulomatous calcification, in which case the calcification is usually eccentric.

The character of the calcification within a solitary pulmonary nodule may be a reliable indicator of the lesion's etiology. For example, a small central *nidus* is the sign of a granulomatous lesion in most cases, *lamination* is almost pathognomonic of a granuloma, usually histoplasmoma, and is the most reliable sign of a benign lesion; *"popcorn-ball"* calcification is characteristic of hamartoma; and *multiple punctate foci* throughout a lesion may be seen in either granulomas or hamartomas (Figure 4–43).[16] Tomography may be necessary in the

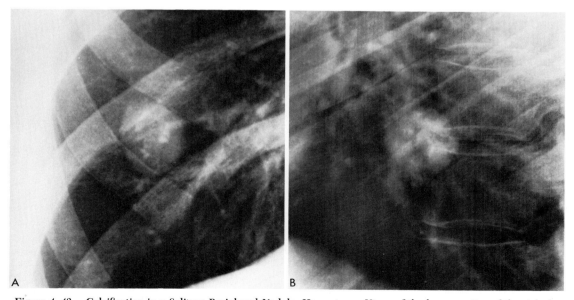

Figure 4–43. Calcification in a Solitary Peripheral Nodule: Hamartoma. Views of the lower portion of the right lung from posteroanterior *(A)* and lateral *(B)* roentgenograms show a solitary nodule in which fairly large calcium deposits are vaguely reminiscent of "popcorn." Proved hamartoma. (Courtesy of Dr. Richard Lesperance, formerly of the Montreal Chest Hospital Center.)

investigation of solitary peripheral nodules to identify calcification not seen or only suggested on plain roentgenograms.

A rare form of local parenchymal calcification occurs when a solitary calcified focus, commonly the result of histoplasmosis, moves by some unknown mechanism from adjacent parenchyma or lymph node into the lumen of a bronchus. Appropriately termed broncholiths, these foci can produce segmental or subsegmental atelectasis and may occasion hemoptysis.

DIFFUSE PARENCHYMAL CALCIFICATION (OR OSSIFICATION). This form may be caused by several conditions, but the pattern in each is usually distinctive. For example, the tiny punctate "calcispherytes" of alveolar microlithiasis present a unique, virtually unmistakable roentgenographic image. Multiple nodular calcifications or ossifications occur in various conditions, including mitral stenosis, silicosis, and certain healed disseminated infectious diseases such as tuberculosis, histoplasmosis, and varicella pneumonitis (Figure 4–44).

Extensive metastatic pulmonary calcification may occur in cases of long-standing hypercalcemia associated with chronic renal disease and secondary hyperparathyroidism, and in other diseases such as diffuse myelomatosis in which the serum calcium level is chronically elevated. Metabolic factors etiologically related to this type of calcification are increased serum calcium and phosphate, relative alkalinity of the site of calcium deposition, and impaired renal function.[17] In some cases the calcification may be so extensive as to cause respiratory failure. The calcific nature of the pulmonary opacities can be readily confirmed by scanning with bone imaging agents such as ^{99m}Tc diphosphonate.[18]

LYMPH NODE CALCIFICATION. This form of calcification is usually amorphous and irregularly distributed throughout the node. It results most commonly from healed granulomatous infection, usually tuberculosis or histoplasmosis, and constitutes part of the Ranke complex. "Eggshell" calcification is uncommon; it consists of a ring of calcification around the periphery of a lymph node and occurs most typically in silicosis, occasionally in sarcoidosis. The various causes of eggshell calcification of lymph nodes has recently been reviewed.[19]

PLEURAL CALCIFICATION. Pleural calcification is most often the result of a remote hemothorax, pyothorax, or tuberculous effusion, and commonly is associated with thickening of the pleura over the entire lung surface. The calcification may be in the form of a broad continuous sheet or of multiple discrete plaques. It usually extends from about the level of the midthorax posteriorly, around the lateral lung margin in a generally inferior direction, roughly paralleling the chief fissure (Figure 4–45). Calcium usually is deposited on the inner surface of the thickened visceral pleura, resulting in a thick tissue layer of unit density between the calcium and the thoracic wall. In contrast to

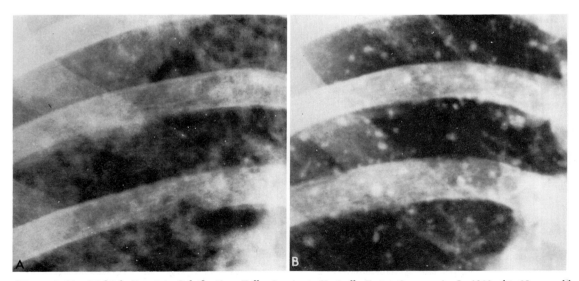

Figure 4–44. Multiple Punctate Calcifications Following Acute Varicella-Zoster Pneumonia. In 1962, this 28-year-old woman developed widespread air-space pneumonia in association with classic cutaneous chickenpox. A chest roentgenogram revealed generalized patchy acinar consolidation, seen to advantage in a magnified view of the right midlung zone (*A*). Eight years later, a posteroanterior roentgenogram (*B*) revealed multiple tiny punctate calcifications throughout both lungs. (Courtesy of Dr. Max Palayew, Jewish General Hospital, Montreal.)

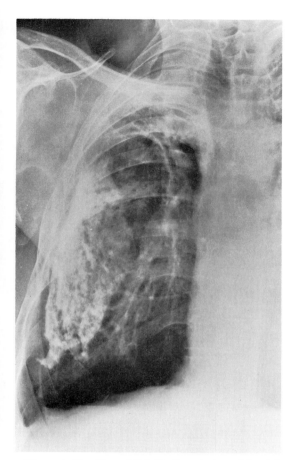

Figure 4–45.   Pleural Calcification. A view of the right hemithorax from a posteroanterior roentgenogram reveals a heavy, broad sheet of calcium situated over the convexity of the lung and oriented in a position roughly corresponding to the axillary line of the chief fissure. There is considerable loss of volume of the right upper lobe as evidenced by elevation of the right hilum and displacement of the trachea. Old fibrotic upper lobe tuberculosis: the pleural calcification resulted from tuberculous empyema.

pleural calcification caused by silicatosis this form is nearly always unilateral.

Pleural calcification of an entirely different form is now recognized as a frequent occurrence in silicatosis, including asbestosis and talcosis. The calcification usually forms in plaques, commonly along the diaphragm, and with extensive thickening of the pleura in some cases; it invariably occurs in the parietal pleura, while when secondary to pyothorax or hemothorax it is found in the visceral pleura. It is almost invariably bilateral. The mediastinum may be involved, but calcification of the interlobar pleura has not been observed.[20]

CALCIFICATION IN OTHER SITES. Calcification of the cartilages of the trachea and major bronchi appears to be a physiologic concomitant of aging; curiously, it is far more common in elderly females than in males.[17]

Calcification of the walls of the central pulmonary arteries occurs in a high percentage of patients with severe long-standing pulmonary arterial hypertension, particularly those with a left-to-right shunt. The calcification may be localized to the main pulmonary artery or may extend into the major hilar and even lobar branches; the arteries invariably are severely dilated.

DISTRIBUTION OF DISEASE WITHIN THE LUNGS (ANATOMIC BIAS)

For several reasons, some known and others obscure, many lung diseases tend to develop predominantly in certain anatomic locations. Knowledge of such anatomic bias is of obvious diagnostic importance; the following selected examples indicate how this sign can be used in differential diagnosis.

Aspiration pneumonia is a typical example in which the influence of gravity largely establishes the anatomic distribution of disease. If aspiration occurs when the patient is supine (during the postoperative period, for instance), the upper lobes are involved more often than the lower and their posterior portions more frequently than their anterior; conversely, if aspiration occurs when the patient is erect, involvement of the lower lobes predominates. Whether the patient is recumbent or erect, aspiration occurs more readily into the right than left lung because of the more direct origin of the right main bronchus from the trachea.

Pulmonary infarction occurs much more frequently in lower than in upper lobes. This anatomic bias probably reflects the more direct flow of blood from the main pulmonary arteries into lower rather than upper lobes. For the same reason, metastatic lesions occur more frequently in lower lobes; a solitary mass in an upper lobe is unlikely to be metastatic.

In contrast to the bias for lower lung zones displayed by metastatic neoplasms, primary bronchogenic carcinoma has an unexplained predilection for upper lung zones. In 250 cases analyzed by Garland,[21] the ratio of upper to lower lobe origin was approximately 2.5 to 1. Cavitary carcinoma similarly shows a strong anatomic bias for the upper lobes.

Pulmonary tuberculosis provides a singular opportunity to employ anatomic bias in differential diagnosis. In postprimary tuberculosis in adults, susceptibility of the apical and posterior bronchopulmonary segments of the upper lobes and the superior segment of the lower lobes is well recognized. These segments of lung are characterized by poor perfusion, diminished respiratory ventilation, and a bronchial distribution favoring bronchogenic spread. The rarity with which the anterior bronchopulmonary segment of an upper lobe is affected *to the exclusion* of other segments is sufficient to make the diagnosis of postprimary tuberculosis in this area extremely unlikely (only one case was reported in the series of 100 cases).[22]

In contrast, *primary tuberculosis* shows an opposite anatomic bias. In the 90 children studied by Frostad,[23] involvement greatly predominated in the anterior segments of the right lung, both in the upper and middle lobes. The reasons for this difference in anatomic distribution in primary and postprimary tuberculosis are not clear.

Pulmonary sequestration occurs almost exclusively in the lower lobes, most commonly in the posterior basilar bronchopulmonary segment, and more commonly on the left side than the right.

Diffuse lung disease frequently shows an anatomic bias, a factor that may be important to differential diagnosis. For example, the ground-glass opacity and reticulation of asbestosis typically is of basal distribution. Chronic idiopathic interstitial fibrosis and interstitial fibrosis of scleroderma frequently are predominantly basal in distribution, particularly in the early stages. Conversely, upper lobe predilection is shown by silicosis, coal-workers' pneumoconiosis, sarcoidosis, and histiocytosis X.

ROENTGENOLOGIC LOCALIZATION OF PULMONARY DISEASE (THE "SILHOUETTE SIGN")

The anatomic location of the great majority of pulmonary diseases that increase local density can be established precisely from posteroanterior and lateral roentgenograms. When only a single PA or AP roentgenogram is available, however, the "silhouette sign"[24] is useful. The mediastinal and diaphragmatic contours are rendered roentgenographically visible by their contrast with contiguous air-containing lung. When consolidation or atelectasis affects any portion of lung adjacent to a mediastinal or diaphragmatic border, that border can no longer be visualized roentgenographically (Fig. 4–46). The corollary is that an opacity within the lungs which does *not* obliterate the mediastinal or diaphragmatic contour cannot be situated within lung contiguous with these structures (Figure 4–47). The silhouette sign is perhaps of greatest use in the differentiation of middle lobe and lingular disease from lower lobe disease, but in many other sites it may show the precise anatomic location—for example, oblit-

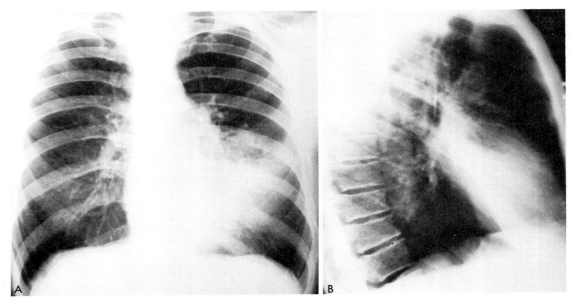

Figure 4–46. The Silhouette Sign. Posteroanterior *(A)* and lateral *(B)* roentgenograms reveal obliteration of the left heart border by an opacity of homogeneous density situated within the lingula; such obliteration inevitably indicates lingular disease (provided there is adequate roentgenographic exposure). Squamous cell carcinoma of the lingular bronchus with distal obstructive pneumonitis.

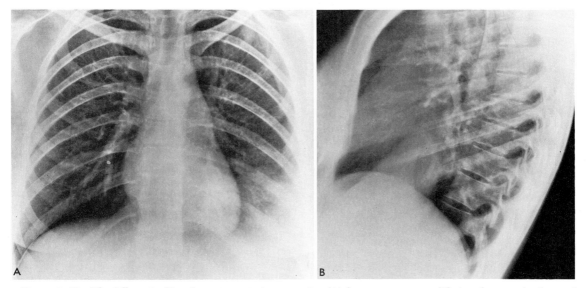

Figure 4–47. The Silhouette Sign. In posteroanterior projection *(A)*, homogeneous consolidation obscures the dome of the left hemidiaphragm from the heart border to the costophrenic sulcus. The left heart border is clearly defined and distinct. This combination of changes implies that the consolidation must lie in a plane behind the heart but contiguous with the left hemidiaphragm in a position tangential to the x-ray beam—that is, the anterior bronchopulmonary segment. If the consolidation was situated more posteriorly, the diaphragmatic dome tangential to the plane of the beam would be contiguous with air-containing lung and thus would be visible. In lateral projection *(B)*, note the precise anatomic localization to the anterior bronchopulmonary segment. In *A*, the segment of the left hemidiaphragm from the heart border medially is obscured by contiguity with the heart—an additional example of the silhouette sign.

eration of the aortic knuckle on the left side by airlessness of the apical-posterior segment of the left upper lobe or obliteration of the posterior paraspinal line by contiguous airless lung in the left posterior gutter.

Although this sign is used chiefly to localize pulmonary disease, we have found it almost as useful for identifying disease processes. For example, it may be very difficult to identify the shadow of minor consolidation or atelectasis in a posterior basal segment of a lower lobe but invisibility of the posterior portion of the hemidiaphragm in lateral projection permits a categorical statement that there is disease in that segment.

THE TIME FACTOR IN ROENTGENOLOGIC DIAGNOSIS

In clinical practice, situations occur relatively frequently in which a lack of specific roentgenologic signs precludes positive diagnosis. In both acute and chronic lung diseases, roentgenographic signs may overlap so that only differential diagnostic possibilities can be suggested at the first examination; if the diagnosis cannot be established by the integrated clinical evidence and results of laboratory and pulmonary

function tests, serial films showing changes over the subsequent days, weeks, or months often provide valuable clues. A few examples illustrate the importance of assessing time relationships in roentgenologic diagnosis.

Acute pneumonia caused by *Streptococcus pneumoniae* or *Mycoplasma pneumoniae* organisms sometimes can be differentiated by their characteristic roentgenographic patterns. If this is not possible immediately, changes evidenced in roentgenograms over the next few days sometimes permit distinction, even without antibiotic therapy (progressive changes despite penicillin therapy might suggest a *Mycoplasma* etiology, indicating the need for administration of a more efficacious antibiotic). The rapidity with which diffuse interstitial pulmonary edema may appear and disappear (often within hours) allows immediate differentiation from irreversible interstitial disease, which it may otherwise closely mimic. Finally, it is surprising how frequently a small area of parenchymal consolidation in an upper lobe, roentgenographically typical of exudative tuberculosis, disappears in about 7 to 10 days, indicating a less significant etiology.

It is not only in the field of acute pulmonary disease that the time relationship is important. Growth characteristics of peripheral pulmonary nodules have been studied a great deal in recent years. The "doubling time"* hypothesis developed by Collins and associates[25] has increased our knowledge of the natural history of bronchogenic carcinoma. For example, in a study of 218 pulmonary nodules, of which 177 were malignant and 41 benign, Nathan and his colleagues[26] concluded that virtually all nodules with a doubling time of 7 days or less are benign. At the other end of the scale, almost all nodules whose volume doubles in 465 days or more are benign. Perhaps the growth rate principle is most useful in assessing solitary nodules in patients over 40 years of age, when the incidence of malignancy increases significantly. In this age group, Nathan and associates found that nearly all solitary nodules that doubled in less than 37 days were benign, and that the longest doubling time of 72 malignant nodules was 200 days. It seems, therefore, that pulmonary nodules whose rate of growth falls outside these "benign" limits should be considered malignant.

LINE SHADOWS

The normal substratum of all chest roentgenograms is formed by line shadows—the vascular markings and interlobar fissures; the roentgenologic appearance of these is described in Chapter 1. The present section describes the many line shadows of varied etiology, seen from time to time in roentgenograms of the chest, which can be grouped most appropriately under this descriptive umbrella. Primary and secondary abnormalities of the pulmonary vasculature form a comprehensive topic in their own right and are considered in detail in Chapter 10.

Linear opacities on a chest roentgenogram fall into six different categories on the basis of pathogenesis: (1) septal lines; (2) tubular shadows (bronchial wall shadows); (3) linear opacities extending from peripheral parenchymal lesions to the hila or visceral pleura; (4) parenchymal scarring; (5) line shadows of pleural origin; (6) horizontal or obliquely oriented linear opacities of unknown nature.

Septal or Lymphatic Lines

In 1933 Kerley[27] described certain linear shadows in the chest roentgenogram that he

ascribed to engorged lymphatics. In 1951 he further categorized three patterns of linear change which he designated "A" lines, "B" lines, and "C" lines.[28]

Kerley A lines are straight or almost straight linear opacities, seldom more than 1 mm thick and 2 to 6 cm long, within the lung substance; their course bears no definite relationship to the anatomic distribution of bronchoarterial bundles (Figure 4–48). Most are situated approximately midway between hilum and pleura and none more peripherally. Trapnell[29] has shown positive correlation between roentgenographic A lines and sheets of connective tissue deep within the lung in which run both veins and anastomotic lymphatics. He showed histologically that the lymphatics contribute one tenth or less to the thickness of the line shadow, and that in certain conditions such as pulmonary edema they may be invisible. As with Kerley B lines, the visibility of A lines depends upon the accumulation of abnormal amounts of edema fluid or other tissue within the perilymphatic connective tissue, and not distention of the lymphatics themselves. Depending upon the disease process that causes them, they may be reversible (as in pulmonary edema) or irreversible (as in pneumoconiosis or lymphangitic carcinoma).

Kerley B lines are less than 2 cm long (shorter than A lines). In contrast to A lines, which lie in the substance of the lungs, B lines are in the periphery; they are short and straight, seldom more than 1 mm thick, and lie roughly perpendicular to the pleural surface (Figure 4–49). Their outer ends invariably abut against the visceral pleura. B lines are caused by increased fluid or tissue in the interlobular septa of the lungs, chiefly in the perilymphatic interstitial tissue. Because of their anatomic location they are sometimes referred to as "septal lines." Their pathogenesis varies widely: one of the commonest causes is interstitial pulmonary edema secondary to pulmonary venous hypertension (as in mitral stenosis or left ventricular failure). When the edema is transient, septal lines appear and disappear sporadically with each episode of decompensation; with repeated insults of this character, or in the presence of chronic and severe pulmonary venous hypertension, fibrosis and hemosiderin deposits within the interlobular septa give rise to permanent, irreversible B lines. Other causes of irreversible septal lines include pneumoconiosis, sarcoidosis, lymphangitic carcinomatosis, lipid pneumonia, and lymphoma.

Kerley C lines consist of a fine network of interlacing linear shadows sometimes seen in

---

*"*Doubling*" refers to volume, not diameter. Assuming a nodule to be spherical, multiply its radius by 1.25 to obtain the radius of a sphere whose volume is double; *e.g.*, the volume of a nodule 2 cm in diameter (1.0 cm radius) is doubled by the time its diameter reaches 2.5 cm.

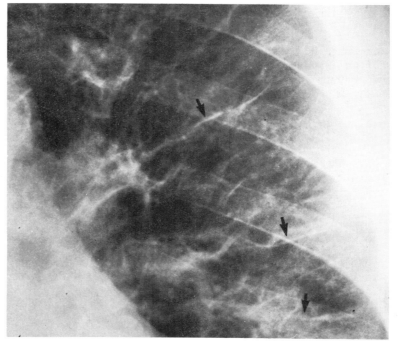

Figure 4–48. Line Shadows; Kerley A Lines. A view of the left lung from a posteroanterior roentgenogram reveals a coarse network of linear strands widely distributed throughout the lung. Several long line shadows measuring up to 4 cm in length can be identified in the central zone approximately midway between the axillary lung margin and the heart *(arrows)*; the orientation of these lines does not conform to the distribution of bronchovascular bundles. These are Kerley A lines and represent edema of central pulmonary septa.

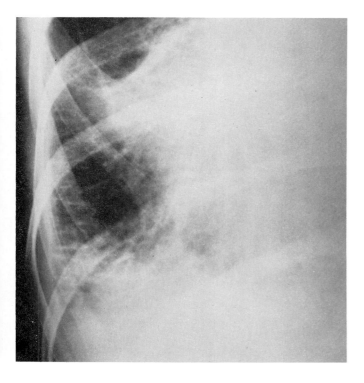

Figure 4–49. Line Shadows: Septal (Kerley B) Lines. A magnified view of the lower portion of the right lung from a posteroanterior roentgenogram reveals several line shadows approximately 1 cm in length oriented in a horizontal plane perpendicular to the axillary pleura. These are Kerley B lines, caused by edema of the interlobular septa.

cases of interstitial pulmonary edema and are caused by the superimposition of many Kerley B lines in the anterior and posterior portions of the lungs. Such a network of shadows is probably a manifestation of severe interlobular edema rather than separate and distinct anatomic involvement of lymphatic channels.

Tubular Shadows (Bronchial Wall Shadows)

Tubular shadows are double-line shadows that may be parallel or slightly tapered as they proceed distally. They are situated outside the anatomic limits of the hila, and always follow the bronchovascular distribution; they may branch in a manner typical of the bronchial tree.

The commonest cause of tubular shadows is bronchiectasis (Figure 4–50), in which the line shadows are roughly parallel and are 1 mm or slightly wider. The width of the air column separating them depends upon the severity of the bronchial dilatation. Morphologically these line shadows are caused by a combination of thickening bronchial walls and peribronchial

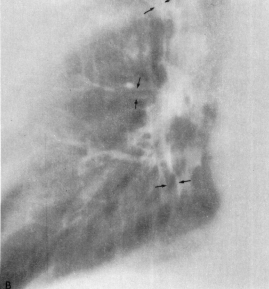

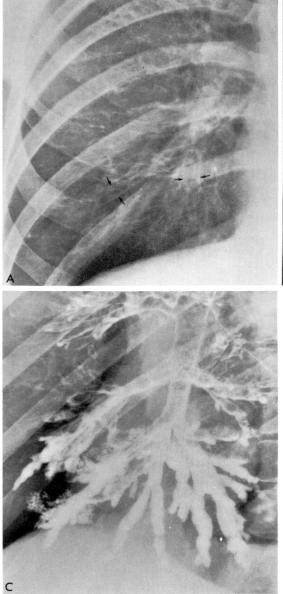

Figure 4–50. Line Shadows: Tubular. A view of the lower half of the right lung from a posteroanterior roentgenogram *(A)* reveals numerous tubular shadows *(arrows)*, some of whose walls are parallel and others divergent; their visualization is improved on tomographic section *(B)*. A right bronchogram *(C)* reveals severe cylindrical and varicose bronchiectasis of all segmental bronchi of the middle and lower lobes, with abrupt termination of the dilated segments suggesting obliterative bronchiolitis. The line shadows are caused by the thickened bronchial walls. This 33-year-old man had been exposed 3 months previously to a heavy concentration of sulfur dioxide fumes with subsequent development of severe obliterative bronchiolitis and bronchiectasis.

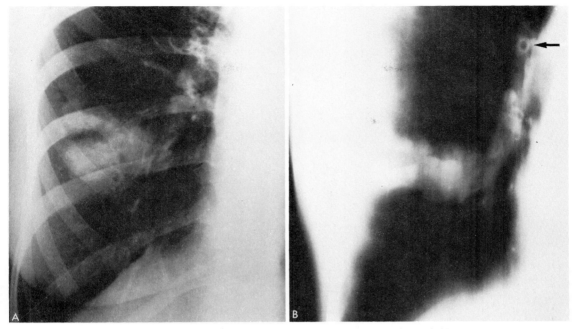

Figure 4–51. **Y-Shaped Opacity Caused by Mucoid Impaction.** Views of the lower half of the right lung from a posteroanterior roentgenogram *(A)* and an anteroposterior tomogram *(B)* reveal a homogeneous opacity composed of a horizontal component and a branched component extending laterally, the whole possessing a Y-configuration. The patient is a 28-year-old woman with long-standing spasmodic asthma and hypersensitivity bronchopulmonary aspergillosis. The opacity is produced by mucoid impaction. Note the markedly thickened bronchial wall in *B (arrow).*

fibrosis and alveolar collapse. When bronchiectatic segments become filled with retained mucus or pus their tubular appearance is transformed into homogeneous bandlike densities which Simon[30] terms the "gloved-finger" shadow. Of a similar nature but more proximal in the bronchial tree are the mucous plugs of mucoid impaction or hypersensitivity bronchopulmonary aspergillosis; these vary from a broad linear shadow to a Y or V configuration, depending on the length of airway involved and whether a bronchial bifurcation is affected (Figure 4–51).

Of a different nature are the "end-on" bronchial shadows roentgenographically identifiable in the parahilar zones of a large percentage of subjects (Figure 4–51). These bronchi represent segmental or subsegmental bronchi in the anterior bronchopulmonary segment of an upper lobe or superior bronchopulmonary segment of a lower lobe. They range in diameter from 3 to 7 mm and thus represent different stages in bronchial subdivision. To assess whether thickening of the walls of bronchi visualized end-on reliably distinguishes the patient with chronic bronchitis from the normal subject, we studied the roentgenograms of 300 persons—roughly equal numbers of patients with established chronic obstructive pulmonary disease and age-matched asymptomatic subjects with normal standard pulmonary function tests.[31] It was concluded that caliper measurement of bronchial wall thickness and subjective assessment of thickening provide suggestive but not conclusive evidence for the presence of chronic bronchitis.

Linear Communications Between Peripheral Parenchymal Lesions and the Hila or Visceral Pleura

Line shadows of varying width are often visible extending from a peripheral parenchymal opacity to the hilum. Usually they are uneven in width and their course may be interrupted for varying distances. Their conformity to the pattern of vascular distribution establishes their anatomic location within bronchovascular bundles. Such communicating strands have been described in both infectious and neoplastic processes. For example, in cavitary tuberculosis the connecting line shadows are produced by an admixture of tubercles, fibrous tissue, thickened lymphatics, and thickened bronchial walls; when tuberculosis becomes chronic and productive, fibrosis is histologically more predominant. In some cases of a peripheral mass or nodule, line shadows extend to the

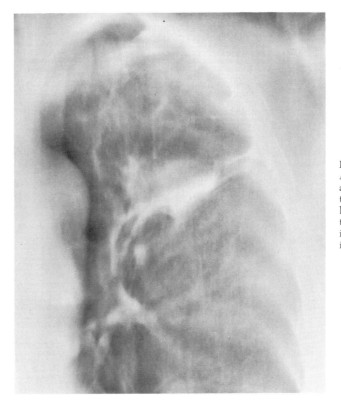

Figure 4–52. Line Shadows: Communication Between a Peripheral Mass and the Visceral Pleura. A view of the upper half of the left lung from an anteroposterior tomogram reveals a rather indistinctly defined homogeneous mass lying in the mid-lung zone. A prominent line shadow extends from the lateral margin of the mass to the pleura, resulting in a V-shaped deformity of the pleura caused by indrawing. Proved exudative histoplasmosis.

hilum; since the sign may be present in both infectious and neoplastic lesions, it is of no value in differential diagnosis.

When a parenchymal mass of almost any etiology is situated near the periphery of the lung, a line shadow is sometimes visible from the mass to the visceral pleura, commonly with a local indrawing of the pleura (Figures 4–52 and 4–53). Rigler[32] observed this sign in 20 of 25 cases of alveolar cell carcinoma and feels that its presence is highly suggestive of the diagnosis; he states further that, although such lines may occur occasionally in cases of peripheral adenocarcinoma, he has not observed them in squamous cell cancer. In several cases of chronic infectious processes in the lung periph-

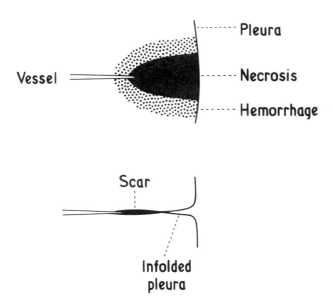

Figure 4–53. Diagrammatic Representation of Indrawn Pleura. Possible mechanism of the production of a line shadow with a pleural component, specifically following an infarct. (Reprinted from Br. J. Radiol., 43:327, 1970, with permission of Dr. Lynne Reid and the editor.)

ery we have visualized line shadows extending from the periphery of the process to the visceral pleura; therefore we do not consider this sign by itself of value in the differential diagnosis of peripheral parenchymal masses, an attitude with which Webb[33] is in complete agreement.

Parenchymal Scarring

A segment of lung that was the site of infectious disease and has undergone healing through fibrosis and scar formation may present as a linear shadow. Again, the width of the shadow largely depends upon the amount of lung originally involved. Healed upper lobe postprimary tuberculosis is a common example of this type of linear shadow. Several shadows may be fairly closely grouped, commonly extending from the hilum to the visceral pleural surface and diverging slightly toward the periphery. In many cases there is compensatory overinflation of adjacent lung parenchyma.

The line shadow created by healed pulmonary infarction represents fibrous scarring secondary to lung necrosis, commonly associated with indrawing of visceral pleura (Figure 4–53).

LINE SHADOWS OF PLEURAL ORIGIN

In addition to the normal interlobar fissure lines and those that occur sporadically in anomalous locations such as the azygos fissure, some line shadows that originate in the pleura constitute important direct or indirect signs of disease. Roentgenographic visibility of fissures not normally seen in a particular projection may be important evidence of otherwise invisible disease. For example, when a lower lobe loses volume, the upper portion of the major fissure sweeps downward and medially, and at a certain stage becomes visible on posteroanterior roentgenograms as an obliquely oriented shadow extending inferiorly and laterally from the lateral aspect of the mediastinum above the hilum, across the shadow of the hilum, to end near the lateral costophrenic sulcus. This evidence of atelectasis may be present even when the density in the lower lobe is not increased.

Line shadows simulating pleural thickening by small effusions may be caused by "subpleural" edema. Since the subpleural connective tissue layer is continuous with the interlobular septa, it is reasonable to assume that when edema fluid accumulates in the latter sites— Kerley B lines—it might also collect in the subpleural space. In such circumstances, it not only thickens the interlobar fissures but also widens the pleural layer along the lung's convex surface.

Fibrous pleural thickening over the anterior or posterior lung surfaces occasionally gives rise to rather broad linear opacities usually situated near the lung bases. These line shadows tend to appear rather "stringy" and commonly are oriented in a horizontal or oblique plane—not unlike the scars of old pulmonary infarction. Their true nature is usually apparent from their association with other signs of pleural fibrosis (such as obliteration of the costophrenic angle) or by the minimal change in their relationship to contiguous ribs during respiration.

Horizontal or Obliquely Oriented Linear Opacities of Unknown Nature

There would be little dispute to the statement that of all pathologic linear opacities observed on chest roentgenograms, by far the most common are those that tend to occur in the lung bases and that for many years have traditionally been called "platelike atelectasis" (*synonyms:* platter atelectasis, discoid atelectasis). Despite the frequency of these lines as a sign of pulmonary disease, their precise pathogenesis remains shrouded in mystery. These linear opacities of unit density range in thickness from 1 to 3 mm and in length from approximately 4 to 10 cm and are situated anatomically in the mid and lower lung zones, most commonly the latter. Although usually oriented in a roughly horizontal plane, they may be obliquely oriented depending upon the zone of lung affected, and in mid-lung zones particularly may be angled more than 45 degrees to the horizontal. They may be single or multiple, unilateral or bilateral.

"Platelike atelectasis" was originally described by Fleischner[34] in 1936 and has come to bear the eponymous designation "Fleischner's lines." Despite the frequency with which these lines are observed, it has proven exceedingly difficult to determine their precise morphologic nature, either because the pathologist is unaware of their presence or because the lesion rarely is found in lungs examined at necropsy. In fact, apart from the two cases on which the original report was based, to the best of our knowledge there have been no subsequent reports that have accurately documented the nature of these lines by roentgenologic/pathologic correlation. Fleischner and his colleagues[35, 36] described the typical gross appearance as a grayish-blue linear band of collapsed lung, slightly depressed below the pleural surface. The small bronchi and bronchioles leading to the collapsed zone showed inflammatory changes of varying degrees of severity and often contained mucous plugs. In personal communication, Fleischner stated that not only were the alveoli collapsed, but they commonly showed "alveolitis," inflammatory exudate lying within the alveoli and alveolar walls. It is probable that the latter changes were intimately involved in the pathogenesis of the process, since it is doubtful whether airway obstruction at this level can by itself result in focal atelectasis: since collateral air drift ostensibly constitutes a potent force in preventing parenchymal collapse at the subsegmental level, and since collateral air drift depends upon the integrity of the pores of Kohn, it would be essential for the pores to be blocked in order for atelectasis to occur and such blockage could effectively occur as a result of inflammatory exudate. To be precise, therefore, the linear opacities should be labeled focal pneumonitis rather than simple atelectasis. This pathogenetic sequence does not take into account the role of surfactant deficit in the development of atelectasis, but it is probable that abnormalities of this agent are operative to some degree.

These linear opacities are almost invariably associated with diseases that diminish diaphragmatic excursion, but it is doubtful whether this factor *per se* is solely responsible. A frequent contributing factor is intra-abdominal disease, usually inflammatory. After abdominal surgery, for example, it is probable that a complex group of changes combine to produce basal linear opacities: (a) restriction of diaphragmatic excursion diminishes ventilation of the lungs, especially in the bases; (b) coughing is inhibited by the pain and discomfort it engenders, resulting in accumulation of bronchial secretions in the dependent portions of the lungs and obstruction of small airways; and (c) stagnation of secretions encourages the development of pneumonia, the resulting inflammatory exudate obstructing the channels of interalveolar communication. The result is focal pneumonitis and atelectasis.

It is important to recognize that the postoperative clinical setting described above is commonly accompanied by an entirely different group of pathologic conditions, those associated with pulmonary thromboembolism. In the late 1960's Simon[37, 38] attributed horizontally or obliquely oriented linear opacities in the mid and lower lung zones to thrombosed arteries and veins, more commonly the latter. Bronchography and tomography, performed simul-taneously in a few patients, failed to show any relationship between the lines and the bronchial tree. His evidence for the vascular nature of these opacities was both inferential and direct—inferential because the direction taken by the linear opacity was identical to that followed by a pulmonary vein, particularly the position of its medial extremity (which coincided with the left atrium), and direct because the position of the line shadow related to that of the vein in subsequent angiography. In recent years, in many cases we have observed line shadows whose anatomic distribution was similar to that reported by Simon; the major clues to their nature are their anatomic position (which shows little or no relationship to bronchovascular distribution) and the position of their medial extremity (which coincides with the left atrium) (Figure 4–54). They range in thickness from 2 to 10 mm, and, in our experience, just as frequently follow the distribution of a major upper lobe vein as of veins draining the middle or lower zones. These shadows cannot be caused purely by blood clot within the vein itself: since the density of blood clot is identical to that of fluid blood, the roentgenographic shadows of clot and vein should be identical. Although pathologic confirmation appears singularly difficult to obtain in these cases, it seems reasonable to suggest that the process is rendered visible by a combination of edema, hemorrhage, and perhaps atelectasis and fibrosis in lung parenchyma surrounding the vein.

Although precise pathologic confirmation is still lacking, the evidence accumulated over the past few years favors the thesis that these shadows represent thrombosed veins (or occasionally arteries) accompanied by reaction in the surrounding parenchyma. We feel that this evidence is now strong enough that their visualization on a chest roentgenogram should alert the referring physician or surgeon to the *possibility* of thromboembolic disease, despite the fact that in many of these cases the patients' clinical histories have given no hint of an acute thromboembolic episode, apart from their being in a postoperative period or confined to bed for other reasons.

LUNG DISEASES THAT DECREASE ROENTGENOGRAPHIC DENSITY

The lung diseases that cause a decrease in roentgenographic density (increase in translucency) can be considered appropriately in the

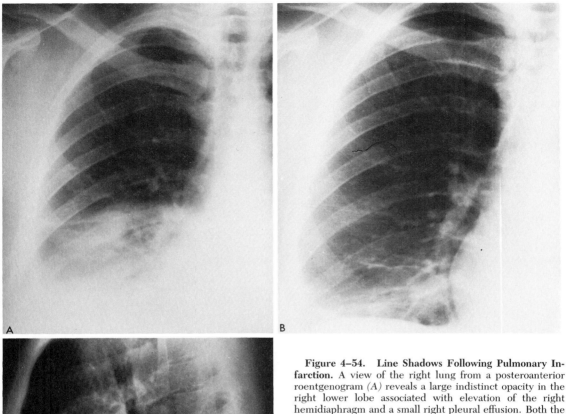

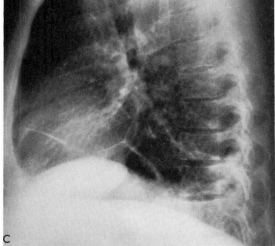

Figure 4–54. Line Shadows Following Pulmonary Infarction. A view of the right lung from a posteroanterior roentgenogram *(A)* reveals a large indistinct opacity in the right lower lobe associated with elevation of the right hemidiaphragm and a small right pleural effusion. Both the clinical presentation and the presence of perfusion defects in other portions of the lungs on lung scan supported the diagnosis of pulmonary embolism and infarction. Nine days later, posteroanterior *(B)* and lateral *(C)* roentgenograms showed two well-defined linear opacities, one in the right middle lobe and the other in the right lower lobe (seen to best advantage in *C*). The anterior extremity of the lower lobe opacity relates to the major fissure and is associated with local posterior displacement of the fissure. It is suggested that this opacity represents a pulmonary vessel (? vein) with reaction in contiguous parenchyma. Both linear opacities had disappeared 3 weeks later. In *C*, the residual opacity from the infarct can be seen in the region of the posterior gutter.

same manner as diseases that increase density, but as their antithesis. Just as density may be increased by a combination of changes in the relative amounts of air, blood, and interstitial tissue, so may decreased density result from alteration of these three elements in the opposite direction. In both groups of diseases, one component seldom is altered to the exclusion of the others, but it is useful to subdivide the diseases on the basis of predominant modification of each component, individually and combined.

It is emphasized that here we are dealing with the diseases of the *lung* that cause reduced roentgenographic density and not of the thorax as a whole. Any assessment of chest roentgenograms must take into consideration the contribution that abnormalities of *extrapulmonary tissue* might make to reduced density. Thus, certain pleural diseases (*e.g.,* pneumothorax) and some congenital and acquired abnormalities of the chest wall (*e.g.,* congenital absence of the pectoral muscles, mastectomy, poliomyelitis, and other neuromuscular disorders that affect one side of the thorax) produce unilateral radiolucency that easily might be mistaken for pulmonary disease unless this possibility is continuously borne in mind.

Accepting that diseases that reduce density are characterized by an altered ratio of the three components of air, blood, and interstitial tissue, four combinations of changes can reduce lung density.

INCREASED AIR BUT UNCHANGED BLOOD AND TISSUE. This group of diseases is exemplified by obstructive overinflation without lung destruction. It may be either *local* (*e.g.,* compensatory overinflation secondary to pulmonary resection or atelectasis) or *general* (*e.g.,* spasmodic asthma, and acute bronchiolitis in infants).

INCREASED AIR WITH DECREASED BLOOD AND TISSUE. This group is epitomized by diffuse obstructive emphysema; not only are the lungs overdistended but also the capillary bed is reduced and the alveolar walls are dissipated. Bullae and thin-walled cysts are examples of local diseases within this category.

NORMAL AMOUNT OF AIR BUT DECREASED BLOOD (AND TISSUE). This group is characterized by lack of pulmonary overinflation but reduced quantities of blood and tissue. *Local* diseases include lobar or unilateral emphysema and pulmonary embolism without infarction. The generalized abnormalities include diseases characterized by diminished pulmonary artery flow (*e.g.,* tetralogy of Fallot) and those affecting the peripheral vascular system (*e.g.,* primary pulmonary hypertension and multiple peripheral pulmonary emboli).

REDUCTION IN ALL THREE COMPONENTS. This condition is rare and probably relates to only one abnormality or variants thereof—unilateral pulmonary artery agenesis. Usually the lung is reduced in volume and derives its vascular supply solely from the systemic circulation; the resultant density is usually but not always reduced.

On the basis of this concept and using the roentgenologic signs to be described, one can fairly confidently diagnose most cases of pulmonary disease that decrease density. In the following section no attempt is made to describe roentgenologic characteristics of individual disease entities; specific affections will be cited only to exemplify points under discussion.

ROENTGENOLOGIC SIGNS

ALTERATION IN LUNG VOLUME

With the exception of the reduction in lung volume that occurs in unilateral pulmonary ar-

tery agenesis, sometimes in unilateral or lobar emphysema (Swyer-James syndrome), and in pulmonary embolism without infarction, all lung diseases that decrease roentgenographic density *in which volume is altered* are characterized by *overinflation.* Before considering the roentgenologic signs of overinflation, it is well to review briefly the mechanisms that keep the lung expanded and the alterations in these mechanisms that increase lung volume. The lung has a natural tendency to collapse and does so when removed from the chest. This tendency stems from its inherent elastic recoil properties, which are partly related to collagenous and elastic fibers that impart an elastic quality similar to that of a coil spring, and partly to alveolar surface tension. When the lung's elastic properties are deranged, as in emphysema, the organ inflates beyond its normal maximal volume; this constitutes *overinflation.* As a result, the lung's compliance—the change in volume per unit change in pressure—is increased; in other words, a given pressure will produce a greater volume change than in normal lung. It is important to recognize that this loss of elastic recoil is the major if not the only factor that permits the lung to overinflate. The loss of recoil may be irreversible, as in emphysema, or temporary and reversible, as in spasmodic asthma; in any event, *unequivocal roentgenographic evidence of pulmonary overinflation implies loss of elastic recoil.*

The roentgenologic signs of overinflation depend upon whether the process is *general* or *local.*

General Excess of Air in the Lungs

Signs to be observed are chiefly those relating to the diaphragm. At total lung capacity the diaphragm is depressed and the normal "dome" configuration is flattened, particularly as viewed in lateral projection (Figure 4–55). The low position of the diaphragm increases the angle of the costophrenic sinuses, sometimes to almost a right angle.

In a study designed to test the accuracy of a variety of measurements from posteroanterior and lateral roentgenograms in discriminating normal and overinflated lungs, Thomson and his colleagues[39] found that the best criterion was obtained from the sum of the height of each diaphragmatic dome in posteroanterior and lateral projection. It was of interest in this preliminary study that some commonly used roentgenologic criteria of pulmonary overinflation, such as the anterior rib count and the distance from the ascending aorta to the sternum, were

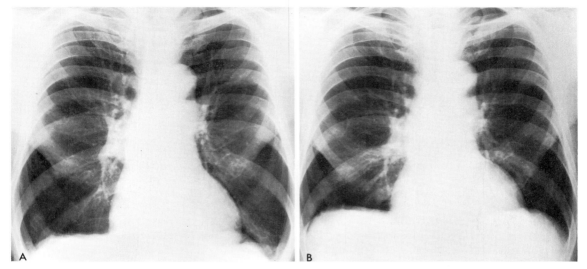

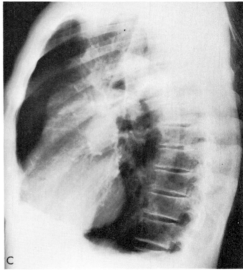

Figure 4–55.   Diffuse Emphysema. Posteroanterior roentgenograms of the chest in inspiration *(A)* and expiration *(B)* reveal a low position and somewhat flattened contour of both hemidiaphragms; excursion of the diaphragm from TLC to RV is reduced. In lateral projection *(C)*, the superior aspect of the diaphragm is concave rather than convex and the retrosternal air space somewhat deepened. The lungs are generally oligemic.

poor discriminants of normal and overinflated lungs.

When the diaphragm is depressed the heart tends to be elongated, narrow, and central in position. This long vertical configuration of the cardiovascular contour is of little value as a roentgenologic sign, but it creates difficulty in the assessment of cardiac enlargement when pulmonary hypertension has given rise to right ventricular hypertrophy and cor pulmonale.

Local Excess of Air

Overinflation of one or more lobes, the remainder of the lungs being normal, occurs in two quite different sets of circumstances—with and without air trapping; distinction between the two is of major diagnostic importance. Over-

inflation *with air trapping* results from obstruction of the egress of air from affected lung parenchyma. It has several causes, in all of which the common pathogenetic denominator is airway obstruction—for example, lobar emphysema in infants and congenital atresia of the left upper lobe bronchus (Figure 4–56). Overinflation *without air trapping* is a compensatory process: parts of the lung assume a larger volume than normal in response to loss of volume elsewhere in the thorax. This may occur after surgical removal of lung tissue or as a result of atelectasis or parenchymal scarring, but in any event the remaining lung contains more than its normal complement of air (thus indicating a loss of elastic recoil, presumably reversible as in asthma). Since there is no airway obstruction, the roentgenologic signs are different from

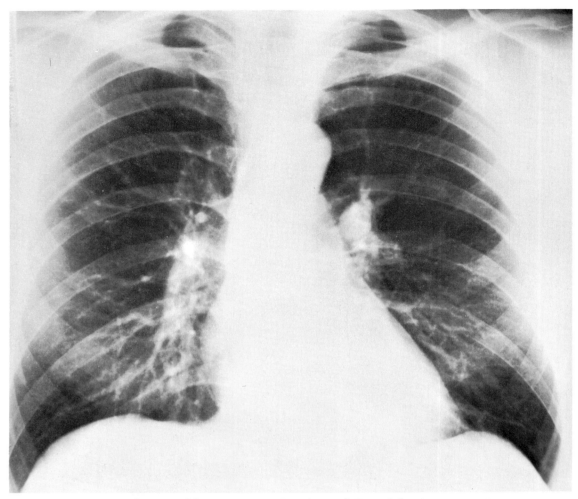

Figure 4–56. Congenital Atresia of the Apicoposterior Bronchus, Left Upper Lobe. A posteroanterior roentgenogram reveals increased radiolucency of the upper half of the left lung due to both excess air and diminished blood. The oval mass related to the upper border of the left hilum represents inspissated mucus within the lumen of the affected bronchus distal to the atresia. The affected bronchopulmonary segment is air-containing owing to collateral air drift from contiguous, normally ventilated segments. Oligemia is the result of hypoxic vasoconstriction secondary to diminished ventilation. (Courtesy of Dr. George Genereux, University Hospital, Saskatoon.)

those of conditions in which air trapping plays a significant role. Thus it is important to consider the roentgenologic signs of local excess of air under two headings—static and dynamic—according to the presence or absence of airway obstruction.

STATIC SIGNS. By "static" is implied the changes apparent on standard roentgenograms exposed at total lung capacity.

1. Alteration in lung density: The fact that the excess of air is local permits comparison with normal density in the remainder of that lung or in the contralateral lung; thus, in contrast to those diseases with generalized excess of air, altered density is a significant and reliable sign. The increased translucency is caused

chiefly by an increase in air in relation to blood content; blood flow to the affected lung is normal or reduced, the only difference being that, in the latter circumstances, translucency is even more increased.

2. Alteration in volume: The volume of the affected lung depends entirely upon whether the excess of air is compensatory (secondary to resection or atelectasis) or caused by airway obstruction. Since compensatory overinflation is the expansion of lung tissue beyond its normal volume to fill a limited space, the volume that the expanded lung tissue occupies cannot exceed the volume for which it compensates. By contrast, the volume of lung parenchyma distal to a partially obstructing endobronchial lesion

varies: in our experience volume is seldom greater than normal *at total lung capacity;* in such circumstances, volume is either normal or, more commonly, less than normal, especially if the partial obstruction exists in a main or lobar bronchus (Figure 4–57). Of major importance in this consideration is that roentgenograms be obtained in maximum inspiration; at any lung volume less than total lung capacity, air will be trapped in the affected lung parenchyma, thus creating a volume that is greater than normal. Thus, it is vital to distinguish the terms "obstructive overinflation" and "air trap-

ping": the former is a static situation and the latter a dynamic one (*see* later on). We feel that this distinction is particularly important in infants and young children who have inhaled foreign bodies; although the commonest roentgenographic abnormality reported in such cases is pulmonary overinflation,[40] we suspect that in many cases roentgenograms are obtained at a phase of respiration less than total lung capacity, chiefly because of technical difficulty. Thus, the roentgenogram is in fact demonstrating air trapping rather than obstructive overinflation.

These statements regarding lung volume be-

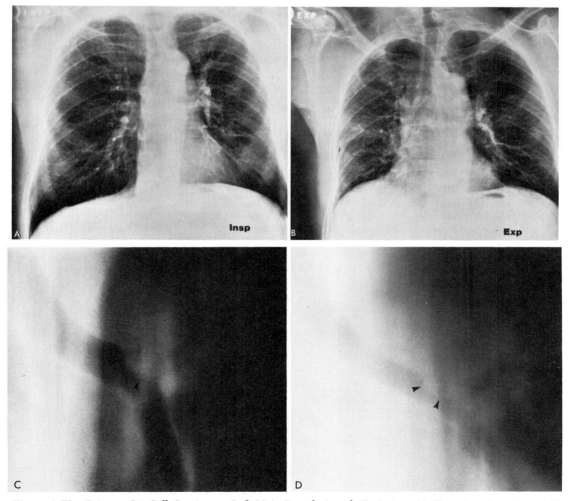

Figure 4–57. Primary Oat-Cell Carcinoma, Left Main Bronchus, with Expiratory Air Trapping. A posteroanterior roentgenogram exposed at full inspiration (*A*) reveals considerable smallness of the left lung compared with the right; the left hemidiaphragm is moderately elevated and the mediastinum is shifted to the left. Despite this loss of volume, no opacities are visualized in the left lung to suggest collapse or airlessness. Left lower lobe vessels are obviously smaller than corresponding vessels on the right, indicating reduced perfusion. A roentgenogram exposed at maximal expiration (*B*) reveals little change in the volume of the left lung from inspiration, indicating air trapping; by contrast, the right hemidiaphragm has elevated considerably and the mediastinum has swung to the right, indicating good air flow from the right lung. Tomograms of the left main bronchus in inspiration (*C*) and expiration (*D*) reveal a smooth, well-defined soft tissue mass protruding into the air column of the bronchus near its bifurcation (*arrowheads*); the caliber of the bronchial air column is markedly reduced on expiration.

yond a partly obstructing endobronchial lesion apply chiefly when the obstruction has existed for only a relatively short period of time (days in the case of an aspirated foreign body, weeks or even a few months in the case of an endobronchial neoplasm). However, if obstruction persists for several months or longer, volume will gradually increase, presumably as a result of progressive loss of elastic recoil (Figure 4–58). The main roentgenologic sign of increased volume is displacement of structures contiguous with overinflated lung, the degree varying with the amount and location of affected lung tissue.

3. Alteration in vascular pattern: The linear markings throughout the affected lung are splayed out in a distribution consistent with the extent of overinflation, and their angles of bifurcation are increased. Provided that blood flow is maintained at normal or near normal levels, vessel caliber is little altered. However, it is important to recognize that the characteristic response of pulmonary vessels to a partly obstructing endobronchial lesion is hypoxic vasoconstriction;[41] thus, even if affected lung volume is less than normal, its density will also be less than normal as a result of oligemia.

DYNAMIC SIGNS. By "dynamic" is implied changes that occur during respiration; they are readily apparent on roentgenograms exposed during full inspiration and maximal expiration.

When local increase in translucency is caused by *compensatory overinflation*, during expiration the volume of the overinflated lobe decreases proportionately with the normal lung tissue: airway obstruction being absent, the affected lung parenchyma deflates normally. Since the overinflated lung tissue contains more air than normal at total lung capacity, it still contains a greater than normal complement of air at residual volume and, therefore, is still relatively more translucent.

When *airway obstruction* is the major pathogenetic mechanism of local overinflation, the roentgenologic signs are different. During expiration, air is trapped within the affected lung parenchyma and volume changes little, whereas the remainder of the lung deflates normally. The roentgenologic signs depend upon both the volume and the anatomic location of affected lung: since during expiration there is negligible change in the amount of air within the obstructed lung parenchyma, density is little altered and the contrast between affected areas and normally deflated lung is maximally accentuated at residual volume (Figure 4–59). Since the overinflated parenchyma occupies space within the hemithorax, contiguous structures are displaced away from the affected lobe during expiration: the mediastinum shifts toward the contralateral side, elevation of the hemidiaphragm is restricted, and the thoracic cage maintains its position of inflation.

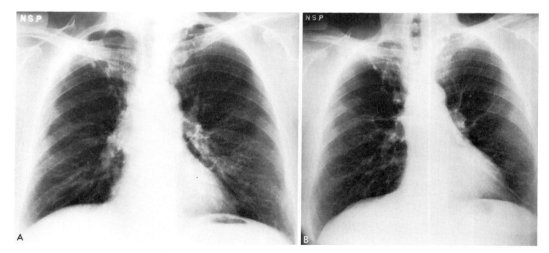

Figure 4–58. Effects on Lung Volume of Long-standing Endobronchial Obstruction. The posteroanterior roentgenogram illustrated in A was obtained in June, 1973, when this 40-year-old woman was discovered to have a partial obstruction of the right main bronchus from tuberculous granulation tissue; note that the volume of the right lung is less than that of the left and that its radiolucency is greater, indicating relative oligemia. Approximately 1 year later (B), the volume of the right lung had increased considerably, to a point in fact where it was greater than that of the left. The relative oligemia persisted but was more evident in the upper half of the lung. This increase in lung volume over a period of a year is a reflection of loss of elastic recoil in response to persistent expiratory air trapping; it indicates that the endobronchial obstruction has not been relieved despite triple antituberculous therapy. Bronchoscopy revealed disappearance of the granulation tissue; however, the lumen of main bronchus was considerably narrowed by a fibrous stricture.

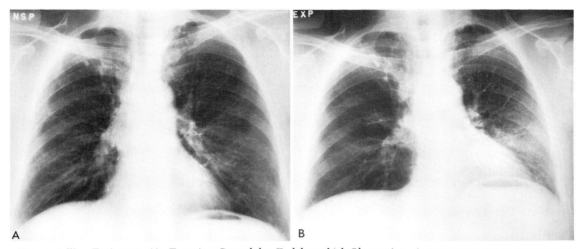

Figure 4–59. Expiratory Air Trapping Caused by Endobronchial Obstruction. A posteroanterior roentgenogram exposed at full inspiration *(A)* shows both the volume and density of the right lung to be less than the left; vessel markings are smaller throughout. Anatomic structures in the right hilum are somewhat obscured. On expiration *(B)*, the left hemidiaphragm has elevated normally while the right has maintained its inspiratory position; the mediastinum has shifted to the left. The small volume and relative oligemia of the right lung on inspiration associated with air trapping on expiration indicate an obstructing lesion in the right main bronchus. This 40-year-old woman had a 4-month history of low-grade fever, cough, retrosternal pain, tightness in the chest, and yellow sputum; coughing brought on wheezing. Physical examination demonstrated rales and muffled breath sounds over the right upper zone and a general wheeze over the whole thorax. Bronchoscopy revealed granulation tissue piled up in the right main-stem bronchus, almost occluding the right upper lobe bronchus and extending up onto the tracheal wall. *M. tuberculosis* was identified on smear and culture. Same patient as in Figure 4–58.

ALTERATION IN VASCULATURE

Just as overinflation may reflect abnormality of the conducting airways of the lung, so may alteration in the vascular pattern indicate abnormality of perfusion. Like overinflation, alteration in lung vasculature may be either general or local; since the roentgenologic signs differ somewhat, it is desirable to describe them separately.

General Reduction in Vasculature

Diffuse pulmonary oligemia is characterized by a reduction in caliber of the arterial tree throughout the lungs. Generally, appreciation of such vascular change is a subjective process based on a thorough familiarity with the normal, and is admittedly subject to considerable observer error. It appears likely that computed tomography will be able to provide much more precise assessment of density patterns in the lungs, as recently suggested.[42]

Since reduction in the size of peripheral vessels constitutes the main criterion of diagnosis of all diseases in this category, reliance must be placed on secondary signs for their differentiation. There are two ancillary signs of major importance: *the size and configuration of the central hilar vessels* and *the presence or absence of general pulmonary overinflation*. Three combinations of changes are possible:

1. *Small peripheral vessels; no overinflation; normal or small hila*. This combination indicates reduced pulmonary blood flow from central causes and is virtually pathognomonic of cardiac disease, usually congenital (Figure 4–60). Such anomalies as the tetralogy of Fallot, Ebstein's anomaly, and, occasionally, isolated pulmonic stenosis, are associated with a reduced pulmonary artery blood flow manifested roentgenographically by small peripheral vessels and hila.

2. *Small peripheral vessels; no overinflation; enlarged hilar pulmonary arteries*. This combination may result from peripheral or central causes. The *peripheral* conditions include primary pulmonary arterial hypertension, and multiple peripheral emboli. In each of these the major changes apparent roentgenographically are the consequence of pulmonary arterial hypertension and consist of enlargement of the hilar pulmonary arteries and diminution of the peripheral vessels. The commonest cause of *central* origin is massive pulmonary artery embolism without infarction.[43] In this situation the reduction in peripheral pulmonary flow results

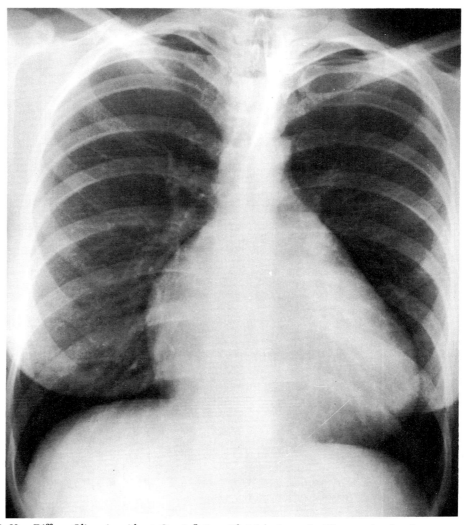

Figure 4–60. Diffuse Oligemia without Overinflation: Ebstein's Anomaly. The peripheral pulmonary markings are diminished in caliber, and the hila are diminutive; the lungs are not overinflated. The contour of the markedly enlarged heart is consistent with Ebstein's anomaly. Proved case.

from mechanical obstruction in the large hilar vessels, the latter being ballooned out by thrombus within them; severe cardiac enlargement caused by acute cor pulmonale is usually present (Figure 4–61).

3. *Small peripheral vessels; general pulmonary overinflation; normal or enlarged hilar pulmonary arteries.* This combination is virtually pathognomonic of diffuse emphysema (Figure 4–62).[44] Enlargement of the hilar pulmonary arteries may be present but is not essential to the diagnosis; it indicates pulmonary arterial hypertension resulting from chronically increased vascular resistance and usually is seen only in the late stages of chronic obstructive emphysema. In such circumstances, the rapid

tapering of pulmonary vessels distally is accentuated by the hilar enlargement.

Local Reduction in Vasculature

The same three combinations of changes apply as in general reduction in vasculature; the major difference lies in their effects on pulmonary hemodynamics. In the following examples the affected portion of lung may be segmental, lobar, or multilobar:

1. *Small peripheral vessels; normal or reduced inflation; normal or small hilum.* This combination is epitomized by lobar or unilateral hyperlucent lung, variously known by the eponyms Swyer-James' syndrome[45] and Macleod's

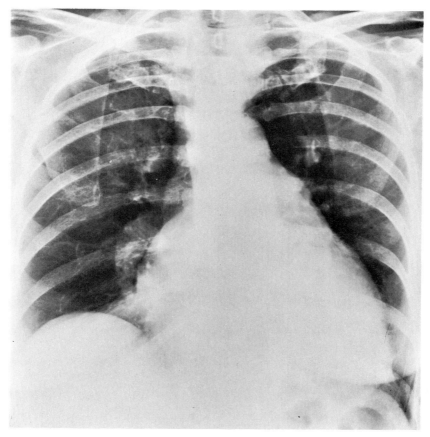

Figure 4–61.   Diffuse Oligemia without Overinflation: Massive Pulmonary Artery Thromboembolism without Infarction. Marked oligemia of both lungs is associated with moderate enlargement of both hila and rapid tapering of the pulmonary arteries as they proceed distally. The cardiac contour is typical of cor pulmonale. There is no overinflation.

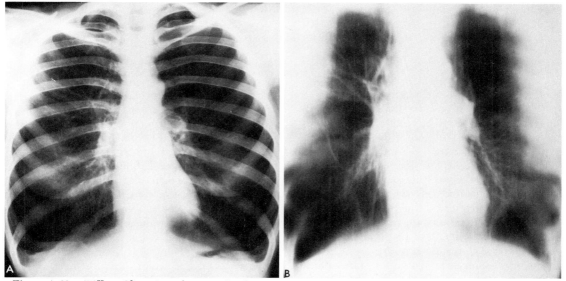

Figure 4–62.   Diffuse Oligemia with Generalized Overinflation: Emphysema. The peripheral vasculature of the lungs is markedly diminished as revealed in both the posteroanterior roentgenogram (A) and the anteroposterior tomogram (B). Despite the severe oligemia, the hilar pulmonary arteries are not enlarged. The lungs are severely overinflated.

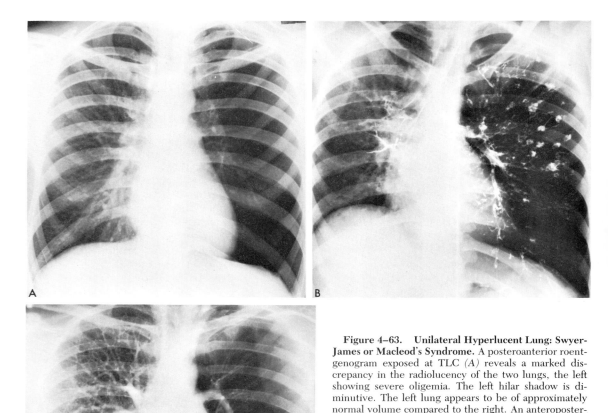

Figure 4–63.   Unilateral Hyperlucent Lung: Swyer-James or Macleod's Syndrome. A posteroanterior roentgenogram exposed at TLC *(A)* reveals a marked discrepancy in the radiolucency of the two lungs, the left showing severe oligemia. The left hilar shadow is diminutive. The left lung appears to be of approximately normal volume compared to the right. An anteroposterior roentgenogram at RV following bronchography *(B)* demonstrates severe air trapping in the left lung, little change in volume having occurred from TLC. Since deflation of the right lung is normal, the mediastinum has swung sharply to the right. In the pulmonary angiogram *(C)*, the discrepancy of blood flow to the two lungs is readily apparent; note that the left pulmonary artery is present although diminutive (differentiation from congenital absence of the left pulmonary artery).

syndrome (Figure 4–63).[46] This unique abnormality is characterized by normal or slightly reduced lung volume at total lung capacity, severe airway obstruction during expiration, greatly reduced circulation (oligemia), and a diminutive hilum. A similar picture may be produced by unilateral pulmonary artery agenesis, in which the pulmonary artery is interrupted in the region of the hilum so that the lung is devoid of pulmonary artery perfusion.[47] Roentgenographic changes identical to those of Swyer-James' syndrome may also result from a clinically more important situation. Consider an endobronchial lesion incompletely obstructing the lumen of a lobar bronchus (Figure 4–57): the reduced ventilation of distal parenchyma

results in local hypoxia, which leads to reflex vasoconstriction[41] and consequent reduced perfusion of affected bronchopulmonary segments. Contrary to common belief and teaching, the volume of affected lung generally is reduced rather than increased. Since the endobronchial lesion invariably causes expiratory air trapping, it may be extremely difficult roentgenologically to differentiate this combination of changes from the much less significant Swyer-James' syndrome. Therefore, whenever this combination of changes is present, it is imperative to exclude an endobronchial lesion (initially by bronchoscopy).

Of considerable interest is the observation that in patients with local hypoventilation as a result of a partly obstructing endobronchial lesion, hypoxic vasoconstriction may be strikingly prolonged following removal of the bronchial obstruction,[48] and that the interval for return of blood flow to normal levels is probably directly related to the duration of the initial airway obstruction. The precise mechanism for this phenomenon is unclear.

2. *Small peripheral vessels; normal lung volume; enlarged hilar pulmonary arteries (or an enlarged hilum).* This combination is nearly always caused by unilateral pulmonary artery embolism without infarction (Figure 4–64). The occluding embolus or thrombus almost invariably leads to enlargement of the involved artery.[49] Since bronchial obstruction is not a feature, there is no overinflation—on the contrary, lung volume may be reduced. A similar roentgenographic picture may be produced by ob-

struction of a pulmonary artery by invasive neoplasm: the hilar enlargement is caused by the original lesion rather than by the vessel, although the overall roentgenographic appearance may be the same.

3. *Small peripheral vessels; overinflation; normal hilar pulmonary arteries.* This combination is distinctive of obstructive emphysema. The roentgenographic appearance of the vascular deficiency of emphysema is often local rather than general. The lower or upper lobes or almost any combination of individual lobes may be predominantly affected. The involved portions of lung show a combination of overinflation and severely diminished peripheral vasculature; less involved areas tend to be pleonemic as a result of redistribution of blood flow to them caused by the increased resistance to flow in emphysematous areas. Since the lack of

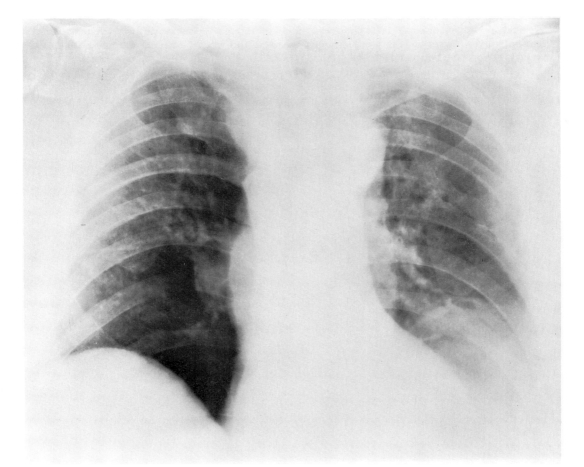

Figure 4–64. Lobar Oligemia without Overinflation: Thromboembolism without Infarction. An anteroposterior roentgenogram exposed in the supine position demonstrates marked increase in the radiolucency of the lower half of the right lung. The vascular markings are diminished in caliber and the descending branch of the right pulmonary artery is dilated and sharply defined; this vessel tapers rapidly as it proceeds distally. Lobar oligemia as a result of thromboembolism without infarction constitutes Westermark's sign.

increase in vascular resistance in uninvolved lung prevents the development of pulmonary artery hypertension, the hilar pulmonary arteries do not enlarge.

PULMONARY AIR CYSTS

This term is used for all thin-walled air-containing intrapulmonary spaces that are roentgenologically visible, regardless of their pathogenesis. One of the most important distinctions to be made is whether an air cyst is a solitary abnormality in otherwise healthy lung or part of generalized pulmonary disease: the implications in terms of the effects on pulmonary function are of obvious importance.

A pulmonary air cyst (bulla or bleb) is an air-containing space ranging in size from 1 cm in diameter to the volume of a whole hemithorax and possessing a smooth wall of minimal thickness (from a hairline to 2 to 3 mm). The space may be unilocular or separated into several compartments by thin septa (Figure 4–65). It may arise *de novo*, when surrounding lung tissue is normal, or may occur secondary to other disease, usually infectious and commonly associated with much parenchymal scarring. Secondary signs may be present, depending upon the size of the cyst; for example, when a huge bulla occupies most of the volume of one hemithorax (Figure 4–66), signs of air trapping are apparent during deep breathing. Cysts are characteristically avascular, an observation that may be facilitated by tomographic examination, particularly with small lesions. These roentgenologic signs conform to the physiologic observations that pulmonary air cysts are poorly ventilated and unperfused.[50] Studies of the mechanical properties of pulmonary cysts and bullae have shown that, during expiration, the cysts inflate while the rest of the lung deflates, a paradox attributed to their high compliance and to air flow restriction by small deficiencies in the walls of the bullae occasioned by loss of alveolar tissue. When the air cyst is filled these communications are compressed, resulting in permanent inflation.

The specific characteristics of thin-walled cystic lesions of the lung have recently been reviewed[51] and are discussed in some detail in Chapter 11. A brief outline of the nomenclature used and of the general characteristics of each lesion is presented here.

Pulmonary air cysts may be *congenital* or *acquired*. The congenital type includes bronchogenic cysts whose fluid contents have been expelled. Acquired disease includes the two

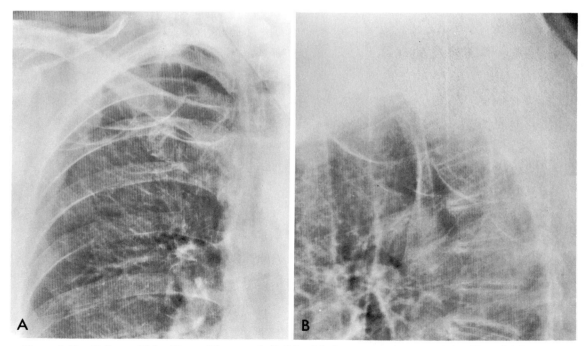

Figure 4–65. Bullae or Blebs. Views of the upper half of the right lung in posteroanterior *(A)* and lateral *(B)* projections reveal several cystic spaces in the lung apex sharply separated from contiguous lung by curvilinear, hairline shadows. The appearance suggests multiple blebs or bullae rather than a single space separated into compartments by thin septa.

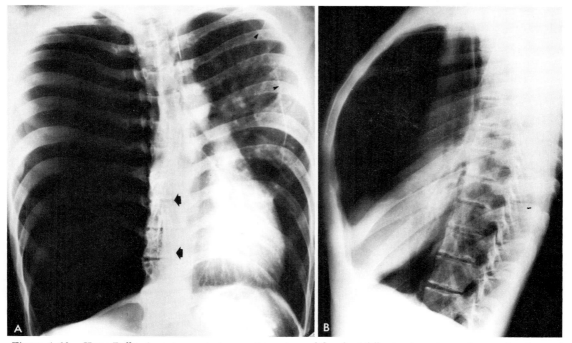

Figure 4–66. Huge Bulla. An anteroposterior roentgenogram of the chest following bronchography reveals a huge air sac completely filling and overdistending the right hemithorax and displacing the anterior mediastinal septum almost as far as the left axillary pleura (the line shadow indicated by *arrowheads* is formed by four layers of pleura). The right lung is compressed into a small nubbin of tissue situated in the midline; note the markedly crowded right bronchial tree (*thick arrows*). In lateral projection (*B*), extension of the bulla across the midline has resulted in marked increase in depth of the retrosternal air space and posterior displacement of the heart and major vessels.

common types of pulmonary air cysts, *blebs* and *bullae*.[52] *Blebs* seldom exceed 1 to 2 cm in diameter; they are either intrapleural or immediately subpleural and most frequently develop over the lung apices. They characteristically have a narrow neck and usually contain only gas, without evidence of alveolar remnants or blood vessels. These lesions are usually regarded as the major cause of spontaneous pneumothorax. *Bullae*, which are intrapulmonary structures, are usually attributed to excessive rupture of alveolar walls. They appear to affect upper and lower lobes equally and may develop in the absence of generalized emphysema. Their walls are composed of compressed parenchymal tissue, and strands of emphysematous lung and intact blood vessels are pathologically identifiable within many of these lesions. Some cysts develop as a sequela of acute lung abscess; resolution of acute pneumonia surrounding the abscess leaves a thin-walled cystic space that is indistinguishable from a bulla arising *de novo* in otherwise healthy lung. These are to be distinguished from so-called *pneumatoceles*, which are large, thin-walled air-containing spaces that develop most frequently as a complication of acute. staphylococcal pneumonia,

particularly in infants and children. Their pathogenesis is believed to relate either to check-valve obstruction of a small bronchus or bronchiole with distention of lung distal to the obstruction in the form of a coalescent cystic space, or to local necrosis of a bronchial wall and distention outward from this point. Such a lesion in a child with acute pneumonia is highly suggestive of a staphylococcal etiology. *Post-traumatic cysts* resulting from lung tissue laceration associated with nonpenetrating chest trauma may present as typical thin-walled air cysts, with or without an air-fluid level.

Finally, bullae frequently occur as a manifestation of diffuse pulmonary emphysema. The cysts are characteristically very thin-walled and usually are distributed widely throughout the subpleural zone.

ROENTGENOLOGIC SIGNS OF PLEURAL DISEASE

Since effusion is by far the commonest and most important abnormality affecting the pleura, it would be worthwhile for the reader to review the forces that govern the formation and absorption of fluid in the normal pleural space (*see* Chapter 1, page 66).

Despite a usually effective combination of forces maintaining the pleural surfaces in a dry (or slightly moist) state, physiologically occurring pleural fluid can be visualized roentgenographically in a significant percentage of normal healthy humans. Using their modification of the lateral decubitus projection with a horizontal x-ray beam, Müller and Löfsted[53] visualized pleural fluid in 15 of 120 healthy adults (12.5 per cent), the smallest amount of fluid identifiable by this technique being 3 to 5 ml; the largest amount found was 15 ml. In a later study of 300 healthy adults, Hessén[54] found conclusive evidence of roentgenologically demonstrable fluid in 12 healthy adults (4.0 per cent) and suggestive evidence in an additional 19 (6.3 per cent). The thickness of the fluid layer ranged from 1 mm to 10 mm and averaged 5 mm. Moskowitz and his colleagues extended these observations in a study of cadavers;[55] they injected 5-ml increments of saline or plasma into the pleural space, and showed that even 5 ml of fluid were clearly visible on roentgenograms exposed in the unmodified lateral decubitus position.

These studies are of obvious practical importance insofar as they indicate that small amounts of pleural fluid may be demonstrated roentgenographically in the absence of disease; thus, they point up a potential source of error in the diagnosis of clinically significant pleural effusion.

Reported figures for the amount of pleural fluid required for roentgenographic demonstration in the erect subject range from 250 to 600 ml.

ROENTGENOLOGIC SIGNS OF PLEURAL EFFUSION

TYPICAL ARRANGEMENT OF FREE PLEURAL FLUID

It will be recalled that the negative pressure within the pleural cavity represents the difference between the elastic forces of the chest wall and of the lungs. Lung tissue has a natural tendency to recoil but is prevented from doing so beyond a certain point by the chest wall's tendency to expand outward with an equal, opposite force. Thus, in the normal state, intimate contact between the visceral and parietal pleural surfaces is maintained. When a buffer medium (*e.g.*, fluid or gas) is introduced into the pleural space, the lung can recoil inward

toward its fixed moorings at the hilum, the amount of retraction depending upon the quantity of buffer. The site of retraction depends upon the position of the buffer medium within the pleural space, as illustrated by the different effects of hydrothorax and pneumothorax: in the upright subject, the effect of gravity causes gas to rise and fluid to fall in the pleural space. When pneumothorax is present or the thoracic cage is opened (thoracotomy or necropsy), the shape of the lung in its completely collapsed state is a miniature replica of its shape in the fully distended form. The effect is the same when pleural effusion or pneumothorax is present, except that the collapse may be local rather than general.

These two influences—gravity and elastic recoil—are the major forces that control the arrangement of free fluid in the pleural space.[54, 56] Fluid gravitates first to the base of the hemithorax, where it comes to lie between the inferior surface of the lung and the hemidiaphragm (Figure 4–67)—particularly posteriorly, where the pleural sinus is deepest. With in-

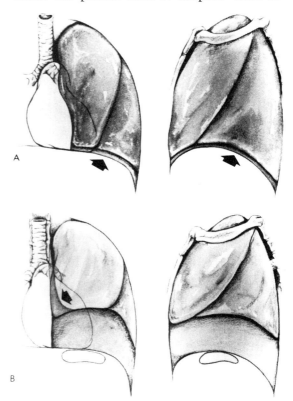

Figure 4–67. Infrapulmonary Accumulation of Pleural Fluid. In these drawings are depicted two degrees of infrapulmonary effusion; in *A*, the situation is "typical" in that it represents the *usual* anatomic location of small amounts of fluid (up to 500 ml); in *B*, the amount of fluid is large (*e.g.*, 1500 ml) and the local infrapulmonary accumulation thus "atypical." *See* text.

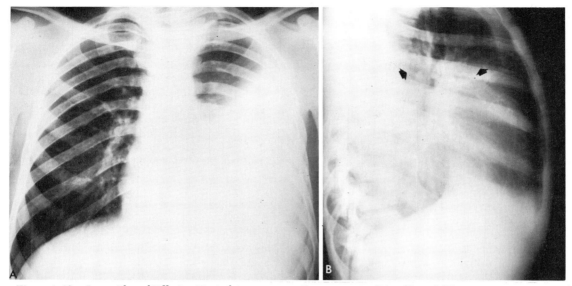

Figure 4–68.   Large Pleural Effusion: Typical Arrangement. Posteroanterior *(A)* and lateral *(B)* roentgenograms exposed in the erect position demonstrate uniform opacification of the lower two thirds of the left hemithorax. The upper level of the fluid is meniscus-shaped in both posteroanterior and lateral projection *(arrows on B)*. Note that only the right hemidiaphragm is visualized in lateral projection, the left being obscured by fluid (the silhouette sign).

creasing amounts, the fluid spills out into the costophrenic sinuses posteriorly, laterally, and, eventually, anteriorly; with further accumulation, it spreads upward in mantlelike fashion around the convexity of the lung, tapering gradually as it assumes a higher position in the thorax. As the thickness of the fluid layer becomes less superiorly, *capillary attraction* between pleural surfaces exerts its effect, constituting the third force affecting the characteristic arrangement of free pleural fluid.

On the basis of this description, it is easy to construct the typical roentgenographic appearance of pleural effusion. Consider the hypothetical situation of a "moderate" pleural effusion (1000 ml) (Figure 4–68): such an amount of fluid will completely obscure the hemidiaphragm and the costophrenic sinuses and will extend upward around the anterior, lateral, and posterior thoracic wall, to about the midportion of the hemithorax. Since the mediastinal surface of the lung possesses relatively less elastic recoil because of its fixation at the hilum and pulmonary ligament, less fluid accumulates along this surface than around the convexity. Thus, in posteroanterior projection, the density of the fluid is high laterally and curves gently downward and medially, with a smooth meniscus-shaped upper border, to terminate along the midcardiac border. In lateral projection, since the fluid has ascended along the anterior and posterior thoracic wall to roughly an equal ex-

tent, the upper surface of the fluid density will be semicircular, being high anteriorly and posteriorly and curving smoothly downward to its lowest point in the midaxillary line. Comparison of the maximal height of the fluid density in the posteroanterior and lateral projections will show that this height is identical posteriorly, laterally, and anteriorly (Figure 4–68); the meniscus shape is caused by the fact that the layer of fluid is of insufficient depth to cast a discernible shadow when viewed *en face*. This typical configuration was excellently reproduced roentgenographically by Fleischner,[56] who constructed paraffin wax models in the shape of half a hollow truncated cone.

Since the distribution of fluid within the free pleural space tends to obey the law of gravity, and since the lung tends to maintain its shape when compressed, the first place fluid accumulates in the erect patient is between the inferior surface of the lower lobe and the diaphragm: in effect, the lung is "floating" on a layer of fluid (Figure 4–67). If the amount of fluid is small it may occupy only this position without spilling over into the costophrenic sinuses—not even the most dependent sinus posteriorly. In such circumstances the configuration of the hemidiaphragm is maintained and the appearance on posteroanterior and lateral roentgenograms suggests no more than slight elevation of that hemidiaphragm. Bearing in mind the individual variation in the height of the diaphragm in normal subjects, it is readily apparent that small accumulations of fluid in the pleural space easily can be missed roentgenologically. It is only if the physician is alert to the possibility of a small pleural effusion that the diagnosis can be confirmed by roentgenography in the lateral decubitus position with a horizontal x-ray beam. Thus, "infrapulmonary" is the *usual* (*not* atypical) distribution in the free pleural space (although it would be reasonable to consider the infrapulmonary accumulation of large amounts of fluid paradoxical or atypical; this subject is dealt with in the section on atypical arrangement of pleural fluid).

With increasing amounts of fluid, the roentgenologic signs develop in predictable fashion: obliteration of the lateral and eventually anterior costophrenic sulci, and extension of fluid up the chest wall in its usual mantle distribution.

Of some importance in the roentgenologic manifestations of pleural effusion is the pattern that develops when the major interlobar fissures are incomplete medially.[57] In such circumstances, fluid that extends into the major fissures creates a sharp concave line, medial to which the lung is of normal or almost normal lucency and peripheral to which the fluid creates a uniform opacity.

The effects on the thorax as a whole of the accumulation of large amounts of fluid in the pleural space depend largely upon the condition of the ipsilateral lung. Even small amounts of

fluid produce "relaxation" atelectasis of contiguous lung, in much the same manner as when air is the buffer medium in pneumothorax. When pleural effusion is massive, collapse of the ipsilateral lung may be almost complete. Despite severe atelectasis, however, the overall effect of a massive effusion almost invariably is that of a space-occupying process, with enlargement of the ipsilateral hemithorax, displacement of the mediastinum to the contralateral side, and severe depression and flattening of the ipsilateral hemidiaphragm; in fact, the hemidiaphragm may be depressed so severely as to be concave superiorly (Figure 4–69). In such circumstances, an air bronchogram should be clearly visible, since there is no bronchial obstruction (Figure 4–70). When one hemithorax is totally opacified, appreciation of the balance of forces between the two sides of the thorax is of obvious importance. If the mediastinum shows no shift and the hemidiaphragm is only slightly depressed, the presence of disease within the ipsilateral lung can be stated with absolute certainty; the conclusion that *must* be reached is that the balance of forces between effusion (a space-occupying process) and parenchymal disease (which reduces volume) ensures that the volume of the hemithorax is not greater than normal. The possibility of an obstructing endobronchial lesion (*e.g.*, bronchogenic carcinoma with pleural metastases) is obvious: in fact, total opacification of one hemithorax without mediastinal or diaphragmatic displacement

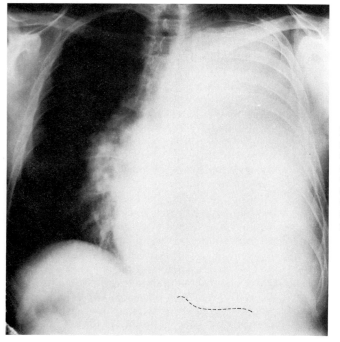

Figure 4–69. Massive Effusion, Underlying Lung Normal. A posteroanterior roentgenogram reveals total opacification of the left hemithorax by a massive pleural effusion. The mediastinum is displaced to the right. The stomach bubble (*dotted line*) is displaced far inferiorly and its upper surface is concave rather than convex, suggesting that the hemidiaphragm possesses the same contour. The underlying lung was normal. Pleural metastases from carcinoma of the maxillary antrum.

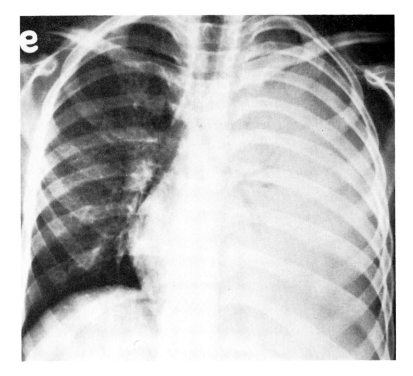

Figure 4–70. Massive Pleural Effusion. Appearances are similar to those in Figure 4–69 except that an air bronchogram is clearly seen in the medial portion of the lung. It can be reasonably assumed that the left lung is almost totally airless as a result of relaxation atelectasis, similar to what would be anticipated if the massive effusion were a large pneumothorax (*see* Figure 4–12*B*).

is highly suggestive of bronchogenic cancer with pleural metastases.

ATYPICAL DISTRIBUTION OF PLEURAL FLUID

The typical arrangement of fluid in the free pleural space requires that the underlying lung be free of disease and thus capable of preserving its shape even while recoiling from the chest wall—that is, it maintains its "form elasticity." An alteration in this uniform recoiling tendency is the influence by which most if not all atypical arrangements of pleural fluid can be explained. Briefly, it can be stated that regardless of its form, any pleural fluid accumulation that does not possess the typical configuration previously described must be associated with underlying pulmonary disease (provided that the fluid is free, not loculated). Thus, the major roentgenologic significance of atypical pleural effusion is that it *alerts the physician to the presence of both parenchymal and pleural disease.* However, it does not necessarily indicate in which lobe or lobes the pulmonary disease is present.

There is disagreement whether *infrapulmonary pleural effusion* (*synonyms:* subpulmonic, diaphragmatic) should be considered atypical, since, as already discussed, this is the site where effusion first accumulates "normally." Usually,

increasing amounts of fluid spill over into the costophrenic sulci and produce the roentgenologic signs described. However, for reasons as yet incompletely understood, fluid sometimes continues to accumulate in an infrapulmonary location without spilling into the costophrenic sulci or extending up the chest wall, producing a roentgenographic configuration in the erect subject that closely simulates diaphragmatic elevation (thus the designation "pseudodiaphragmatic contour") (Figure 4–67). Infrapulmonary pleural effusion occurs in such multifarious conditions of varied etiology (inflammatory, cardiovascular, traumatic, neoplastic, and renal[54, 56]) that it is difficult to cite a specific pathogenetic mechanism. Similarly, the nature and specific gravity of the fluid seem to possess no real significance, since the effusion may be either an exudate or a transudate. "Encapsulation" secondary to fibrous pleural adhesions plays no part in the pathogenesis, since appropriate positioning of the patient invariably shows the fluid spread over the free pleural space.

Some roentgenologic characteristics are common to most cases of infrapulmonary effusion,[54, 56] and any combination of these warrants confirmatory roentgenographic study in lateral decubitus position. All these signs refer to changes observed on posteroanterior and lateral roentgenograms of the erect patient.

1. Infrapulmonary accumulation may be uni-

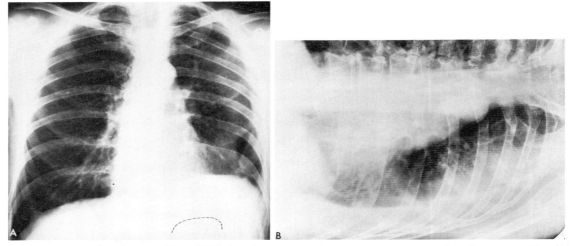

Figure 4–71. Infrapulmonary Pleural Effusion. A posteroanterior roentgenogram exposed in the erect position *(A)* shows a high left pseudodiaphragm whose peak is more laterally situated than that of a normal hemidiaphragm. It is situated several centimeters from the stomach bubble *(dotted line)*. The costophrenic sulcus is sharp. A roentgenogram exposed in the left lateral decubitus position with a horizontal x-ray beam *(B)* shows the fluid to have extended along the axillary lung zone.

lateral or bilateral; when unilateral, it occurs more commonly on the right.

2. In posteroanterior projection (Figure 4–71) the peak of the pseudodiaphragmatic configuration is lateral to that of the normal hemidiaphragm, being situated near the junction of the middle and lateral thirds rather than near the center, and slopes down sharply toward the lateral costophrenic recess.

3. On the left side, the pseudodiaphragmatic contour is separated further than normal from the gastric air bubble (Figure 4–71); the diaphragm and the bubble normally are in contact.

4. Both the lateral and the posterior costophrenic sulci may be sharp and clear, although in many cases the posterior gutter appears blunted because fluid has spilled over into it.

5. In lateral projection a characteristic configuration is frequently seen anteriorly where the upper margin of the fluid meets the major fissure. In many cases the contour anterior to the fissure is flattened, this segment descending abruptly to the costophrenic angle. A small amount of fluid is usually apparent in the lower end of the chief fissure where it joins the infrapulmonary collection.

6. In posteroanterior projection, a thin triangular opacity may be observed in the left paramediastinal zone, with its apex approximately halfway up the mediastinum and its base contiguous with the pseudodiaphragmatic contour inferiorly. This shadow represents mediastinal extension of the infrapulmonary fluid collection. Lateral decubitus roentgenography

with a horizontal beam should be performed in all cases (Figure 4–71), both to confirm the diagnosis and to permit assessment of the quantity of fluid more accurately than is possible with the patient erect.

LOCULATION OF PLEURAL FLUID

Loculated or encysted pleural effusions may occur anywhere in the pleural space, either between parietal and visceral pleura over the periphery of the lung or between visceral layers in the interlobar fissures. Encapsulation is caused by adhesions between contiguous pleural surfaces and, therefore, tends to occur during or following episodes of pleuritis—often pyothorax or hemothorax. Over the convexity of the thorax the loculated effusion appears as a smooth, sharply demarcated, homogeneous opacity protruding into the hemithorax and compressing contiguous lung. Fluoroscopic examination with subsequent roentgenography in tangential projection helps to establish their precise location for subsequent diagnostic or therapeutic thoracentesis, but ultrasonography is a superior technique for this purpose. This procedure not only assesses the amount of fluid loculated in a pleural pocket and indicates the precise anatomic point for thoracentesis but also simplifies the procedure: special aspiration transducers are applied, through which the needle is inserted directly into the specified site. Occasionally CT scanning may be of advantage in distinguishing encapsulated fluid from consolidated lung parenchyma, thereby facilitating diagnostic thoracentesis; it may also be of value in differentiating empyema and a peripheral pulmonary abscess.[58] Mediastinal encysted effusions are uncommon in our experience; they may be situated anteriorly or posteriorly in various locations.

Interlobar encysted effusions are typically elliptical when viewed tangentially, and their extremities blend imperceptibly with the interlobar fissure. In some conditions, particularly cardiac decompensation, the effusion may simulate a mass roentgenographically and be misdiagnosed as a bronchogenic neoplasm (Figure 4–72); however, its distinctive configuration in either posteroanterior or lateral projection should establish the diagnosis. These fluid accumulations occur in the horizontal fissure in up to 80 per cent of cases and tend to absorb spontaneously when the heart failure is relieved and, therefore, have acquired the epithet "van-

ishing tumor" (*synonyms:* "phantom tumor," "pseudo-tumor").

ROENTGENOLOGIC SIGNS OF PLEURAL THICKENING

PLEURAL FIBROSIS

Thickening of the pleural line over the convexity of the thorax is fairly common. The thickness of the pleural line may increase to 1 to 10 mm, usually after an episode of pleuritis and almost exclusively as a result of fibrosis of the visceral pleural surface. (The major exception is the pleural plaque formation characteristic of asbestos-related disease, considered in detail in Chapter 12.) Severe thickening may markedly restrict pulmonary expansion, in which case surgical removal by "peeling" may be curative. Although sometimes local, pleural fibrosis is more often uniform over the whole

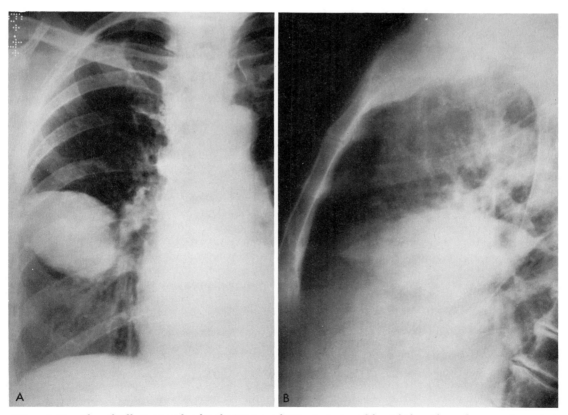

Figure 4–72. Pleural Effusion Localized to the Horizontal Fissure. A view of the right hemithorax from a posteroanterior roentgenogram *(A)* reveals a sharply circumscribed opacity of homogeneous density in the right midlung zone. In lateral projection *(B)*, the true nature of the opacity can be appreciated; the mass is elliptical in shape, its pointed extremities being situated anteriorly and posteriorly in keeping with the position of the minor fissure. This unusual collection of pleural fluid developed during a recent episode of cardiac decompensation. With appropriate therapy, it disappeared completely in 3 weeks; thus the designation "vanishing tumor."

lung surface, presenting as a thin line of unit density separating air-containing lung from contiguous ribs. The costophrenic recesses often are partly or completely obliterated, particularly laterally, and roentgenography in lateral decubitus position may be necessary to differentiate such old fibrous thickening from a small pleural effusion.

A curved shadow of unit density frequently is visualized in the apex of one or both lungs, in the concavity formed by the first and second ribs. Euphemistically called the "apical cap," it is sometimes falsely ascribed to tuberculosis. In one study[59] the commonest pathologic finding (in 20.3 per cent of cases) was nonspecific fibrous scarring of apical lung parenchyma which merged with the visceral pleura. Care should be taken not to fail to recognize apparent apical pleural thickening as an early manifestation of a much more serious disease—apical pulmonary cancer, or Pancoast tumor. The various etiologies of unilateral or bilateral apical caps have recently been reviewed by McLoud and her colleagues.[60]

PLEURAL NEOPLASMS

These are discussed in detail in Chapter 15, and the present section is concerned only with the two roentgenologic signs sometimes of value in distinguishing between diseases that arise in the lung and in the pleura. *Local mesothelial neoplasms* may arise from either the parietal or visceral pleural surface, over the convexity of the lung, or from an interlobar fissure. When they arise from the convexity of the lung these solitary tumors may be either sessile or pedunculated, but in either event they almost invariably form an obtuse angle with the chest wall when viewed in profile. It is important to recognize this obtuse angle: it distinguishes these lesions from those that arise within the lung parenchyma, which tend to form an acute angle with the chest wall. *Diffuse mesothelial neoplasms*, which usually are highly malignant, are commonly accompanied by pleural effusion. Even when the effusion is massive, however, there tends to be little displacement of the mediastinum and diaphragm away from the affected hemithorax. The reasons for this are not clear: in some cases it may result from inability of the lung to expand fully because of extensive neoplastic involvement of the pleural surface; in others, it occurs when neoplastic invasion of the mediastinal surface of the lung has caused bronchial occlusion, resulting in atelectasis. Regardless of mechanism, the lack

of displacement is important to the roentgenologic diagnosis of this highly malignant lesion—although it should be borne in mind that a similar picture may be produced by primary bronchogenic carcinoma with obstructive atelectasis and metastatic pleural effusion.

ROENTGENOLOGIC SIGNS OF PNEUMOTHORAX

A roentgenologic diagnosis of pneumothorax can be made only on identification of the visceral pleural line (*see* Figure 4–12, page 174). Since the lung is partly collapsed by the pneumothorax, it might be anticipated that its density would be increased and that this altered density, compared with that of the normal lung, should be sufficient to suggest the diagnosis; in fact, this is not so. As the lung progressively collapses with increasing size of the pneumothorax, blood flow through it diminishes; therefore the ratio of air and blood is not materially altered and the overall density of the collapsing lung is not changed (Figure 4–73). Undoubtedly the gas in the pleural space anterior and posterior to the collapsed lung makes an important contribution to overall density, but, regardless of the mechanism involved, the empirical observation is valid: roentgenographic density of a collapsing lung changes little until volume is greatly reduced.

The visceral pleural line is usually fairly readily identifiable, even on roentgenograms exposed at total lung capacity. When pneumothorax is strongly suspected clinically but a pleural line is not visualized (possibly obscured by an overlying rib), gas in the pleural space can be identified by either of two procedures: (1) Roentgenography in the erect position in full expiration (the rationale being that lung volume is reduced although the volume of gas in the pleural space is constant, thereby providing a smaller surface of visceral pleura in contact with air). (2) Roentgenography in the lateral decubitus position with a horizontal x-ray beam; the rationale here is obvious—air rises to the highest point in the hemithorax and is more clearly visible over the lateral chest wall than over the apex, where confluence of overlying bony shadows may obscure fine linear shadows.

In the majority of clinical settings, patients with suspected pneumothorax will be radiographed in the erect position, in which case air rises to the apex of the hemithorax and causes collapse of the upper portion of the lung. When patients must be examined in the supine position, as is so often the case with today's prolif-

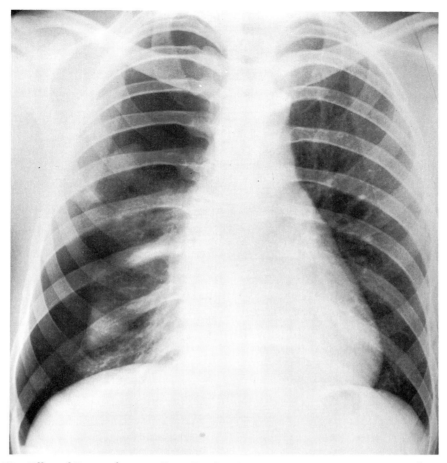

Figure 4–73.   Effect of Pneumothorax on Lung Density. A posteroanterior roentgenogram reveals a moderate right pneumothorax; despite the fact that the right lung has been reduced in volume by approximately 50 per cent, its density (except in local areas) differs little from that of the left lung. *See* text.

eration of intensive care units, gas within the pleural space rises to the highest point in the hemithorax, which frequently is immediately above the diaphragm anteriorly. Thus, gas in the anterior costophrenic sulcus results in an abrupt curvilinear change in density projected over the right or left upper quadrant.[61] A sub-pulmonic accumulation of gas has also been reported as an occasional manifestation of spontaneous pneumothorax in patients with chronic obstructive pulmonary disease.[62]

Hydropneumothorax should be immediately apparent on roentgenograms exposed in the erect position, by dint of the almost invariable air-fluid level. Encapsulated hydropneumothorax may occur as single or multiple encysted collections, some of which may contain air-fluid levels.

"TENSION" PNEUMOTHORAX AND HYDROTHORAX

On the evidence supplied by roentgenograms of the chest at total lung capacity, the detection of increased pressure in a pneumothorax may be exceedingly difficult, especially if the pneumothorax is complete and collapse of the ipsilateral lung total. Shift of the mediastinum away from the side of a pneumothorax of any size is inevitable, pressure in the contralateral (normal) hemithorax being relatively more negative; such a shift must not be mistaken for evidence of "tension" pneumothorax. In fact, the term "tension" is semantically inaccurate. For the volume of a pneumothorax to increase, air must flow from the lung parenchyma (where pressure is atmospheric) through the pleural defect and into the pleural space; obviously such flow cannot occur if pleural pressure is greater than atmospheric, or under "tension." Thus, for a pneumothorax to increase in volume, pressure within the pleural space must be relatively negative *during inspiration:* if a check-valve mechanism exists, allowing air to enter the pleural space during inspiration but preventing its egress during expiration, pressure within the pleural space will be positive only during the latter phase of respiration. Thus the correct term is *"expiratory* tension pneumothorax." On fluoroscopic examination, the situation should be clear: the increased tension prevents mediastinal shift toward the side of the pneumothorax on inspiration and may severely restrict inflation of the normal lung, constituting what may be the major cause of respiratory difficulty.

Tension hydrothorax, although rare, constitutes as much of a danger as expiratory tension pneumothorax—perhaps more so, since the possibility of its occurrence is not generally recognized. It is well to bear the possibility in mind in any patient with a massive pleural effusion, disproportionately increasing symptoms, and progressive deterioration in condition.

REFERENCES

1. Loosli, C. G.: Interalveolar communications in normal and in pathologic mammalian lungs: Review of the literature. Arch. Pathol., 24:743, 1937.
2. Dornhorst, A. C., and Pierce, J. W.: Pulmonary collapse and consolidation: The role of collapse in the production of lung field shadows and the significance of segments in inflammatory lung disease. J. Fac. Radiol., 5:276, 1954.
3. Fraser, R. G., and Wortzman, G.: Acute pneumococcal lobar pneumonia: The significance of non-segmental distribution. J. Can. Assoc. Radiol., 10:37, 1959.
4. Culiner, M. M., and Reich, S. B.: Collateral ventilation and localized emphysema. Am. J. Roentgenol., 85:246, 1961.
5. Hogg, J. C., Macklem, P. T., and Thurlbeck, W. M.: The resistance of collateral channels in excised human lungs. J. Clin. Invest., 48:421, 1969.
6. Schneider, H. J., Felson, B., and Gonzalez, L. L.: Rounded atelectasis. Am. J. Roentgenol., 134:225, 1980.
7. Clements, J. A.: Surface phenomena in relation to pulmonary function. Physiologist, 5:11, 1962.
8. Sutnick, A. I., and Soloff, L. A.: Surface tension reducing activity in the normal and atelectatic human lung. Am. J. Med., 35:31, 1963.
9. Staub, N. C., Nagano, H., and Pearce, M. L.: Pulmonary edema in dogs, especially the sequence of fluid accumulation in lungs. J. Appl. Physiol., 22:227, 1967.
10. Angus, G. E., and Thurlbeck, W. M.: Number of alveoli in the human lung. J. Appl. Physiol., 32:483, 1972.
11. Bateson, E. M.: An analysis of 155 solitary lung lesions illustrating the differential diagnosis of mixed tumours of the lung. Clin. Radiol., 16:51, 1965.
12. Bateson, E. M.: The solitary circumscribed bronchogenic carcinoma: A radiological study of 100 cases. Br. J. Radiol., 37:598, 1964.
13. Rigler, L. G.: The roentgen signs of carcinoma of the lung. Am. J. Roentgenol., 74:415, 1955.
14. Woodring, J. H., Fried, A. M., and Chuang, V. P.: Solitary cavities of the lung: Diagnostic implications of cavity wall thickness. Am. J. Roentgenol., 135:1269, 1980.
15. Bancks, N., and Zornoza, J.: Pseudocavitary granulomas of the lung. Am. J. Roentgenol., 127:251, 1976.
16. Good, C. A.: The solitary pulmonary nodule: A problem of management. Radiol. Clin. North Am., 1:429, 1963.
17. Salzman, E.: Lung Calcifications in X-ray Diagnosis. Springfield, Ill., Charles C Thomas, 1968.
18. Rosenthal, D. I., Chandler, H. L., Azizi, F., and Schneider, P. B.: Uptake of bone imaging agents by diffuse pulmonary metastatic calcification. Am. J. Roentgenol., 129:871, 1977.
19. Gross, B. H., Schneider, H. J., and Proto, A. V.: Eggshell calcification of lymph nodes: An update. Am. J. Roentgenol., 135:1265, 1980.
20. Kiviluoto, R.: Pleural calcification as a roentgenologic sign of non-occupational endemic anthophyllite-asbestosis. Acta Radiol. (Supplement) 194, 1960.
21. Garland, L. H.: Bronchial carcinoma. Lobar distribution of lesions in 250 cases. Calif. Med., 94:7, 1961.
22. Lentino, W., Jacobson, H. G., and Poppel, M. H.: Segmental localization of upper lobe tuberculosis: The rarity of anterior involvement. Am. J. Roentgenol., 77:1042, 1957.
23. Frostad, S.: Segmental atelectasis in children with primary tuberculosis. Am. Rev. Tuberc., 79:597, 1959.
24. Felson, B., and Felson, H.: Localization of intrathoracic lesions by means of the postero-anterior roentgenogram: The silhouette sign. Radiology, 55:363, 1950.
25. Collins, V. P., Loeffler, R. K., and Tivey, H.: Observations on growth rates of human tumors. Am. J. Roentgenol., 76:988, 1956.
26. Nathan, M. H., Collins, V. P., and Adams, R. A.: Differentiation of benign and malignant pulmonary nodules by growth rate. Radiology, 79:221, 1962.
27. Kerley, P.: Radiology in heart disease. Br. Med. J., 2:594, 1933.
28. Shanks, S. C., and Kerley, P.: A Textbook of X-Ray Diagnosis, 4th ed. Philadelphia, W. B. Saunders Co., 1973, Vol. III, p. 271.
29. Trapnell, D. H.: The differential diagnosis of linear shadows in chest radiographs: Radiol. Clin. North Am., 11:77, 1973.
30. Simon, G.: Principles of Chest X-Ray Diagnosis, 3rd ed. London, Butterworth, 1971.
31. Fraser, R. G., Fraser, R. S., Renner, J. W., Bernard, C., and Fitzgerald, P. J.: The roentgenologic diagnosis of chronic bronchitis: A reassessment with emphasis on parahilar bronchi seen end-on. Radiology, 120:1, 1976.
32. Rigler, L. G.: Personal communication, 1965.
33. Webb, W. R.: The pleural tail sign. Radiology, 127:309, 1978.
34. Fleischner, F.: Uber das Wesen der basalan horizontalen Schattenstreifen im Lungenfeld. Wien. Arch. Inn. Med., 28:461, 1936.
35. Fleischner, F., Hampton, A. O., and Castleman, B.:

Linear shadows in the lung (interlobar pleuritis, atelectasis and healed infarction). Am. J. Roentgenol., 46:610, 1941.

36. Fleischner, F. G.: Personal communication, 1967.

37. Simon, G.: The cause and significance of some long line shadows in the chest radiograph. Proc. R. Soc. Med., 58:861, 1965.

38. Simon, G.: Further observations on the long line shadow across a lower zone of the lung. Br. J. Radiol., 43:327, 1970.

39. Thomson, K. R., Eyssen, G. E., and Fraser, R. G.: Discrimination of normal and overinflated lungs and prediction of total lung capacity based on chest film measurements. Radiology, 119:721, 1976.

40. Brown, B. St.J., Ma, H., Dunbar, J. S., and MacEwan, D. W.: Foreign bodies in the tracheobronchial tree in childhood. J. Can. Assoc. Radiol., 14:158, 1963.

41. Allison, D. J., and Stanbrook, H. S.: A radiologic and physiologic investigation into hypoxic pulmonary vasoconstriction in the dog. Invest. Radiol., 15:178, 1980.

42. Rosenblum, L. J., Mauceri, R. A., Wellenstein, D. E., Bassano, D. A., Cohen, W. N., and Heitzman, E. R.: Computed tomography of the lung. Radiology, 129:521, 1978.

43. Ball, K. P., Goodwin, J. F., and Harrison, C. V.: Massive thrombotic occlusion of the large pulmonary arteries. Circulation, 14:766, 1956.

44. Scarrow, G: D.: The pulmonary angiogram in chronic bronchitis and emphysema. Clin. Radiol., 17:54, 1966.

45. Swyer, P. R., and James, G. C. W.: A case of unilateral pulmonary emphysema. Thorax, 8:133, 1953.

46. MacLeod, W. M.: Abnormal transradiancy of one lung. Thorax, 9:147, 1954.

47. Kieffer, S. A., Amplatz, K., Anderson, R. C., and Lillehei, C. W.: Proximal interruption of a pulmonary artery: Roentgen features and surgical correction. Am. J. Roentgenol., 95:592, 1965.

48. Chiorazzi, N., Weiss, H. S., Margouleff, D., Farber, S., and Gulotta, S. J.: Long-term pulmonary blood flow alterations following relief of partial bronchial obstruction. Am. J. Med., 56:559, 1974.

49. Fleischner, F. G : Unilateral pulmonary embolism with increased compensatory circulation through the un-occluded lung: Roentgen observations. Radiology, 73:591, 1959.

50. Laurenzi, C. A., Turino, G. M., and Fishman, A. P.: Bullous disease of the lung. Am. J. Med., 32:361, 1962.

51. Godwin, J. D., Webb, W. R., Savoca, C. J., Gamsu, G., and Goodman, P. C.: Multiple, thin-walled cystic lesions of the lung. Am. J. Roentgenol., 135:593, 1980.

52. Reid, L.: The Pathology of Emphysema. London, Lloyd-Luke (Medical Books) Ltd., 1967.

53. Müller, R., and Löfstedt, S.: The reaction of the pleura in primary tuberculosis of the lungs. Acta Med. Scand., 122:105, 1945.

54. Hessén, I.: Roentgen examination of pleural fluid: A study of the localization of free effusion, the potentialities of diagnosing minimal quantities of fluid and its existence under physiological conditions. Acta Radiol. Suppl. 86, 1951.

55. Moskowitz, H., Platt, R. T., Schachar, R., and Mellins, H.: Roentgen visualization of minute pleural effusion: An experimental study to determine the minimum amount of pleural fluid visible on a radiograph. Radiology, 109:33, 1973.

56. Fleischner, F. G.: Atypical arrangement of free pleural effusion. Radiol. Clin. North Am., 1:347, 1963.

57. Dandy, W. E., Jr.: Incomplete pulmonary interlobar fissure sign. Radiology, 128:21, 1978.

58. Baber, C. E., Hedlund, L. W., Oddson, T. A., and Putman, C. E.: Differentiating empyemas and peripheral pulmonary abscesses. The value of computed tomography. Radiology, 135:755, 1980.

59. Renner, R. R., Markarian, B., Pernice, N. J., and Heitzman, E. R.: The apical cap. Radiology, 110:569, 1974.

60. McLoud, T. C., Isler, R. J., Novelline, R. A., Putman, C. E., Simeone, J., and Stark, P.: The apical cap. Am. J. Roentgenol., 137:299, 1981.

61. Rhea, J. T., vanSonnenberg, E., and McLoud, T. C.: Basilar pneumothorax in the supine adult. Radiology, 133:593, 1979.

62. Christensen, E. E., and Dietz, G. W.: Subpulmonic pneumothorax in patients with chronic obstructive pulmonary disease. Radiology, 121:33, 1976.

5

Pulmonary Abnormalities of Developmental Origin

A complete understanding of developmental anomalies of the lungs requires knowledge of their normal development. Before reading this chapter, therefore, the reader is referred to the section on Development of the Lung in Chapter 1 (*see* page 60).

Developmental anomalies of the lungs are divided into two major groups, depending upon the *predominant* anlage affected: those originating in the primitive foregut or its derivative, the lung bud (bronchopulmonary or foregut anomalies), and those arising from the sixth embryonic arch and its derivative, the pulmonary vasculature.

BRONCHOPULMONARY (FOREGUT) ANOMALIES

These anomalies derive from a developmental defect in the primitive foregut or its ventral diverticulum, the lung bud. They include agenesis, aplasia, and hypoplasia, bronchopulmonary sequestration (intralobar and extralobar), cystic intrathoracic derivatives of the foregut (bronchial cyst), congenital cystic bronchiectasis, congenital cystic adenomatoid malformation of the lung, congenital bronchial atresia, and congenital (neonatal) lobar emphysema. Certainty that one is dealing with a developmental defect rather than an acquired lesion may be lacking at times, particularly in cases of solitary cystic intrapulmonary lesions.

PULMONARY AGENESIS, APLASIA, AND HYPOPLASIA

Factors interfering with the formation of the lungs must be effective between the twenty-fourth day and twenty-fourth week of gesta-

tion—during the embryonic, pseudoglandular, and canalicular periods (although any insult between the twenty-fourth week and term could interfere with development during the terminal sac period and could affect postnatal development up to the age of approximately 8 years). Factors responsible for *major* interference in lung formation must become effective not later than 26 days after conception.[1a–1d] According to Boyden,[2] there are three degrees of arrested development:

1. *Agenesis*, in which there is complete absence of one or both lungs; there is no trace of bronchial or vascular supply or of parenchymal tissue.

2. *Aplasia*, in which there is suppression of all but a rudimentary bronchus, which ends in a blind pouch; there are no vessels or parenchyma.

3. *Hypoplasia*, in which the bronchus is completely formed but is smaller than normal and ends in a fleshy structure that usually lies within the mediastinum.[2] Hypoplasia commonly involves the whole lung. When it affects only one lobe, the clinical and roentgenographic manifestations are different and in many cases the hypoplasia is accompanied by anomalies of the ipsilateral pulmonary artery and the pattern of anomalous pulmonary venous drainage (hypogenetic lung syndrome). The incidence of these anomalies is low, and there is no clear-cut sex or lateral predominance.

The *roentgenographic findings* in cases of agenesis, aplasia, or whole lung hypoplasia are as might be expected, with total or almost total absence of aerated lung in one hemithorax. The markedly reduced volume is indicated by approximation of the ribs, elevation of the ipsilateral hemidiaphragm, and shift of the mediastinum (Figure 5–1). In most cases the contralateral lung is greatly overinflated, and

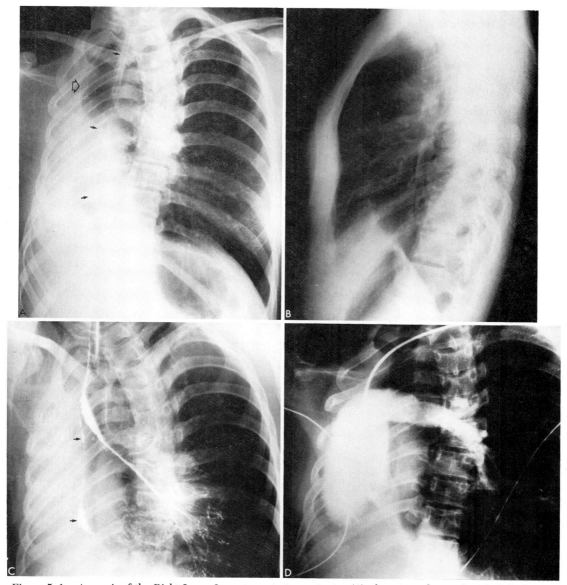

Figure 5–1. Agenesis of the Right Lung. In posteroanterior projection (A), there is evidence of marked displacement of the mediastinum to the right, both the heart and esophagus being entirely within the right hemithorax (the latter indicated by the position of the nasogastric tube—*solid arrows*). The left lung is severely overinflated, as indicated by the displaced anterior mediastinal septum in posteroanterior projection (*open arrow*) and by the large retrosternal air space in lateral projection (B). A bronchogram (C) shows no vestige of a right main bronchus (*arrows* point to contrast medium in the displaced esophagus). A pulmonary angiogram (D) reveals total absence of a right pulmonary artery. (Courtesy of Dr. David Stephen, formerly of the Royal Prince Albert Hospital, Sydney, Australia.)

displaced along with the anterior mediastinal septum into the involved hemithorax. Tomography and angiography may be required to establish the degree of underdevelopment or to differentiate agenesis from other conditions that may closely mimic it, such as total atelectasis from any cause. In some cases, it may be very difficult, even on examination of the pathologic specimen, to establish with certainty that the

lesion is congenital rather than a result of early acquired infection.

About 60 per cent of patients with agenesis of the lung are said to have other congenital anomalies, the most frequent of which are patent ductus arteriosus, tetralogy of Fallot, anomalies of the great vessels, and congenital diaphragmatic hernia. Since the bronchial tree, the diaphragm, and the gut develop rapidly between the eighth and twelfth weeks, interference with one may affect the others; *e.g.*, if the diaphragm fails to close, herniation of abdominal contents (particularly midgut) into the thorax may retard bronchial and bronchiolar subdivision. Thus, the degree of resultant hypoplasia depends on timing—if interference occurs at or after 12 weeks, pulmonary underdevelopment is mild.

Most patients with pulmonary agenesis have no acutely distressing symptoms, and many are totally asymptomatic and live normal lives. However, the anomaly appears to predispose to respiratory infection, and some of these patients die before the second decade of life, whether from the anomaly itself or from other associated congenital malformations.

BRONCHOPULMONARY SEQUESTRATION

Bronchopulmonary sequestration is a congenital pulmonary malformation in which a portion of pulmonary tissue is detached from the remainder of the normal lung and receives its blood supply from a systemic artery. The anomaly may be *intralobar* or *extralobar:* the former lies contiguous to normal lung parenchyma and within the same visceral pleural envelope; the latter is enclosed within its own pleural membrane, usually in close proximity to lung parenchyma but sometimes within or below the diaphragm. Recent reports support a common embryologic origin,[3] and examples have been described that occupy an intermediate position between the two.

The lung bud arises as an outpouching of the foregut in the 3-week-old embryo and shares the splanchnic plexus with the foregut. Normally, when the pulmonary artery elaborates from the sixth embryonic arch and invaginates its branches into the primitive pulmonary anlage, the branches of the splanchnic plexus supplying the lung bud persist as the bronchial arteries. In some fetuses, branches of the splanchnic plexus arising from the aorta persist, resulting in anomalous systemic arterial supply of the lung. Although this anomalous vessel may supply otherwise normal lung,[4] it usually is associated with sequestered, cystic lung. When arrest occurs in the earliest stages of foregut development, the sequestration remains in free communication with the parent esophagus through a muscular, epithelial-lined tube that often shares the anomalous blood supply. In the great majority of these malformations, however, the esophagobronchial diverticulum

is obliterated, the only evidence of the origin of the sequestration being the persistent anomalous blood supply arising from the splanchnic plexus.

INTRALOBAR SEQUESTRATION

This congenital pulmonary malformation is a nonfunctioning portion of lung within the visceral pleura of a pulmonary lobe. It almost invariably derives its arterial supply from the aorta or one of its branches, most commonly the descending thoracic aorta and occasionally the abdominal aorta or one of its branches. Although it has been stated that venous drainage is always via the pulmonary venous system, producing a left-to-left shunt, sporadic cases have been reported of venous drainage into the inferior vena cava or azygos system.[5] In approximately two-thirds of cases the sequestered portion of lung is in the paravertebral gutter, in the posterior bronchopulmonary segment of the left lower lobe; in most others it occupies the same anatomic region in the right lower lobe.[6] The upper lobes are rarely affected. Except for cases in which there is communication with the esophagus or stomach, intralobar sequestration is not associated with other anomalies.

Intrapulmonary sequestration usually is recognized in adulthood as a result of acute pneumonia. Although not reported in neonates at necropsy, sporadic reports have appeared of the anomaly becoming manifest in infancy.

Characteristically, the sequestered segment is a closed system unconnected with the normal bronchial tree; when communication develops it is usually in association with infection in the sequestered lung. All patients with suspected sequestration should undergo examination of the esophagus and stomach with barium to exclude the possibility of communication, although such is uncommon.

Pathologically, the affected segment typically is cystic, the spaces being filled with mucus, or, when infection is present, with pus. In the majority of cases, the lining consists of flattened epithelium lacking cartilage and glands,[4] and in others it is ciliated columnar epithelium indistinguishable from that of a normal bronchus. Typically, the anomalous vessel enters the lung by way of the lower part of the pulmonary ligament and is much larger than might be expected from the volume of tissue supplied. Histologically, this vessel is an elastic artery which, in many cases, shows intimal thickening and arteriosclerotic changes.

The roentgenographic appearance depends largely on whether the sequestered segment has been the site of infection and, as a result, communicates with the airways of contiguous lung tissue. When no communication exists, the anomalous tissue appears as a homogeneous opacity of water density in the posterior portion of a lower lobe (usually the left) and almost invariably contiguous with the diaphragm. It is round, oval, or triangular, and usually is sharply circumscribed.

When infection has resulted in communication with the bronchial tree, the roentgenographic presentation is an air-containing cystic mass with or without air-fluid levels (Figure 5–2). The cysts may be single and very large, but more commonly are multiple. The infectious process often affects the surrounding parenchyma as well, obscuring the underlying anomaly with pneumonic consolidation; the cystic nature of the mass may not become manifest until the pneumonia resolves (Figure 5–2). Typically, a bronchogram reveals the bronchial tree to be festooned around the mass, a distinctive and in fact almost diagnostic finding (Figure 5–2); the bronchial tree is numerically complete.

Although the diagnosis of bronchopulmonary sequestration may be strongly suspected from the preceding findings, definitive diagnosis depends upon opacification of the anomalous vessel by angiography. This is best accomplished by percutaneous aortography, either by flood technique or preferably by selective catheterization of the anomalous vessel.

The clinical picture is nonspecific and a diagnosis cannot be made on clinical grounds alone. Most patients are asymptomatic until the sequestered tissue becomes infected, usually by pyogenic organisms but occasionally by *M. tuberculosis*.[7] In many cases infection does not develop until adulthood.

EXTRALOBAR SEQUESTRATION

This characteristically differs in several respects from the intralobar type. It is often referred to as an accessory lung, since it develops as a complete ectopia of pulmonary tissue enclosed in its own pleura (in contrast to an intralobar sequestered segment, which is enclosed within the visceral pleura of the affected lobe). Anatomically, extralobar sequestration is related to the left hemidiaphragm in 90 per cent of cases; it may be situated between the inferior surface of the lower lobe and the diaphragm, below the diaphragm, within the sub-

stance of the diaphragm, or even in the mediastinum.[8] In contrast to the intralobar variety, it usually drains via the systemic venous system—the inferior vena cava, the azygos or hemiazygos system, or the portal venous system—creating a hemodynamic communication in the form of a left-to-right shunt. The systemic arterial supply is commonly from the abdominal aorta or one of its branches. In contrast to intralobar sequestration, the extralobar anomaly is often seen at necropsy of neonates, in many cases with other congenital anomalies. Eventration or paralysis of the ipsilateral hemidiaphragm may be present, and congenital diaphragmatic hernias have been noted on the left side in approximately 30 per cent of cases.

Since an extralobar sequestered segment is enveloped in its own pleural sac, the chances of its becoming infected are greatly reduced unless there is communication with the gastrointestinal tract.[9] Consequently, its chief mode of presentation, whether intrathoracic or intra-abdominal, is as a homogeneous soft tissue mass.

CONGENITAL BRONCHIAL CYSTS

A bronchial cyst is a rare congenital anomaly resulting from an abnormality of budding or branching of the tracheobronchial tree during its embryologic development. Cystic intrathoracic derivatives of the foregut fall into three distinct embryologic categories: (1) *Posterior mediastinal (enteric) cysts*, commonly associated with spinal anomalies, which arise from gut anlage that has herniated through a split in the notochord. This "split notochord syndrome" may give rise to various abnormal endodermal remnants. (2) *Intramural esophageal cysts or esophageal duplication*, resulting from failure of the originally solid esophagus to vacuolate completely to produce a hollow tube. (3) *Bronchial cysts*, resulting from abnormal budding of the ventral diverticulum of the foregut. Bronchial cysts must appear between the twenty-sixth and fortieth day of intrauterine life, the period of most active tracheobronchial development.

Bronchial cysts develop in the pulmonary parenchyma or mediastinum, or rarely within or beneath the diaphragm. The anomaly appears to have a predilection for males, and also for Yemenite Jews, not only in comparison with Jews from other countries but also with other populations throughout the world.[11]

Pathologically, these thin-walled cysts are

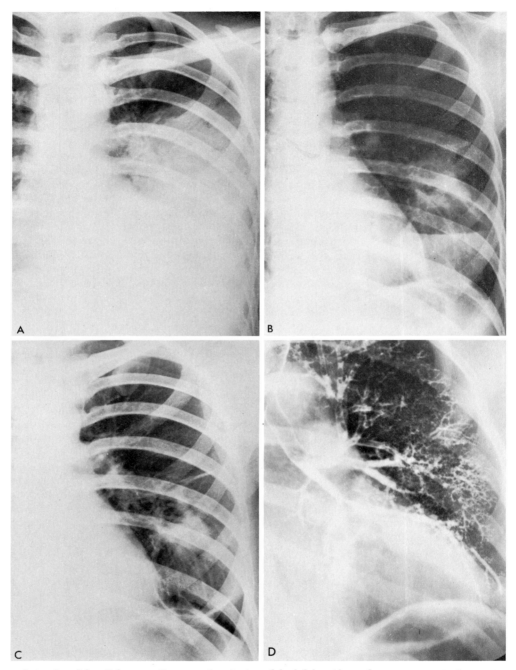

Figure 5–2. Intralobar Pulmonary Sequestration. A view of the left hemithorax from a posteroanterior roentgenogram (A) reveals massive air-space consolidation of the lower two-thirds of the left lung; note the air bronchogram in the upper portion of the consolidation. Three weeks later (B), there is almost complete resolution of the pneumonia, but there remains a rather well-defined mass lying contiguous to the left hemidiaphragm and possessing a prominent air-fluid level. Two months later (C), the fluid has disappeared, leaving a thin-walled cyst measuring several centimeters in diameter and showing an irregular nubbin of tissue in its superior portion. At this time, a bronchogram (D) demonstrates the basal bronchi to be festooned around the cystic space, a finding that is characteristic of intralobar pulmonary sequestration. At thoracotomy, the anomalous systemic vessel was seen to enter the sequestered mass from the diaphragm.

lined with respiratory epithelium and usually filled with mucoid material. Their walls may contain mucous glands, cartilage, elastic tissue, and smooth muscle. They do not communicate with the tracheobronchial tree unless they become infected, in which case the mucus may be replaced by pus or by pus and air.

PULMONARY BRONCHIAL CYSTS

The pulmonary parenchyma is the commonest location for these cysts.[12] There is a preference for the lower lobes with equal distribution in the two lungs.[12] In some cases the cysts are supplied by a systemic vessel and then may just as correctly be regarded as pulmonary sequestration.

The typical roentgenographic appearance is of a sharply circumscribed, solitary, round or oval shadow of unit density, usually in the medial third of the lungs. Characteristically, the lesions do not communicate with the tracheobronchial tree until they become infected. Infections occur eventually in about 75 per cent of cases. When communication is established, the cyst contains air, with or without fluid[12] (Figure 5–3).

It may be difficult to differentiate congenital bronchogenic from acquired cysts; even pathologists may fail to establish the origin with certainty once a congenital lesion has been infected, since the respiratory epithelium that lines the congenital cyst may be destroyed by the infection. Most acquired pulmonary cysts are residua of remote lung abscesses, and a history of an acute respiratory episode may be of help in diagnosis.

The majority of uninfected bronchogenic cysts occasion no symptoms and are discovered by accident on a screening chest roentgenogram. Symptoms, of which hemoptysis is the most common, almost invariably relate to infection in and around the cyst.

MEDIASTINAL BRONCHIAL CYSTS

The majority of mediastinal bronchial cysts are situated in the vicinity of the carina, often attached by a stalk to one of the major airways; in this location even a small cyst can cause symptoms by putting pressure on surrounding structures.[13] In a series of 14 pathologically proved mediastinal bronchial cysts,[12] two (14 per cent) were in the superior mediastinum, five (35 per cent) in the midmediastinum, and seven (50 per cent) in the posterior mediastinum. The vast majority of mediastinal bronchial cysts are solitary.

Roentgenographically, mediastinal bronchial cysts usually present as clearly defined masses of homogeneous density just inferior to the carina and often protruding slightly to the right,

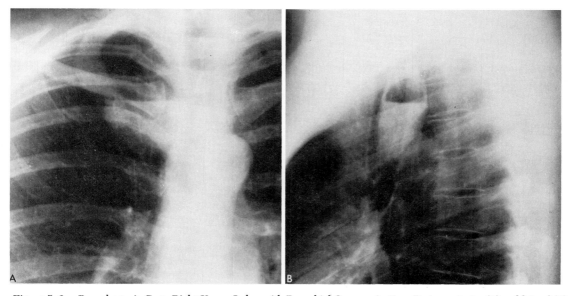

Figure 5–3.   Bronchogenic Cyst, Right Upper Lobe, with Bronchial Communication. Posteroanterior (*A*) and lateral (*B*) roentgenograms of an asymptomatic 30-year-old woman reveal a sharply circumscribed, elliptical mass in the right upper lobe, its medial border contiguous to the mediastinum. A prominent fluid level is present, indicating communication with the bronchial tree. The lesion was resected and proved to be a typical bronchial cyst; pathologically, there was no evidence of infection so that the presence of bronchial communication was unexplained. (Courtesy of Dr. Richard Lesperance, formerly of the Montreal Chest Hospital Center.)

overlapping the right hilar shadow. The majority are oval or round; the shape may vary with inspiration and expiration. They may displace the esophagus. In infants particularly, the intimate relationship of these cysts to the trachea and major bronchi may cause respiratory embarrassment. Unlike pulmonary bronchial cysts, the mediastinal variety seldom communicates with the tracheobronchial tree. They are almost always solitary but some are multiloculated. Calcification of the cyst wall is uncommon.

Mediastinal bronchogenic cysts may become very large without causing symptoms, although those in the carinal area may cause pressure symptoms even when quite small and roentgenographically invisible. Particularly in infants and young children, midmediastinal cysts may compress the major airways and cause severe respiratory distress. Symptoms include dyspnea on effort, stridor, and persistent cough.

CONGENITAL CYSTIC BRONCHIECTASIS

The congenital maldevelopment presenting as cystic bronchiectasis is much rarer than the acquired disease, but their similarities can lead to great difficulty in differentiation. Congenital bronchiectasis and congenital cystic foregut disease probably differ only in the degree of arrest of bronchial development.[3]

If microscopy of a resected portion of lung demonstrates cystic dilatation of bronchi whose walls show no inflammation and an intact muscularis, elastica, and cartilage, the condition is probably congenital and developmental.

CONGENITAL CYSTIC ADENOMATOID MALFORMATION

This anomaly consists of an intralobar mass of disorganized pulmonary tissue best classified as a pulmonary hamartoma. It occurs chiefly in infants. The malformation shows no preference for either lung or any lobe; more than one lobe seldom is affected. The lesions tend to be solid in infants and more cystic in children;[14] they lack a well-defined bronchial system but do communicate with the bronchial tree (distinguishing this anomaly from intralobar sequestration) and are supplied by the pulmonary circulation.

Histologically, the mass is an overgrowth of bronchioles with polypoid changes in the mucosa; the respiratory epithelium contains patches of tall mucoid cells and may show metaplasia.[14] Roentgenologically, the volume of lung affected varies considerably from case to case. The lesion is visualized as a mass composed of numerous air-containing cysts scattered irregularly through tissue of unit density. It is space-occupying, expanding the ipsilateral hemithorax and shifting the mediastinum to the contralateral side. Occasionally, the anomalous tissue can present roentgenographically as a solid homogeneous mass that evolves over time into multiple cysts.[15]

Clinically, the patient may be cyanotic and evidence respiratory embarrassment.[16] Clinical manifestations usually occur during the first days of life and their severity appears to be related to the volume of lung involved.

CONGENITAL BRONCHIAL ATRESIA

This rare anomaly consists of atresia or stenosis of a lobar, segmental, or subsegmental bronchus at or near its origin; the apicoposterior segmental bronchus of the left upper lobe is most commonly affected, followed by bronchi within the right upper lobe, right middle lobe, and, rarely, a lower lobe. The abnormality is probably developmental in origin, a conclusion supported by the report of this defect in very early childhood.[17]

Pathologically, the bronchial tree peripheral to the point of obliteration is patent; the complement of bronchi and bronchioles is normal or near normal. Macroscopically, the involved lung is voluminous as a result of emphysema, and pigmentation is absent or markedly reduced as a reflection of impaired ventilation.[18] Mucus secreted within the patent airways distal to the point of atresia cannot pass the stenosis and accumulates in the form of a plug; depending upon the amount of inspissated mucus, the plug may be linear, branched, ovoid, or cyst-like.

Roentgenographically, a well-circumscribed, somewhat elliptical mass of unit density is situated (in left upper lobe atresia) just above the left hilum in the anatomic position of the apicoposterior bronchus; the mass may be linear or branched. Air can enter the affected bronchopulmonary segments only via collateral channels, creating air drift between obstructed and adjacent normally ventilated segments and causing overinflation and expiratory air trapping.[19] The reduced ventilation results in hypoxic vasoconstriction, thus decreasing perfusion and diminishing vascular markings. The combination of overinflation, expiratory air trap-

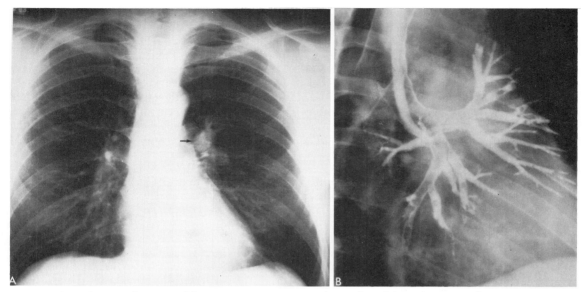

Figure 5–4. **Congenital Atresia of the Apicoposterior Segmental Bronchus of the Left Upper Lobe.** A posteroanterior roentgenogram (*A*) reveals increased radiolucency, overinflation, and sparse vasculature (oligemia) of the upper half of the left lung. An oval mass of homogeneous density is present just above and behind the left hilum (*arrows*). Since the differential diagnosis included a vascular malformation, a pulmonary arteriogram was carried out, but neither the arterial nor venous phase showed evidence of opacification of the mass. A left bronchogram (*B*) shows only the lingular and anterior segmental bronchi arising from the left upper lobe bronchus, there being no evidence of an apicoposterior bronchus. The elliptic mass relates to the expected position of origin of the apicoposterior bronchus and represents inspissated mucus within the lumen of the affected bronchus distal to atresia. The affected bronchopulmonary segment is air-containing as a result of collateral air drift from contiguous, normally ventilated segments. Oligemia is the result of hypoxic vasoconstriction secondary to diminished ventilation. (Courtesy of Dr. George Genereux, University Hospital, Saskatoon, Saskatchewan.)

ping, oligemia, and a well-circumscribed, elliptical, suprahilar mass produces a distinctive roentgenographic picture (Figure 5–4).

Congenital bronchial atresia rarely causes symptoms, the anomaly usually being discovered on a screening chest roentgenogram.

CONGENITAL (NEONATAL) LOBAR EMPHYSEMA

Lobar emphysema in infants is characterized by severe overinflation of a pulmonary lobe, usually causing severe respiratory distress. Only about one-third of cases become manifest at birth,[20] the remainder not being recognized until some weeks later. Developmental origin of the abnormality is supported by the frequent association of congenital cardiac anomalies, estimated by some to occur in approximately 50 per cent of cases. There is no familial incidence; the condition is rare in Negroid peoples.

Infantile lobar emphysema shows some male predominance. There is a distinct predilection for the left upper lobe and a slightly lesser one for the right middle lobe.

The pathogenesis of infantile lobar emphy-

sema can be divided into four groups.[21] (1) *Vascular:* Bronchial obstruction is produced by pressure from an abnormal vessel such as a large patent ductus arteriosus. (2) *Idiopathic:* An unrecognized infection probably antedates the lobar emphysema, which is not identified until some time after birth. (3) *Characterized by absence, hypoplasia, or dysplasia of bronchial cartilage:* Although malformation of bronchial cartilage associated with a redundant intrabronchial mucosal fold has been postulated as responsible for the lobar overinflation and obstruction in this group, only rarely is this abnormality clearly demonstrated in resected specimens.[21] (4) *The polyalveolar lobe,*[22] in which the number of alveoli is greatly increased.

The roentgenographic manifestations of infantile lobar emphysema are distinctive. The cardinal features are overinflation and air trapping, the former manifested by markedly increased volume of the affected lobe, even at TLC, depressing the ipsilateral hemidiaphragm and displacing the mediastinum into the contralateral hemithorax. The distended lobe may lead to compression (relaxation) atelectasis of the lung's other lobes. Vascular markings in the affected lobe tend to be widely separated and attenuated, the lobe appearing more radiolucent than other lung tissue. Identification of vascular markings is important, permitting differentiation from congenital air cysts, postpneumonic pneumatocele, and loculated pneumothorax.

The differential diagnosis includes other causes of lobar overinflation, such as aspiration of a foreign body or partial obstruction of a bronchus by an endobronchial or parabronchial space-occupying lesion.

About 90 per cent of affected infants suffer respiratory distress during the first few days of life (in a small percentage, symptoms are absent), and cyanosis may develop in the more severe cases. Physical examination may reveal thoracic asymmetry caused by unilateral overinflation. The percussion note is increased, breath sounds are much reduced, rales and a local wheeze may be audible, and the respiratory rate is increased. In many cases the course is rapid and progressive, and may end fatally unless the lobe is resected. However, the urgency of treatment depends on the severity of respiratory embarrassment, and the trend in recent years has been toward supportive therapy and a policy of watchful waiting. In many cases the clinical and roentgenographic manifestations regress spontaneously without the need for thoracotomy and lobar resection.[23]

ANOMALIES OF THE PULMONARY VASCULATURE

HYPOGENETIC LUNG SYNDROME

This rare congenital anomaly consists of partial hypoplasia of the right lung and of the right pulmonary artery, anomalies of the right bronchial tree (commonly mirror image), and anomalous pulmonary venous return from the right lung to the inferior vena cava, either below the diaphragm or at the vessel's junction with the right atrium (Figure 5–5). The hypogenetic right lung is supplied partly or completely by systemic arteries, producing a left-to-right (arteriovenous) shunt.

In some cases the anomalous vein is visible roentgenographically as a broad, gently curved shadow descending to the diaphragm just to the right of the heart; this shadow is shaped like a scimitar—thus the designation *scimitar syndrome* (Figure 5–5).[24] Most commonly the entire right lung is drained by the anomalous vein. Associated cardiovascular anomalies are common. Hypogenetic lung syndrome shows considerable variation, both in the amount of lung supplied by the pulmonary and bronchial arteries and in the pattern of venous drainage.

More than half the patients have cardiorespiratory symptoms, similar in many respects to those of large left-to-right shunts and pulmonary

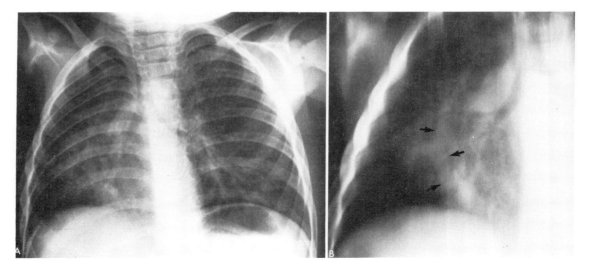

Figure 5–5. Hypogenetic Lung Syndrome. A posteroanterior roentgenogram (*A*) of a 3-year-old white boy reveals moderate loss of volume of the right lung, evidenced chiefly by shift of the mediastinum. Although the vasculature of the right lung is poorly visualized, there is a suggestion of a broad, obliquely oriented vascular shadow in the vicinity of the right cardiophrenic angle. An anteroposterior tomogram (*B*) reveals this shadow to good advantage (*arrows*); it represents an anomalous pulmonary vein draining blood from the right lung to the inferior vena cava. An angiogram was not performed, but the combination of hypoplasia of the right lung and anomalous pulmonary venous drainage to the IVC constitutes convincing evidence of the hypogenetic lung syndrome or the "scimitar syndrome." (Courtesy of Dr. David Lewall, formerly of the Foothills Hospital, Calgary, Alberta.)

arterial hypertension. Some patients have repeated bronchopulmonary infections or hemoptysis. A systolic murmur of moderate intensity usually is heard along the left sternal border, and the electrocardiogram characteristically shows hypertrophy of the right heart chambers.

ANOMALOUS PULMONARY VENOUS DRAINAGE

Both partial and total anomalous pulmonary venous drainage form an extracardiac left-to-right shunt; in addition, total anomalous connection provides a right-to-left shunt through an obligatory septal defect.

The *partial* anomaly incorporates the venous drainage from part or all of one lung via one or more pulmonary veins into the systemic venous system. It is often associated with other cardiovascular anomalies, particularly atrial septal defect. The anomalous vein may be visible on plain roentgenograms, but pulmonary angiography is necessary to confirm the diagnosis and to elucidate the specific anatomic variation.

In *total* anomalous pulmonary venous drainage, the pulmonary veins usually join directly behind the heart before communicating with the systemic venous system.[25] The common pulmonary vein draining the two lungs may terminate at three levels: supracardiac (usually a left superior vena cava), cardiac (usually the right atrium or coronary sinus), or infradiaphragmatic (usually the portal vein). In contrast to partial anomalous pulmonary venous drainage, the total connection rarely is associated with other cardiovascular anomalies, apart from the obligatory atrial septal defect (which may be no more than a patent foramen ovale).

Obstruction of the venous return results in pulmonary venous hypertension and a characteristic roentgenographic combination of interstitial pulmonary edema and a normal-sized heart. Such obstruction is almost invariably of the infradiaphragmatic type when venous return to the inferior vena cava is via the capillary bed of the liver.

The majority of patients with total anomalous pulmonary venous drainage die in infancy.[26] Those who survive to adulthood characteristically have a large septal defect and a short anomalous pathway, drainage being directly into the superior vena cava or right atrium. In adults, the clinical picture may simulate isolated atrial septal defect; the second heart sound is often widely split and there is usually an ejec-tion systolic murmur and gallop rhythm. Since pulmonary venous blood mixes with systemic venous blood at or before the right atrium, oxygen saturation tends to be identical in all heart chambers and the two major vessels.

ABSENCE (PROXIMAL INTERRUPTION) OF THE RIGHT OR LEFT PULMONARY ARTERY

This rare anomaly preferably is designated "proximal interruption" of the right or left pulmonary artery, since the vessels within the lung are usually intact and patent. The ipsilateral lung is hypoplastic and of reduced volume (Figure 5–6): its arterial supply is derived from a hypertrophied bronchial circulation or from extensive intercostal and subdiaphragmatic transpleural collaterals.[27] Despite its reduced volume, the lung usually is hyperlucent—a finding which, when taken in conjunction with the diminutive hilar shadow, may lead to the erroneous diagnosis of the acquired disease known as Swyer-James' or Macleod's syndrome. However, differentiation is usually possible by roentgenography in full expiration—patients with Swyer-James' syndrome show ipsilateral air trapping due to bronchiolar obstruction, a sign that is absent in cases of proximal interruption of a pulmonary artery.

The anomalous pulmonary artery usually occurs on the side opposite the aortic arch.[28] Proximal interruption on the left has a high incidence of associated congenital cardiovascular anomalies, particularly tetralogy of Fallot and septal defects. When the proximal interruption is on the right, associated congenital anomalies are less frequent.

PULMONARY ARTERY STENOSIS OR COARCTATION

This rare anomaly is characterized by single or multiple coarctations of the pulmonary arteries, commonly with poststenotic dilatations.[29] The stenoses may be short or long, peripheral or central, unilateral or bilateral. Associated cardiovascular anomalies are common, consisting of infundibular, valvular, or supravalvular pulmonic stenosis (60 per cent of cases)[30] and atrial septal defects.

Roentgenographically, the pulmonary vasculature may appear normal, diminished, or increased, depending on the presence and nature of associated malformations. The precise

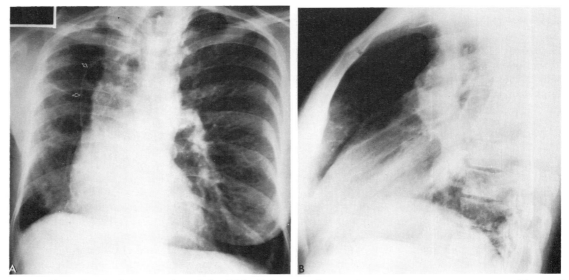

Figure 5–6. Proximal Interruption of the Right Pulmonary Artery. A posteroanterior roentgenogram (A) reveals moderate elevation of the right hemidiaphragm and shift of the mediastinum to the right, indicating considerable loss of volume of the right lung. A right hilar shadow cannot be identified and the vascularity of the right lung is markedly reduced in amount and atypical in pattern. The overinflated left lung is displaced into the right hemithorax, as indicated by the anterior pleural line (*arrows*); note the deep retrosternal air space in lateral projection (B).

morphologic nature of the abnormality may be obscure without selective pulmonary angiography, and this procedure is essential to positive diagnosis.

When the stenosis affects a main branch or branches of the pulmonary artery, the clinical picture is usually that of the associated anomalies: a continuous murmur may not be heard at the site of the pulmonary arterial stenosis, presumably because flow is decreased by the valvular or infundibular stenosis. When the stenoses are peripheral in location, the pulmonic second sound is accentuated and a grade II to IV/VI continuous murmur usually is audible bilaterally over the upper part of the chest anteriorly, radiating to the neck and back.[30] When stenosis is severe, flow may be so reduced that the lesions are acoustically silent.

Familial incidence of the anomaly and its association with the Ehlers-Danlos syndrome have been reported. Its occurrence in association with maternal rubella is well documented.

ANOMALOUS ORIGIN OF THE LEFT PULMONARY ARTERY FROM THE RIGHT

Of the many recognized anomalous origins of the pulmonary arteries,[28] derivation of the left vessel from the right pulmonary artery is particularly interesting because of its effects on the lungs.[31] From its point of origin the aberrant left artery passes posteriorly to the right of the right main bronchus or lower trachea, then turns sharply to the left and passes between the esophagus and trachea in its course to the left hilum. Its intimate relationship to the right main bronchus and to the trachea results in their compression and various degrees of obstructive overinflation or atelectasis of the right or both lungs.[28] Airway obstruction usually becomes manifest shortly after birth and may be severe. The infant or child almost invariably presents with stridor, often with feeding problems, and consequent frequent respiratory tract infections. The demonstration of local posterior displacement of the barium-filled esophagus in the region of the lower trachea makes the diagnosis virtually certain; this can be confirmed by pulmonary angiography, although the diagnosis can usually be made with conviction by conventional roentgenographic methods and computed tomography.[32] Early recognition of the lesion is vital, since surgical correction is feasible and usually results in abatement of respiratory symptoms and signs.

Bronchoscopy should be performed prior to surgery in any patient with anomalous origin of the left pulmonary artery from the right in order to establish whether respiratory difficulty might be caused by an intrinsic tracheal anomaly (ring cartilages) rather than by the vascular anomaly *per se*.

CONGENITAL ANEURYSMS OF THE PULMONARY ARTERIES

These rare lesions are said to be associated almost invariably with other pulmonary abnormalities, such as arteriovenous fistulas or bronchopulmonary sequestration.[28] Aneurysms of the central pulmonary arteries, commonly accompanied by congenital cardiovascular anomalies and present at birth, usually are the result of such disturbed hemodynamics as the jet of blood and turbulence created by pulmonary valvular stenosis. This type of poststenotic dilatation affects the left pulmonary artery much more commonly than the right; in fact, enlargement of the main pulmonary artery and its left branch in conjunction with a normal right hilum should strongly suggest the diagnosis of pulmonary valvular stenosis. A similar type of dilatation may occur as an isolated "anomaly" unassociated with pulmonary stenosis. The dilatation usually is confined to the pulmonary trunk; although often fusiform in nature, it may be saccular.

PULMONARY ARTERIOVENOUS FISTULA

Communication between blood vessels is abnormal in a wide variety of both congenital and acquired diseases of the lungs. Acquired fistulas are more properly designated "vascular shunts," since they occur not only *from artery to vein* (for example, in cases of metastatic carcinoma from the thyroid) but also *from artery to artery* (epitomized by the bronchial artery to pulmonary artery shunts that develop in many pulmonary diseases associated with chronic ischemia or chronic infection, such as bronchiectasis) and *from vein to vein* (such as the bronchial vein to pulmonary vein shunt in advanced pulmonary emphysema). In the present section, discussion is restricted to abnormal communications of congenital origin.

The term "congenital arteriovenous fistula" usually connotes an abnormal vascular communication within the pulmonary circulation—from pulmonary artery to pulmonary vein. Congenital pulmonary arteriovenous fistula or aneurysm is considered to be caused by a defect in the terminal capillary loops that allows dilatation and the formation of thin-walled vascular sacs supplied by a single distended afferent artery and drained by a single distended efferent vein.[33] In addition to this relatively simple arteriovenous communication between a single artery and vein, a more complex aneurysm has been described with multiple feeding arteries and draining veins.

Approximately one-third of cases of pulmonary arteriovenous fistula have multiple lesions in the lungs; some resected specimens contain small fistulas not apparent on plain roentgenograms—a point of obvious importance when resection of a known fistula is contemplated.

From 40 to 65 per cent of patients with arteriovenous fistulas in the lungs have arteriovenous communications elsewhere, including the skin, mucous membranes, and other organs. This condition, known as *hereditary hemorrhagic telangiectasia* or Rendu-Osler-Weber's disease, is of simple, dominant non–sex-linked transmission. Although it is assumed that the vascular defect is present at birth, it seldom becomes manifest clinically until adult life when the vessels have been subjected to pressure over several decades. In one family of 91 individuals known to have this condition,[33] 14 (15 per cent) were found to have arteriovenous fistulas in the lungs, a finding that underlines the need to search thoroughly for pulmonary lesions in all cases of cutaneous or mucous membrane telangiectasis.

Roentgenographically, pulmonary arteriovenous fistulas are seen more commonly in the lower lobes than in the middle or upper lobes[34] and are single in about two-thirds of cases. The classic appearance is of a round or oval homogeneous opacity of unit density, somewhat lobulated in contour but sharply defined, most often in the medial third of the lung, ranging from less than 1 cm to several centimeters in diameter. Identification of the feeding and draining vessels, which is essential to the diagnosis, may be difficult with plain roentgenograms and often requires tomography. The artery and vein usually can be distinguished fairly easily, the artery relating to the hilum and the vein deviating from the course of the artery toward the left atrium. Angiography may be required to confirm the diagnosis (Figure 5–7) but, in any event, is mandatory in any patient for whom resectional surgery is contemplated (Figure 5–8). *Care must be exercised in obtaining angiographic visualization of all portions of both lungs;* it is not enough to perform selective angiography of the lung in question, since lesions may be present in the contralateral lung and may not be visible on the plain roentgenogram (Figure 5–7).

Even without angiography, positive identification of the feeding artery and draining vein establishes the diagnosis beyond reasonable doubt. When such vessels are not clearly de-

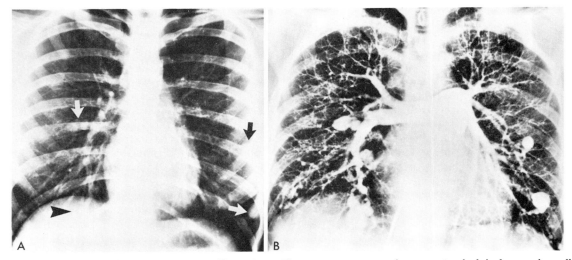

Figure 5–7. Multiple Arteriovenous Malformations. This young woman in her twenties had had several small hemoptyses over the past couple of years and had noticed increasing shortness of breath on exertion. A posteroanterior roentgenogram (*A*) reveals several fairly sharply defined nodular opacities in both lungs (*arrows*). Note that the opacity in the right lower lobe (*arrowhead*) appears to possess an intimate relationship to vessels. A pulmonary angiogram during the arterial phase (*B*) reveals many more large arteriovenous communications than are evident on the standard roentgenogram. (Courtesy of Dr. George Genereux, University of Saskatchewan, Saskatoon, Canada.)

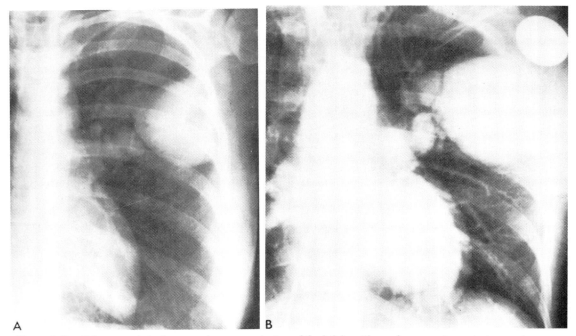

Figure 5–8. Pulmonary Arteriovenous Aneurysm. A view of the left hemithorax from a posteroanterior roentgenogram (*A*) reveals a large, sharply circumscribed, homogeneous opacity in the midlung zone. A broad, serpentine shadow extends from the medial aspect of the mass to the left hilum. A late venous phase of a pulmonary angiogram (*B*) shows uniform opacification of the large mass as well as the broad serpentine structure extending medially. Note the markedly delayed circulation time indicated by the fact that the arteriovenous malformation is uniformly opacified at a time when the right pulmonary veins, the left ventricle, and the aorta are already opacified. The patient is a 28-year-old woman with Osler-Weber-Rendu syndrome. (Courtesy of Dr. Harold Jacobson, Montefiore Hospital, The Bronx, New York.)

monstrable, the differential diagnosis is from any solitary pulmonary nodule.

Clinically, pulmonary arteriovenous fistulas usually are not recognized until the third or fourth decade of life, although approximately 10 per cent are identified in infancy or childhood.[35] They occur twice as frequently in females as in males. The incidence of symptoms varies. In addition to hemoptysis, which is the commonest presenting complaint, the only other common symptom referable to the lungs is dyspnea, which is present in 60 per cent of cases.[34] *Signs* suggestive of pulmonary arteriovenous fistula include cyanosis, finger clubbing, and a continuous murmur or bruit audible over the lesion(s). Telangiectasis in the skin or mucous membranes obviously is an important clue. Although the majority of patients with arteriovenous aneurysms have polycythemia, repeated hemorrhages from the nose or lungs may cause anemia.

Arterial blood gas analysis and cardiac catheterization may provide useful data in confirming the diagnosis: PO_2 and arterial oxygen saturation are decreased, cardiac output is increased, and the pulmonary artery pressure is normal. The electrocardiogram usually is normal, a useful sign in differentiation from congenital heart disease. Blood volume studies reveal increased red blood cell mass in many cases, with normal or near normal plasma volume.

For symptomatic patients for whom surgery is contraindicated for one reason or another, some success has been reported with the technique of transcatheter embolization of multiple pulmonary arteriovenous malformations, either with a nonabsorbable material such as Ivalon (polyvinyl alcohol) or silk[36] or with detachable silicone balloons.[37]

VARICOSITIES OF THE PULMONARY VEINS

This rare abnormality may be either congenital or acquired and consists of abnormal tortuosity and dilatation of a pulmonary vein just before its entrance into the left atrium.[38] It seldom gives rise to symptoms, but hemoptysis and some fatalities have been reported. In most cases the lesion is apparent as a round or oval homogeneous opacity of unit density, somewhat lobulated but well defined, in the medial third of either lung (Figure 5–9). On the left, the

lingular vein usually is affected, and, on the right, a branch of the inferior pulmonary vein in the region of the medial basal segment of the right lower lobe. At least five of the patients reported in the literature had pulmonary venous hypertension, and other associated congenital anomalies have been reported.[39]

Angiography usually is necessary to differentiate this abnormality from arteriovenous aneurysm. In cases of venous varicosity opacification is apparent in the venous phase only (Figure 5–9), whereas in arteriovenous fistula it occurs in the arterial phase also.

ANOMALIES OF THE HEART AND GREAT VESSELS RESULTING IN INCREASED OR DECREASED PULMONARY BLOOD FLOW

Anomalies that cause *increased flow* (considered in greater detail in Chapter 10) include atrial and ventricular septal defect, patent ductus arteriosus, aorticopulmonary window, and anomalous pulmonary venous drainage. Rarely, a congenital aneurysm of the aortic sinus of Valsalva will rupture into the right atrium, right ventricle, or pulmonary artery, immediately increasing pulmonary blood flow. The left-to-right shunt results in some degree of increased pulmonary blood flow.

By far the commonest cause of *decreased flow* is a congenital cardiac anomaly of the right ventricular outflow tract (isolated pulmonic stenosis, tetralogy of Fallot with pulmonary atresia, type IV persistent truncus arteriosus, and Ebstein's anomaly). The caliber of the pulmonary vessels generally reflects the severity of the flow decrease, the hila usually being diminutive and the peripheral vessels correspondingly small (except with valvular pulmonic stenosis, in which poststenotic dilatation may enlarge the main or left pulmonary artery).

Since decreased pulmonary circulation always increases bronchial collateral flow, the pulmonary vascular pattern throughout the lungs may be formed partly or wholly by a greatly hypertrophied bronchial arterial system. This extensive systemic arterial supply is particularly evident in tetralogy of Fallot and in type IV persistent truncus arteriosus. Although pulmonary arterial flow is negligible in these cases, the diminutive vascular markings throughout the lungs may represent the pulmonary arterial tree, being filled through systemic-pulmonary artery anastomoses.

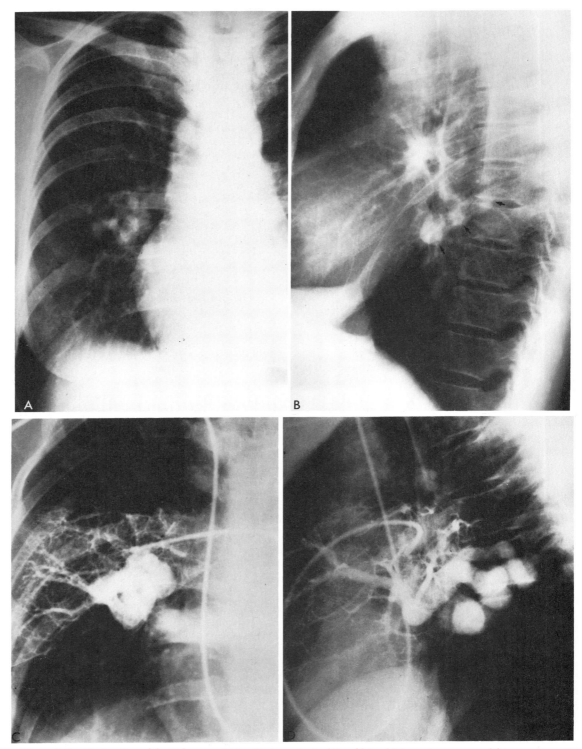

Figure 5–9. Varicosities of the Pulmonary Veins. Posteroanterior (*A*) and lateral (*B*) roentgenograms of this asymptomatic 39-year-old woman reveal a somewhat lobulated opacity projected in the plane of the right hilum and situated slightly posterior to it (*arrows* in *B*). The anterior segmental artery of the right upper lobe was selectively catheterized and contrast medium injected; during the venous phase of this injection (*C* and *D*), dense opacification of several spherical vascular spaces occurred, draining via large dilated veins into the left atrium. (Reprinted from Beamish, W. J.: Canad. Assoc. Radiol., 23:136, 1972, with permission of the author and editor.)

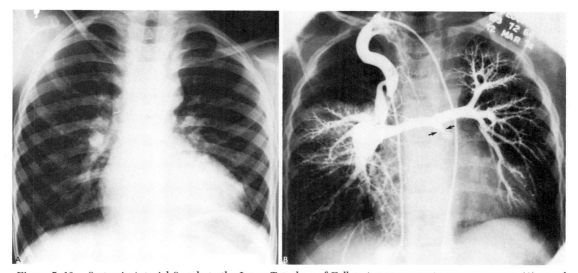

Figure 5–10.   Systemic Arterial Supply to the Lung: Tetralogy of Fallot. A posteroanterior roentgenogram (*A*) reveals an abnormal cardiac configuration, there being a prominent concavity of the left border of the heart in the region of the main pulmonary artery and a somewhat prominent ventricular mass. The hila are normal or slightly enlarged, and the pulmonary vasculature is generally within normal limits. Following selective injection of contrast medium into the right internal mammary artery (*B*), at least 80 per cent of the pulmonary arterial tree has been opacified via a large branch of this artery which joins the pulmonary artery in the right hilum. Note the diminutive main pulmonary artery (*arrows* in *B*). The patient is a six-year-old boy with pulmonary atresia and ventricular septal defect; his course was excellent following establishment of a conduit between the right ventrical and main pulmonary artery and closure of the VSD. (Courtesy of Dr. Kent Ellis, Columbia-Presbyterian Medical Center, New York.)

SYSTEMIC ARTERIAL SUPPLY TO THE LUNG

A portion of lung, which may be normal or dysplastic,[40] may be supplied by a systemic artery arising from the aorta or one of its branches. The commonest form of this anomaly is bronchopulmonary sequestration, but occasionally the bronchial tree and pulmonary arterial distribution to the portion of lung supplied by the systemic vessel are normal, findings incompatible with bronchopulmonary sequestration.[41] Most published examples of systemic arterial supply to the lung have been congenital, although some are acquired; in fact, the incidence of acquired systemic arterialization of the lung is unknown and probably is much higher than is commonly realized. We have seen several cases in which obliteration of the pleural space by fibrous tissue as a result of pleuritis has been accompanied by extension of systemic vessels from the chest wall across the pleura into contiguous lung parenchyma; such transgression probably occurs fairly frequently, especially if the underlying lung has been damaged by the infection (*e.g.,* in bronchiectasis).

In cases of anomalous arterial supply the systemic vessel may arise from the aorta, internal mammary arteries (Figure 5–10), bronchial arteries, intercostal arteries, or even from the celiac plexus. Within the lung, the anomalous vessel communicates with either pulmonary artery or vein with approximately equal frequency. Aortography is usually required for definitive diagnosis (Figure 5–10).

These patients may be asymptomatic or may suffer recurrent hemoptysis, and a murmur may be audible over the defect.

PULMONARY LYMPHANGIECTASIA

This almost invariably fatal abnormality usually becomes manifest at birth. As the name implies, the condition consists of dilatation of the pulmonary lymphatics; in its severest degree this reaches cystic proportions. Felman and his colleagues[42] proposed a classification of this abnormality based on the presence or absence of congenital cardiac malformations. In the first group, patients with a cardiac anomaly (approximately one-third of all cases), there appears to be a close association with obstructed pulmonary venous return: hemodynamic factors tend to keep pulmonary lymphatics dilated and probably play a major role in the pathogenesis of the lymphangiectasia. Group two comprises patients in whom the lymphangiectasia is not associated with cardiac anomalies (approximately two-thirds of all reported cases); the pathogenesis is clearly different. This form is thought to result from abnormal development of the lung between the fourteenth and twentieth weeks of gestation. During this phase the pulmonary lymphatics are large in relation to the remainder of the lung, whereas by the eighteenth and twentieth weeks of intrauterine life the lung's connective tissue elements normally diminish and the lymphatics become much narrower. It has been postulated that congenital lymphangiectasia represents a failure of the lymphatics to undergo regression while lung parenchyma continues to grow. This form of the disease is invariably fatal at an early age: of the ten patients in group two reported by Felman and his colleagues, seven died within 24 hours of birth, two survived for 1 month, and one lived for 2 months. In contrast to those patients who had associated cardiac anomalies, many of the group two patients had congenital abnormalities of other structures. The typical roentgenographic change in this group is marked prominence of septal markings in the form of Kerley A and B lines, simulating interstitial pulmonary edema.

CONGENITAL DEFICIENCY OF THE LEFT SIDE OF THE PARIETAL PERICARDIUM

This absence, which is readily recognizable on standard chest roentgenograms, may be complete or partial; a portion of heart herniates through the defect into the left hemithorax. Complete absence of the left side of the parietal pericardium is a benign condition quite compatible with a normal life span.

The roentgenologic features are as follows:[43] (1) a shift of the heart to the left; (2) an unusual cardiac silhouette, with an elongated left heart border and three convexities: the aortic knob, a long, prominent, sharply demarcated pulmonary artery segment, and a left ventricular segment; (3) a band of radiolucency between the aortic knob and the main pulmonary artery; and (4) a band of radiolucency between the left hemidiaphragm and the base of the heart caused by interposed air-containing lung. Symptoms include nonspecific anterior chest pain, often brought on by exercise or by lying on the left side, and mild shortness of breath on exertion. The apical impulse is in the left axilla and there is a sustained left ventricular thrust; patients almost invariably have systolic ejection murmurs of grade I to III/VI intensity.

REFERENCES

1a. Streeter, G. L.: Developmental horizons in human embryos: Description of age group XI, 13 to 20 somites, and age group XII, 21 to 29 somites. Contrib. Embryol. 30:211, 1942.

1b. Streeter, G. L.: Developmental horizons in human embryos: Description of age group XIII, embryos about 4 or 5 millimeters long, and age group XIV, period of indentation of the lens vesicle. Contrib. Embryol., 31:27, 1945.

1c. Streeter, G. L.: Developmental horizons in human embryos: Description of age groups XV, XVI, XVII, and XVIII. Contrib. Embryol., 32:133, 1948.

1d. Streeter, G. L.: Developmental horizons in human embryos. Description of age groups XIX, XX, XXI, XXII, and XXIII. Contrib. Embryol., 34:165, 1951.

2. Boyden, E. A.: Developmental anomalies of the lungs. Am. J. Surg., 89:79, 1955.

3. Spencer, H.: Pathology of the Lung (Excluding Pulmonary Tuberculosis), 2nd ed. Oxford, Pergamon, 1968.

4. Iwai, K., Shindo, G., Hajikano, H., Tajima, H., Morimoto, M., Kosuda, T., and Yoneuda, R.: Intralobular pulmonary sequestration, with special reference to developmental pathology. Am. Rev. Resp. Dis., 107:911, 1973.

5. Köhler, R.: Pulmonary sequestration. Acta Radiol. [Diagn.] (Stockholm), 8:337, 1969.

6. Ranniger, K. and Valvassori, G. E.: Angiographic diagnosis of intralobar pulmonary sequestration. Am. J. Roentgenol., 92:540, 1964.

7. Schachter, E. N., and Karpick, R. J.: Bronchopulmonary sequestration and pulmonary tuberculosis. Chest, 62:331, 1972.

8. Williams, A. O., and Enumah, F. I.: Extralobar pulmonary sequestration. Thorax, 23:200, 1968.

9. Gerle, R. D., Jaretzki, A., III, Ashley, C. A., and Berne, A. S.: Congenital bronchopulmonary-foregut malformation: Pulmonary sequestration communicating with the gastrointestinal tract. N. Engl. J. Med., 278:1413, 1968.

10. Kirwan, W. O., Walbaum, P. R., and McCormack, R. J. M.: Cystic intrathoracic derivatives of the foregut and their complications. Thorax, 28:424, 1973.

11. Baum, G. L., Racz, I., Bubis, J., Molho, M., and Shapiro, B. L.: Cystic disease of the lung. Report of eighty-eight cases, with an ethnologic relationship. Am. J. Med., 40:578, 1966.

12. Rogers, L. F., and Osmer, J. C.: Bronchogenic cyst: A review of 46 cases. Am. J. Roentgenol., 91:273, 1964.

13. Editorial: Bronchial cysts. Br. Med. J., 2:501, 1973.

14. Moncrieff, M. W., Cameron, A. H., Astley, R., Roberts, K. D., Abrams, L. D., and Mann, J. R.: Congenital cystic adenomatoid malformation of the lung. Thorax, 24:476, 1969.

15. Fasanelli, S., Bellussi, A., Patti, G. L., and Talamo, D.: Congenital cystic adenomatoid malformation. Unusual presentation. RAYS (Roma), 5:43, 1980.

16. Craig, J. M., Kirkpatrick, J., and Neuhauser, E. B. D.: Congenital cystic adenomatoid malformation of the lungs in infants. Am. J. Roentgenol., 76:516, 1956.

17. Tsuji, S., Heki, S., Kobara, Y., and Sato A.: The

syndrome of bronchial mucocele and regional hyperinflation of the lung: Report of four cases. Chest, *64*:444, 1973.

18. Reid, L.: The Pathology of Emphysema. London, Lloyd-Duke Medical Books Ltd., 1967.
19. Genereux, G. P.: Bronchial atresia: A rare cause of unilateral lung hypertranslucency. J. Can. Assoc. Radiol., *22*:71, 1971.
20. Cremin, B. J., and Movsowitz, H.: Lobar emphysema in infants. Br. J. Radiol., *44*:692, 1971.
21. Stovin, P. G. I.: Congenital lobar emphysema. Thorax, *14*:254, 1959.
22. Hislop, A., and Reid, L.: New pathological findings in emphysema of childhood. I. Polyalveolar lobe with emphysema. Thorax, *25*:682, 1970.
23. Roghair, G. D.: Nonoperative management of lobar emphysema: Long-term follow-up. Radiology, *102*:125, 1972.
24. Jue, K. L., Amplatz, K., Adams, P., Jr., and Anderson, R. C.: Anomalies of great vessels associated with lung hypoplasia: The scimitar syndrome. Am. J. Dis. Child., *111*:35, 1966.
25. Elliott, L. P., and Schiebler, G. L.: A roentgenologic-electrocardiographic approach to cyanotic forms of heart disease. Pediatr. Clin. North Am., *18*:1133, 1971.
26. Gathman, G. E., and Nadas, A. S.: Total anomalous pulmonary venous connection. Clinical and physiologic observations of 75 pediatric patients. Circulation, *42*:143, 1970.
27. Kleinman, P. K.: Pleural telangiectasia and absence of a pulmonary artery. Radiology, *132*:281, 1979.
28. Ellis, K., Seaman, W. B., Griffiths, S. P., Berdon, W. E., and Baker, D. H.: Some congenital anomalies of the pulmonary arteries. Semin. Roentgenol., *2*:325, 1967.
29. Gay, B. B., Jr., Franch, R. H., Shuford, W. H., and Rogers, J. V, Jr.: The roentgenologic features of single and multiple coarctations of the pulmonary artery and branches. Am. J. Roentgenol., *90*:599, 1963.
30. Baum, D., Khoury, G. H., Ongley, P. A., Swan, H. J. C., and Kincaid, O. W.: Congenital stenosis of the pulmonary artery branches. Circulation, *29*:680, 1964.
31. Berdon, W. E., and Baker, D. H.: Vascular anomalies and the infant lung: Rings, slings, and other things. Semin. Roentgenol., *7*:39, 1972.
32. Stone, D. N., Bein, M. E., and Garris, J. B.: Anomalous left pulmonary artery: Two new adult cases. Am. J. Roentgenol., *135*:1259, 1980.
33. Hodgson, C. H., Burchell, H. B.,, Good, C. A., and Clagett, O. T.: Hereditary hemorrhagic telangiectasia and pulmonary arteriovenous fistula: Survey of a large family. N. Engl. J. Med., *261*:625, 1959.
34. Moyer, J. H., Glantz, G., and Brest, A. N.: Pulmonary arteriovenous fistulas. Physiologic and clinical considerations. Am. J. Med., *32*:417, 1962.
35. Gomes, M. M. R., and Bernatz, P. E.: Arteriovenous fistulas: A review and ten-year experience at the Mayo Clinic. Mayo Clin. Proc., *45*:81, 1970.
36. Castaneda-Zuniga, W., Epstein, M., Zollikofer, C., Nath, P. H., Formanek, A., Ben-Shachar, G., and Amplatz, K.: Embolization of multiple pulmonary artery fistulas. Radiology, *134*:309, 1980.
37. Kaufman, S. L., Kumar, A. A. J., Roland, J.-M. A., Harrington, D. P., Barth, K. H., Haller, J. A., Jr., and White, R. I., Jr.: Transcatheter embolization in the management of congenital arteriovenous malformations. Radiology, *137*:21, 1980.
38. Ben-Menachem, Y., Kuroda, K., Kyger, E. R, III, Brest, A. N., Copeland, O. P., and Coan, J. D.: The various forms of pulmonary varices. Report of three new cases and review of the literature. Am. J. Roentgenol., *125*:881, 1975.
39. Papamichael, E., Ikkos, D., Alkalais, K., and Yannacopoulos, J.: Pulmonary varicosity associated with other congenital abnormalities. Chest, *62*:107, 1972.
40. Wagenvoort, C. A., Heath, D., and Edwards, J. E.: The Pathology of the Pulmonary Vasculature. Springfield, Ill., Charles C Thomas, 1964.
41. Kirks, D. R., Kane, P. E., Free, E. A., and Taybi, H.: Systemic arterial supply to normal basilar segments of the left lower lobe. Am. J. Roentgenol., *126*:817, 1976.
42. Felman, A. H., Rhatigan, R. M., and Pierson, K. K.: Pulmonary lymphangiectasia: Observation in 17 patients and proposed classification. Am. J. Roentgenol., *116*:548, 1972.
43. Morgan, J. R., Rogers, A. K., and Forker, A. D.: Congenital absence of the left pericardium. Clinical findings. Ann. Intern. Med., *74*:370, 1971.

6

Infectious Diseases of the Lungs

HOST DEFENSE MECHANISMS IN BRONCHOPULMONARY INFECTIONS

A basic understanding of the mechanisms by which the lungs prevent and deal with infection is an essential feature of the diagnostic process. Like the gastrointestinal tract but unlike other mammalian organs, the bronchopulmonary system is relatively accessible to the multifarious microbes of the environment. If contamination of the lower respiratory tract occurs, the invader is confronted by a formidable barrier in the epithelium lining the airways and air spaces and in the mucosecretions that contain specific immunoglobulins and antimicrobials. When this first line of defense fails, and the invader penetrates the tissues and establishes a foothold, there follows a highly complex, integrated sequence of events, termed the inflammatory response.

Although the essential steps in host defense are discussed individually, it must be remembered that success depends upon both phagocytic activity and the *interaction* of humoral and cell-mediated immunity. When these defense mechanisms break down, the host becomes compromised and prone to infection by ordinarily avirulent (opportunistic) microorganisms.

LOCAL DEFENSE MECHANISMS

NONSPECIFIC MECHANISMS

The bronchopulmonary tree is covered by a tightly knit epithelium that presents a first line of defense against invading microorganisms.[1] In its endeavors to prevent penetration by foreign substances, the epithelial barrier is aided by other highly integrated defense mechanisms—the mucociliary transport system and its biological constituents, the alveolar macrophages, and locally produced immunoglobulins.[2]

IMMUNE MECHANISMS

Immunoglobulin A (IgA), which constitutes only a relatively small fraction of the serum immunoglobulins (10 to 15 per cent), is the predominant species in secretions that bathe mucous membranes in communication with the external environment. The final molecule of IgA in the secretions is larger than that of serum IgA because of the addition of a secretory "piece" or "component" by bronchopulmonary epithelial cells.

SELECTIVE IgA DEFICIENCY

This condition is not uncommon: population surveys have recorded isolated IgA deficiency in one per 700 persons in Sweden, one per 500 in England, and one per 1000 in North America. Some individuals lacking IgA appear to be in the best of health, whereas others have recurrent sinopulmonary infections, gastrointestinal disorders, atopy, and autoimmune disease.[3] There is a familial incidence in IgA deficiency,[3] the mode of inheritance probably being an autosomal dominant trait.

Ammann and Hong,[4] who described 30 cases of selective IgA deficiency and reviewed reports of 175 others, found a high incidence of autoimmune disease, including rheumatoid arthritis, lupus erythematosus, pernicious anemia, thyroiditis, and pulmonary hemosiderosis. It has been established that secretory IgA has neutralizing activity against viruses, probably involving interplay with phagocytic systems and cellular mechanisms, as well as with nonimmune substances such as interferon.

It is not known why some persons lacking IgA escape infections and other diseases. It may be that other immunoglobulins (mainly IgM but also IgG) play a role in protection.

IMMUNOLOGIC DEFENSE MECHANISMS

The immune response in host defense results from the introduction into the body of material recognized as foreign; in the context of this chapter such antigens (immunogens) can be considered synonymous with microorganisms.

Since the immune response depends upon the establishment and differentiation of lymphoid tissue, it is pertinent to outline the steps in development of the lymphocyte, leading to the production of immunoglobulins (antibodies) and cell-mediated immunity. The precursor of lymphoid tissue is thought to be a bone-marrow stem cell that travels via the circulation to specific sites, where it differentiates into a cell capable of expressing cell-mediated immune responses or of secreting antibodies and immunoglobulins. In man, the microenvironment for the former type of differentiation is the thymus gland, the cells produced being designated thymus-dependent lymphocytes (T lymphocytes or T cells). The environment leading to the formation of antibody-producing cells (B lymphocytes or B cells) from the lymphoid precursor has not been identified in man. Morphologic, biophysical, and biochemical studies have revealed clear-cut differences that permit categorization of most lymphocytes as either T or B cells. T cells form cellular aggregates (rosettes) with sheep erythrocytes under appropriate experimental conditions. B cells, which have surface immunoglobulin receptors for aggregated IgG and complement components, form rosettes with heterologous erythrocytes coated with antibody and complement. These rosette-forming techniques can be used to enumerate peripheral T and B lymphocytes in vitro.

T LYMPHOCYTES AND CELL-MEDIATED IMMUNITY

T cells are found in blood, thoracic duct lymph, deep cortical areas and centrifugal portions of the follicular structure of lymph nodes, periarteriolar areas of the spleen, and diffusely in virtually all tissues to which lymphocytes have access.[5] About 60 to 85 per cent of thoracic duct and nodal lymphocytes and 30 to 50 per cent of splenic lymphocytes are derived from the thymus. Because of their long life and recirculation, these small lymphocytes are logical candidates for initial antigen recognition and memory retention. T cells somehow potentiate the processing of antigen by the monocyte-macrophage system (see further on) and the recruitment of other lymphocytes into the antigen-specific pathway of differentiation. This recruitment of other lymphocytes is thought to be brought about by transfer factor, one of the chemical mediators produced by T lymphocytes. Biologic activities detectable in supernatant fluids from T lymphocyte cultures include a skin-reactive factor, a lymphocyte-transforming (blastogenic) factor, a chemotactic factor for leukocytes and macrophages, a migration-inhibiting factor that localizes monocytes and macrophages at the inflammatory site, and interferon (a nonantigenic specific substance related to antiviral defense). In the presence of a specific antigen all these biologically active materials can be produced from T lymphocytes from a sensitized person. In addition, T lymphocytes, whether sensitized or not, respond to such nonspecific mitogens as phytohemagglutinin and concanavalin A, producing chemical mediators apparently identical to those produced by sensitized lymphocytes.

Differential leukocyte counts, delayed skin reactions, and in vitro assays for lymphocytic chemical mediators are used to evaluate cellular immunity. Loss of cell-mediated immunity may be evidenced by persistent lymphopenia (1200 per cu mm or less) or by a predominance of medium-sized and large lymphocytes but no small thymus-derived cells in peripheral blood smears.

A study of delayed hypersensitivity in a large hospitalized population[6] showed overall reactivity to one or more of the test antigens in 91 per cent of subjects given combinations of PPD, mumps, *Trichophyton*, and *Candida*, and a similar study in patients with Hodgkin's disease identified mumps antigen and DNCB as the most reliable skin tests to exclude anergy.[7] Blastogenesis of lymphocytes in culture can be measured by exposing the cells to a mitogen or allogenic antigen. This results in increased T cell DNA and RNA synthesis, which can be measured with thymidine incorporation. Some patients who do not evidence blastogenic response to a specific antigen respond to phyto-hemagglutinin. Cultured lymphocytes can be assayed for migration inhibition factor (MIF), using peritoneal macrophages.

A fundamental feature of the role of T lymphocytes in cell-mediated immunity is the recognition and processing of antigenic material. These cells appear to be endowed with "immunologic memory," an ability to react much faster and more vigorously to a second stimulus of the same antigen.

Pure deficiency of either cell-mediated or humoral immunity is relatively uncommon; in most cases, whatever its degree, impairment of immune response is mixed. Nevertheless, because of a preponderance of one or the other defect, individual patients can be expected to lack resistance to specific organisms; for example, a deficiency or loss of CMI increases the tendency to intracellular infection by viruses and fungi. The primary congenital and acquired immunodeficiency states are considered in Chapter 7 (*see* page 394). In the following section on the compromised host, particular attention is paid to patients rendered susceptible to infection because of secondary factors such as malignancy or immunotherapy.

HUMORAL IMMUNITY

In man, the B cells (thymus-independent lymphocytes) mature in the peripheral lymphocytic tissues and become plasma cells, the source of antibody or immunoglobulin production. They constitute a minority of the recirculating pool lymphocytes and seem to have a much shorter life span than T cells—probably of days to weeks rather than months to years.[5] B cells locate in the subcapsular and medullary areas and germinal centers of lymph nodes and in the spleen's peripheral white and red pulp. They play little part in cell-mediated immunity but are largely responsible for humoral antibody synthesis, being stimulated by antigen that has been processed by macrophages. A second signal, produced by interaction of nearby T lymphocytes with antigen, often is required to stimulate B cells to proliferate and transform into antibody-secreting cells. The humoral defense mechanism is assessed by determining serum immunoglobulins and antibody production in response to specific antigens. Patients lacking antibodies tend to have severe recurrent bacterial infections, particularly pneumonia caused by *Streptococcus pneumoniae*, *Str. pyogenes*, *Pseudomonas aeruginosa*, and

Haemophilus influenzae, but are not unduly susceptible to viral infections (except for viral hepatitis, which may be very severe).

INFLAMMATION AND PHAGOCYTOSIS

The passage of an invading microorganism across the threshold into the *milieu intérieur* of the host triggers a complex system of defense mechanisms, largely revolving around the phagocyte. Local reaction in the lung parenchyma depends on the type and virulence of the infecting microorganism and the immunologic status of the host. If the intruder is a stranger, the naive lymphocytes will muster a rather delayed, weak defense, in contrast to "experienced" lymphocytes facing a recognized enemy. For this reason some nonimmune mechanisms must act first at the site of inflammation. Since the major role in host defense is played by the body phagocytes, nonimmune chemotactic factors are extremely important. These are supplied (a) from the bacteria themselves, (b) from the properdin system, by which microorganisms can still produce chemotactic substances from complement when a specific antibody is absent, and (c) from Hageman factor activation, a concomitant of clotting that leads to the formation of two chemotactic agents, kallikrein and plasminogen activator.[8] Furthermore, an impressive group of plasma bactericidins plays a major role in primary defense even before the phagocytes arrive. These substances include lysozyme, properdin, complement, and natural inhibitors of enzymes.

PHAGOCYTOSIS

Phagocytes can be divided into two types, circulating and fixed. The latter constitute the reticuloendothelial system and include splenic macrophages, alveolar macrophages, Kupffer cells, lymph node macrophages, and microglial cells of the brain. The circulating cells include polymorphonuclear leukocyte neutrophils, eosinophils, basophils, and monocytes. All these cells help to combat infection in the presence of bacteremia. However, our primary concern in microbial invasion of the lungs is with the neutrophilic polymorphonuclear leukocytes and mononuclear phagocytes, *i.e.*, blood monocytes and tissue macrophages.

DEVELOPMENT OF PHAGOCYTES. Neutrophils and macrophages, like the lymphoid B cells and T cells, originate from stem cells in the bone

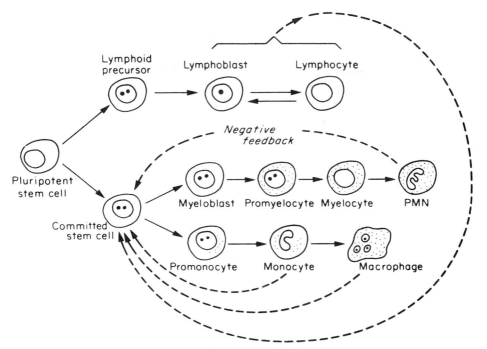

Figure 6–1.   Tentative Scheme of Humoral Regulation of Granulopoiesis. *Arrows* from the monocyte, macrophage, and lymphocyte undergoing blastogenesis indicate stimulation (positive feedback) of the committed stem cell via colony-stimulating activity. *Arrow* from the mature granulocyte (*PMN*) represents negative feedback or inhibition of granulopoiesis at the stem-cell level. (Reprinted from Golde, D. W., and Cline, M. J.: N. Engl. J. Med., *291*:1388, 1974, with permission of the authors and editor.)

marrow. It is believed that erythrocytes, megakaryocytes, granulocytes, and monocyte-macrophages originate from a stem cell with multiple potentialities for differentiation (pluripotent). From this pluripotent stem cell, unipotent stem cells develop that are committed to differentiate along only one pathway (Figure 6–1).[9]

REGULATION OF PHAGOCYTE PRODUCTION. Blood-borne monocytes are believed to be the precursor cells for all macrophagocytic components of the far-flung reticuloendothelial system. Feedback mechanisms that both stimulate and inhibit production from unipotent stem cells have been described. A negative feedback system, like that produced by the action of corticosteroids on the pituitary gland, is thought to result from the action of "hormones" produced by mature neutrophils, reversibly inhibiting cell proliferation (Figure 6–1).[10]

MIGRATION OF PHAGOCYTES. Phagocytes migrate to the site of bacterial invasion in response to (a) substances elaborated by certain bacteria, (b) antigen-antibody complement activation, (c) properdin acting on complement, (d) a factor elaborated from neutrophils themselves, and (e) lymphokines produced by sen-

sitized lymphocytes. Inhibitors also may play a role in phagocytic migration; for example, the MIF of lymphocytes and the neutrophil immobilizing factor[11] aid in defense by preventing the egress of phagocytes that have arrived at the inflammatory site.

RECOGNITION BY PHAGOCYTES. Phagocytes must recognize what to attack. Although little is known about this phase of phagocytosis, it is clear that opsonization of the foreign antigen induces more rapid ingestion. Opsonic activity of serum has both a heat-stable and a heat-labile component. The heat-stable component is due to an IgG antibody and is present in considerable quantity in hyperimmunized subjects; the heat-labile component can be attributed entirely to complement proteins. Many microorganisms, particularly the encapsulated ones, resist ingestion by phagocytes, a characteristic that contributes to their pathogenicity. Particles that have interacted with fresh serum or are coated with enough specific antibody are ingested avidly by phagocytes.

INGESTION BY PHAGOCYTES. Engulfment of the recognized particle is accomplished by extension of pseudopodia that surround the organism and encase it within the phagocytic vesicle or phagosome.

DEGRANULATION OF PHAGOCYTES. Within seconds of engulfment of a microorganism, cytoplasmic organelles (granules) fuse with the phagosome's membranes. These granules contain enzymes that enter the phagosome and to some extent escape into the extracellular space. The cytoplasm of mature human neutrophils contains two types of membrane-bounded granules: (1) *primary granules*, which originate on the proximal face of the Golgi complex in the myelocytic stage of granulocytic development; they contain acid phosphatase, other acid hydrolases, myeloperoxidase, sulfated mucopolysaccharide, and other components; and (2) *secondary granules*, which form on the distal face of the Golgi complex and appear later in the development of the neutrophil; they contain alkaline phosphatase, lactoferrin, and most of the neutrophil's lysozyme. A classic example of a disorder of degranulation is Chédiak-Higashi disease, a hereditary disorder in which giant primary granules fail to fuse with phagosomes (*see* further on).

KILLING BY PHAGOCYTES. When enclosed within the confines of the phagosome or free in extracellular space, microorganisms are usually killed, and in part degraded, by enzymes liberated from primary and secondary granules. In mammalian phagocytes, recognition of the invader results in increased metabolic activity, reflected in an oxygen consumption rate 15 to 20 times that of nonphagocytic cells.[9] This metabolic reaction is accompanied by substantial increases in hydrogen peroxide (H_2O_2) production and in glucose oxidation via the hexosemonophosphate shunt. H_2O_2 itself is microbicidal, a property greatly potentiated by myeloperoxidase in the presence of a halide cofactor such as chloride or iodide ions. The numerous other substances elaborated by human neutrophils that have microbicidal properties include lysozyme, hydrolytic enzymes, lactoferrin, and cationic proteins.

DISORDERS OF PHAGOCYTOSIS

There is considerable overlapping in control of the aforementioned steps that lead to engulfment and death of the microorganism. For this reason, defects in phagocytic function usually reflect more than one deficiency.

With few exceptions, neutropenia alone does not compromise the host; when it is accompanied by impairment of monocyte and macrophage function, however, susceptibility to infection may be greatly enhanced. The accepted figure for neutropenia is ≤ 1500 cells per cu mm. Neutropenia may have serious clinical consequences even when the macrophage system is functional in cases of infection caused by virulent organisms or when it is a manifestation of hypersplenism. When neutropenia is accompanied by a sparsity of mononuclear phagocytes—as in bone-marrow failure and in drug-induced "agranulocytosis," in which all phagocytes are depressed—infectious complications may be severe, and its development in cases of agammaglobulinemia or autoimmune disease compounds the susceptibility to infection.[12]

Phagocytes may migrate abnormally; and sometimes, despite normal random migration, unidirectional cell movement in response to chemical stimulation (chemotaxis) is defective. Normal chemotaxis implies not only the production of appropriate chemical mediators but also cellular response; its impairment often is associated with disturbed phagocytic and bactericidal function, as well as with immunoglobulin deficiency and lack of complement. Although immunoglobulins are required for activity of the classic complement pathway and acceleration of the alternate pathway, studies in some patients with agammaglobulinemia have shown normal chemotaxis, probably reflecting the action of nonspecific proteases and the properdin system on complement components C3 and C5.

Lack of cellular response to chemotactic substances has been noted in patients with Chédiak-Higashi syndrome, myeloproliferative disorders, and diabetes mellitus. Polymorphonuclear leukocytes from patients with such diverse diseases as rheumatoid arthritis, hepatic cirrhosis, and multiple myeloma react abnormally to chemotactic stimulation.

Once attracted to the site of invasion the phagocyte is faced with antigen recognition and ingestion, phases in the process of phagocytosis that basically involve opsonization. Like chemotaxis, this activity requires immunoglobulins, complement components, and properdin. In humoral immunodeficiency with absence of the classic complement system, the properdin system can activate C3 and opsonize microorganisms, although the classic complement system cannot compensate similarly for deficiencies of the properdin pathway. In many patients with sickle-cell anemia and in some neonates the serum is deficient in heat-labile opsonins but has essentially normal classic complement function. This abnormality in the properdin system markedly increases susceptibility to infection, particularly with virulent encapsulated bacteria such as *Str. pneumoniae, Pseudomonas,* streptococci, or *H. influenzae.*

Phagocytic microbicidal activity is rendered defective by disordered degranulation or lack of H_2O_2 production. The former may result from deficiency of either primary or secondary granules or from the granules' inability to secrete their contents into the phagosome. Deficiencies of myeloperoxidase may be inherited or acquired.

Chédiak-Higashi Syndrome

This rare hereditary disorder is characterized by deficient secretion of myeloperoxidase from abnormally large lysosomes. The disease is transmitted as an autosomal recessive trait; a high incidence of consanguinity in affected families has been reported. The neutrophils, monocytes, and lymphocytes contain abnormal cytoplasmic inclusion bodies of deeply staining basophilic appearance, of fairly uniform size, with a fine granular structure similar to that of normal smaller granules except for striations in some instances. The characteristic finding of neutropenia probably reflects intramedullary destruction of granulocytes. Although initial bactericidal activity is compromised, intracellular killing eventually occurs, presumably because of compensatory increased production of hydrogen peroxide.

Few patients with Chédiak-Higashi syndrome survive beyond the age of 10 years,

death in most cases being caused by pneumonia and septicemia. The characteristic clinical features include photophobia, retinal albinism, horizontal nystagmus, recurrent infections, fever, and, terminally, splenomegaly and sometimes hepatomegaly.

Chronic Granulomatous Disease of Childhood

This is the commonest phagocytic deficiency syndrome involving the microbicidal phase. There appear to be two forms. In one, transmission is X-linked and the female carrier is asymptomatic. The other form, which develops in boys or girls with apparently unaffected parents, is inherited as an autosomal recessive trait.

All the microbial species that infect patients with this defect produce catalase; they include *Staphylococcus aureus, Staph. epidermidis,* gram-negative bacteria such as *Klebsiella pneumoniae, Escherichia coli, Serratia marcescens,* and *Proteus* or *Salmonella* species, and fungal infections. The underlying enzyme defect is not known.

The pathologic reaction to infection is usually granulomatous. The cellular response consists of lymphocytes, macrophages, and plasma cells; giant cells are rare. The granulomatous response is thought to be caused by the persistence of intracellular bacteria in mononuclear cells, which in tissue have a life span of weeks, as opposed to polymorphonuclear leukocytes,

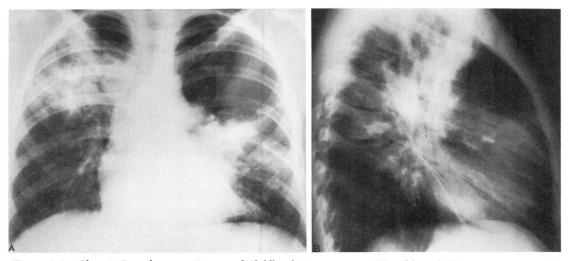

Figure 6–2. Chronic Granulomatous Disease of Childhood. Posteroanterior (*A*) and lateral (*B*) roentgenograms of this young white male reveal extensive patchy consolidation of the right upper lobe and the superior segment of the left lower lobe. At least one cavity is visible in the right upper lobe. Right paratracheal and left hilar lymph node enlargement are present. Culture of the sputum produced a heavy growth of *Staphylococcus aureus.* The nitroblue terazolium test was positive. (Courtesy of Dr. Alex Margulis, University of California, San Francisco.)

which live only hours. In the lung, in addition to local granulomas there may be extensive fibrous thickening of alveolar walls and dense infiltration by lymphocytes and plasma cells. Pigmented lipid histiocytes may be present, frequently in large numbers. Abscesses may occur in the lung, liver, bone, gastrointestinal tract, and elsewhere.

Chronic granulomatous disease (CGD) is usually fatal, death generally resulting from extensive lung involvement but in some cases from liver disease. However, some patients now survive into adulthood.

The roentgenographic hallmark of CGD in children is recurrent pneumonia that typically resolves incompletely or progresses to abscess formation; hilar lymph node enlargement is usually striking (Figure 6–2).

Most patients with CGD have recurrent infections, although some have minimal problems. Hepatosplenomegaly and a seborrheic rash over the postauricular, periorbital, nasal, scalp, axillary, and inguinal areas are common. Suspicion should be aroused whenever a patient, particularly a young male, manifests repeated staphylococcal or gram-negative infections that slowly resolve with antibiotic therapy despite normal or raised immunoglobulins. The diagnosis can be confirmed by the nitroblue tetrazolium (NBT) test. In CGD of the X-linked type, NBT reduction occurs in approximately 50 per cent of neutrophils of female carriers but in only about 5 per cent of neutrophils from homozygous males.

Although disorders of phagocytosis are relatively rare causes of recurrent pneumonia, they should not be overlooked, particularly in patients with no underlying disease that might depress host defenses, and when humoral and cell-mediated immunity are normal. Since the condition of seriously ill patients with abnormal phagocytes may be improved by neutrophil transfusions, recognition of phagocytic defects is important.

THE COMPROMISED HOST

The term "compromised host" describes the person whose defense mechanisms are impaired, rendering him or her more susceptible to infection. Although great emphasis has been placed on defects in the immune response in the pathogenesis of host compromise, defenses may be jeopardized by other factors of equal importance (Table 6–1). The most dramatic examples of increased susceptibility to infection

TABLE 6–1. FACTORS THAT COMPROMISE HOST DEFENSE MECHANISMS*

BASIC DISEASES
  Hodgkin's disease
  Other lymphomas and leukemias
  Multiple myeloma
  Carcinomas and sarcomas
  Inherited and acquired primary immuno-
    deficiency diseases

SUPERIMPOSED CONDITIONS
  Altered physical barriers:
    indwelling intravenous and urethral cath-
      eters
    gastrointestinal mucosal toxicity
    nebulizers with intermittent positive pres-
      sure breathing apparatus
    local mechanical disruption of tissues, mem-
      branes, and blood vessels by tumor
      growth and necrosis
  Altered indigenous microbial flora:
    broad-spectrum antibiotic therapy
  Leukopenia:
    immunosuppressives
    cytotoxic chemotherapy
    irradiation
  Altered leukocyte response:
    decreased migration
    diminished phagocytosis
    decreased bactericidal capacity
  Impaired T and/or B cell–mediated immunity:
    corticosteroid therapy
    cytotoxic chemotherapy
    irradiation
    antilymphocyte globulin

*Reprinted from Bode, F. R., Paré, J. A. P., and Fraser, R. G.: Medicine, 53:255, 1974, with permission of the authors and editor.

occur in patients with primary immunodeficiencies; these may be congenital or acquired and in either case are commonest in children; they represent basic defects in humoral or cell-mediated immunity (or both), in contrast to states in which increased susceptibility is secondary to disease. The primary immunodeficiencies are considered in Chapter 7. Here, we are concerned with diseases that interfere with the body's defenses against infection, and also the significant effect of therapy on protective mechanisms. The next section, concerning the commonest types of opportunistic infections, shows how different diseases have a propensity for certain specific infections.

Reduced defense against infection is most often, but not invariably, irreversible. Some patients, despite careful documentation of humoral or cellular deficiency, do not manifest the expected proneness to infection. Defects, particularly in cell mediated immunity, are transient in some diseases, including rubella, rubeola (measles), infectious mononucleosis, and sarcoidosis. Corticosteroids depress defense function in various ways. Resistance may improve after reduction of immunosuppressive or prednisone therapy in patients with kidney transplants, and the number of granulocytes may increase during remissions of acute leukemia. More often, however, the inability to respond is a consequence of an irreversible progression of primary disease, and there is little hope of improving resistance by eliminating the factor causing susceptibility. In these circumstances it is nevertheless important to determine the etiology of the infections, or at least to know which microorganisms are most likely to be responsible in specific diseases. In treating the growing numbers of patients with malignancies or with renal, hepatic, or respiratory failure, autoimmune disease or organ transplantation, the physician faces a dilemma: with too little therapy the patient may succumb to his or her biologic illness; with too much therapy a new constellation of apparently unrelated but equally ominous pathologic processes may arise. These complications of therapy range all the way from bleeding tendencies to diffuse pulmonary fibrosis caused by drug toxicity, but most often the new problem is infection, usually in the lung and of uncertain etiology.

The patient who is recognized as being compromised because of some underlying disease either shows clinical deterioration or, perhaps just as often, manifests a new abnormality on a chest roentgenogram. Although there might seem little reason for alarm at this stage, experience has shown that this phase usually presages rapid deterioration in the patient's condition within days. Fever may be absent in some cases, probably because of suppression by corticosteroids. If fever is present it may just as readily be ascribed to an exacerbation of the underlying disease as to a superimposed infection. Discussing infections in neoplastic diseases, Armstrong and associates[14] state that, in chronic lymphatic leukemia and multiple myeloma, fever nearly always indicates infection, whereas in 30 to 50 per cent of cases of acute leukemia, Hodgkin's disease, and other lymphomas, fever is not caused by infection. Pyrexia is more likely to be a symptom of infection if the neoplastic disease is severe or of long duration; in patients with renal transplantation, it is equally likely to reflect rejection. Careful analysis of chest roentgenograms is extremely important at this stage, since recognized patterns of progression of underlying diseases are often distinguishable from complicating infection. In a minority of instances a drug reaction involving lung tissue must be considered in the differential diagnosis.

A history of repeated infections, particularly in young people with primary immunodeficiencies, is often the major clue to defective host defenses. Since the inflammatory reaction and granulocytic response are reduced in such patients, the clinical findings may be atypical; e.g., there may be little tenderness, "abscesses" may be unusually soft, and erythema of the skin may be absent. Perirectal abscesses in particular should be sought.

It is much more difficult to diagnose fungal than bacterial infections, chiefly because certain fungi, particularly *Aspergillus* and *Candida*, frequently colonize the oropharynx, especially in patients receiving antibiotics. Growth of a fungus in culture does not necessarily indicate that the developing pneumonia is mycotic, but repeated cultures showing heavy growth of a specific fungus increase the likelihood of its pathogenicity. Perhaps just as frequently sputum cultures are negative in mycotic infections, and other methods of obtaining infected material should be carried out, such as transbronchial biopsy or transthoracic needle aspiration. As in all patients with pneumonia, sputum samples should be smeared and stained; the predominant microorganisms and clinical presentation should dictate the choice of antibiotic to be given until culture results are known. Although tuberculosis is not a common infection in the compromised host, sputum or needle aspirate should be stained for acid-fast organisms.

A differential leukocyte count to determine numbers and morphology of granulocytes, monocytes, and lymphocytes is of fundamental importance in screening for host defense impairment.

In selected cases (for example, young people with recurrent infections), phagocytic activity should be investigated more thoroughly. *In vitro* tests for lymphocyte chemical mediators (blastogenesis, MIF, chemotactic factor, and T lymphocyte rosette formation) should be done in cases of negative delayed skin sensitivity to multiple antigens. The quantity of gamma globulin can be established by electrophoresis, and selective immunoglobulin deficiencies (such as lack of secretory IgA) can be identified by serum assay. In rare instances it may be necessary to determine serum complement and properdin. Other laboratory tests indicated in patients with repeated infections are those that measure organ function, particularly of the liver, kidneys, pancreas, lung, and endocrine glands.

OPPORTUNISTIC INFECTIONS

Microorganisms that take advantage of reduced host defense mechanisms are referred to as opportunistic. They may be traditional pathogens, but much more often are those ordinarily considered nonpathogenic. Many of these ubiquitous, saprophytic, usually nonvirulent commensals are resistant to antibiotics. Although most individuals can live in symbiotic relationship with these organisms, the compromised host is rendered susceptible by one or more of three mechanisms: (1) altered host resistance caused by the basic disease; (2) altered host resistance on account of therapy; and (3) increased inocula of organisms as a result of therapy and the hospital environment. We shall first consider the commoner organisms that demonstrate opportunism and then outline the causes of impaired host defense in specific diseases (untreated and under treatment) and the organisms to which they are unduly susceptible.

ETIOLOGY

Innumerable microorganisms have been reported to cause infections in compromised hosts. Bacterial infections are commonest, closely followed by fungal disease; viral infection and parasitic infestations are much less common.

Bacteria

Pneumonias caused by gram-positive cocci are relatively rare in the compromised host, compared to those of gram-negative etiology. *Staph. aureus*, although still the commonest, is seen less often than formerly. Armstrong and associates[14] found gram-positive bacteremia in patients with lymphoma and leukemia more commonly caused by *Str. pneumoniae* than by staphylococci; the major susceptibility factor appeared to be leukopenia and the prognosis was very poor. Streptococcal infections are rare and may be due to the less pathogenic Lancefield groups B, C, and G.[14]

Most gram-negative infections are acquired while the patient is in the hospital. Although many of these pathogens are lactose fermenting Enterobacteriaceae (*E. coli*, *Klebsiella-Enterobacter-Serratia* group, *Proteus*, and *Acinetobacter*), there is a considerable incidence of nonfermenting organisms, including *Pseudomonas* species (especially *Ps. aeruginosa*), *Mima* and *Herellea*, *Pasteurella multocida*, and *Achromobacter*.

In many cases of hospital-acquired pneumonia caused by gram-negative bacilli the infection is spread from the oropharynx during assisted ventilation or the use of suction equipment, in patients receiving ill-advised prophylactic antibiotics, and in those rendered susceptible by corticosteroid, antimetabolite, or immunosuppressive therapy for neoplastic or autoimmune disease.

In view of the special cultural requirements of anaerobic organisms and the blind use of antibiotic therapy in many of these cases, most such infections undoubtedly go unrecognized and their incidence is grossly underestimated.

Of the higher bacteria, *Nocardia asteroides* causes disseminated infections, particularly in patients with leukemia or lymphoma who are receiving corticosteroids. This organism can occur in the sputum as a saprophyte, and special techniques are required for its culture. Dissemination, usually from the lungs, involves kidneys, subcutaneous tissues, and occasionally the brain.[14]

Fungi

The primary mycotic infections of the lung—histoplasmosis, coccidioidomycosis, and blastomycosis—are rare in compromised hosts. The opportunistic fungi—*Candida*, *Aspergillus*, *Cryptococcus*, and the *Phycomycetes*—are a frequent cause of infection, particularly in patients who have been treated for *Ps. aeruginosa* infection.

Viruses

There is little evidence that viral infections represent a serious threat to the compromised host. As with anaerobic bacterial infections, cultures are not routinely done and a search for viral antibodies usually is overlooked. It is therefore conceivable that viruses may play a larger role than is suggested by present data, in morbidity if not mortality.

Cytomegalovirus infection is common in acute leukemia[14] and immunosuppressed states, and often is found in association with *Pneumocystis carinii* and fungal infections. Inclusion bodies up to 17 μ in diameter may be seen in the nuclei of alveolar lining cells that are greatly enlarged (up to 40 μ in diameter). Viruria is common in asymptomatic carriers;[14] in one study of patients receiving immunosuppressive therapy for organ transplantation,[15] viruria was demonstrated in 65 per cent of patients, although CMV inclusions were present in only one of 51 kidneys at necropsy. Since 60 to 80 per cent of healthy adults have complement-fixing antibodies to CMV, this finding is not useful in diagnosing infection by this virus.

The incidence of varicella-zoster among recipients of renal transplant and patients over the age of 50 years with hematologic neoplasms is not commoner than in noncompromised persons, but morbidity is greater in immunosuppressed patients in whom the disease is more severe and progressive. Patients with defective defenses also appear less able to contain infection caused by herpes simplex, vaccinia, and measles: smallpox vaccination may progress to vaccinia gangrenosa, and measles may result in giant cell pneumonia without a rash.

Parasites

The opportunistic parasites most often encountered are the protozoa *Pneumocystis carinii* and *Toxoplasma gondii. Pneumocystis carinii* pneumonia occurs in patients with organ transplants, in immunosuppressed patients with malignant disease, and in infants, particularly the premature and those with gamma globulin deficiency.

All immunosuppressed patients are at risk from toxoplasmosis, and patients with Hodgkin's disease are particularly susceptible.[14] Increased antibody titers to this organism aid in diagnosis. With the exception of *Strongyloides*, helminths have not been recognized as opportunists. *Strongyloides stercoralis*, which usually involves only the mucosa of the small intestine, may become disseminated, leading to blood-borne pulmonary infection.

HOST-ETIOLOGY RELATIONS IN THE COMPROMISED HOST

Individual defects in host defense mechanisms confer susceptibility to specific organisms. This helps to narrow the diagnostic possibilities, and when the offending invader cannot be identified it provides a rationale for empiric therapy.

NEOPLASTIC DISEASE

Patients with neoplasia, particularly lymphoreticular and hematologic, are prone to opportunistic infections, a propensity that has recently been well reviewed.[16] This susceptibility derives from several factors, including the stage of the disease, derangement of granulopoiesis

through invasion of the bone marrow, and the effects of therapeutic agents such as corticosteroids, cytotoxic and immunosuppressive drugs, and antibiotics.

Hodgkin's Disease and Other Lymphomas

In the early stages, lymphoma patients are probably not abnormally susceptible to infection; as the disease progresses, cell-mediated immunity deteriorates and susceptibility to intracellular invasion by fungi, parasites, and viruses increases. In the later stages, when therapy is intensive, bacterial infections also are common, most often caused by hemolytic *Staph. aureus, Ps. aeruginosa,* and *E. coli.*[14] Patients with Hodgkin's disease appear to be particularly susceptible to infection with *Cryptococcus neoformans*[14] and to a lesser extent to other fungal infections.

Leukemia

Patients with *chronic leukemia* who are under treatment have both humoral and cell-mediated immune deficiencies, making them susceptible to a great variety of opportunistic organisms. In such patients, roentgenologically apparent pulmonary parenchymal disease, with or without fever, is almost certainly due to superimposed infection, since leukemic involvement of the lungs is rarely demonstrable. Patients with *acute leukemia* may be susceptible to bacterial infections as a result of agranulocytosis, but their humoral and cell-mediated immunity apparently remain intact until cytotoxic chemotherapy is instituted. Bacterial infections are common,[14, 17] usually by the spread of gram-negative organisms from the oropharynx and often after administration of absorbable or oral nonabsorbable antibiotics.[17] Fungal infections also are common in leukemia, particularly candidiasis and phycomycosis. The diagnosis usually is evidenced by continuing fever despite antibiotic therapy for assumed or proved gram-negative pneumonia.

Multiple Myeloma

This unrestrained clonal proliferation of plasma cells (plasma cell neoplasm) inevitably impairs humoral immunity. Since most patients with this disease have normal cell-mediated immunity, their antibody deficiency renders them prone to infection from encapsulated bacterial pathogens.

Other Neoplasms

In the later stages of their disease, patients with carcinoma or other nonlymphoreticular malignancies become compromised hosts, perhaps largely because of cytotoxic and steroid therapy.[14]

POST-TRANSPLANT PNEUMONIA

Recipients of organ transplants are particularly vulnerable to infection. Factors increasing risk of infection in these patients include granulocytopenia, corticosteroids and other immunosuppressive drugs that impair T cell and B cell functions, hyperglycemia caused by very high doses of steroids, and renal failure.

In many cases of post-transplant pneumonia the exact etiology is in doubt, particularly in patients who survive; certainly, survival appears to correlate as well with an immediate drastic reduction in immunosuppressive therapy as with administration of specific antimicrobial therapy. Concomitant bacterial, viral, parasitic, and fungal infections are so common that recovery often is ascribed more logically to improvement in host defenses than to such therapy.

In cases with an established diagnosis of *Pneumocystis carinii* pneumonia (based on recovery of the organisms, most often by invasive biopsy), good response is usually obtained to therapy. Systemic fungal infections, particularly candidiasis and aspergillosis, are fairly common after renal transplantation. The latter may be susceptible to therapy with amphotericin B, although most patients die despite therapy. Patients who receive bone marrow transplantation are particularly susceptible to *C. tropicalis*.[18]

OTHER COMPROMISED HOSTS

Several other disorders are known to increase susceptibility to opportunistic infection. Patients with diabetes mellitus and those with renal failure have defective phagocytic function, perhaps largely because of acidosis. Depression of the host defenses in liver disease is engendered by reduction in the circulating T lymphocytes and in respiratory failure by hypoxemia, acidosis, and defective mucociliary transport; in the latter condition, tracheostomy and inhalation therapy enhance the possibility of rapid colonization by opportunistic organisms. Sickle-cell anemia is characterized by increased susceptibility to bacterial, particularly pneumococcal, infections.

PNEUMONIA

GENERAL CONSIDERATIONS

Infection of the lung parenchyma is called pneumonia or pneumonitis. Pneumonia can be divided into three pathogenetic types, each with different morphologic and roentgenologic characteristics that usually permit their differentiation. (1) Some organisms—notably *Str. pneumoniae*—reach the peripheral air spaces of the lung, where they incite inflammatory edema which spreads centrifugally from unit to unit through communicating channels (the pores of Kohn and canals of Lambert). This is designated air-space or alveolar pneumonia (the term "lobar pneumonia," although in common use, is not recommended: only seldom are these pneumonias lobar in extent, and the term gives little indication of the pathogenesis of parenchymal consolidation). (2) Other organisms—for example, *Staph. aureus*—initiate an inflammatory response in the conducting airways of the lung and surrounding parenchyma; this type of pneumonia is designated bronchopneumonia or lobular pneumonia. (3) The viral organisms and *Mycoplasma* tend to affect the interstitial tissues predominantly, producing a pattern that is designated interstitial pneumonia or pneumonitis. Although it is not always possible to fit an individual case into one of these categories, recognition of these patterns is of obvious importance for the prompt institution of specific therapy.

The clinical diagnosis of pneumonia often is suggested by cough, expectoration, chills and fever, and particularly pleural pain. In many cases physical signs indicate the location of the disease, although signs may be absent or limited to fine rales and decreased breath sounds.

In a significant percentage of patients the organism or organisms responsible for the pneumonia are not detectable. Sometimes the reason for this is obvious; for example, before admission to the hospital the patient may have received antibiotics without prior bacteriologic study. Since healthy subjects may harbor pathogenic bacteria in their upper respiratory tracts, isolation of specific pathogens does not *necessarily* indicate the etiology of parenchymal disease, and such bacteriologic findings must be interpreted in the light of clinical features and roentgenographic patterns. Repeated heavy growth of the same organism on culture of purulent expectorated material obviously strengthens the likelihood of that organism being etiologically responsible for the disease, and culture of the same organism from both blood and sputum provides convincing evidence of this.

Failure to isolate a bacterial pathogen from the sputum of patients with pneumonia usually leads to a diagnosis of viral pneumonia which may be confirmed by subsequent isolation of the organism or by a rise in titer of an antibody to a specific virus during the convalescent period. A significant percentage of pneumonias in which aerobic cultures fail to show an accepted pathogen are due to anaerobic infections of the lung and pleural space; this type of infection should be suspected when the history suggests oropharyngeal aspiration and roentgenography demonstrates cavitation.

In many cases, bacterial pneumonia may follow a viral infection. Circumstantial evidence for the development of staphylococcal pneumonia after influenza is overwhelming, and for the development of bronchopneumonia from various organisms after measles.

The majority of pneumonias develop through inhalation or aspiration of the causative organism, and some result from direct infection of the bloodstream from a primary site elsewhere. Gram-positive and more often gram-negative bacterial septicemia may cause severe congestion, edema, hemorrhage, and thrombosis of the pulmonary capillaries, the clinical and roentgenologic picture simulating diffuse pulmonary edema. Since systemic hypotension commonly accompanies this form of infection, the pulmonary involvement has been termed "shock lung" or adult respiratory distress syndrome (ARDS).

Empyema as a complication of pneumonia is much less frequent since the advent of antibiotics. It occurs most commonly in association with pneumonia caused by *Staph. aureus* and only rarely when the causative organism is *Str. pneumoniae*.

A useful approach to the patient with pneumonia is to divide the infections into those that are community (nonhospital)-acquired and those that develop in inpatients (nosocomial).

COMMUNITY-ACQUIRED PNEUMONIA

Pneumonias acquired outside hospitals frequently occur in otherwise healthy persons and usually are caused by viruses, *Str. pneumoniae*, or *Mycoplasma pneumoniae*. Most patients admitted to the hosptial with clinical and roentgenologic evidence of pneumonia already have received antibiotics, virtually eliminating the possibility of finding *Str. pneumoniae* in the sputum.

Of the 292 seriously ill patients with acute pneumonia studied by Sullivan and associates,[20] a specific bacterial etiology was established in 167 (57 per cent); *Str. pneumoniae* was the commonest organism (62 per cent), followed by gram-negative bacilli (20 per cent) and *Staph. aureus* (10 per cent). Four-fifths of the patients had associated diseases. In this group of primary community-acquired pneumonias the mortality was 24 per cent, including 19 per cent of those with pneumococcal pneumonia (32 per cent of those with bacteremia and 6 per cent of those without). These authors concluded that 20 per cent of their cases were caused by gram-negative bacilli; mortality in this group was 79 per cent.

Although pneumonia caused by *Str. pneumoniae* is still the commonest reason for hospital admission, rarer pathogens and opportunistic pulmonary infections should be kept in mind in the case of newly admitted patients with chronic disease, alcoholics, debilitated persons, infants, and the aged. *Staph. aureus* more commonly causes pneumonia in hospitalized patients but should be suspected during influenza epidemics and in debilitated persons recently discharged from the hospital or in contact with such patients.

A considerable percentage of community-acquired pneumonias are caused by anaerobic organisms. Anaerobic pulmonary infections are usually recognizable by the characteristic clinical and roentgenologic findings. Commonly, the patient's oral hygiene is poor and he or she has some disability that occasions loss of consciousness (*e.g.*, epilepsy or alcoholism); an insidious low-grade fever is typical, and the chest roentgenogram demonstrates segmental involvement of dependent areas of the lungs, often with cavitation.

HOSPITAL-ACQUIRED PNEUMONIA

Hospital-acquired pneumonia is usually more serious than that acquired in the community. This is partly because of the impaired resistance of acutely or chronically ill patients, but even more important is the character of the causal organisms. Although lacking in virulence and incapable of infecting healthy persons, *Ps. aeruginosa* and enteric gram-negative bacilli frequently produce uncontrollable sepsis in hospital patients who are devoid of host defenses—and they are resistant to all antibiotics. It is paradoxical that such devastating infections are acquired in the hospital, and deplorable that the physician, by the indiscriminate use of antibiotics and contaminated equipment, fosters their development.

Nosocomial (hospital-acquired) bacterial infections of the respiratory tract occur in 0.5 per cent to 5.0 per cent of inpatients.[21] Over 15 per cent of patients admitted for treatment of pneumonia contract bronchopulmonary superinfections, some of which are fatal. The incidence of pneumonia in intensive care units is particularly disturbing.

During the past three decades there has been a marked change in the organisms responsible for nosocomial pneumonia. Organisms that were etiologically responsible in the 50's—Str. pneumoniae, H. influenzae, and β-hemolytic streptococcus—were rare in the 60's when penicillinase-producing Staph. aureus, and to a lesser extent gram-negative organisms, were the major etiologic agents. By the mid-1970's this situation had again changed: the chief culprits responsible for serious, usually fatal, hospital-acquired pneumonia had become Ps. aeruginosa and the Enterobacteriaceae. In hospital-acquired Pseudomonas pneumonias, even the "best" antibiotic combinations have little effect on mortality—in fact, prolonged gentamicin therapy frequently results in fungal superinfection, as exemplified by one series in which candidiasis developed in 17 per cent of the patients treated with gentamicin (10 of the 13 patients died despite amphotericin B therapy).[22]

Gram-negative bacilli often are isolated from sputum cultures in circumstances that render their clinical significance difficult to evaluate: they may be spurious contaminants, harmless commensals, or opportunistic pathogens. Since colonization of the oropharynx or lower GI tract without invasion of the lung is frequent in patients, an erroneous diagnosis of acute pneumonia is possible when there is concomitant acute air-space consolidation (due to some other cause, such as pulmonary infarction).

Hospital-acquired pneumonias are believed to develop from aspiration of oropharyngeal secretions or GI contents into the lungs. The colonization of the oropharynx is largely the result of contact spread from contaminated personnel or equipment. In a prospective study of 213 patients admitted to a medical ICU,[23] 95 (45 per cent) became colonized with gram-negative organisms, those with primary respiratory illness being the most susceptible. Organisms were isolated as frequently from patients who were colonized but not infected as from those considered infected. Nosocomial respiratory infections developed in 22 (23 per cent) of the colonized patients but in only four (3.3 per cent) of the noncolonized.

Colonization (and presumably infection) with gram-negative organisms appears more likely in patients receiving antibiotics in the hospital. In the study of 38 ICU patients by Johanson and associates,[23] sputum cultures showed colonization by gram-negative bacilli in 21 (55 per cent) before antibiotic therapy and in 30 (79 per cent) during or after therapy, indicating not only a high incidence of colonization before these ICU patients received therapy but also that the incidence was increased by antimicrobial drugs. The major source of colonization is contaminated respiratory therapy equipment. It is now known that the chief culprits are the large-volume nebulizers (Venturi, spinning disk, and ultrasonic): the nidus of contamination is in the nebulizer jet, which apparently is beyond the reach of disinfecting solutions.[24] It is not known how nebulizers become contaminated, but probably this results from the introduction of contaminated fluids into the reservoir or the handling of the inner surface by contaminated personnel.

Indwelling intravenous catheters may be responsible for pulmonary infection caused by hematogenous spread of organisms. The longer the catheter remains in position, the greater the risk of infection.[25]

Measures to reduce the incidence of colonization and hospital-acquired pneumonia have proved successful. These methods of control are particularly warranted in intensive care units where seriously ill patients are clustered and natural barriers to infection are eliminated by tracheostomy and intravenous feeding. Venturi nebulizers should be sterilized by autoclaving with ethylene oxide gas or by soaking in a disinfectant followed by aerosolization with 0.25 per cent acetic acid. Spinning disk nebulizers cannot be sterilized with dilute acetic acid, and daily sterilization with ethylene oxide is necessary to prevent contamination. Ultrasonic nebulizers can be decontaminated by nebulization with 2 per cent acetic acid for 30 min or 7.5 per cent hydrogen peroxide for 20 min. Venous catheters should not be kept in place for more than 2 or 3 days if at all possible, and should be removed immediately if phlebitis develops.

Control of nosocomial staphylococcal pneumonia requires detection of infected personnel and isolation of patients.

In the most susceptible hosts (*e.g.*, patients with acute leukemia receiving chemotherapy), prophylactic oral antibiotics, skin antibiotics, and complete isolation in special units may be required to prevent contamination.

PNEUMONIA CAUSED BY GRAM-POSITIVE AEROBIC BACTERIA

STREPTOCOCCUS PNEUMONIAE

THE CAUSATIVE ORGANISM

Although over 82 serotypes of pneumococci have been identified, the great majority of pneumonias in humans are caused by types 8, 4, 5, 12, 3, 1, 7 and 9, in decreasing order of frequency. The organism is gram-positive and usually is seen on smear in pairs or short chains; its capsule swells when placed in homologous antiserum.

EPIDEMIOLOGY

Although many patients with pneumococcal pneumonia treated with antibiotics are cured or rendered culturally sterile by the time of admission to hospital, Austrian[26] showed that the incidence of bacteremic pneumococcal infections is unchanged, an incidence that has recently been estimated at one-fourth to one-third of patients with this type of pneumonia.[27]

Pneumococcal pneumonia may occur in otherwise healthy people, but it is much more common in vagrants, alcoholics, and other compromised hosts. Pneumococcal pneumonia is generally mild and clinically similar to nonbacterial pneumonias in patients diagnosed and treated from the office or in the home.[28] The risk of pneumococcal infection is greater in patients with hepatic cirrhosis, diabetes mellitus, renal failure, lymphoma or leukemia, multiple myeloma, and sickle-cell disease, and in those lacking a spleen. Type 3 *Str. pneumoniae* appears to show predilection for the elderly, often causing bacteremia and usually pneumonia with a high mortality.[27, 29]

PATHOLOGIC CHARACTERISTICS

Str. pneumoniae is aspirated into the lungs from the upper respiratory tract and flows under the influence of gravity to the most dependent portion of the lungs. Thus, like any aspiration pneumonia, it shows an anatomic bias for the lower lobes and posterior segments of the upper lobes. Organisms penetrate to the most peripheral air spaces of the lung, where initially they incite an outpouring of inflammatory edema that permits rapid multiplication of the organism. Centrifugal propagation of the bacteria-laden exudate proceeds rapidly, with spread from alveolus to alveolus and from acinus to acinus via the communicating pores of Kohn. This centrifugal spread accounts for the homogeneity of consolidation, seen both morphologically and roentgenologically, and for its nonsegmental distribution: the mechanism of spread does not respect segmental boundaries.

ROENTGENOGRAPHIC MANIFESTATIONS

The roentgenographic pattern of acute pneumococcal pneumonia should be readily apparent from the pathologic description. Characteristically, there is homogeneous consolidation of lung parenchyma (Figure 6–3). Since the consolidation begins in the peripheral air spaces of the lung, it almost invariably abuts against a visceral pleural surface, either interlobar or over the convexity. The lack of respect for segmental boundaries is of major importance in differentiating acute air-space pneumonia from bronchopneumonia. Contrary to the implication of the common term "lobar" pneumonia, only seldom is a complete lobe consolidated. An air bronchogram is almost invariable, and its absence should cast doubt upon the diagnosis. Since the pathologic process is one of replacement of air by inflammatory exudate, loss of volume is either slight or absent during the acute stage of the disease; during resolution, however, some degree of atelectasis is common, presumably caused by exudate within airways and resultant obstruction. Most frequently the disease is confined to one lobe, but the infection may develop simultaneously in two or more lobes and then carries a poorer prognosis. Cavitation is rare, although several cases of acute pneumococcal pneumonia have been described in which massive pulmonary gangrene occurred.

The pattern of homogeneous air-space consolidation, although usual, is not the invariable mode of presentation in acute pneumococcal pneumonia. Sometimes the roentgenographic pattern is atypical, being segmental and inhomogeneous in density, conforming to the usual

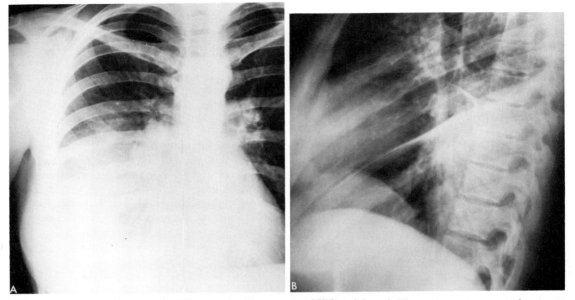

Figure 6–3. Acute Pneumococcal Pneumonia. Posteroanterior (A) and lateral (B) roentgenograms reveal extensive consolidation of the right lower lobe, a portion of the anterior segment being the only volume of lung unaffected. An air bronchogram is visible in the lateral projection. There is little loss of volume. Sputum culture produced a heavy growth of *Streptococcus pneumoniae.*

pattern of acute bronchopneumonia. This pattern is seen most commonly in infants and the elderly and in patients with chronic bronchitis, serious systemic illness, or immunologic deficiency.[27] Similarly, emphysema can alter the typical pattern so that the homogeneity of consolidation is interrupted by a multitude of small air-containing "holes"—presumably large emphysematous spaces that have escaped consolidation. This picture is not unique to acute pneumococcal pneumonia; as might be expected, it may occur in acute air-space pneumonia of any etiology.

In contrast to its frequency before the advent of antibiotics, roentgenographically demonstrable pleural effusion is uncommon today, at least on posteroanterior and lateral roentgenograms exposed in the erect position. However, since no large series of cases of acute pneumococcal pneumonia appears to have been studied by lateral decubitus roentgenography, the true incidence of associated effusion is unknown. Roentgenographic resolution of acute *Streptococcus pneumoniae* pneumonia usually begins promptly with the institution of antibiotic therapy; in fact, progression of consolidation following such institution should raise serious doubt whether *Str. pneumoniae* is the etiologic agent. Complete roentgenographic resolution characteristically takes 8 to 10 weeks.[30] In one series in which 72 patients were followed to complete resolution,[30] it was found that resolution oc-

curred earlier than 8 to 10 weeks in patients less than 50 years old and in the absence of alcoholism and underlying airways disease, but that delayed clearing occurred when these complicating factors were present in patients over 50.

CLINICAL MANIFESTATIONS

The usual clinical presentation of acute pneumococcal pneumonia in hospital patients is abrupt, with fever, shaking chills, cough, slight expectoration, and intense pleural pain. On close questioning many patients admit to an upper respiratory tract infection before the onset of the more dramatic symptoms. Temperature may be as high as 41°C. The cough may be nonproductive at first but soon produces bloody, "rusty," or greenish material. Debilitated and alcoholic patients may be deeply cyanosed and shock may ensue rapidly. Typical findings include decreased breath sounds, crepitation, and impaired percussion over the site of the pneumonia, with bronchial breathing, bronchophony, and whispering pectoriloquy audible on auscultation in a small percentage of patients. During resolution, the creptitations first increase and then slowly disappear as normal breath sounds return. In many cases a friction rub is audible over the consolidated lung.

Formerly fairly common, complications of

acute pneumococcal pneumonia—empyema, meningitis, endocarditis, and pericarditis—are now rarely seen. Patients with sickle-cell disease are particularly prone to serious pneumonia (usually pneumococcal), the incidence being estimated at 20 to 100 times greater than in hematologically normal black children. Jaundice also may occur, caused in most patients by hepatocellular damage but in some by hemolysis. Perhaps the commonest complication is superinfection, usually by gram-negative organisms and commonly in patients who have received huge doses of penicillin or a combination of antibiotics.

Although the diagnosis of acute pneumococcal pneumonia may be strongly suspected from the clinical picture and the roentgenographic pattern, a definitive diagnosis requires isolation of the organism. The demonstration of cocci on a smear is helpful. However, since *Str. pneumoniae* is a common commensal in the oropharynx, a positive smear or culture of expectorate cannot be accepted as absolute confirmation of the diagnosis (by contrast, a pure growth of *Str. pneumoniae* on blood culture is diagnostic).

In the great majority of patients, *Str. pneumoniae* is sensitive to penicillin and tetracycline. Prophylaxis with polyvalent pneumococcal capsular polysaccharide vaccines is indicated in the elderly and in patients with sickle cell anemia, chronic disability, or lymphoreticular and hematologic disorders.[27]

The white cell count usually is over 20,000 per cu mm, in a range of 10,000 to 40,000 per cu mm; polymorphonuclear leukocytosis, with many band forms, is common. However, leukopenia develops in many extremely ill patients. Analysis of arterial blood gas may show mild or even severe hypoxemia during the stage of "red hepatization." In most cases the P_{CO_2} is reduced, and the minute ventilation indicates hyperventilation with small tidal volume.

STAPHYLOCOCCUS AUREUS

THE CAUSATIVE ORGANISM

Staph. aureus is a gram-positive organism which on smear usually appears in clumps; it grows readily on blood agar, usually in a golden-yellow colony surrounded by hemolysis. Among other substances produced by the organism are coagulase, hemolysins, and enterotoxin. Its pathogenicity in man relates chiefly to its ability to produce coagulase (coagulase-negative strains rarely cause human disease).

EPIDEMIOLOGY

Staph. aureus has replaced *Str. pyogenes* as the commonest cause of bronchopneumonia, frequently complicating viral infections or developing in hospital patients whose resistance has been lowered by disease or recent operation. The emergence of the *Staphylococcus* as an important and often virulent pathogen is related to its ability to develop antibiotic resistance and to the contamination of the hospital environment, where the majority of cases occur.

Staphylococcal pneumonia rarely develops in healthy adults and seldom is acquired outside the hospital. More commonly, the pneumonia develops in hospital patients who are debilitated or have recently undergone operation. Those receiving antibiotic therapy, particularly with multiple drugs, are most susceptible. Prolonged stay in the hospital increases the risk of infection. Sometimes the infection follows influenza, a complication that may well be the commonest cause of death during influenzal epidemics.

PATHOLOGIC CHARACTERISTICS

The pathologic findings in staphylococcal pneumonia depend upon the rapidity of the disease's progress. In acute fulminating cases the picture may be one of severe hemorrhagic pulmonary edema: the disease begins in the conducting airways and histologically the bronchi show destruction of epithelium and infiltration with polymorphonuclear leukocytes. The alveoli are filled with proteinaceous material, blood, and a few polymorphonuclear cells; organisms abound in both bronchial and alveolar exudate. In cases of insidious progression of the disease, the pathologic picture is one of consolidation of acinar units surrounding the airways. Peribronchial abscesses form that subsequently communicate with the lumen of the airways, permitting entry of air into the abscess pockets and the development of the characteristic pneumatoceles. These may rapidly become enormous, particularly in children, presumably as a result of check-valve obstruction at the site of perforation.

Pleural effusion is fairly common and may be serous or serosanguineous; more commonly, however, and particularly in infants and children, the pleural reaction is purulent.

ROENTGENOGRAPHIC MANIFESTATIONS

Since the pathogenesis of acute staphylococcal pneumonia is related to the bronchial tree,

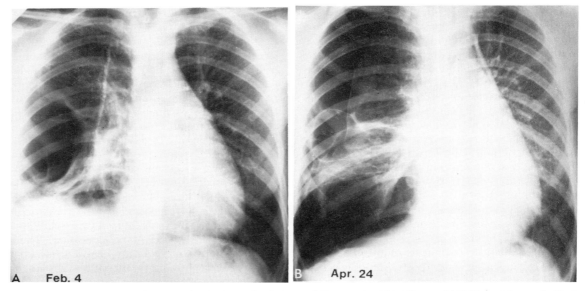

Figure 6–4. Pneumatocele Formation in Acute Staphylococcal Pneumonia. This 16-year-old Eskimo girl was admitted to the hospital with an acute respiratory illness. Her original roentgenogram (A) reveals an inhomogeneous opacity in the lower portion of the right lung associated with a large cystic space (pneumatocele) laterally and several smaller air-containing spaces inferiorly. The mediastinum is shifted to the left. A small pleural effusion is present, probably representing empyema. Resolution of the pneumonia was exceedingly slow. Two-and-one-half months after the onset of the acute illness, she presented again with a moderate-sized right pneumothorax (B), undoubtedly due to rupture of one of the pneumatoceles. Eventual complete recovery.

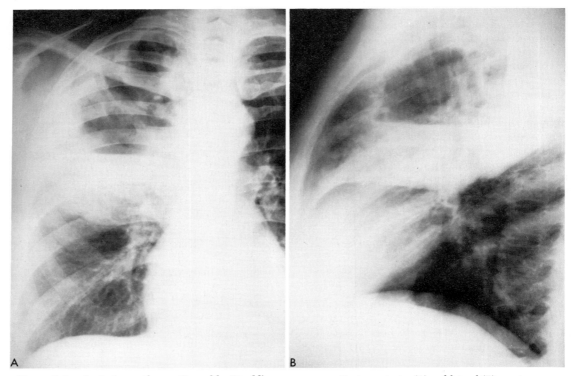

Figure 6–5. Acute Lung Abscess Caused by *Staphlyococcus aureus*. Posteroanterior (A) and lateral (B) roentgenograms reveal massive consolidation of the whole of the right upper lobe, a huge ragged cavity being evident in its center. Volume of the lobe has been increased, as indicated by the posterior bulging of the major fissure. Sputum culture produced a heavy growth of *Staph. aureus*.

resultant parenchyma consolidation typically is segmental in distribution. Depending on the severity of involvement, the process may be patchy or homogeneous; the latter represents confluent bronchopneumonia and in our experience is the commoner presentation. Acute inflammatory exudate fills the airways, so that loss of volume may accompany the consolidation; for the same reason an air bronchogram is seldom observed, and its presence should cast some doubt upon the diagnosis.

The roentgenographic pattern differs somewhat in children and adults. *In children*, consolidation develops very rapidly, usually involves a whole lobe, and may be multilobar. Complicating pneumothorax and empyema are common. A distinctive characteristic is the development of pneumatoceles, which are reported to occur in 40 to 60 per cent of child patients (Figure 6–4). These cystic spaces are commonly thin-walled and are thought to result from check-valve obstruction of a communication between a peribronchial abscess and the lumen of a bronchus. They may be enormous—the size of a hemithorax—in which case they may simulate a large pneumothorax. They may persist for weeks or even months but eventually disappear.

In adults, the disease is bilateral in over 60 per cent of cases. Abscess formation with subsequent communication with the bronchial tree and the appearance of fluid-containing cavities is fairly common, occurring in 25 to 75 per cent. Abscesses characteristically have a very irregular shaggy inner wall (Figure 6–5) and may be multiple. As in children, enlargement of the cavity may occur through check-valve obstruction of the bronchial communication, but is manifested simply by enlargement of the abscess cavity rather than by development of the thin-walled pneumatoceles so characteristic of the disease in infants and children. Resolution commonly takes several weeks; when abscess formation has occurred, a residual thin-walled bulla may remain. Pleural effusion or empyema occurs in approximately 50 per cent of adult patients and is a useful sign in differentiating staphylococcal from other forms of pneumonia.

The common method of development of acute staphylococcal pneumonia is by inhalation or aspiration of the organism, but occasionally organisms reach the lung in septic emboli, frequently from pelvic veins or an infected site of an intravenous catheter. Then the roentgenographic appearance is one of multiple nodular masses throughout the lungs, sometimes with poorly defined borders and often cavitated; they may be confluent and resemble homogeneous consolidation.

CLINICAL MANIFESTATIONS

The clinical picture varies, depending on the patient's age, the degree of debilitation, and whether the pneumonia is superimposed on influenzal infection. In infants, the onset often is abrupt, with high fever, tachypnea, and cyanosis; prompt treatment is necessary to save the patient's life. In children and adults who acquire the infection following influenza or in the very occasional case in which the disease develops outside the hospital in an otherwise healthy subject, the onset is also abrupt, with pleural pain, cough, and the expectoration of purulent yellow or brown material, sometimes streaked with blood.

When the infection develops in the hospital, either after an operation or complicating a chronic disease being treated with corticosteroids or multiple antibiotics, the onset often is insidious and is characterized by cough, fever, and the expectoration of purulent, blood-streaked material, but rarely by chest pain and chills. Physical signs vary; they include signs of consolidation, with bronchial breathing, patchy areas of rales, rhonchi, and decreased breath sounds, usually with signs of pleural effusion.

The diagnosis of staphylococcal pneumonia should be suspected whenever pneumonia develops soon after influenza or in a hospital patient. In infants, the roentgenographic demonstration of pneumonia with pneumatocele formation is almost pathognomonic. In all patients the diagnosis should be confirmed by sputum culture; in the majority, a heavy growth—sometimes pure—of *Staph. aureus* is obtained. The white cell count usually is elevated to between 16,000 and 25,000 per cu mm, with polymorphonuclear leukocytosis, but leukopenia may be present in severely ill patients. Positive results from blood cultures have been obtained in up to 50 per cent of patients, but septicemia is probably less common than in acute pneumococcal pneumonia.

Complications of acute staphylococcal pneumonia include meningitis, metastatic abscesses (particularly to the brain and kidneys), and acute endocarditis, which may develop in patients without valvular disease. Pneumothorax, pyopneumothorax, and empyema occur so frequently that they should be considered manifestations of the disease rather than complications.

STREPTOCOCCUS PYOGENES

THE CAUSATIVE ORGANISM

This gram-positive organism (Lancefield group A β-hemolytic *Streptococcus)* appears on a smear in the form of chains. Culture on blood agar is very rapid, colonies being identifiable microscopically and serologically within 24 hours; typical β-hemolysis surrounds the colonies. The organism may be cultured from the sputum or from the pleural effusion that commonly accompanies the pneumonia. It is very sensitive to penicillin and, unlike *Staph. pyogenes,* has not developed resistant strains.

EPIDEMIOLOGY

Until the advent of antibiotics, *Str. pyogenes* was the commonest cause of bronchopneumonia, a disease that affected predominantly the young and the elderly. Often it followed attacks of measles and pertussis, and in the influenza pandemic following World War I it was a common and serious complication. Acute streptococcal pneumonia rarely is seen nowadays. The infection is commonest during the coldest months. The organism enters the lungs by inhalation and aspiration and under the influence of gravity passes to the most dependent zones; thus the disease is almost invariably localized to the lower lobes. Lancefield group B streptococci may cause opportunistic infection, particularly in patients with diabetes mellitus, and occasionally cause fatal pneumonia.

PATHOLOGIC CHARACTERISTICS

The morphologic characteristics of acute streptococcal pneumonia are almost identical to those of the staphylococcal variety. In the preantibiotic era, many patients with the acute fulminating disease died within 36 hours, necropsy revealing severe serosanguineous pleural effusion and hemorrhagic edema of the lung parenchyma, particularly of the lower lobes.

In patients with less acute disease—commonly associated with whooping cough or measles—the pathologic picture differs and is similar to that of acute staphylococcal pneumonia. Peribronchial consolidation is accompanied by fairly severe bronchial and bronchiolar epithelial damage, and infiltration by polymorphonuclear leukocytes and lymphocytes. The peripheral parenchyma shows both inflammatory edema and atelectasis.

ROENTGENOGRAPHIC MANIFESTATIONS

In most respects the roentgenographic characteristics are indistinguishable from those of acute staphylococcal pneumonia—homogeneous or patchy consolidation in segmental distribution (Figure 6–6) and some loss of volume that typically affects the lower lobes and sometimes is bilateral. The tendency to pneumatoceles or pyopneumothorax found in acute staphylococcal pneumonia is absent, although lung abscesses and cavities may develop and empyema is common (the latter was an inevitable accompaniment before the advent of antibiotics).

CLINICAL MANIFESTATIONS

The onset of acute streptococcal pneumonia is usually abrupt, with pleural pain, shaking chills, fever, and cough productive of purulent and often blood-tinged material. Patchy areas of decreased breath sounds may be heard at the lung bases, together with rales and rhonchi; signs of pleural effusion are usually detectable.

Positive diagnosis depends on culture of the organism from sputum, pleural fluid, or occasionally blood. There is commonly a polymorphonuclear leukocytosis, with a mixture of mature and immature cells.

Complications include significant residual pleural thickening, bronchiectasis (especially in children in whom the disease develops in conjunction with an exanthem), and rarely glomerulonephritis.

BACILLUS ANTHRACIS

B. anthracis is a large, gram-positive, spore-forming, rod-shaped organism that may contaminate the fur of animals and be imported in wool or hides; thus the disease is commonest in sorters and combers in the wool industry. The organism is exceptionally virulent, and laboratory workers who come in contact with it are at considerable risk.

PATHOLOGIC CHARACTERISTICS

The most dramatic pathologic finding in the thorax is the hemorrhagic edema of hilar lymph nodes and surrounding mediastinal tissues. In the lungs, hemorrhagic foci may be found in the peripheral air spaces, and the larger bronchi may be filled with blood and mucus.

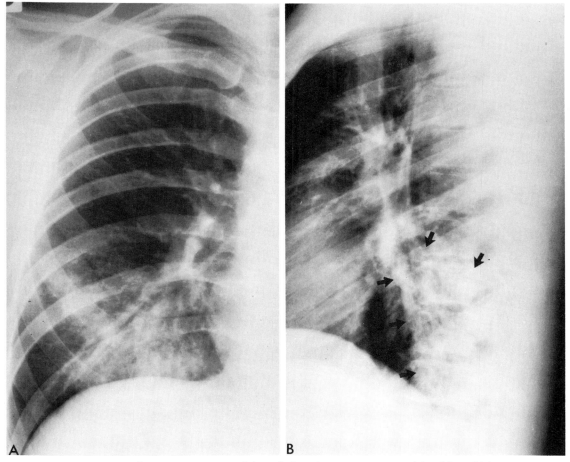

Figure 6–6. Acute Bronchopneumonia. Views of the right lung from posteroanterior (A) and lateral (B) roentgenograms show patchy consolidation of the posterior basal segment of the right lower lobe. The consolidation is inhomogeneous and possesses a roughly triangular configuration in lateral projection (*arrows* in *B*), indicating a true segmental distribution. Sputum culture produced mixed flora but with a predominance of *Streptococcus pyogenes*, which was considered the etiologic agent.

ROENTGENOGRAPHIC MANIFESTATIONS

The characteristic roentgenologic finding is mediastinal widening resulting from lymph node enlargement; this is of particular diagnostic significance if it develops acutely in a patient with a history of occupational exposure. Patchy, nonsegmental opacities may develop throughout the lungs, presumably caused by hemorrhagic edema. Pleural effusion is common.

CLINICAL MANIFESTATIONS

The initial symptoms following the inhalation of spores of *B. anthracis* are those of an acute bronchitis, frequently associated with a sensation of precordial oppression. The second stage, which begins abruptly within a few days, is characterized by acute dyspnea, cyanosis, tachycardia, fever, and sometimes shock. Most patients die within 24 hours after onset of the second stage.

The organism may be cultured on peptone agar from the blood, cerebrospinal fluid, and sputum. However, if life-saving therapy is to be instituted promptly, the diagnosis cannot await positive culture results and must be made on the basis of a history of acute febrile illness in a person occupationally exposed to anthrax spores and showing mediastinal widening roentgenographically.

LISTERIA MONOCYTOGENES

Listeriosis is a rare infectious disease that seldom involves the lungs or pleura. Infection with *Listeria monocytogenes* usually affects the meninges and endometrium, and in the latter location is suspected of being a cause of repeated abortion. Of 18 cases reported in 1967, all had neoplasms, 16 of the reticuloendothelial system.

L. monocytogenes is a gram-positive rod, about 0.5 μ wide by 1 to 3 μ long; it grows well on most standard culture media. The organism closely resembles the diphtheroids and is recognizable by its hemolytic activity on blood agar and its motility when incubated at room temperature. It locates within cells; a histologic picture of cell-mediated resistance develops in immune mice aerogenically infected with this organism.

Listeriosis may develop following the inhalation of, ingestion of, or direct contact with contaminated food or animal products. Pulmonary or pleural involvement, which is rare, presumably occurs via the bloodstream.

PNEUMONIA CAUSED BY GRAM-NEGATIVE AEROBIC BACTERIA

Coincident with the advances in the treatment of gram-positive infections, certain gram-negative bacilli have emerged as important pathogens in the etiology of pneumonia, particularly in hospital environments. The widespread use of penicillin and broad-spectrum antibiotics permits overgrowth of these more resistant organisms, and corticosteroids and immunosuppressive agents intensify the attack on host defense mechanisms, increasing the susceptibility of the chronically ill, elderly, and debilitated patient to pneumonia caused by gram-negative organisms. Infection with these organisms usually is acquired in the hospital.

Although the properties of opportunistic gram-negative bacilli that determine their ability to produce serious disease are not well defined, bacterial endotoxin has been suspected of playing a major role in the manifestations of bacillemia.

Aerobic gram-negative bacilli that cause pneumonia are described next. The two major families are the Pseudomonadaceae and the Enterobacteriaceae. The former consists of the nonfermenting gram-negative bacilli and includes the genus *Pseudomonas*, of which the species *Ps. aeruginosa* is the commonest agent to cause pneumonia in the western world; *Ps. pseudomallei* and *Ps. mallei* are relatively infrequent causes of lung infection. The Enterobacteriaceae, the nonspore-forming gram-negative bacilli (coliforms), include the *Klebsiella-Enterobacter-Serratia* group, *Escherichia coli*,

and the various species of *Proteus* and *Salmonella*. Mimeae, a very uncommon family of aerobic gram-negative organisms, occasionally cause pneumonia in compromised hosts, the specific organisms being *Herellea vaginicola* (*Bacterium anitratum*) and *Mima polymorpha*. Pneumonia may also be caused by small aerobic gram-negative bacilli, including *Legionella pneumophila* and related organisms, *Haemophilus influenzae*, *Bordetella pertussis*, *Francisella tularensis*, *Pasteurella multocida* (*septica*), *Yersinia* (*Pasteurella*) *pestis*, *Brucella* species, and *Vibrio fetus*.

PSEUDOMONADACEAE

PSEUDOMONAS AERUGINOSA

EPIDEMIOLOGY

Because of the resistance of these organisms to almost all antibiotics, pulmonary infections caused by *Ps. aeruginosa* have become the most dreaded of pneumonias acquired in hospitals.

The organism is a gram-negative bacillus that occasionally can be cultured from the sputum of healthy subjects, particularly those who have received antibiotic therapy recently. Most cases of pneumonia occur in the young or in elderly patients with debilitating disease; infection is frequently acquired in the hospital.

Most patients who acquire the disease either have been in contact with a heavily infected source, such as patients with wounds, burns, urinary tract infections, and, particularly, respiratory tract involvement, or have inhaled large numbers of bacilli through contamination of saline soap, antiseptic solutions, creams, jellies, or other substances used in the care of tracheostomy sites or as repositories for suction catheters. In our experience, the commonest source of infection in hospital patients is heavily contaminated nebulizers attached to artificial ventilators.

In the adult, most infections develop in patients suffering from chronic lung disease, congestive heart failure, diabetes mellitus, alcoholism, or kidney disease; patients with tracheostomies are particularly susceptible, especially in the early postoperative period.

In summary, *Pseudomonas* pneumonia is most likely to develop in hospital patients with debilitating disease, usually on multiple antibiotic and often corticosteroid therapy, with a tracheostomy—especially when frequent suction is required or ventilatory aids are introduced. It is equally true, however, that the disease develops in only a proportion of patients fulfilling these criteria, indicating the survival of some natural defense mechanism(s) in the respiratory tract of even the critically ill. Entry of the organism into the body may be directly via the bloodstream, usually secondary to contamination at the site of an indwelling intravenous catheter.

PATHOLOGIC CHARACTERISTICS

At necropsy, patients who have acquired their disease through aspiration usually show affection of the posterior segments of the lower lobes. Microabscesses may be identified in the peribronchial tissues, with necrosis of the alveolar walls within the lung parenchyma. These abscesses may be walled off and contain many polymorphonuclear cells. Foci of atelectasis and emphysema may be present; hemorrhagic or purulent pleural effusion is almost invariable.

A somewhat different pathologic picture is found in those patients in whom pneumonia resulted from *Pseudomonas* bacteremia.[31] Nodular infarcts develop, with massive gram-negative bacillary infiltration of arterial and venous walls. A distinctive skin lesion known as *ecthyma gangrenosa* may develop which begins as a vesicle and later becomes necrotic; these lesions range from a few millimeters to several centimeters in diameter and their center is black.

ROENTGENOGRAPHIC MANIFESTATIONS

The roentgenographic pattern of acute *Ps. aeruginosa* pneumonia is unlike that of other gram-negative pneumonias and more closely resembles the pattern of acute staphylococcal pneumonia.[31] There is a definite lower lobe predilection, and both lungs are affected in the vast majority of patients. There are three main roentgenographic patterns of parenchymal abnormality, depending at least partly on whether the organisms reach the lung parenchyma via the tracheobronchial tree by aspiration or via the bloodstream by bacteremia.

1. *Extensive bilateral parenchymal consolidation.* The early stage is manifested by poorly defined, patchy shadows of homogeneous density that appear simultaneously in both lungs. The shadows extend rapidly, despite vigorous antibiotic therapy, and coalesce; ultimately, the major portions of both lungs are massively consolidated.

2. *Patchy areas of parenchymal consolidation with abscess formation.* In every reported series, almost all the lung abscesses exceeded 2 cm in diameter. These abscesses, which undoubtedly are the result of lung necrosis, differ greatly from the numerous tiny translucencies throughout the consolidated parenchyma.[32] Although it has been suggested that these small radiolucent foci may be the roentgenographic counterpart of the microabscesses seen at necropsy, Renner and colleagues[32] concluded on the basis of roentgenologic-pathologic correlation in several cases that they represent either unaffected secondary pulmonary lobules or small areas of lobular emphysema caused by check-valve obstruction of small airways.

3. *Widespread patchy or nodular shadows diffuse throughout both lungs.* This roentgenographic pattern probably reflects bacteremia. The numerous tiny translucencies that may be observed throughout areas of consolidation are probably not true microabscesses, but areas of air-containing parenchyma unaffected by inflammatory edema. Small effusions are visualized in many cases and are an almost invariable finding at necropsy.

In addition to acute pneumonia of other etiology, the main conditions to be considered in differential diagnosis include pulmonary oxygen toxicity (the majority of these patients are mechanically ventilated), cardiogenic pulmonary edema, and possibly pulmonary embolism and infarction.

CLINICAL MANIFESTATIONS

Most patients with *Pseudomonas* pneumonia acquire the infection in the hospital, and almost invariably they have underlying disease that has reduced their resistance. An upper respiratory tract infection may precede the pneumonia, whose onset is typically abrupt, with chills, fever, severe dyspnea, and cough productive of copious yellow or green, occasionally blood-streaked, sputum. Although empyema is common, pleural pain is said to be infrequent. Bradycardia is the rule. The temperature curve is unusual in that it peaks in the mornings rather than the evenings. The white cell count usually is normal in the early stages but commonly rises to an average of about 20,000 per cu mm.

In the bacteremic form of the disease, diagnosis may be extremely difficult during the early stages and only the appearance of circulatory collapse or the typical skin lesions may suggest the etiology. When the disease is secondary to inhalation, the diagnosis usually is made by repeated culture of heavy—sometimes pure—growths of *Ps. aeruginosa*. Blood cultures should be made whenever the diagnosis is suspected.

PSEUDOMONAS PSEUDOMALLEI

The Causative Organism

Pseudomonas pseudomallei, like *Ps. aeruginosa*, is a motile, pleomorphic gram-negative rod with one or two flagella at one pole and no capsule. It can be isolated aerobically and anaerobically on all culture media. Its specific enzyme reactions and sugar fermentation permit its differentiation from *Ps. mallei*, the organism responsible for glanders.

Epidemiology

Melioidosis, the disease caused by *Ps. pseudomallei*, occurs principally in rodents, cats, and dogs, and is endemic in Ceylon, India, Burma, and the East Indies, where the organism has been found in the soil. In endemic areas, serologic tests have shown infection to be of widespread distribution, most patients being asymptomatic. Humans are believed to acquire melioidosis through damaged skin, by inhalation, or by the ingestion of food contaminated by animal excreta; person to person transmission does not occur.

Pathologically, multiple small abscesses are found throughout the lungs, spleen, lymph nodes, liver, and kidneys.

Roentgenographic Manifestations

Both roentgenographically and clinically, two distinct patterns have been described—the acute and the chronic. The more common—the acute—is characterized by a roentgenographic pattern consisting of irregular nodular opacities, 4 to 10 mm in diameter, widely disseminated throughout both lungs. These have indistinct borders and tend to enlarge, coalesce, and cavitate as the disease progresses.

The chronic form of the disease is said to simulate tuberculosis. Roentgenographically demonstrable pleural effusion does not occur.

Clinical Manifestations

The onset of acute melioidosis is usually abrupt but may be preceded by a brief period of malaise, anorexia, and diarrhea. The symptoms of high fever, chills, cough, expectoration of purulent blood-streaked material, dyspnea, and pleuritic pain may be followed rapidly by evidence of bacteremic dissemination, including miliary visceral and osseous abscesses, leading to prostration and resulting in death within a few days. In chronic cases the lungs appear to be the organs predominantly involved; however, many patients have abscesses in viscera, bones, joints, and skin. Underlying disease increases susceptibility to the infection. There have been reports of asymptomatic service personnel returning from Vietnam in whom the infection has recurred months to years later, usually concomitant with other illnesses or surgical procedures.

The white cell count may be normal or may show moderate leukocytosis with neutrophilia. Cultures should be made of sputum, urine, blood, and, if symptoms indicate meningeal spread, cerebrospinal fluid. There is no specific skin test; an agglutination test may aid in diagnosis when cultures are negative.

MALLEOMYCES MALLEI

This organism is the cause of glanders, a disease primarily of horses and rarely of humans. *M. mallei* is a gram-negative bacillus; it grows on ordinary culture media and is antigenically separable from *Ps. pseudomallei*, the organism responsible for melioidosis.

The disease should be suspected in persons residing in Asia or South America who are exposed to horses and in whom oral and nasal ulcers develop, with nodules along the lymphatics, and acute or chronic pneumonia. Agglutination and complement-fixation tests are available, and a skin test using a sterile culture filtrate known as mallein is highly specific.

ENTEROBACTERIACEAE

KLEBSIELLA, ENTEROBACTER, AND SERRATIA GENERA

The *Klebsiella*, *Enterobacter* (*Aerobacter*), and *Serratia* genera have been grouped together on the basis of colonial morphology and biochemical tests and are known as the

Klebsielleae. Those organisms that are encapsulated, nonmotile, gram-negative rods are usually designated *Klebsiella pneumoniae*, whereas the motile variety belongs to the genus *Enterobacter*. *Serratia*, a motile, gram-negative, aerobic, nonsporulating bacillus, is differentiated from *Klebsiella* and *Enterobacter* on biochemical testing.[33] Pneumonia caused by *Klebsiella* is almost always sensitive to cephalothin, although this organism rapidly develops resistance. The *Enterobacter* and *Serratia* genera produce cephalosporinase, which renders them resistant to the cephalosporins. Most of the gram-negative Klebsielleae bacilli found in hospitals belong to the genus *Klebsiella*. *K. pneumoniae* can cause acute fulminating air-space pneumonia and is responsible for 1 to 5 per cent of all acute alveolar pneumonias. Although serotypes are not identified in most cases of pneumonia, types 1 to 6 are most often isolated from respiratory sources and are those found in typical Friedländer's pneumonia.[34] Other serotypes of *K. pneumoniae* may be isolated from the lungs in pure culture in cases of more chronic respiratory infection, usually with a clinical picture of bronchopneumonia. Similarly, *Enterobacter* (usually *E. aerogenes*) may cause a less fulminant form of pneumonia that may cavitate. Most instances of *Klebsiella-Enterobacter-Serratia* (KES) infections occur in elderly hospital patients who have been compromised by major medical or surgical illnesses. In contrast, most cases of pneumonia caused by *Klebsiella* types 1, 3, 4, and 5 develop in alcoholic or otherwise debilitated patients and are rarely hospital acquired.[34] The mortality from KES infections with bacteremia is approximately 50 per cent, death occurring usually within 48 hours of onset of the disease.

Serratia marcescens is a common saprophyte of soil, water, and sewage. Most infections are hospital acquired by elderly, debilitated patients, the majority of whom have been receiving antibiotic therapy.[33] Most strains are slow lactose fermenters or nonfermenters, and in a few patients produce a red pigment in expectorated material that simulates blood (pseudohemoptysis).[33]

PATHOLOGIC CHARACTERISTICS

As with other organisms, such as *Str. pneumoniae*, that cause acute air-space pneumonia, *Klebsiella* gains entry by inhalation and flows by gravity to the most dependent portions of the lung. Acute pneumonia usually is unilateral and most frequently involves the right lung. Grossly, the consolidated lung is reddish-gray, with cavitation in many cases. Histologically, the peripheral air spaces are filled with edema fluid containing many gram-negative bacilli; mononuclear cells present initially are replaced by polymorphonuclear leukocytes. Extension to the pleura with resultant empyema is common. Massive lung necrosis may lead to the formation of huge cavities.

ROENTGENOGRAPHIC MANIFESTATIONS

As an acute air-space pneumonia, *Klebsiella* pneumonia presents as homogeneous parenchymal consolidation containing an air bronchogram but showing no precise segmental distribution. Three features of acute *Klebsiella* pneumonia aid its differentiation from acute pneumococcal pneumonia: (1) a tendency for the formation of such voluminous inflammatory exudate that the volume of affected lung becomes supranormal, with resultant bulging of interlobar fissures; (2) a tendency to abscess and cavity formation; and (3) a greater frequency of pleural effusion and empyema. Abscesses and unilocular or multilocular cavities usually develop rapidly if the patient survives the initial 48 hours. This complication occurs in as many as half of those who survive, and in most can be recognized within 4 days of onset of the illness. The separation of large masses of necrotic lung into an abscess cavity—massive lung gangrene (Figure 6–7)—is rare, with about the same frequency as in acute pneumococcal pneumonia.

Roentgenographically, *Serratia* pneumonia causes a somewhat different picture than *Klebsiella*: in a recent review of 18 patients who died of *Serratia marcescens* infection,[35] the predominant radiologic findings were focal bronchopneumonia in 13, lobar consolidation in two, and diffuse inhomogeneous opacities in 10; small radiolucent areas were identified within the opacities in five patients, a large pulmonary abscess in one, and pleural effusion in seven.

CLINICAL MANIFESTATIONS

Acute pneumonia caused by *Klebsiella* is seen predominantly in men in their sixth decade of life, most being chronic alcoholics. Chronic bronchopulmonary disease, and to a lesser extent diabetes mellitus, appear to predispose to *Klebsiella* pneumonia.[36]

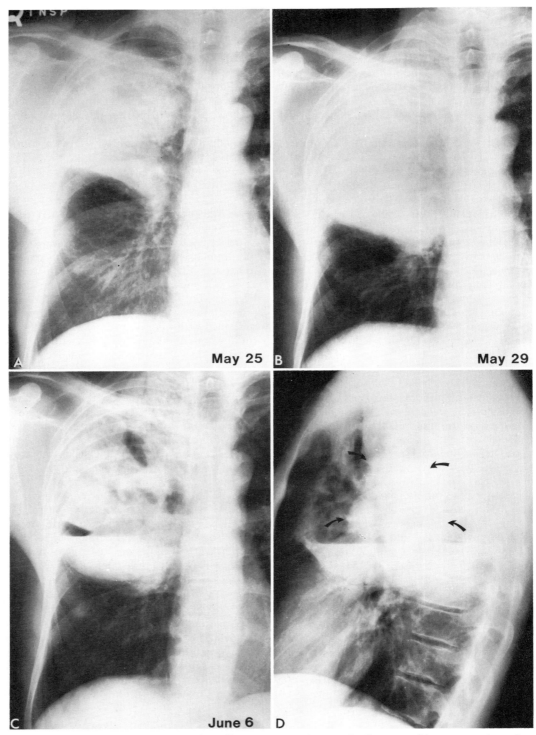

Figure 6–7. Acute Lung Gangrene in *Klebsiella* Pneumonia. This acutely ill 50-year-old man was admitted to the hospital with a 5-day history of fever, increasing dyspnea, right-sided pleuritic chest pain, and cough productive of tenacious brown sputum. The admission chest roentgenogram (*A*) showed extensive air-space pneumonia. *Klebsiella pneumoniae* was cultured from the sputum. Four days after admission and despite antibiotic therapy, the pneumonia had worsened considerably, to a point at which the upper lobe had now expanded considerably (*B*); note the concave configuration of the lower border of the consolidated lobe where it relates to the horizontal fissure. One week later, roentgenograms in posteroanterior (*C*) and lateral (*D*) projection show a hugh ragged cavity within the consolidated lobe, possessing a prominent air-fluid level in its lower portion and a large irregular mass in its center (seen to best advantage in *D* as indicated by *arrows*). At thoracotomy 23 days after admission, a right pneumonectomy was required because of involvement of all three lobes of the right lung by the necrotizing process.

The onset usually is abrupt, with prostration, pain on breathing, cyanosis, moderate fever, and severe dyspnea; expectoration usually is greenish, purulent, and blood-streaked, and occasionally brick red and gelatinous.[36] Physical signs usually are those of parenchymal consolidation; breath sounds are decreased when pus in the airways results in bronchial obstruction.

The white cell count usually is moderately elevated; when it is normal or reduced the prognosis is most unfavorable. Bacteremia has been reported to occur in about 25 per cent of cases.[36]

The diagnosis should be suspected from the clinical picture and roentgenographic findings. If a sputum smear shows a preponderance of gram-negative bacilli, antibiotic therapy should be instituted immediately; to await the results of culture is to court disaster. Extrapulmonary manifestations are uncommon.

Pneumonia caused by S. *marcescens* in compromised hosts is usually fatal.

ESCHERICHIA COLI

E. coli is a rare cause of bronchopneumonia. It chiefly affects debilitated patients and occasionally neonates, in the latter presumably via aspirated amniotic fluid. In patients with chronic lung disease, or chronic extrapulmonary diseases such as diabetes mellitus or renal or cardiovascular conditions, the organism may penetrate to the lower respiratory tract and incite acute or subacute pneumonia. Many patients have gastrointestinal or genitourinary disease, suggesting that lung involvement is usually, although not invariably, secondary to bacteremia.

Morphologically, necropsy of patients who die within 48 hours after onset reveals hemorrhagic pneumonia, usually of the lower lobes.

Roentgenographically, the usual pattern is one of acute air-space pneumonia; involvement is usually multilobar, with a strong lower lobe anatomic bias. Cavitation is uncommon, but pleural effusion is frequent. Acute *E. coli* pneumonia in infants may give rise to pneumatoceles during resolution, presumably in the same manner as the more commonly associated acute staphylococcal pneumonia.

Clinically, the usual history is of existing chronic disease, with abrupt onset of fever, chills, dyspnea, pleuritic pain, cough, and expectoration of yellow—rarely blood-tinged—sputum. Gastrointestinal symptoms, including nausea, abdominal pain, dysphagia, diarrhea, and vomiting, may be present. The onset may be fulminating, with shock leading rapidly to death. The classic signs of consolidation are lacking, the sole finding on physical examination being basal rales; empyema may lead to decreased breath sounds and dullness or flatness on percussion. The white cell count may be decreased or may be increased to over 20,000 per cu mm.

Diagnosis requires a predominant or pure growth of *E. coli* on culture; occasional colonies are of no significance, particularly in patients receiving antibiotic therapy. A positive culture from the blood or pleural fluid is strong evidence that the organism is pathogenic.

BACILLUS PROTEUS

Many patients who develop pneumonia from this organism have chronic pulmonary disease and some have chronic extrathoracic disease such as diabetes mellitus or alcoholism. Like *E. coli*, *Proteus* is more commonly a cause of kidney infection.

The organism is thought to gain entry to the lungs by inhalation. *Both morphologically and roentgenographically*, the picture is one of acute air-space pneumonia similar in most respects to that of *Str. pneumoniae* and more particularly the *Klebsiella* organisms. Abscess formation is frequent.

Clinically, the onset and course of acute *Proteus* pneumonia is more insidious than is usual in the other gram-negative pneumonias. For several weeks before admission to the hospital, patients may complain of a general lack of well-being and worsening of the symptoms of their chronic pulmonary disease; as these symptoms become more severe, pleural pain develops, with cough productive of purulent yellow sputum that sometimes is blood-streaked. There is moderate fever but no evidence of shock. Physical signs of pulmonary consolidation are invariably present; a moderate leukocytosis with a shift to the left is common.

SALMONELLA SPECIES

Salmonella, which are gram-negative bacteria of the family Enterobacteriaceae, rarely affect the lungs. Although they are more commonly pathogens in the gastrointestinal tract, any of these organisms may cause bronchopneumonia secondary to aspiration, or diffuse pneumonitis secondary to bacteremia. Infections usually develop during the warm months, but sporadic cases may occur at any time. Patients with disseminated malignant disease are predisposed to the infection.

Morphologic characteristics depend largely on the mode of infection, aspiration of organisms causing focal bronchopneumonia, and bacteremia resulting in diffuse bilateral suppurative disease. Suppuration and necrosis lead to cavity formation and empyema.

Roentgenographically, the pattern is one of segmental bronchopneumonia if the organism gains entry by aspiration; cavitation and pleural effusion (empyema) are common. An acute miliary pattern has been described in cases of proved *Salmonella* bacteremia.

Clinically, the course of the disease usually is prolonged, with chills, fever, and pleural pain. The white cell count varies from leukopenic to moderately leukocytic.

ACINETOBACTER

The genus *Acinetobacter* includes two species of clinical importance, *Mima* and *Herellea*, which frequently are found in sputum cultures and are not always indicative of disease; however, two species, *Mima polymorpha* and *Herellea vaginicola (Bacterium antitratum)*, occasionally cause bronchitis, pneumonia, lung abscess, and pleural effusion. These organisms are polymorphic, gram-negative, encapsulated, and nonmotile. They appear as diplococci on solid media and as rods in liquid media. They can be readily differentiated from Enterobacteriaceae by their negative nitrate reaction, but can be confused with *Neisseria* because of their morphologic resemblance.

In the lungs, *H. vaginicola* can produce severe acute air-space pneumonia, usually in patients with underlying disease. Empyema is frequent. Patients complain of pleural pain, fever, nausea, vomiting, and purulent expectoration; leukocytosis is usual.

SMALL AEROBIC GRAM-NEGATIVE BACILLI

LEGIONELLA PNEUMOPHILA AND RELATED MICROORGANISMS

In July, 1976, the National Convention of the American Legion was held in Philadelphia, and by the end of August, 180 cases of an acute respiratory illness could be related to attendance at the convention or to presence in the headquarters' hotel; 29 patients died. In the vast majority of patients, this "new" infectious entity was characterized by acute pneumonia; not unexpectedly, it became known euphemistically as legionnaires' disease.[37] In the following months, the etiologic agent, *Legionella pneumophila* was identified at the Centers for Disease Control (CDC) in Atlanta.[38] In addition, in a retrospective study of stored serum obtained from patients seen in previously unsolved outbreaks of respiratory disease, the CDC found that *L. pneumophila* was not an uncommon cause of minor "epidemics."[38] Subsequent to the recognition of legionellosis in Philadelphia, a number of common source outbreaks were identified throughout the United States, Canada, and Europe,[39] and by the end of September, 1979, over 1000 cases of sporadic legionellosis had been described in the United States alone.[40] The epidemiology of the many outbreaks of the disease in the United States was summarized by Meyer in 1980.[41]

The recognition of *L. pneumophila* aroused interest in identifying other fastidious, pneumonia-causing microorganisms, many of which had already been cultured in yolk sacs and had tentatively been described as rickettsia-like agents. A number of such microorganisms have now been identified as weakly staining, gram-negative bacteria phenotypically similar to but genetically different from *L. pneumophila;* they have been isolated from patients with pneumonia and from natural sources such as water in air-conditioning cooling towers. In common with *L. pneumophila*, they grow on charcoal yeast extract medium. At the time of writing, only a few cases of pneumonia caused by Legionella-like microorganisms have been described; however, it seems probable that future studies will show that these bacilli are not uncommon causes of the one-half to one million cases of pneumonia of undetermined etiology seen yearly in the United States. Published reports of Legionella-like bacteria include descriptions of the "Pittsburgh pneumonia agent,"[42-44, 285] the Tatlock, HEBA, WIGA, and Tex-K1 bacteria.[45-47]

THE CAUSATIVE ORGANISM

L. pneumophila is a fastidious, pleomorphic bacillus, 0.4 to 0.8 μm in width and 2 to 4 μm in length. The fine structure of the *L. pneumophila* bacillus has been described by a number of authors.[48-50] The organism stains weakly negative with a Gram stain but is seen to much better advantage on Giménez or Dieterle silver-impregnation stains of lung specimens. In common with a number of other Legionella-like bacteria, flagella may be demonstrated using a simplified Leifson flagellar stain.[51] The most reliable method of identifying the organism is by direct immunofluorescent staining of respiratory tract secretions or tissue.[52] The organism is weakly oxidase- and catalase-positive and grows best at 35°C in an atmosphere containing from 2.5 to 5.0 per cent carbon dioxide. Charcoal yeast extract is the medium of choice for culturing *L. pneumophila* from blood, pleural fluid, tissue, or transtracheal aspirate, although this is not an effective means of isolating the organism from sputum, since contaminating bacteria from the oropharynx tend to overgrow the medium.[52]

At the time of this writing, *L. pneumophila* has been identified as occurring in six separate serogroups, the great majority of reported cases falling into group I (84 per cent of the 1005 sporadic cases reported to the CDC in the United States).[40]

EPIDEMIOLOGY

The patient becomes infected by inhaling organisms in the atmosphere, not by person-to-person contact. Approximately 75 per cent of cases occur during the summer months from June through October. Most victims are middle-aged or elderly, although the range of ages of patients involved has been very broad (2 to 84 years).[41] Among sporadic cases, men outnumber women in a three-to-one ratio.[41] Men who are heavy drinkers and smokers are particularly susceptible. Many patients who develop the disease are immunosuppressed or have advanced renal or pulmonary disease, diabetes mellitus, or cancer; it is not surprising, therefore, that outbreaks frequently are hospital-associated. Even among sporadic cases seen in the community, approximately 5 per cent will give a history of recent hospitalization. Other factors that appear to increase the likelihood of infection include overnight traveling, living in close proximity to construction or excavation sites, and recent attendance at a convention.[40] In outbreak-associated disease, *L. pneumophila* and related organisms appear to possess an affinity for water: in several instances, bacteria have been recovered from air-conditioning cooling towers, evaporative condensers, or streams and silt.[39, 53] Such an association has not been detected to the same extent in sporadic cases.

The incubation period of the pneumonic form of legionnaires' disease ranges from 2 to 10 days. In the rare nonpneumonic type, the incubation period is much shorter (24 to 48 hours), and the disease lasts for only two to seven days.[39]

PATHOLOGIC CHARACTERISTICS

The pathologic picture is not in any way unique or characteristic, consisting of a necrotizing type of infection that should be suspected when the usual bacterial stains fail to demonstrate organisms.[54] The pulmonary reaction has been described both as an acute fibrinopurulent bronchopneumonia.[55] and as a nonsegmental air-space pneumonia.[56] Abscess formation is seen occasionally.[56] Tissue stained with the Dieterle silver-impregnation method reveals a myriad of small pleomorphic rods. Rarely, *L. pneumophila* may be found in extrapulmonary sites.[57] Following prolonged illness, examination of tissue removed by biopsy or necropsy reveals organization of inflammatory lesions.[58]

ROENTGENOGRAPHIC MANIFESTATIONS

In the original Philadelphia outbreak, chest roentgenograms were abnormal in 90 per cent of 182 patients with the disease.[37] Of the 1005 cases of sporadic legionellosis reported in the United States in 1981,[40] 984 had roentgenographically documented acute pneumonia (of the remainder, three patients were reported to have had normal chest roentgenograms and the rest had not been radiographed).

The characteristic roentgenographic pattern is one of air-space consolidation. A feature that is seldom seen in the usual form of acute air-space pneumonia, such as that caused by *Str. pneumoniae*, is the tendency for the consolidation to progress following its initial discovery, sometimes despite appropriate therapy (Figure 6–8).[41] Spread is usually rapid, a zone of consolidated lung (sometimes rounded[59]) spreading to involve most of a lobe in three to four days.[60]

In most cases, the pneumonia is unilateral when first seen,[40, 41, 59, 60] although there is a tendency to bilateral involvement at the peak of the disease. For example, of the 24 patients reported by Dietrich and his colleagues,[59] the pneumonia was unilateral in 68 per cent at the onset but was bilateral in 65 per cent at the peak of the disease (10 days after the first occurrence of symptoms). There is a distinct lower lobe predilection. Abscess formation is exceedingly uncommon, although at least one well-documented case has been reported.[61]

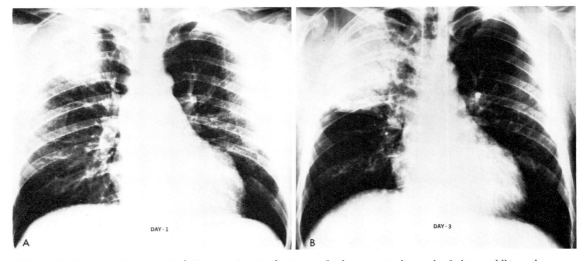

Figure 6–8. Acute Legionnaires' Pneumonia. At the time of admission to hospital of this middle-aged man, a posteroanterior roentgenogram (A) revealed a rather poorly defined homogeneous consolidation in the right upper lobe characteristic of acute air-space pneumonia. He was promptly placed on penicillin therapy but two days later, a roentgenogram (B) revealed marked extension of the acute pneumonia to involve most of the volume of the right upper lobe. An air bronchogram was now evident. By this time, *Legionella pneumophila* had been identified in the patient's sputum and he was placed on more appropriate therapy with eventual complete recovery. (Courtesy Dr. Fred Valdmanis, Pennock Hospital, Hastings, Michigan.)

Lymph node enlargement does not occur. The frequency of pleural effusion varies widely in reported series, being observed in half of the patients in one series[41] but in only 2 of 17 patients in another.[60] Pleural effusion may occasionally antedate the roentgenographic appearance of pneumonia.[41, 62]

In contrast to its occurrence in acute *Klebsiella* pneumonia, lobar expansion is a rare manifestation of legionnaires' pneumonia. That the disease can appear in very atypical form is illustrated by the recent report of a solitary pulmonary nodule approximately 2 cm in diameter from which *L. pneumophila* organisms were recovered from a transthoracic needle aspirate.[63] Of similar nature were the roentgenographic findings in seven patients with pneumonia caused by the Pittsburgh pneumonia agent, *L. micdadei*:[285] in addition to consolidation involving part or all of one or more lobes, there were observed single or multiple nodules that tended to undergo rapid growth.

With appropriate therapy, roentgenographic resolution tends to be fairly rapid, occurring in two weeks or less.[41, 60]

CLINICAL MANIFESTATIONS

The earliest symptoms are malaise, muscle aches, and slight headache, followed usually within 24 hours by fever, shaking chills, and a nonproductive cough. Pleuritic chest pain oc-

curs in approximately 35 per cent of patients. Dyspnea occurs as the pneumonia becomes more extensive.

The incidence of prodromal symptoms suggesting upper respiratory tract infection is controversial, some[64] regarding such symptoms as a useful feature differentiating legionellosis from other pneumonias, and others[65] regarding the *absence* of such symptoms as a useful criterion for diagnosis. However, there appears to be general agreement that symptoms reflecting other organ involvement, notably the gastrointestinal, renal, and central nervous systems, are much more common in legionnaires' pneumonia that in pulmonary infections caused by other microorganisms; patients complain of diarrhea and abdominal pain, and many become confused and even obtunded.[37, 64-66] Hematuria and proteinuria may be present, and liver function tests are often abnormal.

Pneumonia caused by *L. pneumophila* is a serious disease, with one-third of patients requiring assisted ventilation and one-fifth dying.[40] In patients who survive, fever has been shown to break by lysis, even when there is good response to antibiotics.[37] The white blood cell count is below 15,000 per cu mm in the great majority of patients; lymphopenia is frequent, the lymphocyte count being 1000 or less.[37] Hyponatremia may be present, and the BUN and liver enzymes are slightly elevated in many instances.

In the majority of cases, the diagnosis of legionellosis has been made on the basis of a fourfold increase in indirect immunofluorescent antibody or by direct fluorescent staining of the bacillus in tissue. A microhemagglutination technique for the detection of antibodies appears to be promising.[67] Only 3 per cent of sporadic cases have been diagnosed by direct fluorescent staining or culture of secretions.[40] A cross-reaction of seropositivity with *Mycoplasma pneumoniae* has been described.[68]

HAEMOPHILUS INFLUENZAE

The upper respiratory tract of healthy persons yields nonencapsulated strains of *H. influenzae* so commonly that in this location these organisms can be regarded as normal flora. Carriers of encapsulated strains are extremely rare.[69]

Nonencapsulated strains of *H. influenzae* are the commonest organisms cultured from purulent expectoration of patients with chronic pulmonary disease, although their pathogenicity is still in doubt. The six strains that are encapsulated can be differentiated into types a to f, according to the nature of their capsular polysaccharides. Type b strains are those that usually cause disease in humans.[70]

Infants are protected for up to about 2 months by passive immunity acquired from their mothers. Those most susceptible to *H. influenzae* infection are infants and children aged 2 months to 3 years, although the incidence of infection in adults is increasing,[69] probably because prompt antibiotic treatment of infections prevents the development of protective antibodies.

H. influenzae can cause meningitis, epiglottitis, bronchitis, bronchiolitis, and segmental bronchopneumonia in very young children.[69, 70] As a primary pathogen, it usually causes acute inflammation of the mucous membranes of the airways, although when it follows respiratory virus disease, it may penetrate the bronchial wall and cause an inflammatory reaction in the peribronchiolar tissues—typical bronchopneumonia. *H. influenzae* pneumonia in adults most often is seen in compromised hosts.

Roentgenographically, acute bronchopneumonia usually occurs in the lower lobes and may be bilateral.[71] In adults the organism occasionally induces acute air-space pneumonia simulating that caused by *Str. pneumoniae*.[71] Empyema is frequent. The white cell count may be normal or may reveal moderate leukocytosis. The organism may be cultured from the sputum, blood, or pleural fluid.

BORDETELLA (HAEMOPHILUS) PERTUSSIS

This gram-negative organism causes whooping cough (pertussis). Although it has been assumed that this disease was largely eradicated by immunization, recent studies suggest that immunity may not be very long-lasting and that the disease may be occurring in more adults. Pathologically, acute pertussis is characterized by endobronchitis and endobronchiolitis, which may progress to peribronchitis, interstitial pneumonitis, ulceration of the bronchial epithelium, and bronchial obstruction.

In a review of the chest roentgenograms of 556 children with pertussis, Fawcitt and Parry[72] found various combinations of atelectasis, segmental pneumonia, usually in the lower lobes or middle lobe, and hilar lymph node enlargement. A fairly common but not distinctive feature of the pulmonary disease is its tendency to conglomerate contiguous to the heart, obscuring the cardiac borders.

Acute pertussis is commonest in children under 2 years of age. The characteristic clinical picture is of paroxysmal cough ending in a whoop. Adults rarely show the full-blown picture of "whoop" and vomiting, usually manifesting no more than a short-lived mild paroxysmal cough; thus, the condition may be more difficult to diagnose in adults. Acute pertussis engenders moderate to severe lymphocytosis. Diagnosis depends on positive culture from nasopharyngeal swabbing on Bordet-Gengou medium; a fluorescent antibody technique is a useful aid to diagnosis in questionable cases.

It is probable that some cases of "whooping cough" are not caused by the Bordet-Gengou bacillus but by types 1, 2, 3, or 5 adenovirus.[73, 74]

FRANCISELLA TULARENSIS

Francisella tularensis is responsible for tularemia, a disease that is commonest in rodents and small mammals; insects act as both reservoirs and vectors. The organism is a gram-negative, nonmotile bacillus that grows best on blood glucose–cysteine agar or after inoculation of purulent material into mice. Acute pulmonary tularemia is rare compared to other bacterial pneumonias but has been reported from all areas of the United States, Canada, and Scandinavia. Humans may be infected via various routes: the organism may gain entry through an open sore on one's hands while skinning infected rabbits or muskrats; certain insects (ticks, deer flies, and mosquitoes) may transmit the disease from animal to human through a bite (in addition, the tick may pass the organism on to its offspring); or the disease may be acquired by the ingestion of contaminated meat from infected animals or the inhalation of culture material in the laboratory. The majority of cases in the U.S. have been reported from four states (Missouri, Oklahoma, Arkansas, and Utah), areas in which ticks and deer flies are the predominant vector for tularemia in humans.

Four forms of the disease have been described, depending on pathogenesis: (1) *the ulceroglandular form*, consisting of ulcerated cutaneous lesions and regional lymph node enlargement; (2) *the oculoglandular form;* (3) *the typhoidal form*, which is associated with bacteremia and occurs chiefly following the ingestion of contaminated meat; and (4) *the pulmonary form*, which results from the inhalation of organisms, chiefly by laboratory workers.

Pathologically, the pulmonary form is manifested in the peripheral parenchyma. The regional lymph nodes usually are enlarged and contain abscesses. *Histologically*, there is widespread necrosis surrounded by an inflammatory zone containing mononuclear cells and polymorphonuclear leukocytes. Arteritis and thrombosis are apparent in the pulmonary arteries.

Roentgenographically, the pattern is said to be distinctive: homogeneous consolidation occurs within the substance of any lobe, tends to be oval, and has been likened to an acute lung abscess before cavitation develops. Oval areas of parenchymal consolidation averaging approximately 2 × 8 cm were identified in 15 of 17 cases described by Overholt and his colleagues;[75] in 12 cases the lesions were solitary, without lobar predilection, and in three they were multiple. Hilar lymph node enlargement occurs in 25 to 50 per cent of cases, and pleural effusion occurs with about the same frequency. The hilar node enlargement is characteristically ipsilateral. Cavitation is rare. In contrast to the generally accepted prevalence of an oval homogeneous opacity in tularemia, this "characteristic" pattern was observed in only two of 29 well-documented cases studied by Miller and Bates:[76] the roentgenographic features were highly variable, consisting of bronchopneumonia in 17 cases, hilar adenopathy in 13, pleural effusion in six, consolidation in four, apical "infiltrate" in four, oval opacity in two, mediastinal mass in one, miliary pattern in one, and lung abscess in one. A highly variable pattern was also noted by Rubin in a review of 50 patients with proven pleuropulmonary tularemia.[77]

Tularemia may be suspected first because of occupational exposure: a butcher, a hunter, or a laboratory worker gives a history of recently skinning wild rabbits or muskrats, or a patient reports being bitten recently by a tick. Exposure is followed by the development of peripheral cutaneous ulcers, enlarged draining lymph nodes, acute pulmonary infection, and typhoid-like symptoms. Ulcers range in size from 2.5 to 4.0 cm, and regional lymph nodes may enlarge to 2 to 3 cm. Pneumonia develops in about one-third of patients with the ulceroglandular form of the disease and three-quarters of those with the typhoidal form. The disease should be suspected in any patient with the typical symptoms and signs who lives in or has been exposed recently to an endemic area.

The primary pneumonic form of tularemia is commonest in laboratory workers. Symptoms appear within 1 to 14 days of exposure and consist of high septic fever (temperature usually is over 40° C), chills, malaise, weakness, and headaches. The throat frequently is affected, ranging from simple pharyngitis to ulcerative tonsillitis. Physical findings in the chest are minimal in most patients.

Cultures can be made directly from skin lesions, lymph nodes, or sputum (blood culture findings rarely are positive). Inoculation into mice or guinea pigs produces necrotic foci in the liver, spleen, and lymph nodes, and cultures should be made from these organs on blood glucose–cysteine agar. The white cell count usually is normal or low, but mild leukocytosis may occur; in the series reported by Miller and Bates[76] the leukocyte count was over 10,000 per cu mm in 16 of the 29 patients. Serial agglutination tests, with or without positive cultures, permit positive diagnosis, the antibody titer rising 8 to 10 days after onset of infection.

There is a highly specific tuberculinlike delayed-reaction skin test, which becomes positive during the first week of the disease.

YERSINIA PESTIS

This organism is the cause of plague, which used to occur in worldwide pandemics but has been largely controlled by public health measures. *Yersinia (Pasteurella) pestis* is a short, ovoid, bipolar gram-negative bacillus containing a potent endotoxin; it grows rather slowly on blood agar and is highly virulent in mice and guinea pigs.

Endemic areas still remain in Asia, Africa, and South America. Epidemics in humans usually are preceded by an outbreak of plague in the local rodent population, usually in rats. Fleas (usually the rat flea, *Xenopsylla cheopis*) from infected rodents disseminate the disease in humans: after a blood meal and while still adherent to the host they regurgitate large numbers of bacilli, which give rise within 1 to 5 days to a local lesion, usually on the leg. Regional lymph nodes become enlarged and extremely tender, and the overlying skin becomes firm and purplish. This is known as bubonic plague. Bacteremia and septicemia resulting from these infected buboes may lead to secondary pneumonia; once the organism has gained entry to the lungs the infection can be passed from person to person by airborne transmission.

Pathologically, plague pneumonia is characterized by severe bronchitis and alveolitis; patchy areas of parenchymal disease tend to become confluent, forming large areas of nonsegmental homogeneous consolidation. Microscopically, severe hemorrhagic pulmonary edema is seen, the alveolar exudate containing polymorphonuclear leukocytes, macrophages, and many organisms; hyaline membranes may be present.

Roentgenographically, the pattern is one of nonsegmental, homogeneous, parenchymal consolidation, which may be extensive and occasionally simulates diffuse bilateral pulmonary edema but does not cavitate. In a recent review of 42 proved cases in New Mexico,[78] the roentgenographic manifestations in the more severely involved patients simulated disseminated intravascular coagulation or ARDS; it was emphasized that in an endemic area and in the proper clinical setting, patients with this type of roentgenographic abnormality should be considered to have pneumonic plague until proved otherwise by epidemiologic studies. Pleural effusion may be present. Roentgenographic manifestations within the thorax may be restricted to hilar and paratracheal lymph node enlargement.

Until the advent of antibiotics, plague pneumonia was invariably fatal within 2 to 4 days. Antibiotic therapy now results in complete resolution in the majority of cases. Bubonic plague should be suspected from the combination of confluent pneumonia, enlarged mediastinal lymph nodes, tender enlarged peripheral lymph nodes, and a history of contact with rats in an endemic area. Primary pneumonic plague is fulminating, with high fever, dyspnea, cyanosis, and a rapid downhill course. Cough and the expectoration of bloody, frothy material may occur. Pleural pain is common.

The diagnosis can be established by culture of the sputum, blood, or material aspirated from an enlarged lymph node; similarly, mouse or guinea pig inoculation provokes a diagnostic reaction. Most patients have mild to moderate leukocytosis. Antibodies are present during the second week of the illness and may be demonstrated by agglutination or complement-fixation tests.

PASTEURELLA MULTOCIDA

This organism usually affects domestic, farm, and wild animals, which may rarely infect humans through a bite or scratch. *P. multocida* (*P. septica*) is a small, gram-negative, bipolar staining nonmotile rod which grows slowly on ordinary media.

When isolated in humans, the organism is usually in the sputum of patients with bronchiectasis; thus the roentgenographic features are nonspecific. The diagnosis can be made by culture of a heavy growth of the organism from patients with chronic lung disease who have a history of close contact with dogs, cats, cattle, or sheep.[79]

BRUCELLA SPECIES

Brucella organisms (*B. melitensis, B. abortus, B. suis*) rarely cause pneumonia. In a recent study of 160 patients with brucellosis who worked in an Iowa abattoir, none showed roentgenographic abnormality of lungs or pleura, although 23 per cent complained of cough.

Brucella organisms are gram-negative rods that require exposure to 10 per cent carbon dioxide for culture. The species can be differentiated biochemically and serologically. *Brucella* organisms may penetrate the abraded skin, be absorbed after ingestion, or inhaled.

Symptoms of brucellosis include musculoskeletal pain, sweats, chills, and malaise. Splenomegaly and peripheral lymph node enlargement are found in 50 per cent of patients. The white cell count is normal or low. Agglutination and skin tests are dependable and specific.

OTHER PNEUMONIAS CAUSED BY AEROBIC BACTERIA

NEISSERIA MENINGITIDIS

In recent years it has been suggested that this large, gram-negative coccus often is not recognized now as the etiologic agent in pneumonia because it is eradicated rapidly by antibiotics and is difficult to culture from expectorated material. It can be isolated from the blood of patients with pneumonia without meningitis or, in patients with negative blood cultures, from transtracheal aspirates. Y is the serotype most commonly found. Most cases have occurred in adults with clinical, cultural, or serologic evidence of prior adenovirus[80] or influenza virus infection.

The published reproductions of chest roentgenograms show a pattern of acute air-space pneumonia, although some are described as segmental in distribution. Cavitation has not been described, but bilateral pulmonary disease and pleural effusion may occur.

Young adults in military service appear to be most susceptible to primary meningococcal pneumonia, perhaps because of their close contact with carriers of *N. meningitidis* and the greater likelihood of their acquiring adenoviral or influenza virus infections. The typical history is of gradually increasing fever for 2 to 3 weeks, followed by pleural pain.[80]

LEPTOSPIROSIS

The spirochete serotypes responsible for most cases of this infection include *Leptospira icterohaemorrhagiae, L. canicola, L. pomona, and L. autumnalis.* A 1973 report described approximately 60 per cent of cases of leptospirosis as occurring in children, students, and housewives, and only 16.7 per cent in patients occupationally exposed.[81] This may reflect increasingly frequent acquisition of the disease from family pets.[81] Although pulmonary involvement in leptospirosis is overshadowed by the more dramatic symptoms and signs of kidney and liver failure, roentgenographically evident pneumonia was present in 39 (11 per cent) of 345 cases in one series.[82] The pattern has been described as peripheral, nonsegmental, patchy or diffuse air-space consolidation, without pleural effusion or hilar enlargement; pathologic correlation has shown that this represents hemorrhage and edema without inflammation.

The clinical manifestations include headache, muscular pain, chills, nausea, and vomiting, pyuria and hematuria, jaundice, and hepatomegaly. Respiratory symptoms include cough, occasional hemoptysis, and chest pain (which may be more muscular than pleural in origin).[82] Signs of meningitis, usually aseptic, may be evident, and in severe cases hemorrhage may occur into the GI tract or skin.

Leptospirosis may be suspected from the clinical picture and information that house pets have been exposed to rats. Diagnosis is confirmed by the culture of organisms from blood and urine and by serologic testing.

PNEUMONIA CAUSED BY ANAEROBIC ORGANISMS

Anaerobic pulmonary infections are less common now, as a result of improved oral hygiene. Nevertheless, increasing attention has been paid to this entity in recent years because of improved diagnostic techniques. New culture methods have been formulated,[83] and contamination of specimens by oropharyngeal microorganisms can now be avoided by transtracheal aspiration (TTA). TTA and modern culture techniques have established that anaerobic lung infection has characteristic features that should permit confident diagnosis on clinical grounds alone. It is important that the physician be familiar with this clinical picture, to avoid falsely attributing the etiology to commensal microorganisms reported on aerobic cultures, and to obviate the requirements for TTA with its inherent potential complications.[84]

Anaerobic pulmonary infection is referred to by some as "aspiration pneumonia,"[83] a term also used to describe pulmonary disease resulting from aspiration of gastric juice or solid particles of vomit. To avoid this semantic confusion, we recommend returning to basic descriptive terminology, calling anaerobic infection of the lungs simply "anaerobic pneumonia" (with or without cavitation).

Bartlett and Finegold[85] differentiate between pneumonitis and abscess formation (single or multiple), with or without empyema, in their description of anaerobic infections of the lung and pleura. In our opinion the formation of cavities and the development of empyema represent stages in the natural history of untreated anaerobic pulmonary disease and any attempt to separate these entities serves little purpose.

Anaerobic organisms may be considered pathogenic only if isolated from a closed space such as the pleural or peritoneal cavities, subcutaneous or intra-abdominal abscesses, the blood, or the trachea (by TTA). Positive cultures from these sources usually reveal mixed anaerobes, alone or with aerobes, and only rarely is a pure culture of a single anaerobe obtained. Anaerobic lung infection may develop as a result of aspiration from the oropharynx, or in association with bacteremia (if the latter, the source of infection is usually the gastrointestinal tract or, in females, the genitourinary tract).

In cases of pneumonia caused by aspiration of organisms from the oropharynx in which contamination of the specimen can be excluded, the chief anaerobes are *Fusobacterium nucleatum*, *Bacteroides melaninogenicus*, peptostreptococci, peptococci, and the anaerobic, non-spore-forming gram-positive *Eubacterium* bacilli;[86] less common are *B. fragilis* and microaerophilic streptococci.[83] In such cases the flora are usually polymicrobial, averaging three bacterial species per case. In more than 50 per cent of cases the isolates are exclusively anaerobic.[85, 86]

By contrast, the commonest anaerobe on blood culture in cases of bacteremia is *B. fragilis*. *Bacteroides* bacteremia usually is associated with abdominal surgery or gynecologic and obstetric conditions.

Anaerobic bacteria commonly are isolated from empyemas and, when proper precautions are taken, have been demonstrated to be a common cause of acute purulent sinusitis.[87]

The *pathologic* findings of anaerobic bacterial pneumonia are acute inflammation and necrosis involving air spaces and bronchi.

Roentgenographically, the distribution of pneumonia from inhalation of anaerobically infected material reflects gravitational flow, affecting posterior segments of the upper lobes or superior segments of the lower lobes (aspiration in the recumbent position), or basal segments of the lower lobes (aspiration when erect). The right lung is affected approximately twice as often as the left. Tracheobronchial deposition of anaerobic organisms results in segmental homogeneous consolidation and in some instances in a peripheral mass. In a recent review of the roentgenographic findings in 69 patients with bacteriologically proven anaerobic infections in the thorax,[88] the initial radiographs showed the disease to be confined to the lung parenchyma in 50 per cent and to the pleura in 30 per cent of patients; the remaining 20 per cent had combined pleural and parenchymal disease. Over 50 per cent of the cases with pneumonia showed abscess formation on the initial presentation. Pleural effusion tended to

progress very rapidly and always proved to be empyema. Many empyemas occurred without recognizable pneumonia. In occasional cases, the characteristic pattern of pulmonary gangrene is evident as a more or less homogeneous mass within a large cavity.

Clinically, in contrast to the acute fulminating aerobic pneumonias, pulmonary disease from aspirated infectious anaerobes has a protracted, insidious course. The mean duration of symptoms before admission to hospital appears to be from two to three weeks,[85, 86] although in some cases it may be several months.[83] Male patients outnumber females in a ratio of 3:1. Many are alcoholics or epileptics with poor oral hygiene, accounting for the location of the disease in most instances in regions most accessible to gravitational flow in the recumbent position. When looked for, peridontitis and gingivitis are found in two-thirds of patients with lung abscesses. Dyphagia also may be a predisposing cause, commonly in association with multiple sclerosis, vascular or malignant brain disease, and esophageal disease.

Patients with anaerobic pulmonary infection may be virtually asymptomatic. The majority do not appear seriously ill when first seen, although in occasional patients the disease runs a fulminant course leading to death. Fever occurs in 70 to 80 per cent of cases. Cough is usual and often is productive of purulent material, the amount of which increases with abscess formation and cavitation. Putrid expectoration has been reported in 40 to 75 per cent of cases, starting 7 to 10 days or more after the onset of infection and most often when discharge from cavitary lesions is profuse.[83] Foul-smelling sputum always indicates anaerobic organisms. Pleural pain occurs in approximately 50 per cent of cases and hemoptysis in 25 per cent, the latter not necessarily in association with purulent expectoration. Physical findings are those of pneumonia. Clubbing is common when the infection is chronic and insidious.

In contrast to inhalation anaerobic infection, *Bacteroides* bacteremia commonly occurs in already ill patients. Leukocytosis is common in aspiration anaerobic pneumonias and lung abscesses, ranging in one series[83] from 7800 to 32,000 per cu mm (mean peak, 17,000). Anemia, which commonly accompanies weight loss, further testifies to the frequent chronicity of this infection.[85]

The diagnosis of anaerobic infection of the lung is based on finding an insidious infection in a patient with poor oral hygiene, cough productive of blood with or without putrid material, and a clinical history leading to a suspicion of aspiration. Roentgenographic visualization of lung abscess in the posterior segments of a lung strongly supports the diagnosis. Sputum smears are probably of more value than sputum cultures and reveal large numbers of microorganisms. Cultures of blood and pleural effusion are important. Although in the absence of a positive culture of blood or pleural fluid a definitive diagnosis can be made only with TTA, we consider that this invasive procedure seldom is indicated, since anaerobic infections respond to penicillin therapy even when the organisms isolated include *B. fragilis*.

Penicillin should be given in moderate doses over a prolonged period, usually for 2 months. With response to therapy cavity closure occurs steadily but may take many months to complete.

MYCOBACTERIAL INFECTIONS OF THE LUNGS

Various species of the genus *Mycobacterium* can cause disease of the lungs and pleura, and by far the most important of these is *M. tuberculosis*, which is responsible for 95 to 99 per cent of pulmonary mycobacterial infections. With the control of *M. tuberculosis* and the improvement in methods of culture in recent years, several other nontuberculous mycobacteria have been recognized as infrequent causes of pulmonary disease. The pathologic and roentgenographic changes they produce are virtually identical to those of *M. tuberculosis*.

MYCOBACTERIUM TUBERCULOSIS

EPIDEMIOLOGY

Although according to the U.S. National Tuberculosis Association any mycobacterial disease of the lungs other than that caused by *M. leprae* can be designated as tuberculosis, the term usually implies and sometimes is restricted to infections caused by *M. tuberculosis*. Tuberculosis is worldwide in distribution but occurs most often in conditions of crowding and poverty. At the turn of the century it was the commonest cause of death in the United States, but the subsequent progress in both diagnosis and therapy has greatly reduced both the rate of infection and the mortality, particularly the latter. The true magnitude of the impact of tuberculosis on society is more clearly evi-

denced by a consideration of the situation in countries such as India. Whereas less than 20 per cent of the U.S. population in 1965 had positive tuberculin skin tests, in India 27 per cent of children under the age of 5 years are positive reacters and 90 per cent of the 40-year-olds are strong reactors to tuberculin. Of even greater significance is the observation that 1.5 per cent of the population of India is estimated to have tuberculosis on the basis of roentgenographic abnormalities in the chest.

Although active pulmonary tuberculosis may develop at any age, infants, pubertal adolescents, and the aged are particularly susceptible. Negroes appear much more susceptible to infection than Caucasians. In women the incidence tends to level off or even fall slightly after the childbearing period, whereas in men it increases gradually into the late fifties. In recent years the older male has been recognized as a frequent source of tuberculous infection. Undoubtedly these patients represent the survivors of a child population that was heavily infected early in the twentieth century and is now showing endogenous reactivation of the disease. Studies in a number of major U.S. cities categorized the patient with active tuberculosis in the 1970's as a male at the bottom of the socioeconomic scale, between 35 and 65 years of age, living alone or homeless, and probably an alcoholic, who has failed to complete an adequate course of prescribed chemotherapy. A greater incidence of infection and active disease also is found in certain ethnic groups, such as among recent Asian immigrants. The likelihood of nurses and other hospital employees acquiring infection has been greatly reduced in recent years. In a study of active tuberculosis in hospital employees in Ontario during 1966 to 1969, Ashley and Wigle[89] found a very low morbidity rate in student nurses, active disease occurring largely in foreign-born students who had lived in Canada for less than 5 years; most of these had a positive tuberculin reaction at the time of employment and undoubtedly represented examples of reactivation of prior infection rather than new infection from contact with patients.

PATHOGENESIS

Mycobacteria are aerobic, nonmotile rods. They possess an affinity for certain aniline dyes (particularly carbol-fuchsin) which are not removed on exposure to acid—thus, they are acid-fast. Enrichment of ordinary laboratory media with egg, potato, blood, or albumin is required to produce growth on culture. Growth is slow, taking 2 to 8 weeks. Humans acquire pulmonary tuberculosis by inhalation of droplets carrying this organism. In most cases, this means repeated or constant contact with a person who has cavitary disease and whose sputum is highly positive for the bacilli. The organisms are phagocytosed by alveolar macrophages, but many remain viable and may even multiply within these cells. Bacilli spread through the lymphatic channels and bloodstream to more distant sites, where they replicate until overcome by host defense mechanisms. In the majority of patients immunity prevents multiplication and symptoms do not develop, but in those with inadequate immune mechanisms the active disease can develop, usually in the upper lobes (progressive primary tuberculosis). Others who are infected may remain asymptomatic for years before reactivation develops in an old focus of primary infection (postprimary or reactivation tuberculosis).

Most active disease in adults represents reactivation of an endogenous focus acquired in childhood, although occasionally an exogenous source causes superinfection which overwhelms the immunity acquired from earlier tuberculous infection.

ALLERGY AND IMMUNITY

Reaction of the body to the tubercle bacillus depends upon the host's natural immunity, tissue hypersensitivity, and acquired immunity. The tissues of a person never previously infected show an entirely different response to tuberculoprotein than those of a previously infected person who is "reinfected," either from reactivation of dormant bacilli within his or her body or, rarely, from an exogenous source. These differences are governed by the still vague and controversial properties of allergy and immunity in relation to tuberculoprotein.

If a person or an appropriate animal is infected with tubercle bacilli or is vaccinated with attenuated organisms such as BCG (bacillus Calmette-Guérin), the tissues become sensitive to the protein (tuberculin) of the organism: this represents *hypersensitivity* or *allergy*. When such a person or animal is later injected with tuberculoprotein,* edema develops (with or

without erythema) at the site of the intradermal injection; this area, which measures 10 mm or more in diameter, indicates reaction to the organism. Some authorities believe that acquired immunity is just another manifestation of delayed hypersensitivity. Others[90] contend that delayed hypersensitivity and immunity to tuberculosis are different responses to various components of the tubercle bacillus. In contrast to the nonimmunized, the immunized host resists infection through increased bactericidal action of activated macrophages, which prevent multiplication of tubercle bacilli within the phagocytes. These macrophages are activated by lymphocytes sensitized to specific antigen (in this case, tubercle bacillus). Chemical mediators (lymphokines) capable of enhancing the bactericidal properties of macrophages can be extracted *in vitro* from the supernatant fluid of lymphocytes from immunized animals stimulated with PPD. The production of various chemical mediators from lymphocytes, including the lymphokines presumed responsible for delayed hypersensitivity and immunity and the specific and nonspecific cytotoxins of sensitized lymphocytes, suggests a multiplicity of T cell (and B cell?) activities responsible for the cellular-type immune responses associated with both hypersensitivity and immunity.

The tissue response in patients sensitized by previous infection or vaccination is "caseous necrosis." Although this reaction is usually considered allergic in type, it also destroys numerous mycobacteria, thus providing a useful defensive role. This property of sensitivity and immunity acquired from previous infection also appears to act by localizing the disease process.

The mechanism of acquired immunity in tuberculosis and its relationship to allergy is still not clear, and even less is known about the property of *natural resistance* to tuberculous infections. It seems that natural resistance to tuberculosis is considerably greater in whites than in blacks, and appears to vary with age, since infants and pubertal adolescents are more prone to the infection.

Since patients exposed for the first time have pathologic, roentgenologic, and clinical features different from those who are superinfected or have reactivation of previous disease, it is logical to consider the disease processes under the separate headings of "primary tuberculosis" and "postprimary tuberculosis." It should be remembered, however, that the pathologically and roentgenologically apparent changes produced by postprimary tuberculosis are conditioned by allergy and acquired immunity; since these qualities of tissue reaction develop within

*PPD (purified protein derivative), prepared from a single strain of *M. tuberculosis* and precipitated with ammonium sulfate; or OT (old tuberculin), prepared by heat sterilization of cultures of tubercle bacilli in liquid medium and subsequent evaporation of the filtrate to one-tenth its volume.

4 to 6 weeks after primary infection, the post-primary type of response may occur from the primary infection itself if this is not promptly checked by the body's natural defense mechanisms. Progression of the primary complex to chronic destructive or postprimary tuberculosis without a latent interval has been called progressive primary tuberculosis.[91]

PRIMARY PULMONARY TUBERCULOSIS

Primary pulmonary tuberculosis occurs predominantly in children and is particularly prevalent in geographic areas in which control measures are inadequate. However, since reduction in the incidence of the disease is resulting in an ever-increasing nonsensitized population, this form of disease is becoming much commoner in adults.

PATHOLOGIC CHARACTERISTICS

The reaction to the tubercle bacillus in a previously uninfected host depends upon both the number of organisms aspirated and the inherent resistance of the host. The initial reaction is exudative and consists of dilation of capillaries, swelling of endothelial and alveolar lining cells, and an outpouring of fibrin, macrophages, and polymorphonuclear leukocytes into the alveolar spaces. With the onset of hypersensitivity—2 to 10 weeks after initial infection—caseous necrosis develops in the center of the lesion. Coincident with caseation (which tends to remain solid), the numerous microorganisms present during the exudative phase tend to disappear. Once caseation has occurred healing begins, with invasion by fibroblasts, progressive hyalinization, and, if the lesion is sufficiently large, calcification and occasionally ossification.

Extension of the parenchymal infection to regional lymph nodes via lymphatic channels is common, so that their enlargement is a frequent manifestation; organisms from the involved nodes may gain access to the bloodstream. Hematogenous dissemination probably is common, but in most cases the full-blown clinical picture of miliary or extrapulmonary tuberculosis is prevented by the limited number of organisms and the host's natural immunity.

The disease may spread into the pleural or pericardial cavities from caseous foci in lung parenchyma adjacent to these serous membranes. Lymphatic spread may occur from the pleura, usually to the upper lumbar vertebrae.

In a minority of patients, primary disease may progress directly to a chronic destructive form of postprimary tuberculosis.

ROENTGENOGRAPHIC MANIFESTATIONS

Primary tuberculous infection within the thorax usually affects one or more of four structures—the pulmonary parenchyma, the mediastinal and hilar lymph nodes, the tracheobronchial tree, and the pleura. In 1968, Weber and associates[92] reported a detailed analysis of the roentgenologic changes of primary tuberculosis in a 6-year study. Of 235 children with primary tuberculosis admitted to a large sanatorium in Massachusetts, 85 had positive cultures for M. tuberculosis; chest roentgenograms of 83 were available for analysis.

Parenchymal Involvement

In Weber and coworkers'[92] study, the upper lobes were affected slightly more often than the lower, but there were no significant differences between left and right lungs or between anterior and posterior segments. The parenchymal reaction typically is that of air-space consolidation, ranging in diameter from 1 to 7 cm (Figure 6–9). The consolidation tends to be homogeneous in density and to have ill-defined margins, except where it abuts against a fissure. Parenchymal involvement in primary disease in adults appears to differ little from that seen in children.

Cavitation is a rare manifestation of pulmonary tuberculosis in infants and children, at least in Caucasians living in communities where they have long been exposed to the tubercle bacillus; for example, Weber and associates[92] observed only one instance of cavitation in the 83 children they studied. Fulminating disease and cavitation are much commoner in infants and children raised in communities in which tuberculosis has been introduced comparatively recently and who are unable to localize the primary lesion.

Lymph Node Involvement

Hilar or paratracheal lymph node enlargement is the roentgenographic finding that clearly differentiates primary from postprimary tuberculosis. Of the 83 cases of primary tuberculosis studied by Weber and his colleagues,[92] 80 showed clear roentgenographic evidence of hilar or paratracheal lymph node enlargement, or both. In 13 of the 80 cases, node enlargement

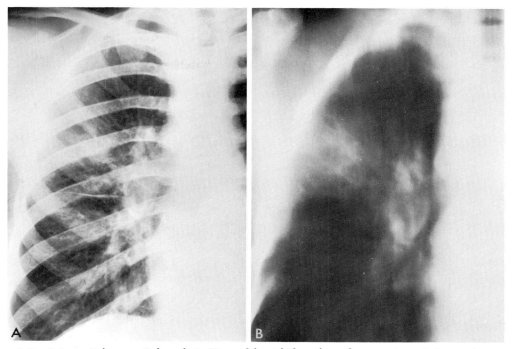

Figure 6–9.   Primary Pulmonary Tuberculosis. Views of the right hemithorax from a posteroanterior roentgenogram (*A*) and an anteroposterior tomogram (*B*) reveal relatively homogeneous consolidation of the axillary zone of the right upper lobe, seen to better advantage in the tomogram. There is enlargement of the right bronchopulmonary lymph nodes and of the tracheobronchial (azygos) node. This 19-year-old man had noted increasing weakness during the previous month, with recurrent right-sided chest pain for 2 weeks; *M. tuberculosis* was recovered from the sputum.

was bilateral and hilar, in 34 it was predominantly unilateral and hilar, and in 33 it was unilateral and both hilar and paratracheal, predominantly on the right side.

Although lymph node enlargement as a manifestation of primary tuberculosis is much more common in children, it can also be the presenting roentgenographic abnormality in adults, particularly in young black women.[93–95] Of the 33 patients studied by Dhand and associates,[93] the node enlargement was bilateral paratracheal in 75 per cent, unilateral hilar in 45 per cent, combined paratracheal and hilar in 48 per cent, and bilateral hilar in 15 per cent. Positive diagnosis requires lymph node biopsy in the majority of cases, particularly because of possible confusion with sarcoidosis.

Airway Involvement

Tracheobronchial disease is common and usually the result of compression of bronchi by enlarged lymph nodes; less commonly, tuberculous granulation tissue may accumulate in the bronchial mucosa and be visible at bronchoscopy. Weber and his coworkers[92] identified tracheobronchial changes in 23 (28 per cent) of

their 85 patients and atelectasis in 25 (30 per cent). Atelectasis in primary tuberculosis characteristically affects the anterior segment of an upper lobe or the medial segment of the middle lobe. This distribution probably reflects the anatomic relationships of lymph nodes to the bronchial tree on the right side. Provided that bronchial occlusion has not persisted too long, perforation of a lymph node into the bronchial tree usually causes the atelectasis to disappear, presumably by relieving the compression.[96]

Although transient bacteremia is common, it is rarely accompanied by evidence of miliary spread. Clinically and roentgenologically diagnosed hematogenous dissemination was found in only two (2.5 per cent) of 83 patients reported by Weber and his colleagues.[92] The great majority of children and adults have neither symptoms nor roentgenographic signs of disease after initial exposure to tubercle bacilli, the sole evidence of infection being a positive tuberculin test. In the small proportion with roentgenographic evidence of the disease, this usually clears within 6 months to 2 years after institution of therapy. Complete resolution without residua is roentgenographically apparent in the majority of cases: only 15 (32 per cent) of the

47 patients who were followed up long enough by Weber and associates[92] had residual scarring. Decrease in size of enlarged lymph nodes usually parallels resolution of the pulmonary lesions. Despite clearing of the active parenchymal infection, however, in some cases atelectasis remains, owing to residual lymph node enlargement.

Pleural Involvement

Pleural effusion as a manifestation of primary tuberculosis occurs more commonly in adults than in children. Weber and coworkers[92] observed effusion in only 10 per cent of their child patients.

Calcification

Calcification in both pulmonary lesions and lymph nodes was surprisingly uncommon in Weber and his colleagues' series of 85 children with bacteriologically proved primary pulmonary tuberculosis.[92] Of the 58 patients with adequate follow-up, calcification occurred in the pulmonary lesion in only 10 (17 per cent) and in the lymph nodes in 21 (36 per cent). If these figures are truly representative, it is apparent how seldom chest roentgenography can detect the primary Ranke complex, indicating previous tuberculous infection.

CLINICAL MANIFESTATIONS

Very few patients with primary pulmonary tuberculosis have clinical evidence of the disease. Symptoms are seldom striking, consisting of fever, cough, anorexia, weight loss, excessive perspiration, chest pain, lethargy, and dyspnea. More severe symptoms may develop as a result of complications or of progressive primary disease in patients with impaired resistance (as in infants or in patients with other illnesses); the more severe symptoms and signs may be due to spread of the disease to extrathoracic locations, including (rarely) the meninges. Involvement of extrathoracic structures by tuberculosis is not necessarily accompanied by roentgenographic abnormality in the chest. In studies of children with tuberculous meningitis, the chest roentgenogram was normal in 43 per cent of 180 cases (only 23 per cent had roentgenographic evidence of miliary tuberculosis).[97]

In a small minority of children and perhaps more commonly in adults, primary pulmonary tuberculosis may progress to the clinical and roentgenographic picture of the postprimary disease. The local exudative lesion may increase to form large, homogeneous areas of consolidation, which may cavitate, or the primary exudative focus may shrink while other lesions develop elsewhere in the lungs, usually the apical segments.[91]

POSTPRIMARY TUBERCULOSIS

Postprimary or "reactivation" tuberculosis is used to describe a clinical and roentgenographic pattern of disease that can be correlated pathogenetically with acquired hypersensitivity and immunity. Nearly all cases of postprimary tuberculosis occur in adults either as a result of reactivation of a focus of infection acquired in childhood or as an initial infection from virulent organisms in individuals vaccinated with BCG. A minority of cases represent continuation of the active disease since the original infection, the postprimary pattern becoming evident with the attainment of cell-mediated immunity. Even less commonly, postprimary tuberculosis is exogenous superinfection on an inactive or even active original infection—true reinfection.

PATHOLOGIC CHARACTERISTICS

The morphologic appearance of postprimary tuberculosis differs considerably from that of primary disease in that the tissue reaction appears directed toward localizing the infection and destroying the tubercle bacilli causing it. The disease tends to be limited mainly to the apical and posterior segments of the upper and the superior segment of the lower lobes. Histologically, the exudative phase consists of foci of caseous necrosis with surrounding edema, hemorrhage, and mononuclear cell infiltration. These caseous foci may liquefy and empty into a bronchus, disseminating tubercle bacilli through the airways into other areas of the lungs, giving rise to a multitude of small foci of air-space disease roentgenologically visible as acinar shadows. Caseous necrosis and subsequent cavity formation probably result from sensitivity to tuberculoprotein.[98] Like caseous necrosis, the *tubercle* is a hallmark of postprimary tuberculosis. Tubercles, which usually develop at the periphery of a necrotic lesion, are accumulations of mononuclear macrophages that have swollen and become pale (epithelioid cells). Also, Langhans' giant cells, which develop in the margins of tubercles, are believed to originate from mononuclear macrophages. The tubercle is surrounded by lymphocytes, fibroblasts, and collagenous tissue. Although necrosis is not necessarily seen in all granulomas, central caseation inevitably develops with time. In fulminating disease, the exudative lesion predominates and the picture may be one of acute tuberculous pneumonia with consolidation of an entire lobe. More commonly the pattern is one of progressive disease, presumably as a result of dissemination of liquefied caseous material within the airways.

Healing occurs by fibrosis and contracture. The terms "fibrocaseous" and "productive" tuberculosis denote cavitation with surrounding thickened fibrotic walls, slow formation of tubercles, and fibrotic replacement. Examination of resected lungs at necropsy reveals some degree of healing in almost all cases of postprimary tuberculosis, even when the disease is progressing in other areas. Commonly, fibroblasts slowly invade the areas of caseous necrosis and around them, reducing the extent of involvement and walling off the caseous foci, preventing dissemination via the airways. Calcium deposits in caseous foci are less common in postprimary than in primary tuberculosis. Since viable tubercle bacilli may be recovered from calcified lesions, calcification is no proof of cure. Chemotherapy tends to accelerate healing and, in fact, the roentgenographic disappearance of acute exudative disease may be so rapid as to simulate resolution of nontuberculous pneumonia. Open cavities often contain no viable organisms; the relapse rate of these "open negative" cavities is virtually nil with modern chemotherapy.

ROENTGENOGRAPHIC MANIFESTATIONS

Anatomic Distribution

A characteristic although not unique manifestation of postprimary tuberculosis is a tendency to localize in the apical and posterior segments of the upper lobes. It has been postulated that this location relates to the high Po_2 in these zones, the result of high ventilation-perfusion ratios. Postprimary tuberculosis rarely is situated *solely* in an anterior segment of an upper lobe, a useful clue in differentiating tuberculosis from other granulomatous diseases, such as histoplasmosis, which often affect the anterior segment. The right lung is involved more often than the left. The lower lobes are affected in 7 per cent or less of patients with active tuber-culosis. Disease of the lower lobe basal bronchopulmonary segments tends to predominate in women, particularly in pregnant women, and in Negroes and diabetics. This may represent primary rather than postprimary tuberculosis. Women thus affected tend to be in the younger age group, and in an unusually high percentage of cases the disease is complicated by cavitation.

Caution should be used in labeling tuberculous foci as active or inactive. We prefer to use qualifying phrases such as "having the appearance of" or "compatible with," terms that connote the element of fallibility so often innate in roentgenologic interpretation.

Several roentgenographic patterns can be identified in postprimary tuberculosis and any one case may show one or more of these patterns; they include local exudative lesions, local fibroproductive lesions, cavitation, bronchogenic spread and acute tuberculous pneumonia, miliary tuberculosis, bronchiectasis, bronchostenosis, tuberculoma, and tuberculous pleurisy and empyema (the last named are discussed in Chapter 15).

Local Exudative Tuberculosis

The roentgenographic pattern is of air-space (acinar) consolidation, patchy or confluent in nature, in specific anatomic regions—apical and posterior segments of an upper lobe or the superior segment of a lower lobe. Individual shadows commonly are indistinctly defined and homogeneous. There is frequently an accentuation of the drainage markings toward the ipsilateral hilum. Cavitation may be present (Figure 6–10). Lymph node enlargement is not a feature. The shadows may disappear rapidly following the institution of chemotherapy or, if the disease is untreated, may progress to acute tuberculous pneumonia. Even with inadequate therapy, exudative lesions may regress but become "productive" or "fibroproductive."

Local Fibroproductive Tuberculosis

The relatively poor definition of the exudative lesion is replaced by a more sharply circumscribed shadow, usually somewhat irregular and angular in contour. Although the shadow may be homogeneous, its density is no greater than that of the exudative lesion—thus, the terms "soft" and "hard" to describe the shadows of pulmonary tuberculosis are meaningless. Caseation necrosis becomes evident only when necrotic material calcifies or is expelled into an

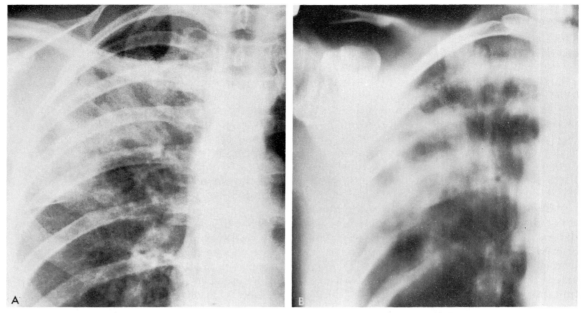

Figure 6–10. Exudative Pulmonary Tuberculosis with Cavitation. Views of the upper half of the right hemithorax from a posteroanterior roentgenogram (*A*) and an anteroposterior tomogram (*B*) show inhomogeneous consolidation of much of the right upper lobe. A fairly large cavity is present, possessing a smooth, although somewhat nodular inner lining. This 28-year-old woman had had the abrupt onset of symptoms suggesting acute pneumonia approximately 1 week prior to these studies; *Mycobacterium tuberculosis* was isolated from the sputum.

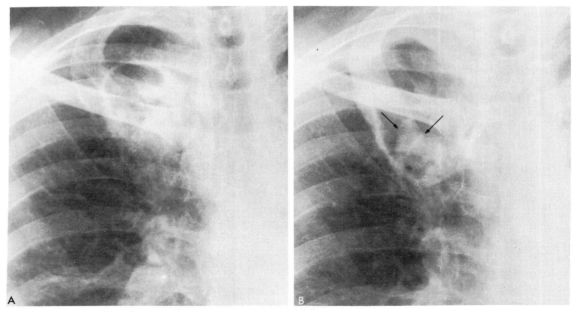

Figure 6–11. Tuberculous Cavitation: Mycetoma. A view of the upper half of the right lung from a posteroanterior roentgenogram (*A*) shows a well-defined cavitary lesion measuring approximately 4 cm in diameter. The wall of the cavity is thin but sharply circumscribed. An air-fluid level is not present. Sputum culture was positive. Six weeks later (*B*), the cavity is much larger and now relates to the apical and mediastinal pleura; its wall is somewhat thicker, particularly inferiorly and laterally. A well-defined intracavitary structure can now be identified (*arrows*) which on further study was seen to move freely within the cavity. Proved mycetoma or intracavitary fungus ball in a tuberculous cavity. Increase in the thickness of a cavity wall has been reported to occur frequently in association with a developing mycetoma.

airway and produces a cavity. The latter may occur even in a lesion that roentgenographically appears largely "fibrotic." Healing occurs by replacement of the tuberculous granulation tissue by fibrous tissue; the resultant cicatrization may result in considerable loss of volume. If the volume of affected lung is sufficient, compensatory signs of loss of volume become evident in elevation of the ipsilateral hilum, overinflation of the rest of the affected lung, and in some cases in bulla formation.

Cavitation

When lysis of semisolid caseous material occurs—through some process as yet unknown—the liquefied caseous material may be expelled from the center of the lesion into the bronchial tree, with resultant cavity formation. The evacuated material may be expectorated in the sputum or aspirated into other bronchial segments. The wall of an untreated tuberculous cavity is moderately thick, and its inner surface usually is fairly smooth (Figure 6–11). An air-fluid level seldom is seen. With adequate therapy, a cavity may disappear; sometimes its wall becomes paper thin but it remains an air-filled cystic space. Such persistent cavitation after chemotherapy does not necessarily indicate active disease. Tomography may be of value in identifying cavities, even those not suspected on plain roentgenograms. Caseous material in a tuberculous focus may simulate cavitation roentgenographically, because of its high lipid content and the fact that its density is slightly less than that of the cavity wall (so-called pseudocavitation).

Bronchogenic Spread and Acute Tuberculous Pneumonia

When caseation necrosis liquefies and communicates with the bronchial tree, infective material may disseminate widely to other bronchial segments and establish new foci of infection in the same lobe or in other lobes of either lung. Characteristically, such dissemination leads to the formation of multiple small shadows whose appearance is typical of acinar shadows, an appearance that in our experience is almost pathognomonic of bronchogenic spread of tuberculosis. Extension of the disease through surrounding air spaces may result in acute confluent air-space pneumonia, indistinguishable from that caused by *Streptococcus pneumo-*

niae. Clues to tuberculosis as the cause are the finding of an open cavity in that or the other lung, or of fairly discrete acinar shadows in parts of the lung remote from the massive consolidation. We have never seen the latter in acute air-space pneumonia of other etiology.

Miliary Tuberculosis

Although hematogenous dissemination of tubercle bacilli throughout the body is common in primary tuberculosis, there is seldom clinical or roentgenographic evidence of miliary spread or multiple organ involvement, presumably because of the resistance of the host and the small number of bacilli causing the bacteremia. If large numbers of tubercle bacilli enter the bloodstream, however, there is widespread invasion of tissues and organs. In the lung this is manifested by tiny discrete foci, widely and uniformly distributed throughout both lungs (Figure 6–12). The interval between dissemination and the development of roentgenographic evidence of disease probably is 6 weeks or more, during which time the foci are too small for roentgenographic visualization. When first visible they measure little more than 1 mm in diameter; in the absence of adequate therapy they may reach 2 to 3 mm before the patient dies.

With appropriate treatment, clearing may be extremely rapid, sometimes even faster than in nonhematogenous pulmonary tuberculosis. Resolution is usually complete, without residua, the chest roentgenogram returning to normal in the majority of cases by 16 weeks.[99] Without treatment, the major cause of death is respiratory failure. Although the development of the adult respiratory distress syndrome is not widely recognized as a complication of miliary tuberculosis, it has been shown that the prompt institution of antituberculous therapy can result in a reversal of the respiratory failure and eventual cure.[100]

Although the source of dissemination of tubercle bacilli usually is apparent clinically or roentgenographically (Figure 6–12), in some cases of miliary tuberculosis the primary focus is not obvious, even at necropsy.[99]

Tuberculous Bronchiectasis

Two mechanisms may give rise to tuberculous bronchiectasis: (1) the bronchial wall is infected during active disease, and the fibrosis and ci-

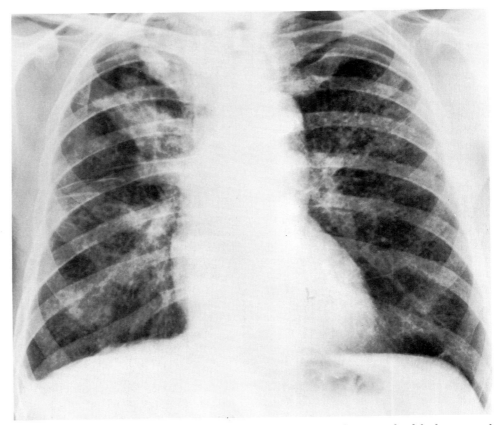

Figure 6–12. Miliary Tuberculosis. A posteroanterior roentgenogram reveals a pattern of widely disseminated, nodular shadows throughout both lungs; the shadows are perfectly discrete and uniformly distributed. A rather large area of parenchymal consolidation is present in the right upper lobe, representing the source for the hematogenous dissemination; such evidence is the exception rather than the rule in miliary tuberculosis.

catrization that occur during healing lead to irreversible bronchial dilatation; (2) a segmental bronchus is obstructed by compression by enlarged lymph nodes in primary tuberculosis, or by bronchostenosis secondary to endobronchial disease, resulting in obstructive pneumonitis and subsequent bronchiectasis. Since the vast majority of cases of postprimary tuberculosis affect apical and posterior segments of an upper lobe, facilitating bronchial drainage, bronchiectasis usually is asymptomatic. Hemoptysis occurs in some cases.[101]

Tuberculous Bronchostenosis

In postprimary tuberculosis, endobronchial involvement is fairly common and occurs particularly in airways that drain a pulmonary cavity. Ulceration of the bronchial mucosa leads eventually to fibrosis and cicatricial bronchostenosis. Of considerable importance is the fact that tuberculous bronchitis may occur in the absence of roentgenographically demonstrable abnormality; ulceration of the bronchial mucosa can be the source of positive sputum culture. Persistent respiratory wheeze may suggest the diagnosis.

Tuberculoma

A tuberculoma, which may be a manifestation of either primary or postprimary tuberculosis, is a round or oval lesion situated most commonly in an upper lobe, the right more often than the left. Tuberculomas range from 0.5 to 4.0 cm or more in diameter and typically are smooth and sharply circumscribed.[102] Small discrete shadows in the immediate vicinity of the main lesion—"satellite" lesions—may be identified in as many as 90 per cent of cases.

The majority of these lesions remain stable for a long time and many calcify. The larger the lesion, the more likely it is to be active (Figure 6–13).

CLINICAL MANIFESTATIONS

Most cases of tuberculosis come to medical attention following the discovery of disease on a screening chest roentgenogram. When the diagnosis has been suggested as the result of such a procedure, and the tuberculin reaction is positive, further investigation and follow-up reveal inactive disease in the majority of cases. Most of these patients have no history indicative of active disease, although some will recollect a severe bout of "pneumonia" with a rather protracted course and persistent pleuritic pain and fever, but not documented by chest roentgenography. In many cases one or both of the patients' parents suffered from the disease or died from it.

Even when disease detected on a screening chest roentgenogram is active, the majority of patients are well, deny symptoms, and often are somewhat incredulous of the diagnosis. Symptoms when present are usually nonspecific and do not direct the attention of the patient or the physician to the lungs—tiredness, weakness, anorexia, weight loss, and a low-grade fever in the afternoon or evening. Direct questioning may elicit a history of recent onset of unproductive or mildly productive cough. Less commonly, patients present with respiratory symptoms, most often a cough that has persisted since an upper respiratory tract infection and which may be mildly productive and occasionally associated with hemoptysis. In some the initial complaint is pleuritic chest pain, fre-

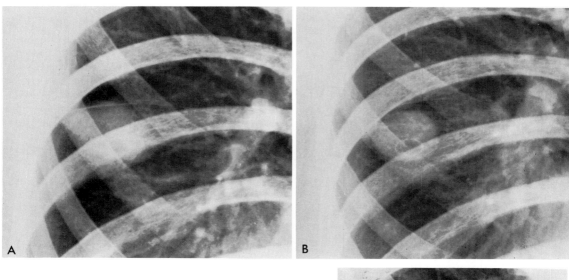

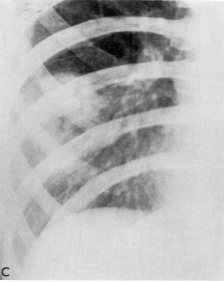

Figure 6–13. Tuberculoma with Breakdown. A view of the right midlung from a posteroanterior roentgenogram (A) reveals a sharply circumscribed, oval shadow measuring approximately 3 cm in diameter; a small, calcific ring shadow can be identified in the center of the lesion. The surrounding lung parenchyma is normal. Two years later (B), the shadow is slightly smaller in size and the central ring calcification more evident. Two years later, the patient developed an abrupt onset of an acute respiratory illness; a roentgenogram at that time (C) revealed breakdown of the tuberculoma and the development of acute air-space disease in the surrounding parenchyma. The lobe was resected; proved exudative tuberculosis.

quently with fever, and although this symptom is more common in adults, a majority of these patients are believed to have primary tuberculosis. Hoarseness, usually a manifestation of laryngeal involvement, indicates active disease and in most cases is associated with a positive sputum culture.

A history of contact, usually in the family, is common. Inmates of prisons or mental institutions are at increased risk, and patients with chronic disabling diseases such as diabetes, alcoholism, and silicosis, and those receiving corticosteroid therapy, are highly susceptible. Acute tuberculous infection may develop in association with granulocytopenia; miliary dissemination is said to occur in 3 to 4 per cent of patients with myeloid leukemia. In a study of 129 patients maintained on hemodialysis for an average of 1.4 years, five cases of active tuberculosis developed—an estimated 15 times the expected incidence.

Every patient with suspected pulmonary tuberculosis should undergo a complete physical examination, with particular attention given to the possibility of extrapulmonary lesions. Examination of the chest itself is unrewarding in many cases and rarely provides information helpful in diagnosis. If an apical lesion is identified on the chest roentgenogram, post-tussic rales on auscultation strongly suggest activity. Physical signs in acute tuberculous pneumonia are the same as in air-space pneumonia of other causes.

Miliary tuberculosis presents a clinical picture different from that of other types of pulmonary involvement. Men over 60 years of age, Negroes, and pregnant women appear to be particularly susceptible to this form of the disease.[99] The onset of miliary tuberculosis is insidious. The mean duration of symptoms in one series[103] was 15.7 weeks and over half the patients had had symptoms for more than 8 weeks, but we have seen patients who have been unwell for only 1 to 2 weeks. Symptoms are usually nonspecific. Cough, weight loss, weakness, anorexia, and night sweats are common. Headache and abdominal pain suggest spread to the meninges and peritoneum. Signs ascribed to meningeal involvement occur late; funduscopic examination reveals choroidal tubercles in 30 to 60 per cent of patients when a diligent search is made.[103] Tuberculin testing with 5 TU is negative in at least 25 per cent of patients.

The diagnosis of miliary tuberculosis should be considered in any patient who has both fever and a miliary roentgenographic pattern. Other subacute or chronic pulmonary diseases may show a similar roentgenographic picture but seldom are associated with pyrexia.

Clinical Course

Although the incidence of tuberculosis has shown an almost linear decrease in every industrialized country during the last century, the death rate did not alter appreciably until the introduction of chemotherapy.

In North America, active tuberculosis most often is seen in positive tuberculin reactors whose chest roentgenograms are abnormal and whose disease is considered to represent endogenous reactivation. Clinically apparent disease rarely develops in tuberculin-positive persons with normal chest roentgenograms.

Parenchymal disease rarely develops in patients with tuberculous pleural effusion that has been treated with chemotherapy.[104]

Chemotherapy rapidly renders the patient with positive sputum noninfectious. The number of bacilli is reduced by 95 per cent after 2 weeks and by 99.75 per cent after 4 weeks of treatment. The incidence of primary resistance of the tubercle bacillus to drugs—a major problem in developing countries because of high rates of default and meager facilities for treatment—ranges between 2 per cent and 4 per cent of cases in the United States,[105] although in children in ghetto areas it may be as high as 10 per cent.

Tuberculosis is now managed largely on an ambulatory basis and frequently by internists in general hospitals. However, well-trained internists have had so little contact with the disease that it is hardly surprising that cases now go unrecognized, not only to the detriment of patients but also those involved in their care.

Relationship Between Pulmonary Tuberculosis and Bronchogenic Carcinoma

The coexistence of pulmonary tuberculosis and bronchogenic carcinoma has been reported by several authors, and a pathogenetic relationship has been implied. However, certain aspects of these two diseases suggest that their coexistence may be no more than coincidental; for example, both bronchogenic carcinoma and tuberculosis tend to involve predominantly the upper lobes; similarly, the incidence of tuberculosis is increasing in older patients, who are also more prone to bronchogenic carcinoma. Of perhaps even greater importance are the observations of Snider and Placik[106] based on a study of 124 patients with both diseases who were matched by race, sex, and age with 124 patients who had bronchogenic carcinoma alone. They observed that the carcinoma could reactivate the pulmonary tuberculosis by eroding encapsulated caseous foci or by engendering cachexia and debilitation, and they emphasized that the recovery of acid-fast bacilli from patients with suspected bronchogenic carcinoma should not delay procedures aimed at detecting neoplasm.

Relationship Between Pulmonary Tuberculosis and Sarcoidosis

Most specialists in pulmonary disease have encountered one or more patients who, despite a typical clinical and pathologic picture of sarcoidosis, subsequently have acid-fast organisms in their sputum. *M. tuberculosis* is isolated from the sputum of more patients thought to have sarcoidosis than can be accepted as purely coincidental, and it is likely that this represents tuberculosis as a complication of sarcoidosis.

EXTRAPULMONARY TUBERCULOSIS

Despite the annual reduction in the number of new cases of pulmonary tuberculosis during the past decade in the United States, there has been no corresponding decrease in the number of new cases of extrapulmonary tuberculosis. The reason for this discrepancy is not clear, but probably reflects the lack of a simple means, equivalent to the chest roentgenograms, to detect the disease in other areas of the body. Nonpulmonary tuberculosis often presents as a chronic febrile illness, particularly in Negroes.

Hematogenous dissemination is a frequent complication of primary tuberculosis and many years may elapse before the involvement of other tissues and organs becomes clinically manifest. Perhaps the commonest form of extrapulmonary tuberculosis in adults is genitourinary. Although formerly common in children, bone and joint involvement, from hematogenous dissemination or from direct extension via the lymphatic system from the pleura to the thoracic and lumbosacral spine, is rarely seen today. Involvement of the hilar and mediastinal lymph nodes is almost invariable in primary tuberculosis. Control of *Mycobacterium bovis* has markedly reduced the frequency of cervical lymph node involvement (scrofula), which now is most often caused by atypical mycobacteria. Tuberculous meningitis causes headache, somnolence, irritability, vomiting, and sometimes neck stiffness; the diagnosis is made by culture of the tubercle bacillus in cerebrospinal fluid. Chemotherapy has largely averted the involvement of the upper respiratory and gastrointestinal tracts. The gastrointestinal tract usually is affected in the ileocecal area or around the rectum, in the latter instance leading to perianal or ischiorectal abscesses.

LABORATORY PROCEDURES IN DIAGNOSIS

TUBERCULIN SKIN TEST. Diagnostic skin testing for mycobacterial infections is described in Chapter 3 (*see* p. 144).

BACTERIOLOGIC INVESTIGATION. Although definitive diagnosis of pulmonary tuberculosis requires culture of *M. tuberculosis*, a smear showing acid-fast organisms is virtually diagnostic in a patient with clinical and roentgenographic findings suggestive of the disease. However, in the absence of this evidence an acid-fast smear is likely to be a false positive finding, at least in a population with a low prevalence of tuberculosis. Material for diagnosis comes from sputum, gastric and bronchial lavage, or a laryngeal swab. Sputum is the most valuable source of organisms. In patients who do not expectorate spontaneously, inhalation of a warmed solution of propylene glycol may induce production. Specimens of sputum obtained immediately after bronchoscopy are particulary valuable. Material smeared on a glass slide should be stained by the Ziehl-Neelson method, which reveals the organisms to be gram-negative and acid-fast; since certain diphtheroids and *Nocardia* species also may be acid-fast, culture is required for final identification.

Material for culture should consist of at least one early morning specimen per day collected on 3 consecutive days. A pooled specimen collected over 12 to 24 hours or even 48 hours may be helpful when other methods are not effective or appropriate. Smears are made on egg yolk and potato media and are incubated at 37° C for up to 8 weeks. The characteristics of the colony serve to differentiate *M. tuberculosis* from other mycobacteria. Every biopsy specimen should be submitted for both pathologic and bacteriologic study; although caseous necrosis in a granuloma may strongly support a diagnosis of tuberculosis, mycotic infections also may show a similar histologic appearance. Pleural granulomas imply tuberculosis. Although positive cultures are obtained in about two-thirds of cases of miliary tuberculosis, the seriousness of this form of tuberculosis may necessitate direct lung biopsy while awaiting results of culture. Our policy is to assume that a patient with pyrexia and a miliary pattern on a chest roentgenogram has miliary tuberculosis, which warrants immediate treatment; lung biopsy is performed 2 to 3 weeks later to confirm the diagnosis, especially if specimens of sputum or gastric washings obtained for culture are considered inadequate. The detection of tubercle bacilli in suspected cases of miliary tuberculosis by bone-marrow aspiration or biopsy has been disappointing.[103]

HEMATOLOGIC AND BIOCHEMICAL INVESTIGATION. The leukocyte count in tuberculosis is usually within normal limits but may be increased to 10,000 to 15,000 per cu mm; in miliary tuberculosis there is often a shift to the left with a relative polymorphonuclear leukocytosis and lymphocytopenia. Pancytopenia (with or without anaplastic bone marrow) and leukemoid reactions resembling leukemia are rare in miliary disease. Anemia occurs particularly in more chronic pulmonary disease and in miliary tuberculosis.[103]

Hyponatremia develops in some cases of pulmonary tuberculosis but is more common in tuberculous meningitis; it probably represents the effect of inappropriate antidiuretic hormone secretion, an explanation supported by the findings of elevated antidiuretic activity in extracts from tuberculous lung tissue.

Bronchoscopy should be performed in any patient with tuberculosis who manifests evidence of tracheobronchial involvement—rhonchi, a positive sputum culture without roentgenographic abnormality, local atelectasis, or obstructive pneumonitis.

PULMONARY FUNCTION TESTS. In the absence of chronic bronchitis and emphysema, patients with pulmonary tuberculosis—even when this is advanced—show little impairment of respiratory function. Pulmonary function tests are useful in assessing patients before surgery and to determine objectively the degree of disability in patients with diffuse chronic destructive tuberculosis. In miliary tuberculosis, pulmonary function tests show a diffuse restrictive pattern most clearly apparent as reduction of the diffusing capacity. With treatment and restoration of the chest roentgenogram to normal, the diffusing capacity may remain considerably below predicted normal values.

NONTUBERCULOUS MYCOBACTERIA

A small but perhaps increasing proportion of mycobacterial infections of the lung are caused by organisms other than *M. tuberculosis* and *M. bovis;* these are referred to variously as "anonymous," "atypical," "chromogenic," or "unclassified" mycobacteria, but are perhaps best designated "nontuberculous."

THE CAUSATIVE ORGANISMS

Characteristics common to nontuberculous mycobacteria include ready growth of almost all strains on culture at 25 or 37° C (in contrast to *M. tuberculosis*, which grows only at 37° C) and their nonpathogenicity in guinea pigs. Based on cultural characteristics—morphology, presence or absence of pigment, and rate of growth—Runyon classified these organisms into four groups.

GROUP I—THE PHOTOCHROMOGENS. This group includes three organisms that can cause disease in man: *M. kansasii, M. marinum,* and *M. simiae.* In culture, colonies turn yellow when exposed to light.

GROUP II—THE SCOTOCHROMOGENS. The disease-producing organisms in this group are *M. scrofulaceum,* which characteristically produces a scrofulalike picture and rarely causes pulmonary disease, and *M. szulgai,* which has been identified by lipid chromatography and serologic testing as the responsible agent in five cases of pulmonary disease. Characteristically, in culture, colonies are pigmented yellow, but turn orange on exposure to light.

GROUP III—AVIUM-INTRACELLULARE GROUP. Several species have been reported to cause disease in humans: *M. avium, M. intracellulare* (Battey bacillus), and *M. xenopei* can cause pulmonary disease, whereas *M. ulcerans* produces tropical skin ulcers. In culture, colonies characteristically are white to beige and, with the exception of *M. xenopei,* are nonpigmented; full growth takes 2 to 4 weeks.

GROUP IV—NONCHROMOGENS. (These are known also as "rapid growers," since these organisms take only 3 to 5 days to reach full growth in culture.) Species recognized as causing human disease include *M. fortuitum, M. chelonei* and *M. abscessus.* All produce skin abscesses, and *M. fortuitum* is rarely a pathogen in the lungs. In culture, coloring characteristically is identical to that of group III; the two groups are most readily differentiated by their rate of growth.

Specific organisms within these groups can be identified by serologic testing[107, 108] and by lipid[108] and pyrolysis liquid chromatography.[109] In particular, classification by seroagglutination is receiving greater acceptance, and since considerable variation in cultural characteristics occurs between strains recognized as closely related serotypes, colony culture pigmentation or nonpigmentation now appears to be of secondary importance.[110] Variable pigmentation and the similarity of biochemical reactions and surface antigens seen in the *M. avium-intracellulare* complex and the *M. scrofulaceum* species has led some investigators to group these organisms together under the name *M. avium-intracellulare-scrofulaceum* (MAIS complex).[111,112]

EPIDEMIOLOGY

In North America, the nontuberculous species account for less than 1 per cent of mycobacterial pulmonary disease. The incidence varies geographically: *M. kansasii* is more prevalent in the southern and midwestern states and the Battey bacillus in the southeastern states. Mycobacterial disease caused by nontuberculous acid-fast bacilli is more common in adults than in children; white males over the age of 50 with underlying pulmonary disease appear to be particularly susceptible.[113]

Nontuberculous mycobacteria considered to be saprophytes, commensals, or contaminants have been identified in approximately 5 per cent of patients in hospitals and sanatoria.

Nontuberculous mycobacteria have frequently been isolated from water, soil, and dust, and from fish that contaminate both fresh and salt water with *M. marinum*.[110, 114] Mycobacteria recovered from raw milk include rapidly growing strains and those of the *M. avium-intracellulare-scrofulaceum* complex. *M. kansasii* is rarely cultured from nonhuman material but has been isolated from water. Other sources of potential infection in humans include domestic and wild animals and birds, and since person-to-person transmission rarely has been confirmed, it seems reasonable to conclude that humans may become infected from the environment.[110]

There is considerable cross-reactivity (low specificity) between antigens isolated from various mycobacterial serotypes used in intradermal testing. Therefore, it is perhaps wise to assume that a reaction to a nontuberculous mycobacterial antigen represents infection with this type of organism only when the induration is 5 mm larger than that produced by a simultaneous test with PPD-S or OT.[107, 110]

PATHOLOGIC CHARACTERISTICS

The pathologic characteristics of pulmonary disease caused by nontuberculous mycobacteria

and by *M. tuberculosis* are virtually identical, although a higher incidence of severe endobronchitis has been reported in pathologic specimens from patients whose disease was caused by *M. kansasii*.

ROENTGENOGRAPHIC MANIFESTATIONS

The roentgenographic pattern of pulmonary disease caused by nontuberculous mycobacteria cannot be accurately differentiated from that produced by *M. tuberculosis*, although the changes usually indicate advanced disease.[115, 116] Certain features, however, seem more suggestive of nontuberculous mycobacterioses: (a) there is a greater tendency to cavitation; of 184 cases of pulmonary *M. kansasii* infection studied by Christensen and his colleagues[117] 96 per cent manifested cavitation of their pulmonary disease; cavities tend to be multiple and thin-walled; (b) exudative lesions are very uncommon; (c) hematogenous dissemination is rare; (d) pleural effusion is rare; and (e) there is a strong association with pre-existing pulmonary disease, particularly emphysema and pneumoconiosis.[118]

CLINICAL MANIFESTATIONS

The clinical picture of the nontuberculous mycobacterioses is indistinguishable from that of tuberculosis,[115] although middle-aged and elderly persons appear to be more commonly affected, particularly those with associated disease such as chronic bronchitis and emphysema, and pneumoconiosis.[110, 113, 119, 121] The diagnosis of nontuberculous pulmonary mycobacterioses should be based on at least three positive cultures of the organisms (in the absence of other mycobacteria) and a chest roentgenogram indicating unstable chronic disease. Strong supportive evidence is provided when skin tests with atypical antigens cause induration at least 5 mm larger than the reaction to an equivalent dose of PPD-S. There is underlying disease, particularly alcoholism, in one-quarter to one-third of cases.[113]

There are many well-documented cases of primary pulmonary disease caused by *M. intracellulare* and *M. kansasii*,[113] but other atypical mycobacteria rarely cause pulmonary disease. There are a few fairly well-documented cases of lung infection by pathogenic *M. fortuitum*;[122, 123] a strong association of this infection with aspiration secondary to esophageal disease has been demonstrated.[124] Cases of pulmonary disease caused by *M. xenopei* were originally described in Europe[125, 126] but now have been reported in the United States.[127] Cases of lung infection by other atypical mycobacteria include ten caused by *M. szulgai*[110, 128] and one caused by *M. simiae*.[129] Lymphadenitis in children can be caused by nontuberculous mycobacterial organisms, particularly of the MAIS complex. Cutaneous mycobacterial disease is usually due to *M. marinum* and various "rapid-growers." Disseminated nontuberculous mycobacterioses can develop in compromised hosts, with an almost invariably fatal outcome.[110, 130]

MYCOTIC INFECTIONS OF THE LUNG

Recognition of the frequency of fungal lung infections is increasing, an awareness that probably derives from two factors: an apparent increase in the incidence of these diseases, notably histoplasmosis, and the relatively recent discovery of chemotherapeutic agents, particularly amphotericin B, which are highly effective in combating these diseases. Some of these organisms—such as *Histoplasma capsulatum*, *Coccidioides immitis*, and *Blastomyces dermatitidis*—can cause infection in otherwise healthy subjects, whereas others—such as *Aspergillus fumigatus* and *Candida albicans*—are nearly always saprophytic or "opportunistic," affecting susceptible individuals who are already ill, especially those receiving antibiotic, corticosteroid, immunosuppressive, or antineoplastic therapy. The majority of fungal infections produce benign illness, often without symptoms, and may be recognized only in retrospect after a positive skin reaction to a specific mycotic antigen. In some instances, however, fungi may rapidly disseminate throughout the body and produce acute, subacute, or chronic disease that may be fatal.

Most fungi live in two forms—mycelial and yeast—changing from one to another with changes in environment. The filamentous (mycelial) phase occurs in nature and grows in culture at room temperature; a parasitic form exists in host tissues and grows in culture at body temperature. The source of contamination is almost invariably the soil; apart from *Coccidioides immitis*, which grows best in dry compact soil, most fungi thrive in moist areas. *H. capsulatum* and *B. dermatitidis* inhabit river valleys, the former being cultured with relative ease and the latter with difficulty from the soil. Some fungi, particularly *H. capsulatum* and *Cryptococcus neoformans*, grow well in soil

contaminated by bird and bat excreta. In contrast to most fungi, *Candida* and *Actinomyces* are commensals in the buccal cavity of man and invade the lungs when host defense mechanisms are impaired.

The Actinomycetaceae, which include *Actinomyces israelii* and *Nocardia* species, are presently classified as bacteria.

Pathologically, fungi in the lungs, as elsewhere, produce granulomas that are nonspecific in type and in no way different from those of tuberculosis or sarcoidosis. Pathologic diagnosis depends on finding the organisms in tissue but is only as valid as the uniqueness of the organism's morphology. The yeastlike cells of *H. capsulatum*, *Sporothrix (Sporotrichum) schenkii*, *Torulopsis glabrata*, and *Candida*, as well as *Paracoccidioides*, *Blastomyces*, and even *Coccidioides*, cannot always be differentiated histologically. Definitive diagnosis nearly always requires culture of the organism, although identification in tissue, together with positive serologic findings and clinical features, may lead to a strong presumptive diagnosis. A subcommittee of the American College of Chest Physicians has made recommendations for obtaining suitable material and for its staining, processing, and culturing.

HISTOPLASMOSIS

THE CAUSATIVE ORGANISM

Histoplasma capsulatum, in its mycelial form, is a saprophyte in moist soil of appropriate chemical composition. It gains entry into humans by inhalation and then assumes its yeast form and resides in cellular cytoplasm; it is oval and measures 3 to 5 μ in diameter. Histoplasmosis is seldom diagnosed as a result of identification of the organism in smears of expectorated material, pleural fluid, or bone marrow. Culture is more reliable, and in suspected cases the body fluids, bone marrow, or tissue should be cultured both on glucose agar at 30° C and on cysteine blood agar at 37° C; growth usually takes 2 to 3 weeks. Final identification depends on the demonstration of tuberculate spores in mycelial growth. Cultures of sputum or gastric aspirate are more often positive in the cavitary form of the disease; blood, bone marrow, and tissue from biopsies are the major sources of the fungus in cases of disseminated disease.

Pathologically, *H. capsulatum* produces granulomas, sometimes with central caseation. Biopsy or necropsy material should be stained with the periodic acid–Schiff (PAS) method, or with one of the tissue silver stains, the best of which appears to be Gomori's methenamine–silver nitrate.

EPIDEMIOLOGY

Most reports of the disease have come from North America, particularly the central and eastern portions and notably in the Ohio, Mississippi, and St. Lawrence River valleys, which are regarded as endemic areas. It has also been reported from South and Central America, India, Malaya, and Cyprus; it is rare in Europe and Australia and almost nonexistent in England and Japan.

In Africa, a somewhat different clinical picture is produced by an organism that some consider quite distinct from *H. capsulatum* and that has been called *Histoplasma duboisii*. This variety appears to involve mainly the skin and bones and seldom the lungs, suggesting a different mode of entry.[131]

In endemic areas, the histoplasmin skin tests may be positive in up to 80 per cent of the population. Sometimes a positive skin test will revert to negative but will subsequently become positive again on re-exposure to the antigen.[132] Serial postmortem examinations have revealed splenic calcification in 50 per cent of cases, possibly indicating a benign insidious dissemination.

The infection is unevenly distributed, even in highly endemic areas, probably reflecting "point sources" of heavily contaminated soil in areas of bird or bat roosts or congregations of chickens or pigeons. The excreta of birds and bats are considered to foster growth of the organism in the soil, and heavily contaminated soil may prove to be a source of infection even in nonendemic areas.

Persons of all ages may be affected, but the disease is particularly virulent in infants, the elderly, and patients with lymphoma or on corticosteroid therapy. Histoplasmosis is particularly common as a symptom-producing disease in Caucasian males and extremely uncommon in Negroes, but skin test surveys indicate that probably the infection is equally common in Negroes and females.

Symptoms and roentgenographic manifestations probably relate to the degree of exposure. An incubation period of 18 days has been roughly determined from dramatic instances of exposure in "epidemic histoplasmosis."

Histoplasmosis is manifested in fairly well-defined clinical presentations and roentgenographic patterns. These varieties can be grouped into three categories: (1) primary disease, usually benign; (2) chronic disease or reinfection; and (3) disseminated histoplasmosis.

PRIMARY HISTOPLASMOSIS

BENIGN TYPE. This common form of histoplasmosis frequently is discovered on a screening chest roentgenogram or, in retrospect, when calcified nodules in the lung periphery and calcification in draining hilar lymph nodes are found to be associated with a positive histoplasmin skin test. Onset of the disease may be ushered in by mild respiratory symptoms such as fever or erythema nodosum. In 1970, an epidemic of nonspecific "flulike" symptoms occurred in 384 (40 per cent) of the students and staff of a school 5 to 15 days after the Earth Day activities, which consisted of cleaning up a courtyard that was heavily contaminated with *H. capsulatum*.[133] Positive skin and serologic reactions developed in 85 to 90 per cent of students and staff, much higher rates than in comparison groups. Symptoms in this epidemic consisted of fever, headache, and nonpleuritic chest pain; anorexia, nausea, and cough also were present in half the patients. Chest roentgenographic findings were not described in this series, but in the benign form of the disease are said to consist of one or more ill-defined nonsegmental opacities, more often in lower than in upper zones (Figure 6–14). Hilar lymph node enlargement may be present; unlike tuberculosis, histoplasmosis rarely gives rise to pleural effusion. Despite the mild or asymptomatic response to the invasion of this microorganism, widespread dissemination may occur.

PNEUMONIC TYPE. This form of the disease is more acute. It is characterized roentgenographically by homogeneous parenchymal consolidation of nonsegmental anatomic distribution, and thus may simulate acute bacterial airspace pneumonia. Unlike the latter, however, the disease tends to clear in one area and appear in another. Hilar lymph node enlargement is common. The symptoms include cough with mucopurulent sputum and sometimes hemoptysis, and headaches, pleuritic pain, or pain in the limbs and back. Fever may be present. Physical signs include rales, a friction rub, and occasionally signs of consolidation.

HISTOPLASMOMA. This relatively common form of pulmonary histoplasmosis is usually a solitary, sharply circumscribed, nodular

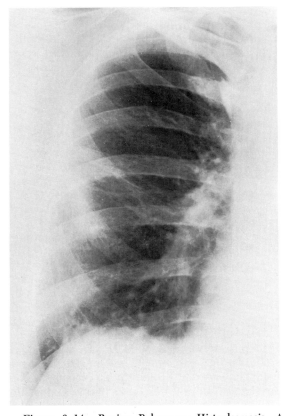

Figure 6–14. Benign Pulmonary Histoplasmosis. A view of the right lung from a posteroanterior roentgenogram reveals an indistinctly defined, hazy consolidation of the axillary portion of the right lung, situated within the middle lobe. There is slight enlargement of hilar lymph nodes. This 41-year-old man had mild symptoms consisting of unproductive cough and anorexia; a histoplasmin skin test was strongly positive. The illness occurred during a mild epidemic of acute histoplasmosis.

shadow, seldom more than 3 cm in diameter.[134] In most cases the lesion is in a lower lobe, often with satellite lesions nearby; many calcify, producing the "target" lesion that is virtually pathognomonic of this disease. Hilar lymph node calcification is common. Histoplasmomas seldom exceed four or five in number and often differ considerably in size; serial roentgenograms over months or years may reveal moderate growth, even to a point at which a metastatic etiology may be entertained. Goodwin and Snell[134] postulated that the original necrotic focus of histoplasmosis, measuring no more than 2 to 4 mm, eventually develops a fibrous capsule that progressively enlarges as a reactive phenomenon. A central nidus of calcification, or a concentric calcific ring, does not necessarily mean that a lesion is "healed": in hyper-respon-

sive individuals calcified lesions may grow, suggesting continued reaction to an antigenic stimulus.[132] A histoplasmoma usually is discovered by chance; it probably represents a residual lesion from an active primary focus and may cavitate.

LYMPH NODE INVOLVEMENT. Histoplasmosis sometimes is manifested by unilateral or bilateral enlargement of hilar, mediastinal, or intrapulmonary lymph nodes, without roentgenographic evidence of parenchymal disease. This form is particularly common in children, in whom it may produce tracheal obstruction. Most patients are asymptomatic during the active phase of the disease; however, with healing and subsequent calcification, extrinsic pressure of enlarged nodes on the airways, particularly the right middle lobe bronchus, may cause obstruction and resulting distal infection or atelectasis. Calcification of lymph nodes, usually of the bronchopulmonary group, may cause erosion into the bronchial lumen—*broncholithiasis*. Cough and hemoptysis usually result.

MEDIASTINAL INVOLVEMENT. Various clinical and roentgenologic presentations may result from mediastinal lymph node involvement or from actual extension of the pulmonary infection into the mediastinal space with production of granulomatous and fibrotic mediastinitis. There are four main types of involvement.

Pericarditis. Pericardial effusion may be apparent roentgenologically as enlargement of the cardiovascular silhouette. Mediastinal lymph node enlargement is common. Calcification of the pericardium or constrictive pericarditis may develop.

Esophageal Encroachment. During either the active or the healed stage, enlarged posterior mediastinal lymph nodes may encroach upon the esophagus and displace or partially obstruct it. Healing of the affected lymph nodes may create cicatrices on the esophagus, leading to traction diverticulum.

Superior Vena Cava Obstruction. Encroachment on the superior vena cava by enlarged mediastinal nodes may result in the classic picture of the superior vena cava syndrome. Angiography is usually required for proper assessment (Figure 6–15).

Pulmonary Arterial and Venous Obstruction. In a few cases, severe mediastinitis with granuloma formation and fibrosis results in obstruction of pulmonary arteries and veins as they leave and enter the mediastinum. The effects on the lungs, more commonly local than general, are predictable: oligemia, or the manifestations of pulmonary venous hypertension.

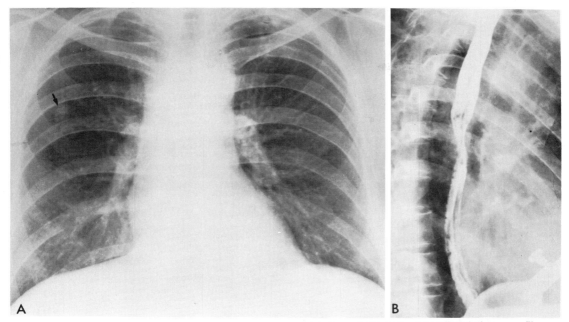

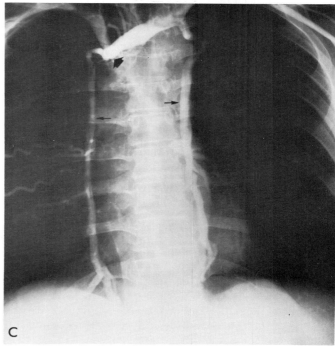

Figure 6–15. Mediastinal Histoplasmosis: Superior Vena Cava Obstruction. A posteroanterior roentgenogram (A) shows a somewhat widened upper mediastinum possessing a smooth contour. A partly calcified nodule can be identified in the upper portion of the right lung (*arrow*). This 51-year-old man presented with a typical picture of obstruction of the superior vena cava. In addition to the typical symptoms and signs referable to the head and neck and upper extremities, the patient complained of "hemoptysis," which on further questioning and examination was found to arise from the esophagus rather than the lungs and to be caused by "downhill" esophageal varices (B). A roentgenogram of the thorax following the rapid injection of contrast medium into an antecubital vein (C) reveals complete obstruction of the superior vena cava just proximal to the junction of the right and left innominate veins (*thick arrow*). Filling of the internal mammary veins can be identified on both sides (*thin arrows*), representing part of the extensive collateral circulation. Note the multiple small calcifications throughout the spleen; this finding, in addition to a strongly positive histoplasmin skin test, constituted highly suggestive evidence for the diagnosis of mediastinal histoplasmosis.

ACUTE DIFFUSE NODULAR DISEASE. This is the "epidemic" form of the disease, which typically develops in groups of people heavily exposed to organisms in caves inhabited by bats or in a locale where soil is heavily contaminated by bird excreta. Symptoms may be very mild and, in fact, exposure may not be recognized until many years later when multiple calcific nodules are seen roentgenologically in the lungs. On the other hand, overwhelming exposure may result in severe illness and death. Following heavy exposure and despite symptoms, the roentgenogram may show no abnormalities for a week or more; eventually, widely disseminated, fairly discrete nodular shadows appear throughout the lungs, individual lesions measuring up to 3 or 4 mm in diameter,[135] with hilar lymph node enlargement in the majority of cases. These shadows may clear completely in 2 to 8 months or may fibrose and eventually calcify.

CHRONIC OR REINFECTION HISTOPLASMOSIS

In contrast to the types already mentioned, the chronic form of the disease is thought to result from reinfection. It is not known whether reinfection is principally endogenous or exogenous. Two fairly well-defined groups are recognizable: early chronic pulmonary histoplasmosis and a more advanced cavitary type.

EARLY CHRONIC DISEASE. Roentgenographically, this form of the disease is characterized by fairly sharply circumscribed zones of parenchymal consolidation, usually in the upper lobes and tending to involve one area after another; considerable loss of lung volume may result. Symptoms include mild fever, weight loss, malaise, anorexia, cough, and chest pain.

CHRONIC CAVITARY DISEASE. Cavitation occurs most commonly in men over the age of 40 with centrilobular emphysema.[132] The roentgenographic appearance closely simulates reinfection tuberculosis, and in some cases the diseases coexist. One or more cavities may be identified, usually in the upper lobes, with varying degrees of surrounding parenchymal consolidation. A calcified primary lesion may be apparent in a remote location. The prognosis in this form of the disease is dependent upon the severity of the underlying emphysema.[132]

Disseminated Histoplasmosis. The widespread dissemination of *H. capsulatum* via the bloodstream may be unrecognized until multiple punctate calcifications are identified throughout the spleen or lung, long after the primary infection. In some cases, however, disseminated disease is virulent and many of these patients die if not adequately treated.[136, 137] In either the primary or reinfection type of the disease, virulent dissemination is commonest in infants under the age of 1 year and in adults over 40;[137] it affects white males more often than females, in a ratio of about 7:1,[136, 137] presumably because of occupational exposure as farmers.[136, 137] The lungs usually are affected; roentgenographic manifestations include cavitation, a miliary pattern (Figure 6–16), and hilar lymph node enlargement.[136] Underlying disease that impairs host defense mechanisms is found in a small number of patients. Symptoms are relatively nonspecific; they include fever, cough, dyspnea, weakness, anorexia, and weight loss; hepatomegaly and splenomegaly are common, as are lesions of the oropharyngeal mucous membrane. About 50 per cent of patients with disseminated histoplasmosis develop Addison's disease,[136] and many have anemia, leukopenia, and thrombocytopenia. The organism usually is found in the sputum and often is cultured from blood, urine, and bone marrow.

LABORATORY STUDIES

Hematology

The white cell count usually is normal but may increase to 13,000 per cu mm in the acute "epidemic" form. Leukopenia and anemia develop in approximately 50 per cent of cases of disseminated disease.

Serology

In many cases the diagnosis must be based on serologic tests, including agglutination, precipitation, and complement-fixation tests. Serologic tests become positive about a month after primary infection. A difference in titer in serial determinations is more significant than the result of a single test, but values of 1:4 for mycelial and 1:16 for yeast antigens are strong evidence of activity. Unlike the series of events in cocidioidomycosis, the degree of dissemination of histoplasmosis does not necessarily relate to the height of antibody formation—benign primary cases may have levels as high as 1:2048. The more severe and persistent infections in histoplasmosis frequently are associated with a relatively low titer of activity which fails to fall to normal over a period of months.

As in tuberculosis, the histoplasmin skin test indicates only that the patient has been exposed to *H. capsulatum* at some time and that an allergic reaction has developed. Since skin testing itself may produce antibodies, blood should be drawn at the time of skin testing—or at least within the next 4 or 5 days—to provide a "control" sample and avoid false positive serologic results. When active disease is strongly suspected, it is perhaps wise to forgo skin testing so that the true pattern of antibody levels can be determined by sequential testing. Because of the likelihood of cross-reactions, skin testing should be done simultaneously with histoplasmin, tuberculin, blastomycin, and coccidioidin, the strongest reaction indicating the likely cause of the disease.

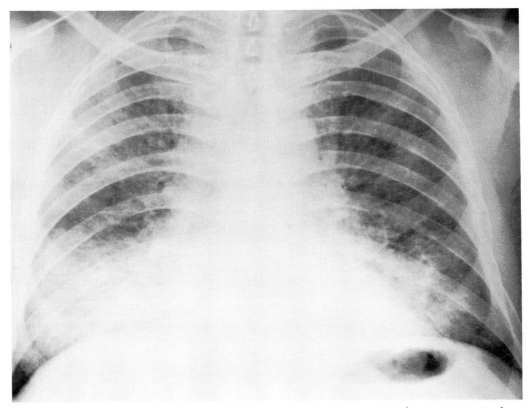

Figure 6–16. Acute Disseminated Histoplasmosis. A posteroanterior roentgenogram shows extensive involvement of both lungs by a process characteristic of air-space consolidation. In most areas, the shadows are confluent; an air bronchogram can be identified. This 40-year-old man had had proved Hodgkin's disease for many years, manifested roentgenologically by hilar and mediastinal lymph node enlargement. He was receiving high doses of corticosteroids and antineoplastic drugs at the time of onset of acute disseminated histoplasmosis; it is clear that the dissemination occurred from an endogenous source although the site was not discovered.

COCCIDIOIDOMYCOSIS

This highly infectious mycotic disease is usually but not always localized in the lungs. It appears to be limited to the western hemisphere, particularly the southwestern United States.

THE CAUSATIVE ORGANISM

The etiologic agent of coccidioidomycosis is the pathogenic soil fungus *Coccidioides immitis*. In tissue, the fungus has the form of a spherule—a round, thin-walled cell 20 to 80 μ in diameter and containing a multitude of endospores about 2 to 4 μ. The spherules rarely are found in the sputum, but may be identified in abscess and tissue specimens cultured on Sabouraud's glucose medium at 30° C. Mycelial growth appears as hyphae-containing rectangular arthrospores in 2- to 8-day cultures and may occur in cavities *in vivo*. If mycelia grown from culture are inoculated into mice or guinea pigs, spherules develop in the animal and may be found in exudate. Spherulation also can be produced by culture in liquid synthetic medium in 1 to 8 days, and in mice in 5 to 15 days.

EPIDEMIOLOGY

Coccidioidomycosis is endemic in the southwestern United States, notably in California, central southern Arizona, western Texas, southern New Mexico, southwestern Utah, and the southern tip of Nevada. In California, although endemicity is greatest in the San Joaquin valley, cases have been documented from just north of San Francisco to the Mexican border; a few cases have been reported from Central and South America. The disease is acquired by inhalation of the organism from contaminated soil. Even in endemic areas there are local pockets where arthrospores of *C. immitis* are concentrated, as has been shown by skin testing of young men working in adjacent work camps.[138]

Proliferation of the mycelial form of the fungus requires an alkaline soil free from severe frost and a dry season following a wet one. The mycelia produce arthrospores, which become airborne and are inhaled. Epidemics may occur following earth-moving for construction and therefore can be kept to a minimum by dust control. The disease is not spread from person to person. An "epidemic" occurrence of the disease has been reported in a group of non-immune college students who had been digging for native American artifacts in California.[139]

The incidence of infection is very high in endemic areas: 25 per cent of persons newly arrived in such an area may be expected to have positive skin tests at the end of 1 year, and 50 per cent at the end of 4 years. Most of these conversions from negative to positive skin tests take place without recognizable symptoms.

Data from several series indicate that of approximately 6000 cases of infection, 2000 give rise to symptoms; 1 per cent of these (20 patients) have illness lasting weeks or months, and the disease becomes disseminated in one patient. Disseminated disease is thus very uncommon—one in 6000 cases; it occurs 20 times more frequently in Filipinos and Negroes than in Caucasians. The incubation period is 1 to 4 weeks.

Coccidioidomycosis may be manifested by various clinical pictures and roentgenographic patterns, which are best considered under the headings *benign* and *disseminated* disease. On the basis of an extensive review of the literature and the addition of 90 cases of primary coccidioidomycosis and 43 cases of disseminated disease, McGahan and his colleagues[140] have recently reviewed the classic and contemporary imaging of coccidioidomycosis, including manifestations identified on computed tomography and radionuclide imaging as well as on conventional roentgenography.

BENIGN COCCIDIOIDOMYCOSIS

ASYMPTOMATIC AND "FLULIKE" DISEASE. It has been estimated that 60 to 80 per cent of cases are asymptomatic. The frequency with which the disease is recognized probably depends on how closely it is looked for and also to some extent on the degree of exposure. Some patients have influenza-like episodes, with fever, cough, and myalgia, in some cases with arthralgia, conjunctivitis, and a maculopapular rash.[139]

Roentgenographically, the changes are said to consist of "fleeting" areas of parenchymal consolidation, usually in the upper lobes, which tend to leave thin-walled cavities.

PNEUMONIC TYPE. Parenchymal consolidation occurs mainly in the lower lobes; it may be homogeneous or mottled, segmental or non-segmental. In approximately half of the patients, pneumonia is the sole roentgenographic abnormality, and in the remainder it is combined with other abnormalities such as pleural effusion or hilar or mediastinal lymph node enlargement.[141] Pleural effusion is rarely the sole roentgenographic finding, and hilar node enlargement alone occurs in less than 10 per cent of patients.[142] Symptoms include fever, dry cough, occasional bloody expectoration, chills, muscle and joint pains, and pleuritic pain. Rales and rhonchi may be heard on auscultation, but signs of consolidation in the lower lobes are rare. Toxic cutaneous erythemas may develop; erythema nodosum or multiforme occurs in 5 to 20 per cent of patients. Pneumonia caused by this organism may be very persistent and can even end fatally, usually in immunocompromised hosts in whom the disease is confined to the lungs. Less commonly, chronic progressive coccidioidal pneumonia may develop, the roentgenographic pattern simulating chronic cavitary tuberculosis or histoplasmosis. Sometimes resolving pneumonia evolves into nodules that may or may not cavitate.[139]

NODULAR LESIONS (WITH OR WITHOUT CAVITATION). Well-defined nodules, 0.5 to 3.0 cm in diameter, may occur singly or in groups. The nodules are not roentgenographically distinguishable from other granulomas. Few calcify, and then as soon as 1 year after their discovery. These nodules are the residue of active parenchymal infection, probably the equivalent of reinfection-type histoplasmosis. As in histoplasmosis, chronic disease probably indicates exacerbation from an endogenous source rather than exogenous reinfection. Dissemination seldom occurs, even when the lesion is active locally.

In 10 to 15 per cent of cases, nodules excavate to form thin- or thick-walled cavities (Figure 6–17). Thin-walled cavities have a strong tendency toward rapid inflation and deflation, presumably reflecting changes in their check-valve communication with the bronchial tree. Cavities often constitute the initial or sole manifestation of the disease. Cavitation occurs predominantly in the upper lobes, and unlike in tuberculosis it may develop in the anterior segment. Pneumothorax and empyema develop in only about 2 per cent of cases with cavitation.

Many patients are asymptomatic—even

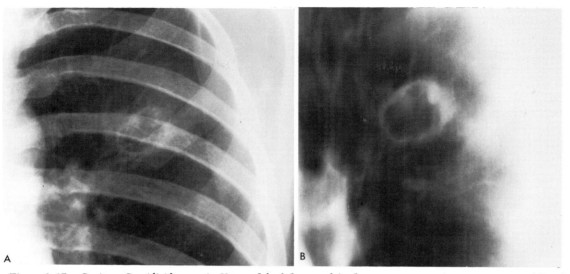

A   B

Figure 6–17. Cavitary Coccidioidomycosis. Views of the left upper lobe from a posteroanterior roentgenogram (A) and an anteroposterior tomogram (B) reveal a fairly sharply circumscribed cavitary lesion measuring 16 × 24 mm. The wall is thin except laterally, where a small protuberance exists on the inner wall. Proved coccidioidomycosis. The patient is a 43-year-old woman, resident of Arizona. (Courtesy of Dr. Paul Capp, University of Arizona Medical Center, Tucson.)

those with cavitary disease—and the nodules may not be discovered for months or years after the patient has left an endemic area. Approximately 10 per cent of symptomatic patients with coccidioidomycosis have tuberculosis; this creates problems in diagnosis and management, particularly if both lesions are located in the same lobe and especially in the same cavity.

LYMPH NODE INVOLVEMENT. Enlargement of lymph nodes in the hilar or paratracheal regions may be unilateral or bilateral, even in the absence of parenchymal disease, and may not give rise to symptoms. Involvement of paratracheal nodes may indicate imminent dissemination of the disease.

DISSEMINATED COCCIDIOIDOMYCOSIS

The "miliarylike" roentgenographic pattern of acute histoplasmosis caused by inhalation of large numbers of organisms does not occur in coccidioidomycosis. A diffuse micronodular pattern indicates widespread dissemination via the bloodstream, as in tuberculosis (Figure 6–18); it usually is seen early in the course of the infection and rarely more than 2 months after onset.[143] Among the southwestern American Indians, the prognosis for those with disseminated disease is unfavorable in the young (under 5 years) and persons over 50 years of age. Miliary involvement of the lungs is not invariable in disseminated disease, which usually can be suspected, 4 weeks after onset, from weight loss, persistent fever, slow clearing of local lesions

on the chest roentgenogram, and clinical signs of extrapulmonary spread. Lymph nodes, skin, and subcutaneous tissues may be involved, with sinus formation in some cases, and spread may occur to the meninges, liver, spleen, kidneys, adrenals, bone (with formation of osteolytic lesions), and occasionally the endocardium and pericardium.

LABORATORY STUDIES

Hematology

The hemoglobin value is decreased in many cases of disseminated disease. The white cell count is normal or moderately elevated in most patients, often with a significant degree of eosinophilia, particularly in those with erythema nodosum.

Serology

Serologic tests include agglutination, complement fixation (CF), immunodiffusion (ID), and latex particle agglutination (LPA) tests; the last two are invaluable for screening sera. The agglutination and precipitation reactions become positive 1 to 3 weeks after exposure, and CF usually a little later; however, the latter never becomes positive in a large percentage of cases of primary infection with positive precipitin reactions. If these remain positive after 6 months, or the CF titer rises above 1:16, dissemination has *probably* occurred. Serologic

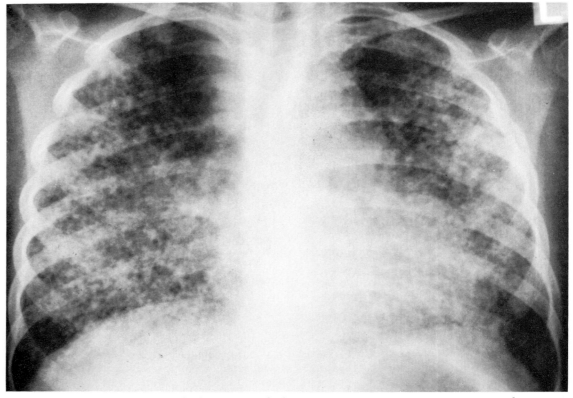

Figure 6–18. **Disseminated Coccidioidomycosis.** Multiple punctate opacities measuring up to 2 mm in diameter are scattered widely throughout both lungs, in some areas being so numerous as to be almost confluent. This represents miliary spread of the disease. This child had acute leukemia and was receiving antineoplastic therapy; he was thus a compromised host. On appropriate therapy, he recovered from his acute coccidioidomycosis but subsequently died from his primary disease. (Courtesy of Dr. Paul Capp, University of Arizona Medical Center, Tucson.)

tests are positive in 92 per cent of symptomatic patients with benign disease and in 60 per cent of those with residual lesions. Skin testing can be done with either spherulin (antigen prepared from the sporangium of *C. immitis*) or coccidioidin (antigen from mycelial filtrate), spherulin being the more sensitive; 0.1 ml of a 1:100 solution is used and the reaction is read at 24 and 48 hours. In the benign nondisseminated form of the disease the skin test is positive in virtually all patients within 3 weeks of the onset of infection; it may revert to negative within 2 years but can remain positive for as long as 10 years. In disseminated disease the skin test is usually negative (70 per cent of patients); a combination of this finding with a CF titer of more than 1:16 is practically pathognomonic.

NORTH AMERICAN BLASTOMYCOSIS

North American blastomycosis is a granulomatous mycotic infection caused by the fungus *Blastomyces dermatitidis*. The name of the disease is a misnomer, since it also has been reported in Central and South America and in Africa. The major target organs are the skin and lungs; bone and other organs are involved in some cases.

THE CAUSATIVE ORGANISM

B. dermatitidis, a dimorphic organism, occurs in mycelial phase in the soil and in yeast phase in mammals. On Sabouraud's glucose agar it grows slowly as mycelia, its oval or round conidia being attached to hyphae or carried on short lateral conidiophores. On blood agar at 37° C it grows as yeast with single buds having a thick-necked attachment to a doubly refractile walled parent cell.[144] Organisms may be identified in tissue stained with PAS, Gridley, Gomori, or Bauer stains.

EPIDEMIOLOGY

The precise incidence of North American blastomycosis is unknown, but the infection is much less common than histoplasmosis, which occurs in roughly the same geographic areas. Middle-aged males are most commonly infected, male predominance being 6:1 to 15:1.[145] It has been suggested[144] that this incidence reflects the male predominance of hunting in wooded areas; bird dogs of hunters have also been shown to have a high incidence of infection.[144] There appears to be no racial predominance. The disease is confined largely to the western hemisphere, mainly the central and southeastern United States.[145]

The fungus is believed to reside in the soil, and most cases occur in heavily exposed persons.[145] Point sources of infection have not been proved, even in rare reports of epidemics.[146] Most incidences of the disease in persons in close contact almost certainly reflect a common source of infection.[146]

Although *B. dermatitidis* is considered to be a primary pathogen and not an opportunistic fungus, many affected persons have underlying disease; for example, in one report,[145] 34 of 40 patients had what might be considered predisposing conditions.

ROENTGENOGRAPHIC MANIFESTATIONS

The roentgenographic findings in pulmonary blastomycosis are entirely nonspecific, none of the changes being characteristic or diagnostic.[145] The usual pattern is one of acute air-space pneumonia, most often nonsegmental; consolidation is usually homogeneous but may be patchy, and the upper lobes are affected more frequently than the lower, in a ratio of about 3:2. Cavitation occurs in no more than 15 per cent of cases.[145]

A solitary pulmonary mass is not an unusual manifestation of this disease and may closely mimic primary carcinoma, especially when associated with unilateral lymph node enlargement or bone destruction. In fact, a pulmonary mass was the commonest roentgenologic finding in a series of 36 cases in central Canada.[147] A widely disseminated nodular or miliary pattern is infrequent. One report of 51 cases[148] described the chest roentgenographic findings as follows: acute air-space consolidation (22 patients); mass (2), chronic cavity (9), fibronodular disease simulating other chronic granulomatous processes (14), miliary disease with or without associated consolidation (5), and diffuse homogeneous consolidation (2); hilar nodes were enlarged in 3 patients. Hilar and mediastinal lymph node enlargement and pleural effusion are very uncommon, and the latter invariably

connotes concomitant parenchymal disease. Osteolytic lesions in the thoracic skeleton usually are associated with superficial abscesses.

CLINICAL MANIFESTATIONS

Like histoplasmosis and coccidioidomycosis, blastomycosis is probably most often a primary infection, occurring without symptoms or with mild fever, cough, and malaise.[146, 149] The prevalence of this presumed initial infection cannot be documented because of the unreliability of skin and serologic testing. Most reported cases are therefore symptomatic and probably represent reinfection from endogenous or exogenous sources. Although the portal of entry is believed to be the lungs in almost all cases, the pulmonary lesion may not cause symptoms and often is discovered roentgenographically during investigation of symptomatic extrapulmonary disease.[150] Symptoms of pulmonary disease occur in only one-third to one-half of cases and consist of cough, expectoration of purulent and sometimes bloody sputum, and occasionally chest pain. Low-grade fever is rare.[145] Rales and rhonchi may be heard in some cases. Pleural effusion is said to occur in 2 per cent of patients. Bone lesions develop in about 25 per cent of cases,[145] sometimes by direct extension from the pleura to the ribs.

Skin lesions are just as common as lung lesions and tend to resemble neoplasms.[145] A remarkable hyperplasia of the epidermis results in verrucous granulomas and subcutaneous nodules that may develop into chronic draining sinuses and ulcerative lesions.[145] The genitourinary system is involved in 10 per cent of male patients. The central nervous system is affected in some cases, and rare reports of adrenal insufficiency have appeared.

If untreated or inadequately treated, the course of North American blastomycosis is one of frequent remissions and exacerbations. Approximately 30 per cent of patients die, but therapy with amphotericin B greatly improves the prognosis.

The leukocyte count is normal or only moderately raised in most patients. Anemia may develop in cases of chronic disease.[145]

The yeast-phase CF test and serologic and skin tests, using mycelial and yeast antigens, are of no practical value in most cases.[145] Cross-reactions with histoplasmin and coccidioidin are frequent, and a positive blastomycin test should be considered significant only when its reaction is stronger than that to histoplasmin and coccidioidin.

SOUTH AMERICAN BLASTOMYCOSIS (PARACOCCIDIOIDOMYCOSIS)

Paracoccidioidomycosis, a granulomatous fungal infection caused by *Paracoccidioides (Blastomyces) brasiliensis*, is rare in the United States but common along the east coast of South America. It is thought to be exogenous in origin, but its natural site is unknown. The disease shows a striking male predominance of 10:1. Animal-to-human and human-to-human transmissions have not been reported. In Brazil, paracoccidioidin skin test surveys have shown that primary disease ·may be asymptomatic. However, as with the other major mycotic infections, progressive or disseminated disease is thought to represent reinfection from endogenous foci.

It is a systemic infection, as evidenced by granulomatous lesions in the skin, mouth, lung, and other viscera, although doubtless the organism gains access to the body via the respiratory tract.

In tissues or exudates cultured on media at 37° C, the organism is a multiple-budding yeast form 2 to 16 μ in diameter. Culture on Sabouraud's glucose-agar medium at <30° C grows mycelia with branching hyphae and conidia. The organism is large and multinucleated and, with its multiple buds, readily recognizable. There are no practical serologic methods for indirect diagnosis or screening.

In a review of the pathologic characteristics in 25 patients,[152] the lungs were involved in 96 per cent, lymph nodes in 76 per cent, oropharynx in 64 per cent, and adrenal glands in 52 per cent. The initial lesion consists of an inflammatory reaction in the alveolar septae surrounding infected blood vessels; leukocytic and histiocytic infiltration occurs, with proliferation of reticulin fibers; granulomas develop later, with giant cells, focal suppuration, and caseous necrosis.[152] It is now generally believed that *Paracoccidioides brasiliensis* enters the body by inhalation, the lungs being the site of the primary lesion, and then disseminates hematogenously to other viscera and the skin. In one series of 41 laborers over 30 years of age residing in a subtropical forest region,[153] 29 had ulcers, either in the mouth or (occasionally) on the skin, and 28 of these had pulmonary involvement. *P. brasiliensis* was found in the sputum in 27.[153] Symptoms and physical signs were scanty and pulmonary involvement was not generally suspected. The remaining 12 patients presented with pulmonary disease only. Fungemia may lead to involvement of the liver and spleen and also the lungs, a miliary pattern being roentgenographically apparent in many cases.

CRYPTOCOCCOSIS

Cryptococcosis (torulosis, European blastomycosis) is a granulomatous disease caused by the organism *Cryptococcus neoformans*, a unimorphic fungus that exists in yeast form in soil and in animals and humans.

THE CAUSATIVE ORGANISM

The yeast cell of *C. neoformans* is a spherical, single-budding, doubly-refractile organism 4 to 15 μ in diameter. Except for its thick capsule, the organism could be confused with mononuclear leukocytes or erythrocytes. It can be identified in sputum, cerebrospinal fluid, or urine which has been mixed with a drop of India ink and examined wet under a coverslip. Hematoxylin and eosin stain of tissue material is often unsatisfactory, but the organism stains jet black with the silver chromate technique.

Positive sputum cultures of this organism in pathologically proved cases are rare;[154] spinal fluid culture is more rewarding. Glucose or blood agar is used as culture medium (the latter being useful in differentiating pathogenic from nonpathogenic strains)[155] and produces growth in from 48 hours to several weeks. Mice are highly susceptible; their organs should be cultured 2 to 4 weeks after intraperitoneal inoculation.

Although clinically the central nervous system is most frequently involved, neocropsy studies have shown that *C. neoformans* occurs as frequently in the lungs.

The granulomatous lesion has a caseous necrotic center surrounded by moderately well-developed connective tissue containing groups of lymphocytes and occasional giant cells and plasma cells.

EPIDEMIOLOGY

C. neoformans is of worldwide distribution.[155] It lives in soil, particularly that contaminated by pigeon excreta.[155] There is no proof of transmission from animal to human or from human to human. Although not a common saprophyte in man, colonization is most frequent in patients with other chronic pulmonary disease. The disease may affect persons of any age, but is commonest in middle-aged males;[154] in one series of 101 pulmonary cases, 82 per cent were males and 87 per cent Caucasian.[154] The respiratory tract is the portal of entry in most if not all cases. The organism has a particular affinity for the central nervous system.[155]

As with blastomycosis, a benign asymptomatic form of disease is suspected but not proved. *C. neoformans* is a relatively uncommon primary pathogen but may occur as an opportunistic invader in compromised hosts, particularly in patients with terminal Hodgkin's disease and, to a lesser extent, with lymphosarcoma, lymphatic or myeloid leukemia, lupus erythematosus, and chronic pulmonary conditions.[155]

ROENTGENOGRAPHIC MANIFESTATIONS

The most common form of pulmonary involvement roentgenographically is a fairly well-circumscribed mass, 2 to 10 cm in diameter (Figure 6–19).[155–157] The lesions are usually single and may closely mimic primary bronchogenic carcinoma. In the majority of cases, the disease is confined to one lobe.[154] Well-defined lobar or segmental consolidation was noted in nine of the 26 cases reported by Gordonson and colleagues.[157] Cavitation is relatively uncommon compared with its incidence in other mycoses.[154, 156] Widely disseminated disease may give rise to a miliary pattern or multiple, diffuse, ill-defined shadows. Hilar and mediastinal lymph node enlargement is unusual. Calcification is extremely rare. Pleural effusion is uncommon and rarely develops secondary to primary pulmonary cryptococcosis.

Six of Gordonson and coworkers' 26 patients[157] had lung disease and 12 had predisposing *systemic* disease, chiefly chronic alcoholism, disseminated tuberculosis, and systemic lupus erythematosus.

CLINICAL MANIFESTATIONS

Pulmonary involvement frequently is asymptomatic, and since sputum cultures usually are

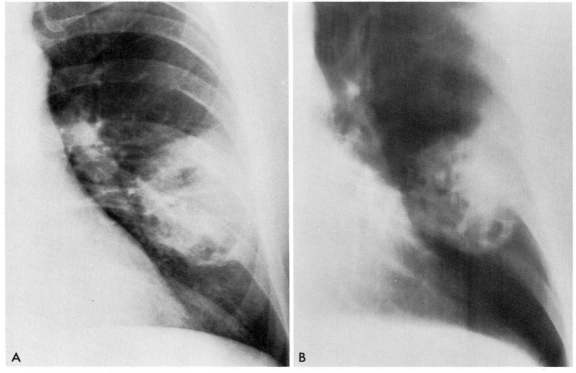

Figure 6–19. Pulmonary Cryptococcosis. Views of the left hemithorax from a posteroanterior roentgenogram (A) and an anteroposterior tomogram (B) reveal a well-circumscribed mass situated in the axillary portion of the left lower lobe; its lateral aspect abuts against the visceral pleura. Several irregular areas of radiolucency are present throughout the mass, representing multiple foci of cavitation. The appearance of the mass is quite characteristic of cryptococcosis, although the cavitation is somewhat unusual. *Cryptococcus neoformans* was cultured from the sputum.

unrewarding,[154] the diagnosis of pulmonary cryptococcosis is often made histologically from tissue removed at thoracotomy.[154, 156] When disease confined to the lungs causes symptoms these are usually mild; they include cough, scanty mucoid and rarely bloody sputum, with chest pain and low-grade fever in some cases.[154, 156] A history of exposure to pigeon excreta may suggest the diagnosis.[155] Physical examination of the chest occasionally reveals rales and rhonchi and rarely signs of consolidation. Extrapulmonary spread is most common in patients with underlying chronic disease, particularly of the reticuloendothelial system.[154]

A common clinical presentation is low-grade meningitis, with a normal chest roentgenogram in some; the cerebrospinal fluid contains leukocytes and cryptococci, the latter easily mistaken for lymphocytes or red blood cells, and has a low sugar and high protein content. Cryptococcal meningitis, formerly 100 per cent fatal, now has a 60 per cent survival rate when treated with amphotericin B.

Skin tests are not very helpful because of an extreme degree of cross-reactivity with other fungi. Serologic tests for both antigens and antibodies show considerable promise.[158] Circulating antigens indicate continuing disease and are highly specific for cryptococcosis; antibodies are found only after therapy, when the serum or cerebrospinal fluid has become culturally negative and the antigen titer has decreased.[158] The CF test appears to be more sensitive than either a modified latex fixation or a slide agglutination test.[158]

CANDIDIASIS (MONILIASIS)

Pulmonary infection with *Candida* species is rare and almost invariably occurs in infants, the elderly, or persons debilitated by chronic disease.[159] It is a common saprophyte of the upper respiratory tract. A high yield of positive cultures in patients receiving antibiotic therapy is well recognized.

The lung is a relatively rare site of candidal infection, the oropharynx, vagina, and skin being much more commonly affected. Fungemia develops in susceptible individuals, disseminating the organism throughout the body and forming granulomas in the tissues. Debilitated patients following multiple abdominal operations[159] or on prolonged gentamicin therapy for hospital-acquired *Pseudomonas* pneumonia are particularly prone to disseminated, fatal candidiasis.

THE CAUSATIVE ORGANISM

In humans, almost all of these infections are due to *Candida albicans.* Wet preparations with potassium hydroxide under a coverslip show the budding yeastlike fungus to be 2 to 4 μ in diameter and to have a thin wall. *Candida* is a dimorphic fungus and is thought by some[160] to be more likely a pathogen if both yeast and mycelial forms are isolated from body fluids or tissues. The organism may be identified in tissue stained with hematoxylin and eosin or with PAS. *Candida albicans* is readily identifiable by its cultural characteristics on cornmeal agar, on which it produces thick-walled chlamydospores.

ROENTGENOGRAPHIC MANIFESTATIONS

Roentgenographic patterns in candidiasis are nonspecific. The commonest is patchy, segmental inhomogeneous consolidation;[161] nonsegmental air-space consolidation also occurs. Miliary dissemination has been described,[161] as well as cavitation in consolidated lung, with or without a fungus ball.

CLINICAL MANIFESTATIONS

There is nothing distinctive about the clinical picture of pulmonary candidiasis. The diagnosis should be considered in immunocompromised patients with roentgenographic evidence of acute or chronic pulmonary disease who have repeated, heavy growth of *C. albicans* in sputum that is otherwise pathogen-free. Suspicion should be increased when blood culture is positive and there is an increasing titer of *Candida* antibodies. However, since the organism is ordinarily a respiratory tract saprophyte, and transient candidemia can occur without tissue dissemination, conclusive diagnosis requires demonstration of the organism in tissues;[160] thus, percutaneous aspiration, transbronchial brushing, or even open lung biopsy may be indicated. The symptoms of pulmonary involvement include cough, purulent expectoration, and hemoptysis.

Candidemia may reflect only a transient contamination of the bloodstream and does not always result in tissue invasion.[162] Repeated positive blood culture in association with likely clinical states strongly indicates dissemination, particularly when the organism is isolated from a catheter specimen of urine.[162]

Agglutinating and precipitating antibodies can be detected in patients with disseminated candidiasis and may prove useful in establishing a diagnosis. Periodic serologic studies should be performed on patients at high risk for mycotic infections (such as those with acute leukemia) to detect a rise in antibody titer. There is evidence that the survival rate can be improved only by frequent culture for fungi and repeated search for antibodies.[159]

TORULOPSIS GLABRATA

Like *Candida* and cryptococci, this organism is a member of the family Cryptococcaceae. A nonspore-forming yeast, it reproduces by budding but fails to produce septate hyphae. It is widely distributed in nature and is saprophytic in many mammals, including humans. The characteristic pinpoint, clear, nonhemolytic colonies that grow on sheep blood agar within 24 to 72 hours may enable early species identification. Infections in humans are opportunistic and usually involve the urinary tract. Pulmonary involvement is rare.

ACTINOMYCOSIS

In humans, actinomycosis is caused by *Actinomyces israelii*, a pleomorphic organism that exists in rod-shaped bacterial form as a commensal in the mouth and tonsillar crypts and in mycelial form in tissues.

The organism is found commonly in dental caries and at gingival margins in persons with poor oral hygiene, and pulmonary infection in such individuals is believed to occur through aspiration of the organism. Before the advent of antibiotics, actinomycosis was the most commonly diagnosed pulmonary fungal disease, presenting a fairly typical clinical picture of empyema and sinus tracts in the chest wall. This advanced stage is rarely seen now; in fact, the incidence of thoracic involvement has declined markedly.

The great majority of infections are caused by *A. israelii* (a frequent oral inhabitant of healthy people). Despite the many similarities in clinical presentation of actinomycosis and fungal infections, the actinomycetes have been firmly established as bacteria rather than fungi. However, tradition and the similarities to the mycoses in clinical and roentgenographic presentation led us to include actinomycosis with diseases of fungal etiology.

The finding of white or yellow "sulfur granules" in the sputum or in exudate from sinus tracts is highly suggestive of the diagnosis. These granules are 1 to 2 mm in diameter; they consist of mycelial clumps, with very thin hyphae that have peripheral radiations, with or without clubbing at the ends. Acid-fast stain helps to differentiate this organism from *Nocardia*, which is more likely to be acid-fast; however, some stains of *Actinomyces* also are acid-fast if a weak decolorizing solution is used.

Despite the highly suggestive nature of sulfur granules, culture is required to confirm the diagnosis.[163] Anaerobic conditions are necessary for culture, using an enriched agar plate or Brewer's thioglycollate medium for incubation at 37° C.

Actinomycosis affects both humans and cattle. In the former, the organism attacks the mandibulofacial area, intestinal tract, and lung, in this order of frequency. It is a worldwide disease, and no age or race is immune; men are affected slightly more often than women, without occupational predilection or seasonal variation.[163]

The typical *roentgenographic* pattern in the fulminating variety of the disease is of acute airspace pneumonia, without recognizable segmental distribution, commonly in the periphery of the lung and with a predilection for the lower lobes. Sometimes the presentation is in the form of a mass, with or without cavitation,[164] and in such cases the resemblance to bronchogenic carcinoma not infrequently leads to inappropriate surgical resection. Extension across the pleural fissures and into the chest wall occurs sometimes but is not unique to this disease—it may also occur in blastomycosis, cryptococcosis, and, of course, tuberculosis. The manifestations of chest wall involvement include a soft tissue mass, which was seen in almost half the patients with this type of involvement in one series,[164] sometimes without pulmonary spread; periosteal proliferation along the ribs may have a peculiar wavy configuration; frank rib destruction may occur,[164] and very occasionally vertebral destruction.

In those patients in whom the pleuropulmonary disease becomes chronic, extensive fibrosis in and about the lung can become a prominent roentgenographic feature; the result is severe distortion of normal anatomic structures.[164]

The initial *clinical* manifestations of pulmonary involvement are nonproductive cough and low-grade fever; the cough later becomes productive of purulent and, in many cases, blood-streaked sputum. The patient's temperature rises, and pain on breathing develops as the infection spreads to the pleura and chest wall. Rarely, a sinus tract infection may result in a bronchocutaneous fistula, or the infection may penetrate through the diaphragm or into the mediastinum, causing such complications as pericarditis. Although most cases of pulmonary disease are the result of aspiration of infected material from the oropharynx, some result from extension of the disease through the esophagus or diaphragm from primary sites in the gastrointestinal tract.

The leukocyte count is normal or moderately increased. Examination of the chest may reveal signs of consolidation and in some cases a soft tissue mass in the chest wall. As the disease progresses, weight loss, anemia, and finger clubbing may occur.[163] The development of pleural effusion almost certainly indicates an empyema.

NOCARDIOSIS

Nocardia species inhabit the soil throughout the world; in tropical and subtropical climates, some species are the main cause of mycetoma of the foot (Madura foot or maduromycosis). In North America, the organism chiefly responsible for pulmonary disease is *Nocardia asteroides*. Both the clinical picture and the morphologic appearance of the mycelium in tissue closely resemble that of actinomycosis. In tissue section *Actinomyces israelii* forms "sulfur granules," which helps in differentiation from systemic nocardiosis. *Nocardia* strains are more commonly acid-fast than *A. israelii*.

N. asteroides is an uncommon laboratory contaminant,[165] and, whereas formerly it was seen almost exclusively as a primary pulmonary pathogen, it is now more frequently recognized as an opportunistic invader in patients with chronic disease, particularly those receiving glucocorticosteroids.[165] Human nocardiosis has recently been the subject of an excellent review.[166]

There is a male sex predominance of 2:1 but no apparent predilection for race or age group in nocardiosis. Humans presumably contract the disease from exposure to contaminated soil; spread does not occur from animal to person or from person to person.

As with the *Actinomyces*, the *Nocardia* species formerly were classified as mycoses but now are considered bacteria. Because of their similarity to the fungi, the disease is considered here. *N. asteroides* is a gram-positive organism with delicate, branching, filamentous hy-

phae; it is sometimes acid-fast but this characteristic may be affected during tissue fixation. The organism may be identified on smears or cultures of exudate from the lung, subcutaneous abscesses, and occasionally the joints. Aerobic culture is made on glucose agar at 30° C or on blood agar at 37° C; colonies may take up to 4 weeks to appear. The pathologic lesion is a combination of granuloma formation and suppuration; morphologically, in tissue the organism is indistinguishable from *Actinomyces*.

The *roentgenologically* apparent changes vary but in most respects are similar to those of actinomycosis. The most frequent manifestation is air-space pneumonia, usually homogeneous and nonsegmental,[167] but sometimes patchy and inhomogeneous. Cavitation is frequent,[165, 168] and as with actinomycosis the infection may extend into the pleural space and cause empyema. Chest wall involvement and widespread dissemination now are rare. The organism can form solitary nodules.[167]

The *clinical* manifestations include cough, purulent sputum (sometimes blood-streaked), pleural pain, and night sweats. Examination may reveal rales over the affected area, and signs of consolidation or pleural effusion in some cases.[167, 168] The course is usually chronic but in patients with lowered resistance an acute, fulminating, nocardial pneumonia may develop. The infection may spread to other areas of the body, most often forming abscesses in the brain[168] or subcutaneous tissue. Empyema and rib osteomyelitis develop in a small percentage of cases.[168]

Since in most cases this infection is superimposed on some other disease, the signs and symptoms of the primary disease may confuse the clinical picture. Although nocardiosis may coexist with any chronic condition,[165, 168] patients with disease of the reticuloendothelial system—and, for reasons not known, with alveolar proteinosis—appear to be the most susceptible.[165] Patients receiving immunosuppressive therapy after organ transplantation are particularly vulnerable. Most strains of *N. asteroides* are susceptible to sulfonamides; therefore, since the early institution of therapy appears to improve the prognosis, transtracheal aspiration, bronchial brushing, and aspiration lung biopsy are warranted (and often necessary) to establish a diagnosis, particularly in immunosuppressed patients.

The white cell count usually is moderately elevated, with neutrophilia; lymphocytosis or leukopenia develops in a few cases.[167] Animal inoculation and serologic tests do not aid diagnosis.

ASPERGILLOSIS

Aspergillosis is a mycotic disease caused by species of the dimorphic fungus *Aspergillus*. Although many of these species can cause disease in humans, the responsible organism is almost invariably *Aspergillus fumigatus*. *Aspergillus* species are ubiquitous in nature and occur as saprophytes in the upper respiratory tract and as contaminants in the laboratory. The organisms are found more commonly in the sputum of patients with bronchial asthma than in the general population. In one series, its isolation was considered more than a coincidental finding in 50 per cent of cases.[169]

The disease is of worldwide distribution but is more commonly reported from France and England than from North America. It shows a male sex predominance of about 3:1. There is no evidence of transmission from animal to person or from person to person. When resident in the lung, the organism is usually a saprophyte in residual cavities or in mucous plugs in sensitized patients. When this normally saprophytic fungus invades tissues, almost invariably there is underlying disease or reduced resistance.[170]

THE CAUSATIVE ORGANISM

Microscopically, all species of *Aspergillus* are characterized by conidiophores which expand into large vesicles. The mycetoma is composed of intertwined hyphae matted together with fibrin, mucus, and cellular debris. The organisms may be absent or sparse in the sputum of patients with intracavitary disease or bronchial asthma productive of mucous plugs.

Conclusive diagnosis of aspergillosis in those forms of the disease other than pulmonary mycetoma may be difficult. Infection may be strongly suspected if this organism and no other pathogens can be cultured repeatedly from the sputum, but definite evidence that an *Aspergillus* species is playing the role of a pathogen necessitates microscopic demonstration of tissue invasion.

Tissue reaction to *Aspergillus* consists of a granuloma similar in many respects to that caused by other fungi. When the organism is more invasive, acting either as a primary pathogen or as an opportunistic microorganism, necrosis occurs in addition to the granulomatous process.

Infections caused by *Aspergillus* may be divided into "primary" and "secondary," the former representing the invasion of tissues in a previously healthy person and the latter an infection superimposed upon a condition that has reduced host resistance. It is emphasized that these terms, here and in the literature, do not connote "original infection" and "reinfection" as understood in relation to pulmonary tuberculosis. The thoracic manifestations of aspergillosis have recently been reviewed.[171–173]

PRIMARY ASPERGILLOSIS

Primary infection with *Aspergillus* is exceedingly rare. In most of the few reported instances of aspergillosis in otherwise healthy persons there was no history of significant occupational exposure.

The *roentgenographic* pattern of primary aspergillosis is of nonsegmental, homogeneous consolidation that may progress to abscess formation; in the absence of cavitation, the appearances are indistinguishable from those of acute pneumococcal pneumonia.

Clinically, the picture is one of chronic granulomatous infection, with low-grade fever, cough, sometimes purulent expectoration, hemoptysis, and chest pain. Thoracic tissues, including the mediastinum, may be extensively involved.

SECONDARY ASPERGILLOSIS

Pulmonary Mycetoma

A mycetoma can be defined as a conglomeration of intertwined fungal hyphae matted together with fibrin, mucus, and cellular debris, within a pulmonary cavity (*see* Figure 6–11, page 294). In the great majority of cases the fungus is present as a pure saprophyte: (1) almost invariably the underlying cavity can be ascribed to other causes, such as bronchiectasis, sarcoidosis, tuberculosis, histoplasmosis, bronchial cysts, chronic bacterial abscess, or carcinoma;[169, 174] (2) invariably the organism is in a mycelial form; and (3) the cavity wall does not evidence invasion by the organism. The diagnosis is readily apparent in the typical roentgenographic features but can be confirmed only after surgical removal of the specimen, since few patients with this form of aspergillosis expectorate the fungi.

The invariable *roentgenographic appearance* of pulmonary mycetoma is a solid rounded mass of unit density within a spherical or ovoid cavity, separated from the wall of the cavity by a crescent-shaped air space. Fluid levels are not seen within the cavities.[174] The intracavity fungus ball occurs much more commonly in upper than in lower lobes, probably because it

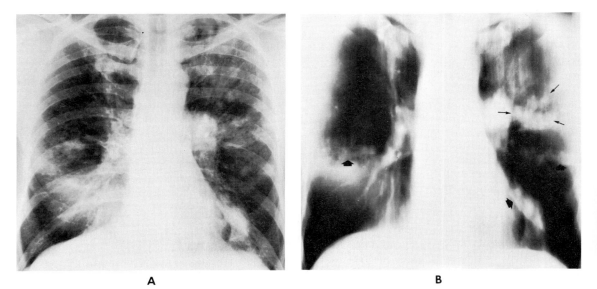

A   **B**

Figure 6–20. Hypersensitivity Aspergillosis. A posteroanterior roentgenogram (A) reveals extensive bilateral pulmonary disease, all lobes of the lung being affected by a process possessing an unusual mixed pattern. In the left upper lobe, the pattern appears to be one of air-space consolidation, confluent shadows of homogeneous density being associated with an air bronchogram; the medial segment of the right middle lobe shows a combination of atelectasis and consolidation; broad areas of consolidation extend into the anterior basal segment of the left lower lobe and the anterior segment of the left upper lobe. A full lung tomogram in anteroposterior projection (B) shows numerous broad-band shadows bilaterally, each measuring approximately 1 cm in diameter and extending in a distribution compatible with the bronchovascular bundles (*thick arrows*). In the midportion of the left lung, one of these shadows possesses a Y-configuration (*thin arrows*). These band shadows are caused by inspissated mucus within markedly dilated bronchi; the Y-shaped shadow in the left midlung represents a bifurcating bronchus impacted with mucus. Note that with the exception of the right middle lobe, all impacted bronchi are unassociated with consolidation or atelectasis of the lung distal to them, presumably as a result of effective collateral air drift. This 42-year-old man had an industrial exposure to powdered casein, samples of which grew *Aspergillus fumigatus*. He presented with fever, productive cough, and dyspnea; there was a moderate peripheral eosinophilia. *Aspergillus fumigatus* was recovered from the sputum.

so frequently occupies a tuberculous cavity.[174, 175] Most of the cavities are thin-walled.[174] They are often contiguous to a pleural surface, which may be thickened. The fungus ball should move when the patient changes position. Calcification of the mycelial mass may occur. The size of the ball may vary or may remain constant for many years.[174] The differential diagnosis should include a fragment of tissue in a carcinoma that has undergone necrosis, a mass of necrotic lung in an abscess, a disintegrating hydatid cyst, and an intracavitary blood clot. A precipitin test usually permits differentiation.

Thickening of the walls of tuberculous cavities has been described as an early roentgenographic sign of secondary aspergillosis, antedating the formation of a fungus ball. There have been occasional reports of mycetomas developing in apical fibrotic lesions in patients with advanced ankylosing spondylitis[176] and in association with hypersensitivity and invasive pulmonary aspergillosis.[176]

Clinically, most patients with intracavitary aspergilloma are healthy. Cough and expectoration are common; hemoptysis has been re-

ported in up to 70 per cent of cases.[174] The affected lobe should be resected in patients with copious hemoptysis, since the hemorrhage may proceed to fatal exsanguination. Mycetomas lyse spontaneously in approximately 10 per cent of cases, and some disappear when pyogenic infection of the cavity develops.

Hypersensitivity Aspergillosis

This form of the disease is characterized by mucous plugs containing aspergilli and eosinophils in segmental bronchi. Most patients give a history of long-standing bronchial asthma.

The *roentgenographic pattern* of this form of aspergillosis is identical to that of mucoid impaction.[177] Homogeneous, fingerlike shadows of unit density lie in a precise bronchial distribution, usually involving the upper lobes and almost always in the more central segmental bronchi rather than the peripheral branches (Figure 6–20).[177] The impacted bronchi may relate to atelectatic areas; in our experience, atelectasis often is notable by its absence, a fact explained by collateral airdrift. The shadows tend to be transient but may persist unchanged for weeks or even months or may enlarge. Resolution of the lesion leaves cylindrical or saccular dilatation of the bronchi at the site of mucoid impaction. These lesions tend to recur in the same segmental bronchi, suggesting that bronchial damage predisposes locally to further episodes. Limited tissue invasion has been reported in patients treated with corticosteroids.[177]

Clinically, these patients have fever, cough, purulent expectoration (sometimes with hemoptysis), and expectoration of mucous plugs. Dyspnea may be very severe and leukocytosis with eosinophilia develops in most cases. The fungus appears to be more than a saprophyte, since many patients with a positive skin reaction to *Aspergillus* extract have a positive reaction to the precipitation test for antibodies;[169] many also have aspergilli in their sputum at the time of the first attack of bronchospasm.

Aspergillosis with Chronic Debilitating Disease

In patients with impaired host defenses, aspergilli may extend beyond a pre-existing cavity or the bronchial wall, invading pulmonary tissue and even disseminating throughout the body. Virtually all patients with invasive and disseminated disease have malignancy (the majority hematologic or lymphoreticular)[178] or have recently had organ transplantation. Usually they are receiving corticosteroids or other immunosuppressive medication, antineoplastic chemotherapy, or antibiotics directed against a gram-negative organism.[170] Patients with acute leukemia in relapse and with granulocytopenia are particularly susceptible.[178] Occasionally, fatal invasive pulmonary aspergillosis may follow acute viral infection that depresses T-cell function.[179] Dissemination is to the gastrointestinal tract, brain, liver, kidneys, and heart;[170, 178] rarely, it occurs in the absence of lung involvement.[178]

The *pathologic changes* in the lung are combined granulomatous and pyogenic infection, with extension to neighboring vessels and consequent hemorrhagic infarction. Since sputum and blood cultures are seldom positive, in the vast majority of patients the diagnosis is made only after death.[178]

The *roentgenographic pattern* is of single or multiple areas of pneumonic consolidation, with or without cavitation (Figure 6–21).[170, 178] An unusual radiographic pattern of invasive aspergillosis has recently been described,[180] important to recognize because of its highly suggestive nature: single or multiple areas of parenchymal consolidation are associated with air crescents suggesting the presence of cavities containing loose bodies (these are not necessarily fungus balls as illustrated by one of the patients reported by Curtis and her colleagues[180] in whom it proved pathologically to be a sequestrum of lung tissue). We have recently seen one example of this unique roentgenographic presentation. *Aspergillus* infection may be superimposed on bacterial pneumonia and, if the latter has abscessed, may present as a mycetoma. Miliary spread thoughout the lungs is very rare.

Clinically, these patients characteristically present with unremitting fever which responds poorly or not at all to antibiotic therapy.

SEROLOGY

The results of skin testing and serologic studies implicate *Aspergillus* as a pathogen rather than a saprophyte.[169, 181] Nearly all patients with pulmonary aspergillomas have positive precipitin reactions. After resection of a mycetoma, the precipitin test becomes weaker but rarely reverts to negative. Sera from patients with allergic bronchopulmonary aspergillosis also may contain precipitins to *Aspergillus;* in one series of patients with transient pulmonary opacities and eosinophilia, positive results were obtained in 63 per cent.[181]

Immediate and late Arthus skin reactions occur in a large percentage of patients with hypersensitivity aspergillosis, but rarely in patients with pulmonary mycetoma.[181]

Serum IgE levels, measured by radioimmunoassay, are markedly elevated in patients with allergic pulmonary aspergillosis, especially during the acute phase of pulmonary opacification. Young and Bennett[182] could not detect antibodies to *A. fumigatus* in sera from 15 patients with widespread invasive aspergillosis, most of whom were receiving immunosuppressive therapy intermittently for malignant disease.

MUCORMYCOSIS

Although this disease commonly is referred to as mucormycosis, it includes infections caused by other members of the class Zygomycetes, order Mucorales—*Absidia, Rhizopus,* and *Mucor* species.[183] These fungi appear to be worldwide in distribution and are found on bread and fruit and in soil. Infection is probably exogenous, the spores entering the

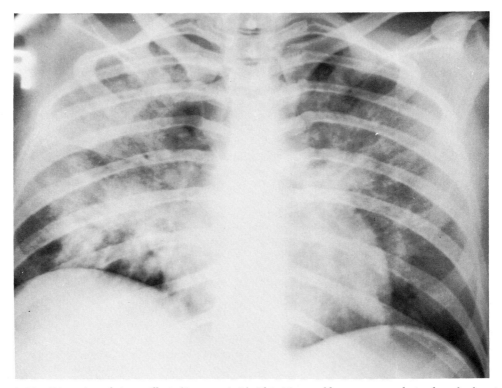

Figure 6–21. Disseminated Aspergillosis (Opportunistic). This 27-year-old woman was admitted to the hospital with complaints referable to multiple systems which eventually proved to be due to systemic lupus erythematosus. For this she received corticosteroid therapy, to which were added high doses of antibiotics when she developed clinical and roentgenologic evidence of pneumonia. This anteroposterior roentgenogram reveals extensive bilateral pulmonary disease characterized by confluent air-space consolidation; a well-defined air bronchogram can be identified in most areas. The patient's clinical condition rapidly deteriorated and she died in severe respiratory distress 4 days after this roentgenogram. At necropsy, in addition to the characteristic findings of systemic lupus erythematosus, there was evidence of multisystem involvement by *Aspergillus fumigatus*, most pronounced in the lungs, heart, and kidneys.

paranasal sinuses and lung by inhalation. The disease occurs almost invariably in patients with underlying disease,[184] especially during treatment with corticosteroids or antibiotics. The commonest primary diseases are diabetes (present in 21 of 55 cases in one series[184]), lymphoma, and leukemia.[184]

The organism has a distinctive appearance in tissue—wide, nonseptate hyphae—but culture is required for confirmation of diagnosis. Growth occurs readily on Sabouraud's glucose agar. Microscopy reveals hyphae bearing large globular sacs 100 μ in diameter; these sacs, known as sporangia, contain round or elliptic spores measuring 6.0 to 8.5 μ. The organism is a common laboratory contaminant. Mucormycetous hyphae invade blood vessels; the massive growth of fungi, or thrombus formation on a tangled mass of hyphae, occludes the vessels and causes infarction and infection; many of these areas cavitate.[185]

Roentgenographically, lung involvement is usually segmental and homogeneous, reflecting the vascular obstruction.[184] Cavitation is frequent.

The only distinctive part of the *clinical picture* is the tendency to involvement of the paranasal sinuses, particularly in patients with diabetes mellitus. Extension may occur to the orbits and cranium, causing orbital cellulitis and meningoencephalitis. Almost all patients with diabetes who present with this clinical picture evidence pulmonary disease. Mucormycetes infection is rarely diagnosed before death; the outcome is almost invariably fatal,[185] but rare cases have been reported of cure with amphotericin B therapy and surgery.[183]

GEOTRICHOSIS

This rare fungal infection may exist in either a bronchial or pulmonary form. The causative organism (*Geotrichum* species) is usually detected as a saprophyte in the sputum of patients with chronic pulmonary disease. *Geotrichum candidum* is a ubiquitous, yeastlike fungus which is found in soil and dairy products and is a normal inhabitant of the intestinal tract.[186]

The sputum may contain large, rectangular arthrospores 4 to 6 by 8 to 12 μ in diameter, with rounded ends. Culture on Sabouraud's glucose agar may grow hyphae attached to the elongated arthrospores; these may become oval or spherical when separated from the hyphae. *Geotrichum* stains well with Gram or PAS stains.

The chest roentgenogram is not distinctive. The bronchial form of the disease may show no roentgenographic abnormalities or merely an accentuation of basal pulmonary markings.[187] The pulmonary form usually is evidenced by parenchymal consolidation of the upper lobes, frequently with thin-walled cavities.

Clinically, the bronchial type is associated with bronchitis or asthma, with eosinophilia in some cases.[187] In both bronchial and pulmonary forms of geotrichosis, purulent expectoration may be copious and the sputum may be very gelatinous.[186] Fever and hemoptysis are present in most cases of the pneumonic form. Rales, rhonchi, and occasionally signs of consolidation may be detected. A skin test and agglutination test are available and are useful in diagnosis.

SPOROTRICHOSIS

Sporotrichosis in humans is caused by *Sporotrichum schenckii,* a dimorphic fungus of worldwide distribution. It is a saprophyte in soil, sphagnum, peat moss, decaying vegetable matter, and on thorns, but not in the human respiratory tract.[188] There is a distinct occupational hazard to farmers, laborers, and florists, and thus a significant male sex predominance. Animals also can be infected, and the disease can be transmitted from animals to humans.[189]

The organism is readily isolated from the sputum and may be seen on smear. Culture at 30° C on Sabouraud's agar reveals delicate hyphae supporting conidiophores terminating in clusters of pyriform conidia. Enriched media at 37° C or mouse tissues may support a growth of the cigar-shaped, gram-positive, yeastlike forms. *S. schenckii* stains well with methionine silver.[189]

Primary pulmonary disease is extremely rare, about 40 authenticated cases having been reported.[188–190]

Roentgenographically, the disease may be manifest in any portion of the lung, and the number of variations in its presentation are almost as great as the number of cases reported. Changes include isolated nodular masses, which may cavitate, leaving thin-walled cavities;[189] segmental parenchymal consolidation; hilar lymph node enlargement, which occurs in a high percentage of cases and may cause bronchial obstruction;[189] and, in some cases, pulmonary disease spreading through the pleura into the chest wall, creating a sinus tract.[189] The reaction to the organism in the tissues is usually suppurative but may be granulomatous.

Clinical manifestations vary from mild acute bronchitis to pneumonia, which may be associated with severe malaise, cough, and fever. In humans most infections are cutaneous, with spread to regional lymph nodes. Commonly, a pustule forms on the hand and the infection spreads along the lymphatic channels, forming nodules that may ulcerate; bones and joints may be directly involved from cutaneous and lymph node spread, and bloodstream invasion has been reported. Anemia and polymorphonuclear leukocytosis may develop. Best therapeutic results are obtained with a supersaturated solution of potassium iodide.[190]

Agglutination and complement-fixation tests sometimes aid diagnosis, and a skin test is available.

ALLESCHERIASIS AND MONOSPOROSIS

The fungus *Allescheria boydii* and its asexual form (*Monosporium apiospermum*) cause maduromycosis and sometimes opportunistic infection in the lungs.[191] The roentgenographic pattern is one of cavitation with or without a fungus ball inside.[191] The patient may be asymptomatic, may suffer repeated hemoptysis, or may have symptoms and signs of underlying disease. The fungus can be cultured from sputum or blood, and precipitating antibodies are found in the serum.[191]

LUNG INFECTIONS CAUSED BY VIRUSES, MYCOPLASMA PNEUMONIAE, AND RICKETTSIAE

Many respiratory tract infections caused by viruses and by *Mycoplasma pneumoniae* begin in the upper respiratory passages. Some viruses, including certain enteroviruses and the chickenpox and measles viruses, frequently propagate in the upper respiratory tract and disseminate throughout the body without producing respiratory symptoms. Others typically remain confined to the respiratory mucous membrane, where they cause a spectrum of diseases ranging from mild, virtually asymptomatic rhinitis to widely disseminated, sometimes fatal, air-space pneumonia. Specific respiratory viruses tend to produce fairly well-defined clinical syndromes; but each can produce any of the respiratory syndromes, depending upon the inoculum's characteristics and the host's resistance. The virulence and dose of the organism are important in determining whether the infection is confined to the nose and throat or spreads to the upper and lower respiratory tract. Experimental work has indicated that the size of the virus-carrying aerosol particle may be a major factor in determining the site of infection;[192] large aerosol particles tend to deposit in the nasopharynx, resulting in an influenzalike infection with little or no involvement of the lower respiratory tract; small aerosol particles measuring 3 μ or less are carried deep into the lungs, where they produce clinical and roentgenographic evidence of acute bronchitis, bronchiolitis, or pneumonia.

The resistance of the host is important in that it affects not only the ability to cope with the infection but also the extent to which the affecting agent may penetrate the defenses of the respiratory tract. The host's age also partly determines the extent of infection, resistance in the very young and old being limited by immunologic and constitutional factors. Debilitating diseases such as the reticuloendothelioses and specific immunoglobulin and cellular deficiency states also may increase individual susceptibility to respiratory viral infection. The influence of exposure and cold in reducing host resistance has long been debated, but it seems fairly certain that temperature and humidity have little effect on susceptibility to viral disease.

Local factors probably play an even greater role than constitutional factors in modifying the extent of viral penetration of the respiratory tract. Normally, the lower part of the tract is sterile, and experimental studies have demonstrated a remarkable ability of the healthy lung to rid itself of microorganisms. Their rapid clearance depends largely on a healthy mucous membrane and active cilia and an appropriate consistency of the mucus that lines the respiratory tract; it also appears to relate to IgA in mucous secretion. These local defense mechanisms can be diminished by the inhalation of fumes—particularly chemical and cigarette smoke—or aerosols that damage respiratory tract epithelium and inhibit ciliary activity. Although infections with respiratory viruses usually are restricted to the upper respiratory tract, pneumonia may develop when the organism appears in epidemic form, such as when civilian and military personnel are grouped closely together.

RESPIRATORY SYNDROMES

CORYZA

Acute coryza (the common cold) is a syndrome that includes rhinorrhea, nasal obstruction, and occasionally cough and sore throat. Although it has been known for many years that coryza can be caused by several respiratory viruses, it was not until 1965 that the rhinoviruses were recognized as the major cause. A small percentage of cases of coryza are caused by other viruses, including influenza, parainfluenza (especially types 1 and 3), the adenoviruses, respiratory syncytial virus, Coxsackievirus A21, some ECHO viruses, *Mycoplasma pneumoniae*, and especially coronovirus.[193]

Despite these multiple etiologies, in a substantial number of cases of common cold the responsible organism defies identification.

ACUTE PHARYNGITIS-TONSILLITIS INFECTIONS

The most common etiologic agent in this group is not a virus but a bacterium, β-hemolytic streptococcus of the Lancefield group-A type, which is said to be responsible for 25 to 35 per cent of cases. The etiologic agent is unknown in approximately 30 per cent of clinical cases. Acute pharyngitis and tonsillitis clinically identical to streptococcal infection are most commonly caused by the adenoviruses and Coxsackieviruses.

ACUTE RESPIRATORY DISEASE (ARD)

This is an ill-defined group of upper respiratory tract infections that cannot be classified as one of the other respiratory syndromes because the nose does not run enough, the throat is not sore or red enough, and the cough is not severe or paroxysmal enough. Fever is a constant feature, and malaise and generalized aching occur in most cases. Physical signs are sparse, but redness of the throat and occasional rales are common. Fifteen to 30 per cent of cases are believed to be caused by influenza virus, 2 to 9 per cent by parainfluenza virus, approximately 4 per cent by the respiratory syncytial virus, and 3 per cent by adenovirus. The last named appears to be responsible for a large percentage of cases of ARD in military recruits.

ACUTE LOWER RESPIRATORY TRACT DISEASE

This term includes acute laryngotracheobronchitis (croup), tracheobronchitis, bronchiolitis, bronchopneumonia, and primary atypical pneumonia. Most of these syndromes are easily recognized by symptoms, signs, and roentgenologic findings, but it is probable that, in the absence of symptoms in "mild upper respiratory tract" infections, involvement of the small bronchioles is a common pathologic denominator. The evidence for this lies in disturbed pulmonary function. Although virtually all viruses and *M. pneumoniae* have been found responsible for each of these syndromes, specific viruses tend to produce a distinctive clinical pattern. In infants, under the age of two, laryngotracheobronchitis usually is caused by parainfluenza viruses and less commonly by respiratory syncytial (RS) virus; similarly, acute bronchiolitis in early life (a highly virulent disease) is commonly caused by RS virus and sometimes by parainfluenza virus type 3. Acute bronchiolitis and bronchopneumonia caused by RS virus frequently occur in epidemic form. In older children and adults, acute nonbacterial lower respiratory tract disease presents as bronchitis or pneumonia; responsible organisms are *Mycoplasma pneumoniae* (the etiologic agent in 25 to 60 per cent of all nonbacterial pneumonias), the adenoviruses, and parainfluenza virus type 3.

Primary Atypical Pneumonia (PAP)

General Comments and Epidemiology

Approximately 30 years ago it was recognized that a certain percentage of cases of pneumonia did not respond to sulfonamides and penicillin, and that this group possessed clinical and roentgenographic manifestations which set them apart from the usual bacterial pneumonias. The

demonstration of cold agglutinins (serum macro-gammaglobulins that agglutinate human type O cells at 0° C but not at 37° C) in such patients led to the inclusion of this finding as one of the criteria for diagnosis of this type of pneumonia, called primary atypical pneumonia (PAP). In 1944, Eaton and his colleagues[194] isolated a specific agent on culture embryos that appeared responsible for at least some cases of PAP. In 1957, Liu[195] identified the responsible organism in the sputum of patients by an antigen-antibody reaction, using fluorescein-labeled antibody on frozen sections of infected chick embryo lung. Subsequent studies revealed that the Eaton agent was a pleuropneumonialike organism (PPLO), since designated *Mycoplasma pneumoniae*. Cold agglutinins usually develop in the second week of illness and reach maximal titer in the third or fourth week, after which they usually disappear. A titer of 1:32 or greater usually is considered positive, and a fourfold or greater rise during convalescence is required for demonstration of activity. In one series of cases of primary atypical pneumonia,[196] 43 per cent were considered caused by *M. pneumoniae*, 7 per cent by adenovirus, and the remainder were of undetermined etiology; a cold agglutinin titer of 1:32 or higher was found in 57 per cent, 17.6 per cent, and 43 per cent, respectively. A fourfold rise in titer was seen in 59 per cent of patients with *Mycoplasma* infections, in none of the adenovirus cases, and in only 29 per cent of those in whom the cause was undetermined. Other organisms that may produce the generally accepted clinical and roentgenographic features of PAP are influenza, parainfluenza, and RS viruses, as well as the etiologic agents responsible for psittacosis, Q fever, and histoplasmosis.

Although primary atypical pneumonia may occur at any time of year, cases due to *M. pneumoniae* show a peak incidence in the late summer and autumn and those due to adenovirus occur predominantly during the winter months.[196]

Pathologic Characteristics

The pathology of pneumonias caused by viral and viruslike organisms differs somewhat from that of bacterial pneumonia, presumably because of intracellular invasion by viruses. The process is predominantly interstitial, the acute inflammatory reaction in the peribronchial and peribronchiolar tissues extending along blood vessels and lymphatics into interlobular septa;[197] there is proliferation of respiratory epithelium

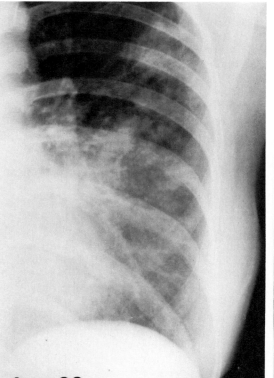

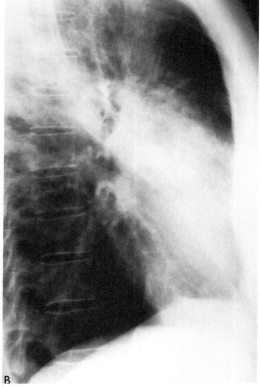

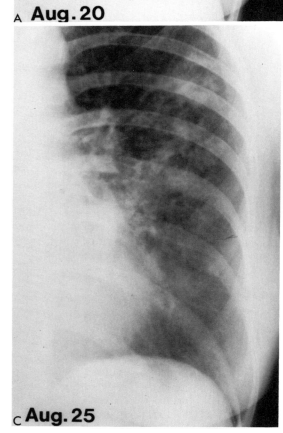

Figure 6–22. Acute Pneumonia Caused by *My-coplasma pneumoniae*. Views of the left lung from posteroanterior (*A*) and lateral (*B*) roentgenograms reveal patchy air-space consolidation in the distribution of the lingular and posterior segments of the left upper lobe. The consolidation is not homogeneous as would be anticipated in acute bacterial pneumonia due to, for example, *Streptococcus pneumoniae*. Immuno-fluorescence microscopy of sputum revealed *M. pneumoniae* organisms. Five days later (*C*), considerable resolution had occurred, particularly in the lingula.

of the bronchi, bronchioles, and alveoli and infiltration of mononuclear cells in the bronchial walls and peribronchiolar tissues. This inflammatory reaction may extend to the alveolar walls.

In some of the cases described by Conte and associates[197] severe chronic interstitial fibrosis was the latest change, and the authors postulated that many instances of so-called idiopathic chronic interstitial fibrosis may represent the end result of viral infection.

Roentgenographic Manifestations

Primary atypical pneumonia tends to involve the lower lobes, more often the left, and is limited to a single lobe in about 50 per cent of cases. Our experience with 36 patients with proved *Mycoplasma* or viral pneumonia[198] revealed a sequence of changes that we regard as highly suggestive of the diagnosis. The early change is a fine reticular pattern of segmental distribution seldom involving more than one lobe; this pattern corresponds to a phase of acute interstitial inflammation. In the second phase, the inflammation extends to the air spaces of the lung, producing patchy areas of air-space consolidation in which individual acinar shadows may be identified (Figure 6–22). The third phase indicates the early stage of resolution: signs of air-space consolidation disappear, but the reticular pattern that represents interstitial inflammation persists. Pleural effusion occurs in roughly 20 per cent of patients[199] but may require lateral decubitus roentgenography for its demonstration.

Clinical Manifestations

Symptoms usually are unimpressive, in many cases creating a marked discrepancy between their mildness and the severity of the roentgenographic changes.[200] Fever usually is low grade but temperature may rise to 39.4° C. Cough is usual and may be either dry or productive of mucoid or purulent material; the patient may complain of symptoms relating to the upper respiratory tract. Hemoptysis and pleural pain are most uncommon, although intercostal or retrosternal pain may be complained of on coughing. Findings usually consist of a local decrease in breath sounds, a few rales, and occasionally frank signs of consolidation with bronchial breathing.

PAP rarely gives rise to leukocytosis; in 75 to

80 per cent of cases reported by George and his associates,[196] the white cell count was below 10,000 per cu mm.

PNEUMONIA CAUSED BY MYCOPLASMA PNEUMONIAE

General Comments and Epidemiology

Although the pleuropneumonialike organism (PPLO), *Mycoplasma pneumoniae*, is not a true virus and is more correctly included among the bacteria, it is generally accepted as the commonest cause of "nonbacterial" pneumonia (10 to 33 per cent of all pneumonias in civilian populations and approximately one-third in marine recruits[201]).

Mycoplasma pneumoniae grows readily on enriched agar or beef broth and has been cultured in tissue and in chorioallantoic membrane of chick embryos.[200]

Unlike adenovirus pneumonia, which occurs almost exclusively during the winter months, infections with *M. pneumoniae* occur throughout the year, with a peak during the autumn and early winter.[196, 201, 202] *Mycoplasma* pneumonia is most common in the age group ranging from 5 to 19 years, infection in younger children usually producing no symptoms. It shows a slight bias for males.[201, 202]

Although nearly all infections with this organism are mild, careful inquiry into family groups usually reveals symptoms in the majority of affected persons. Despite the presence of circulating antibody and the administration of tetracycline, shedding of *Mycoplasma* organisms may continue after the patient has recovered from infection. These "carriers" have been found in military populations, student groups, and civilian communities. Infection is acquired by droplet inhalation and has been produced by this means in volunteers. Transmission of infection occurs after prolonged contact in close communities, and probably school children are the major sources of infection. The incubation period is 1 to 3 weeks.[201]

Pathologic Characteristics

The benign nature of this disease has limited pathologic description. The inflammatory reaction is predominantly interstitial but in severe cases extends into the alveoli. No specific morphologic features distinguish *Mycoplasma* from acute viral pneumonia on macroscopic or light microscopic examination but electron microscopy may reveal the organism *in situ*.[203] The organism is filamentous, with special terminal structures attached to ciliated epithelial cells.[203]

Roentgenographic Manifestations

The pattern of acute *Mycoplasma* pneumonia is indistinguishable from that of many viral pneumonias. In the early stages, the acute interstitial inflammation is apparent as a rather fine reticular pattern. This is followed by signs of air-space consolidation of patchy distribution, sometimes with acinar shadows. With resolution, the process is reversed, the air-space consolidation disappearing first. In a study of 116 cases followed serially,[196] roentgenographic resolution averaged 11 days and was complete in all cases within 25 days.

In contrast to the nonsegmental distribution of acute bacterial air-space pneumonia, *Mycoplasma* pneumonia tends to be segmental. In a series of 79 cases[202] only two had a roentgenographic picture that could be confused with bacterial pneumonia, and both of these were readily identified clinically and from the leukocyte count as of *Mycoplasma* or viral origin.

Involvement is predominantly of the lower lobes. Hilar lymph node enlargement is rare in adults.

From a study of 100 patients with serologically proved *Mycoplasma* pneumonia, Putman and his colleagues[204] recognized two distinct clinical and roentgenographic presentations. The largest group (48 patients) presented with symptoms of short duration characteristic of acute pneumonia: nonpleuritic chest pain, cough, myalgias, and fever. Roentgenologically, there was segmental or lobar consolidation associated with an air bronchogram and sometimes with atelectasis; pleural effusion was evident on erect posteroanterior and lateral roentgenograms in nine cases (19 per cent), in four of which it was hemorrhagic. The second group (28 patients) presented with symptoms of malaise, lethargy, and dyspnea ranging in duration from 1 to 4 weeks; in contrast to the first group, most of these patients were afebrile and were free from cough, myalgia, and chest pain. Roentgenologically, they manifested a diffuse, bilateral reticulonodular pattern (Figure 6–23), sometimes associated with septal (Kerley B) lines; none showed lobar or segmental consolidation. Pleural effusion was observed in only one patient. The remaining 24 patients (group

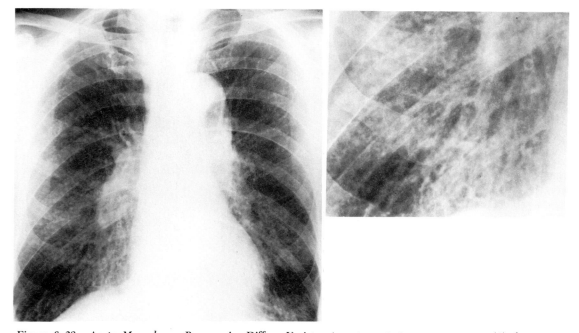

Figure 6–23. Acute *Mycoplasma* Pneumonia, Diffuse Variety. A posteroanterior roentgenogram (*A*) shows an extensive coarse reticulonodular pattern throughout both lungs associated with moderate pulmonary overinflation. The pattern is seen to better advantage in a magnified view of the lower portion of the right lung (*B*). This 70-year-old man was admitted to the hospital with an acute respiratory illness; pulmonary function studies revealed changes consistent with extensive obstruction of small airways. Proved *Mycoplasma* infection.

3) had clinical and roentgenographic manifestations midway between the other two groups and were not easily categorized one way or the other. Blood gas analysis showed more severe derangement in group 2 patients with widespread disease: hypoxemia ($PO_2 < 75$ mm Hg) was found in only four (28 per cent) of 14 patients in group 1 but in 13 (68 per cent) of 19 patients in group 2.

Clinical Manifestations

Pneumonia caused by *M. pneumoniae* usually is more prolonged and severe than that caused by the viruses, lasting an average of 2 to 3 weeks. Symptoms include cough, usually nonproductive but sometimes associated with mucoid expectoration, headache, malaise, fever, and sometimes chills. Upper respiratory tract involvement, characterized by sore throat and nasal symptoms, is noted in about 50 per cent of cases[196, 201] and is indistinguishable from disease caused by respiratory tract viruses.[201] Among the upper respiratory symptoms and signs of particular interest is bullous myringitis, a manifestation originally described in volunteers infected with Eaton agent but since described in a few cases with naturally acquired infections. A maculopapular rash develops over the trunk and back of some patients. Physical examination of the lungs usually reveals rales and decreased breath sounds at the lung bases, and signs of frank consolidation have been described.[196] A relatively rare but fulminating syndrome associated with this microorganism is acute bronchiolitis leading to profound hypoxemia and symptoms and signs of obstructive disease with carbon dioxide retention.

Complications of *M. pneumoniae* infections are not common but may be very serious. In addition to the myringitis (a manifestation of the disease rather than a complication), meningoencephalitis or meningitis may develop.[201] Other complications include hemagglutination or hemolysis (presumably due to the cold agglutinins) and peripheral thrombophlebitis with subsequent pulmonary thromboembolic disease. These complications appear to occur only in patients with very high titers of cold agglutinins. Arthritis and arthralgia may accompany significant rises in CF antibodies to *M. pneumoniae*, usually affecting multiple joints.

Other rare complications include thrombocytopenic purpura and skin eruptions, the most important of which is erythema multiforme (the Stevens-Johnson syndrome).

STEVENS-JOHNSON SYNDROME. The term "erythema multiforme" was coined by Hebra in 1866[205] to describe the red or violet macules, papules, vesicles, or bullae usually distributed widely and symmetrically over most of the body surface and sometimes the mucous membranes. The syndrome described by Stevens and Johnson[206] in 1922 usually is reserved for the more severe cases of erythema multiforme, which have a systemic reaction including high fever, stomatitis, ophthalmia, and occasionally involvement of the lungs. Ludlam and associates[207] were the first to report positive complement fixation for *Mycoplasma pneumoniae* in patients with this syndrome. *M. pneumoniae* has been isolated from the nasopharynx and from blister fluid in patients with erythema multiforme. Not all patients have roentgenographic evidence of pneumonia. When pneumonia is present, the roentgenographic pattern is identical to that of *Mycoplasma* pneumonia.

Evidence that has accumulated to date suggests that the Stevens-Johnson syndrome is related to infection with *M. pneumoniae* in some cases and to drug therapy in others.[208] The age range of patients with Stevens-Johnson syndrome and *M. pneumoniae* infection is virtually identical.[208] The multiple etiologies and clinical presentation of this syndrome strongly suggest an immunologic mechanism.

The white cell count in *Mycoplasma* pneumonia averages less than 10,000 per cu mm.[196] Since culture of *M. pneumoniae* on agar or in broth takes 2 weeks to 3 months, and recovery always occurs within this period, this procedure is useful only to confirm the diagnosis. Similarly, a fourfold rise in specific antibody titer may take several weeks and therefore is of little diagnostic use during the acute phase of the disease. A fourfold rise in cold agglutinin titer during acute illness has been considered a useful indication of primary atypical pneumonia. However, although *M. pneumoniae* infection is the commonest respiratory cause of cold agglutinin production, these are found in not more than 50 per cent of cases.[196, 201] Furthermore, they develop in viral pneumonia also; in fact, approximately one-quarter of cold agglutinin–positive pneumonias are not caused by *M. pneumoniae*.[201]

Of much greater diagnostic value are the techniques that show specific antibodies to *M. pneumoniae*, including immunofluorescence microscopy and CF tests. The former reveals antibodies and the latter a fourfold rise in their titer in virtually every culturally proved case of *Mycoplasma* pneumonia.

RESPIRATORY INFECTIONS CAUSED BY VIRUSES

The respiratory viruses can be divided into two large groups according to the type of nucleic acid they contain. The viruses and rickettsiae are composed of an outer coat of protein and inner core of ribose nucleic acid (RNA), or deoxyribose nucleic acid (DNA), or both. The RNA group includes the myxoviruses, picornaviruses, and reoviruses; the DNA group includes adenoviruses and herpesviruses. The rickettsiae and the etiologic agent of ornithosis contain both types of nucleic acid.

MYXOVIRUS RESPIRATORY INFECTIONS

The myxoviruses capable of producing respiratory infections include influenza, parainfluenza, respiratory syncytial virus, and measles (rubeola) virus. *Influenza virus* infection usually involves only the upper respiratory passages, including the trachea and major bronchi, and chiefly affects school children and young adults. However, in a small percentage of patients—particularly the aged or chronically ill—it may be responsible for fulminating pneumonia. *Parainfluenza viruses* are the cause of croup; in infants and young children they may cause severe bronchiolitis and bronchopneumonia; adults show a strong resistance to infection. The *respiratory syncytial virus* also tends to affect infants and small children; in some it causes severe bronchiolitis and bronchopneumonia. *Measles virus* can cause pneumonia also, although probably the majority of pneumonias in measles represent secondary bacterial infection.

INFLUENZA VIRUS INFECTION

General Comments and Epidemiology

Influenza is an acute infectious disease caused by the inhalation of influenza virus into the upper respiratory tract. Clinically, it is characterized by fever, myalgia, nonproductive cough, protracted weakness and lethargy, and often upper respiratory symptoms. The influenza virus can be divided into groups A, B, and C, each with a specific antigen demonstrable by CF testing. Almost all severe outbreaks of influenza are caused by group A viruses. Group A virus has on its surface two structurally, functionally, and genetically distinct glycoproteins, hemagglutinin (H) and neuraminidase (N). Taking advantage of the fact that the influenza epidemic of 1957 (H_2, N_2) and Hong Kong

outbreak of influenza A in 1968 (H_3, N_2) had similar N but immunologically distinct H antigens, investigators[209] showed that the frequency and severity of response to the 1968 Hong Kong virus related to the level of serum anti-N antibody acquired from the 1957 infection. In patients not completely protected from infection, anti-N antibodies significantly suppressed clinical expression of the infection, and it was concluded that antibody against the neuraminidase of the influenza virus prevented or modified infection when antibodies to the H_3 antigen were lacking. The influenza A virus is responsible for most cases of pneumonia.

Influenza is very contagious, and during epidemics and pandemics the majority of the population contract it in some degree, from asymptomatic infection to fulminating pneumonia and death.

Although the influenza A virus generally has been considered to be an obligate human parasite transmitted from human to human by droplet infection, it is now evident that the virus which caused the Hong Kong influenza epidemic of 1968 can infect a wide range of animals, and that they in turn may act as a reservoir for viral influenza and a milieu for genetic recombination (reassortment of genes), leading to new endemic strains of influenza A virus in humans. The incubation period of influenza virus infection is 24 to 48 hours, allowing rapid spread of the disease. Antibody formation to specific strains by infection or vaccination confers immunity for 1 to 2 years.

Pneumonia is an uncommon but dreaded complication of influenza infection, usually group A; although often localized and of mild to moderate severity, it is sometimes fatal. In perhaps one-third of cases of severe pneumonia, the illness develops abruptly in apparently healthy persons,[209] but the majority have a predisposing condition such as heart disease (particularly rheumatic mitral stenosis), pregnancy, chronic bronchitis, diabetes, or nephrosis.[209]

In the 1918–1919 influenza pandemic, hemolytic *Streptococcus* was a common cause of superinfection. In the pandemic of 1957–1958, *Staphylococcus aureus* replaced the *Streptococcus* and undoubtedly was the pathogen that contributed to the fatal outcome in a large proportion of cases. A fatal outcome can occur without superinfection, however; the influenza virus alone can produce overwhelming pneumonitis, which may prove fatal within 24 hours. In at least some patients, recovery of the virus from extrapulmonary organs postmortem indicates viremia.[210]

Pathologic Characteristics

The influenza virus causes proliferation and necrosis of epithelial cells lining the respiratory tract. Initially, changes consist of destruction of bronchial epithelium including ciliated cells, goblet cells, and many of the bronchial mucous gland secretory cells. The superficial cells necrose, exposing the basal layer. The bronchial walls are edematous and infiltrated with lymphocytes; edema and inflammation extend into the peribronchial tissues and alveoli, which are infiltrated with mononuclear cells also. The changes extend to the respiratory bronchioles and alveolar ducts and may be associated with capillary thrombosis, necrosis, aneurysm formation, and hemorrhage. In the small percentage of cases in which fulminating air-space pneumonia is fatal within 48 hours, in addition to the changes in the airways the alveoli are filled with edema fluid, red blood cells, fibrin, mononuclear cells, and in many cases hyaline membranes.[210]

Roentgenographic Manifestations

The pattern varies, depending upon the virulence of the organism, the resistance of the host, and the presence or absence of superinfection. Involvement may be local or general. The former usually is in the form of segmental consolidation, which may be homogeneous or patchy,[211] most commonly in the lower lobes, and either unilateral or bilateral. In one series[211] the disease was unilateral and bilateral in approximately equal incidence, and widely disseminated in roughly a quarter of the latter cases. Roentgenographically there was diffuse, patchy air-space disease resembling pulmonary edema (Figure 6–24). Pleural effusion is comparatively rare.[211] Resolution averages about 3 weeks.[211]

Clinical Manifestations

The symptoms of influenza are a dry cough, pain in the back and leg muscles, chills, headache, conjunctivitis, sometimes substernal burning pain, and fever for 3 to 5 days. Rhinorrhea and pharyngitis are not major clinical manifestations. When pneumonia develops, symptoms and signs depend on the nature and extent of the affection.

Louria and associates[212] described three distinct lower respiratory tract syndromes in influenza. The mildest is believed to represent bronchiolitis and produces no roentgenographic abnormality in the chest. The second form is more common and occurs when superinfection with staphylococci, pneumococci, *H. influenzae*, or streptococci develops within 2 weeks after

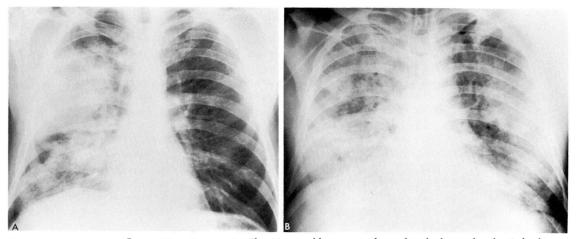

Figure 6–24. Acute Influenza Virus Pneumonia. This 32-year-old man was admitted to the hospital with a 3-day history of progressive dyspnea, cough productive of whitish-yellow sputum, right-sided pleuritic chest pain, chills, and fever. His white cell count was 3,500, consisting of 54 per cent lymphocytes and 46 per cent neutrophils. A posteroanterior roentgenogram on the day of admission (A) reveals extensive homogeneous air-space consolidation of the right upper lobe, with patchy shadows of air-space consolidation of the right lower lobe; the left lung is clear. Two days later (B), consolidation of the right lower lobe has become almost uniform and there has occurred extension of the air-space disease throughout the whole of the left lung; at this time, the roentgenographic appearance would be compatible with diffuse pulmonary edema. Shortly after admission, the patient became comatose and never regained consciousness; even with assisted ventilation on 100 per cent oxygen, the P_{O_2} was below 40 and P_{CO_3} between 80 and 90. Virologic studies revealed a titer of 1:128 CFT for influenza A_2 and of 1:32 CFT for influenza B; a hemagglutination inhibition test was positive to a titer of 1:160 for influenza A_2, Hong Kong variant. In addition, respiratory syncytial virus and influenza virus were cultured from the blood, the sputum, and directly from the lung at necropsy. (Courtesy of Dr. Adolf Glay, St. Mary's Hospital, Montreal.)

the initial viral infection. These patients expectorate purulent sputum that may be rusty or bloody and may complain of pleural pain. The third form, a much more fulminating type of pneumonia, develops within 12 to 36 hours after the initial symptoms and may be caused by the virus alone or by staphylococcal superinfection. These patients are extremely ill: dyspnea and cyanosis develop rapidly, and culture of the frothy, blood-stained sputum may yield a pure growth of coagulase-positive *Staph. aureus*. Most of these patients have mitral stenosis or chronic bronchitis and/or are pregnant.

Various complications of influenza virus infection have been reported. Neurologic sequelae (including transverse myelopathy) are thought to be due to autoimmunity or hypersensitivity, since influenza virus has not been isolated from the brain. Severe myositis has been described[213] as a complication of influenzal infection in 26 young children, in whom acute bilateral lower limb weakness and tenderness developed after the acute respiratory symptoms abated (unlike the simple myalgia that commonly develops during the acute stage); leg pain and weakness were so severe that many of the children could not walk. There have been reports of myoglobinuria associated with influenza A virus infection accompanied by muscle tenderness and swelling.

The white cell count is usually normal in uncomplicated influenza, but leukopenia develops in some cases, and, when severe, indicates a poor prognosis. Overwhelming infection commonly results in a neutrophilia of 20,000 or more per cu mm. The influenza group responsible for the infection can be identified by CF testing, and the subgroup by the demonstration of specific hemagglutination inhibition, neutralization, or antineuraminidase antibodies. The fluorescent antibody technique on nasal secretions is a rapid diagnostic method. The virus can be isolated by culture of the sputum in monkey kidneys or chick embryos, growth occurring in 3 to 21 days.

The majority of patients with mild, uncomplicated influenza have small airway disease, as evidenced by slightly but consistently decreased flow rates at low lung volumes and an increased alveolar-arterial gradient for oxygen.

PARAINFLUENZA VIRUS INFECTION

The parainfluenza or hemadsorption viruses (types 1, 2, 3, and 4) cause predominantly mild upper respiratory tract disease and pharyngitis; in adults it is responsible for a small percentage of cases of coryza, and in infants and young children for the majority of cases of severe croup. Some cases of lower respiratory tract disease are caused by this virus.[214] Parainfluenza virus infections occur predominantly in the winter months and may assume epidemic proportions; in such circumstances they may account for a high proportion of cases of pneumonia, croup, and acute bronchiolitis in nursery outbreaks. Five cases of parainfluenza-related pneumonia requiring hospitalization have been described in naval recruits,[215] the diagnosis being established by a rise in antibody titers. The disease presumably is transmitted by inhalation of microorganisms in droplet form. Pathologic characteristics have not been described, since virtually all these infections are mild and self-limiting.

Roentgenographic changes in the chest are relatively nonspecific, consisting of diffuse or local accentuation of lung markings caused by peribronchial and peribronchiolar infiltration in the lower lobes.[215]

In children the symptoms are those of croup, sometimes with intermittent rales indicating bronchiolitis; the usual manifestation in adults is acute pharyngitis and tonsillitis. The white cell count usually is normal but in croup or pneumonia it may increase to 15,000 per cu mm. The organism can be isolated by the culture of sputum on monkey tissue; growth requires 3 to 21 days. As in influenza infections, immunofluorescent antibody is most useful in identifying the virus in nasopharyngeal secretions. Serologic diagnosis can be achieved by agglutinin neutralization and complement-fixation tests, and hemadsorption with guinea pig erythrocytes.

RESPIRATORY SYNCYTIAL VIRUS (RSV) INFECTION

The RSV is responsible for a small percentage of cases of coryza in children and adults and is a major cause of severe bronchiolitis and bronchopneumonia in infants and small children.[216] Infections occur predominantly during the winter months and early spring; the incubation period is 3 to 5 days.[217]

Infants and children under the age of two are particularly susceptible to RSV infection;[216] it is estimated that the disease is fatal in 2 to 6 per cent of children. The lower respiratory tract is affected in one-third to one-half of the patients. Infections in adults are usually extremely mild, presumably denoting immunity as a result of childhood infection; however, serologic testing of a group of Dutch military recruits with acute respiratory disease[218] showed pulmonary infection to be caused by respiratory syncytial virus in 6 per cent, M. pneumoniae in 25 per cent, and adenovirus in 19 per cent. A recent study during an epidemic indicated the RSV is an important pathogen in the elderly and chronically ill.[219]

The extreme damage to bronchioles in this disease may represent a hypersensitivity reaction by complexes of RS virus to maternal IgG serum antibodies in infants who have no local IgA antibody of their own to intercept the virus and prevent its combination with IgG deeper in the bronchial wall. This hypothesis could explain the disastrous effects in some infants in whom infection due to RS virus develops after they receive killed RS parenteral vaccines; the illness is much more severe than in those not given the vaccine or who have acquired active immunity by natural infection.[220]

It has been postulated that the essential process in bronchiolitis is a widespread allergic reaction (type 1 or 3) dependent upon a second encounter with RSV antigen, whereas in RSV pneumonia the mucosal necrosis and alveolar and interstitial inflammation result from direct viral damage to the lung parenchyma.

A disparity has been noted between the severity of respiratory symptoms and the relative paucity of roentgenographic changes. In infants, the chest roentgenogram is reported to show patchy areas of consolidation interspersed with zones of overinflation.

Symptoms include severe rhinitis, cough, and fever, with mild pharyngitis or conjunctivitis.[217] In the presence of bronchiolitis or pneumonia, wheezing, dyspnea, cyanosis, and retraction of the rib cage are noted, in addition to signs of parenchymal consolidation.

Infection with this organism appears to confer excellent immunity, since adults who are challenged with the virus usually manifest no symptoms or signs or, at most, symptoms of a mild common cold.[217] The infection can be detected by complement-fixation and neutralization tests, and the diagnosis can be established early with immunofluorescent antibody methods.

MEASLES (RUBEOLA) RESPIRATORY INFECTION

Segmental pneumonia and atelectasis are common in patients with measles and in the majority are the result of bacterial superinfec-

tion; however, by inducing pathologic changes in the epithelial cells lining the airways and the alveoli, the measles virus itself may affect the lung directly. This virus is the commonest if not the only organism that causes giant cell pneumonia. The incidence of pneumonia as a complication of childhood measles ranges from 7 to 50 per cent.

Pathologically, predominant changes in giant cell pneumonia are degeneration and hyperplasia of the epithelial cells of the bronchi and bronchioles. Inflammatory exudate appears in the alveolar septa adjacent to the bronchi and bronchioles, the cellular infiltration consisting largely of lymphocytes and plasma cells. Multinucleated epithelial giant cells containing intracytoplasmic inclusion bodies may be found in the respiratory epithelium at all levels of the airways. The measles virus is the only organism isolated to date in cases of true giant cell pneumonia in humans.[222]

Roentgenographically, primary giant cell pneumonia caused by measles virus produces a reticular pattern throughout the lungs, indicating the location of the disease in the interstitium and airways. Hilar lymph node enlargement is usual.[222] Pneumonia due to bacterial superinfection typically is segmental in distribution and usually affects one or both of the lower lobes; atelectasis is very common. The organisms most often responsible are *Str. pneumoniae, Staph. aureus, H. influenzae,* and *Str. hemolyticus.*

An entirely different form of pulmonary reaction appears to occur in children in whom measles develops or who receive live measles virus vaccine[223] after being immunized with killed measles vaccine. In this "altered or atypical measles syndrome," 51 examples of which were reported by Gokiert and Beamish,[224] there is a maculopapular rash, which appears first on the extremities and spreads centripetally, with limb edema and moderate eosinophilia in some cases. Many children who received killed measles vaccine are now adolescent or young adults, and the complication of altered measles syndrome has become very pertinent to the internist. Recent publications[225, 226] have stressed the importance of recognizing the prodromal symptoms of fever, malaise, myalgia, headache, nausea, vomiting, coryza, sore throat, conjunctivitis, photophobia, nonproductive cough, pleuritic pain, and the hemorrhagic and vesicular nature of the peripheral limb rash. Roentgenographically, there is extensive parenchymal consolidation, usually bilateral and consistently nonsegmental. In our experience the pattern frequently consists of one or more pulmonary nodules measuring up to 6 cm in diameter. The parenchymal consolidation may resolve and the effusions absorb very rapidly,[224] in contrast to the pneumonia of typical measles but reminiscent of Loeffler's syndrome and of pulmonary edema due to aspiration of irritants. Hilar lymph node enlargement and pleural effusion are common. Residual nodules may persist for 1 to 2 years after the acute illness.[227]

Although the precise mechanisms of these pathologic changes in atypical measles pneumonia are unknown, their roentgenographic appearance and rapid clearing suggest an immune response, either a type 3 Arthus reaction or type 4 delayed hypersensitivity. The reaction appears to be similar to the atypical illness reported to occur in infants given killed respiratory syncytial virus vaccine.

Clinically, giant cell pneumonia characteristically develops before or coincident with the peak of the measles exanthem, usually in patients with reticuloendothelial disease. Measles virus has been isolated at necropsy in patients with giant cell pneumonia who had had no signs or symptoms of rubeola. Although most cases of measles pneumonia (either primary or superinfection) occur in children, adults (particularly armed forces recruits) may be affected; in some, the super-infecting organism has been shown to be *Neisseria meningitidis*.

The bacterial pneumonia usually develops several days after the rash and when the patient's condition has begun to improve. It should be suspected when cough, purulent expectoration, tachycardia, rise in temperature, and sometimes pleural pain develop during early convalescence.

The white cell count in giant cell pneumonia usually is normal but may be low; in the presence of secondary bacterial pneumonia, polymorphonuclear leukocytosis commonly develops. The measles virus can be isolated on tissue cultures of throat washings or blood, and giant cells may be identified on throat smears and in urine sediment.

PICORNAVIRUS RESPIRATORY INFECTION

The picornaviruses are a group of small RNA-containing organisms; the enteroviruses, which are a subgroup, include the Coxsackie, ECHO, and poliovirus strains. These organisms inhabit the intestinal tract and are transmitted predominantly by the fecal-oral route; children and young adults are most commonly affected. The incubation period ranges from 7 to 12 days. In temperate climates, illnesses caused by the enteroviruses occur chiefly in the late summer and autumn months, but in the tropics they occur at any time. Respiratory infection caused by the Coxsackie and ECHO viruses is usually limited to the upper tract and tends to be mild; pneumonia is rare.

COXSACKIEVIRUS RESPIRATORY INFECTION

The Coxsackieviruses can be divided into two major groups: *group A*, which contains 24 serologic subtypes and is differentiated by its ability to induce flaccid paralysis in mice; and *group B*, which contains six serologic subtypes and causes spastic paralysis in mice. Group A Coxsackieviruses (particularly A10) typically produce vesicular and ulcerative lesions on the soft palate, occasionally aseptic meningitis, and rarely coryza. Group B Coxsackieviruses cause a great variety of clinical patterns, including aseptic meningitis, Bornholm disease, myocarditis, pericarditis, acute meningoencephalitis, and orchitis. Constrictive pericarditis may complicate group B Coxsackievirus infection.

Coxsackievirus infections occur in local or widespread epidemics, usually during the summer months and early autumn. Pneumonia rarely develops in association with Coxsackievirus A infection[228] or with pleurodynia caused by Coxsackievirus B (Bornholm disease). The B5 strain can cause basal linear opacities and pleural effusion.

The pathology of Coxsackievirus infection has not been described, since the disease is not fatal.

In the few reported cases of Coxsackievirus pneumonia, the roentgenographic pattern is said to consist of fine perihilar "infiltration;"[228] parenchymal consolidation in the lung bases may develop when pleurodynia is present.

Symptoms may be limited to the upper respiratory tract, with rhinitis, pharyngitis, and a dry cough, or may relate to epidemic pleurodynia and consist of severe aching and gripping pain in the lower thoracic and upper abdominal regions. Pleurodynia usually is accompanied by difficulty in breathing and by fever, temperature ranging from 37.7 to 39.4° C. We have seen several cases of pleurodynia with persistent widespread bilateral pleural friction rub. The disease is characterized by remissions and by exacerbations that may last several weeks. The white cell count ranges from slight leukopenia to mild leukocytosis. The organism may be isolated by culture on monkey kidney of material from throat or rectal swabs or of serum, cerebrospinal fluid, urine, or stool.[229] Strain-specific neutralization antibody tests are available.

ECHO Virus Respiratory Infection

The enteric cytopathic human orphan (ECHO) viruses include some 28 to 30 strains that cause multifarious clinical manifestations, usually in infants, including fever, diarrhea, maculopapular and petechial rashes, aseptic meningitis, and occasionally pneumonia.[230] In adults, respiratory disease usually simulates the common cold, but a few cases have been described of pleurodynia and acute carditis caused by type 6 and type 19 ECHO viruses.

Involvement of the lung by this organism produces a roentgenographic pattern of increased bronchovascular markings and bilateral hilar lymph node enlargement.[230]

The white cell count usually is within normal limits, with relative lymphocytosis; leukocytosis develops in some cases. Diagnosis depends upon demonstration of the organism on human and simian cell tissue culture, or a fourfold increase in titer of neutralization and complement-fixation antibodies.

Poliovirus Respiratory Infection

The effects of the polioviruses on, the thorax are indirect only; paralysis of the muscles of respiration results in alveolar hypoventilation and respiratory failure. Since chest roentgenograms are normal, this subject is dealt with in the chapter on respiratory disease associated with a normal chest roentgenogram.

Rhinovirus Respiratory Infection

This member of the picornavirus group has at least 89 serotypes and is responsible for over 50 per cent of cases of coryza. Lower respiratory tract rhinovirus infections, including acute bronchitis, croup, bronchiolitis, and bronchopneumonia have been described in children, and rhinovirus is the causal organism in a small percentage of cases of atypical pneumonia in adults; in most cases the disease is localized to one or more segments of a lower lobe.[231]

REOVIRUS RESPIRATORY INFECTION

There have been sporadic reports of pneumonia caused by reoviruses.[232]

ADENOVIRUS RESPIRATORY INFECTION

The adenoviruses are one of the two major groups that contain DNA and are responsible for respiratory infections (the other group is the herpesviruses). The infections they cause range from the common cold to severe pneumonia. Twenty-eight immunologically distinct members of this group have been described, but most respiratory infections are caused by types 3, 4, or 7, frequently in epidemic proportions. Epidemics are most frequent among military populations. In nonepidemic outbreaks, types 1, 2, and 5 are most common: in Britain during 1970 they accounted for 74 per cent of 699 typed adenovirus isolates, and 3, 4, and 7 (epidemic types) for only 21 per cent; 81 per cent of the patients were under 5 years of age.[233]

All types of adenoviruses have a common complement-fixing antibody, and they can be differentiated by serum neutralization tests.

Lower respiratory infection with adenovirus is fairly common and may give rise to epidemics.[234] In one epidemic of adenovirus type 7 disease, 16 per cent of the patients had pneumonia and 67 per cent had acute bronchiolitis.

One of the most extensive reviews of adenoviral pneumonia and its complications in infancy and childhood, by Gold and his associates,[235] reported a five-year study of 69 patients. Forty-six (67 per cent) of the patients were North American Indian, métis, or Eskimo, and the majority were less than 1 year old. Histologic examination of necropsy and biopsy material showed a striking necrotizing bronchiolitis, progressing to obliterative bronchiolitis in the chronic stages of the disease. The usual roentgenographic findings were diffuse bilateral "bronchopneumonia" and severe overinflation. Lobar collapse was a frequent complication, in the right upper lobe in 20 instances and the left lower lobe in six, and re-expansion did not occur in 10. In uncomplicated cases, the roentgenographic changes resolved within 2 weeks, but of particular importance was the incidence of subsequent chronic pulmonary disease: of the 58 children adequately followed up, 31 (53 per cent) had some form of chronic pulmonary disease. The incidence of chronic disease was considerably higher (approximately 64 per cent) in children under 2 years of age at the time of the acute illness than in the older patients (27 per cent). The precise form of the chronic pulmonary disease was not detailed in all cases, but bronchiectasis, obliterative bronchiolitis, interstitial fibrosis, and "unilateral hyperlucent lung syndrome" were prominently mentioned. Etiologically, the last-named disorder appears closely related to acute adenoviral pneumonia. Unilateral hyperlucent lung (Swyer-James' or Macleod's syndrome) was detected[236] in six infants who were under 18 months of age when they had contracted viral pneumonia 7 to 30 months previously; in four of the six the diagnosis had been established by serologic identification of adenovirus.

Pneumonia usually is mild and always is associated with typical upper respiratory symptoms as well as those due to the pneumonia.[237] The pneumonia may be severe, with productive cough in the later stages; pleural pain rarely occurs. Physical findings include pharyngitis, which frequently is exudative and closely resembles that produced by streptoccal infection, and diffuse rales and rhonchi indicative of bronchiolitis but in some cases with definite signs of consolidation.[237] Adenoviral infection occasionally presents clinically as whooping cough that is indistinguishable from the classic disease.

Adenoviruses grow readily in tissue culture of human and simian cells, producing a distinctive destruction of tissue (cytopathogenesis). The white cell count usually is normal but may be slightly increased, and in very ill patients may exceed 30,000 per cu mm. Although the cold agglutination test usually gives negative results,[237] titers of 1:32 or higher may be recorded but seldom rise to a fourfold increase.

HERPESVIRUS RESPIRATORY INFECTION

The herpesviruses, the second group of DNA-containing organisms, include varicella-zoster (chickenpox) virus, variola virus (smallpox), cytomegalovirus (the etiologic agent of cytomegalic inclusion disease), and herpes simplex virus. The last-named may cause fatal disease in infants who acquire the infection from mothers who have recurrent herpetic vulvovaginitis. The Epstein-Barr virus (EBV), which is believed to be the etiologic agent of infectious mononucleosis, is morphologically a herpesvirus.

VARICELLA-ZOSTER RESPIRATORY INFECTION

The virus of varicella-zoster may invade the lungs and cause diffuse pneumonia. The pneumonia can be severe and rapidly fatal or relatively mild. The overall incidence of pneumonia in chickenpox appears to be about 14 per cent,[238] but in adults admitted to hospital it may be as high as 50 per cent. About 90 per cent of affected patients are aged 19 years or over, and more than 75 per cent of cases occur in the third to fifth decades of life.[238, 239]

In both adults and children, pre-existing reticuloendothelial disease and corticosteroid and broad-spectrum antibiotic therapy may predispose patients to primary varicella pneumonia. Similarly, both the incidence of such pneumonia and mortality from it are much higher in pregnant women.[238, 239] In one review[238] the mortality was 11.4 per cent in male and nonpregnant female patients but 41 per cent in pregnant women.

There is no race or sex predilection.[238, 239] Varicella tends to occur during the colder months and is thought to be transmitted by droplet infection. Viremia develops promptly following deposition of the virus in the upper respiratory tract. The incubation period averages 14 days (range, 3 to 21 days).

The varicella virus shows an affinity for epithelial cells and may invade any organ. In the lungs it causes swelling, proliferation, and desquamation of alveolar septal cells, and predominantly mononuclear cell infiltration. Fibrinous exudate fills the alveoli and sometimes forms "hyaline membranes." Focal hemorrhages are common. Intranuclear inclusion bodies are present in many cells. The skin shows papules, vesicles, and pustules which, in cases of pneumonia, almost invariably extend into the oropharynx, trachea, and larger bronchi.

The characteristic roentgenographic pattern is patchy, diffuse, air-space consolidation. The acinar shadows usually are fairly discrete in the lung periphery but tend to coalesce near the hila and in the lung bases (Figure 6–25).[238, 239] Hilar lymph node enlargement may be present but may be difficult to appreciate because of contiguity of the consolidation in the perihilar parenchyma.[238, 239] Roentgenographic clearing may take from 9 days to several months.

An apparently unique manifestation of acute chickenpox pneumonia consists of tiny widespread calcifications throughout both lungs in persons who, many years before but in adulthood, had chickenpox. The calcifications vary in size and number but seldom exceed 2 to 3 mm in diameter; they predominate in the lower half of the lungs. Hilar lymph nodes do not calcify. In a survey of 16,894 persons, 463 (2.7 per cent) had a history of chickenpox as adults; only eight (1.7 per cent) of these had diffuse calcifications presumed caused by chickenpox pneumonia.

Acute chickenpox pneumonia is most common in adults with severe cutaneous manifes-

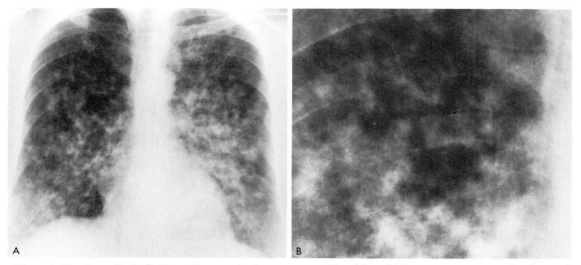

Figure 6–25. Acute Varicella-Zoster Pneumonia. Posteroanterior (A) and lateral (B) roentgenograms reveal widespread pulmonary disease possessing a pattern characteristic of patchy air-space consolidation. The magnified view of the right upper zone (C) reveals a multitude of acinar shadows, some of which are discrete and others coalescent. The patient, a 42-year-old woman, was a compromised host because of non-Hodgkin's lymphoma, for which she was being treated with antineoplastic agents.

tations of the disease. Symptoms, signs, and roentgenographic changes develop 2 to 3 days after the appearance of the vesicular eruption, and in most cases there is a history of contact with an affected child 3 to 21 days before onset of the acute illness. The onset often is marked by high fever, which may precede the rash by 2 to 3 days. In the rare cases of pneumonia in association with herpes zoster, the vesicles and papules are limited to one side of the body, with a peripheral nerve distribution.

The symptoms of pneumonia consist of cough, dyspnea, hemoptysis, tachypnea, pleuritic chest pain, and cyanosis with temperature as high as 40° C. Expectoration is not purulent.[238, 239] Despite the extensive roentgenographic changes, in many cases the physical findings are slight or absent. In nearly all cases the temperature returns to normal within 4 days. Clinical improvement usually antedates roentgenographic clearing by several weeks. A mortality as high as 11 per cent has been reported,[238] and patients with acute pneumonia may die suddenly without warning indications.[239]

In approximately one-third of cases the white cell count exceeds 10,000 per cu mm and is associated with polymorphonuclear leukocytosis. Complement fixing, neutralizing, and fluorescent antibodies are found in both varicella and herpes zoster infections, from about the fifth day of illness; paired titers (in the acute and convalescent stages) can be used to confirm the diagnosis.[238] Arterial oxygen saturation may be reduced, as in two of seven reported cases. The survival of such patients may depend upon assisted ventilation with large tidal volumes and positive end-expiratory pressure (PEEP). Herpes zoster may be complicated by unilateral diaphragmatic paralysis.

VARIOLA PNEUMONIA

A diffuse pneumonia identical to that caused by the virus of varicella-zoster has been reported in a group of nurses who had been immunized against smallpox.[240] This disease was originally thought to represent a manifestation of extrinsic allergic alveolitis, but follow-up roentgenographic studies revealed diffuse micronodular calcifications similar to those seen following varicella-zoster pneumonia, leading to the conclusion that the disease was much more likely an infection associated with necrosis.[240]

CYTOMEGALOVIRUS RESPIRATORY INFECTION

The cytomegalovirus (CMV) is the cause of cytomegalic inclusion disease (CID), a condition predominantly affecting neonates and small infants. Adults with reticuloendothelial disease or immunologic deficiencies, or receiving immunosuppressive therapy, are at increased risk,

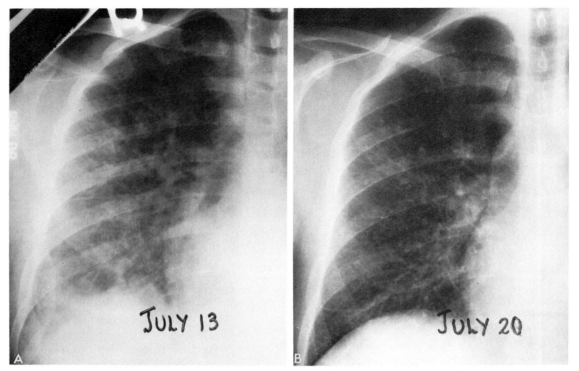

Figure 6–26.   Acute Pneumonia Caused by Cytomegalovirus. One week following the onset of a mild acute respiratory illness in this 23-year-old renal transplant recipient, a view of the right lung from an anteroposterior roentgenogram (A) reveals extensive disease whose pattern suggests involvement of both interstitial and air-space components of the parenchyma. The pleural line is moderately thickened in the vicinity of the costophrenic sulcus, indicating pleural effusion. CMV was isolated from the sputum. One week later (B), marked improvement had occurred although the pulmonary markings were still indistinct, indicating residual interstitial abnormality. The pleural effusion had absorbed.

and the infection is being recognized with increased frequency in recipients of transplanted kidneys and in patients who have had extracorporeal circulation during surgery or exchange transfusions. The virus can exist as a commensal or saprophyte in man, even though it can also cause pathologic changes that may be fatal.

Congenital cytomegalic inclusion disease is acquired *in utero* from a mother who harbors asymptomatic CMV infection. The infants are jaundiced, and develop hepatosplenomegaly and thrombocytopenic purpura; those who survive usually have cerebral damage.[241] As with the asymptomatic "carrier" mothers, adults and small children also may have latent virus whose activity is triggered by a lack of host response.

Histologically, the characteristic change caused by cytomegalovirus infection is the presence of intranuclear and intracytoplasmic inclusion bodies in the parenchymal cells of the salivary glands, liver, kidneys, adrenals, and lungs. In the last named, both the bronchiolar and alveolar epithelial cells become greatly enlarged and eventually are detached so as to lie

in the bronchiolar and alveolar lumen. The alveoli are filled with a serosanguinous exudate and the interstitium of the lung shows edema and mononuclear cell infiltration.[241] Abundant hyaline membranes have been described[241] and inclusion bodies have been reported to occur in large numbers in the mediastinal lymph nodes.[241]

The usual *roentgenographic pattern* of CMV lung infection consists of a diffuse loss of definition of lung markings, indicating predominant interstitial lung involvement (Figure 6–26). Air-space consolidation may be evident as acinar shadows, but not as prominantly as in *Pneumocystis carinii* pneumonia—one of the main conditions to be differentiated.[241] Pleural effusion is uncommon (Figure 6–26).

In small children and adults, *symptoms* caused by pulmonary invasion include progressive dyspnea and cyanosis; paroxysms of coughing and hemoptysis have been reported.[241] A postperfusion syndrome closely resembling infectious mononucleosis and consisting of fever, malaise, hepatosplenomegaly, lymph node enlargement, jaundice, atypical lymphocytosis, and occasionally eosinophilia and anemia has been reported following extracorporeal circulation and multiple blood transfusions.

Although pneumonia is not a common manifestation of CMV mononucleosis, it can occur in previously healthy adults;[242, 243] similarly, the organism is a common commensal in compromised hosts, in whom it can cause serious pneumonia. CMV may be isolated from the urine or sputum. In the absence of leukemia, the white cell count is low normal or leukopenic. Complement-fixation and agglutination tests are useful in diagnosis[241] and may reveal high titers even in immunosuppressed patients.

EPSTEIN-BARR MONONUCLEOSIS

The Epstein-Barr virus (EBV), first discovered in cultures of Burkitt's lymphoma cells, is believed to be the cause of infectious mononucleosis. This conclusion is based on the coincidental development of antibodies to various components of the EBV, the classic picture of infectious mononucleosis in persons previously shown to lack antibody to this virus,[244] and the detection of EBV in the oropharynx early in the illness.[245] Using the indirect immunofluorescence technique, Niederman and his associates[244] found a prevalence rate of antibody to EBV in 26 to 87 per cent of 1084 young adults, depending on age and geographic area. In a prospective study of 150 Yale students, these authors found that 53 had EBV antibody on entering the university, and they demonstrated seroconversion in 43 of the others during the next 4 to 8 years—28 with clinical infectious mononucleosis and 15 with inapparent or unidentified illness. The virus has been detected in the blood of patients with infectious mononucleosis[245] and like CMV can be transmitted by blood transfusion or extracorporeal circulation. However, contagion is much more likely, from human to human, by close oral contact.[245] Cell-mediated immunity is depressed during the acute stage of infectious mononucleosis and returns to normal in the convalescent period.

The roentgenographic findings in 59 cases of infectious mononucleosis were described by Lander and Palayew[246] as follows: hilar lymph node enlargement in eight patients (13 per cent); a diffuse reticular pattern indicating interstitial disease in three patients (5 per cent), one of these also showing an acinar pattern; small bilateral pleural effusions in two; and a moderate unilateral effusion in one. The commonest roentgenologic finding was splenomegaly, observed in 28 patients (47 per cent), and the authors suggest that this finding, in association with hilar node enlargement, pleural effusion, or a diffuse reticular pattern, should alert the radiologist to the possibility of infectious mononucleosis.

In children, marked enlargement of the adenoids, tonsils, or prevertebral cervical soft tissues can occasion severe dysphagia and dyspnea.[247]

CHLAMYDIA (BEDSONIA) RESPIRATORY INFECTIONS

Members of this group of organisms are perhaps more correctly regarded as small bacteria than as viruses. In contrast to the myxoviruses and picornaviruses (which contain RNA) and the adenoviruses and herpesviruses (which contain DNA), the *Chlamydia* viruses contain both RNA and DNA. These organisms cause ornithosis (psittacosis), lymphogranuloma venereum, and trachoma.

ORNITHOSIS (PSITTACOSIS)

Ornithosis results from the inhalation of dry excreta containing *Chlamydia psittaci* from infected birds of any type, including poultry and domestic and wild birds. The disease is diagnosed infrequently, and it is probable that many cases are labeled as primary atypical pneumonia despite the fact that careful history-taking and serologic testing should permit ready differentiation. The incidence is low; in a study of 539 patients with serologically proved "viral" pneumonia,[248] only 29 (5 per cent) fulfilled the criteria of ornithosis. The disease occurs sporadically and in epidemics, the latter usually among poultry workers.[249] The estimated mortality ranges from 10 to 40 per cent,[249] the parrot and turkey strains being most virulent for humans.

In most cases of ornithosis the patient gives a history of exposure to parakeets, pigeons, budgerigars, or poultry.[249] The bird or birds responsible may have been obviously ill or may have died from disease, but not necessarily. The disease may be acquired from an infected bird recently purchased from a dealer who, having acquired immunity, remains healthy. Transmission can occur from human to human.[250]

The *pathologic changes* in ornithosis are similar to those of other viral pneumonias, although considerable hemorrhagic consolidation may occur in the more severe cases. Regional lymph nodes may be enlarged. Proliferation, necrosis, and desquamation of epithelial cells lining bronchi, bronchioles, and alveoli occur, and the alveolar septa become congested and edematous.

The *roentgenographic pattern* varies: it includes a homogeneous "ground-glass" opacity, sometimes containing small areas of radiolucency,[250] a patchy reticular pattern radiating out from the hilar areas or involving the lung bases,[248] and in some cases segmental or lobar consolidation with or without atelectasis. Enlargement of hilar lymph nodes was a common feature in one series of 29 patients.[248]

Roentgenographic resolution often is delayed for many weeks after clinical cure has occurred. In 29 cases the roentgenographic abnormality was still apparent at 6 weeks in 48 per cent and for more than 9 weeks in 17 per cent.[248]

The *clinical picture* of ornithosis ranges from a mild febrile episode to severe pneumonia indistinguishable from acute bacterial pneumonia. In the more severe cases the clinical presentation tends to simulate typhoid and may include bradycardia and even "rose spots."[250] The patient may have fever but no clinical or roentgenographic local signs in the chest. Cough usually is dry but may produce nonpurulent mucoid material;[249, 250] hemoptysis occurs in few cases and pleuritic pain is uncommon. Dyspnea may be very severe in cases of overwhelming infection. Systemic symptoms and signs include malaise, anorexia, shaking chills, nausea and vomiting, polyarthritis, myalgia, headache, abdominal pain, delirium, and unconsciousness.[251] Physical signs may consist only of basal crepitations,[250] but signs of frank parenchymal consolidation have been described, and a friction rub may be heard. Hepatosplenomegaly occurs, and superficial lymph node enlargement and erythema nodosum have been noted.

The white cell count ranges from normal to moderately increased,[250] with or without eosinophilia. Proteinuria may occur and liver function may be disturbed. The organism may be recovered from the sputum during the first 2 weeks of illness or from the blood during the first 4 days. Complement-fixation antibodies appear in the second to fourth week of the disease. In one series five of 27 patients had positive Wassermann or Kahn reactions. Electrocardiographic abnormalities are frequent.

RESPIRATORY INFECTIONS CAUSED BY RICKETTSIAE

The major respiratory disease caused by the rickettsiae is Q-fever pneumonia. Pneumonia occurs occasionally in endemic or scrub typhus but is an inconstant finding in other forms of rickettsial disease, such as epidemic typhus and Rocky Mountain spotted fever. (However, of 20 patients with Rocky Mountain spotted fever in one report,[252] six [30 per cent] exhibited roentgenographic abnormalities in the thorax.) *Rickettsiae* are both intracellular and extracellular organisms.

Q-FEVER PNEUMONIA

Infection with the rickettsial organism *Coxiella burnetii* produces a febrile illness that often simulates influenza or typhoid. The chest roentgenogram is abnormal in one-third to one-half of clinically recognized cases.[253] Q fever appears rare, but probably many sporadic cases are missed, the diagnosis being made most commonly when an epidemic occurs among abattoir workers or laboratory assistants handling specimens.[253] The disease is worldwide in distribution, having been described originally in Australia (Queensland fever) and subsequently in the United States and Europe.

The organism has been isolated from insects, arachnids, birds, rabbits, and domestic animals, apparently being transmitted by the bite of a diseased tick or mite. A few cases in humans may result from the bite of a tick or mite, but the usual mode of transmission is by inhalation of contaminated dust particles. The disease is not transmitted from person to person.

The *pathologic changes* are similar to those of viral pneumonia and are not in any way diagnostic. Both the interstitium and alveoli show edema, mononuclear cell infiltration, and extravasation of red blood cells. In some cases, *Rickettsiae* are identified in the alveolar spaces and within desquamated cells.

Roentgenographically, homogeneous parenchymal consolidation, segmental in distribution, affects predominantly the lower lobes.[253] Pleural effusion occurs in some cases. The hilar lymph nodes are not enlarged.

Clinically, onset of the disease is usually insidious, with malaise for several days. Then fever develops, with headaches, chills, severe myalgia, arthralgia, and in a minority of cases nausea, vomiting, and diarrhea. The incubation period is 1 to 5 weeks, averaging about 14 days.[253, 254]

Involvement of the upper respiratory tract is common, causing troublesome dry cough. Physical examination of the lungs commonly reveals little abnormality despite fairly extensive parenchymal disease roentgenographically.[254] Fever is frequently remittent; it may last for several weeks but averages 8 to 12 days.[254] Endocarditis, usually of the aortic valve, appears to be the commonest nonrespiratory form of presentation. Phlebitis may occur, and complications from this may be more prolonged and disabling than the original infection.[254] The illness may relapse and recur.[253] Of 50 cases in one series, one-third had a white cell count above 13,000 per cu mm, exceeding 15,000 in only one patient. The organism may be isolated from the urine, blood, sputum, or pleural fluid. Complement-fixing and agglutinating antibodies appear within 2 to 3 weeks, and the titer is maximal approximately 30 days after onset of clinical symptoms.[253]

PARASITIC INFESTATION OF THE LUNG

Parasitic diseases of the thorax may be manifested either as a hypersensitivity reaction—a variety of eosinophilic lung disease—or as changes resulting from direct invasion of the pleura or lungs. Although pulmonary parasitic disease is rarely encountered and much more rarely acquired in most industrialized countries, because of an ever-increasing amount of travel to countries in which parasitic infestations are endemic and the migration of people from such countries, knowledge of these diseases and their diagnostic features is required. In the Near and Far East, Africa, and South America, parasitic diseases vary in type from country to country, and, because of lack of public health measures, are more common in rural than in urban areas.

In most cases, parasitic disease is suspected because of the finding of peripheral blood eosinophilia in a patient who has resided in an endemic zone. Confirmation of pleuropulmonary involvement requires the demonstration of ova or larvae in the sputum or pleural fluid; strong circumstantial evidence is the finding of ova or larvae in the stools, or positive serologic tests. Often, the chest roentgenogram shows a pattern that is either strongly suggestive or even diagnostic of a specific parasitic disease.

PROTOZOAN INFESTATION

AMEBIASIS

Amebiasis is predominantly a disease of the colon—amebic dysentery—following ingestion of the cysts of *Entamoeba histolytica*. The organism may embolize either to the liver via the portal vein or, rarely, directly to the lungs via hemorrhoidal veins or the lymphatics. Within the liver, the liberation of cytolytic enzyme gives rise to abscesses which may extend into the subdiaphragmatic space or penetrate the diaphragm into the pleural cavity or lung. Pleuropulmonary disease develops in about 15 to 20 per cent of patients with liver involvement.[255]

Amebic dysentery is of worldwide distribution, with areas of high endemicity, especially where hygiene and therapeutic measures are inadequate. Amebic colitis shows no age or sex predominance, but (for reasons unknown) pleuropulmonary involvement occurs most frequently between the ages of 20 and 40 years and is 10 to 15 times more common in men.[256]

Over 95 per cent of amebic lung abscesses are contiguous with the diaphragm and in 75 per cent an extension is pathologically demonstrable from the liver through the diaphragm into the lungs. On section, a lung abscess is filled with dark reddish-brown liquid resembling anchovy or chocolate sauce. Histologically, in the acute stage an inflammatory exudate containing polymorphonuclear leukocytes may surround the area of necrosis, but in well-established or chronic abscesses the cells become lymphocytic and histiocytic in type; there may be minimal fibrosis. *Entamoeba histolytica* may be identified in the margin of the abscess contiguous with normal lung.

Right-sided pleural effusion combined with basal pulmonary disease constitutes the usual picture of pleuropulmonary amebic infection. The pleural effusion is most commonly a sterile exudate secondary to subdiaphragmatic amebic abscess, but in a small percentage of cases it results from direct invasion of the pleura by organisms that have breached the diaphragm. Pulmonary parenchymal involvement usually consists of ill-defined homogeneous consolidation of the right lower or middle lobes. Some of these progress to abscess formation and, later, cavitation.[257] In a small percentage of cases, parenchymal consolidation, with or without cavitation, develops in a site remote from the diaphragm, such as the upper lobes, presumably by direct involvement of the lungs from the colon and without intermediate liver abscess.

The possibility of pleuropulmonary amebiasis should be suspected in any patient, formerly resident in an endemic area, who has symptoms and signs of amebic dysentery and who complains of right upper quadrant abdominal pain and a dry cough. The dry cough may become productive of "chocolate-sauce" material, indicating hepatobronchial communication, and may be accompanied by severe cachexia, suggesting the possibility of tuberculosis or cancer. Empyema may develop in the pleural or pericardial space, or both.

Leukocytosis is usually moderate and eosinophilia may occur. A positive diagnosis can be made by the demonstration of trophozoites in the sputum or pleural exudate. A presumptive diagnosis can be made in cases of pleuropulmonary disease if the stools contain trophozoites or cysts. An amebic etiology should be suspected if adequate antibiotic therapy for basal pleuropulmonary disease has produced no obvious response, and confirmation of the diagnosis may lie in the patient's response to specific therapy.

TOXOPLASMOSIS

Toxoplasmosis is caused by *Toxoplasma gondii*, a crescent-shaped protozoan of the order of Coccidia. *T. gondii* is an obligate intracellular organism, 4 to 7 by 2 to 4 μ; its nucleus stains red and its cytoplasm blue with Romanowsky-type stain. The organism multiplies intracellularly and after a few days to weeks forms cysts containing 50 to 3000 organisms.[258] Toxoplasmosis is worldwide in distribution; as many as one-third of all adults in the United States have specific antibodies to the organism.

There are four main clinical forms of toxoplasmosis—congenital, ocular, lymphatic, and generalized. In humans, the commonest form of the disease is congenital, resulting from intrauterine transmission of the organism from a mother who has acquired the infection during the first two trimesters of pregnancy. Most cases of the acquired disease probably result from ingestion of contaminated or poorly cooked meat, although a high incidence of antibodies has been reported in human vegetarians and in herbivorous animals and birds.[258] Congenital toxoplasmosis usually damages the central nervous system severely, giving rise to conditions such as hydrocephalus, microcephalus, and chorioretinitis; pulmonary involvement during

widespread dissemination of the organism is rare.

From a study of 31 patients with high titers of IgM immunofluorescent antibodies against *T. gondii*, Dorfman and Remington[259] described histologic changes in toxoplasmic lymphadenitis which they considered sufficiently distinctive for firm diagnosis of acute acquired toxoplasmosis. In the lung, the alveolar lining cells proliferate and may desquamate; some alveoli contain gelatinous exudate in which parasites may be identified. The interstitial tissues are infiltrated with plasma cells, lymphocytes, and a few eosinophils, and in some cases have areas of necrosis. In the compromised host[260] the thickened alveolar septa may contain a sparse round-cell infiltrate and show hyaline membrane formation. Large, prominent alveolar lining cells and macrophages containing encysted parasites ("*Toxoplasma* cells") may be seen. In cases of disseminated disease, myocarditis appears to be a constant finding, usually with involvement of the brain, liver, and spleen.[260, 261]

Pulmonary toxoplasmosis is part of a general infestation. *Roentgenographically,* it usually produces a focal reticular pattern resembling acute viral pneumonia, with air-space consolidation in some cases. Hilar lymph node enlargement is common.

Clinically, toxoplasmosis in adults most commonly resembles infectious mononucleosis caused by EB virus. It may occur in previously healthy persons or compromised hosts. The patients may be asymptomatic, or may manifest low-grade fever and lymph node enlargement, with or without a rash, for several weeks or months. Anemia and lymphocytosis are common. Widely disseminated disease usually occurs in compromised hosts, mostly patients with leukemia or lymphoma,[260, 261] but occasionally in those with other malignancies or autoimmune disease.[260] The commonest symptoms are fever, disorientation, confusion, and headache, along with the clinical findings of myocarditis and interstitial pneumonia. However, these clinical presentations are uncommon. Toxoplasmosis in adults is usually a latent infection, in most cases acquired by inhalation of the organism; there are no distinctive clinical manifestations.[262]

The congenital form of the disease commonly damages the central nervous system severely, causing permanent blindness and mental retardation in some cases; death may result from widespread dissemination.

Four readily available serologic tests are used in the diagnosis of toxoplasmosis: the Sabin-

Feldman dye test, complement fixation, hemagglutination, and the IgM fluorescent antibody test.[258, 262]

PNEUMOCYSTIS CARINII INFESTATION

Pneumonia caused by this organism was originally described in Europe as a disease limited to infants—interstitial plasma cell pneumonia—but later shown to be due to *Pneumocystis carinii* and to occur (less often) in older children and adults also. *P. carinii* usually is classified as a protozoan, although all attempts at culture have failed; the manner in which it divides, by giving rise to new daughter parasites, is more suggestive of fungus-type nuclear division.[256]

Pneumocystis carinii is a saprophyte found in the lungs of many animals. It may be found in the lungs of patients dying from malignancy or glomerulonephritis, or after rejection of renal transplant, in the absence of clinically or roentgenographically apparent pulmonary disease.[263, 264] *P. carinii* can cause pneumonia in compromised hosts. Abnormalities may appear initially in the chest roentgenogram in patients in whom corticosteroid therapy is being reduced but other immunosuppressive therapy is being maintained.[264]

The age and sex characteristics of patients with *P. carinii* pneumonia reflect the epidemiologic features of underlying conditions. Most affected infants are born prematurely and first evidence the infection at 2 to 5 months of age; in such cases, the disease is usually institutional, occurring sporadically and in small epidemics in children's hospitals and nurseries. Many children in whom the disease develops during the first year of life have primary immune-deficiency disorders—and, since these are often X-linked, males are most commonly affected. In children over 1 year of age, acute lymphatic leukemia is frequently responsible for the lack of host defense. In early and middle adulthood, most patients have Hodgkin's disease or are recipients of renal transplants who are receiving immunosuppressive therapy; and most patients over 50 years of age have chronic lymphatic or lymphoreticular malignancy (which shows a predilection for males).[265] Other less commonly associated diseases include solid malignant neoplasms and collagen or connective tissue disorders. The route of infection in man is almost certainly by inhalation, since *P. carinii* parasitemia is rare. In one study involving patients with kidney transplantations staying in two different hospitals, 10 patients in the same

hospital developed this infection, suggesting that colonization of this commensal may occur.[263]

Pneumocystis carinii is the commonest cause of interstitial pneumonia in immunosuppressed patients. Grossly, the lungs are pinkish-white and bulky. There is considerable variation in the severity of changes seen histologically. Mild cases may show only minimal alveolar septal infiltration with lymphocytes and occasional plasma cells, with proliferation of alveolar lining cells and a few *P. carinii* organisms within edema fluid in the alveolar spaces. In more severely affected cases, the changes consist of widespread interstitial and alveolar edema, with lymphocytic and plasma cell infiltration, necrosis of alveolar walls, and many masses of *P. carinii* in the alveoli.[256] The organisms stain with periodic acid–Schiff (PAS) or Gomori's-methenamine silver stain, but not with hematoxylin and eosin. Systemic dissemination of the organism has been found at necropsy in a few cases, but in the great majority of patients the infection is confined to the lungs. Simultaneous cytomegalovirus infection is common.

Roentgenographically, in the early stages of the disease a granular or reticulogranular pattern is apparent, particularly in perihilar areas.[264, 266] In later stages the pattern progresses to air-space consolidation, patchy areas of homogeneous consolidation being interspersed with foci of atelectasis and emphysema, particularly in peripheral zones (Figure 6–27). The changes are diffuse and may resemble those of pulmonary edema. Terminally, the lungs may be massively consolidated, to a point of almost complete airlessness. The hilar lymph nodes do not enlarge. Roentgenographic evidence of pleural effusion is very uncommon.

In a review of the roentgenographic features of 30 cases of *P. carinii* infestation, Doppman and his associates[268] found that at least one atypical finding during the course of the disease was frequent; such findings included marked unilateral predominance (in four), lobar or segmental consolidation in addition to diffuse involvement (in two), a pseudonodular pattern simulating metastases (in two), basal atelectasis (in two), and formation of a single cavity (in one). A classic roentgenographic presentation was seen in only 13 (43 per cent) of the 30 patients.

Clinically, in premature infants, the course may be very stormy, with severe dyspnea, tachypnea, and cyanosis, and in a high percentage of cases ends in sudden death within a few hours or days. In adults, the course is usually

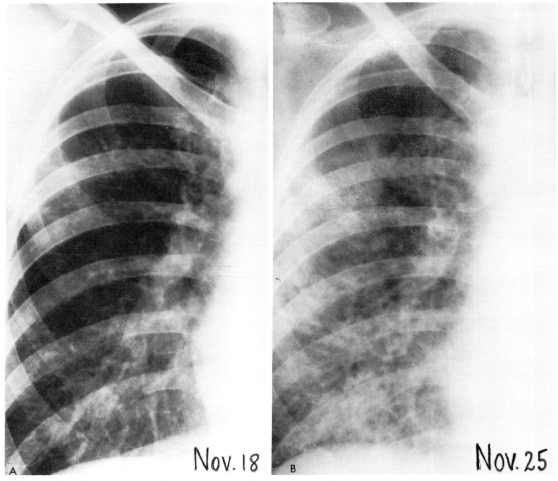

Figure 6–27.   Acute *Pneumocystis carinii* Pneumonia. This 32-year-old renal transplant patient was receiving immuno-suppressive and corticosteroid therapy. Several months after the transplant, he was readmitted with a low-grade fever and dry hacking cough. A roentgenogram (A) revealed the lungs to be diffusely abnormal, the pattern consisting of loss of definition of vessel markings characteristic of diffuse interstitial disease. One week later (B), the pattern had changed to one of diffuse patchy air-space consolidation, indicating extension of the disease from the interstitium into the alveoli. *Pneumocystis carinii* organisms were identified in material obtained by direct needle aspiration of the lung.

more insidious, with a dry, hacking cough, cyanosis, dyspnea, and little or no fever; pleural pain and hemoptysis do not occur. Dyspnea may develop very rapidly, with decreased Po_2 and Pco_2, and increased alveolar-arterial oxygen gradient. This impairment in gas transfer may be present despite a normal chest roentgenogram. Physical signs are minimal and include a few scattered rales or rhonchi. The white cell count is slightly to moderately increased, with polymorphonuclear leukocytes predominating. Lymphopenia occurs in 50 per cent of patients. In one large series,[265] 15 of 17 patients with severe leukopenia died.

Although the disease may be strongly suspected from the roentgenologic findings, the severe cyanosis and dyspnea, and the lack of other symptoms or clinical signs, definitive diagnosis requires demonstration of the organism. The importance of establishing the diagnosis cannot be overemphasized, since specific therapy may cure the infection, particularly if instituted in the early stages. Identification of *P. carinii* is rarely possible in sputum or in aspirate from the tracheobronchial tree and nearly always requires invasive procedures. Open lung biopsy gives the greatest yield; false negatives do not occur but complications are common and may be fatal.[265] Closed cutting needle biopsy and lung aspiration frequently yield diagnostic material,[264, 265] but also produce false negative results[264, 265] and complications, particularly in platelet-depleted patients. Procedures that show promise and carry less risk include transbronchoscopic lung biopsy, endobronchial brush biopsy, and selective bronchopulmonary lavage.

METAZOAN INFESTATION

NEMATHELMINTH (ROUNDWORM) INFESTATION

ASCARIASIS

The adult *Ascaris* worm lives in the small intestine, where it produces eggs which are passed in the feces. The first two larval stages develop within the egg after it has reached soil. Humans contract the disease by ingesting eggs in water or food, or more commonly from contaminated soil under the fingernails. Larvae hatch within the small intestine, then enter the bloodstream and pass to the lung capillaries; they migrate into the alveolar spaces, move up the airways to the larynx, and are swallowed; on reaching the small bowel, they complete their odyssey by developing into mature worms. The parasite usually involved in human infestation is *Ascaris lumbricoides*, although four cases have been reported of infestation with *A. suum*.[269]

Pulmonary disease is caused by the third-stage larvae in their passage through the lungs; the response is allergic in type and invariably gives rise to blood eosinophilia. Since the disease is benign, pathologic data are not available. Roentgenographically, patchy areas of homogeneous consolidation are visible; in many cases they are transient and without clear-cut segmental distribution in the characteristic pattern originally described by Loeffler. With more severe involvement, the shadows tend to confluence and assume a lobular pattern.

Symptoms consist of unproductive cough, substernal chest pain, a pruritic skin eruption (occasionally), and, in more severe cases, hemoptysis and dyspnea. Low-grade fever may be present, and scattered rhonchi and rales may be heard over the lungs. Leukocytosis of 20,000 to 25,000 per cu mm is common, with an eosinophilia of 30 to 70 per cent.

The diagnosis of pulmonary ascariasis is made by the discovery of larvae in the sputum or gastric aspirate; the identification of adult worms or typical mammillated outer-shelled ova in the stools strongly supports the diagnosis, particularly in a patient with leukocytosis and eosinophilia.

STRONGYLOIDIASIS

Strongyloides stercoralis is a nematode whose life cycle includes a larval stage that causes pulmonary disease during migration through the lungs. The disease is worldwide in distribution, being endemic in rural areas where the climate is warm and the soil moist.

As with the hookworms, *Ancylostoma duodenale* and *Necator americanus*, the filariform larvae infect man through penetration of the skin; consequently, the disease is seen in those geographic areas in which barefoot people walk on soil contaminated by feces. After penetrating the skin, the larvae reach the lung by way of the bloodstream, migrating from the capillaries into the alveoli and then climbing the bronchi and trachea to descend into the bowel via the esophagus. Within the bowel, *Strongyloides* develops rhabditiform larvae that may be passed as such in the stool or may progress to the next stage—filariform larvae. Thus, autoinfection may occur through penetration of the intestinal mucosa or perianal skin and the establishment of a cycle within the host. The pulmonary disease in man is associated with migration of the worm from pulmonary capillaries into the alveolar space. *Strongyloides* may exist independently of the human host as free-living forms in the soil.

In recent years, deaths have resulted from overwhelming *Strongyloides* infestation of compromised hosts, permitting identification of pathologic pulmonary changes caused by microfilariae.[256, 270] These include alveolar hemorrhage, edema, bronchopneumonia, pleural effusion, and pulmonary infarction. Roentgenographically, the findings are no different from those in ascariasis or hookworm infestation—nonsegmental, patchy areas of homogeneous consolidation.

Clinically, larval penetration of the skin may produce erythematous papular eruptions. Abdominal pain is the most common symptom, often with diarrhea alternating with constipation; anemia may be present. Severe infestation is most common in compromised hosts, in whom it is usually fatal; it develops chiefly in tropical countries, but some cases have been reported in patients living in temperate climates.[270] Most of these patients have nausea, vomiting, colicky abdominal pain, dyspnea, and hemoptysis, and may evidence bronchospasm. A mild to moderate leukocytosis, with eosinophilia, develops in the peripheral blood. The diagnosis is made by finding larvae in the sputum, stool, or gastric washings.

ANCYLOSTOMIASIS (HOOKWORM DISEASE)

The nematodes *Ancylostoma duodenale* and *Necator americanus* exist in a filariform larval stage in soil. They infect humans by penetrating the skin so that, as with *Strongyloides*, a combination of warm climate, moist contaminated soil, poor hygiene, and bare feet is required for completion of the life cycle. The larvae reach the pulmonary capillaries by way of the systemic veins, then migrate into the alveoli, and then by way of the bronchi and trachea into the esophagus and small intestine. In the small bowel they mature into adult hookworms that produce eggs which are passed in the feces.

The major manifestation of hookworm disease is anemia, caused by the worms' tendency to feed mainly on blood. Pulmonary disease appears less common than in *Strongyloides* infestation, but severe infection may give rise to transient cough and hemoptysis, and nonsegmental homogeneous consolidation may be apparent roentgenographically. Patients typically are pale, weak, and emaciated, with anemia and eosinophilia. The diagnosis is made by finding ova or mature worms in the stools.

FILARIASIS

Filariasis results from infection of the blood, skin, and lymph nodes by threadlike nematodes. The commonest is *Wuchereria bancrofti*, which produces a variety of clinical manifestations related to lymphatic obstruction. Patients with pulmonary disease caused by microfilariae do not usually manifest these changes but present with two rather characteristic syndromes—tropical pulmonary eosinophilia, and "coin" lesions caused by the larvae of *Dirofilaria immitis*.

Tropical Pulmonary Eosinophilia

This is a disease confined to the tropics—the Indian subcontinent, Malaysia, southern Asia, North Africa, and certain areas in South America. The clinical presentation is one of bronchial asthma with moderately severe leukocytosis and eosinophilia; the chest roentgenogram shows a diffuse reticulonodular pattern. Most cases occur in adults between the ages of 20 and 40 years, predominantly in males.[271] Indians and Pakistanis appear particularly susceptible, even in geographic areas where they constitute a minority of the population; Caucasians are rarely affected.

The pathogenesis of the disease is still incompletely understood. It seems that most if not all cases are caused by microfilariae which, for reasons unknown, do not pass through the full cycle to the mature worm, as is generally the case in Bancroft's filariasis. Humans are infected from the bite of a mosquito which introduces filariform larvae into the skin; mature worms develop and discharge microfilariae.

Pathologically, microfilariae of *W. bancrofti* type have been identified in the centers of pulmonary lesions removed surgically. In the early stages there is an outpouring of histiocytes into the alveolar spaces and interstitial tissues; later, the lung tissue develops a hypersensitivity reaction, with eosinophilic infiltration. Six months to 5 years after the onset of symptoms, eosinophils have disappeared and there is histiocytic infiltration with fibrosis; debris may be present, surrounded by foreign body giant cells.[271] Roentgenographically, lung involvement is diffuse and symmetric. There is a general increase in linear markings, in many cases with nodules 2 to 5 mm in diameter, predominantly involving the mid and lower lung zones. Hilar lymph node enlargement occurs in some cases.[271] The chest rentgenogram may show complete clearing with appropriate therapy, but the changes may be permanent, indicating the fibrotic interstitial reaction observed by Udwadia.[271]

The main symptom is cough. Attacks of coughing and dyspnea may be so severe as to suggest status asthmaticus. Weight loss, fatigue, low-grade fever, and slight enlargement of the liver and spleen are frequent. There may be physical signs of bronchospasm. Leukocytosis is usually severe—60,000 white cells per cu mm is not unusual—with eosinophilia, sometimes as high as 60 per cent.

The diagnosis may be suspected from the clinical picture combined with a diffuse reticulonodular pattern roentgenographically in a patient who has resided in an endemic zone. Confirmation may be provided by complement fixation and a skin test using *D. immitis* antigen; microfilariae may be identified in a lung biopsy or (rarely) in nocturnal specimens of blood.

Dirofilaria Immitis Pulmonary Nodule

By late 1975, 42 cases of *Dirofilaria immitis* (the "heart worm of the dog") in excised solitary pulmonary nodules had been reported.[272, 273] In the dog the parasite is worldwide in distribution. Most human cases in the United States have been reported from the southeastern states, in an adult population most likely to undergo screening chest roentgenography. It is thought that a mosquito (*Aedes* sp., *Culex pipiens*) transmits the microfilariae from a fur-bearing animal, usually a dog or cat, to the human host. The developing larvae migrate to the heart or lungs. Man is an unnatural and uncommon host for *D. immitis*; the worm cannot complete its life cycle, and the majority die before reaching sexual maturity. Dirofilarial microfilariae have never been demonstrated in human peripheral blood.

Roentgenographically, the typical manifestation is a solitary, spherical, well-circumscribed nodule 1 to 2 cm in diameter, although bilateral pulmonary nodules have been described. The nodule's spherical shape is probably due to the granulomatous and fibrotic reaction to antigen elaborated by the degenerating worm and permeating surrounding tissue. Diagnosis requires identification of the immature parasite within the lumen of a thrombosed pulmonary artery or arteriole in the middle of the lesion. Special silver (Gomori) and elastic tissue (Verhoeff) stains greatly facilitate location and identification of the worm, which is 100 to 300 μ in cross-section diameter.[273]

Most patients are asymptomatic, the diagnosis being made after pulmonary resection because of suspicion of bronchogenic carcinoma, but some have cough, chest pain, and hemoptysis.[272] Systemic eosinophilia is uncommon. Skin and serologic tests are not reliable or useful.

PULMONARY LARVA MIGRANS

This disease results from infestation by larvae of the dog or cat roundworm, *Toxocara canis* or *T. cati*. It is worldwide in distribution but the majority of reports have come from North America, England, Australia, and Mexico. The disease occurs predominantly in children who swallow soil containing eggs passed in the feces of dogs and cats. The eggs develop into larvae in the intestine, pass into the bloodstream, and are carried to the liver, brain, eyes, lungs, cardiac muscle, lymph nodes, and other tissues (visceral larva migrans). Multiple lesions are found in many organs; they consist of granulomatous foci containing eosinophils, lymphocytes, epithelial cells, and giant cells surrounding the larvae.

Roentgenographically, the chest shows local or diffuse patchy areas of ill-defined pneumonitis.

Children with this disease may be asymptomatic or may complain of cough, wheezing, dyspnea, cyanosis, abdominal pain, and neurologic symptoms. Hepatosplenomegaly is usual. Leukocytosis of 40,000 or more white cells per cu mm is common, usually with eosinophilia of at least 30 per cent. The skin test and immunofluorescent antibody test are considered practical and reliable.[274]

PLATYHELMINTH (FLATWORM) INFESTATION

ECHINOCOCCOSIS (HYDATID DISEASE)

General Comments and Epidemiology

Hydatid disease is caused by the parasite *Echinococcus granulosus*, of the class Cestoda (tapeworm). *E. granulosus* is a small tapeworm whose definitive host is chiefly the dog or wolf and whose intermediate host is a variety of mammals, including humans. There are two types of hydatid disease: the *pastoral* variety, in which the usual intermediate host is the sheep or cow, and the *sylvatic* form, in which the deer and moose are the usual intermediate hosts. Pastoral echinococcosis is particularly common in the sheepraising Mediterranean regions, and in the USSR, Africa, Argentina, Chile, Uruguay, and Australasia. Although endogeneous cases are very uncommon in the United States, they have been reported from 15 states, primarily those in the lower Mississippi valley. The majority of cases of hydatid disease in the United States and southern Canada occur in immigrants. Sylvatic echinococcosis is seen primarily in Alaska and northern Canada, where the disease is endemic. Most Indians and Eskimos living north of the fifty-eighth parallel are hunters and trappers who eat the products of their hunting—thus the high incidence of cysts in this group In both forms of the disease, males are slightly more commonly affected than females.[275]

The minute tapeworm, *E. granulosus*, 3 to 6 mm in length, lives within the small intestine of the definitive host, most commonly the dog but also the wolf, coyote, fisher, and Arctic fox. Millions of ova are passed on to pastures where sheep and cattle may be grazing (in the pastoral variety) or on to ground vegetation and water, from which they are ingested by moose, white-tailed deer, coast deer, reindeer, elk, caribou, or bison (sylvatic form). These animals, and occasionally humans, ingest the ova, which develop into larvae in the duodenum. The larvae enter the bloodstream and pass to the liver and lungs; if they penetrate these two capillary sieves they may reach the spleen, kidneys, brain, or skeleton. Only a few larvae survive the natural defenses of the host, and it may be as long as 20 years before these give rise to symptoms due to a hydatid cyst. The life cycle of the parasite is completed when the definitive host, the dog, feeds on the remains of an intermediate host—sheep or cattle—harboring the larval or cystic stage of the disease, and thereby permits the development of adult worms.

Pathologic Characteristics

Thoracic hydatid cysts occur predominantly within the lung parenchyma, only 2 to 5 per cent developing in the mediastinum, pleural cavity, or diaphragm. In its early stages, the cyst is a spherical or oval mass surrounded by a layer of fibrous tissue formed by the host and sometimes known as the pericyst. The hydatid cyst itself is composed of two layers, a laminated layer which forms the chitinous outer membrane of the cyst (the exocyst) and a thin inner lining formed by a syncytium of cells (the germinal layer or endocyst), from which daughter cysts grow and protrude into the fluid-filled cyst cavity.

Pulmonary hydatid cysts may rupture into surrounding bronchi, expelling the cyst contents and replacing them with air. Sometimes only the pericyst is eroded, permitting communication between the bronchial tree and the potential space between exocyst and pericyst; when this occurs, air accumulates around the exocyst so that the germinal layer tends to collapse. Rupture of a cyst into a bronchus is commonly followed by secondary infection, which tends to kill the parent cyst but permits the daughter cysts to survive. Rarely, a cyst ruptures into the pleural cavity, producing pyopneumothorax.

Roentgenographic Manifestations

Characteristically, pulmonary echinococcal cyst presents as a solitary, sharply circumscribed, spherical or oval mass of unit density surrounded by normal lung.[275, 276] Cysts are multiple in 20 to 30 per cent of patients.[275, 276] Their size ranges from 1 cm to over 10 cm in diameter; the larger cysts usually are of the pastoral type, the sylvatic variety rarely exceeding 10 cm.[277] In a study of the growth rate characteristic of hydatid cysts in 10 patients, the doubling time was 16 to 20 weeks.[276]

The majority of pulmonary hydatid cysts are in the lower lobes, more often posterior than anterior, and somewhat more common on the right.[275] Some hydatid cysts are of bizarre, irregular shape, attributed by some to the fact that, as the cyst grows, it impinges on relatively rigid structures such as bronchovascular bundles, becoming indented and lobulated.[276] The fluid content of a cyst may be evidenced by a change in shape on roentgenograms exposed in maximal inspiration and expiration or in erect and recumbent positions.[275]

Communication between some portion of the cyst and the bronchial tree may occur in two ways, each of which has distinctive roentgenographic characteristics. Rupture may occur between the pericyst and exocyst, permitting air entry between these layers, and producing the appearance of a thin crescent of air around the periphery of the cyst—the "meniscus sign," the "double-arch sign," the "moon sign," or the "crescent sign."[275, 276] Despite the emphasis that has been placed on this sign in the literature, McPhail and Arora[275] observed it in only 5.4 per cent of their 49 patients. The second form of bronchial communication occurs directly with the endocyst (Figure 6–28) when the expulsion of cyst contents produces an air-fluid level roentgenographically; cyst fluid in surrounding parenchyma may simulate pneumonic consolidation.[275] Occasionally, both forms are manifest—an air-fluid level within the cyst and a "crescent sign" around its periphery. After the cyst has ruptured into the bronchial tree, its membrane may float on the fluid within the cyst, giving rise to the classic "water lily sign" or the "sign of the camalote."[276] This sign may also be seen in pleural fluid after rupture of the cyst into the pleural space has resulted in hydropneumothorax or pyopneumothorax. The sylvatic form shows a strong tendency to rupture spontaneously into the bronchial tree, with subsequent complete cure in most instances. By contrast, the pastoral form of hydatid cyst rarely disappears completely after rupture, a residual cavity commonly remaining that often becomes infected. One report[275] recorded spontaneous disappearance of a pastoral cyst after rupture in only 10 per cent of cases.

Calcification of pulmonary hydatid cysts is extremely rare,[276] presumably because growth is so rapid and rupture so frequent that calcification has no chance to develop.

Mediastinal echinococcosis is relatively rare compared with the pulmonary form; cysts develop most commonly in the posterior mediastinum, where they tend to cause erosion of bone.

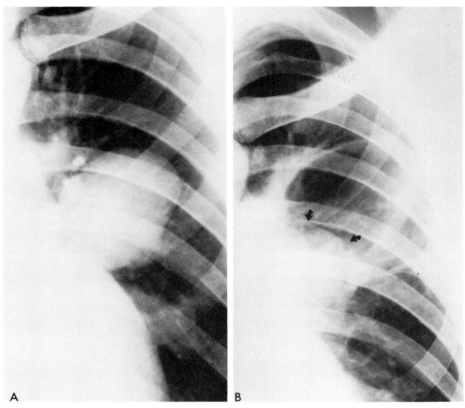

Figure 6–28. Hydatid Cyst with Rupture. In *A*, a sharply circumscribed homogeneous mass is visible in the left mid-lung, possessing a smooth but somewhat lobulated contour. Four years later (*B*), the cyst had expelled all of its liquid contents into the tracheobronchial tree and is now air-containing; an irregular mass is present at the bottom of the cyst (*arrows*), representing collapsed membranes. (Courtesy of Dr. Hal Luke, Alfred Hospital, Melbourne, Australia.)

Clinical Manifestations

The majority of intact pulmonary hydatid cysts, particularly the sylvatic form, occasion no symptoms. When a cyst ruptures, spontaneously or as a result of secondary infection, there is an abrupt onset of cough, expectoration, and fever; an acute hypersensitivity reaction may develop, with urticaria, pruritus, and in some cases hypotension. The patient may complain of chest pain, and the sputum may become purulent and contain fragments of hydatid membrane; rarely, microscopic examination of the sputum reveals hooklets from the scolices. Hydatid cysts arising in the posterior mediastinum may produce pain from bone erosion; those in the anterior mediastinum may cause severe dyspnea from tracheal compression; and the rare involvement of the middle mediastinum may cause catastrophic hemorrhage due to erosion of great vessels.

Unlike many other parasitic diseases, eosinophilia is uncommon in echinococcosis, occurring in less than 25 per cent of cases. Laboratory aids to diagnosis include the occasional identification of hooklets from scolices in the sputum, serologic tests, and a skin test (the Casoni test) using an antigen made from hydatid fluid. Serologic examinations are said to be more reliable than the Casoni skin test.

CYSTICERCOSIS

Cysticercosis is a parasitic infestation caused by various tapeworms, particularly *Taenia solium*, of the class Cestoda. The disease is common in Africa, the Indian subcontinent, and China.[278] Humans occasionally serve as the intermediate host. The eggs lose their shells in the upper small bowel; emerging oncospheres penetrate the mesenteric veins and are carried to various organs and tissues, particularly muscle, brain, and eyes; over a period of 60 to 70 days, the oncospheres metamorphose into cysticerci *(Cysticercus cellulosae)*. Thoracic involvement results from deposition of the cysticerci in respiratory muscles, where their presence may occasion pain. Roentgenographically, they appear as oval, calcified shadows, 3 by 10 mm; they are usually multiple.

PARAGONIMIASIS

Paragonimiasis is caused by the fluke *Paragonimus westermani (Distoma pulmonale)*, of the class Trematoda. This parasite has been shown to be the cause of human lung disease in Korea, Taiwan, Japan, parts of China, the Philippine Islands, Indonesia, New Guinea, Southeast Asia, and certain countries in Africa and South America. The disease occurs in patients of all ages, but tends to be most severe in young children.

The life cycle of *Paragonimus westermani* is one of the most fascinating of all parasites. Within the lungs of humans or animals the larval forms (metacercariae) develop into adult flukes, which deposit eggs in burrows in lung parenchyma. The eggs are coughed up or are swallowed and excreted in the feces. Under suitable moist conditions, the eggs develop into ciliated miracidia which infest freshwater snails. Within the snail, further larval forms develop that after about 2 months are liberated as cercariae; these actively motile parasites penetrate the soft periarticular tissues of certain species of crayfish and crabs. Humans are infected by eating raw or undercooked crabs or crayfish or by drinking water contaminated by them. Metacercariae are liberated in the jejunum, from where they penetrate the wall of the small bowel into the peritoneal cavity, burrow through the diaphragm into the pleural space, and finally into the lung. Within the lung—usually the lower lobe—the metacercariae mature into adult flukes; these produce ova to repeat the cycle. The mature parasite lives for many years in the lung, producing ova continuously.

Since the disease is usually mild and seldom fatal, there are few data on its pathology. Spencer[256] described three forms of reaction within the lung: nonsuppurative, chronic granulomatous reaction, containing numerous ova; a suppurative lesion with caseation; and a chronic ulcerative condition. Ova can be identified throughout the lung tissue. Both flukes and ova may be carried to the brain, resulting in fatal encephalitis.

A comprehensive report of the roentgenographic changes in pulmonary paragonimiasis is that by Ogakwu and Nwokolo.[279] Four roentgenographic patterns were observed: (1) a poorly defined, somewhat hazy, inhomogeneous shadow; (2) shadows of homogeneous density with better defined margins; (3) one to four smoothly outlined cystic areas, 4 to 20 mm in diameter, within the shadows; and (4) a similar type of shadow as described in (1) and (2) but containing "linear streaks." In some cases, all four types of shadows were observed in varying combinations on one roentgenogram.

A somewhat different roentgenographic presentation was observed[280] in a study of 38 patients in an endemic area in Thailand, in which the predominant pattern was of ring shadows or thin-walled cysts 6 mm to 5 cm in diameter, mostly with a crescent-shaped opacity along one aspect of the inner lining. A characteristic feature was irregular tracks or burrows joining two cysts, with a lumen up to 5 mm in diameter (compared with the expected bronchial diameter of 2 to 3 mm).

Hemoptysis is almost invariable and may occur sporadically for months or years in the absence of other signs of illness. There may be dyspnea, mild fever, anorexia, and weight loss; and if pleural effusion or pneumothorax develops, there may be pleural pain. Neither leukocytosis nor eosinophilia is usual, although both may develop temporarily when the metacercariae enter the pleural cavity. Some of the patients are anemic. The diagnosis is made by the finding of typical operculated eggs in the sputum or stool.

SCHISTOSOMIASIS

Three blood flukes (class Trematoda) cause disease in man—*Schistosoma mansoni*, *S. japonicum*, and *S. haematobium*. Two forms of pulmonary disease may be recognized: a transitory process simulating Loeffler's syndrome that occurs coincidentally with the passage of cercariae through the pulmonary capillaries, and pulmonary arterial hypertension, occasionally acute and fulminating but more commonly insidious and chronic, the result of dissemination of *Schistosoma* eggs throughout the pulmonary vascular tree. Schistosoma infestations must be seriously considered as the etiologic agent of cor pulmonale in any person residing in an endemic area.

Both *S. mansoni* and *S. haematobium* are endemic in Egypt and Africa, and the former in the West Indies and South America also; *S. japonicum* is found in China, Japan, and the

Philippines. The great majority of patients with schistosomiasis seen in the United States and Canada are Puerto Ricans infested with *S. mansoni*. It has been estimated that 11 per cent of all Puerto Ricans have schistosomiasis.

The eggs of *S. mansoni* and *S. japonicum* are deposited primarily in the liver, so that symptoms and signs of cirrhosis and hepatosplenomegaly predominate. By contrast, *S. haematobium* affects the urinary bladder chiefly, and hematuria is the major symptom. Pulmonary involvement occurs in approximately one-third of patients with *S. haematobium* and *S. mansoni* infestation; however, despite the presence of eggs in the lungs, cor pulmonale is clinically apparent in only 2 to 6 per cent of these patients.[281]

The life cycle of the blood fluke is complex. Man acquires the infestation by drinking, swimming, working, or washing in fresh water containing the infective cercariae. The larvae penetrate the skin or, less commonly, the mucosa of the mouth or pharynx, and pass via the venous circulation to the pulmonary capillaries; they flow through the pulmonary capillary sieve to the systemic circulation and, in order to survive, must traverse the mesenteric vessels into the intrahepatic portion of the portal system. There they develop into adolescent worms, which migrate against the portal blood flow to the mesenteric, bladder, and pelvic venules. The adult male and female worms copulate in these venules, and then the females migrate to smaller venous channels in the submucosa and mucosa of the bowel and bladder and lay their eggs.[282] Many of these eggs are extruded into the lumen of the bowel and urinary bladder and are passed in the feces or urine; those that reach fresh water develop into larvae which enter snails. Several transformations take place within the snail, infective cercariae eventually emerging; penetration of the skin of a person in contact with the contaminated water completes the odyssey. Some of the eggs deposited by the female worm in the mucosa and submucosa of the bowel and bladder enter the venous system: the eggs of *S. mansoni* and *S. japonicum* are deposited in the liver and those of *S. haematobium* in the lungs. Affection of the lungs by eggs of *S. mansoni* and *S. japonicum* is thought to occur only when the liver has become cirrhotic as a result of schistosomal reaction and has established anastomotic channels that permit migration of the ova between the portal and systemic venous systems.[282, 283]

Pathologic Characteristics

In their passage through the lung capillaries, the metacercariae may incite a local tissue reaction. This is evidenced by transient petechial hemorrhages and foci of eosinophilic and leukocytic infiltration, a picture that fits the usually accepted pathologic criteria of Loeffler's syndrome.[283] Much later in the cycle, eggs deposited in venules of the mucosa and submucosa of the bowel and urinary bladder traverse the systemic veins and right side of the heart and become impacted in pulmonary arterioles that are 50 to 100 μ in diameter. The ova measure 40 to 70 by 100 to 170 μ.[281] After the ovum becomes lodged in a pulmonary vessel, it digests its way through the vessel wall, producing a focal obliterative arteriolitis. The ovum finally reaches the perivascular tissues, where it initiates a tissue reaction which ultimately results in the formation of a granuloma. Infiltration with histiocytes, eosinophilic leukocytes, lymphocytes, and multinucleated giant cells occurs in the tissues surrounding the extruded egg, and this inflammatory reaction eventually becomes fibrotic.[281, 282] When vascular lesions are widespread, a diffuse obliterating endarteritis occurs which restricts the capacity of the pulmonary vascular bed and results in increase in pulmonary artery pressure. Recanalization of obstructed arterioles may lead to the appearance of angiomatoid lesions characteristic of any form of pulmonary hypertension.[256, 281]

Roentgenographic Manifestations

Pulmonary arterial hypertension caused by pulmonary schistosomiasis is indistinguishable from that due to any other cause, there being a marked degree of dilatation of the main pulmonary artery and its branches with rapid tapering toward the periphery.[281] Some cases, perhaps the majority, show a diffuse miliary or reticulonodular pattern presumably produced by the migration of ova through vessel walls and subsequent reaction to this foreign body.[281] The appearance of the chest roentgenogram varies considerably, depending upon the number of eggs that reach the lung and the time of roentgenography in relation to the formation of perivascular granulomas following extrusion of the eggs.

Clinical Manifestations

Extrathoracic symptoms caused by involvement of the urinary and intestinal tracts include dysuria and terminal hematuria, and diarrhea mixed with blood, pus, and mucus. Showers of eggs reaching the pulmonary arterioles produce dry cough, dyspnea, and palpitations. With the development of pulmonary hypertension, expected variations in heart sounds and right-sided valvular murmurs may appear. Hepatosplenomegaly develops in patients with *S. mansoni* and *S. japonicum* infestation.

In addition to the late manifestations due to cor pulmonale, a Loefflerlike syndrome has been described, with transient pulmonary consolidation and eosinophilia, presumably caused by the passage of metacercariae through the pulmonary capillaries.[282, 283]

In patients with suspected schistosomiasis, concentrated specimens of stool and urine should be examined repeatedly for ova. Infestation is demonstrable in many cases by the finding of eggs in biopsy specimens of the rectal and bladder mucosa, but examination of the sputum seldom reveals ova, and lung biopsy usually is required to establish the presence of pulmonary involvement.

The ova of the three varieties of schistosoma have specific characteristics that permit ready differentiation; specific skin tests and precipitin tests are available.[283] Moderate leukocytosis and eosinophilia are usual, the latter to as high as 33 per cent.[281] In patients with cor pulmonale, the electrocardiogram reveals right axis deviation, right ventricular hypertrophy, and incomplete right bundle branch block.[281]

Pulmonary function tests in pulmonary schistosomiasis with cor pulmonale may yield normal results even when catheterization reveals high pulmonary artery pressure. Compliance is reduced, presumably as a result of interstitial fibrosis and destruction of lung elasticity.

ARTHROPOD INFESTATION

PENTASTOMIASIS

The tongue worms *Linguatula serrata* and *Armillifer armillatus* are arachnids whose larval stage may infest man. *L. serrata* is said to be present on every continent.[284] The larval hosts include rabbits and hares, domestic animals, and, occasionally, humans. The eggs hatch when swallowed by the larval host; four- to six-legged larvae emerge in the intestine and migrate to the liver, spleen, lymph nodes, and lungs, where they are transformed into nymphs, which become encapsulated and eventually calcified.

Chest roentgenograms in these patients reveal numerous discrete calcifications 4 to 6 mm in diameter, usually in the form of an incomplete ring shadow.[284] The infestation apparently does not produce symptoms in humans.

REFERENCES

1. Sorokin, S. P.: Properties of alveolar cells and tissues that strengthen alveolar defenses. Arch. Intern. Med., 126:450, 1970.
2. Rylander, R.: Studies of lung defense to infections in inhalation toxicology. Arch. Intern. Med., 126:496, 1970.
3. Tomkin, G. H., Mawhinney, H., and Nevin, N. C.: Isolated absence of IgA with autosomal dominant inheritance. Lancet, 2:124, 1971.
4. Ammann, A. J., and Hong, R.: Selective IgA deficiency: Presentation of 30 cases and a review of the literature. Medicine, 50:223, 1971.
5. Richter, M., and Algom, D.: The heterogeneity of lymphocytes: A consideration of future developments and their impact on clinical medicine. Med. Clin. North Am., 56:305, 1972.
6. Heiss, L. I., and Palmer, D. L.: Anergy in patients with leukocytosis. Am. J. Med., 56:323, 1974.
7. Young, R. C., Corder, M. P., Haynes, H. A., and DeVita, V. T.: Delayed hypersensitivity in Hodgkin's disease. A study of 103 untreated patients. Am. J. Med., 52:63, 1972.
8. Stossel, T. P.: Phagocytosis. N. Engl. J. Med., 290:717, 1974.
9. Cline, M. J., Craddock, C. G., Gale, R. P., Golde, D. W., and Lehrer, R. I.: Granulocytes in human disease. Ann. Intern. Med., 81:801, 1974.
10. Golde, D. W., and Cline, M. J.: Regulation of granulopoiesis. N. Engl. J. Med., 291:1388, 1974.
11. Goetzl, E. J., Gigli, I., Wassermann, S., and Austen, K. F.: A neutrophil immobilizing factor derived from human leukocytes. II. Specificity of action on polymorphonuclear leukocyte mobility. J. Immunol., 111:938, 1973.
12. Stossel, T. P.: Phagocytosis (third of three parts). N. Engl. J. Med., 290:833, 1974.
13. Quie, P. G.: Infections due to neutrophil malfunction. Medicine, 52:411, 1973.
14. Armstrong, D., Young, L. S., Meyer, R. D., and Blevins, A. H.: Infectious complications of neoplastic disease. Med. Clin. North Am., 55, 729, 1971.
15. Hill, R. B., Jr., Rowlands, D. T., Jr., and Rifkind, D.: Infectious pulmonary disease in patients receiving immunosuppressive therapy for organ transplantation. N. Engl. J. Med., 271:1021, 1964.
16. Pagani, J. J., and Libshitz, H. I.: Opportunistic fungal pneumonias in cancer patients. Am. J. Roentgenol., 137:1033, 1981.
17. Sickles, E. A., Young, V. M., Greene, W. H., and Wiernik, P. H.: Pneumonia in acute leukemia. Ann. Intern. Med., 79:528, 1973.
18. Wingard, J. R., Merz, W. G., Saral, R.: *Candida tropicalis*: A major pathogen in immunocompromised patients. Ann. Intern. Med., 91:539, 1979.
19. Winston, D. J., Schiffman, G., Wang, D. C., Feig, S. A., Lin, C.-H., Marso, E. L., Ho, W. G., Young, L. S., and Gale, R. P.: Pneumococcal infections after human bone-marrow transplantation. Ann. Intern. Med., 91:835, 1979.

20. Sullivan, R. J., Jr., Dowdle, W. R., Marine, W. M., and Hierholzer, J. C.: Adult pneumonia in a general hospital. Etiology and host risk factors. Arch. Intern. Med., 129:935, 1972.

21. Sanford, J. P., and Pierce, A. K.: Current infection problems—respiratory. In Proceedings of the International Conference on Nosocomial Infections, Center for Disease Control. Chicago, American Hospital Association, August 3–6, 1970, pp. 77–81.

22. Graybill, J. R., Marshall, L. W., Charache, P., Wallace, C. K., and Melvin, V. B.: Nosocomial pneumonia. A continuing major problem. Am. Rev. Resp. Dis., 108:1130, 1973.

23. Johanson, W. G., Jr., Pierce, A. K., Sanford, J. P., and Thomas, G. D.: Nosocomial respiratory infections with gram-negative bacilli. The significance of colonization of the respiratory tract. Ann. Intern. Med., 77:701, 1972.

24. Pierce, A. K., and Sanford, J. P.: Bacterial contamination of aerosols. Arch. Intern. Med., 131:156, 1973.

25. Freeman, R., and King, B.: Infective complications of indwelling intravenous catheters and the monitoring of infections by the nitroblue-tetrazolium test. Lancet, 1:992, 1972.

26. Austrian, R.: Current status of bacterial pneumonia with especial reference to pneumococcal infection. J. Clin. Pathol., 21(suppl. 2):93, 1968.

27. Finland, M.: Pneumonia and pneumococcal infections, with special reference to pneumococcal pneumonia. The 1979 J. Burns Amberson lecture. Am. Rev. Resp. Dis., 120:481, 1979.

28. Foy, H. M., Wentworth, B., Kenny, G. E., Kloeck, J. M., and Grayston, J. T.: Pneumococcal isolations from patients with pneumonia and control subjects in a prepaid medical care group. Am. Rev. Resp. Dis., 111:595, 1975.

29. Mufson, M. A., Kruss, D. M., Wasil, R. E., and Metzger, W. I.: Capsular types and outcome of bacteremic pneumococcal disease in the antibiotic era. Arch. Intern. Med., 134:505, 1974.

30. Jay, S. J., Johanson, W. G., Jr., and Pierce, A. K.: The radiographic resolution of Streptococcus pneumoniae pneumonia. N. Engl. J. Med., 293:798, 1975.

31. Tillotson, J. R., and Lerner, A. M.: Characteristics of nonbacteremic Pseudomonas pneumonia. Ann. Intern. Med., 68:295, 1968.

32. Renner, R. R., Coccaro, A. P., Heitzman, E. R., Dailey, E. T., and Markarian, B.: Pseudomonas pneumonia: A prototype of hospital-based infection. Radiology, 105:555, 1972.

33. Meltz, D. J., and Grieco, M. H.: Characteristics of Serratia marcescens pneumonia. Arch. Intern. Med., 132:359, 1973.

34. Steinhauer, B. W., Eickhoff, T. C., Kislak, J. W., and Finland, M.: The Klebsiella-Enterobacter-Serratia division: Clinical and epidemiologic characteristics. Ann. Intern. Med., 65:1180, 1966.

35. Balikian, J. P., Herman, P. G., and Godleski, J. J.: Serratia pneumonia. Radiology, 137:309, 1980.

36. Pierce, A. K., and Sanford, J. P.: Aerobic gram-negative bacillary pneumonias. Am. Rev. Resp. Dis., 110:647, 1974.

37. Fraser, D. W., Tsai, T. R., Orenstein, W., Parkin, W. E., Beecham, H. J., Sharrar, R. G., Harris, J., Mallison, G. F., Martin, S. M., McDade, J. E., Shepard, C. C., Brachman, P. S., and the Field Investigation Team: Legionnaires' disease. Description of an epidemic of pneumonia. N. Engl. J. Med., 297:1189, 1977.

38. McDade, J. E., Shepard, C. C., Fraser, D. W., Tsai, T. R., Redus, M. A., Dowdle, W. R., and the Laboratory Investigation Team: Legionnaires' disease. Isolation of a bacterium and demonstration of its role in other respiratory disease. N. Engl. J. Med., 297:1197, 1977.

39. Fraser, D. W.: Legionnaires' disease: Four summers' harvest. Am. J. Med., 68:1, 1980.

40. England, A. C., III, Fraser, D. W., Plikaytis, B. D., Tsai, T. F., Storch, G., and Broome, C. V.: Sporadic legionellosis in the United States: The first thousand cases. Ann. Intern. Med., 94:164, 1981.

41. Meyer, R. D.: Legionnaires' disease update: Be prepared for this summer. J. Resp. Dis., 1:12, 1980.

42. Pasculle, A. W., Myerowitz, R. L., Rinaldo, C. R., Jr.: New bacterial agent of pneumonia isolated from renal-transplant recipients. Lancet, 2:58, 1979.

43. Hébert, G. A., Thomason, B. M., Harris, P. P., Hicklin, M. D., and McKinney, R. M.: "Pittsburgh pneumonia agent": A bacterium phenotypically similar to Legionella pneumophila and identical to the TATLOCK bacterium. Ann. Intern. Med., 92:53, 1980.

44. Thomason, B. M., Ewing, E. P., Jr., Hicklin, M. D., Harding, S. A., and Donowitz, G. R.: TATLOCK bacterium (Pittsburgh pneumonia agent) presumptively identified in five cases of pneumonia. Ann. Intern. Med., 92:510, 1980.

45. Hébert, G. A., Moss, C. W., McDougal, L. K., Bozeman, F. M., McKinney, R. M., and Brenner, D. J.: The rickettsia-like organisms TATLOCK (1943) and HEBA (1959): Bacteria phenotypically similar to but genetically distinct from Legionella pneumophila and the WIGA bacterium. Ann. Intern. Med., 92:45, 1980.

46. Thomason, B. M., Harris, P. P., Hicklin, M. D., Blackmon, J. A., Moss, C. W., and Matthews, F.: A Legionella-like bacterium related to WIGA in a fatal case of pneumonia. Ann. Intern. Med., 91:673, 1979.

47. Lewallen, K. R., McKinney, R. M., Brenner, D. J., Moss, C. W., Dail, D. H., Thomason, B. M., and Bright, R. A.: A newly identified bacterium phenotypically resembling, but genetically distinct from, Legionella pneumophila: An isolate in a case of pneumonia. Ann. Intern. Med., 91:831, 1979.

48. Keel, J. A., Finnerty, W. R., and Feeley, J. C.: Fine structure of the Legionnaires' disease bacterium. In-vitro and in-vivo studies of four isolates. Ann. Intern. Med., 90:652, 1979.

49. Chandler, F. W., Cole, R. M., Hicklin, M. D., Blackmon, J. A., and Callaway, C. S.: Ultrastructure of the Legionnaires' disease bacterium. A study using transmission electron microscopy. Ann. Intern. Med., 90:642, 1979.

50. Neblett, T. R., Riddle, J. M., and Dumoff, M.: Surface topography and fine structure of the Legionnaires' disease bacterium. Ann. Intern. Med., 90:648, 1979.

51. Chandler, F. W., Thomason, B. M., and Hébert, G. A.: Flagella on Legionnaires' disease bacteria in the human lung. Ann. Intern. Med., 93:715, 1980.

52. Edelstein, P. H., Meyer, R. D., and Finegold, S. M.: Laboratory diagnosis of Legionnaires' disease. Am. Rev. Resp. Dis., 121:317, 1980.

53. Band, J. D., LaVenture, M., Davis, J. P., Mallison, G. F., Skaliy, P., Hayes, P. S., Schell, W. L.,

Weiss, H., Greenberg, D. J., and Fraser, D. W.: Epidemic Legionnaires' disease. Airborne transmission down a chimney. J.A.M.A., 245:2404, 1981.

54. Chandler, F. W., Hicklin, M. D., and Blackmon, J. A.: Demonstration of the agent of Legionnaires' disease in tissue. N. Engl. J. Med., 297:1218, 1977.

55. Carrington, C. B.: Pathology of Legionnaires' disease. Ann. Intern. Med., 90:496, 1979.

56. Winn, W. C., Jr., Glavin, F. L., Perl, D. P., and Craighead, J. E.: Macroscopic pathology of the lungs in Legionnaires' disease. Ann. Intern. Med., 90:548, 1979.

57. Watts, J. C., Hicklin, M. D., Thomason, B. M., Callaway, C. S., and Levine, A. J.: Fatal pneumonia caused by *Legionella pneumophila*, serogroup 3: Demonstration of the bacilli in extrathoracic organs. Ann. Intern. Med., 92(Part 1):186, 1980.

58. Blackmon, J. A., Harley, R. A., Hicklin, M. D., and Chandler, F. W.: Pulmonary sequelae of acute Legionnaires' disease pneumonia. Ann. Intern. Med., 90:552, 1979.

59. Dietrich, P. A., Johnson, R. D., Fairbank, J. T., and Walke, J. S.: The chest radiograph in Legionnaires' disease. Radiology, 127:577, 1978.

60. Storch, G. A., Sagel, S. S., and Baine, W. B.: The chest roentgenogram in sporadic cases of Legionnaires' disease. J.A.M.A., 245:587, 1981.

61. Venkatachalam, K. K., Saravolatz, L. D., and Christopher, K. L.: Legionnaires' disease. A cause of lung abscess. J.A.M.A., 241:597, 1979.

62. Meyer, R. D., Edelstein, P. H., Kirby, B. D., Louie, M. H., Mulligan, M. E., Morgenstein, A. A., and Finegold, S. M.: Legionnaires' disease: Unusual clinical and laboratory features. Ann. Intern. Med., 93:240, 1980.

63. Carter, J. B., Wolter, R. K., Angres, G., and Saltzman, P.: Nodular Legionnaire disease. Am. J. Roentgenol., 137:612, 1981.

64. Miller, A. C.: Early clinical differentiation between Legionnaires' disease and other sporadic pneumonias. Ann. Intern. Med., 90:526, 1979.

65. Helms, C. M., Viner, J. P., Sturm, R. H., Renner, E. D., and Johnson, W.: Comparative features of pneumococcal, mycoplasmal, and Legionnaires' disease pneumonias. Ann. Intern. Med., 90:543, 1979.

66. Sharrar, R. G., Friedman, H. M., Miller, W. T., Yanak, M. J., and Abrutyn, E.: Summertime pneumonias in Philadelphia in 1976. An epidemiologic study. Ann. Intern. Med., 90:577, 1979.

67. Edson, D. C., Stiefel, H. E., Wentworth, B. B., and Wilson, D. L.: Prevalence of antibodies to Legionnaires' disease. A seroepidemiologic survey of Michigan residents using the hemagglutination test. Ann. Intern. Med., 90:691, 1979.

68. Grady, G. F., and Gilfillan, R. F.: Relation of *Mycoplasma pneumoniae* seroreactivity, immunosuppression, and chronic disease to Legionnaires' disease. A twelve-month prospective study of sporadic cases in Massachusetts. Ann. Intern. Med., 90:607, 1979.

69. Robbins, J. B., Schneerson, R., Argaman, M., and Handzel, Z. T.: *Haemophilus influenzae* type b: Disease and immunity in humans. Ann. Intern. Med., 78:259, 1973.

70. Holdaway, M. D., and Turk, D. C.: Capsulated *Haemophilus influenzae* and respiratory tract disease. Lancet, 1:358, 1967.

71. Goldstein, E. D., Daly, A. K., and Seamans, C.: *Haemophilus influenzae* as a cause of adult pneumonia. Ann. Intern. Med., 66:35, 1967.

72. Fawcitt, J., and Parry, H. E.: Lung changes in pertussis and measles in childhood. A review of 1894 cases with a follow-up study of the pulmonary complications. Br. J. Radiol., 30:76, 1957.

73. Connor, J. D.: Evidence for an etiologic role of adenoviral infection in pertussis syndrome. N. Engl. J. Med., 283:390, 1970.

74. Connor, J. D.: Pertussis syndrome (letter). N. Engl. J. Med., 283:1174, 1970.

75. Overholt, E. L., and Tigertt, W. D.: Roentgenographic manifestations of pulmonary tularemia. Radiology, 74:758, 1960.

76. Miller, R. P., and Bates, J. H.: Pleuropulmonary tularemia. A review of 29 patients. Am. Rev. Resp. Dis., 99:31, 1969.

77. Rubin, S. A.: Radiologic spectrum of pleuropulmonary tularemia. AJR, 131:277, 1978.

78. Alsofrom, D. J., Mettler, F. A., Jr., and Mann, J. M.: Radiographic manifestations of plague in New Mexico, 1975–1980. Radiology, 139:561, 1981.

79. Ellis, R. H.: *Pasteurella septica* infection in respiratory disease. Thorax, 22:79, 1967.

80. Irwin, R. S., Woelk, W. K., and Coudon, W. L., III: Primary meningococcal pneumonia. Ann. Intern. Med., 82:493, 1975.

81. Feigin, R. D., Lobes, L. A., Jr., Anderson, D., and Pickering, L.: Human leptospirosis from immunized dogs. Ann. Intern. Med., 79:777, 1973.

82. Heath, C. W., Jr., Alexander, A. D., and Galton, M. M.: Leptospirosis in the United States (concluded). Analysis of 483 cases in man, 1949–1961. N. Engl. J. Med., 273:915, 1965.

83. Bartlett, J. G., Gorbach, S. L., and Finegold, S. M.: The bacteriology of aspiration pneumonia. Am. J. Med., 56:202, 1974.

84. Tuazon, C. U.: Aspiration pneumonia and anaerobic lung infections. Primary Care, 5:487, 1978.

85. Bartlett, J. G., and Finegold, S. M.: State of the art. Anaerobic infections of the lung and pleural space. Am. Rev. Resp. Dis., 110:56, 1974.

86. Gorbach, S. L., and Bartlett, J. G.: Anaerobic infections. (second of three parts). N. Engl. J. Med., 290:1237, 1974.

87. Frederick, J., and Braude, A. I.: Anaerobic infection of the paranasal sinuses. N. Engl. J. Med., 290:135, 1974.

88. Landay, M. J., Christensen, E. E., Bynum, L. J., and Goodman, C.: Anaerobic pleural and pulmonary infections. AJR, 134:233, 1980.

89. Ashley, M. J., and Wigle, W. D.: The epidemiology of active tuberculosis in hospital employees in Ontario, 1966–1969. Am. Rev. Resp. Dis., 104:851, 1971.

90. Youmans, G. P.: Relation between delayed hypersensitivity and immunity in tuberculosis. Am. Rev. Resp. Dis., 111:109, 1975.

91. Stead, W. W., Kerby, G. R., Schlueter, D. P., and Jordahl, C. W.: The clinical spectrum of primary tuberculosis in adults: Confusion with reinfection in the pathogenesis of chronic tuberculosis. Ann. Intern. Med., 68:731, 1968.

92. Weber, A. L., Bird, K. T., and Janower, M. L.: Primary tuberculosis in childhood with particular emphasis on changes affecting the tracheobronchial tree. Am. J. Roentgenol., 103:123, 1968.

93. Dhand, S., Fisher, M., and Fewell, J. W.: Intrathoracic tuberculous lymphadenopathy in adults. J.A.M.A., 241:505, 1979.

94. Amorosa, J. K., Smith, P. R., Cohen, J. R., Ramsey, C., and Lyons, H. A.: Tuberculous mediastinal

lymphadenitis in the adult. Radiology, *126*:365, 1978.

95. Liu, C.-I., Fields, W. R., and Shaw, C.-I.: Tuberculous mediastinal lymphadenopathy in adults. Radiology, *126*:369, 1978.

96. Frostad, S.: Segmental atelectasis in children with primary tuberculosis. Am. Rev. Tuberc., *79*:597, 1959.

97. Zarabi, M., Sane, S., and Girdany, B. R.: The chest roentgenogram in the early diagnosis of tuberculous meningitis in children. Am. J. Dis. Child., *121*:389, 1971.

98. Medlar, E. M.: The behavior of pulmonary tuberculous lesions: A pathological study. Am. Rev. Tuberc., *71*:1, 1955.

99. Biehl, J. P.: Miliary tuberculosis. A review of sixty-eight adult patients admitted to a municipal general hospital. Am. Rev. Tuberc., *77*:605, 1958.

100. Dee, P., Teja, K., Korzeniowski, O., and Suratt, P. M.: Miliary tuberculosis resulting in adult respiratory distress syndrome: A surviving case. AJR, *134*:569, 1980.

101. Stinghe, R. V., and Mangiulea, V. G.: Hemoptysis of bronchial origin occurring in patients with arrested tuberculosis. Am. Rev. Resp. Dis., *101*:84, 1970.

102. Sochocky, S.: Tuberculoma of the lung. Am. Rev. Tuberc., *78*:403, 1958.

103. Munt, P. W.: Miliary tuberculosis in the chemotherapy era: With a clinical review in 69 American adults. Medicine, *51*:139, 1972.

104. Pines, A.: The results of chemotherapy in the treatment of tuberculous pleural effusions. Br. Med. J., *2*:863, 1957.

105. Byrd, R. B., Kaplan, P. D., and Gracey, D. R.: Treatment of pulmonary tuberculosis. Chest, *66*:560, 1974.

106. Snider, G. L., and Placik, B.: The relationship between pulmonary tuberculosis and bronchogenic carcinoma. A topographic study. Am. Rev. Resp. Dis., *99*:229, 1969.

107. Lincoln, E. M., and Gilbert, L. A.: Disease in children due to mycobacteria other than *Mycobacterium tuberculosis*. Am. Rev. Resp. Dis., *105*:683, 1972.

108. Jenkins, P. A., Marks, J., and Schaefer, W. B.: Lipid chromatography and seroagglutination in the classification of rapidly growing mycobacteria. Am. Rev. Resp. Dis., *103*:179, 1971.

109. Reiner, E., Hicks, J. J., Beam, R. E., and David, H. L.: Recent studies on mycobacterial differentiation by means of pyrolysis-gas-liquid chromatography. Am. Rev. Resp. Dis., *104*:656, 1971.

110. Wolinsky, E.: Nontuberculous mycobacteria and associated diseases. Am. Rev. Resp. Dis., *119*:107, 1979.

111. Reznikov, M., and Dawson, D. J.: Serological examination of some strains that are in the *Mycobacterium avium-intracellulare-scrofulaceum* complex but do not belong to Schaefer's serotypes. Appl. Microbiol., *26*:470, 1973.

112. Codias, E. K., and Reinhardt, D. J.: Distribution of serotypes of the *Mycobacterium avium-intracellulare-scrofulaceum* complex in Georgia. Am. Rev. Resp. Dis., *119*:965, 1979.

113. Yeager, H., Jr., and Raleigh, J. W.: Pulmonary disease due to *Mycobacterium intracellulare*. Am. Rev. Resp. Dis., *108*:547, 1973.

114. Wolinsky, E.: Nontuberculous mycobacterial infections of man. Med. Clin. North Am., *58*:639, 1974.

115. Curry, Francis J.: Atypical acid-fast mycobacteria. N. Engl. J. Med., *272*:415, 1965.

116. Heitzman, E. R., Bornhurst, R. A., and Russell, J. P.: Disease due to anonymous mycobacteria: Potential for specific diagnosis. Am. J. Roentgenol., *103*:533, 1968.

117. Christensen, E. E., Dietz, G. W., Ahn, C. H., Chapman, J. S., Murry, R. C., and Hurst, G. A.: Radiographic manifestations of pulmonary *Mycobacterium kansasii* infections. AJR, *131*:985, 1978.

118. Anderson, D. H., Grech, P., Townshend, R. H., and Jephcott, A. E.: Pulmonary lesions due to opportunist mycobacteria (review includes 30 cases of *M. kansasii* infections). Clin. Radiol., *26*:461, 1975.

119. Johanson, W. G., Jr., and Nicholson, D. P.: Pulmonary disease due to *Mycobacterium kansasii*. An analysis of some factors affecting prognosis. Am. Rev. Resp. Dis., *99*:73, 1969.

120. Bailey, W. C., Brown, M., Buechner, H. A., Weill, H., Ichinose, H., and Ziskind, M.: Silico-mycobacterial disease in sandblasters. Am. Rev. Resp. Dis., *110*:115, 1974.

121. Wolinsky, E.: The role of scotochromogenic mycobacteria in human disease. Ann. N.Y. Acad. Sci., *106*:67, 1963.

122. Robakiewicz, M., and Grzybowski, S.: Epidemiologic aspects of nontuberculous mycobacterial disease and of tuberculosis in British Columbia. Am. Rev. Resp. Dis., *109*:613, 1974.

123. Nicholson, D. P., and Sevier, W. R.: *Mycobacterium fortuitum* as a pathogen. A case report. Am. Rev. Resp. Dis., *104*:747, 1971.

124. Burke, D. S., and Ullian, R. B.: Megaesophagus and pneumonia associated with *Mycobacterium chelonei*. A case report and a literature review. Am. Rev. Resp. Dis., *116*:1101, 1977.

125. Boisvert, H.: *Mycobacterium xenopei* (Marks et Schwabacher, 1965) mycobactérie scotochromogène, thermophile, dysgonique, éventuellement pathogène pour l'homme. Ann. Inst. Pasteur (Paris), *109*(Suppl.): 447, 1965. (Fr.)

126. Engbaek, H. C., Vergmann, B., Baess, I., and Will, D. W.: *M. xenopei*. A bacteriological study of *M. xenopei* including case reports of Danish patients. Acta. Pathol. Microbiol. Scand., *69*:576, 1967.

127. Tellis, C. J., Beechler, C. R., Ohashi, D. K., and Fuller, S. A.: Pulmonary disease caused by *Mycobacterium xenopei*. Two case reports. Am. Rev. Resp. Dis., *116*:779, 1977.

128. Schaefer, W. B., Wolinsky, E., Jenkins, P. A., and Marks, J.: *Mycobacterium szulgai*—a new pathogen. Serologic identification and report of five new cases. Am. Rev. Resp. Dis., *108*:1320, 1973.

129. Krasnow, I., and Gross, W.: *Mycobacterium simiae* infection in the United States. A case report and discussion of the organism. Am. Rev. Resp. Dis., *111*:357, 1975.

130. Fraser, R. G., and Paré, J. A. P.: Diagnosis of Diseases of the Chest, 2nd ed., vol. II. Philadelphia, W. B. Saunders, 1978, pp. 764, 765.

131. Cockshott, W. P., and Lucas, A. O.: *Histoplasmosis duboisii*. Q. J. Med. (New Series), 33:223, 1964.

132. Goodwin, R. A., Jr., and Des Prez, R. M.: Histoplasmosis. Am. Rev. Resp. Dis., *117*:929, 1978.

133. Brodsky. A. L., Gregg, M. B., Loewenstein, M. S., Kaufman, L., and Mallison, G. F.: Outbreak of histoplasmosis associated with the 1970 earth day activities. Am. J. Med., *54*:333, 1973.

134. Goodwin, R. A., Jr., and Snell, J. D., Jr.: The

enlarging histoplasmona: Concept of a tumor-like phenomenon encompassing the tuberculoma and coccidioidoma. Am. Rev. Resp. Dis., *100*:1, 1969.

135. Furcolow, M. L., and Grayston, J. T.: Occurrence of histoplasmosis in epidemics. Etiologic studies. Am. Rev. Tuberc., *68*:307, 1953.

136. Reddy, P., Gorelick, D. F., Brasher, C. A., and Larsh, H.: Progressive disseminated histoplasmosis as seen in adults. Am. J. Med., *48*:629, 1970.

137. Smith, J. W., and Utz, J. P.: Progressive disseminated histoplasmosis. A prospective study of 26 patients. Ann. Intern. Med., *76*:557, 1972.

138. Rao, S., Biddle, M., Balchum, O. J., and Robinson, J. L.: Focal endemic coccidioidomycosis in Los Angeles County. Am. Rev. Resp. Dis., *105*:410, 1972.

139. Drutz, D. J., and Catanzaro, A.: Coccidioidomycosis. Part 1. Am. Rev. Resp. Dis., *117*:559, 1978.

140. McGahan, J. P., Graves, D. S., Palmer, P. E. S., Stadalnik, R. C., and Dublin, A. B.: Classic and contemporary imaging of coccidioidomycosis. AJR, *136*:393, 1981.

141. Greendyke, W. H., Resnick, D. L., and Harvey, W. C.: The varied roentgen manifestations of primary coccidioidomycosis. Am. J. Roentgenol., *109*:491, 1970.

142. Werner, S. B., Pappagianis, D., Heindl, I., and Mickel, A.: An epidemic of coccidioidomycosis among archeology students in northern California. N. Engl. J. Med., *286*:507, 1972.

143. Colwell, John A., and Tillman, S. P.: Early recognition and therapy of disseminated coccidioidomycosis. Am. J. Med., *31*:676, 1961.

144. Sarosi, G. A., and Davies, S. F.: Blastomycosis. Am. Rev. Resp. Dis., *120*:911, 1979.

145. Witorsch, Philip, and Utz, J. P.: North American blastomycosis: A study of 40 patients. Medicine, *47*:169, 1968.

146. Tosh, F. E., Hammerman, K. J., Weeks, R. J., and Sarosi, G. A.: A common source epidemic of North American blastomycosis. Am. Rev. Resp. Dis., *109*:525, 1974.

147. Kepron, M. W., Schoemperlen, C. B., Hershfield, E. S., Zylak, C. J., and Cherniack, R. M.: North American blastomycosis in Central Canada. A review of 36 cases. Can. Med. Assoc. J., *106*:243, 1972.

148. Rabinowitz, J. G., Busch, J., and Buttram, W. R.: Pulmonary manifestations of blastomycosis. Radiological support of a new concept. Radiology, *120*:25, 1976.

149. Recht, L. D., Philips, J. R., Eckman, M. R., and Sarosi, G. A.: Self-limited blastomycosis: A report of thirteen cases. Am. Rev. Resp. Dis., *120*:1109, 1979.

150. Sarosi, G. A., Hammerman, K. J., Tosh, F. E., and Kronenberg, R. S.: Clinical features of acute pulmonary blastomycosis. N. Engl. J. Med., *290*:540, 1974.

151. Restrepo, A., Calles, G., and Restrepo, M.: South American blastomycosis in Colombia. Rev. Lat. Am. Microbiol., *4*:131, 1961.

152. Murray, H. W., Littman, M. L., and Roberts, R. B.: Disseminated paracoccidioidomycosis (South American blastomycosis) in the United States. Am. J. Med., *56*:209, 1974.

153. Londero, A. T., and Ramos, C. D.: Paracoccidioidomycosis. A clinical and mycologic study of forty-one cases observed in Santa Maria, RS, Brazil. Am. J. Med., *52*:771, 1972.

154. Campbell, G. D.: Primary pulmonary cryptococcosis. Am. Rev. Resp. Dis., *94*:236, 1966.

155. Littman, M. L.: Cryptococcosis (torulosis): Current concepts and therapy. Am. J. Med., *27*:976, 1959.

156. Geraci, J. E., Donoghue, F. E., Ellis, F. H., Jr., Witten, D. M., and Weed, L. A.: Focal pulmonary cryptococcosis: Evaluation of necessity of amphotericin B therapy. Mayo Clin. Proc., *40*:552, 1965.

157. Gordonson, J., Birnbaum, W., Jacobson, G., and Sargent, E. N.: Pulmonary cryptococcosis. Radiology, *112*:557, 1974.

158. Walter, J. E., and Jones, R. D.: Serodiagnosis of clinical cryptococcosis. Am. Rev. Resp. Dis., *97*:275, 1968.

159. Gaines, J. D., and Remington, J. S.: Diagnosis of deep infection with *Candida*. A study of *Candida* precipitins. Arch. Intern. Med., *132*:699, 1973.

160. Kozinn, Philip J., and Taschdjian, C. L.: *Candida albicans:* Saprophyte or pathogen? A diagnostic guideline. J.A.M.A., *198*:170, 1966.

161. Greer, Alvis, E.: Disseminating Fungus Diseases of the Lung. Springfield, Ill., Charles C Thomas, 1962.

162. Ellis, C. A., and Spivack, M. L.: The significance of candidemia. Ann. Intern. Med., *67*:511, 1967.

163. Harvey, J. C., Cantrell, J. R., and Fisher, A. M.: Actinomycosis: Its recognition and treatment. Ann. Intern. Med., *46*:868, 1957.

164. Flynn, M. W., and Felson, B.: The roentgen manifestations of thoracic actinomycosis. Am. J. Roentgenol., *110*:707, 1970.

165. Raich, R. A., Casey, F., and Hall, W. H.: Pulmonary and cutaneous nocardiosis. The significance of the laboratory isolation of *Nocardia*. Am. Rev. Resp. Dis., *83*:505, 1961.

166. Curry, W. A.: Human nocardiosis. A clinical review with selected case reports. Arch. Intern. Med., *140*:818, 1980.

167. Hathaway, B. M., and Mason, K. N.: Nocardiosis. Study of fourteen cases. Am. J. Med., *32*:903, 1962.

168. Murray, J. F., Finegold, S. M., Froman, S., and Will, D. W.: The changing spectrum of nocardiosis. A review and presentation of nine cases. Am. Rev. Resp. Dis., *83*:315, 1961.

169. Campbell, M. J., and Clayton, Y. M.: Bronchopulmonary aspergillosis. A correlation of the clinical and laboratory findings in 272 patients investigated for bronchopulmonary aspergillosis. Am. Rev. Resp. Dis., *89*:186, 1964.

170. Finegold, S. M., Will, D., and Murray, J. F.: Aspergillosis. A review and report of twelve cases. Am. J. Med., *27*:463, 1959.

171. Klein, D. L., and Gamsu, G.: Thoracic manifestations of aspergillosis. AJR, *134*:543, 1980.

172. Greene, R.: The pulmonary aspergilloses: Three distinct entities or a spectrum of disease. Radiology, *140*:527, 1981.

173. Libshitz, H. I., and Pagani, J. J.: Aspergillosis and mucormycosis: Two types of opportunistic fungal pneumonia. Radiology, *140*:301, 1981.

174. Levin, E. J.: Pulmonary intracavitary fungus ball. Radiology, *66*:9, 1956.

175. Joynson, D. H. M.: Pulmonary aspergilloma. Brit. J. Clin. Prac., *31*:207, 1977.

176. Aslam, P. A., Eastridge, C. E., and Hughes, F. A., Jr.: Aspergillosis of the lungs—An eighteen-year experience. Chest, *59*:28, 1971.

177. Henderson, A. H.: Allergic aspergillosis. Review of 32 cases. Thorax, *23*:501, 1968.

178. Meyer, R. D., Young, L. S., Armstrong, D., and Yu, B.: Aspergillosis complicating neoplastic disease. Am. J. Med., 54:6, 1973.

179. Fischer, J. J., and Walker, D. H.: Invasive pulmonary aspergillosis associated with influenza. J.A.M.A., 241:1493, 1979.

180. Curtis, A. McB., Smith, G. J. W., and Ravin, C. E.: Air crescent sign of invasive aspergillosis. Radiology, 133:17, 1979.

181. Longbottom, J. J., and Pepys, J.: Pulmonary aspergillosis: Diagnostic immunological significance of antigens and C-substance in Aspergillus fumigatus. J. Pathol. Bacteriol., 88:141, 1964.

182. Young, R. C., and Bennett, J. E.: Invasive aspergillosis, absence of detectable antibody response. Am. Rev. Resp. Dis., 104:710, 1971.

183. Lehrer, R. I., Howard, D. H., Sypherd, P. S., Edwards, J. E., Segal, G. P., and Winston, D. J.: Mucormycosis. Ann. Intern. Med., 93(Part 1):93, 1980.

184. McBride, R. A., Corson, J. M., and Dammin, G. J.: Mucormycosis. Two cases of disseminated disease with cultural identification of rhizopus; review of literature. Am. J. Med., 28:832, 1960.

185. Meyer, R. D., Rosen, P., and Armstrong, D.: Phycomycosis complicating leukemia and lymphoma. Ann. Intern. Med., 77:871, 1972.

186. Fishbach, R. S., White, M. L., and Finegold, S. M.: Bronchopulmonary geotrichosis. Am. Rev. Resp. Dis., 108:1388, 1973.

187. Ross, J. D., Reid, K. D. G., and Speirs, C. F.: Bronchopulmonary geotrichosis with severe asthma. Br. Med. J., 1:1400, 1966.

188. Mohr, J. A., Patterson, C. D., Eaton, B. G., Rhoades, E. R., and Nichols, N. B.: Primary pulmonary sporotrichosis (case report). Am. Rev. Resp. Dis., 106:260, 1972.

189. Trevathan, R. D., and Phillips, S.: Primary pulmonary sporotrichosis. Case report. J.A.M.A., 195:965, 1966.

190. Mohr, J. A., Griffiths, W., and Long, H.: Pulmonary sporotrichosis in Oklahoma and susceptibilities in vitro. Am. Rev. Resp. Dis., 119:961, 1979.

191. Hainer, J. W., Ostrow, J. H., and Mackenzie, D. W. R.: Pulmonary monosporosis: Report of a case with precipitating antibody. Chest, 66:601, 1974.

192. Spickard, A.: The common cold. Past, present and future research. Survey of the literature. Dis. Chest, 48:545, 1965.

193. Hendley, J. O., Fishburne, H. B., and Gwaltney, J. M., Jr.: Coronavirus infections in working adults. Eight-year study with 229 E and OC 43. Am. Rev. Resp. Dis., 105:805, 1972.

194. Eaton, M. D., Meiklejohn, G., and Van Herick, W.: Studies on the etiology of primary atypical pneumonia: A filterable agent transmission to cotton rats, hamsters and chick embryos. J. Exp. Med., 79:649, 1944.

195. Liu, C.: Studies on primary atypical pneumonia. I. Localization, isolation, and cultivation of a virus in chick embryos. J. Exp. Med., 106:455, 1957.

196. George, R. B., Ziskind, M. M., Rasch, J. R., and Mogabgab, W. J.: Mycoplasma and adenovirus pneumonias. Comparison with other atypical pneumonias in a military population. Ann. Intern. Med., 65:931, 1966.

197. Conte, P., Heitzman, E. R., and Markarian, B.: Viral pneumonia: Roentgen pathological correlations. Radiology, 95:267, 1970.

198. Rosmus, H. H., Paré, J. A. P., Masson, A. M., and Fraser, R. G.: Roentgenographic patterns of acute Mycoplasma and viral pneumonitis. J. Can. Assoc. Radiol., 19:74, 1968.

199. Fine, N. L., Smith, L. R., and Sheedy, P. F.: Frequency of pleural effusions in Mycoplasma and viral pneumonias. N. Engl. J. Med., 283:790, 1970.

200. Rytel, M. W.: Primary atypical pneumonia: Current concepts. Am. J. Med. Sci., 247:84, 1964.

201. Purcell, R. H., and Chanock, R. M.: Role of mycoplasmas in human respiratory disease. Med. Clin. North Am., 51:791, 1967.

202. Alexander, E. R., Foy, H. M., Kenny, G. E., Kronmal, R. A., McMahan, R., Clarke, E. R., MacColl, W. A., and Grayston, J. T.: Pneumonia due to Mycoplasma pneumoniae: Its incidence in the membership of a co-operative medical group. N. Engl. J. Med., 275:131, 1966.

203. Collier, A. M., and Clyde, W. A., Jr.: Appearance of Mycoplasma pneumoniae in lungs of experimentally infected hamsters and sputum from patients with natural disease. Am. Rev. Resp. Dis., 110:765, 1974.

204. Putman, C. E., Curtis, A. McB., Simeone, J. F., and Jensen, P.: Mycoplasma pneumonia. Clinical and roentgenographic patterns. Am. J. Roentgenol., 1242:417, 1975.

205. Hebra, F.: On Diseases of the Skin, Including the Exanthemata. London, The New Sydenham Society, 1866.

206. Stevens, A. M., and Johnson, F. C.: A new eruptive fever associated with stomatitis and ophthalmia. Report of two cases in children. Am. J. Dis. Child., 24:526, 1922.

207. Ludlam, G. B., Bridges, J. B., and Benn, E. C.: Association of Stevens-Johnson syndrome with antibody for Mycoplasma pneumoniae. Lancet, 1:958, 1964.

208. Bianchine, J. R., Macaraeg, P. V. J., Jr., Lasagna, L., Azarnoff, D. L., Brunk, S. F., Hvidberg, E. F., and Owen, J. A., Jr.: Drugs as etiologic factors in the Stevens-Johnson syndrome. Am. J. Med., 44:390, 1968.

209. Monto, A. S., and Kendal, A. P.: Effect of neuraminidase antibody on Hong Kong influenza. Lancet, 1:623, 1973.

210. Oseasohn, R., Adelson, L., and Kaji, M.: Clinicopathologic study of thirty-three fatal cases of Asian influenza. N. Engl. J. Med., 260:509, 1959.

211. Galloway, R. W., and Miller, R. S.: Lung changes in the recent influenza epidemic. Br. J. Radiol., 32:28, 1959.

212. Louria, D. B., Blumenfeld, H. L., Ellis, J. T., Kilbourne, E. D., and Rogers, D. E.: Studies on influenza in the pandemic of 1957–1958. II. Pulmonary complications of influenza. J. Clin. Invest., 38:213, 1959.

213. Middleton, P. J., Alexander, R. M., and Szymanski, M. T.: Severe myositis during recovery from influenza. Lancet, 2:533, 1970.

214. Gardner, P. S., McQuillin, J., McGuckin, R., and Ditchburn, R. K.: Observations on clinical and immunofluorescent diagnosis of parainfluenza virus infections. Br. Med. J., 2:7, 1971.

215. Wenzel, R. P., McCormick, D. P., and Beam, W. E., Jr.: Parainfluenza pneumonia in adults. J.A.M.A., 221:294, 1972.

216. Glezen, W. P., and Denny, F. W.: Epidemiology of acute lower respiratory disease in children. N. Engl. J. Med., 288:498, 1973.

217. Knight, V., Kapikian, A. Z., Kravetz, H. M., Chan-

ock, R. M., Morris, J. A., Huebner, R. J., Smadel, J. E., and Evans, H. E.: Ecology of a newly recognized common respiratory agent RS-virus. Combined clinical staff conference at the National Institutes of Health. Ann. Intern. Med., 55:507, 1961.

218. Hers, J. F. Ph., Masurel, N., and Gans, J. C.: Acute respiratory disease associated with pulmonary involvement in military servicemen in the Netherlands. A serologic and bacteriologic survey, January 1967 to January 1968. Am. Rev. Resp. Dis., 100:499, 1969.

219. Mathur, U., Bentley, D. W., and Hall, C. B.: Concurrent respiratory syncytial virus and influenza A infections in the institutionalized elderly and chronically ill. Ann. Intern. Med., 93(Part 1):49, 1980.

220. Hobson, D.: Acute respiratory virus infections. Br. Med. J., 2:229, 1973.

221. Gardner, P. S., McQuillin, J., and Court, S. D. M.: Speculation on pathogenesis in death from respiratory syncytial virus infection. Br. Med. J., 1:327, 1970.

222. Quinn, J. L., III: Measles pneumonia in an adult. Am. J. Roentgenol., 91:560, 1964.

223. Leading Article: Pneumonia in atypical measles. Br. Med. J., 2:235, 1971.

224. Gokiert, J. G., and Beamish, W. E.: Altered reactivity to measles virus in previously vaccinated children. Can. Med. Assoc. J., 103:724, 1970.

225. Martin, D. B., Weiner, L. B., Nieburg, P. I., and Blair, D. C.: Atypical measles in adolescents and young adults. Ann. Intern. Med., 90:877, 1979.

226. Hall, W. J., and Hall, C. B.: Atypical measles in adolescents: Evaluation of clinical and pulmonary function. Ann. Intern. Med., 90:882, 1979.

227. Mitnick, J., Becker, M. H., Rothberg, M., and Genieser, N. B.: Nodular residua of atypical measles pneumonia. AJR, 134:257, 1980.

228. Lerner, A. M., Klein, J. O., Levin, H. S., and Finland, M.: Infections due to Coxsackie virus group A, type 9, in Boston, 1959, with special reference to exanthems and pneumonia. N. Engl. J. Med., 263:1265, 1960.

229. Herrmann, E. C., Jr., Person, D. A., and Smith, T. F.: Experience in laboratory diagnosis of enterovirus infections in routine medical practice. Mayo Clin. Proc., 47:577, 1972.

230. Cramblett, H. G., Rosen, L., Parrott, R. H., Bell, J. A., Huebner, R. J., and McCullough, N. B.: Respiratory illness in six infants infected with a newly recognized ECHO virus. Pediatrics, 21:168, 1958.

231. George, R. B., and Mogabgab, W. J.: Atypical pneumonia in young men with rhinovirus infections. Ann. Intern. Med., 71:1073, 1969.

232. Tillotson, J. R., and Lerner, A. M.: Reovirus type 3 associated with fatal pneumonia. N. Engl. J. Med., 276:1060, 1967.

233. Adenovirus infections. Br. Med. J., 2:719, 1971.

234. Dascomb, H. E., and Hilleman, M. R.: Clinical and laboratory studies in patients with respiratory disease caused by adenoviruses (RI-APC-ARD agents). Am. J. Med., 21:161, 1956.

235. Gold, R., Wilt, J. C., Adhikari, P. K., and MacPherson, R. I.: Adenoviral pneumonia and its complications in infancy and childhood. J. Can. Assoc. Radiol., 20:218, 1969.

236. MacPherson, R. I., Cumming, G. R., and Chernick, V.: Unilateral hyperlucent lung: A complication of viral pneumonia. J. Can. Assoc. Radiol., 20:225, 1969.

237. Adams, J. M., and Loosli, C. G.: Viral pharyngitis, laryngitis and pneumonitis. The myxoviruses, adenoviruses and enteroviruses in respiratory disease. Med. Clin. North Am., 43:1335, 1959.

238. Triebwasser, J. H., Harris, R. E., Bryant, R. E., and Rhoades, E. R.: Varicella pneumonia in adults. A report of seven cases and a review of literature. Medicine, 46:409, 1967.

239. Burton, G. G., Sayer, W. J., and Lillington, G. A.: Varicella pneumonitis in adults: Frequency of sudden death. Dis. Chest, 50:179, 1966.

240. Evans, W. H. M., and Foreman, H. M.: Smallpox handler's lung. Proc. Roy. Soc. Med., 56:274, 1963.

241. Medearis, D. N., Jr.: Observations concerning human cytomegalovirus infection and disease. Bull. Hopkins Hosp., 114:181, 1964.

242. Klemola, E., Stenström, R., and von Essen, R.: Pneumonia as a clinical manifestation of cytomegalovirus infection in previously healthy adults. Scand. J. Infect. Dis., 4:7, 1972.

243. Case Records of the Massachusetts General Hospital. Case 37–1981. N. Engl. J. Med., 305:627, 1981.

244. Niederman, J. C., Evans, A. S. Subrahmanyan, L., and McCollum, R. W.: Prevalence, incidence, and persistence of EB virus antibody in young adults. N. Engl. J. Med., 228:361, 1970.

245. Pereira, M. S., Field, A. M., Blake, J. M., Rodgers, F. G., Bailey, L. A., and Davies, J. A.: Evidence for oral excretion of E.B. virus in infectious mononucleosis. Lancet, 1:710, 1972.

246. Lander, P., and Palayew, M. J.: Infectious mononucleosis—a review of chest roentgenographic manifestations. J. Can. Assoc. Radiol., 25:303, 1974.

247. Sato, S., and Dunbar, J. S.: Abnormalities of the pharynx and prevertebral soft tissues in infectious mononucleosis. Am. J. Roentgenol., 134:149, 1980.

248. Stenström, R., Jansson, E., and Wager, O.: Ornithosis pneumonia with special reference to roentgenological lung findings. Acta Med. Scand., 171:349, 1962.

249. Yow, E. M., Brennan, J. C., Preston, J., and Levy, S.: The pathology of psittacosis. A report of two cases with hepatitis. Am. J. Med., 27:739, 1959.

250. Barrett, P. K. M., and Greenberg, M. J.: Outbreak of ornithosis. Br. Med. J., 2:206, 1966.

251. Wood, W. H., Jr., and Felson, H.: A case of lymphogranuloma venereum associated with atypical pneumonia. Ann. Intern. Med., 24:904, 1946.

252. Lees, R. F., Harrison, R. B., Williamson, B. R. J., and Shaffer, H. A., Jr.: Radiographic findings in Rocky Mountain spotted fever. Radiology, 129:17, 1978.

253. Johnson, J. E., III, and Kadull, P. J.: Laboratory-acquired Q fever: A report of 50 cases. Am. J. Med., 41:391, 1966.

254. Ramos, H. S., Hodges, R. E., and Meroney, W. H.: Q fever: Report of a case simulating lymphoma. Ann. Intern. Med., 47:1030, 1957.

255. Daniels, A. C., and Childress, M. E.: Pleuropulmonary amebiasis. Calif. Med., 85:369, 1956.

256. Spencer, H.: Pathology of the Lung. 2nd ed., Oxford, Pergamon, 1968.

257. Ducloux, J. M., Ducloux, M., Calvez, F., Astruc, R., and Fournier, H.: Les pleuro-pneumopathies amibiennes. Étude radiologique. (Amebic pleuro-pneumopathies. A radiologic study.) Ann. Radiol. (Paris), 10:341, 1967.

258. Quinn, E. L., Fisher, E. J., Cox, F., Jr., and Madhavan, T.: The clinical spectrum of toxoplasmosis in the adult. Cleve. Clin. Q., 42:71, 1975.

259. Dorfman, R. F., and Remington, J. S.: Value of lymph-node biopsy in the diagnosis of acute ac-

quired toxoplasmosis. N. Engl. J. Med., *289*:878, 1973.

260. Gleason, T. H., and Hamlin, W. B.: Disseminated toxoplasmosis in the compromised host. A report of five cases. Arch. Intern. Med., *134*:1059, 1974.

261. Carey, R. M., Kimball, A. C., Armstrong, D., and Lieberman, P. H.: Toxoplasmosis: Clinical experiences in a cancer hospital. Am. J. Med., *54*:30, 1973.

262. Feldman, H. A.: Toxoplasmosis. N. Engl. J. Med., *279*:1370, 1431, 1968.

263. Rifkind, D., Faris, T. D., and Hill, R. B., Jr.: *Pneumocystis carinii* pneumonia: Studies on the diagnosis and treatment. Ann. Intern. Med., *65*:943, 1966.

264. Burke, B. A., and Good, R. A.: *Pneumocystis carinii* infection. Medicine, *52*:23, 1973.

265. Walzer, P. D., Perl, D. P., Krogstad, D. J., Rawson, P. G., and Schultz, M. G.: *Pneumocystis carinii* pneumonia in the United States. Epidemiologic, diagnostic, and clinical features. Ann. Intern. Med., *80*:83, 1974.

266. Feinberg, S. B., Lester, R. G., and Burke, B.: The roentgen findings in *Pneumocystis carinii* pneumonia. Radiology, *76*:594, 1961.

267. Geary, L., Kashlan, M. B., Hunker, F. D., and Fraser, R. G.: Diffuse lung disease in a compromised host. Invest. Radiol., *15*:85, 1980.

268. Doppman, J. L., Geelhoed, G. W., and De Vita, V. T.: Atypical radiographic features in *Pneumocystis carinii* pneumonia. Radiology, *114*:39, 1975.

269. Phils, J. A., Harrold, A. J., Whiteman, G. V., and Perelmutter, L.: Pulmonary infiltrates, asthma and eosinophilia due to *Ascaris suum* infestation in man. N. Engl. J. Med., *286*:965, 1972.

270. Cruz, T., Reboucas, G., and Rocha, H.: Fatal strongyloidiasis in patients receiving corticosteroids. N. Engl. J. Med., *275*:1093, 1966.

271. Udwadia, F. E.: Tropical eosinophilia—a correlation of clinical, histopathologic and lung function studies. Dis. Chest, *52*:531, 1967.

272. Dayal, Y., and Neafie, R. C.: Human pulmonary dirofilariasis. A case report and review of the literature. Am. Rev. Resp. Dis., *112*:437, 1975.

273. Goodman, M. L., and Gore, I.: Pulmonary infarct secondary to dirofilaria larvae. Arch. Intern. Med., *113*:702, 1964.

274. Woodruff, A. W.: Toxocariasis. Br. Med. J., *3*:663, 1970.

275. McPhail, J. L., and Årora, T. S.: Intrathoracic hydatid disease. Dis. Chest, *52*:772, 1967.

276. Bloomfield, J. A.: Protean radiological manifestations of hydatid infestation. Australas. Radiol., *10*:330, 1966.

277. Wilson, J. F., Diddams, A. C., and Rausch, R. L.: Cystic hydatid disease in Alaska. A review of 101 autochthonous cases of *Echinococcus granulosus* infection. Am. Rev. Resp. Dis., *98*:1, 1968.

278. Faust, E. C., and Russell, P. F.: Craig and Faust's Clinical Parasitology. 7th ed., Philadelphia, Lea & Febiger, 1964.

279. Ogakwu, M., and Nwokolo, C.: Radiological findings in pulmonary paragonimiasis as seen in Nigeria: A review based on one hundred cases. Br. J. Radiol., *46*(Part 2):699, 1973.

280. Suwanik, R., and Harinsuta, C.: Pulmonary paragonimiasis. An evaluation of roentgen findings in 38 positive sputum patients in an endemic area in Thailand. Am. J. Roentgenol., *81*:236, 1959.

281. Farid, Z., Greer, J. W., Ishak, K. G., El-Nagah, A. M., LeGolvan, P. C., and Mousa, A. H.: Chronic pulmonary schistosomiasis. Am. Rev. Tuberc., *79*:119, 1959.

282. Macieira-Coelho, E., and Duarte, C. S.: The syndrome of portopulmonary schistosomiasis. Am. J. Med., *43*:944, 1967.

283. deLeon, Estrella P., and Pardo de Tavera, M.: Pulmonary schistosomiasis in the Philippines. Dis. Chest, *53*:154, 1968.

284. González de Vega, N., Gómez-Moreno, C., and Rodriguez Aguilar, M.: Some cases of probable pulmonary linguatulosis (pentastomiasis, porocephalosis). Enferm. Tórax, *11*:381, 1962.

285. Pope, T. L., Jr., Armstrong, P., Thompson, R., and Donowitz, G. R.: Pittsburgh pneumonia agent: Chest film manifestations. Am. J. Roentgenol., *138*:237, 1982.

7

Diseases of Altered Immunologic Activity

IMMUNOLOGIC DISEASES OF THE THORAX

GENERAL CHARACTERISTICS OF IMMUNE REACTIONS

When an antibody reacts with an antigen, an immune response occurs. This immune response may be beneficial to the host, as in immunization, or it may be harmful, resulting in a variety of immunopathologic mechanisms that constitute the immune diseases. Immune reactions are generally protective in character. These protective (host defense) mechanisms are stimulated not only by infectious agents (previously discussed in detail in Chapter 6), but also by a variety of foreign materials that enter the body through the respiratory and alimentary tracts or develop within the body through cell mutation.

The commonest host response to immunogens within the thorax (excluding those due to infectious agents) is acute bronchospasm, resulting in the clinical picture of spasmodic asthma. (Since the chief manifestation of this disease is airway obstruction, it is described in Chapter 11, which deals with diseases of the airways.) Less common but of growing importance are a number of bronchopulmonary disorders whose immunopathologic origin derives from a variety of specific viable and inert organic materials in the atmosphere—thus they are of *extrinsic* origin (*e.g.*, hypersensitivity bronchopulmonary aspergillosis). In addition, there exist a number of immunologic diseases in which antigenic stimulation arises from within the body itself—the *intrinsic* alveolitides or collagen-vascular diseases. The term "autoimmune" is frequently applied to this category of

disorders, implying an immunologic response to self-antigens, but there is now reasonably convincing evidence that inhaled viruses may alter or assume host cell antigenicity that provokes antibody formation and complement activation resulting in tissue destruction. Nevertheless, the concept of autoimmunity appears valid in certain clinical states (notably Goodpasture's syndrome, in which autoantibody is produced against the basement membranes of the renal glomerulus and pulmonary alveolus).

In 1968, Gell and Coombs[1] classified hypersensitivity or allergic reactions into four types based on different immunopathogenetic mechanisms and morphologic changes (Table 7–1).

Type I Immune Reaction

This reaction requires antibody participation and constitutes the IgE-dependent immune response (Table 7–1). In susceptible individuals, inhalation challenge with appropriate antigens produces bronchospasm within minutes, an "immediate" reaction which is duplicated by introduction of the antigen into the skin (the immediate wheal and flare reaction). IgE is a skin-sensitizing antibody (formerly called reagin), which can transfer skin sensitivity from one person to another (the Prausnitz-Küstner reaction).

Type II Immune Reaction

This occurs when components of the host's tissues stimulate antibody formation; the diseases that result are thus autoimmune and the antibodies are cytotoxic tissue-specific antibodies. The presence of autoantibodies does not necessarily indicate autoimmune disease; it is

TABLE 7–1. IMMUNOPATHOLOGIC REACTIONS

REACTION TYPE	REACTION TIME	IMMUNOPATHOGENESIS	PATHOLOGY	DISEASES
Type I	Minutes	Inhaled or circulating antigen plus IgE attach to mast cells or sensitized leukocytes, with release of histamine, SRS-A, kinins, and ECF-A	Smooth muscle contraction, hypersecretion from mucous glands, vasodilatation, and edema	Asthma
Type II	Variable	Cell or tissue antigen plus autoantibodies (IgM or IgG) plus complement lyse host tissues	Cellular and tissue damage and death	Goodpasture's syndrome
Type III	4–6 hours	Antigen-antibody (IgM, IgG) complexes plus complement are entrapped beneath capillary endothelium. Polymorphonuclear cells are attracted and release lysosomal enzymes	Inflammation and/or necrosis of blood vessels and adjacent structures	Lupus erythematosus and other connective tissue diseases; extrinsic allergic alveolitis; bronchopulmonary aspergillosis
Type IV	Delayed: 48–72 hours	Antigen plus sensitized T lymphocytes lead to formation of lymphocytic chemical mediators that are directly cytotoxic and attract phagocytes; these, in turn, release lysosomal enzymes	Accumulation of mononuclear cells around venules; cell destruction with caseation and/or granuloma formation	Infectious and noninfectious granulomatous diseases including extrinsic allergic alveolitis

only when a disturbance of sufficient magnitude in regulatory mechanisms results in their excessive production that pathologic changes occur (as in type III hypersensitivity reactions). It is believed that viruses can stimulate autoantibody production, either by altering host cell constituents or because their envelopes contain antigenic properties similar to those of host cells; in such circumstances, the host immune system may be incapable of recognizing such antigens as "self." Such a sharing of antigenic determinants has been postulated as the reason for an increased incidence of Goodpasture's syndrome during an influenza epidemic.

Type III Immune Reaction

This reaction consists of the union of antigen and antibody in the form of immune complexes that activate complement, with resulting tissue damage of various types including vasculitis, pneumonitis, and granulomatosis. It is thus called immune complex disese. When these large molecular aggregates (>19 S) of circulating antigen-antibody are soluble, antigen being in excess over antibody, the result is disease exemplified by serum sickness (urticaria, arthritis, arthralgias, proteinuria with abnormal urine sediment, and vasculitis). By contrast,

when antibody is in excess of antigen, insoluble complexes are formed which are rapidly cleared by the reticuloendothelial system, resulting in a group of diseases exemplified by systemic lupus erythematosus (SLE). Necrosis due to this reaction is fibrinoid in type; collagen fibers are swollen and fragmented, and the ground substance is structureless and eosinophilic in appearance and increased in amount, resembling fibrin. In many of these diseases immunodiffusion studies of pathologic material reveal bound complement and antibody, commonly IgG but occasionally IgM.

Most studies suggest that overall T cell function is disturbed only in the late stages of collagen diseases (see further discussion in the section on SLE) and that a subgroup of T cells known as suppressor cells is deficient. Freed from the control of the suppressor T cells, B cells produce autoantibody. Evidence that antigen-antibody complexes bound with complement are responsible for the connective tissue disorders is purely circumstantial but is nevertheless reasonably convincing, particularly in SLE. For example, striking clinical and immunochemical improvement has been reported in SLE patients when their serum, containing high levels of circulating immune complexes, was subjected to plasmapheresis.

In addition to serum sickness and the collagen-vascular disorders, type III immune reactions include bronchopulmonary aspergillosis (sometimes associated with a type I reaction), hypersensitivity pneumonitis (extrinsic allergic alveolitis), and possibly a group of disorders characterized by parenchymal fibrosis, such as fibrosing alveolitis.

Type IV Immune Reaction

This is mediated by sensitized T lymphocytes and neither circulating antibodies nor complement is involved. The hypersensitivity is delayed in type, and since it can be transferred by living lymphocytes but not by serum, it is designated cell-mediated immunity and is exemplified by the tuberculin skin test. Most observers consider the granuloma an integral part of the type IV reaction, although some regard it as a separate immunopathologic mechanism. Although the antigen most commonly responsible for the type IV reaction is an infectious agent, experimental studies have shown that nonviable organic material can produce lung damage in previously sensitized animals; immune reactions of this type could explain the pathologic changes observed in extrinsic allergic alveolitis that appears to be more consistent with a type IV than a type III reaction.

Although both electron microscopy and immunofluorescent labeling have shown distinct differences among the four types of immunopathologic mechanisms outlined by Gell and Coombs,[1] in some diseases more than one type of reaction appears to be responsible.

Primary Immunodeficiency

The immunodeficiencies—whether primary or secondary, humoral or cellular—are associated with an increased incidence of both malignancy and autoimmune disease,[2, 3, 4] an association that appears to result from a defect in the "immune surveillance" system. Immune surveillance is believed to be a function of T lymphocytes, and when these cells are lacking or deficient, impaired tolerance to self-antigens and enhancement of tumor growth occur. In patients with selective IgA deficiency as well, there is a distinct increase in the incidence of rheumatoid arthritis, SLE, pernicious anemia, and thyroiditis. This is believed to be caused by increased absorption of antigen, which alters or assumes host cell antigenicity with consequent excessive autoantibody formation and the development of autoimmune disease.

GOODPASTURE'S SYNDROME AND IDIOPATHIC PULMONARY HEMORRHAGE

GENERAL CHARACTERISTICS

Although it is likely that these two diseases are separate entities,[5] the fact that their thoracic manifestations are identical justifies their simultaneous consideration in a book on chest disease. Both diseases are of unknown etiology and are characterized by repeated episodes of pulmonary hemorrhage, iron-deficiency anemia, and, in long-standing cases, pulmonary insufficiency. Goodpasture's syndrome includes renal disease in addition to the pulmonary manifestations.

The incidence of these diseases differs. Idiopathic pulmonary hemorrhage (IPH) occurs most commonly in children, usually below the age of 10 years; in this age group there is no sex predominance. When it develops in adults, it occurs twice as often in men as in women. By contrast, Goodpasture's syndrome is a disease of young adults over the age of 16 years and shows a striking male predominance. A review of the literature between 1964 and 1970[6] revealed reports on 56 patients, 44 male and 12 female, with an average age of onset of 26.8 years.

PATHOGENESIS

It is now generally accepted that Goodpasture's syndrome is an autoimmune disease. Circulating antibodies against glomerular and alveolar basement membrane have been found repeatedly in patients with this disease, and immunofluorescent studies have demonstrated deposition of IgG (frequently with complement and occasionally with IgA[7]) in a characteristic linear pattern in the kidney glomeruli and, less commonly, in the pulmonary alveoli. Cessation of hemoptysis and hematuria in patients with Goodpasture's syndrome who received immunosuppressive drugs and plasma exchange lend considerable support to the hypothesis of an autoimmune pathogenesis.

It is believed that the renal and pulmonary lesions in Goodpasture's syndrome are mediated by an antiglomerular basement membrane antibody cross-reacting with lung basement membrane. It is generally assumed that the primary target organ is the kidney, pulmonary alveoli being involved on the basis of cross-reactivity; this concept is supported by the relatively greater affinity of glomeruli for IgG anti–basement membrane antibody. There is substantial evidence that bilateral nephrectomy usually but not always results in cessation of further episodes of pulmonary hemorrhage in patients with Goodpasture's syndrome.

On the basis of the foregoing discussion, it is apparent that the diagnosis of IPH should not be based solely on clinical evidence of hemoptysis and iron-deficiency anemia in patients without renal disease, but also on the absence of anti–glomerular basement membrane antibody on immunofluorescent staining.

PATHOLOGIC CHARACTERISTICS

At the time of an acute episode of IPH, histologic examination of either biopsy or necropsy material from the lungs reveals intraalveolar hemorrhage that may be very extensive. Hemorrhage typically is confined to the peripheral air spaces; in fact, massive blood loss can occur into the lungs without hemoptysis, and the trachea and major bronchi may contain little or no blood. Soergel and colleagues[8] reviewed the morphologic findings in 17 patients in whom either biopsy or necropsy studies were carried out 2 months to 10 years after onset of the disease. In addition to fresh hemorrhages within the alveoli and hemosiderin granules and fibrosis in the interstitial tissue, hyperplasia, degeneration, and shedding of alveolar epithelial cells were observed, with marked alveolar capillary dilation and tortuosity. Diffuse interstitial fibrosis, hemosiderosis, degeneration of the elastic fiber network, and dilation and moderate subendothelial sclerosis of pulmonary arteries and veins were also present in most cases. In contrast to other pulmonary and pulmonary-renal syndromes considered to be hyperimmune in nature (such as polyarteritis nodosa and Wegener's granulomatosis), vasculitis is not an invariable pathologic feature of IPH or Goodpasture's syndrome and when present is usually limited to the relatively minor changes described.[8]

In Goodpasture's syndrome the morphologic changes in the lung observed during light microscopy are similar or identical to those of IPH.[5]

The ultrastructure of the lungs and kidneys in Goodpasture's syndrome and IPH has been described by a number of workers. Linear deposits of IgG and complement are bound to the basement membranes of glomeruli and alveoli, findings demonstrable only by immunofluorescent microscopy. Most studies suggest that IPH can be differentiated from Goodpasture's syndrome not only by the lack of renal involvement, but also by the absence of an antigen-antibody reaction. Donald and associates[9] consider that the two diseases can be accurately distinguished by electron microscopy.

The ultrastructure of the glomeruli in Goodpasture's syndrome is similar to that observed in subacute or chronic glomerulonephritis, although the quantity of fibrin appears to be greater in the former. A rather curious associated morphologic finding reported in several patients with IPH has been diffuse nonspecific myocarditis.[8]

ROENTGENOGRAPHIC MANIFESTATIONS

The changes apparent in the chest roentgenogram in both diseases are identical and depend in large measure on the number of hemorrhagic episodes that have occurred in the past. In the early stages of the disease, the pattern is one of diffuse mottled opacities characteristic of patchy air-space consolidation scattered fairly evenly throughout the lungs (Figure 7–1). Distribution usually is widespread but may be more prominent in the perihilar areas and in the middle and lower lung zones. The opacities are confluent in many areas, but individual "rosettes" or acinar shadows may be identifiable. An air bronchogram should be visualized in areas of major air-space consolidation. At this stage the roentgenographic pattern may simulate pulmonary edema (Figure 7–1).

Serial roentgenograms obtained over the several days after an acute episode usually reveal a highly predictable progressive change in the pattern (Figure 7–1): the fluffy deposits characteristic of acinar consolidation disappear within 2 to 3 days and are replaced by a reticular pattern whose distribution is identical to that of the air-space disease.[10] This transition represents a stage in which the alveolar contents have been transported by macrophages to the interstitial space and lymphatics. This reticular pattern gradually diminishes during the next several days, and the appearance of the chest roentgenogram usually returns to normal in 10 days or less after the original acute episode.

With repeated similar episodes, increasing amounts of hemosiderin are deposited within the interstitial tissue and there is progressive interstitial fibrosis. In the majority of cases the chest roentgenogram shows only partial clearing after each fresh hemorrhage, revealing persist-

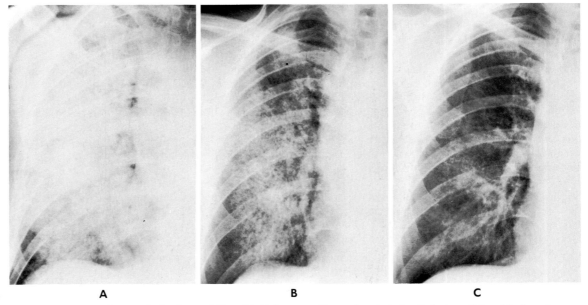

Figure 7–1. Goodpasture's Syndrome (Idiopathic Pulmonary Hemorrhage). A detailed view of the right lung from a posteroanterior roentgenogram *(A)* of a 49-year-old man reveals extensive consolidation of the right lung, in most areas confluent (the left lung was similarly affected). A well-defined air bronchogram is visualized. The distribution and homogeneity of the disease indicate air-space consolidation, from either edema or hemorrhage; in view of the normal heart size, the latter was considered the more likely possibility. Ten days after the initial episode *(B)*, the pattern has become distinctly reticular. Six days later *(C)*, only a fine reticular pattern remains in an anatomic distribution identical to the original involvement. One month later, a fresh episode of massive pulmonary hemorrhage resulted in death from respiratory insufficiency; at necropsy, there was massive pulmonary hemorrhage, subacute glomerulonephritis, and necrotizing arteritis and thrombosis of small splenic arteries; the final diagnosis was Goodpasture's syndrome. The sequence of roentgenologic changes illustrated by this patient is typical of massive pulmonary hemorrhage.

ence of a fine reticular pattern indicative of the chronic irreversible interstitial change. Once these irreversible changes have developed, fresh episodes of pulmonary hemorrhage will usually cause the typical pattern of air-space consolidation to be superimposed upon the diffuse interstitial disease.[5, 10] Rather uncommonly, pulmonary hypertension and chronic cor pulmonale develop as a result of diffuse pulmonary fibrosis.[5]

Hilar lymph nodes may be enlarged, especially during the acute stage, an observation that has been confirmed at necropsy. Septal lines (Kerley B lines) do not develop.

CLINICAL MANIFESTATIONS

Although the morphologic and roentgenographic manifestations of IPH and Goodpasture's syndrome in the lungs are almost identical, there are some important differences in their clinical manifestations. Mention has already been made of differences in age and sex incidence: IPH tends to occur in young children of either sex, whereas Goodpasture's syndrome

occurs more commonly in young adult males.[5, 10]

The onset of IPH may be insidious, with anemia, pallor, weakness, lethargy, and sometimes a dry cough; typical changes of air-space hemorrhage may be apparent roentgenographically without a clear-cut episode of hemoptysis. Rarely, patients present with episodic cough and dyspnea or unexplained iron-deficient hypochromic anemia without a history of hemoptysis and without abnormality on their chest roentgenograms.[11] In some cases the onset is acute, with fever and hemoptysis.

Physical examination during the acute stage of pulmonary hemorrhage may reveal fine rales and dullness to percussion over the affected areas of lung; the liver, spleen, and lymph nodes are palpably enlarged in 20 to 25 per cent of cases.[5] Finger clubbing and hepatosplenomegaly usually are regarded as late manifestations of the disease. Myocarditis develops in a few cases.

Laboratory findings may be normal in children but are abnormal in most older patients. Iron-deficiency anemia usually develops but may not be detectable when intrapulmonary hemorrhage is small and does not severely deplete the bone marrow iron stores. Although bilirubinemia, predominantly of the indirect fraction, and the excretion of excessive amounts of urobilinogen are often present and suggest a hemolytic process, the serum iron values and the iron-binding capacity are characteristic of a severe iron-deficiency anemia, and it is generally agreed that hemolysis does not occur in this disease.[5] Peripheral eosinophilia was present in 12 per cent of cases, and cold agglutinins were detected in ten of the 20 cases tested in Soergel and Sommers' series.[5]

Little is known of the pulmonary function characteristics of either IPH or Goodpasture's syndrome. Several of our patients have had a predominantly restrictive pattern, with decreased diffusing capacity and with or without a fall in resting Po_2. Such a pattern has been said to persist in both diseases even after the chest roentgenogram has returned to normal.[9]

In Goodpasture's syndrome, hemoptysis commonly precedes by several months the clinical manifestations of renal disease. It is seldom as copious as in IPH and may occur late in the course of the disease or be absent altogether.[5] Other presenting symptoms include dyspnea, fatigue, weakness, lassitude, pallor, cough, and hematuria, the last named being noted in only 6 of 51 patients in one series. Physical findings are similar to those of IPH: hepatosplenomegaly, hypertension, and retinal hemorrhages and exudates have been described in approximately 10 per cent of cases.[6] Although the initial urinalysis may be normal, proteinuria, hematuria, and cellular and granular casts almost invariably develop at some stage. In the occasional patient whose urinary sediment is normal, the presence of renal involvement can only be established by biopsy.[9]

Of 51 cases in one review,[6] anemia was present in all and leukocytosis (with a shift to the left) in 50 per cent.

DIAGNOSIS AND PROGNOSIS

Although the diagnosis of IPH may be strongly suspected in young patients who manifest recurrent episodes of hemoptysis, iron-deficiency anemia, and the typical roentgenographic changes, definitive diagnosis may require lung biopsy. Biopsy specimens may be obtained by needle or transbronchial techniques or by limited thoracotomy.

The diagnosis of Goodpasture's syndrome should be suspected when a young patient presents with a combination of hemoptysis and renal disease; it is confirmed by the demonstration on immunofluorescence of circulating or tissue-bound anti–basement membrane antibodies. Confusion may arise occasionally when a patient with renal failure from other causes develops terminal hemoptysis, a complication which, in some instances, has been attributed to disseminated intravascular coagulation. The combination of hemoptysis and renal dysfunction may also occur in the early stages of the collagen-vascular diseases (type III or immune complex disease) before the classic clinical features become manifest.

The prognosis in IPH varies. In the series published by Soergel and Sommers,[5] the average interval from onset of symptoms until death was only two and a half years, whereas individual cases are known to have survived for as long as 18 to 20 years. The prognosis in Goodpasture's syndrome is even worse; 24 of the 25 patients reported by Soergel and Sommers[5] died within an average of 6 months (range, 2 weeks to 3 years) after the appearance of the first symptom. However, some individual case reports have indicated prolonged survival to 6 years and as long as 12 years. Corticosteroid therapy has been employed widely, with disappointing results in most cases, but in some cases there have been indications of arrest of the disease. Cytotoxic and immunosuppressive drugs appear to be more promising therapeutic agents, particularly if therapy is instituted before severe impairment of renal function becomes manifest.

COLLAGEN-VASCULAR DISEASES OF THE LUNG

The collagen-vascular diseases comprise a widely divergent group of disorders whose common denominator is fibrinoid necrosis of connective tissue. The clinical, roentgenologic, and pathologic patterns observed in the thorax alone may be sufficiently type-specific to indicate the diagnosis; however, the overlap among different entities usually necessitates integration of the changes in all organ systems before one can place a specific diagnostic label on any symptom complex.

Histologically, connective tissue is made up of cells, fibrils, and ground substance. The predominant cell is the fibroblast, but macrophages, mast cells, lymphocytes, and leukocytes also are present. The fibrils, which are composed of elastin, collagen, and reticulin, lie in an amorphous ground substance whose composition varies according to its location in soft tissue, cartilage, or synovium. Alteration in the chemical composition and physical constitution of the ground substance, with consequent changes in staining reaction, lead to the edema, fibrinoid degeneration, and vascular lesions that are the pathologic characteristics of this group of diseases. In the lung, connective tissues are found in the walls of the bronchi and of the pulmonary and bronchial vessels, in the bronchovascular and parenchymal interstitium, and in the pleura. Predominant involvement of one or more of these areas produces a clinical, roentgenologic, and pathologic picture which in most cases can be regarded as an "entity." There is some evidence that a symptom complex that includes features of a variety of different connective-tissue disorders may represent a distinct entity. Patients with this "mixed connective-tissue disease" manifest clinical features combining those of SLE, scleroderma, and polymyositis; most are responsive to corticosteroid therapy. Their serum has a high concentration of hemagglutinating antibody to an extractable nuclear antigen consisting mainly of protein and ribonucleic acid; it also contains high titers of fluorescent antinuclear antibody in a speckled pattern. The high titers of antibody to extractable nuclear antigen and its sensitivity to ribonuclease differentiate this complex syndrome from SLE.

The collagen diseases that affect the thorax include systemic lupus erythematosus, rheumatoid pleuropulmonary disease, scleroderma, dermatomyositis and polymyositis, Sjögren's syndrome, and eosinophilic lung disease associated with angiitis or granulomatosis (Wegener's and allergic granulomatosis, and polyarteritis nodosa). Loeffler's syndrome and erythema nodosum are not strictly collagen-vascular diseases, but because of their close relationship are included in this section.

The frequency of involvement of thoracic structures in collagen disease is considerable; two-thirds of 109 patients reported by Nice and colleagues[12] showed roentgenologic changes in the lungs, pleura, or heart; pathologic lesions within the thorax were found at necropsy in 28 of 34 cases.

Classification and discussion of the collagen-vascular diseases can be based either on clinical manifestations in which "entities" or overlap syndromes are defined, or on pathologic findings in which specific components such as the presence of vasculitis or tissue eosinophilia are stressed. This section will deal first with accepted clinical entities and then with a consideration of those collagen-vascular and other immunologically determined diseases that result in blood or tissue eosinophilia or both. The pulmonary vasculitic syndromes will not be discussed as a group, although the presence or absence of vasculitis in each disease entity will be noted in the section on pathologic considerations.

SYSTEMIC LUPUS ERYTHEMATOSUS

EPIDEMIOLOGY

Systemic lupus erythematosus has replaced acute rheumatic fever as the most prevalent of the potentially grave collagen diseases. Characteristically it affects women during the childbearing age, with a female-to-male predominance of about 10 to 1. In a survey of patients from New York City and Jefferson County, Alabama, the incidence, prevalence, and death rates were about three times higher in black than in white women.[13]

Although the connective tissues of any viscus may be affected, there is a tendency to involvement of the vascular system, the skin, and the serous and synovial membranes. In recent years the diagnostic criteria proposed by the American Rheumatism Association Committee for the classification of SLE have been generally adopted (Table 7–2).

TABLE 7–2. CLINICAL CRITERIA FOR THE CLASSIFICATION OF SLE*

1. Facial erythema	8. Lupus erythematosus cells
2. Discoid lupus erythematosus	9. Chronic false positive serologic tests for syphilis
3. Raynaud's phenomenon	10. Profuse proteinuria with protein loss greater than 3.5 g/day
4. Alopecia	11. Cellular casts
5. Photosensitivity	12. Pleuritis and/or pericarditis
6. Oral or nasopharyngeal ulceration	13. Psychosis and/or convulsions
7. Arthritis without deformity	14. Hemolytic anemia and/or leukopenia and/or thrombocytopenia

*Proposed by the American Rheumatism Association Committee for the Classification of SLE (from Cohen, A. S., Reynolds, W. E., Franklin, E. C., Kulka, J. F., et al.: Bull. Rheum. Dis., *21*:643, 1971).

The clinical course usually is prolonged, with frequent remissions and exacerbations; the onset of the disease and subsequent relapses may be precipitated by exposure to sunlight or drugs, emotional upsets, or infection. A familial predisposition has been demonstrated. The lungs and pleura are involved more frequently in SLE than in any other collagen disease, the incidence ranging from 30 to 70 per cent of patients in different series.

PATHOGENESIS

Patients with SLE may show a variety of serologic abnormalities, including a positive reaction to the Coombs test, a falsely positive reaction to the Wassermann test, and antibodies to blood-clotting factors and to a number of nuclear materials including histone, RNA, nucleoprotein, and antigenic components of cytoplasm. The most important of these serum constituents is antibody to the nuclear antigen DNA, especially native DNA, which is considered to be almost specific for SLE. The antigen-antibody complexes engulfed by polymorphonuclear neutrophils are the basis for the *in vitro* lupus erythematosus (LE) cell test. The majority of studies, in both experimental animals and affected patients, incriminate either viruses or genetic susceptibility or both as determinants of this immune complex disorder. A number of studies have shown elevated antibody titers to certain viruses in the serum of SLE patients;[13, 14] also, viruslike particles (referred to as tubular reticular structures or microtubules) have been found in the endoplasmic reticulum of glomerular endothelial cells and in endothelial cells from the skin.[13, 14] A strong genetic component in pathogenesis is indicated by the occurrence of the disease in monozygotic sets of twins, the common finding of certain types of histocompatibility antigens in patients with SLE,[13, 15] and an incidence of approximately 1 to 2 per cent of clinical SLE in first-degree relatives of SLE patients.[14]

In patients with severe, active SLE, skin test reactivity and lymphocyte transformation responses to a variety of antigens *in vitro* are significantly reduced or absent, whereas in patients with mild or inactive SLE these reactions are similar to those observed in control groups. Patients with active SLE have a reduction in both T and B lymphocytes, with increased proportion of "null cells" (cells that lack B and T markers); when blood from such patients was exposed to thymosin, the null cells decreased in number and T cells increased coincidentally.[16] Similar findings have been reported in New Zealand black/white (NZB/W) mice, the animal model for human SLE, in which thymosin administraton enhanced the cell function and decreased the autoimmune features of the experimental model, suggesting the development of suppressor T cells that inhibited antibody formation.[17, 18]

The SLE syndrome, including the presence of antinuclear antibodies and positive LE cell tests, can be induced by certain drugs: those that have been implicated on good evidence include hydralazine, procainamide (Pronestyl), isoniazid, and phenytoin (and other similar antiepileptic drugs); a number of other medications have shown a less convincing association.[13, 19] There are a number of important differences between drug-induced and idiopathic SLE. In the former most patients are older; the bias for females and Negroes does not exist; the kidneys are rarely involved; withdrawal of the drug results in cure; and most patients do not manifest hypocomplementemia or antibodies to native DNA. Patients with active hydralazine-induced lupus have been shown to have circulating antibodies to hydralazine and to native DNA as well as lymphocyte transformation *in vitro* on stimulation with the drug.[19]

In summary, available evidence points to a multifactorial basis for the pathogenesis of SLE.[15] Although the final pathway seems to involve immunologic events, genetic influence may determine whether the disease will develop in response to antigenic stimuli, either autologous or environmental. By altering or simulating tissue or cell antigen, viruses can be implicated in promoting autoantibody formation. Certain drugs may induce a lupus syndrome almost identical to the idiopathic form, although the pathogenesis is unclear. Good correlation exists between the amount of DNA antibody and circulating DNA–anti-DNA complexes, and activity and severity of idiopathic SLE; similarly, a reduction in the number of these antibodies and complexes with immunosuppressive therapy and plasmapheresis correlates well with clinical remission.

PATHOLOGIC CHARACTERISTICS

The hematoxylin body is the *in vivo* equivalent of the *in vitro* LE cell and is found in the tissues of many organs; it represents nuclear damage as a result of cellular anoxia, the altered nucleus reacting with antinuclear antibodies with the development of a purple-staining globule. Other pathologic changes include fibrinoid lesions in the ground substance and an epithelioid reaction in which giant cells enclose fibrinoid necrotic material. Kidney glomeruli show a characteristic "wire-loop" appearance caused by fibrinoid thickening of the basement membrane; in the later stages, the pathologic picture in the kidneys cannot be differentiated from glomerulonephritis.

The pleural lesions generally seen during the course of this disease are usually manifested pathologically by a fibrinous pleuritis. Pathologic changes in the lungs generally are nonspecific and localized and may be caused by sepsis or uremia; they include interstitial pneumonitis, focal alveolar hemorrhage, bronchopneumonia, acute vasculitis, and arteriosclerosis.[20, 21] Immune complexes composed of DNA, anti-DNA antibody, and complement have been reported in two patients with lupus pneumonitis.[22]

ROENTGENOGRAPHIC MANIFESTATIONS

Roentgenologic abnormalities may be seen in the lungs, the pleura, and in the cardiovascular structures, alone or in combination. Of 32 cases reported by Garland and Sisson,[23] 21 showed roentgenologic changes in the thorax, including cardiac enlargement (5), pericardial effusion (5), pleural effusion (13), and various pulmonary parenchymal lesions (10).

In the lungs, the changes usually are nonspecific and commonly consist of rather poorly defined patchy areas of increased density (Figure 7–2), usually in the lung bases and situated

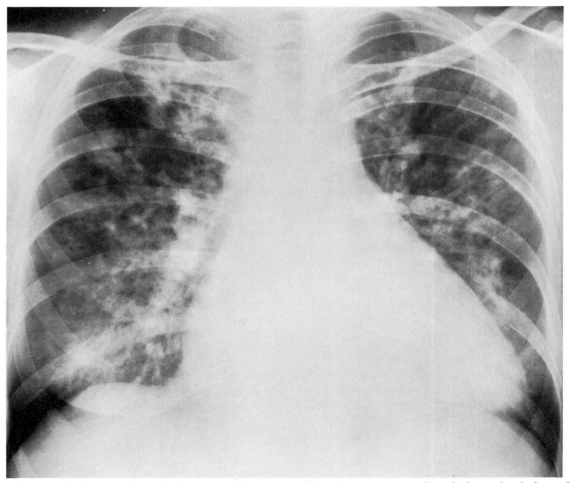

Figure 7–2. Systemic Lupus Erythematosus. A posteroanterior roentgenogram reveals multiple patchy shadows of homogeneous density distributed widely throughout both lungs; the cardiac shadow is moderately enlarged and possesses a contour consistent with pericardial effusion. The precise nature of these pulmonary shadows is in doubt; they could conceivably represent patchy areas of either pneumonitis or edema. It is of some significance that institution of corticosteroid therapy resulted in complete roentgenographic resolution in one week, suggesting a diagnosis of lupus pneumonitis.

peripherally. These changes often are acute and probably represent small areas of pneumonitis. Acute lupus pneumonitis appears to be very uncommon, and the term should probably be restricted to pulmonary opacities that are unaccompanied by evidence of infection and respond to corticosteroid and azathioprine therapy but not to antibiotics.[24]

Horizontal line shadows, usually in both bases and often migratory and fleeting, are of unknown nature although they are usually attributed to platelike atelectasis. Many patients complain of dyspnea and have considerable impairment of pulmonary function without manifesting parenchymal abnormality roentgenologically. In some of these cases, sequential roentgenologic studies show progressive loss of lung volume, a "shrinkage" that may be associated with an elevated sluggish diaphragm.[24] Diffuse interstitial lung disease is uncommon and its nature controversial: whereas it has been stated that not even one case of diffuse interstitial pulmonary fibrosis has been well documented,[24] Eisenberg and his colleagues[25] reported 18 patients with SLE and diffuse interstitial lung disease, in all of whom pulmonary function findings were those common to restrictive lung disease. In the latter series, histopathologic findings were those of nonspecific interstitial fibrosis and chronic inflammation in two cases, fibrosis consistent with healed infarcts in one, and multifocal areas of alveolar epithelial hyperplasia in one. Half of the 18 patients had small lung volumes, which could have contributed at least in part to their restrictive insufficiency.

Massive pulmonary hemorrhage confirmed by pathologic examination occurred in three of 12 patients with SLE in one study.[26] Cavitary pulmonary nodules are rare, and in a recent study of six patients with cavitary nodules and SLE,[27] the disease in five of the patients was proved to be the result of infection or pulmonary embolism.

Pleural effusions are frequently bilateral; they are usually small but may be massive.[28, 29] Winslow and his colleagues[30] stressed the importance of pleuritis as an early manifestation of SLE: of 57 cases reported by these authors, pleural effusion occurred in 42; in three of these, pleuritis appeared as an isolated first sign, and in 16 others it was associated with only minor antecedent symptoms. In 23 of the 42 cases the effusion was bilateral, either simultaneously or alternately, and in 13 of the 19 cases of unilateral effusion it was on the left.

Cardiovascular changes frequently occur in association with other symptoms and signs; increase in the size of the cardiac silhouette is generally the result of pericardial effusion, which usually is relatively small but may be massive (Figure 7–2).[28, 29] Both cardiomegaly and pulmonary edema may be caused by primary lupus myocardiopathy.

The roentgenographic manifestations of drug-induced SLE are no different from those of the idiopathic or primary disease. By contrast, patients with scleroderma or SLE overlap syndrome may manifest roentgenographic changes that reflect coexistence of the two diseases.

CLINICAL MANIFESTATIONS

Clinical manifestations vary from patient to patient. Diagnosis may be difficult in the early stages of the disease if only one organ system is affected, but suspicion usually is aroused when progression of the disease through several exacerbations indicates widespread tissue and organ involvement. Symptoms referable to the respiratory tract include cough with or without mucoid sputum, dyspnea, and pleuritic pain which may be unilateral or bilateral; hemoptysis is very rare but when present may be massive. Pleuritis occurs in 35 to 75 per cent of patients.[31-33] Fever may be a presenting symptom and occasionally is associated with a chill. In patients with advanced disease, renal failure, or on corticosteroid therapy, pyrexia is more likely to be a manifestation of superimposed infection than of primary disease; similarly, leukocytosis with neutrophilia suggests the presence of infection, whereas leukopenia indicates primary disease.[34] In the presence of diaphragmatic dysfunction, patients may complain of dyspnea even though the chest roentgenogram reveals no abnormality other than reduced lung volume.[33] Cutaneous manifestations are seen in 81 per cent of patients and include "butterfly" rash, discoid lupus, alopecia, and photosensitivity. Arthritis and arthralgia are the commonest clinical manifestations of SLE, being observed in 95 per cent of patients;[31, 32] they may be associated with the periarticular subcutaneous nodules usually considered characteristic of rheumatoid disease. Raynaud's phenomenon occurs in 15 to 20 per cent of patients.[31, 32] Patients rarely if ever present with neuropsychiatric complaints, although seizures or psychotic episodes may develop subsequently in almost half of all patients;[31] a similar percentage eventually develop renal disease. Miscellaneous clinical findings include endocarditis, myocarditis, lymph node enlargement, splenomegaly, and purpura. Drug-induced SLE is associated with symptoms and signs similar to those of the idiopathic variety.

The majority of patients eventually have anemia, usually caused by impaired erythropoiesis but occasionally by increased hemolysis. Leukopenia and elevated levels of serum gamma globulins are almost invariable, and thrombocytopenia has been described. The most specific laboratory tests for the confirmation of the diagnosis of SLE are the demonstration of antibodies to deoxyribonucleic acid (DNA) and of the presence of circulating DNA–anti-DNA complexes; the latter finding is a better indication of activity and is often associated with marked hypocomplementemia. The LE cell test and the demonstration of antinuclear antibodies are also useful diagnostic procedures. In one series of 150 SLE patients,[31] the following laboratory abnormalities were found: antinuclear antibodies (present in 87 per cent), positive LE cell preparations (78 per cent), hypergammaglobulinemia (77 per cent), anemia (hemoglobin less than 11 gm per 100 ml, 73 per cent), leukopenia (white blood cells less than 4500 per cu mm, 66 per cent), a positive direct Coombs test (27 per cent), a biologic false positive test for syphilis (24 per cent), positive rheumatoid factor (21 per cent), and thrombocytopenia (platelets less than 100,000 per cu mm, 19 per cent).

Pleural effusion is usually yellow and possesses a high protein and normal glucose concentration typical of an exudate. LE cells may be found in pleural fluid and complement may be absent.

A characteristic of the function values in SLE (seen also in scleroderma) is a severity of impairment out of proportion to the rather mild changes usually apparent clinically and roentgenographically.[35, 36] This dissociation was stressed by Huang and Lyons, who found evidence of impaired function in patients with normal chest roentgenograms and in whom no history could be elicited of previous pulmonary or pleural disease; in this series, however, function was more severely impaired in cases with a history of pleuropulmonary disease. Dyspnea, unexplained by findings on physical or roentgenographic examination, is frequently associated with tachypnea and occasionally with orthopnea and usually is related to severe pulmonary dysfunction.[37] Lung function studies reveal a decrease in lung volume without convincing evidence of airway obstruction; diffusing capacity and arterial oxygen saturation are usually reduced, with low or normal P_{CO_2}, compensated respiratory alkalosis, and reduced lung compliance.[35, 36] Severe diaphragmatic dysfunc-

tion is associated with ventilatory failure and CO_2 retention.

PROGNOSIS

The 10-year survival rates in SLE have been variously reported as 60 per cent[31] and 90 per cent.[32] Only a minority of patients present with a fulminating form of the disease which can prove rapidly fatal because of renal failure or superimposed infection, even when patients are receiving high doses of prednisone. More commonly, the clinical course is chronic, being punctuated with acute exacerbations, and death occurs after many years from renal failure, CNS involvement, or myocardial infarction.[31]

RHEUMATOID DISEASE OF THE LUNGS AND PLEURA

The frequency with which rheumatoid arthritis is associated with extra-articular manifestations—in 76 per cent of one series of 127 patients[38]—clearly justifies the concept of rheumatoid *disease*. In contrast to the female sex predominance characteristic of rheumatoid arthritis, extra-articular manifestations of rheumatoid disease are more common in males. Extra-articular features are present in patients with the most severe joint involvement and include subcutaneous nodules, pleuropulmonary disease, digital vasculitis, skin ulceration, lymph node enlargement, neuropathy, splenomegaly, episcleritis, and pericarditis.[38] The incidence of pleuropulmonary disease in reported series ranges from 5 per cent to over 75 per cent, depending on the criteria for diagnosis and on the presence or absence of positive rheumatoid factor.[39]

The majority of these patients with pleuropulmonary disease have clinical evidence of rheumatoid arthritis, and in about 80 per cent of cases the sheep cell agglutination or latex fixation tests are positive for rheumatoid factor.[33] In some cases, however, rheumatoid arthritis may not be clinically evident when pleuropulmonary abnormality becomes manifest; in such circumstances the diagnosis may be suggested on the basis of positive serologic tests or may not be suspected until the rheumatoid arthritis becomes manifest at some future date.[40, 41] In fact, pleural and pulmonary changes pathologically identical to those of full-blown rheumatoid arthritis may develop without overt evidence of arthritis other than positive sheep cell agglutination or latex fixation tests.

The pleuropulmonary manifestations of rheumatoid disease may be conveniently considered under six headings:[42] diffuse interstitial fibrosis, pleural effusion, the necrobiotic nodule, Caplan's syndrome, rheumatoid disease with pulmonary arteritis and hypertension, and rheumatoid disease with diffuse patchy bronchiolitis.[43] Although these changes may be present in any combination, each is sufficiently distinctive clinically, pathologically, and roentgenographically to warrant separate consideration.[42]

PATHOGENESIS

Rheumatoid disease is of unknown etiology but probably represents a disturbance in immunologic mechanisms. Most patients show high titers of antiglobulin antibody (rheumatoid factor), many have antinuclear antibodies, and in some, LE cell preparations are positive.[38, 44] The circulating autoantibody in rheumatoid disease is largely of the IgM variety,[44] concentrations of IgG and IgA being considerably smaller. In addition to the role played by autoantibodies in the pathogenesis of rheumatoid arthritis, there is good evidence that cell-mediated immune mechanisms may be involved, at least in the pathogenesis of synovitis.[44]

DIFFUSE INTERSTITIAL PULMONARY FIBROSIS

This condition (*synonym:* diffuse interstitial "pneumonitis") was originally described by Ellman and Ball[45] in 1948. It has been estimated that about 20 per cent of recorded cases are caused by rheumatoid disease. In a recent study of 25 patients with established rheumatoid arthritis,[46] 80 per cent were found to have histopathologic evidence of interstitial lung disease.

The morphologic changes in the early stages of the disease consist of nonspecific interstitial pneumonia with mononuclear cell infiltration; as the disease progresses the active inflammatory change is replaced by mature fibrous tissue which, in its most advanced stage, leads to a pathologic picture of "honeycomb lung," with bronchiolectasis and gross distortion of lung architecture. The minute rheumatoid granulomas, often with central necrosis (*see* further on), that develop in many cases distinguish this form of diffuse interstitial fibrosis from that described by Hamman and Rich.[47]

The roentgenographic pattern in the early "subacute" stage of the disease[48] has been described as punctate or nodular; when small it bears some resemblance to miliary tuberculosis, and when larger it is similar to the pattern of sarcoidosis or pneumoconiosis (Figure 7–3).[40] In the later (fibrotic) stage the pattern changes to medium-to-coarse reticulation, often more prominent in the bases than elsewhere and virtually indistinguishable from the pattern seen in late scleroderma or idiopathic pulmonary fibrosis; in our experience a "honeycomb" pattern may be simulated (Figure 7–3). Serial roentgenographic studies may reveal progressive loss of lung volume through cicatrization. Pleural effusion may coexist.[49]

Clinically, the most common symptom is

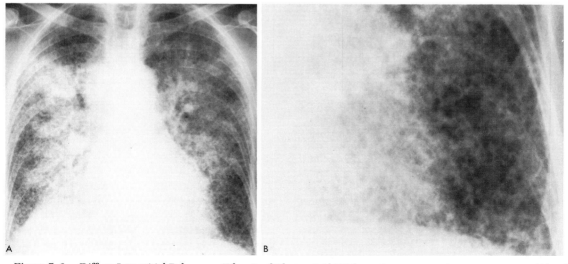

Figure 7–3.   Diffuse Interstitial Pulmonary Fibrosis of Rheumatoid Etiology. A posteroanterior roentgenogram *(A)* and a magnified view of the left lower zone *(B)* reveal a very coarse reticular pattern with some basal and mid-zonal predominance. In the bases, particularly, the pattern is honeycomb in nature. This is a 71-year-old woman with well-established rheumatoid arthritis of several years' duration.

dyspnea on effort, sometimes associated with cough and pleuritic pain. Gross finger clubbing occurs in 50 to 75 per cent of patients,[33] is not uncommonly associated with cor pulmonale, and may antedate the onset of respiratory symptoms. Anemia and slight lymphocytosis develop in some advanced cases. Pulmonary fibrosis occurs more often in the presence of subcutaneous rheumatoid nodules.

Pulmonary function tests show a restrictive ventilatory defect; the diffusing capacity is commonly reduced, even in patients with normal chest roentgenograms, as is the case in patients with SLE or scleroderma.

PLEURITIS AND PLEURAL EFFUSION

Pleural abnormality probably is the most frequent manifestation of rheumatoid disease in the thorax.[40] For reasons as yet unknown, pleural effusion in association with rheumatoid disease has a predilection for males,[49] despite the fact that rheumatoid arthritis occurs predominantly in females, in a ratio of 2 to 1. Middle-aged patients are most often affected, the average age of 52 years in one large series being identical to that usually reported for rheumatoid arthritis as a whole.[49]

The pleural fluid is an exudate with a high protein content and is pale yellow to yellowish-green. Characteristically, the sugar content is very low (20 to 25 mg or less per 100 ml), despite normal blood sugar levels, and does not rise following intravenous infusion of glucose,[49] a finding that aids in differentiation from tuberculous pleural effusion in which the characteristically low sugar content does rise with intravenous administration. When the pleural fluid is nonpurulent, contains no bacteria on smear and culture, and shows no malignant cells on cytologic examination, rheumatoid disease is the likely diagnosis, especially if the possibility of tuberculosis has been excluded by pleural biopsy. It has been estimated that pleural fluid glucose levels below 30 mg per 100 ml are found in 70 to 80 per cent of patients.[50] Cells in the pleural fluid are predominantly lymphocytes. The level of lactate dehydrogenase (LDH) may be much higher in the pleural fluid than in the serum.[51] Rheumatoid factor often is elevated in pleural fluid as in blood, and in some cases the etiology is indicated by the presence of rheumatoid arthritis cells (leukocytes with dense black granules in the cytoplasm). Complement levels in pleural fluid may be decreased. Rheumatoid pleural effusion usually has a protein content greater than 4 gm per 100 ml and may have a milky appearance due to high concentrations of fat and cholesterol, a nonspecific finding that may be seen in any chronic pleural effusion.[50] Empyema is surprisingly common in rheumatoid pleuropulmonary disease;[52] the most plausible causes for its development include a lack of host defense, the discharge into the pleural cavity of necrotic material from rheumatoid nodules situated in the subpleural parenchyma, and perhaps most commonly as a complication of corticosteroid therapy. Pleural biopsy usually is noncontributory, showing only nonspecific inflammatory changes;[49] granulomatous lesions identical to subcutaneous rheumatoid nodules are occasionally identified, however.[51]

The only unique characteristic of the pleural effusion roentgenographically is its tendency to remain relatively unchanged for many months or even years.[48, 49] Of 25 cases of rheumatoid effusion,[49] 23 were unilateral (14 on the right and nine on the left). In the great majority of cases the effusion is the sole abnormality roentgenographically apparent in the thorax; in fact, it has been suggested that the presence of associated parenchymal disease suggests a nonrheumatoid etiology.[49] As with diffuse pulmonary interstitial fibrosis, pleural effusion in association with rheumatoid disease occurs in a significantly greater percentage of cases with subcutaneous nodules than in those without this complication.

The effusion may be entirely unsuspected because of lack of symptoms, and in approximately 50 per cent of cases in one series it was found by chance during roentgenographic examination.[49] The effusion may antedate clinical evidence of rheumatoid arthritis or may occur when joint disease is only mild in degree; in many cases it is associated with episodic exacerbations of arthritis[49, 51] and in some with pericarditis. The development of empyema typically occasions high fever and chills.[52]

THE NECROBIOTIC NODULE

A necrobiotic nodule is a well-circumscribed nodular mass in the lungs, pleura, or pericardium, identical in all respects to a subcutaneous rheumatoid nodule. It is a relatively rare manifestation of pleuropulmonary rheumatoid disease and usually is associated with advanced rheumatoid arthritis and with multiple subcutaneous nodules over the elbows or elsewhere.[53]

These lesions are identical to the subcutaneous rheumatoid nodule. There is a central zone of fibrinoid necrosis surrounded by pali-

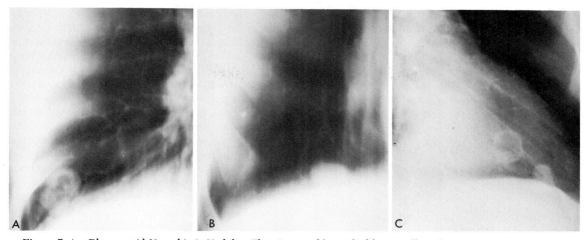

Figure 7–4. Rheumatoid Necrobiotic Nodules. This 41-year-old man had been well until one year prior to admission, when he developed fleeting pains in the shoulders and hips which, in succeeding months, extended to the hands, knees, and neck. The pain in the hands and knees was associated with considerable swelling and morning stiffness. Tomographic sections of the right base at different levels (A and B) show at least two nodules just above the costophrenic angle (one of which is cavitated) and a third nodule of homogeneous density more posteriorly situated. Six years later, an oblique roentgenogram of the lower portion of the left lung (C) reveals two nodules, one of which presents as a ring shadow and the other as a nodule of homogeneous density. (Courtesy of the Montreal General Hospital.)

sading cells—presumably young fibroblasts—whose axis is at right angles to the zone of central necrosis. Surrounding the palisade is a stroma of granulation tissue that may be highly cellular or densely sclerotic.

The necrobiotic nodule represents a relatively rare cause of solitary or multiple nodules in the lungs. Typically they present as well-circumscribed masses, usually multiple, ranging from 3 mm to 7 cm in diameter, commonly situated in the periphery of the lung deep to the pleura (Fig. 7–4).[53] They may be very numerous and resemble metastases. Cavitation is common, the walls being thick and with a smooth inner lining. The nodules may wax and wane in concert with the subcutaneous nodules. During remission of the arthritis the cavities may become thin-walled and gradually disappear.

The lesions tend to occasion no symptoms unless they grow large or become infected.[53] Blood eosinophilia of 10 to 50 per cent is not uncommon.

CAPLAN'S SYNDROME

Caplan originally described this syndrome in 1953 in coal miners in South Wales.[54] It is characterized by single or multiple well-defined spherical opacities in the lungs, ranging from 0.5 to 5.0 cm in diameter. In·contrast to the slow development of progressive massive fibrosis in coal-worker's pneumoconiosis, these lesions usually develop rapidly and tend to appear in "crops." In many cases the background of simple pneumoconiosis is slight or even absent. Since Caplan's original description of the disease in coal workers, the number of pneumoconioses with which these lesions may be associated has grown to include many relating to industries in which silica or silicates are a hazard. It has been hypothesized that these lesions represent a hypersensitization reaction to irritating dust particles in the lungs of rheumatoid patients who are already hyperimmune.

Morphologically, individual nodules measure 1 to 2 cm in diameter and consist of a central necrotic zone surrounded by an active inflammatory layer with cellular infiltration by macrophages and, frequently, polymorphonuclear leukocytes. Some of the macrophages in the inflammatory zone contain dust, and when these disintegrate the dust is deposited, resulting in a characteristic darkened concentric ring surrounding the central core; it is this pigmented ring that differentiates Caplan's nodule from the necrobiotic nodule of rheumatoid arthritis unassociated with pneumoconiosis. Multinucleated giant cells are present in some instances, lying within a zone of fibroblasts situated outside the inflammatory zone; the fibroblasts are typically oriented in a palisade pattern, with their long axis perpendicular to the zone of necrosis and surrounded by a zone of collagen.

Roentgenographically, there is little to distinguish the nodular lesions of Caplan's syndrome from the necrobiotic nodules of rheumatoid arthritis without pneumoconiosis. The nodules may increase in number, remain unchanged, or calcify; cavitation may occur and may be followed by fibrosis or disappearance of the lesion.[54]

The opacities may appear before, coincident with, or after the clinical onset of arthritis, and there is no apparent relationship between the severity of the arthritis and the extent and type of roentgenographically apparent change in the lungs.

RHEUMATOID DISEASE WITH PULMONARY ARTERITIS AND HYPERTENSION

Although arteritis of the pulmonary vessels frequently develops in association with other forms of pleuropulmonary rheumatoid disease, in some patients the principal morphologic manifestation of the disease is in the pulmonary vasculature; first the endothelium of the affected artery is separated from the intima by edema, and then the edema is replaced by fibroelastoid intimal proliferation. Perivascular cuffing with lymphocytes may be seen in the smaller vessels.

Narrowing of the lumen of the pulmonary vessels secondary to the arteritis often leads to pulmonary hypertension and eventually to cor pulmonale.[48] Rheumatoid vasculitis is commonly associated with circulating immune complexes and responds to cyclophosphamide therapy.[55]

OBLITERATIVE BRONCHIOLITIS

The sixth pleuropulmonary manifestation of rheumatoid disease has been recognized only in recent years[43] and consists of diffuse bronchiolitis and patchy fibrotic bronchiolar obliteration. In the original description,[43] only women were involved, all with rheumatoid arthritis. We have seen this disorder in a nonsmoking middle-aged woman with rheumatoid arthritis whose course was rapidly progressive to respiratory failure. In a surprising number of the few cases that have been reported, patients were receiving penicillamine at the time of onset of symptoms.[57]

DIFFUSE SYSTEMIC SCLEROSIS (SCLERODERMA)

GENERAL CHARACTERISTICS

Diffuse systemic sclerosis is a collagen disease characterized by atrophy and sclerosis of the skin, gastrointestinal tract, musculoskeletal system, heart, and lungs. The majority of patients are affected in the fourth, fifth, or sixth decade of life. There is a female sex predominance of the order of 3 to 1, but no significant racial predominance. The prognosis is very unfavorable: in two series of 236[58] and 198[59] patients, five-year survival rates were reported at 49 and 67 per cent, respectively. The cause of death may be cardiovascular, pulmonary, or renal.[59]

Ninety per cent of patients with scleroderma show morphologic and functional evidence of pulmonary fibrosis, but only a minority have an abnormal chest roentgenogram. A review of 800 patients revealed positive roentgenologic changes in the lungs in only 25 per cent and pulmonary symptoms in only 16 per cent.[60]

PATHOGENESIS

Evidence that autoimmunity plays a role in the pathogenesis of scleroderma is considerably less than in most other collagen-vascular diseases. There may be a mild degree of hypergammaglobulinemia; positive serologic tests for syphilis have been reported in 5 per cent of 363 patients, and rheumatoid factor has been identified in the serum of 35 per cent of 265 patients. The prevalence of antinuclear factors ranges from 30 to 80 per cent in different series,[61] and the predominant pattern of fluorescence is speckled.

PATHOLOGIC CHARACTERISTICS

In the early stages of the disease the pathologic changes consist of edema and lymphocytic infiltration of the connective tissues of the body, including muscle and skin. Subsequently this reaction is replaced by a proliferation of fibrous tissue with an increase in the number of collagen fibrils and consequent induration; atrophy occurs as a final stage. In the lungs the process is one of diffuse interstitial fibrosis. Pulmonary vascular lesions are common and, in fact, can predominate to the extent that patients may present with cor pulmonale without roentgenologic or pathologic evidence of interstitial fibrosis.

The late stages of the disease are characterized by gross distortion of lung architecture. The parenchyma is replaced by multiple microcysts separated by irregularly thickened walls of mature collagen and much proliferated muscle, giving rise to a striking morphologic "honeycomb" appearance. The cysts may be lined with cuboidal and columnar epithelium whose tendency to mucous secretion results in the retention of considerable amounts of mucoid material within the microcysts. The vessels may show a severe degree of medial thickening and intimal proliferation. The histologic characteristics are indistinguishable from those of chronic idiopathic interstitial fibrosis, and knowledge of the morphologic changes in other organs is required for differentiation. Morphologic evidence of lung involvement is common; in fact, extensive changes have been found pathologically in patients who have shown no clinical or roentgenologic manifestations.

ROENTGENOGRAPHIC MANIFESTATIONS

Roentgenographic abnormalities may be observed in the lungs, gastrointestinal tract, musculoskeletal system, and teeth, and usually the combination of findings is diagnostic.

The Lungs

The roentgenographic pattern is one of diffuse interstitial disease manifested at different stages of the disease by variations of the reticular or reticulonodular pattern. There is a tendency for predominant involvement of the lower lung zones. In the early stages the pattern is typically a fine reticulation (Figure 7–5); as the disease progresses the reticulation tends to be-

come coarser. Serial roentgenograms over a period of 2 to 3 years may show progressive and uniform loss of lung volume; we have been impressed repeatedly by the tendency for both pulmonary scleroderma and idiopathic interstitial pulmonary fibrosis to show this progressive loss of volume, in contrast to other causes of diffuse interstitial fibrosis. Small cysts up to 1 cm in diameter may be identified in the lung periphery, particularly in the bases. In contrast to other collagen diseases, pleural involvement is uncommon.

Abnormalities of the lungs may not be caused entirely by the primary disease; the disturbance of esophageal motility may result in the retention of food and lead to aspiration pneumonia.

The Gastrointestinal Tract

The most characteristic finding is esophageal dilatation and aperistalsis; the esophagus is reported to be involved clinically and roentgenologically in over 50 per cent of cases. Although the majority of patients who have roentgenographic evidence of esophageal involvement complain of dysphagia, this association is not invariable. Whereas the presence or absence of esophageal aperistalsis must be assessed by fluoroscopic study and barium swallow (preferably in the horizontal position), the atrophy and atony of the esophagus that result in aperistalsis also lead to dilatation, which may be manifested

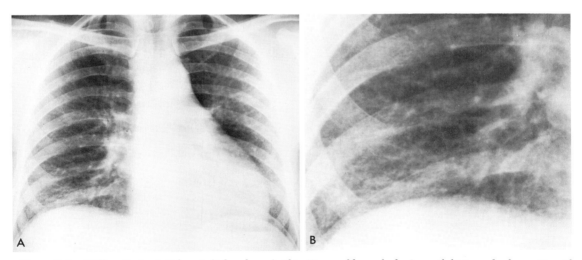

Figure 7–5. Diffuse Systemic Sclerosis (Scleroderma). This 42-year-old man had a 3-month history of polyneuritis with transient episodes of weakness in both legs. A posteroanterior roentgenogram (A) and magnified view of the right lower lung (B) reveal a fine reticular pattern more or less uniformly distributed throughout both lungs although slightly more prominent in the bases; there is no hilar lymph node enlargement or pleural effusion. Examination with barium showed esophageal aperistalsis associated with a small hiatus hernia and free gastroesophageal reflux; the small bowel showed evidence of dilatation, segmentation, and dysperistalsis. Physical examination revealed typical changes of scleroderma in the skin. Although by itself the roentgenographic pattern in the lungs is not in any way diagnostic, its association with the GI manifestations and cutaneous changes is pathognomonic of scleroderma.

on plain roentgenograms as an "air esophagogram." Although an air-containing esophagus may be seen in other diseases, such as mediastinitis and achalasia, the association of this finding with the lung changes described previously is virtually pathognomonic of diffuse systemic sclerosis.

Hiatus hernia is a frequent complication of the esophageal fibrosis and atrophy, and the resulting gastroesophageal reflux may give rise to esophagitis. Other changes in the gastrointestinal tract include irregular dilatation and disturbed motility of the small and large bowel.[62]

The Musculoskeletal System

The roentgenographically apparent changes are chiefly those associated with Raynaud's phenomenon, which is a component of the syndrome in many cases of diffuse systemic sclerosis. In advanced cases absorption of the distal phalanges of the fingers, particularly when associated with calcinosis of the terminal pulp, is frequent and is highly suggestive of the diagnosis. Calcinosis, which usually is seen only in the presence of cutaneous sclerosis, occurs in other sites also, particularly over pressure areas such as the elbows and ischial tuberositis. Arthritis of the interphalangeal joints of the hands is not uncommon, and in approximately 25 per cent of cases the roentgenographic and clinical picture is indistinguishable from that of rheumatoid arthritis.[58]

The Teeth

Uniform widening of the periodontal space is reported to occur in 7 per cent of cases;[60] this is a useful but not diagnostic sign, which is seen also in other conditions (*e.g.*, Paget's disease).

CLINICAL MANIFESTATIONS

In addition to the symptoms and signs referable to the skin and GI tract and to Raynaud's phenonenon, patients may manifest weight loss and low-grade fever. Pulmonary involvement may cause a slightly productive cough and progressive dyspnea; it is usually a late feature of widespread systemic disease and may be present without demonstrable abnormality on the chest roentgenogram. Basilar rales occur in approximately 50 per cent of cases.

Cardiac decompensation may develop as a result of cor pulmonale, sclerosis of the cardiac muscle, or a combination of the two. The most common electrocardiographic finding is right-sided heart strain; a prolonged P–R interval or a left or right bundle branch block may indicate myocardial fibrosis.[60]

Raynaud's phenomenon occurs in the majority of cases of diffuse systemic sclerosis, *e.g.*, in 22 of 27 patients in one series.[60] In fact, it may precede skin changes and may antedate or occur simultaneously with clinical or function test evidence of pulmonary parenchymal involvement.

The patient with advanced scleroderma presents a characteristically distressing picture that is dominated by the skin changes, with a thickened inelastic and waxy appearance most prominent about the face and extremities. The skin is frequently bronzed and sometimes contains calcium deposits.[58]

Esophageal involvement can be suspected if the patient complains of difficulty in swallowing, but esophageal dilatation and disturbed motility can be detected in some patients by manometry and fluoroscopic examination before dysphagia becomes clinically manifest.

Arthralgia, particularly of the hands, is common, rheumatic complaints appearing in 50 to 80 per cent of patients at some stage in the course of the disease. Clinical evidence of renal involvement has been reported in approximately 25 per cent,[60] although at necropsy the kidneys are found to be diseased in the great majority of cases. Impotence has been reported and is possibly related to vascular or autonomic nervous system alterations.[63] Hypothyroidism and thyroid gland fibrosis have been observed more frequently in patients with progressive systemic sclerosis than in age- and sex-matched controls.[64]

Pulmonary Function Tests

Pulmonary function is almost invariably disturbed, even when the chest roentgenogram is normal. Functional aberrations consist of a restrictive insufficiency with decreased vital capacity and residual volume, the latter diminishing progressively with increasing fibrosis. Except in heavy cigarette smokers, flow rates are usually reduced only in proportion to the reduction in vital capacity; both diffusing capacity and lung compliance are almost invariably decreased.[60] Hypoxia is common with exercise and sometimes at rest.

Relationship to Other Diseases

There is considerable overlap with other collagen diseases in a minority of these patients.[60]

There seems little doubt that scleroderma is associated with an increased incidence of lung cancer and with both coal-miner's pneumoconiosis and silicosis.

The "CREST" Syndrome

This syndrome, whose characteristics were detailed by Winterbauer in 1964,[65] comprises a group of five abnormalities for which the word "CREST" constitutes an acronym—calcinosis of the skin, Raynaud's phenomenon, esophageal dysfunction, sclerodactyly, and telangiectasia. Although it was originally considered to be a benign variant of diffuse systemic sclerosis, more recent studies have indicated that the combination of findings represents a distinct serologic entity with anti-centromere antibodies.[66] Its benign nature also is open to question, since pulmonary vascular obliteration can eventually lead to lethal pulmonary hypertension.[67]

The telangiectatic lesions are identical in appearance and distribution to those of hereditary telangiectasia but are said to appear later and to cause hemorrhage less frequently. When pulmonary lesions occur, they are identical to those of diffuse systemic sclerosis.

In a study that compared the varied manifestations in 13 patients with the CREST syndrome with those of 26 patients with progressive systemic sclerosis,[68] no significant differences were found in the age of onset of Raynaud's phenomenon, ulcerations of the fingers, sclerodactyly, or in the frequency of abnormal esophageal peristalsis or dysphagia. However, the CREST patients had a significantly lower frequency of arthralgia (54 per cent) and arthritis (15 per cent) than did those with scleroderma (88 per cent and 65 per cent, respectively).

Syndrome of Pulmonary Hypertension and Raynaud's Phenomenon

This combination, several cases of which have been reported,[69] is found most commonly in middle-aged women. Although the vascular changes are considered by some to represent peripheral pulmonary arterial vasospasm—and, hence, primary pulmonary hypertension[69]— their association with other abnormalities, such as arthritis, arteritis, and abnormal serum globulins has led some observers to believe that the syndrome may be part of a general "collagen" disease. Changes apparent on the plain roentgenogram are those of primary pulmonary hypertension, with severe diminution in the peripheral vasculature of the lungs, enlargement of central pulmonary arteries, and little or no overinflation; other signs of pulmonary disease are absent.

DERMATOMYOSITIS AND POLYMYOSITIS

These terms include a group of disorders generally considered autoimmune in nature. They are characterized by weakness and sometimes pain in the proximal limb muscles and occasionally in the muscles of the neck; in about half the reported cases they are associated with a characteristic violaceous skin rash and in a minority of cases with neoplastic disease. Although the clinical picture differs considerably from case to case, the common denominator is muscular weakness which, when it affects the thorax, may be associated with atelectasis, pneumonia, aspiration pneumonitis due to pharyngeal muscle paresis, and attendant respiratory failure.

The disease is worldwide in distribution and occurs twice as often in females as in males; it shows two peak age incidences, the first during the first decade and the second in the fifth and sixth decades.[70, 71]

Most studies suggest an abnormality of cell-mediated immunity. Tests for antiglobulin and antinuclear and anti–DNA antibodies are negative except in patients who have symptoms and signs of an associated collagen-vascular disorder.[70] Human muscle homogenates have been shown to cause blastogenesis when incubated with lymphocytes of patients with polymyositis, but not with those of controls. Peripheral lymphocytes of patients with active polymyositis have been found to be cytotoxic to human fetal muscle cultures and to produce lymphotoxin when incubated with autologous muscle.

Histologic examination of muscle biopsy in patients with polymyositis reveals necrosis of type I and type II fibers. Pathologic changes in the lung consist of widespread fibrosis with thickening of the alveolar walls and infiltration by lymphocytes and plasma cells. It has been suggested that the response to glucocorticoid therapy is influenced by both the cellularity of the interstitial infiltration and the degree of fibrosis of alveolar septae.[73] In contrast to what is seen in adults, childhood polymyositis and dermatomyositis are associated with vasculitis.[70, 72]

The discovery of a malignancy at necropsy is rare, and it is very likely that the association of these diseases with cancer has been overemphasized because of a tendency to publish such cases and because of some clinical confusion with the myopathies.[70]

In our experience the chest roentgenogram may show one of several patterns, depending upon the nature of the collagen-vascular disease and the muscle groups that are paralyzed. Many patients have normal chest roentgenograms. In others, a diffuse reticular or reticulonodular pattern is seen, involving predominantly the lung bases; histologic examination of biopsy material reveals infiltration by lymphocytes and plasma cells and, in some, considerable fibrosis.[72]

When polymyositis involves the muscles of respiration, particularly the diaphragm, diaphragmatic elevation and small volume lungs are apparent, often in conjunction with basal linear opacities, suggesting "plate atelectasis." When pharyngeal muscle paralysis is present, unilateral or bilateral segmental atelectasis or pneumonia may result from aspiration of food and oral secretions.

Patients present with symmetric weakness of the proximal limb muscles which progresses rapidly over a period of weeks or months rather than years, as is characteristic of the muscular "dystrophies." In some patients muscle destruction is extremely rapid and is associated with diffuse, profound weakness, pain, tenderness, and swelling of muscle groups.[70] In patients whose disease tends to be more chronic, muscle weakness is often ascribed to a catabolic protein losing condition or to concomitant steroid therapy.[72] Symptoms and signs of associated connective-tissue disorders range from Raynaud's phenomenon to full-blown examples of the various accepted clinical entities. Manifestations of visceral involvement in polymyositis and dermatomyositis include interstitial pneumonitis and fibrosis, hypomotility of the distal esophagus and small bowel, and cardiac arrhythmias and heart block.[70] Pulmonary interstitial disease sometimes causes dyspnea and this may be the major presenting symptom; more often, however, extensive disease is unassociated with symptoms and is discovered on a screening chest roentgenogram. In fact, only a minority of patients manifest symptoms and signs referable to the respiratory system; Rose and Walton[71] found respiratory muscle weakness severe enough to cause respiratory embarrassment in only six of their 89 patients with polymyositis.

The clinical picture of advanced polymyositis may be indistinguishable from that of late onset muscular dystrophy, in which case electromyography and measurement of serum creatine phosphokinase may be of differential value.

Patients with pharyngeal paralysis may present a pathetic picture of drooling, dyspnea, ineffective cough, and an inability to lie flat. Respiratory muscle paralysis may result in extreme dyspnea and cyanosis; cough is usually ineffective. Fever resulting from associated pneumonia is present in many cases.

The incidence of coexistent carcinoma probably is not nearly as great as is often assumed, being 6 per cent in one series[74] and 16 per cent in another.[70] Carcinomas of a wide variety of sites have been found associated with polymyositis, including the stomach, prostate, pancreas, and ovary. It is important that this association be distinguished from the myasthenia-like syndrome and myopathy that occur in conjunction with bronchogenic carcinoma.

Measurement of serum enzyme levels, particularly creatine phosphokinase and aldolase and, to a lesser extent, SGOT, SGPT, and LDH, is more useful in establishing the diagnosis than in assessing the results of therapy, but values may be within normal limits even in patients with active myositis and muscle atrophy resulting from severe long-standing disease. Muscle biopsy results are reported to be normal in 10 to 50 per cent of cases.[75]

Pulmonary function tests show no abnormality in most patients; in those in whom diffuse interstitial fibrosis has developed, findings are identical to those of scleroderma. When the respiratory muscles are paralyzed, the vital capacity is decreased, flow rates are reduced, and hypoxemia develops, with or without a rise in P_{CO_2}.

SJÖGREN'S SYNDROME

In 1933, Sjögren[76] described a triad consisting of keratoconjunctivitis sicca, xerostomia, and recurrent swelling of the parotid gland. More recently it has been established that Sjögren's syndrome is frequently associated with other collagen-vascular diseases and that the "sicca syndrome"—dryness of the mucous membranes, particularly of the mouth (xerostomia), eyes (xerophthalmia), and nose (xerorhinia)—represents less than half the cases of Sjögren's syndrome, the remainder being patients with other collagen-vascular diseases that manifest sicca components,[77] usually rheumatoid arthritis. It appears that the sicca features are present to some extent in virtually every case of collagen-vascular disease. Sjögren's syndrome shows a remarkable female sex predominance (90 per cent).[78, 79] The mean age in one series of 171 patients was 57.2 years.

Evidence for autoimmunity in Sjögren's syndrome is equally as strong as in SLE. Genetic factors have also been implicated in the pathogenesis, as evidenced by the occurrence of the disease in families; the hereditary factor appears to be expressed as a depression in immune surveillance, which permits increased antibody responses and the development of lymphoproliferative malignancies. Hypergammaglobulinemia, usually polyclonal in type, is common and may result in serum hyperviscosity with all its complications. Rheumatoid factor and antinuclear antibodies or both are present in 70 to 100 per cent of patients; specific autoantibodies for Sjögren's syndrome have been described.[80] Widespread disease has been linked to decreased clearance of immune complexes by a defective reticuloendothelial system.[81] Levels of serum immunoglobulins of all types, particularly IgG and IgM, are increased; lymphocytes infiltrating the salivary glands actively synthesize IgG and IgM, including rheumatoid factor.[78] The association of Sjögren's syndrome with a broad spectrum of lymphoproliferative disorders ranging from benign disease, through nonmalignant extraglandular lymphoproliferation (pseudolymphoma), to frankly malignant disease (presenting as macroglobulinemia or the lymphomas) suggests cellular immunologic imbalance.

Pathologically, lymphoid infiltrates, sometimes associated with atrophy, are present in the lacrimal glands, the mucus-secreting glands of the conjunctivae, nasal cavity, pharynx, larynx, trachea, and bronchi, and occasionally in the sweat glands and vagina.[79] Alveolar walls may be infiltrated by mononuclear cells and may show an increase in fibrous tissue; the pathologic changes in the lungs have been said to bear a strong resemblance to those in Hashimoto's thyroiditis. Biopsy of the nasal mucous membrane and of the minor salivary glands of the lower lip has proved useful in elucidating the pathology of Sjögren's syndrome and, when performed serially, in reflecting response to therapy. Pseudolymphoma, histiocytic or lymphocytic lymphoma, or Waldenström's macroglobulinemia may develop in a small number of patients, usually those with severe and long-standing sicca syndrome.

In one study of 58 patients with Sjögren's syndrome,[79] roentgenograms of the chest were available for 42, and of these, 14 (33 per cent) showed a reticulonodular pattern similar to that of other collagen diseases characterized by vasculitis (Figure 7–6). Pneumonitis and atelectasis are two complications commonly seen in patients with Sjögren's syndrome and are manifested roentgenographically as patchy parenchymal consolidation.[79] Joint changes are roentgenographically similar to those in rheumatoid or psoriatic arthritis.

The chief symptoms of Sjögren's syndrome are grittiness or burning sensation of the eyes, dryness of the mouth, nose, and skin, and sometimes dyspareunia.[82] Involvement of the nasal and nasopharyngeal mucous membrane may lead to obstruction of the eustachian tubes, with resultant persisting otitis media and deafness.[82] Involvement of the larynx and tracheobronchial mucous glands may result in hoarseness and a persistent cough productive of thick,

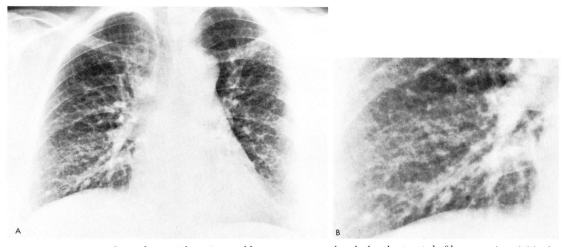

A

B

Figure 7–6. Sjögren's Syndrome. This 45-year-old woman presented with the classic triad of keratoconjunctivitis sicca, xerostomia, and recurrent swelling of the parotid glands. Her roentgenogram (A) reveals a diffuse, coarse reticular pattern throughout both lungs, seen to better advantage in the magnified view of the right lower zone (B). Note also the enlargement of the left lobe of the thyroid.

tenacious sputum. Interstitial cellular infiltration and fibrosis of the lungs may be associated with dyspnea. Renal tubular acidosis is found in some patients and has been ascribed to hyperglobulinemia; however, characteristic histologic changes of Sjögren's syndrome may be present in the kidney in the absence of hyperglobulinemia. Approximately one-half to two-thirds of patients with Sjögren's syndrome will manifest symptoms and signs of an associated collagen-vascular disease.[77, 79]

Xerostomia and keratoconjunctivitis are usually not associated with enlargement of salivary and lacrimal glands. Physical signs of pulmonary involvement include those of complicating pneumonia, and in some patients with diffuse interstitial disease crepitations may be heard at the lung bases. Purpura hyperglobulinemia is a rare manifestation of Sjögren's syndrome.[77, 78]

Although the diagnosis of Sjögren's syndrome is usually based on characteristic clinical manifestations, it may be substantiated by tests of glandular secretory function and by the detection of various serum antibodies.[80] The former include Shirmer's test for the measurement of tear formation and by scintillation scanning or radionuclide excretion studies for assessment of salivary gland function; their structure can be evaluated by parotid sialography and by lip biopsy for histologic examination of the morphology of the minor salivary glands.

Patients with Sjögren's syndrome who de-

velop one of the lymphomas generally manifest a severe sicca syndrome and an increased incidence of lymph node enlargement, splenomegaly, leukopenia, vasculitis, neuropathy, Raynaud's phenomenon, and purpura hyperglobulinemia; gammopathy may be of the monoclonal rather than the more common polyclonal type and is usually of the IgM variety.[82]

EOSINOPHILIC LUNG DISEASE

Pulmonary disease affecting the major airways or parenchyma (or both) associated with blood or tissue eosinophilia (or both) comprises a group of conditions so diverse as to render logical classification exceedingly difficult. Efforts to understand these diseases and their interrelationships have been hampered by two major influences. (1) Since the common denominator is the presence of excess eosinophils in tissue or blood or both, and since a wide variety of influences can lead to such excess, the pathogenesis of the individual entities is of necessity diverse: extrinsic influences (certain drugs, fungi, and parasites), intrinsic influences (various hypersensitivity or autoimmune states), and finally a group of disorders in which the influences are unknown (Loeffler's syndrome, chronic eosinophilic pneumonia). (2) The use of terms such as "pulmonary infiltration with eosinophilia" (the PIE syndromes) has led to con-

TABLE 7–3. EOSINOPHILIC LUNG DISEASE

MAIN CLASSIFICATION	SUBCLASSIFICATION	DISEASE
(A). *Idiopathic eosinophilic lung disease*	Transient (benign) pulmonary eosinophilia	Loeffler's syndrome
	Prolonged pulmonary eosinophilia	Chronic eosinophilic pneumonia
		Hypereosinophilic syndrome
(B). *Eosinophilic lung disease of specific etiology*	Drug-induced	Nitrofurantoin
	Parasite-induced	Ascariasis Strongyloidiasis Ancylostomiasis Tropical pulmonary eosinophilia Pulmonary larva migrans Schistosomiasis
	Fungus-induced	Hypersensitivity bronchopulmonary aspergillosis Bronchocentric granulomatosis
(C). *Eosinophilic lung disease associated with angiitis and/or granulomatosis*	Collagen-vascular disease	Wegener's granulomatosis Limited form Lymphomatoid variant Allergic granulomatosis Polyarteritis nodosa Necrotizing "sarcoidal" angiitis and granulomatosis

fusion because it denotes excess eosinophils in the peripheral blood, a finding which is by no means always the case in this group of diseases.

The eosinophilic lung diseases vary widely in severity. The more benign conditions are exemplified by Loeffler's syndrome, the intermediate by eosinophilic pneumonia, and the more malignant by hypersensitivity angiitis or polyarteritis nodosa. Pathologic changes in the lungs range from local tissue edema and eosinophilia to granuloma formation and vasculitis with thrombosis and infarction.

The classification we have employed (Table 7–3) is a modification and extension of the one formulated by Citro and associates,[83] and includes three general groups of conditions whose etiologic, clinical, roentgenologic, and pathologic features differ. It is emphasized that this section does not include all pulmonary diseases associated with eosinophilia but only those in which the pathogenesis appears to be predominantly allergic or immunogenic.

IDIOPATHIC EOSINOPHILIC LUNG DISEASE

LOEFFLER'S SYNDROME

Loeffler's syndrome may be defined as a state in which local nonsegmental areas of parenchymal consolidation, usually transient, are associated with blood eosinophilia. Although the diagnosis can be made only on the basis of positive roentgenologic findings, it should be suspected whenever blood eosinophilia develops in a patient with a background of atopy. The syndrome may occur without any exciting extrinsic factor or may have its onset in relation to infections, infestations with parasites, or drug therapy,[84] in which circumstances we prefer to use the more precise etiologic designations listed in Table 7–3 (*e.g.*, drug-induced eosinophilic lung disease). In a group of 5702 patients with bronchial asthma, Ford[85] found 20 cases of Loeffler's syndrome, one-third of them with no obvious extrinsic cause. When caused by an identifiable extrinsic agent, the disease usually is acute and transitory and responds readily to removal of the offending organism or drug. When no obvious cause is detectable, the pulmonary consolidation and eosinophilia tend to be more prolonged and persistent.

Because of its benign and transient nature, the pathology of the parenchymal consolidation has been only rarely documented; in the few cases in which biopsy was reported, interstitial and alveolar edema contained a large number of eosinophilic leukocytes.[85]

The pattern of roentgenologic changes is diagnostic when serial roentgenograms reveal the transitory and migratory character of the parenchymal consolidations. Areas of consolidation may be single or multiple; they are characteristically homogeneous in density, ill-defined, and nonsegmental in distribution in the lung periphery (Figure 7–7). Peirce and his colleagues[86] were the first to point out the characteristic peripheral location of the consolidation; they described a peculiar unilateral or bilateral consolidative process running more or less parallel to the lateral chest wall which they regarded as highly suggestive of Loeffler's syndrome. The transient and shifting nature of the consolidation is a characteristic feature. Reduction in the size of one area of parenchymal consolidation over a 24-hour period, if associated with a new area of consolidation elsewhere, should be highly suggestive.

To our knowledge cavitation has not been described, nor have associated pleural effusion, lymph node enlargement, or cardiomegaly (although pericardial effusion has been reported in some cases).

Of importance in roentgenologic differential diagnosis are the various entities in which a specific etiologic agent can be implicated. It is also important to differentiate the more chronic and serious form of eosinophilic lung disease, chronic eosinophilic pneumonia,[87] whose roentgenographic manifestations are very similar although more protracted. It is probable that cases of mucoid impaction (with or without hypersensitivity bronchopulmonary aspergillosis) also have been misdiagnosed as Loeffler's syndrome.[84] However, the distinction is apparent in the majority of these cases by the strictly segmental distribution of mucoid impaction compared with the nonsegmental and peripheral nature of involvement in Loeffler's syndrome.

In some cases the syndrome is unassociated with symptoms, and its presence may be detected only when the patient is referred for roentgenographic examination in the investigation of bronchial asthma. Conversely, symptoms may be severe, with high fever and dyspnea requiring immediate corticosteroid therapy for relief.

Leukocytosis is common, to a total white cell count of more than 20,000 per cu mm. An increase in eosinophils is responsible for most of this elevation. When pulmonary parenchymal involvement is extensive, even in an asthmatic patient,[85] results of function tests usually indi-

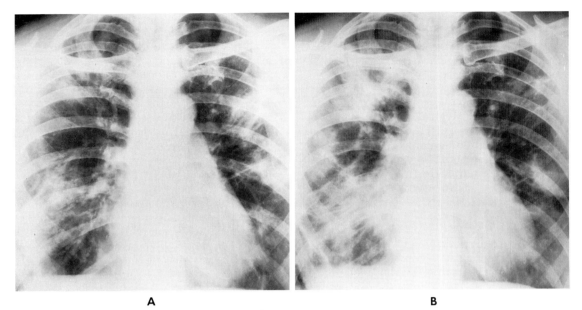

A   **B**

Figure 7–7. Loeffler's Syndrome. This 61-year-old woman was admitted to the hospital for the first time with a 2-month history of anorexia, a 10-pound weight loss, afternoon fever, and mild cough productive of greenish phlegm occasionally flecked with blood; there was no history of allergies. On admission, a posteroanterior (A) roentgenogram revealed numerous shadows of homogeneous density in both lungs, occupying no precise segmental distribution; note particularly the broad shadow of increased density along the lower axillary zone of the right lung. At this time her total white cell count was 11,000 per cu mm with 1,700 (15 per cent) eosinophils. One week later (B), the anatomic distribution of the shadows had changed considerably, being more extensive in the right upper and lower lobes and less extensive in the left upper lobe; at this time the total white cell count was 14,000 per cu mm with 20 per cent eosinophils. The institution of ACTH therapy resulted in prompt remission of symptoms and roentgenographic abnormalities.

cate restrictive insufficiency, with arterial oxygen unsaturation and a decrease in diffusing capacity.

CHRONIC EOSINOPHILIC PNEUMONIA

This term was originally coined by Christoforidis and Molnar[88] in 1960. Although the condition appears to have a predilection for women and has a more protracted clinical and roentgenologic course than Loeffler's syndrome, it possesses so many similarities to that condition that it could justifiably be regarded as a variant of Loeffler's syndrome. In our experience and that of others[87] there appears to be an unusual association with therapeutic desensitization to a variety of allergens. In one report of eight patients, an association with penicillin allergy was noted in four.[89]

The pathologic characteristics have been established chiefly from biopsy material, since fatalities are rare. The predominant finding is one of massive infiltration of alveolar walls and sacs by mature eosinophils, macrophages, histiocytes, lymphocytes, and polymorphonuclear granulocytes. In some cases a mild angiitis, affecting chiefly small venules, and granuloma formation with or without necrosis and cavitation, have been observed.[87]

Roentgenologically, the pattern is identical to that of Loeffler's syndrome, consisting of nonsegmental homogeneous consolidation in the lung periphery (Figure 7–7). This has led some observers to apply the designation "reversed pulmonary edema pattern" because of its confinement to the lung periphery in contrast to the perihilar or central distribution of pulmonary edema.[87] Cavitation has been described.[89] Compared with the transitory and migratory character of the consolidations in Loeffler's syndrome, the lesions of chronic eosinophilic pneumonia tend to persist unchanged for many days or even weeks unless corticosteroid therapy is instituted.

Clinically, chronic eosinophilic pneumonia is associated with high fever, malaise, weight loss, dyspnea, and hypoxia.[87] Response to corticosteroid therapy is characteristically dramatic, with roentgenographic resolution and clinical improvement occurring within three to seven days.[87] Follow-up studies have indicated that corticosteroid therapy may have to be continued for months or years; even then, symptoms and roentgenographic abnormalities may recur on cessation of treatment.[89]

Laboratory investigation reveals blood eosinophilia in most patients. In some cases pulmonary function tests have been reported to show restrictive malfunction and lowered diffusing capacity.

HYPEREOSINOPHILIC SYNDROME

This rare condition (*synonyms*: eosinophilic leukemia, disseminated eosinophilic collagen disease, and Loeffler's fibroblastic endocarditis) is characterized by infiltration of a number of organs by mature eosinophils and an increase in collagen connective tissue, particularly in the myocardium. It occurs almost exclusively in males.[90] The pulmonary parenchyma may be strikingly infiltrated with eosinophils; pulmonary hypertension has been reported.[90] It has been stated that both clinical symptoms and roentgenographic abnormalities are caused more often by cardiac decompensation than by eosinophilic infiltration of lung parenchyma.[91]

EOSINOPHILIC LUNG DISEASE OF SPECIFIC ETIOLOGY

DRUG-INDUCED EOSINOPHILIC LUNG DISEASE

Two quite different patterns of pulmonary disease occur in response to drug therapy: a Loeffler-like pattern caused by a variety of drugs, and a diffuse reticular pattern caused specifically by nitrofurantoin. Drugs that cause the transient nonsegmental peripheral consolidation characteristic of Loeffler's syndrome include penicillin; the sulfonamides, administered either orally or as a vaginal cream; mecamylamine; mephenesin; aminosalicylic acid; para-aminosalicylic acid; the tricyclic antidepressants (imipramine and trimipramine); hydrochlorothiazide; and even cromolyn sodium, a drug used in the treatment of asthma.

NITROFURANTOIN-INDUCED EOSINOPHILIC LUNG DISEASE

Nitrofurantoin (Furadantin) therapy can give rise to pulmonary changes whose pathogenesis is probably similar to that of Loeffler's syndrome but whose roentgenographic manifestations are entirely different.[92] The chest roentgenogram characteristically reveals a diffuse reticular pattern with some basal predominance.[92] When considered along with the rapidity with which the roentgenographic changes clear following drug withdrawal, it is possible that interstitial edema caused by increased microvascular permeability may play a considerable role in the production of the roentgenographic opacities. Pleural effusion may be present.

The commonest clinical presentation is acute and consists of dry cough, chills, fever, and moderate or severe dyspnea beginning a few hours to 3 or 4 days after the institution of therapy. Less commonly the disease is chronic and its onset insidious,[93, 94] pulmonary symptoms persisting for weeks to years and the interval between the initial dose of the drug and the onset of pulmonary symptoms ranging from 6 months to 6 years.[93] In patients with the acute presentation, eosinophilia of considerable degree is usually present in the peripheral blood; although the roentgenographic patterns of the acute and chronic forms of the disease are identical, the latter may not be associated with peripheral eosinophilia.[93] Lung biopsies on patients with the chronic form of the disease have been reported to show changes indistinguishable from desquamative interstitial pneumonia[94] or idiopathic interstitial pulmonary fibrosis.[93] Physical examination may reveal crepitations at the lung bases, suggesting pulmonary edema.[94]

In both forms of the disease, the pulmonary function pattern is restrictive. In the acute variety, withdrawal of the drug results in prompt clinical, roentgenographic, and functional clearing; in the chronic type, some functional improvement occurs despite persistence of roentgenographic evidence of diffuse interstitial disease.[93, 94]

PARASITE-INDUCED EOSINOPHILIC LUNG DISEASE

Parasitic infestation represents a common cause of Loeffler's syndrome in developing countries but is uncommon in the western hemisphere. All these infestations are metazoan and by far the majority result from roundworms (nemathelminths). These diseases have been described in detail in Chapter 6; they include ascariasis (page 343), strongyloidiasis (page 343), ancylostomiasis (page 344), tropical pulmonary eosinophilia (page 344), pulmonary larva migrans (page 345), and schistosomiasis (page 348). Parasite-induced eosinophilic lung disease is the result of migration of larvae through the lungs and characteristically is associated with marked leukocytosis and eosinophilia. With one exception, symptoms may be minimal, often being

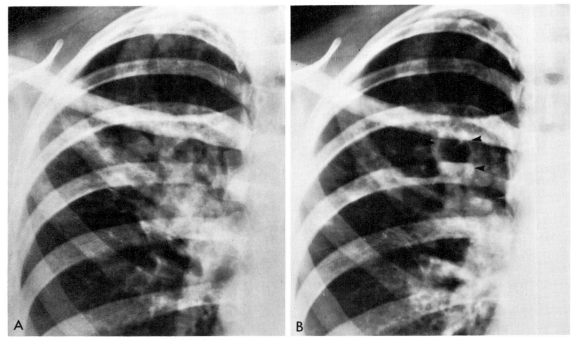

Figure 7–8. Mucoid Impaction (Hypersensitivity Bronchopulmonary Aspergillosis). A view of the upper half of the right hemithorax from a posteroanterior roentgenogram *(A)* demonstrates multiple fingerlike opacities extending upward and outward from the right hilum and occupying the central and mid zones of the right upper lobe; distribution is consistent with subdivisions of the bronchial tree. The peripheral lung shows no evidence of collapse or obstructive pneumonitis despite the major degree of bronchial obstruction that must be present. This picture is highly suggestive of mucoid impaction. One month later *(B)*, the opacities have largely disappeared, leaving in their wake markedly dilated proximal bronchi (one of these is indicated by *arrowheads*). Note that this bronchiectasis is central rather than peripheral. This is the same patient shown in Figure 7–10 (page 387) several years earlier.

limited to an urticarial skin rash, with or without mild bronchospasm; the chest roentgenogram reveals transitory patchy areas of nonsegmental consolidation. The exception is tropical pulmonary eosinophilia, which is a more chronic process associated with asthmatic symptoms and a diffuse reticulondular pattern roentgenographically.

FUNGUS-INDUCED EOSINOPHILIC LUNG DISEASE

The majority of fungus-induced hypersensitivity diseases of the lung are caused by *Aspergillus fumigatus*. There are two forms of the disease, hypersensitivity bronchopulmonary aspergillosis and bronchocentric granulomatosis, both of which have been described in detail elsewhere in the book (*see* pages 386 and 388, respectively). Hypersensitivity bronchopulmonary aspergillosis is characterized by the presence in segmental bronchi of mucous plugs containing aspergilli and eosinophils. The roentgenographic pattern is identical to that of mucoid impaction: homogeneous fingerlike opaci-

ties of unit density are situated in a precise bronchial distribution, almost always in central segmental bronchi (Figure 7–8). Most patients give a history of long-standing bronchial asthma. Bronchocentric granulomatosis is closely related to bronchopulmonary aspergillosis but affects asthmatics and nonasthmatics with approximately equal frequency. In contrast to bronchopulmonary aspergillosis, the disease affects small bronchi and bronchioles rather than larger segmental bronchi. Roentgenographic manifestations include linear patterns and opacities attributable to the abnormal airways.

EOSINOPHILIC LUNG DISEASE ASSOCIATED WITH ANGIITIS OR GRANULOMATOSIS

WEGENER'S GRANULOMATOSIS

GENERAL CHARACTERISTICS

Both Wegener's and "allergic" granulomatosis usually are included within the group characterized by transient pulmonary shadows with eosinophilia, although in fact the former seldom gives rise to either blood eosinophilia or any significant degree of tissue eosinophilia. In its typical form, Wegener's granulomatosis is manifested by a triad of upper respiratory tract lesions, pulmonary disease, and glomerulonephritis; however, Carrington and Liebow[95] reported 16 cases in which the typical pulmonary changes were present without evidence of lesions in the other two systems. The disease affects males and females equally, usually in the fourth or fifth decade. Unlike the allergic variety (see further on), Wegener's granulomatosis usually is not associated with a background of atopy.

PATHOGENESIS

Although Wegener's granulomatosis is a disease of undetermined etiology, both immunologic and pathologic manifestations suggest a fulminant hypersensitivity or autoallergic process, a concept supported by the dramatic therapeutic response to cytotoxic drugs in many cases. Immunoglobulin and complement deposits of the coarse granular type have been described in some cases.[96] Levels of serum complement are normal or elevated in contrast to the hypocomplementemia characteristic of SLE.[96] Serum IgA levels are increased[96, 97] and rheumatoid factor[96] and smooth muscle autoantibodies[97] have been demonstrated. Although cell-mediated immunity may be depressed in advanced or therapeutically immunosuppressed cases,[97] delayed hypersensitivity skin reactions are positive if patients are tested prior to therapy.[96]

PATHOLOGIC CHARACTERISTICS

The lesions may involve many organs of the body, including the central nervous system, skin, joints, and spleen, as well as the structures affected in the typical clinical triad. In the *upper respiratory tract*, thickening of the mucous membrane of the paranasal sinuses occurs in the early stages and may progress to destruction of bone and cartilage; the middle ear and orbital cavity may be involved. In the *lungs*, involvement is characterized by granulomas situated in relationship to the bronchi but usually independent of vascular lesions.[98] In almost every case, vasculitis is present within or adjacent to the nodular granulomas or at some distance from them. Small pulmonary arteries and veins are infiltrated with plasma cells, a few eosino-

phils and lymphocytes, and infrequent polymorphonuclear leukocytes. Microscopic examination of the granulomas reveals epithelioid cells[98] surrounded by plasma cells, lymphocytes, scattered eosinophils, and occasional multinucleated giant cells of either the foreign body or Langhans' type.[99] Central necrosis is present in many of the granulomas.[98] In the *kidneys*, the characteristic change is a glomerulitis, consisting of necrosis and thrombosis of the capillary tufts, and eosinophilic fibrinoid degeneration similar to the focal glomerulitis associated with subacute bacterial endocarditis and polyarteritis nodosa.[99]

Although Wegener's granulomatosis and polyarteritis nodosa undoubtedly are related within the group of collagen diseases, the incidence of pulmonary involvement is quite different: lung involvement probably is a *sine qua non* in the former but occurs relatively infrequently in the latter.[100]

ROENTGENOGRAPHIC MANIFESTATIONS

The typical roentgenographic pattern in the lungs in Wegener's granulomatosis is that of rounded opacities, usually sharply circumscribed, ranging from a few millimeters to 9 cm in diameter (Figure 7–9). They are commonly bilateral and widely distributed, with no predilection for any lung zone. The nodules are usually multiple but may be solitary. Cavitation occurs eventually in one-third to one-half of cases. The cavities are thick-walled and tend to have an irregular, rather shaggy inner lining; the thickness of the walls may diminish gradually until the cavities become thin-walled cystic spaces. Acute air-space pneumonia is fairly common and varies widely in extent, sometimes involving a whole lobe. Pleural effusion is uncommon but may be massive. Maguire and his colleagues[101] have drawn attention to the occurrence of endobronchial disease that can result in local airway narrowing and can even lead to atelectasis of a lobe or a whole lung.

Roentgenographic abnormalities may clear fairly rapidly with cytotoxic and immunosuppressive therapy, and the chest roentgenogram may remain clear while disease activity is suppressed.[102]

CLINICAL MANIFESTATIONS

Wegener's granulomatosis typically affects adults in their fifth decade, males slightly more commonly than females.[96] The onset of the

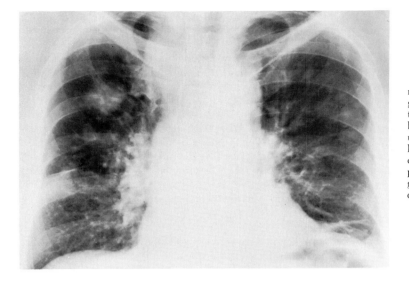

Figure 7–9. Wegener's Granulomatosis. A posteroanterior roentgenogram of a 63-year-old man reveals multiple well-defined nodules throughout both lungs, at least one of which has undergone cavitation. During the following 2 weeks, many of these nodules cavitated. Corticosteroid and azathioprine (Imuran) therapy resulted in gradual disappearance of these shadows over the subsequent months.

disease may be acute and its course fulminating, although more commonly the onset is insidious. The majority of patients present with complaints referable to the nose, paranasal sinuses, or chest. Thoracic symptoms consist of intractable cough, sometimes with hemoptysis and pleuritic pain;[96] rarely, hemoptysis may be massive. Renal manifestations occur in the majority of patients at some time in the course of the disease. Occasionally, skin ulceration, symptoms referable to the joints, eyes, or middle ear, or constitutional complaints such as fever, weakness, weight loss, anorexia, or malaise may cause the patient to seek medical advice. The incidence of organ system involvement in 18 patients in one series was as follows: respiratory tract (100 per cent), urinary tract (83 per cent), joints (56 per cent), skin and muscle (44 per cent), eyes or middle ear (39 per cent), heart or pericardium (28 per cent), and nervous system (22 per cent). Neurologic involvement is primarily due to vasculitis and may be central or peripheral, the latter manifested as mononeuritis multiplex or as polyneuritis.[96] Occasionally, necrotizing coronary vasculitis and pancarditis can result in sudden death.[96] Laboratory findings include anemia, thrombocytosis,[96] and leukocytosis, occasionally with eosinophilia.

Until fairly recently the clinical course was rapidly downhill, death occurring within six months from uremia or occasionally from respiratory failure. In recent years, therapy with cytotoxic drugs, either alkylating agents or purine antagonists, has not only resulted in clinical remission of the disease but has led to apparent cures, even in patients with renal involvement.[96, 102]

THE "LIMITED" FORM OF WEGENER'S GRANULOMATOSIS

In 1966, Carrington and Liebow[95] reported 16 cases of Wegener's granulomatosis in which the predominant manifestations were pulmonary, with little or no systemic involvement; 11 had no extrapulmonary manifestations. Prognosis in patients with the limited form of the disease is somewhat better than in patients with the classic triad of symptoms.

THE LYMPHOMATOID VARIANT OF WEGENER'S GRANULOMATOSIS

This condition, first described by Liebow and Carrington in 1969,[103] possesses histologic characteristics that are difficult to differentiate from reticuloendothelial neoplasms, although a prominent vasculitis and an absence of lymph node involvement may serve as distinguishing features from lymphoma.[104] It is noteworthy that four patients who were originally diagnosed as having the lymphomatoid variant of Wegener's granulomatosis subsequently developed malignant lymphoma.[104] The lymphomatoid variant is a systemic disease that involves primarily the lungs but also the kidneys, skin, and central nervous system.[105] The roentgenographic manifestations in the lungs are virtually identical to those of Wegener's granulomatosis;[33] however, the paranasal sinuses are rarely involved. The disease termed by Israel and associates "benign lymphocytic angiitis and granulomatosis"[106] probably represents an early stage of lymphomatoid granulomatosis.

It is difficult to know where the recently

described entity known as *angioimmunoblastic lymphadenopathy* fits into this rather diverse group of conditions. This disease appears to lie somewhere between a lymphoma and an atypical immunoblastic reaction, and although its etiology has not been established, an abnormal immune state is suggested. Histologic features in lymph nodes consist of effacement of architecture, lymphocyte depletion, a pleomorphic cellular infiltrate (including prominent histiocytes, plasma cells, and immunoblasts), vascular proliferation, and the presence of amorphous eosinophilic interstitial material. The roentgenographic manifestations have been described by Zylak and his colleagues.[107] Initially, a rather coarse reticulonodular pattern indicates filling of the interstitial space, followed subsequently by extensive air-space consolidation caused by progressive involvement of the alveoli. Clinically, the disorder is characterized by fever, sweats, weight loss, rash, pruritis, generalized lymph node enlargement, and hypergammaglobulinemia.[107]

ALLERGIC GRANULOMATOSIS

Churg and Strauss[108] described a granulomatous disease involving many organs, associated with considerable blood and tissue eosinophilia and restricted to patients with a history of asthma. As in Wegener's granulomatosis, lesions may occur in the lungs, with or without a perivascular distribution; unlike that disease, however, allergic granulomatosis shows a high incidence of cardiac, gastrointestinal, skin, and central nervous system involvement.[108, 109]

Necrotizing lesions of the upper respiratory tract are uncommon, although rhinorrhea and nasal polyps are frequent manifestations.[109] In contrast to Wegener's granulomatosis, allergic granulomatosis and angiitis are associated with prominent tissue and blood eosinophilia and with granulomas that show fibrinoid rather than coagulative or liquefactive necrosis. Roentgenographic manifestations in the lungs include transient patchy air-space consolidation, pulmonary nodules without cavitation, and diffuse interstitial disease.[33, 109] In the Mayo Clinic series of 30 patients,[109] 15 died within less than five years of diagnosis; cardiac disease was the major cause of death.

POLYARTERITIS NODOSA

Polyarteritis nodosa is a collagen disease characterized by an inflammatory and necrotizing reaction involving all layers of the walls of medium-sized and small arteries and arterioles. Although the tissue surrounding the diseased vessels may be affected by the same pathologic change—hence the synonym *periarteritis nodosa*—the more significant lesion is of the vessel walls themselves, so that the term "polyarteritis" is more appropriate. Typically, many organ systems are involved, and in at least 50 per cent of cases the diagnosis is made by histologic examination of a muscle biopsy.[110] It is difficult to estimate the frequency with which this disease involves the lungs, since many series include cases in which the findings are more suggestive of Wegener's or allergic granulomatosis, or even Loeffler's syndrome.[100, 110] In a recent review of the subject by Hunninghake and Fauci,[33] it was concluded that lung involvement occurs rarely if at all in classic polyarteritis nodosa.

Allergic and Wegener's granulomatoses and polyarteritis nodosa have many clinical and pathologic features in common. It is clear that a syndrome of severe necrotizing vasculitis may occur in which features of allergic granulomatosis and polyarteritis nodosa overlap.[111]

The roentgenographic changes in the thorax are highly variable, and appearances are seldom, if ever, sufficiently characteristic to indicate the diagnosis. The chest roentgenogram revealed abnormality in 19 of 28 patients with polyarteritis nodosa described by Garland and Sisson.[23] There were four cases of cardiac enlargement or pericardial effusion, four of pleural effusion, and 14 (50 per cent) with pulmonary changes, this last group comprising pulmonary venous engorgement in six, massive pulmonary edema in one, accentuated lung markings (particularly to the middle and lower lung zones) in three, and parenchymal nodules and patchy consolidation in four. Hennell and Sussman[112] stated that the most characteristic roentgenographic pattern is one of fleeting, patchy consolidation of nonsegmental distribution identical to the pattern of Loeffler's syndrome. The angiographic demonstration of multiple arterial aneurysms in one or more abdominal organs is considered virtually diagnostic of this disease.

Commonly the predominant symptoms in polyarteritis nodosa are those caused by involvement of systems other than the cardiorespiratory, particularly the gastrointestinal tract, the kidneys, and the nervous system. Renal involvement is said to occur in 80 per cent of cases, and systemic hypertension is a common clinical manifestation, particularly as a consequence of healing of renal arterial lesions. Symptoms from involvement of the thorax are nonspecific and include cough, wheezing, occasionally hemoptysis, and pain due to pleural effusion.

The pathogenetic relationship between polyarteritis nodosa and hepatitis B antigenemia has now been well established.[113, 114]

NECROTIZING "SARCOIDAL" ANGIITIS AND GRANULOMATOSIS

In his 1973 J. Burns Amberson Lecture, Liebow[115] defined five forms of pulmonary angiitis and granulomatosis not produced by known infectious agents and not associated with rheumatoid disease; four of these have already been described. The fifth is necrotizing sarcoidal granulomatosis, of which Liebow described 11 examples. This rare form of granulomatous angiitis, which affects young or middle-aged adults of equal sex distribution, is associated with marked infiltration of the lungs by sarcoid tubercles and is distinguished from ordinary sarcoidosis by the presence of severe arteritis. The majority of patients manifest roentgenologic evidence of multiple well-defined nodules or ill-defined opacities and present clinically with symptoms of cough, fever, sweats, malaise, dyspnea, and pleuritic pain. Present evidence suggests that the course of necrotizing sarcoidal granulomatosis is relatively benign and that the condition is responsive to corticosteroid therapy.

BRONCHOPULMONARY HYPERSENSITIVITY TO ORGANIC DUSTS

The polluted air of industrial areas contains many chemicals in aerosol form that exert a nonspecific irritative effect on the tracheobronchial tree of all exposed individuals and especially those with hyperactive bronchi and obstructive airway disease. In addition to these atmospheric chemical pollutants, a variety of inhaled organic particles may cause bronchopulmonary disease by inciting hypersensitivity reactions. The reaction depends in large measure on the size of the inhaled particles. Large particles (pollens, certain fungi, and some animal and insect epithelial emanations) impinge on the tracheobronchial mucosa, where they incite a local hypersensitivity response, usually in persons with an atopic background; the diseases produced include extrinsic asthma, hypersensitivity aspergillosis (with mucoid impaction), bronchocentric granulomatosis, and byssinosis. Smaller organic particles (less than 5 μ in diameter) tend to escape deposition on the major airways and reach the alveoli, where they initiate an acute hypersensitivity reaction—extrinsic allergic alveolitis or hypersensitivity pneumonitis.[116]

The pathogenesis of this group of diseases is incompletely understood, but there is little question that immunologic mechanisms are predominant.

TRACHEOBRONCHIAL HYPERSENSITIVITY

In the four diseases that come under this heading—spasmodic asthma, hypersensitivity aspergillosis with mucoid impaction, bronchocentric granulomatosis, and byssinosis—the target tissue is the respiratory airways. Patients usually have a history of atopic reactions, and the clinical picture is one of bronchospasm or "asthma" mediated by nonprecipitating reaginic antibodies.[116] Extrinsic (spasmodic) asthma is discussed in detail in Chapter 11 and will not be further considered here.

HYPERSENSITIVITY BRONCHOPULMONARY ASPERGILLOSIS WITH MUCOID IMPACTION

Although it is probable that some cases of hypersensitivity (allergic) aspergillosis are not associated with mucous impaction of second-order bronchi, there is no doubt that mucoid impaction is the commonest morphologic manifestation. The majority of affected patients have a history of early onset asthma and peripheral eosinophilia. The association with asthma or chronic bronchitis has been noted in several studies,[117] but not all patients have pre-existing chronic bronchial disease and, in fact, some have no respiratory symptoms.

The pathogenesis is incompletely understood, but it is most probable that the primary abnormality lies in a constitutional defect resulting in abnormal bronchial secretions, and that the obstructive airway disease renders inspissation of these secretions more likely. The role played by *Aspergillus* species is inconclusive, since not all patients demonstrate microbiologic or serologic evidence of aspergillosis. It may be that *Aspergillus* mycelia increase the consistency of mucus whose viscosity is already

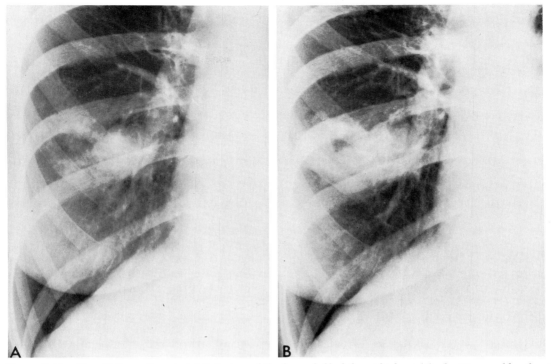

Figure 7–10.   Mucoid Impaction. A detailed view of the lower half of the right lung (A) of a 29-year-old asthmatic woman reveals an opacity possessing a Y configuration, the two prongs facing laterally. This represents mucoid impaction in dilated branching bronchi. Two years later (B), the shadow had increased considerably in size. Note that the peripheral parenchyma is air-containing, despite the total bronchial obstruction that must be present.

greater than normal because of chronic bronchial disease.

Mucoid impaction, first described by Shaw in 1951,[118] consists of the plugging with inspissated mucus of one or more orders of bronchi distal to the lobar bronchus, with resultant dilatation and severe distortion.

Knowledge of the pathology of the disease has come from the study of lobes removed because of a clinical suspicion of bronchogenic carcinoma. The second-, third-, and fourth-order bronchi distal to the lobar bronchus are filled with hard, rubbery, brown to greenish-gray mucous plugs of puttylike consistency, ranging from 2.5 to 6.0 cm in length and up to 3 cm in width.[117, 119] The peribronchial area may contain abundant eosinophils as well as lymphocytes, plasma cells, lipophages, and occasional foreign body giant cells. In many cases the changes in the bronchi are permanent, consisting of loss of cartilaginous and smooth muscle elements and replacement of normal respiratory epithelium by squamous epithelium. Anatomic distribution shows a clear-cut upper lobe predominance.[119, 120]

Roentgenologically, the shadows created by the dilated mucus-filled bronchi are distinctive (Figure 7–10). The plugs appear as round, oval, or elliptical opacities, usually in the upper lobes and seldom in the main-stem or first-order bronchi. When several second-order bronchi in one region are involved, the appearance may resemble a cluster of grapes. When a bronchus and both limbs of its bifurcation are involved simultaneously, the shadow has a distinctive "Y" configuration, the leg of the Y pointing toward the hilum (Figure 7–10); a variation of this is the V-shaped shadow that results when two branches are plugged. In many cases tomography defines precisely such distinctive shadows.

When plugs are expectorated, residual bronchiectatic segments should be clearly visible, particularly with tomography. It is important to recognize the "proximal" nature of the bronchiectasis, which differentiates this condition from the "usual" form of bronchiectasis in which more peripheral bronchi are chiefly affected; in mucoid impaction the peripheral tree is characteristically normal. In cases manifesting typical mucoid impaction, the character of the lung distal to the obstructed segments varies. Since the bronchus is completely obstructed, it might reasonably be assumed that lung segments distally would manifest atelectasis or obstructive pneumonitis; in fact, lobar or segmental atelectasis is seen in only a minority of patients (in six of 14 patients in one series),[121] its absence clearly being the result of collateral air drift from contiguous ventilated segments. Cavitation occurs in roughly 15 per cent of cases and may be associated with mycetoma formation.[120]

Clinically, symptoms consist of a productive cough, which results in the expectoration of mucous plugs or bronchial casts in up to one-half of cases. Fever and chest pain may be present, but an important feature of the clinical picture in most patients is the total absence of symptoms or the mild symptomatology sometimes associated with extensive pulmonary disease.[117, 120] Aerosol inhalation of acetylcysteine usually results in liquefaction and expectoration of mucous plugs[119] and may constitute a valuable diagnostic and therapeutic test.

A confident diagnosis of allergic bronchopulmonary aspergillosis with mucoid impaction can usually be made on the basis of the typical roentgenographic appearance, especially if mucoid impaction is associated with evidence of proximal bronchiectasis in remote areas of the lungs. A history of spasmodic asthma and the presence of peripheral eosinophilia virtually clinch the diagnosis. In the presence of such a clinical-roentgenographic presentation, all patients should be tested for hypersensitivity to *Aspergillus fumigatus*, including both a skin test and a search for precipitating antibodies in the serum. Specific IgG or IgE to *Aspergillus fumigatas* is usually present, and an increase in the latter may indicate the formation of a mucous plug.[122]

BRONCHOCENTRIC GRANULOMATOSIS

This condition was first described by Liebow in 1973 and by 1975,[115] 23 cases had been recognized.[123] The clinical and roentgenographic manifestations of the disease are very similar to those of bronchopulmonary aspergillosis and mucoid impaction, and the disease may simply represent a variant of this entity.

Pathologically, the major changes occur in the small bronchi and bronchioles, which are filled with yellow-white cheesy material associated with necrotic granulomata surrounded by palisaded epithelioid cells. The bronchocentric nature of the lesions is demonstrated by elastic stains, which in many cases reveal remnants of bronchial elastic tissue within the granulomatous reaction. Cellular reaction is predomi-

nantly eosinophilic in asthmatic patients but consists mainly of plasma cells in nonasthmatics. In many instances, the alveoli behind obstructed bronchioles are filled with foamy macrophages, constituting the entity of cholesterol (endogenous lipid) pneumonitis. In the more proximal bronchi, the submucosa is infiltrated by plasma cells, lymphocytes, and variable numbers of eosinophils; granulomas are also identified here. Four of the 23 cases showed mucoid impaction in larger bronchi.

Roentgenographically, the manifestations are similar to those of bronchopulmonary aspergillosis and mucoid impaction except more peripherally situated; they may consist of segmental consolidation and atelectasis, irregular masses, linear opacities, and shadows due to abnormal bronchi. As in the more common mucoid impaction, the disease was unilateral in 75 per cent of the cases and showed definite upper lobe predilection.

Clinically, 10 of the 23 patients were asthmatic, with an average age of 22 years; by contrast, the 13 nonasthmatics noted the onset of symptoms much later, at an average age of 50 years. Symptoms were present in the majority of patients and included dyspnea, cough, hemoptysis, malaise, and fever. Nine of the 10 asthmatic but only two of the nonasthmatic patients had blood eosinophilia. The presence of noninvasive fungi within the bronchial mucus of the asthmatic patients suggested the possibility of hypersensitivity reactions to these organisms.

BYSSINOSIS

This disease occurs in workers engaged in the initial processing of cotton, retted flax, and hemp fibers.[124] Most of the reports come from the United Kingdom and continental Europe, but in recent years the disease has been recognized with increasing frequency in North America. The incidence is highest in cardroom and blowroom workers, although virtually any worker exposed to cotton dust is susceptible.

The mechanism by which bronchoconstriction develops in these patients is still not fully understood. At a recent international symposium on byssinosis,[125] a number of substances were implicated as potential exciting agents in the causation of bronchospasm, including a histaminelike substance from cotton bracts, gram-negative bacterial contamination of organic cotton and flax fibers, and a polyphenol compound extracted from cotton mill dust. The decrease in expiratory flow rates that characteristically follows exposure can be prevented by the administration of either a bronchodilator or an antihistaminic substance.[124] Atopic patients exposed to air-borne cotton dust in textile mills may show rapid and severe impairment of pulmonary function, although even patients without a history of previous sensitization may develop symptoms and lung function changes on exposure. In contrast to tobacco, cotton dust has been implicated in the development of chronic bronchitis but not emphysema.[126, 127]

Roentgenographic changes in the chest are negligible during reversible stages of the disease and, in fact, the chest roentgenograms in symptomatic patients are indistinguishable from those of control subjects. The roentgenologic and pathologic findings in the third stage of the disease are those of chronic bronchitis, with nothing specific to suggest the diagnosis of byssinosis.

The clinical history of patients with byssinosis is characterized by the gradual onset of dyspnea during the first day at work after an absence, usually a Monday, and is accompanied by cough, tightness in the chest, and general malaise. The increase in dyspnea on a Monday correlates well with decrease in the FEV_1; in fact, in some persons, exposure to the dust may result in a drop in FEV_1 without the development of symptoms.[124] Three clinical stages have been described:[124] (1) the development of dyspnea on Mondays, disappearing later in the week and associated with a decrease in flow rates; (2) symptoms present throughout the week although usually more severe on Mondays; and (3) irreversible ventilatory insufficiency. In the last, the clinical picture may be indistinguishable from chronic bronchitis and emphysema and may progress to cor pulmonale. The third stage develops only after long exposure to cotton, flax, or hemp dust, and is associated with severe ventilatory insufficiency.

ALVEOLAR HYPERSENSITIVITY

GENERAL CHARACTERISTICS

The term "alveolar hypersensitivity" (*synonyms:* hypersensitivity pneumonitis, extrinsic allergic alveolitis) denotes a group of diseases characterized by a response of the lungs to specific antigens contained in a wide variety of organic dusts of such fine particle size that they can penetrate to the most distal lung parenchyma. The list of diseases and the antigens associated with them has increased steadily since "farmer's lung" was first clearly described

in 1924[128] and now contains a multitude of conditions. Regardless of the name of the disease and the specific exposure involved, striking similarities exist among the clinical, pathologic, and roentgenologic features of all these diseases, although it must be emphasized that the immunopathology and the exact criteria required to make the diagnosis are by no means clearly defined. The following list includes those criteria generally accepted for the establishment of a positive diagnosis.

1. Exposure to an organic dust of sufficiently small particle size ($<6\mu$) to penetrate to the most distal lung parenchyma.

2. Episodes of dyspnea, frequently accompanied by a dry cough, fever, and malaise, occurring some hours after exposure to the relevant antigen.

3. Auscultatory evidence of bilateral crepitations heard best over the lung bases bilaterally.

4. Roentgenologic evidence of a diffuse reticulonodular or nodular pattern, commonly associated in the acute stage with an air-space component. The result of repeated or long-term exposure is the "end-stage" lung, sometimes manifested by a honeycomb pattern roentgenologically.

5. Pulmonary function tests indicating restrictive lung disease. There is little or no evidence of airway obstruction.

6. Intracutaneous injection of the appropriate antigen resulting in "late" (Arthus) or delayed hypersensitivity reactions.

7. The presence in the serum of precipitins against the suspected antigen.

8. The demonstration *in vitro* of blastogenesis and the production of migration inhibitory factor on stimulation of lymphocytes with specific antigens.

9. The development, some hours after aerosol provocation by the specific antigen, of appropriate symptoms, with or without impairment of pulmonary function and the appearance of abnormalities on the chest roentgenogram.

10. Histopathologic features on lung biopsy that, while not diagnostic, are sufficiently characteristic to be compatible with the diagnosis.

11. In most cases, resolution of the episodic systemic and respiratory symptoms after cessation of exposure to the antigen and, in time, disappearance of precipitins from the serum. In some cases, the persistence of exertional dyspnea, abnormal pulmonary function test values, and roentgenographic changes indicates irreversible interstitial pulmonary fibrosis.

Although the great majority of cases of allergic alveolitis are occupational in nature, exciting causes have also been found within the home or office, originating in heating systems, humidifiers, or air conditioners.

As more and more cases of alveolar hypersensitivity are reported, involving an ever-increasing variety of organic antigens, it is becoming clear that the diagnosis must be based primarily on clinical findings and that meticulous history-taking may be required to uncover environmental or atmospheric exposure coincident with the development of acute respiratory symptoms. In fact, it is now known that in some cases the chest roentgenogram can be normal and serum precipitins can be absent. In cases in which the etiology is in doubt, supporting evidence may be obtained clinically by challenging the patient with an aerosol of the antigen under suspicion or by documenting clinical remission coincident with removal of the patient from the environment. It is obvious that the diagnosis will be more secure if there is roentgenographic evidence of a diffuse reticulonodular pattern and if there is impairment of pulmonary function, particularly reduced diffusing capacity or pulmonary compliance.

PATHOGENESIS AND IMMUNOLOGIC CHARACTERISTICS

In persons exposed to various organic dust antigens, the development of symptoms and signs 4 to 6 hours after exposure has suggested both a causal relationship and an immunologic mechanism. Such a "late" onset is characteristic of immune-complex disease, classified by Gell and Coombs as an Arthus type III immunologic reaction. Although serum titers of specific IgG, IgA, and IgM precipitating antibodies are high in many patients with hypersensitivity pneumonitis and decrease with clinical improvement, there is considerable variation in the reported incidence of positive precipitation reactions in patients with clinically diagnosed farmer's lung. For example, it has been shown that most if not all patients with acute disease but only about half those with the more chronic form have serum precipitins, and it is now known that the presence of precipitating antibodies to organic dust reflects nothing more than exposure to that dust. The majority of patients who have been exposed to organic dust and whose sera contain precipitins are asymptomatic.[129]

Despite the common occurrence of serum precipitins in exposed asymptomatic persons, there is a good deal of evidence that the type III immune reaction plays a role in the pathogenesis of hypersensitivity pneumonitis. In some of the extrinsic allergic alveolitides, the time interval required for the development of a positive skin test suggests a late Arthus reaction. Both the prick test (employed for the identification of IgE) and the intracutaneous test (used to identify the "late" or "dual" reactions) may be positive when other allergens, particularly material obtained from birds, are employed. The term "dual reaction" describes an immediate wheal and flare (IgE-mediated), followed 3 to 4 hours later by the development of erythema and swelling at the site of puncture; the skin reaction usually resolves within 24 to 48 hours. Although in atopic individuals the immediate intracutaneous reaction is due to IgE, it is thought that in nonatopic persons it may result from short-term IgG. Hargreaves and Pepys[129] found that "late" responses correlated closely with both clinical disease and the presence of precipitating antibodies; in patients exposed to avian antigens and showing serum precipitins, positive "late" reactions were observed in 84 per cent of those with symptoms and signs and in none of those who were asymptomatic.

A useful diagnostic procedure considered to reflect both type I and type III immune reactions is the allergen inhalation (provocation) test or challenge test. Reactions to aerosolized extracts of the appropriate antigen may be immediate, late, or dual in terms of their time of appearance, being manifested early in their course as bronchospasm but later more likely as a restrictive defect.[129]

Almost all patients who manifest either dual or late reactions to inhalation challenge have serum precipitins to the appropriate antigen. Positive responses to inhalation challenge with specific antigens correlate closely with results of skin testing and are further evidence for a hypersensitivity state in this group of diseases.[129]

It is now generally believed that not all the clinical and morphologic features of extrinsic allergic alveolitis can be explained solely on the basis of an Arthus reaction in the lungs associated with the formation of precipitating antigen-antibody complexes and activation of the complement cascade, and there is increasing evidence that the type IV delayed hypersensitivity response must also be invoked.

PATHOLOGIC CHARACTERISTICS

The histologic features of the many different varieties of extrinsic allergic alveolitis are strikingly similar and, with few exceptions, do not permit differentiation. As might be anticipated, the pathologic characteristics depend partly on the intensity of exposure to the allergen and partly on the stage of the disease at which the biopsy is taken. Three stages may be recognized—acute, subacute, and chronic.

The Acute Stage

There is little doubt that bronchiolitis is a common feature of this disease, ranging in incidence from 25 to 100 per cent of cases.[130–132] In some cases, the bronchiolar lesions have been described as obstructive and organizing, presenting the appearance of bronchiolitis obliterans. In an immunofluorescent study of lung tissue from four patients with farmer's lung, Wenzel and colleagues[130] found high concentrations of antibody to *Micropolyspora faeni* in the walls of bronchioles in the lungs of two of the patients who were acutely ill but not in the two with more chronic disease.

The Subacute Stage

Biopsies examined at a slightly later stage (1 to 2 months after the onset of the acute stage) reveal noncaseating "histiocytic" granulomas, closely resembling those seen in sarcoidosis. The granulomas are present in the peribronchiolar tissues and cause localized thickening of alveolar walls. There may be a striking interstitial pneumonitis of mononuclear cells. There is generally no evidence of fibrosis in the interstitial tissues, although reticulin may be increased. Giant cells of Langhans and of foreign body types[132] are often seen, the latter frequently containing birefringent material. During this stage, intra-alveolar exudation may be present. Although sarcoidlike granulomas have been shown to arise as a result of the formation of antigen-antibody complexes, they are more commonly associated with type IV allergy.

The Chronic Stage

Over the course of the next several months, lesions become nonspecific as the granulomas disappear and fibrosis supervenes.[132] Interstitial pneumonitis and doubly refractile material persist. The degree of ensuing fibrosis is variable, the upper zones being affected most. The end result is a variable mixture of scarring, pneumonitis, honeycombing, and emphysema.

ROENTGENOGRAPHIC MANIFESTATIONS

As with the pathologic manifestations, the roentgenographic changes vary with the stage of the disease. Early in the course of the acute stage, the chest roentgenogram may show no discernible abnormality. Once roentgen changes are visible, however, they usually parallel the severity of the clinical symptoms. They consist of granular or nodular mottling scattered diffusely throughout both lungs, without zonal predominance although commonly less evident in the apices and bases. The individual nodules range from 1 mm or less up to several mm in diameter. They may be quite discrete, although usually they are poorly defined. The pattern may be predominantly reticular or reticulonodular (Figure 7–11).

This fine nodular or reticular pattern is characteristic of the subacute stage of the disease, usually visualized between acute episodes. In the acute stage (shortly after heavy exposure to the appropriate antigen), acinar shadows are commonly visualized, particularly in the lower lung zones (Figure 7–11). Air-space consolidation may be quite extensive and may obscure the reticular or nodular pattern characteristic of the subacute stage (Figure 7–11). Within a few days the acinar pattern resolves, once again permitting visualization of the irreversible reticulonodular pattern. This sequence of roentgenologic changes should strongly suggest the diagnosis of hypersensitivity pneumonitis—diffuse involvement of both lungs as evidenced by a persistent reticular or nodular pattern, superimposition of an acinar pattern with acute exacerbations, and resolution of the latter pattern within a few days of the initial acute clinical presentation. In our experience, hilar lymph node enlargement is variable. Neither its presence nor its absence can be used as a useful diagnostic criterion for distinguishing this disease from sarcoidosis.

The subsequent course of the roentgenographic changes depends on whether exposure to the antigen is continued. If the patient is removed from the environment, the chest roentgenogram may return to normal in from 10 days to several weeks.[131] If exposure is continued or repeated, the diffuse nodular pattern characteristic of the acute and subacute stages is replaced by changes characteristic of diffuse interstitial fibrosis—a medium to coarse reticular pattern, loss of lung volume, a honeycomb pattern, and sometimes compensatory overinflation of lung zones that are least affected. The loss of lung volume (cicatrization atelectasis) tends to show a striking upper zone predominance. Ring shadows measuring 5 to 8 mm in diameter characterize the late stages of interstitial fibrosis, creating a honeycomb pattern indistinguishable from the late stages of fibrosing alveolitis.

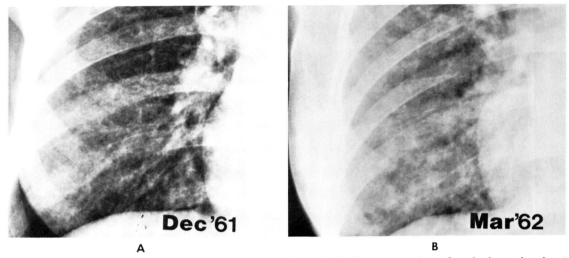

Figure 7–11. Farmer's Lung. This 25-year-old woman, the wife of a farmer, was admitted to the hospital with a 2-week history of moderate dyspnea, mildly productive cough, and daily temperature rise to 103° F; on examination she was slightly cyanotic. A detailed view of the lower half of the right lung *(A)* reveals a coarse reticulonodular pattern. She was placed on antibiotic therapy, and over the next 5 or 6 days her temperature gradually returned to normal; she was discharged without a diagnosis. Three months after her original acute episode, she was admitted for a second time following the acute onset of dyspnea, cough, and high fever. The chest roentgenogram at this time *(B)* revealed definite extension of the disease, an acinar pattern being superimposed on the reticulonodular pattern seen earlier. This was regarded as evidence of involvement of the air spaces of the lung and was felt to represent an acute exacerbation subsequent to re-exposure. (Courtesy of Dr. John Silny, Sherbrooke, Quebec.)

In any study of a disease in which the basic criteria for diagnosis are clinical, it is not unusual for a number of patients to show no roentgenographic abnormalities of the chest. By contrast, roentgenographic abnormalities consistent with the diagnosis may be present in the absence of clinical symptoms.

CLINICAL MANIFESTATIONS

Intermittent exposure of susceptible individuals to high concentrations of antigen is accompanied by recurrent episodes of fever, chills, dry cough, and dyspnea, whereas continuous exposure to lower concentrations characteristically results in gradually progressive dyspnea in the absence of other detectable systemic symptoms.[133] The diagnosis of farmer's lung is easily made when a patient presents with a history of recurrent systemic and respiratory symptoms that appear several hours after he has entered a barn containing moldy hay. In many cases, however, patients may experience no more than slowly increasing dyspnea, cough, and weight loss, which they may attribute to cigarette smoking; in such circumstances, they may delay seeking medical advice until the disease has progressed to an irreversible fibrotic stage.[133] In a small percentage of patients, usu-

ally those with a history of allergy, the clinical presentation may suggest "asthmatic bronchitis"; the acute asthmatic episode develops within a few minutes of exposure, subsides slowly, and may be repeated as a "late" response some 4 to 6 hours after the initial episode of bronchospasm—the Arthus reaction.

Pulmonary function tests may be very useful in both the assessment of functional impairment in the naturally occurring disease and the determination of the response to aerosol challenge. It is usual to find a slight to moderate reduction in FEV_1 which is proportional to a decrease in vital capacity. The overall pattern is one of restrictive disease.

Removal of patients from their hazardous environment frequently results in restoration of pulmonary function to normal, but in some cases function may continue to be impaired even after the chest roentgenogram has returned to normal.

NOTES ON SPECIFIC DISEASES

FARMER'S LUNG. This is the earliest described and most thoroughly understood of the many conditions causing hypersensitivity pneumonitis. Although it may have been recognized for centuries, the earliest clear descriptions in

English appeared in 1924.[128] Farmer's lung is the prototype of extrinsic allergic alveolitis and the bulk of the material in this section originates from studies of farmers exposed to thermophilic actinomycetes. More recent studies have shown that many farmers have the clinical syndrome without exhibiting all the immunologic and roentgenologic manifestations commonly associated with the disease.[134] The prevalence of the syndrome among farmers in different communities ranges from less than 1 per cent to 10 per cent.[134]

Pepys and Jenkins[135] found that approximately 90 per cent of patients with farmer's lung had precipitating antibodies to thermophilic actinomycetes, 87 per cent to *Micropolyspora faeni*, and the remaining 3 per cent to other actinomycete strains. Other workers[134] have found positive precipitins to actinomycete species in approximately 50 per cent of patients with chronic disease and in up to 100 per cent of those with acute disease. A significant number of patients have serum precipitins to thermophilic actinomycetes other than *M. faeni*, and some even to *Aspergillus fumigatus*.

Farmer's lung typically affects males between 40 and 50 years of age and has a peak incidence during the season when stored hay is used for feeding cattle. The clinical picture varies according to the degree of exposure to antigens in the moldy hay and to the degree of sensitivity of the subject. The classic acute onset occurs in perhaps no more than a third of cases, the more common form being insidious and characterized by a gradual progression of dyspnea, cough, and weight loss, and by fever, chills, malaise, and aches and pains.

BIRD-FANCIER'S LUNG. Although this hypersensitivity disease (*synonyms:* pigeon-breeder's lung, bird-breeder's lung) is commonly associated with budgerigars and pigeons, it was originally described as occurring in a breeder of parakeets[136] and has since been shown to occur in persons handling various other species of birds, including parrots, hens, ducks, and geese. Thus, the name bird-fancier's lung is now favored. The antigen consists of protein contained in bird sera, droppings, or feathers. The major source is probably bird serum that is secreted into the lumen of the gut, excreted, and inhaled in the form of droppings.

MUSHROOM-WORKER'S LUNG. The specific antigens, *Micropolyspora faeni* and *Micromonospora vulgaris*, are the same as in farmer's lung. The culture of mushrooms requires a process of steam pasteurization to destroy mi-

croorganisms; temperatures during this process rise to 60° C at 100 per cent humidity, which encourages the rapid growth of thermophilic actinomycetes. Subsequently, the compost is spread on trays and mixed with mushroom mycelia grown on manure and grain. This process, which is called "spawning," gives rise to clouds of dust. The clinical and immunologic features of this disease are very similar to those of farmer's lung.

BAGASSOSIS. This disease occurs from inhalation of bagasse fibers contaminated by the specific microorganism *Thermoactinomyces sacchari*.[137] Bagasse is a fibrous material that remains after the sugar-containing juice has been extracted from sugar cane and is composed almost entirely of cellulose and other complex plant carbohydrates. Bagassosis is more likely to occur as a result of exposure to freshly produced bagasse or bagasse fibers stored indoors than to moldy bagasse stored outside.

HYPERSENSITIVITY PNEUMONITIS DUE TO FORCED-AIR EQUIPMENT. Equipment used to heat, humidify, or cool air may harbor microorganisms responsible for extrinsic allergic alveolitis.[138] In the majority of cases the causative agents are thermophilic actinomycetes, particularly *Thermoactinomyces candidus*.[138] Since the disease is acquired in the office or home, it may be very difficult to diagnose, particularly if the clinical presentation is insidious rather than intermittent and acute. The diagnosis is made on the basis of a combination of clinical and laboratory findings; in some cases, suspicion may be aroused by the presence of a diffuse reticulonodular pattern on the chest roentgenogram. Supporting evidence for the diagnosis may be provided by the demonstration of serum precipitins, the presence of appropriate pulmonary function test abnormalities, and positive results from histologic studies, particularly the identification of antigen by immunofluorescence. The diagnosis can usually be confirmed by inhalation challenge with the suspected antigen or by clinical remission coincidental with removal of the patient from the suspected site of contamination.

MALT-WORKER'S LUNG. Heavy exposure to the fungus *Aspergillus clavatus* has been shown to result in the typical clinical picture of hypersensitivity pneumonitis in a small percentage of malt workers.[139] As with many of the other extrinsic allergic alveolitides, precipitating antibodies may be present in the serum in the absence of symptoms of the disease.[139]

MAPLE BARK DISEASE. This rare disease was originally described[140] in 36 sawmill workers.

The responsible antigen appears to be the spore of the fungus *Cryptostroma corticale (Coniosporium corticale)*, which lies deep in the bark of the maple tree. Spores have been identified in lung biopsies, and precipitating antibodies have been found in patients' sera.

PITUITARY SNUFF-TAKER'S LUNG. Powdered extract of pig or ox pituitary glands may be administered by nasal insufflation in the treatment of diabetes insipidus, and four separate reports have appeared of lung disease resulting from this treatment.

SUBEROSIS. To the best of our knowledge, this respiratory disease of cork workers has been reported only from Portugal.[141] The sera of patients with the disease contain high levels of precipitins to moldy cork dust but not to extracts of clean cork dust.[141]

IMMUNOLOGIC DEFICIENCY SYNDROMES

Patients with undue susceptibility to respiratory infection often have a similar lack of resistance to infection elsewhere in the body. Immune deficiency diseases may be *primary* (resulting from genetic abnormalities in the development of immune maturity) or *secondary* (associated with diseases that interfere with the expression of a mature immune system). Although the vast majority of patients with primary deficiency of their immunologic mechanisms are infants and young children, most of whom die of infection before reaching adulthood, as a result of newer knowledge permitting recognition of milder cases and the availability of antibiotic and replacement therapy for recognized cases, more adults are now being seen with immunologic host defense disorders. Seven varieties of deficiency states can be recognized: (1) decrease or absence of all immunoglobulins; (2) decrease or absence of a specific immunoglobulin; (3) lack of complement; (4) inability to recognize or deal with various antigens; (5) defect in leukocyte function; (6) the presence of various serum inhibitors of essential components of immune defense; and (7) various combinations of these abnormalities. Although the clinical and roentgenographic manifestations are sufficiently characteristic in many cases to arouse suspicion of the presence of immune deficiency, elucidation of the precise nature of the defect(s) usually requires a variety of laboratory procedures.

The diseases leading to secondary immunodeficiency and those associated with phagocyte dysfunction have already been described. In this section we will deal with the primary immunodeficiencies of genetic origin, divided into three groups: (a) humoral (B cell) incompetence; (b) cell-mediated (T cell) incompetence, and (c) quantitative and qualitative impairment of both systems (by far the largest group).

DISEASES PRIMARILY OF HUMORAL DEFICIENCY

This term includes the agammaglobulinemias, the hypogammaglobulinemias, and the dysgammaglobulinemias. Immunologic techniques that differentiate the various gammaglobulinemias have shown that one immunoglobulin may be deficient while others may show a proportional increase; thus, gammaglobulin deficiency can easily be missed if looked for simply on the basis of protein determination by electrophoretic pattern. Five immunoglobulin molecules have been recognized: IgG, IgA, IgM, IgD, and IgE.

THE AGAMMAGLOBULINEMIAS

TRANSIENT HYPOGAMMAGLOBULINEMIA

IgA and IgM molecules do not traverse the placental barrier into the fetal circulation to any extent, whereas IgG molecules are found in similar concentrations in both fetus and mother. IgM and IgA globulins are synthesized slowly by newborn infants, and adult levels may not be reached until the age of 1 to 2 years; also, by the end of the third month the infant has largely catabolized his store of maternal IgG and must begin manufacturing his own. Delay in the onset of manufacture of any of these immunoglobulins results in increased susceptibility to infection until adequate gammaglobulin synthesis occurs (usually by 9 to 15 months of age); infections contracted at this time usually are gram-positive.

CONGENITAL AGAMMAGLOBULINEMIA

The commonest form of congenital agammaglobulinemia (*synonyms:* Bruton's agammaglobulinemia, infantile sex-linked agammaglobulinemia) is transmitted as an X-linked recessive trait and thus is seen exclusively in males. Symptoms usually have their onset late in the first year of life, after passive immunity has worn off. These male infants are particularly susceptible to infection with staphylococci, pneumococci, streptococci, and *Haemophilus influenzae*, there being little if any increased susceptibility to gram-negative bacilli, viruses, fungi, or protozoa.[142, 143] The clinical picture often is similar to that of rheumatoid arthritis; atopic allergy is not infrequent.

The lymphoid tissues of patients with agammaglobulinemia are devoid of plasma cells, and draining lymph nodes do not tend to enlarge in the normal way in response to local infection. This lack of reaction in lymphatic tissue may be manifested roentgenographically by virtual absence of the shadow of adenoid tissue in the posterior nasopharynx (Neuhauser's sign).[143] As the child grows older, lymph nodes may become evident as a result of hyperplasia of reticulum cells or of lymphocyte T cells or B cells incapable of producing immunoglobulins.[142, 143]

"ACQUIRED" OR COMMON VARIABLE AGAMMAGLOBULINEMIA

This deficiency state is seen in both sexes of all ages. Although the designation "acquired" implies that patients manifest symptoms of the disease after an asymptomatic period in earlier life, it is now generally believed that the deficiency is of genetic origin. There is a high incidence of other immunologic abnormalities in the relatives of many of these patients, and multiple cases have been described in a single kindred. B cells may be normal in number but tend to be defective in function; they either are incapable of developing into plasma cells and producing immunoglobulins, or fail to secrete immunoglobulins once they are produced.

These patients have a particular susceptibility to infection of the lungs[144] and paranasal sinuses. Noncaseating granulomas develop in the lungs, spleen, liver, and skin with resultant hepatosplenomegaly and superficial lymph node enlargement. Nodular lymphoid hyperplasia of follicles within the lamina propria of the small intestine may result in a spruelike disorder.

Chest roentgenographic patterns are highly variable: acute air-space pneumonia, bronchopneumonia, atelectasis, and bronchiectasis result in opacities that may be segmental or nonsegmental, homogeneous or inhomogeneous.

THE DYSGAMMAGLOBULINEMIAS

Immunoelectrophoretic techniques have resulted in a more precise definition of the immunoglobulins and have permitted identification of individuals who are deficient in one or two immunoglobulin groups and have normal or elevated levels of others.[143] These combinations categorize the dysgammaglobulinemias. Perhaps the most common form of selective deficiency of immunoglobulin is that due to an absence of IgA. Although an isolated absence of IgA is found in a small but significant proportion of the normal population, it may also play a role in the pathogenesis of infantile atopy by permitting various antigens to penetrate the respiratory and intestinal mucosa.

CELL-MEDIATED DEFICIENCIES

Selective deficiencies of T cell function are rare. Congenital absence of the thymus gland (Di George's syndrome) includes aplasia of the parathyroid glands as well[145, 146] and is due to embryonic maldevelopment of the third and fourth pharyngeal cleft pouches; malformations of the face, ears, and nose are inevitable and cardiovascular anomalies are frequent accompaniments. The parathyroid aplasia leads to tetany during the first few days of life and the thymic aplasia to increased susceptibility to infection. Serum levels of immunoglobulins are normal, but delayed hypersensitivity does not develop. Most other varieties of cell-mediated immune deficiency have in addition some impairment of immunoglobulin production.

COMBINED IMMUNODEFICIENCIES

SWISS-TYPE AGAMMAGLOBULINEMIA

This abnormality of immunologic response (*synonym:* autosomal recessive alymphopenic agammaglobulinemia) occurs in both sexes and is associated with a high incidence of consanguinity in the parents of affected infants; it is transmitted as an autosomal recessive characteristic. The basic abnormality is a failure of embryonic differentiation of the thymus gland. Death usually occurs before the age of 2 years. Delayed hypersensitivity reactions are totally lacking. Lymphoid tissue is strikingly decreased or absent, and agammaglobulinemia or some form of dysgammaglobulinemia and lymphopenia is found in most cases.

WISKOTT-ALDRICH SYNDROME

This X-linked recessive disorder, first described by Aldrich and associates in 1954,[147] is characterized by the triad of thrombocytopenia, intractable eczema during the first year of life (often followed by the development of bronchial asthma), and an extraordinary susceptibility to infection.[148] The majority of patients die of overwhelming infection during the first few years of life; those who survive the multiple infections either bleed to death or succumb to lymphoreticular neoplasia.[148] The basic immunologic defect in Wiskott-Aldrich syndrome is cellular, but many patients show an impairment of humoral immunity also. Immunoglobulin levels are normal or nearly so, IgM sometimes being slightly decreased and IgA slightly increased.[148]

ATAXIA-TELANGIECTASIA

This is a developmental disease affecting many organ systems in which there is defective interaction among primitive ectoderm, endoderm, and mesoderm. Most patients present with cerebellar ataxia (related to enlarged venules and chronic degenerative changes in the cerebellum) associated with scleral and cutaneous telangiectasia.[56] Recurrent paranasal sinusitis and acute pneumonia are common as a result of profound defects in cellular and humoral immunity; the respiratory infections frequently result in pulmonary insufficiency. At necropsy the thymus gland is either absent or small and deficient in lymphocytes and Hassall's corpuscles. Histologic examination of the lungs reveals dilatation and epithelial ulceration of the bronchioles and an inflammatory exudate containing lymphocytes, plasma cells, and polymorphonuclear cells in the walls of the bronchi, bronchioles, and alveoli.[56] These histologic changes may be manifested roentgenographically by a prominent, symmetric, thicketlike branching linear pattern in the lungs.

REFERENCES

1. Gell, P. G. H., and Coombs, R. R. A.: Clinical Aspects of Immunology. Oxford, Blackwell Scientific Publications, 1968.
2. Ammann, A. J., and Hong, R.: Selective IgA deficiency: Presentation of 30 cases and a review of the literature. Medicine, 50:223, 1971.
3. Fudenberg, H. H.: Genetically determined immune deficiency as the predisposing cause of "autoimmunity" and lymphoid neoplasia. Am. J. Med., 51:295, 1971.
4. O'Loughlin, J. M.: Immunologic deficiency states. Med. Clin. North Am., 56:747, 1972.
5. Soergel, K. H., and Sommers, S. C.: Idiopathic pulmonary hemosiderosis and related syndromes. Am. J. Med., 32:499, 1962.
6. Proskey, A. J., Weatherbee, L., Easterling, R. E., Greene, J. A., and Weller, J. M.: Goodpasture's syndrome: A report of five cases and review of the literature. Am. J. Med., 48:162, 1970.
7. Border, W. A., Baehler, R. W., Bhathena, D., and Glassock, R. J.: IgA antibasement membrane nephritis with pulmonary hemorrhage. Ann. Intern. Med., 91:21, 1979.
8. Soergel, K. H., and Sommers, S. C.: The alveolar epithelial lesion of idiopathic pulmonary hemosiderosis. Am. Rev. Resp. Dis., 85:540, 1962.
9. Donald, K. J., Edwards, R. L., and McEvoy, J. D. S.: Alveolar capillary basement membrane lesions in Goodpasture's syndrome and idiopathic pulmonary hemosiderosis. Am. J. Med., 59:642, 1975.
10. Hodson, C. J., France, N. E., and Gordon, I.: Idiopathic juvenile pulmonary haemosiderosis. J. Fac. Radiol., 5:50, 1953.
11. Ognibene, A. J., and Johnson, D. E.: Idiopathic pulmonary hemosiderosis in adults. Report of case and review of literature. Arch. Intern. Med., 111:503, 1963.
12. Nice, C. M., Jr., Menon, A. N. K., and Rigler, L. G.: Pulmonary manifestations in collagen diseases. Am. J. Roentgenol., 81:264, 1959.
13. Wallace, S. L., Diamond, H., and Kaplan, D.: Recent advances in rheumatoid diseases: The connective tissue diseases other than rheumatoid arthritis—1970 and 1971. Ann. Intern. Med., 77:455, 1972.
14. Block, S. R., and Christian, C. L.: The pathogenesis of systemic lupus erythematosus. Am. J. Med., 59:453, 1975.
15. Decker, J. L., Steinberg, A. D., Reinertsen, J. L., Plotz, P. H., Balow, J. E., and Klippel, J. H.: Systemic lupus erythematosus: Evolving concepts. Ann. Intern. Med., 91:587, 1979.
16. Scheinberg, M. A., Cathcart, E. S., and Goldstein, A. L.: Thymosin-induced reduction of "null-cells" in peripheral-blood lymphocytes of patients with systemic lupus erythematosus. Lancet, 1:424, 1975.
17. Dauphinee, J. M., and Talal, N.: Alterations in DNA synthetic response of thymocytes from NZB mice of different ages. Proc. Natl. Acad. Sci., 70:3769, 1973.
18. Gershwin, M. E., Ahmed, A., Steinberg, A. D., Thurman, G. B., and Goldstein, A. L.: Correction of T cell function by thymosin in New Zealand mice. J. Immunol., 113:1068, 1973.
19. Hahn, B. H., Sharp, G. C., Irvin, W. S., Kantor, O. S., Gardner, C. A., Bagby, M. K., Perry, H. M., Jr., and Osterland, C. K.: Immune responses to hydralazine and nuclear antigens in hydralazine-induced lupus erythematosus. Ann. Intern. Med., 76:365, 1972.
20. Gross, M., Esterly, J. R., and Earle, R. H.: Pulmonary alterations in systemic lupus erythematosus. Am. Rev. Resp. Dis., 105:572, 1972.
21. Olsen, E. G. J., and Lever, J. V.: Pulmonary changes in systemic lupus erythematosus. Br. J. Dis. Chest, 66:71, 1972.
22. Inoue, T., Kanayama, Y., Ohe, A., Kato, N., Horiguchi, T., Ishii, M., Shiota, K.: Immunopathologic studies of pneumonitis in systemic lupus erythematosus. Ann. Intern. Med., 91:30, 1979.
23. Garland, L. H., and Sisson, M. A.: Roentgen findings in the "collagen" diseases. Am. J. Roentgenol., 71:581, 1954.
24. Hoffbrand, B. I., and Beck, E. R.: "Unexplained" dyspnoea and shrinking lungs in systemic lupus erythematosus. Br. Med. J., 1:1273, 1965.

25. Eisenberg, H., Dubois, E. L., Sherwin, R. P., and Balchum, O. J.: Diffuse interstitial lung disease in systemic lupus erythematosus. Ann. Intern. Med., 79:37, 1973.

26. Marino, C. T., and Pertschuk, L. P.: Pulmonary hemorrhage in systemic lupus erythematosus. Arch. Intern. Med., 141:201, 1981.

27. Webb, W. R., and Gamsu, G.: Cavitary pulmonary nodules with systemic lupus erythematosus: Differential diagnosis. Am. J. Roentgenol., 136:27, 1981.

28. Bulgrin, J. G., Dubois, E. L., and Jacobson, G.: Chest roentgenographic changes in systemic lupus erythematosus. Radiology, 74:42, 1960.

29. Taylor, T. L., and Ostrum, H.: The roentgen evaluation of systemic lupus erythematosus. Am. J. Roentgenol., 82:95, 1959.

30. Winslow, W. A., Ploss, L. N., and Loitman, B.: Pleuritis in systemic lupus erythematosus: Its importance as an early manifestation in diagnosis. Ann. Intern. Med., 49:70, 1958.

31. Estes, D., and Christian, C. L.: The natural history of systemic lupus erythematosus by prospective analysis. Medicine, 50:85, 1971.

32. Fessel, W. J.: Systemic lupus erythematosus in the community. Arch Intern. Med., 134:1027, 1974.

33. Hunninghake, G. W., and Fauci, A. S.: Pulmonary involvement in the collagen vascular diseases. Am. Rev. Resp. Dis., 119:471, 1979.

34. Stahl, N. I., Klippel, J. H., and Decker, J. L.: Fever in systemic lupus erythematosus. Am. J. Med., 67:935, 1979.

35. Huang, C.-T., and Lyons, H. A.: Comparison of pulmonary function in patients with systemic lupus erythematosus, scleroderma, and rheumatoid arthritis. Am. Rev. Resp. Dis., 93:865, 1966.

36. Huang, C.-T., and Lyons, H. A.: Respiratory abnormalities in systemic lupus erythematosus: A neglected parameter of study. Clin. Res., 11:397, 1963.

37. Gibson, G. J., Edmonds, J. P., and Hughes, G. R. V.: Diaphragm function and lung involvement in systemic lupus erythematosus. Am. J. Med., 63:926, 1977.

38. Gordon, D. A., Stein, J. L., and Broder, I.: The extra-articular features of rheumatoid arthritis. A systematic analysis of 127 cases. Am. J. Med., 54:445, 1973.

39. Fraser, R. G., and Paré, J. A. P.: Diagnosis of Diseases of the Chest, 2nd Ed., vol. II. Philadelphia, W. B. Saunders Co., 1978, p. 921.

40. Rubin, E. H.: Pulmonary lesions in "rheumatoid disease" with remarks on diffuse interstitial pulmonary fibrosis. Am. J. Med., 19:569, 1955.

41. Lee, F. I., and Brain, A. T.: Chronic diffuse interstitial pulmonary fibrosis and rheumatoid arthritis. Lancet, 2:693, 1962.

42. Burrows, F. G. O.: Pulmonary nodules in rheumatoid disease: A report of two cases. Br. J. Radiol., 40:256, 1967.

43. Geddes, D. M., Corrin, B., Brewerton, D. A., Davies, R. J., and Turner-Warwick, M.: Progressive airway obliteration in adults and its association with rheumatoid disease. Quart. J. Med., 46:427, 1977.

44. DeHoratius, R. J., Abruzzo, J. L., and Williams, R. C., Jr.: Immunofluorescent and immunologic studies of rheumatoid lung. Arch. Intern. Med., 129:441, 1972.

45. Ellman, P., and Ball, R. E.: "Rheumatoid disease" with joint and pulmonary manifestations. Br. Med. J., 2:816, 1948.

46. Cervantes-Perez, P., Toro-Perez, A. H., and Rodriguez-Jurado, P.: Pulmonary involvement in rheumatoid arthritis. J.A.M.A., 243:1715, 1980.

47. Popper, M. S., Bogdonoff, M. L., and Hughes, R. L.: Interstitial rheumatoid lung disease. A reassessment and review of the literature. Chest, 62:243, 1972.

48. Locke, C. B.: Rheumatoid lung. Clin. Radiol., 14:43, 1963.

49. Carr, D. T., and Mayne, J. G.: Pleurisy with effusion in rheumatoid arthritis, with reference to the low concentration of glucose in pleural fluid. Am. Rev. Resp. Dis., 85:345, 1962.

50. Lillington, G. A., Carr, D. T., and Mayne, J. G.: Rheumatoid pleurisy with effusion. Arch. Intern. Med., 128:764, 1971.

51. Campbell, G. D., and Ferrington, E.: Rheumatoid pleuritis with effusion. Dis. Chest, 53:521, 1968.

52. Jones, F. L., Jr., and Blodgett, R. C., Jr.: Empyema in rheumatic pleuropulmonary disease. Ann. Intern. Med., 74:665, 1971.

53. Sienewicz, D., J., Martin, J. R., Moore, S., and Miller, A.: Rheumatoid nodules in the lung. J. Can. Assoc. Radiol., 13:73, 1962.

54. Caplan, A.: Certain unusual radiological appearances in the chest of coal-miners suffering from rheumatoid arthritis. Thorax, 8:29, 1953.

55. Abel, T., Andrews, B. S., Cunningham, P. H., Brunner, C. M., Davis, J. S., IV, and Horwitz, D. A.: Rheumatoid vasculitis: Effect of cyclophosphamide on the clinical course and levels of circulating immune complexes. Ann. Intern. Med., 93:407, 1980.

56. Centerwall, W. R., and Miller, M. M.: Ataxia, telangiectasia, and sinopulmonary infections: A syndrome of slowly progressive deterioration in childhood. J. Dis. Child., 95:385, 1958.

57. Murphy, K. C., Atkins, C. J., Offer, R. C., Hogg, J. C., and Stein, H. B.: Obliterative broncholitis in two rheumatoid arthritis patients treated with penicillamine. Arthritis Rheum., 24:557, 1981.

58. Farmer, R. G., Gifford, R. W., Jr., and Hines, E. A., Jr.: Prognostic significance of Raynaud's phenomenon and other clinical characteristics of systemic scleroderma. A study of 271 cases. Circulation, 21:1088, 1960.

59. Medsger, T. A., Jr., Masi, A. T., Rodnan, G. P., Benedek, T. G., and Robinson, H.: Survival with systemic sclerosis (scleroderma). Life-table analysis of clinical and demographic factors in 309 patients. Ann. Intern. Med., 75:369, 1971.

60. Bianchi, F. A., Bistue, A. R., Wendt, V. E., Puro, H. E., and Keech, M. K.: Analysis of twenty-seven cases of progressive systemic sclerosis (including two with combined systemic lupus erythematosus) and a review of the literature. J. Chron. Dis., 19:953, 1966.

61. Clark, J. A., Winkelmann, R. K., and Ward, L. E.: Serologic alterations in scleroderma and sclerodermatomyositis. Mayo Clin. Proc., 46:104, 1971.

62. Battle, W. M., Snape, W. J., Jr., Wright, S., Sullivan, M. A., Cohen, S., Meyers, A., and Tuthill, R.: Abnormal colonic motility in progressive systemic sclerosis. Ann. Intern. Med., 94:749, 1981.

63. Lally, E. V., and Jimenez, S. A.: Impotence in progressive systemic sclerosis. Ann. Intern. Med., 95:150, 1981.

64. Gordon, M. B., Klein, I., Dekker, A., Rodnan, G. P., and Medsger, T. A., Jr.: Thyroid disease in progressive systemic sclerosis: Increased frequency

of glandular fibrosis and hypothyroidism. Ann. Intern. Med., 95:431, 1981.

65. Winterbauer, R. H.: Multiple telangiectasia, Raynaud's phenomenon, sclerodactyly, and subcutaneous calcinosis: A syndrome mimicking hereditary hemorrhagic telangiectasia. Bull. Johns Hopkins Hosp., 114:361, 1964.

66. Fritzler, M. J., and Kinsella, T. D.: The CREST syndrome: A distinct serologic entity with anticentromere antibodies. Am. J. Med., 69:520, 1980.

67. Salerni, R., Rodnan, G. P., Leon, D. F., and Shaver, J. A.: Pulmonary hypertension in the CREST syndrome variant of progressive systemic sclerosis (scleroderma). Ann. Intern. Med., 86:394, 1977.

68. Velayos, E. E., Masi, A. T., Stevens, M. B., Shulman, L. E.: The "CREST" syndrome. Comparison with systemic sclerosis (scleroderma). Arch. Intern. Med., 139:1240, 1979.

69. Celoria, G. C., Friedell, G. H., and Sommers, S. C.: Raynaud's disease and primary pulmonary hypertension. Circulation, 22:1055, 1960.

70. Bohan, A., and Peter, J. B.: Polymyositis and dermatomyositis (first of two parts). N. Engl. J. Med., 292:344, 1975.

71. Rose, A. L., and Walton, J. N.: Polymyositis: A survey of 89 cases with particular reference to treatment and prognosis. Brain, 89:747, 1966.

72. Thomson, P. L., and MacKay, I. R.: Fibrosing alveolitis and polymyositis. Thorax, 25:504, 1970.

73. Salmeron, G., Greenberg, S. D., and Lidsky, M. D.: Polymyositis and diffuse interstitial lung disease. A review of the pulmonary histopathologic findings. Arch. Intern. Med., 141:1005, 1981.

74. Winkelmann, R. K., Mulder, D. W., Lambert, E. H., Howard, F. M., Jr., and Diesner, G. R.: Course of dermatomyositis-polymyositis: Comparison of untreated and cortisone-treated patients. Mayo Clin. Proc., 43:545, 1968.

75. Bohan, A., and Peter, J. B.: Polymyositis and dermatomyositis (second of two parts). N. Engl. J. Med., 292:403, 1975.

76. Sjögren, H.: Zur Kenntnis der Keratoconjunctivitis sicca (keratitis filiformis bei Hypofunktion der Tränendrüsen). (Keratoconjunctivitis sicca [keratitis filiformis with hypofunction of the lacrimal glands].) Acta Ophthalmol. (Suppl.), 2:1, 1933.

77. Whaley, K., Williamson, J., Chisholm, D. K., Webb, J., Mason, D. K., and Buchanan, W. W.: Sjögren's syndrome in progressive systemic sclerosis (scleroderma). Am. J. Med., 57:78, 1974.

78. Whaley, K., Webb, J., McEvoy, B. A., Hughes, G. R. V., Lee, H. P., MacSween, R. N. M., and Buchanan, W. W.: Sjögren's syndrome: 2. Clinical associations and immunological phenomena. Q. J. Med., 42:513, 1973.

79. Silbiger, M. L., and Peterson, C. C., Jr.: Sjögren's syndrome. Its roentgenographic features. Am. J. Roentgenol., 100:554, 1967.

80. Martinez-Lavin, M., Vaughan, J. H., and Tan, E. M.: Autoantibodies and the spectrum of Sjögren's syndrome. Ann. Intern. Med., 91:185, 1979.

81. Hamburger, M. I., Moutsopoulos, H. M., Lawley, T. J., and Frank, M. M.: Sjögren's syndrome: A defect in reticuloendothelial system Fc-receptor-specific clearance. Ann. Intern. Med., 91:534, 1979.

82. Hughes, G. R. V., and Whaley, K.: Sjögren's syndrome. Br. Med. J., 4:533, 1972.

83. Citro, L. A., Gordon, M. E., and Miller, W. T.: Eosinophilic lung disease (or how to slice P.I.E.). Am. J. Roentgenol., 117:787, 1973.

84. Israel, H. L., and Diamond, P.: Recurrent pulmonary infiltration and pleural effusion due to nitrofurantoin sensitivity. N. Engl. J. Med., 266:1024, 1962.

85. Ford, R. M.: Transient pulmonary eosinophilia and asthma. A review of 20 cases occurring in 5,702 asthma sufferers. Am. Rev. Resp. Dis., 93:797, 1966.

86. Peirce, C. B., Crutchlow, E. F., Henderson, A. T., and McKay, J. W.: Transient focal pulmonary edema. Am. Rev. Tuberc., 52:1, 1945.

87. Carrington, C. B., Addington, W. W., Goff, A. M., Madoff, I. M., Marks, A., Schwaber, J. R., and Gaensler, E. A.: Chronic eosinophilic pneumonia. N. Engl. J. Med., 280:787, 1969.

88. Christoforidis, A. J., and Molnar, W.: Eosinophilic pneumonia: Report of two cases with pulmonary biopsy. J.A.M.A., 173:157, 1960.

89. Pearson, D. J., and Rosenow, E. C., III: Chronic eosinophilic pneumonia (Carrington's). A follow-up study. Mayo. Clin. Proc., 53:73, 1978.

90. Clinicopathologic Conference: Disseminated eosinophilic collagen disease. Ann. J. Med., 56:221, 1974.

91. Epstein, D. M., Taormina, V., Gefter, W. B., and Miller, W. T.: The hypereosinophilic syndrome. Radiology, 140:59, 1981.

92. Bahk, Y. W.: Pulmonary paragonimiasis as a cause of Loeffler's syndrome. Radiology, 78:598, 1962.

93. Rosenow, E. C., III, DeRemee, R. A., and Dines, D. E.: Chronic nitrofurantoin pulmonary reaction: Report of five cases. N. Engl. J. Med., 279:1258, 1968.

94. Bone, R. C., Wolfe, J., Sobonyar, R. E., Kerby, G. R., Stechschulte, D., Ruth, W. E., and Welch, M.: Desquamative interstitial pneumonia following chronic nitrofurantoin therapy. Chest, 69(Suppl.):296, 1976.

95. Carrington, C. B., and Liebow, A. A.: Limited forms of angiitis and granulomatosis of Wegener's type. Am. J. Med., 41:497, 1966.

96. Fauci, A. S., and Wolff, S. M.: Wegener's granulomatosis: Studies in eighteen patients and a review of the literature. Medicine, 52:535, 1973.

97. Shillitoe, E. J., Lehner, T., Lessof, M. H., and Harrison, D. F. N.: Immunological features of Wegener's granulomatosis. Lancet, 1:281, 1974.

98. McGregor, M. B. B., and Sandler, G.: Wegener's granulomatosis. A clinical and radiological survey. Br. J. Radiol., 37:430, 1964.

99. Townley, R. G., Martin, J. C., and Souders, C. R.: Wegener's granulomatosis. Am. Rev. Resp. Dis., 85:576, 1962.

100. Rose, G. A., and Spencer, H.: Polyarteritis nodosa. Q. J. Med., 26:43, 1957.

101. Maguire, R., Fauci, A. S., Doppman, J. L., and Wolff, S. M.: Unusual radiographic features of Wegener's granulomatosis. Am. J. Roentgenol., 130:233, 1978.

102. Raitt, J. W.: Wegener's granulomatosis: Treatment with cytotoxic agents and adrenocorticoids. Ann. Intern. Med., 74:344, 1971.

103. Liebow, A. A., and Carrington, C. R. B.: The lymphomatoid variant of "limited Wegener's granulomatosis" (Abstract). Am. J. Pathol., 55:78-A, 1969.

104. Smith, S. R., Smith, J. W., and Theros, E. G.: Wegener's granulomatosis, lymphomatoid variant. Radiology, 98:439, 1971.

105. Liebow, A. A., Carrington, C. R. B., and Friedman, P. J.: Lymphomatoid granulomatosis. Human Pathol., 3:457, 1972.

106. Israel, H. L., Patchefsky, A. S., and Saldana, M. J.:

Wegener's granulomatosis, lymphomatoid granulomatosis, and benign lymphocytic angiitis and granulomatosis of lung. Recognition and treatment. Ann. Intern. Med., 87:691, 1977.

107. Zylak, C. J., Banerjee, R., Galbraith, P. A., and McCarthy, D. S.: Lung involvement in angioimmunoblastic lymphadenopathy (AIL). Radiology, 121:513, 1976.

108. Churg, J., and Strauss, L.: Allergic granulomatosis, allergic angiitis, and periarteritis nodosa. Am. J. Pathol., 27:277, 1951.

109. DeRemee, R. A., Weiland, L. H., and McDonald, T. J.: Respiratory vasculitis. Mayo Clin. Proc., 55:492, 1980.

110. Rose, G. A.: Clinical features of polyarteritis nodosa with lung involvement. Br. J. Tuberc., 51:113, 1957.

111. Fauci, A. S.: Vasculitis: New insights amid old enigmas. Am. J. Med., 67:916, 1979.

112. Hennell, H., and Sussman, M. L.: The roentgen features of eosinophilic infiltrations in the lungs. Radiology, 44:328, 1945.

113. Case Records of the Massachusetts General Hospital. Case 40-1981. N. Engl. J. Med., 305:814, 1981.

114. Pear, B. L.: Radiologic recognition of extrahepatic manifestations of hepatitis B antigenemia. Am. J. Roentgenol., 137:135, 1981.

115. Liebow, A. A.: Pulmonary angiitis and granulomatosis. Am. Rev. Resp. Dis., 108:1, 1973.

116. Editorial: Allergic alveolitis. Br. Med. J., 3:691, 1967.

117. Greer, A. E.: Mucoid impaction of the bronchi. Ann. Intern. Med., 46:506, 1957.

118. Shaw, R. R.: Mucoid impaction of bronchi. Thorac. Surg., 22:149, 1951.

119. Urschel, H. C., Paulson, D. L., and Shaw, R. R.: Mucoid impaction of the bronchi. Ann. Thorac. Surg., 2:1, 1966.

120. McCarthy, D. S., Simon, G., and Hargreave, F. E.: The radiological appearance in allergic bronchopulmonary aspergillosis. Clin. Radiol., 21:366, 1970.

121. Gefter, W. B., Epstein, D. M., and Miller, W. T.: Allergic bronchopulmonary aspergillosis: Less common patterns. Radiology, 140:307, 1981.

122. Rosenberg, M., Patterson, R., Roberts, M., and Wang, J.: The assessment of immunologic and clinical changes occurring during corticosteroid therapy for allergic bronchopulmonary aspergillosis. Am. J. Med., 64:599, 1978.

123. Katzenstein, A.-L., Liebow, A. A., and Friedman, P. J.: Bronchocentric granulomatosis, mucoid impaction, and hypersensitivity reactions to fungi. Am. Rev. Resp. Dis., 111:497, 1975.

124. Brouhuys, A.: Byssinosis in textile workers. Trans. N.Y. Acad. Sci. (Series II), 28:480, 1966.

125. Weill, H. (ed.): International Conference on Byssinosis. Chest, 79(Suppl.):1981.

126. Pratt, P. C.: Comparative prevalence and severity of emphysema and bronchitis at autopsy in cotton mill workers vs controls. Chest, 79(Suppl.):49S, 1981.

127. Rooke, G. B.: The pathology of byssinosis. Chest, 79(Suppl.):67S, 1981.

128. Cadhan, F. T.: Asthma due to grain rusts. J.A.M.A., 82:27, 1924.

129. Hargreave, F. E., and Pepys, J.: Allergic respiratory reactions in bird fanciers provoked by allergen inhalation provocation test. J. Allergy Clin. Immunol., 50:157, 1972.

130. Wenzel, F. J., Emanuel, D. A., and Gray, R. L.: Immunofluorescent studies in patients with farmer's lung. J. Allergy, 48:224, 1971.

131. Seal, R. M. E., Hapke, E. J., and Thomas, G. O., with Meek, J. C., and Hayes, M.: The pathology of the acute and chronic stages of farmer's lung. Thorax, 23:469, 1968.

132. Emanuel, D. A., Wenzel, F. J., Bowerman, C. I., and Lawton, B. R.: Farmer's lung. Clinical, pathologic and immunologic study of twenty-four patients. Am. J. Med., 37:392, 1964.

133. Pepys, J.: Pulmonary hypersensitivity disease due to inhaled organic antigens. Ann. Intern. Med., 64:943, 1966.

134. Grant, I. W. B., Blyth, W., Wardrop, V. E., Gordon, R. M., Pearson, J. C. G., and Mair, A.: Prevalence of farmer's lung in Scotland: A pilot survey. Br. Med. J., 1:530, 1972.

135. Pepys, J., and Jenkins, P. A.: Precipitin (F.L.H.) test in farmer's lung. Thorax, 20:21, 1965.

136. Pearsall, H. R., Morgan, E. H., Tesluk, H., and Beggs, D.: Parakeet dander pneumonitis, acute psittacokerato-pneumoconiosis. Report of a case. Bull. Mason Clin., 14:127, 1960.

137. Salvaggio, J., Arquembourg, P., Seabury, J., and Buechner, H.: Bagassosis. IV, Precipitins against extracts of thermophilic actinomycetes in patients with bagassosis. Am. J. Med., 46:544, 1969.

138. Fink, J. N., Banaszak, E. F., Barboriak, J. J., Hensley, G. T., Kurup, V. P., Scanon, G. T., Thiede, W. H., and Unger, G. F.: Interstitial lung disease due to contamination of forced air systems. Ann. Intern. Med., 84:406, 1976.

139. Channell, S., Blyth, W., Lloyd, M., Weir, D. M., Amos, W. M. G., Littlewood, A. P., Riddle, H. F. V., and Grant, I. W. B.: Allergic alveolitis in maltworkers. A clinical, mycological, and immunological study. Q. J. Med., 38:351, 1969.

140. Towey, J. W., Sweany, H. C., and Huron, W. H.: Severe bronchial asthma apparently due to fungus spores in maple bark. J.A.M.A., 99:453, 1932.

141. Avila, R., and Villar, T. G.: Suberosis. Respiratory disease in cork workers. Lancet, 1:620, 1968.

142. Margulis, A. R., Feinberg, S. B., Lester, R. G., and Good, R. A.: Roentgen manifestations of congenital agammaglobulinemia. Radiology, 69:354, 1957.

143. Rosen, Fred S., and Janeway, C. A.: The gamma globulins. III. The antibody deficiency syndromes. N. Engl. J. Med., 275:709, 1966.

144. Dukes, R. J., Rosenow, E. C., III, and Hermans, P. E.: Pulmonary manifestations of hypogammaglobulinaemia. Thorax, 33:603, 1978.

145. Cooper, M. S., Peterson, R. D. A., and Good, R. A.: A new concept of the cellular basis of immunity. J. Pediatr., 67:907, 1965.

146. Rosen, F. S.: The lymphocyte and the thymus gland—congenital and hereditary abnormalities. N. Engl. J. Med., 279:643, 1968.

147. Aldrich, R. A., Steinberg, A. G., and Campbell, D. C.: Pedigree demonstrating a sex-linked recessive condition characterized by draining ears, eczematoid dermatitis and bloody diarrhea. Pediatrics 13:133, 1954.

148. Cooper, M. D., Chase, H. P., Lowman, J. T., Krivit, W., and Good, R. A.: Wiskott-Aldrich syndrome. An immunologic deficiency disease involving the afferent limb of immunity. Am. J. Med., 44:499, 1968

8

Neoplastic Diseases of the Lungs

BENIGN NEOPLASMS

Primary neoplasms of the lung other than bronchogenic carcinoma are uncommon. For example, bronchial adenomas constitute almost half of all "benign" neoplasms of the respiratory tract[1] but less than 6 to 10 per cent of all primary lung neoplasms.[1] In fact, in two large series, each spanning over 20 years, the incidence of bronchial adenoma among all bronchial neoplasms was 35 in 2953 cases (1.2 per cent).[2]

This section deals with all neoplasms other than bronchogenic and bronchiolo-alveolar carcinoma that originate from epithelial or mesenchymal lung tissues. Although these neoplasms usually appear benign histologically, many are potentially malignant. Their morphologic, roentgenographic, and clinical manifestations within the lung are varied, depending almost entirely upon the relationship of the neoplasm to an airway. Thus, if they occur in the lung periphery, near the hilum, or within the medulla and they are nonobstructive, they may cause no symptoms or signs and may be discovered only during mass screening. If, however, they obstruct a bronchial lumen—the more usual mode of presentation—they cause atelectasis and obstructive pneumonitis, with bronchiectasis and abscess formation distal to the neoplasm. In these cases the clinical picture is more obvious, with cough, hemoptysis, wheezing, and repeated respiratory infections. Some of these patients have been considered clinically to have bronchial asthma, often for years, before the correct diagnosis is made by roentgenography or bronchoscopy.

BRONCHIAL ADENOMA

Bronchial adenomas arise from the duct epithelium of bronchial mucous glands. Although the term "adenoma" implies a benign epithelial lesion, bronchial adenomas are in reality neoplasms of low-grade malignancy. Pathologically, they can be divided into two distinct groups— *carcinoid* and *salivary gland types*. The latter can be subdivided into *cylindromas, mucoepidermoid adenomas*, and *pleomorphic adenomas* (mixed tumors). The carcinoid type accounts for 85 to 95 per cent of bronchial adenomas.[3] This neoplasm is at least as common in females as in males, and most series indicate a higher incidence in the former.[1] Ninety per cent of patients are less than 50 years of age, the mean age being the late 30's or early 40's.

PATHOLOGIC CHARACTERISTICS

Approximately 80 per cent of bronchial adenomas arise from the major bronchi and, therefore, are situated centrally.[1, 3, 4] Most present as well-circumscribed masses in the submucosa of larger bronchi. Overlying bronchial mucosa is usually intact unless secondary infection has resulted in ulceration. The degree of protrusion of the tumor into the bronchial lumen varies from complete obstruction to an "iceberg" effect in which much of the tumor extends into contiguous tissues and causes little deformity of the lumen.

Carcinoid adenomas consist of regular cuboidal cells, with fine granular cytoplasm and round or oval deeply staining nuclei, usually arranged in sheets, strands, or islands. Mitotic figures are virtually absent. In most cases the stroma is highly vascular.

Cylindromas occur in the trachea and major bronchi;[1] they usually recur after removal and are more malignant and locally invasive than the carcinoid type.[1] Cylindromas originate in mixed serous and mucous glands and are composed of small pleomorphic and stellate cells, with darkly staining nuclei, mostly arranged in trabeculae or interlacing cylinders or tubes.

Mucoepidermoid tumors consist of anastomosing cellular columns and masses separated by fine sheets of delicate connective tissue. The cells are cylindric and pseudostratified. As the name indicates, there are distinct areas of squamous cells together with mucus-secreting columnar cells.

Most bronchial adenomas have a well-defined capsule and appear benign, but a small percentage invade local areas. The incidence of metastases ranges from none, even with long-term follow-up,[3] to 10 per cent with metastatic spread to regional lymph nodes or remote areas.[4]

ROENTGENOGRAPHIC MANIFESTATIONS

These depend largely upon the location of the adenoma. Since 80 per cent of these lesions are located centrally in major or segmental bronchi, bronchial obstruction is the commonest morphologic and roentgenographic finding. Lesions that arise in the trachea may occasion airway obstruction for long periods of time before being discovered, as was the case in the patient illustrated in Figure 8–1. In most cases of bronchial origin, obstruction is complete, with peripheral atelectasis and obstructive

pneumonitis. Thus, the characteristic roentgenographic pattern is of homogeneous increase in density confined precisely to a lobe or to one or more segments, usually with considerable loss of volume (Figure 8–2). Segmental atelectasis and pneumonitis may show periodic exacerbations and remissions, presumably reflecting intermittent relief of the obstruction. However, recurrent infections distal to the neoplasm inevitably result in bronchiectasis and lung abscesses.

Although massive collapse is fairly common,[1, 27] collateral air drift may prevent atelectasis even with complete obstruction of a major bronchus. We have seen one patient whose left lower lobe bronchus was completely obstructed by a carcinoid adenoma and in whom both the volume of the lobe and its roentgenographic density were reduced, indicating decreased ventilation and resultant diminished perfusion. The phenomena of reflex vasoconstriction and resultant oligemia in response to reduced ventilation and local hypoxia are now well recognized;[5, 6] it was illustrated in dramatic fashion by a patient we have recently seen in whom a

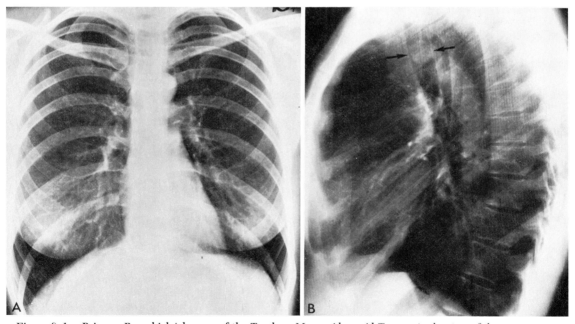

Figure 8–1.   Primary Bronchial Adenoma of the Trachea, Mucoepidermoid Type.   At the time of the roentgenogram illustrated in *A*, this 32-year-old woman presented with a 4-year history of sporadic attacks of acute shortness of breath that had been diagnosed and treated by her family physician as spasmodic asthma. A number of roentgenographic examinations of the chest during this period had been interpreted as normal. This posteroanterior roentgenogram reveals mild to moderate overinflation of both lungs, consistent with a diagnosis of asthma. However, note that the mediastinum is intolerably underpenetrated, to a point at which the tracheal air column is not visualized. In lateral projection *(B)*, a smooth, sharply demarcated mass can be identified in the plane of the tracheal air column *(arrows)*. The mass is almost completely occluding the tracheal air column. Following resection, the patient experienced an uneventful recovery. This case illustrates graphically the often repeated observation that the tracheal air column tends to be a "blind area" for many radiologists. (Courtesy of Dr. Michael Lefcoe, Victoria Hospital, London, Ontario.)

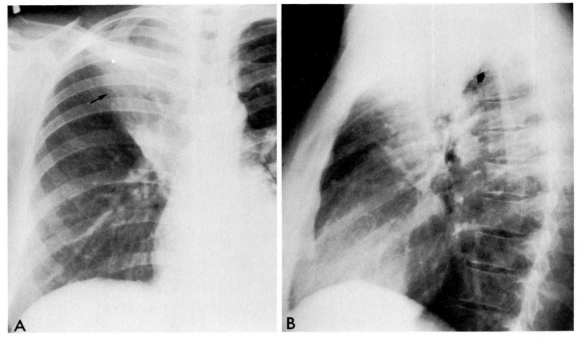

Figure 8–2. Bronchial Adenoma (Carcinoid Type). Views of the right hemithorax from posteroanterior (A) and lateral (B) roentgenograms demonstrate a roughly triangular shadow of homogeneous density occupying the superomedial portion of the right lung. The inferolateral border of the shadow is formed by the upward displaced minor fissure (*arrow* in A) and the posterior border by the anteriorly displaced major fissure (*arrow* in B). This shadow represents combined consolidation and atelectasis of the right upper lobe due to an endobronchial obstructing lesion (obstructive pneumonitis). The lobe was resected; proved bronchial adenoma, carcinoid type.

large carcinoid adenoma almost completely obstructed the orifice of the right main bronchus, resulting in reduced volume of the right lung at TLC, marked expiratory air trapping, and severe oligemia.

Bronchial adenomas arising peripherally (roughly 20 per cent) do not cause bronchial obstruction and appear roentgenographically as solitary nodules. They are usually homogeneous in density, sharply circumscribed, round or oval,[4] and in many cases slightly lobulated. They average about 4 cm in diameter (range, 1 to 10 cm)[4] and occur most often in the right upper and middle lobes and the lingula.[4] Calcification and ossification are rare.

Tomography may be helpful in determining morphologic characteristics of these neoplasms, particularly centrally placed tumors likely to cause deformity of a contiguous bronchial air column. Osseous metastases develop in few cases, and are more often osteolytic than osteoblastic.[7]

CLINICAL MANIFESTATIONS

Most peripheral adenomas occasion no symptoms, but the majority of endobronchial lesions give rise to symptoms and signs stemming from atelectasis and pneumonitis secondary to bronchial obstruction. Symptoms include cough, expectoration, fever, wheezing, and chest pain. Hemoptysis occurs in at least 50 per cent of patients,[1, 3] reflecting the highly vascular nature of these neoplasms. Physical signs depend upon the degree of obstruction, the size of the bronchus obstructed, and whether peripheral infection has developed.

Some carcinoid adenomas give rise to symptoms and signs of the *carcinoid syndrome* (*see* page 418). Patients with the clinical picture of the carcinoid syndrome invariably have widespread metastatic disease, usually involving the liver.[8] *Cushing's syndrome* also may develop in patients with bronchial carcinoids; by 1973, 18 such cases had been described.[9]

Overall prognosis in patients with bronchial adenoma is good; in one series,[10] actuarially assessed survival of 71 patients who underwent surgical resection was 75 per cent at 15 years.

PULMONARY HAMARTOMA

A hamartoma is a "tumor" composed of the tissues that normally constitute the organ in which it occurs, but the tissue elements are not organized. Despite the concept that this tumor originates from an embryologic rest, it seldom becomes roentgenographically visible until adulthood. In fact, the peak incidence is in the sixth decade and only 6 per cent occur in patients under the age of 30.[11] In Bateson's review of 2958 solitary lung lesions,[12] 5.7 per cent were hamartomas.

Pathologically, unlike bronchial adenomas, nearly all hamartomas lie in the peripheral parenchyma. Only about 10 per cent are endobronchial,[12] although even the peripheral tumors are thought to arise in the connective tissues of small bronchi. They tend to be well circumscribed and slightly lobulated. Cartilage is almost invariably present and often predominates. Other tissues often present include epithelium (seldom ciliated), fibrous connective tissue, smooth muscle, adipose tissue, and sometimes bone. The tissues are arranged haphazardly with complete lack of organization. Hamartomas are benign.

Roentgenographically, pulmonary hamartomas typically are well-circumscribed solitary nodules, the majority smaller than 4 cm in diameter,[11, 12] without lobar predominance.[13] Calcification is less common than formerly thought, being identified on the preoperative roentgenogram in only two of 65 lesions removed surgically.[13] The roentgenographic pattern of calcification most often resembles popcorn, a finding that is almost diagnostic. Serial films may reveal slow or, rarely, rapid growth of these lesions,[14] increasing the difficulty in differentiation from bronchogenic carcinoma. In only a small percentage of cases, bronchial obstruction leads to atelectasis, obstructive pneumonitis, and progressive peripheral lung destruction.

Clinically, because of their peripheral location, hamartomas are unlikely to cause symptoms. Hemoptysis is rare. In the absence of calcification, the differential diagnosis of peripheral hamartoma must be from bronchogenic carcinoma, and thoracotomy is required for definitive diagnosis.

PAPILLOMA

Papillomas are the commonest laryngeal tumors in children but are rare in adults. They may be single or multiple and, when multiple, may extend down the tracheobronchial tree into the lungs, obstructing the airways. Distal spread occurs in about 2 per cent of cases of juvenile laryngeal papillomatosis, usually limited to the trachea.[15] Bronchial papillomas very rarely develop in the absence of laryngeal or tracheal lesions.[16]

Pathologically, papillomas contain a core of vascular connective tissue covered by stratified squamous epithelium and occasionally by a surface layer of ciliated respiratory columnar epithelium.[15] The lesions probably are viral in origin. Malignant change occurs in some.[15]

Roentgenographically, papillomas characteristically obstruct airways, resulting in peripheral atelectasis and obstructive pneumonitis; cavitation and bronchiectasis are frequent.[17] Multiple papillomas deep in the smaller bronchi and alveolar ducts may be visualized as multiple nodular lesions, frequently associated with cavitation[15] and often resembling advanced cystic bronchiectasis.

Clinically, the diagnosis should be suspected in any patient with a history of recurrent papillomas of the larynx in whom cough, hemoptysis, asthmalike symptoms, recurrent pneumonia, and atelectasis develop.

LEIOMYOMA AND MULTIPLE PULMONARY FIBROLEIOMYOMAS

Leiomyomas arise from the smooth muscle of the lung periphery or from the walls of the trachea or bronchi and are as often malignant (leiomyosarcoma) as benign.[18]

Morphologically, leiomyomas are usually found in the lung periphery. They range from 2.5 to 13 cm in diameter and are encapsulated. They tend to be rather fibrous in consistency and perhaps should be termed "fibroleiomyoma;" they may show hyaline degeneration and calcification. Leiomyosarcomas usually occur in large bronchi, range in size from 1 to 4 cm, and may be invasive; they metastasize by way of the bloodstream, not to regional lymph nodes.

Roentgenographic manifestations vary with the location and number of tumors. Peripheral lesions usually present as solitary nodules of various sizes.[18] Those that arise from the wall of a major or segmental bronchus may obstruct the lumen, causing atelectasis and obstructive pneumonitis.

Clinically, the peripheral lesions usually occasion no symptoms. Centrally located benign and malignant varieties may give rise to cough, hemoptysis, dyspnea, chest pain, atelectasis, and obstructive pneumonitis.[18] The clinical picture may simulate asthma.

Multiple pulmonary fibroleiomyomas appear to be a distinct entity. Since most, if not all, patients have had "benign" uterine fibroids, and the lesions are invariably multiple and occur only in women, these tumors may be metastases from well-differentiated, slow-growing leiomyosarcomas.[19] In fact, there would appear to be some justification in abandoning the term "benign metastasizing leiomyoma" in favor of "metastatic well-differentiated leiomyosarcoma" on the strength of four cogent observations:[19] (1) there is a frequent association with uterine smooth muscle neoplasms; (2) cases with equally benign appearing histology have shown lymph node metastases; (3) the nonmesenchymal elements have been shown to represent engulfed bits of adjacent pulmonary tissue; and (4) the histologic distinction between the benign and malignant nature of mesenchymal neoplasms is known to be unreliable in some cases. However this unusual condition is classified, it should not be confused with pulmonary lymphangiomyomatosis, a diffuse dysplasia of smooth muscle that may occur alone or as one manifestation of tuberous sclerosis (*see* Chapter 14).

Multiple pulmonary fibroleiomyomas are well-differentiated, noninvasive bundles of smooth muscle cells interspersed with bands of fibrous tissue and cystic or tubular formations, lined by cuboidal or columnar epithelium; neither cartilage nor bone is present. They present roentgenographically as nodules 0.5 to 4.5 cm in diameter; they may increase in both size and number or new nodules may appear while others shrink and actually disappear.[20]

OTHER MESENCHYMAL AND RELATED NEOPLASMS

Fibroma is a benign fibrous tissue neoplasm of the lung whose malignant counterpart is fibrosarcoma. This tumor may arise from the peripheral parenchyma or from the walls of the trachea or bronchi. The roentgenographic appearance is not distinctive. Peripheral fibromas present as solitary nodules, and endobronchial lesions cause segmental or lobar atelectasis.

Lipoma is a benign neoplasm composed of adipose tissue. Thoracic lipomas are usually solitary and may arise in the parenchyma of the lung, the tracheobronchial tree, the pleura, or in tissues immediately external to the parietal pleura. Approximately 80 per cent arise in the wall of the tracheobronchial tree and sometimes cause atelectasis and pneumonitis as a result of bronchial obstruction. The parenchymal, subpleural, and small endobronchial lipomas typically present as solitary nodules. The majority of intrapleural lipomas lie in the right cardiophrenic angle.

Chondroma is an extremely rare benign lesion that arises in the parenchyma or in a bronchial wall. It consists of cartilage covered with epithelium, without glands or other elements. Most endobronchial lesions lie in the medial third of either lung, adjacent to a large bronchus. Roentgenographic and clinical signs depend on the presence or absence of airway obstruction.

Hemangioma is a benign tumor consisting of a mass of proliferated thin-walled vessels with little surrounding stroma. The lesion may sclerose, forming hyalinized connective tissue— thus, the designation "sclerosing hemangioma." Some authors[21] do not accept all sclerosing hemangiomas as vascular in origin and refer to such lesions as fibrous histiocytomas. Hemangiomas usually develop in the peripheral parenchyma, commonly subpleural. They appear roentgenographically as single or multiple nodules. No connection is visible between the lesion and the pulmonary vasculature. Hemoptysis is very common.

Hemangiopericytoma is a neoplasm that may arise anywhere in the body. It originates in the capillary pericyte, a cell now considered to be multipotential and capable of developing into other cell types. In the lungs, the lesions are usually large, and about 50 per cent are malignant. They are usually centrally situated and encapsulated but may grow so large as to reach the visceral pleura. Microscopically they are highly vascular. The roentgenographic appearance is that of a clearly demarcated nodule or mass.

Neurogenic tumors are exceedingly rare in the lungs although not uncommon in the mediastinum. They may occur in a benign state as neurilemomas or neurofibromas, or in a malignant form as neurogenic sarcomas. These neoplasms may arise in the peripheral lung parenchyma or (rarely) in a bronchial wall.

Chemodectoma is a nonchromaffin paraganglioma; unlike chromaffin paragangliomas (pheochromocytoma), this neoplasm has no hormonal activity. It occurs much more frequently in the mediastinum than in the lungs, as aortic or carotid body tumors. Most pulmonary chemodectomas are solitary and may be very large.

Granular cell "myoblastoma" is a neoplasm that most often arises in the tongue, skin, subcutaneous breast tissue, and sometimes in the lungs. It is almost invariably benign. The origin of this neoplasm has not been established. It develops almost invariably in the walls of large bronchi and may present roentgenographically as a solitary nodule or with atelectasis and obstructive pneumonitis, depending upon whether a bronchus is obstructed.

Pulmonary blastoma is a rare malignant neoplasm sometimes designated "carcinosarcoma."[22] Characteristically it is situated in peripheral lung parenchyma, often subpleurally. It is a mixed tumor with malignant epithelial and connective-tissue components that possess a distinctive histologic appearance resembling fetal lung. There are no specific clinical or roentgenologic features of this neoplasm that help to distinguish it from any other peripheral pulmonary mass. Overall prognosis is poor.

Endometriosis develops rarely in the thorax, usually in the parenchyma but sometimes endobronchially. The origin of endometrial tissue in the lung is not known. In the few cases reported, the roentgenographic appearance is of a solitary nodule measuring up to 4 cm in diameter. Recurrent pneumothorax is an unusually frequent complication and tends to occur simultaneously with menstrual periods (catamenial pneumothorax); the pneumothorax is almost always right-sided. Clinically, the diagnosis may be strongly suspected from the history alone when hemoptysis or pneumothorax occurs coincidentally with menstrual periods.

Pulmonary teratoma is a very uncommon benign tumor within the thorax and almost invariably develops in the mediastinum rather than the lung. This tumor contains nonmalignant tissue from one or more of the three germ layers, including skin, hair, and other dermal appendages, and pancreatic and osteoid tissue. Presenting clinical features are hemoptysis and, rarely, expectoration of hair.

Primary pulmonary pseudolymphoma is a term that derives from cases in which pulmonary parenchymal consolidation has closely resembled malignant lymphoma histologically but in which follow-up studies after surgical extirpation have shown no recurrence. An additional differential factor is noninvolvement of lymph nodes. This benign condition consists histologically of a mixed cellular infiltration, with mature lymphocytes predominating. The commonest roentgenographic presentation is of segmental parenchymal consolidation that tends to stop short of the pleural surface;[23] an air bronchogram is invariable.

In recent years, a variety of disorders of the chest have been recognized in which a common histologic feature is the presence of mature-appearaing lymphocytes.[24, 25] These lymphoid disorders involve the lung parenchyma or the mediastinal or hilar lymph nodes and include pseudolymphoma, lymphocytic interstitial pneumonitis, lymphomatoid granulomatosis, giant lymph node hyperplasia (Castleman's disease), and well-differentiated lymphocytic lymphoma. Distinction between these disorders can be of considerable importance therapeutically and prognostically.

Inflammatory pseudotumor is an ill-defined entity that has several synonyms, the most familiar of which are plasma cell granuloma and histiocytoma. Although its precise etiology is unknown, it is considered by most pathologists to represent a reparative process of an inflammatory lesion. The lesions are usually well circumscribed, up to 7 cm in diameter. Histologically, reactive fibroblasts predominate in a mixture of inflammatory cells including plasma cells, lymphocytes, foreign body giant cells, histiocytes, and foam cells. Roentgenographically, this benign tumor presents as a solitary pulmonary nodule or as a homogeneous area of consolidation that may mimic primary or metastatic neoplasm. Some patients give a history of an acute respiratory illness, which suggests that the process represents a stage in the resolution of acute pneumonia—so-called unresolved pneumonia or carnified lung. Typically, long-term follow-up shows no change in size or configuration of these lesions.

MALIGNANT NEOPLASMS

BRONCHOGENIC CARCINOMA

INCIDENCE

Even taking into account the increased longevity and the wider use of better methods of diagnosis, the incidence of bronchogenic carcinoma has increased progressively since the turn of the century. Formerly a relatively rare neoplasm, it is now the commonest fatal malignancy in males, at least in the western hemisphere. The 1966 statistics for the United Kingdom show that, in men, 39 per cent of all deaths attributable to cancer and 8 per cent of all deaths from all causes were due to bronchogenic carcinoma.[26] More recent statistical analyses in Canada indicate that by the year 1985, of individuals aged 45 to 64 years who smoke 25 or more cigarettes a day, lung cancer will develop in approximately one in 20 men and one in 50 women.[27] Cigarette consumption by women has increased considerably in recent years, to the extent that if present trends continue, within the next decade bronchogenic carcinoma will become the number one cause of death from cancer in women.[28]

Overall, 75 to 90 per cent of patients with bronchogenic carcinoma are male and 75 per cent of cases occur in the fifth and sixth decades.[30] The disease is rare before the age of 35.

EPIDEMIOLOGY

Although, as with most neoplasms in humans, the etiology of bronchogenic carcinoma remains obscure, statistical evidence suggests that prolonged inhalation of carcinogenic substances may be a major cause. It is probable also that familial or racial predisposition exists, and that immunologic status plays a role in determining susceptibility.

Influence of Cigarette Smoking

There is now a vast amount of statistical evidence incriminating cigarette smoking as a causative factor in bronchogenic carcinoma. The incidence is four to ten times more frequent in cigarette smokers as a whole than in nonsmokers,[31] and the incidence in heavy smokers is 15 to 30 times higher than in nonsmokers.[32] More than 30 retrospective studies in 10 countries and seven prospective studies in Canada, the United Kingdom, and the United States have shown that the risk of lung cancer increases directly in proportion to the number of cigarettes smoked.[31, 32]

The rising curve of incidence appears to have reached a plateau for males, which correlates well with the assumption that patients in whom the diagnosis is now being made first smoked maximally as young men after World War I.[33] The curve for women continues to rise, presumably because women did not smoke heavily until the early 1930's.[33]

Although the correlation between cigarette smoking and bronchogenic carcinoma was formerly thought to apply particularly to the squamous-cell and oat-cell types,[34] there is increasing evidence that adenocarcinoma also is related to this habit.[34, 35]

Influence of Industrial Exposure

Various substances in mining and industry have been cited as causes of bronchial neoplasm. Undoubtedly the major one is *asbestos*, a substance of worldwide distribution and extensive industrial use. The risk of lung cancer among asbestos workers is calculated to be six to ten times that of the population at large,[36, 37] and one report recorded an astounding incidence (13.8 per cent) of squamous-cell lung carcinoma in cases of asbestosis.[38] Not only is the incidence of lung cancer increased with asbestos exposure; of equal importance is the highly significant correlation of asbestos fiber inhalation and the development of pleural and peritoneal neoplasms.[39]

Other substances that have been incrimi-
nated as being potentially carcinogenic include radioactive materials, nickel ore, chloromethyl methyl ether[40] and bischloromethyl ether, bichromates, hematite, arsenic, silica, coal dust, toxic gases, and combinations of these substances; a study in Ontario, Canada, suggests that less than 1 per cent of cancer is caused by occupational factors, over 80 per cent of these being pleuropulmonary in origin.[41]

All carcinogenic agents have in common a long induction period or a long interval between cessation of exposure and the appearance of the neoplasm, indicating that the carcinogenic stimulus is weak. The histologic type of neoplasm thought to result from inhaled carcinogens is predominantly squamous-cell or undifferentiated in type and less commonly glandular. The finding of a greater incidence of bronchogenic carcinoma in urban than in rural populations leads inevitably to the conclusion that carcinogens in city air probably play some role in the development of many cases of bronchogenic carcinoma, perhaps in association with cigarette smoking.[42]

Influence of Concomitant Disease

Some workers accept without question that cancer of the lung can originate in a scar. In a review of 1186 cases of lung cancer, Auerback and his colleagues[43] found 15 per cent to originate in the periphery of the lung and 45 per cent of these to occur in relationship to a scar. These authors observed an increasing incidence of scar cancer over a 21-year period; 72 per cent of the scar cancers were adenocarcinomas, 18 per cent squamous-cell carcinomas, and none was oat-cell or small cell in type. No relationship was found between smoking habits and scar cancer.

The association of tuberculosis and carcinoma in the same area of lung has been reported frequently enough to suggest that this combination may be more than coincidental.[44] In some cases the malignancy appears to originate in tuberculous scars, suggesting that the hyperplasia and metaplasia associated with healing may relate to the later development of neoplasia. Such scars may be inconspicuous, the first evidence of neoplasia being metastases or nonmetastatic extrapulmonary manifestations. In two large series of patients with both tuberculosis and bronchogenic carcinoma, the association appeared purely coincidental;[45, 46] in another series of 24 patients, 21 had lesions in the same lung but in only three were the lesions contiguous.[47] Of the 82 peripheral cancers related to scars reported by Auerback and his associates,[43] over three-quarters were found in the upper lobes and more than half were related to infarcts; if a cause and effect relationship truly exists between scars and cancer, the observation regarding infarcts is indeed surprising, since both infarcts and scars occur more frequently in lower lobes.

Other conditions in which a possible carcinogenic effect is operative include diffuse interstitial pulmonary fibrosis (fibrosing alveolitis),[48] the end-stage lung,[49] and scleroderma.[50]

Influence of Genetics and Immunologic Status

In 1954, by demonstrating a familial clustering that could be dissociated from environmental factors, Tokuhata[51] showed that susceptibility to lung cancer can be inherited. More recently it has been shown[52] that this genetic factor lies in an inducible membrane-bound enzyme, aryl hydrocarbon hydroxylase (AHH), whose activity can be increased by adding polycyclic hydrocarbons and other substrates.

Antibody production and cell-mediated immunity may play major roles in the host's response to antigenic neoplastic cells.[53] A study of delayed cutaneous hypersensitivity in 219 patients with bronchogenic carcinoma[54] showed correlation between the degree of differentiation of cell type, stage of the disease, response to chemotherapy, and prognosis and survival; many patients with anergy had advanced, undifferentiated cell tumors that failed to respond to therapy and were rapidly fatal. Cellular immunity in cancer appears to relate to the organ in which the neoplasm originates, as well as to tumor anaplasia and clinically advanced disease.[55]

PATHOLOGIC CHARACTERISTICS

The various histologic types of primary bronchogenic carcinoma produce different clinical and roentgenographic patterns and have dissimilar prognoses. The classification of neoplasms is intrinsically subjective, and pathologists have been shown to disagree on as many as 25 per cent of cases. Of major importance in histopathologic labeling is the adequacy of specimens; for example, a biopsy specimen may not be representative of the predominant cell type, since any neoplasm may contain regional histologic differences. Thus, any large series includes cases that cannot be classified precisely.

Although differences of opinion still exist as to the proper classification of lung neoplasms, that proposed by the World Health Organiza-

TABLE 8–1. WHO INTERNATIONAL HISTOLOGIC CLASSIFICATION OF LUNG TUMORS (1977)*

I. EPITHELIAL TUMORS

A. BENIGN
  1. Papillomas
    a. Squamous-cell papilloma
    b. "Transitional" papilloma
  2. Adenomas
    a. Pleomorphic adenoma ("mixed" tumor)
    b. Monomorphic adenoma
    c. Others
B. DYSPLASIA
   CARCINOMA IN SITU
C. MALIGNANT
  1. Squamous-cell carcinoma (epidermoid carcinoma)
     Variant:
    a. Spindle-cell (squamous) carcinoma
  2. Small cell carcinoma
    a. Oat-cell carcinoma
    b. Intermediate cell type
    c. Combined oat-cell carcinoma
  3. Adenocarcinoma
    a. Acinar adenocarcinoma
    b. Papillary adenocarcinoma
    c. Bronchiolo-alveolar carcinoma
    d. Solid carcinoma with mucous formation
  4. Large cell carcinoma
     Variants:
    a. Giant cell carcinoma
    b. Clear cell carcinoma
  5. Adenosquamous carcinoma
  6. Carcinoid tumor
  7. Bronchial gland carcinomas
    a. Adenoid cystic carcinoma
    b. Mucoepidermoid carcinoma
    c. Others
  8. Others

II. SOFT TISSUE TUMORS

III. MESOTHELIAL TUMORS

A. BENIGN MESOTHELIOMA
B. MALIGNANT MESOTHELIOMA
  1. Epithelial
  2. Fibrous (spindle-cell)
  3. Biphasic

IV. MISCELLANEOUS TUMORS

A. BENIGN
B. MALIGNANT
  1. Carcinosarcoma
  2. Pulmonary blastoma
  3. Malignant melanoma
  4. Malignant lymphomas
  5. Others

V. SECONDARY TUMORS

VI. UNCLASSIFIED TUMORS

VII. TUMORLIKE LESIONS

A. HAMARTOMA
B. LYMPHOPROLIFERATIVE LESIONS
C. TUMORLET
D. EOSINOPHILIC GRANULOMA
E. "SCLEROSING HEMANGIOMA"
F. INFLAMMATORY PSEUDOTUMOR
G. OTHERS

*From WHO report on meeting on the histological classification of lung tumors. Geneva, October 24–28, 1977.

tion in a 1977 meeting (Table 8–1) appears to be the most widely accepted by pathologists. Many of the neoplasms listed were considered in the section on benign and potentially malignant lung tumors; this section deals primarily with groups I to V and group IX (neoplasms that histopathologically have both sarcomatous and carcinomatous features).

Incidence Based on Cell Type

A review of 662 necropsies[57] may reflect a realistic picture of present-day pathologic criteria: 35.2 per cent of the neoplasms were designated epidermoid (squamous-cell) carcinoma, 24.6 per cent were small cell carcinoma, 25.2 per cent were adenocarcinoma, and 14.2 per cent were large cell undifferentiated carcinoma. Rare varieties of primary lung neoplasms include giant cell and syncytial cell carcinoma and the carcinosarcomas.

Classification Based on Cell Type

In a comprehensive review of the histology of about 1000 cases of bronchogenic carcinoma at the Mayo Clinic during 1950 to 1957, the neoplasms were classified into four types: squamous-cell carcinoma, adenocarcinoma, and large cell and small cell anaplastic carcinomas.[58] The following paragraphs summarize the criteria used for cell type identification.

SQUAMOUS-CELL CARCINOMA. This neoplasm is characterized histologically by keratin production, the presence of intercellular bridges or keratohyaline granules, and a fairly characteristic growth pattern of sizable islands of large, rather sharply outlined, neoplastic cells. Poorly differentiated squamous-cell carcinomas merge imperceptibly into a pattern of completely anaplastic or undifferentiated large cell carcinoma.

ADENOCARCINOMA. Histologic criteria for diagnosis of adenocarcinoma include a recognizable glandular architecture, or the production of mucus by the neoplasm, or both. In some cases, neoplastic cells line the alveoli, particularly at the outer margin of the growth, simulating bronchiolo-alveolar carcinoma.

LARGE CELL UNDIFFERENTIATED CARCINOMA. This type shows no recognizable differentiation toward squamous-cell or adenocarcinoma and contains no cells of the small or oat-cell variety.

SMALL CELL UNDIFFERENTIATED (OAT-CELL) CARCINOMA. This type is characterized by extremely small cells completely lacking differentiation. The cells are mostly round or oval, with some spindle-shaped. The largest cells are two to three times the diameter of a lymphocyte. There is very little cytoplasm, and mitotic figures are common. These tumor cells contain neurosecretory type granules in their cytoplasm, similar to those in intestinal argentaffin cells, adrenal medullary cells, sympathetic nerve endings, and cells of bronchial carcinoid tumors.[59] Oat-cell pulmonary cancer and bronchial carcinoid tumors may be closely related[59]—perhaps they are the malignant and locally malignant varieties, respectively, of tumors derived from Kulchitsky-type cells normally found throughout the bronchial tree.

Studies have shown a considerable degree of interobserver disagreement in the classification of lung tumors, which, it is hoped, may be reduced by the revision of the 1967 WHO criteria proposed in 1977.[60]

Roentgenographic Patterns Based on Cell Type

The Mayo Clinic survey of approximately 1000 cases[61–64] (Table 8–2) clearly indicated that certain roentgenographic patterns are more characteristic of certain cell types. We have tried to draw some conclusions that may help in the assessment of the most likely cell type in individual cases.

1. As the sole roentgenographic abnormality, a hilar mass is the commonest finding in small cell carcinoma and is virtually nonexistent in adenocarcinoma.

2. A mass 4 cm or less in diameter is most likely adenocarcinoma.

3. A mass more than 4 cm in diameter is most unlikely to be a small cell carcinoma but is a relatively common finding in the other three types, particularly large cell carcinoma.

4. Apical tumors are uncommon and, when the sole finding, usually are squamous-cell carcinoma.

5. Multiple masses are very rare.

6. Overinflation due to air trapping did not occur in the Mayo series.

7. Atelectasis, as a single manifestation or combined with other findings, strongly indicates squamous-cell carcinoma.

8. Consolidation (*i.e.,* homogeneous opacification of a lung, lobe, or segment, *without decrease in volume*) is extremely rare in all cell types.

9. Pneumonitis (*i.e.,* a nonhomogeneous opacity with a hazy outline, without decrease in volume) as the *only* finding suggests squa-

TABLE 8–2. ROENTGENOGRAPHIC PATTERNS BASED ON CELL TYPE:
600 CASES OF BRONCHOGENIC CARCINOMA*

ROENTGENOGRAPHIC ABNORMALITY	SQUAMOUS-CELL CARCINOMA (263 cases)		ADENO-CARCINOMA (126 cases)		LARGE CELL CARCINOMA (97 cases)		SMALL CELL CARCINOMA (114 cases)	
	Sole Abnormality (%)	*Other Abnormalities Present (%)*	*Sole Abnormality (%)*	*Other Abnormalities Present (%)*	*Sole Abnormality (%)*	*Other Abnormalities Present (%)*	*Sole Abnormality (%)*	*Other Abnormalities Present (%)*
Hilar								
Prominence	0.0	5.3	0.0	2.4	0.0	7.2	0.9	6.1
Hilar mass	6.5	16.5	0.8	8.7	6.2	12.4	14.9	50.0
Peripheral mass	6.5	5.3	4.0	1.6	4.1	2.0	4.4	1.7
Pulmonary Parenchymal								
Small mass (4.0 cm or less)	8.2	0.7	38.9	6.3	12.4	5.1	7.0	14.0
Large mass (larger than 4.0 cm)	15.2	3.4	17.4	8.7	27.8	13.4	4.4	3.5
Apical mass	2.7	0.4	0.8	0.0	1.0	3.0	1.7	0.9
Multiple masses	0.4	0.0	2.4	0.0	1.0	1.0	0.9	0.0
Hypertranslucency	0.0	0.0	0.0	0.0	0.0	0.0	0.0	0.0
Collapse	16.7	19.7	3.2	7.1	1.0	12.4	3.5	14.0
Consolidation	0.7	3.0	0.0	0.8	0.0	1.0	0.0	0.9
Pneumonitis	4.9	11.3	2.4	11.9	1.0	22.6	0.9	21.9
Cavitation	6.8		2.4		4.1		0.0	
Intrathoracic Extrapulmonary								
Mediastinal mass or widening	0.4	0.4	1.6	0.8	4.1	6.2	0.0	13.1
Chest wall	0.0	0.0	0.0	0.0	0.0	0.0	0.0	0.0
Pleural effusion	0.4	3.0	0.8	4.0	0.0	2.0	0.0	5.3
Hemidiaphragm elevation	0.4	0.7	0.0	4.0	0.0	1.0	0.0	3.5

*Adapted from Lehar, T. J., Carr, D. T., Miller, W. E., et al.: Am. Rev. Resp. Dis., 96:245, 1967, and Byrd, R. B., Miller, W. E., Carr, D. T., et al.: Mayo Clin. Proc., 43:327, May, 1968.

mous-cell type, but when accompanied by other findings commonly indicates large or small cell undifferentiated carcinoma.

10. Cavitation is most common in squamous-cell type, less common in large cell and adenocarcinoma, and nonexistent in small cell carcinoma.

11. Mediastinal widening almost certainly indicates spread from small cell undifferentiated carcinoma.

12. Chest wall involvement did not occur in this series.

ROENTGENOGRAPHIC MANIFESTATIONS

Anatomic Location

A ratio of 6 to 4 applies to both right versus left lung and upper versus lower lobe predominance.[65] In the upper lobes the anterior segment is most often affected.[65] Both squamous-cell and oat-cell carcinomas occur centrally and peripherally, but adenocarcinoma almost invariably develops in the periphery. Excluding neo-

plasms arising in peripheral parenchyma, the site of origin within the bronchial tree shows a striking predominance (60 to 80 per cent) for the segmental bronchi;[65] the remainder arise in main and lobar bronchi. Bronchogenic carcinoma arising in the trachea is rare, amounting to no more than 1 per cent of cases. Approximately 4 per cent arise in the extreme apex of the upper lobes (the superior pulmonary sulcus)—Pancoast tumors.

Roentgenographic Patterns

It has been estimated that when a neoplasm of the lung is first detectable roentgenographically it has completed three-quarters of its "natural" existence.[66] The roentgenographic manifestations of bronchogenic carcinoma are related both to the size of the lesion and, perhaps more importantly, to its anatomic location, particularly in its relationship to an airway. Since 60 to 80 per cent (excluding the peripheral neoplasms) arise in segmental bronchi, the earliest roentgenographic sign is not the lesion itself but the consequences of obstruction of the airway in which the lesion is situated.

AIRWAY OBSTRUCTION. Most observers consider the effects of airway obstruction the commonest roentgenographic manifestation of bronchogenic carcinoma. Chief among these is *atelectasis*. The collapse is most often segmental but may be lobar and, very occasionally, of a whole lung. Since obstruction of the bronchus is usually a slowly progressive process, infection is common distal to the obstruction and, when the bronchus becomes totally occluded, inflammatory exudate prevents complete collapse of distal parenchyma. Thus, the roentgenographic appearance ranges from total collapse (*see* Figure 4–17, page 178), to a minor decrease in volume limited by distal infection, bronchiectasis, and abscess formation—obstructive pneumonitis (*see* Figure 4–10, page 173). However, some degree of atelectasis is almost invariable. Since air cannot pass the obstruction, an air bronchogram is absent, a sign virtually pathognomonic of an endobronchial obstructing lesion and of utmost importance in differential diagnosis. Clinically, such patients may present with acute pneumonia; subsidence of the acute inflammation with antibiotic therapy may open the airway, so that air may be visible roentgenographically in distorted channels within the obstructed segment. In these circumstances, the pneumonia may resolve partially, in which case the lesion may be misdiagnosed as a slowly resolving pneumonia. For this reason, any pneumonia should be followed roentgenographically to complete resolution, particularly in patients in the "cancer age group."

Although overinflation of lung distal to an endobronchial lesion as a result of check-valve obstruction is frequently cited as an important sign in the early diagnosis of bronchogenic carcinoma, it is in fact a rare manifestation. Overinflation of the lung at TLC must be distinguished from air trapping on expiration (resulting in overinflation at RV). The former, whether local or general, implies loss of elastic recoil (either reversible, as in spasmodic asthma, or irreversible, as in emphysema). Loss of this recoil is usually a lengthy process, hardly commensurate with an aggressive condition such as bronchogenic carcinoma. *In our experience, the volume of lung behind an obstructing endobronchial lesion is usually reduced at full inspiration* (*see* Figure 4–57, page 217). Despite this smaller volume, however, the density of affected parenchyma typically is *less* than the opposite lung rather than greater as might be anticipated. This is caused by reduction in perfusion (oligemia), resulting almost always from hypoxic vasoconstriction in response to hypoventilation. *Air trapping* during expiration is a dynamic event resulting from air flow obstruction as the bronchial caliber reduces to embrace the endobronchial lesion.

Primary carcinoma of the trachea is rare, accounting for no more than 1 per cent of bronchogenic cancers. It is not generally appreciated that the site of origin of a tracheal neoplasm strongly influences the clinical presentation. Since the intrathoracic portion of the trachea dilates on inspiration and narrows on expiration, a lesion arising in this segment will be characterized clinically by *expiratory* airway obstruction, often simulating asthma (*see* Figure 8–1, page 401), and roentgenographically by expiratory air trapping. Conversely, the cervical portion of the trachea narrows on inspiration and dilates on expiration, so that symptoms and signs of expiratory airway obstruction are lacking (Figure 8–3).

HILAR ENLARGEMENT. Unilateral enlargement may be the earliest roentgenographic manifestation of bronchogenic carcinoma.[30] It may represent a primary carcinoma that has arisen in the major hilar bronchus, or enlarged bronchopulmonary lymph nodes that are the site of metastases from a very small primary lesion in adjacent or peripheral parenchyma. Enlargement of hilar lymph nodes by metastasis from a remote neoplasm is particularly characteristic of oat-cell carcinoma, which may give rise to bulky nodes (Figure 8–4) and even bilateral distribution (*see* Table 8–2). Abnormality in a hilum may be evidenced not only by enlargement but also by increased density; the mass, even when too small to enlarge the hilum, may reveal itself by altering hilar density.

MEDIASTINAL LYMPH NODE INVOLVEMENT. Although uncommon, enlargement of mediastinal lymph nodes other than bronchopulmonary may be the main or sole abnormality roentgenographically[30] and almost always indicates spread from an anaplastic carcinoma (*see* Table 8–2). The chief roentgenographic sign is mediastinal widening, usually with an undulating or lobular contour. Involvement of the bifurcation (carinal) or posterior mediastinal nodes may displace the esophagus, and adequate contrast study of the esophagus is essential when bronchogenic carcinoma is suspected; in fact, dysphagia is occasionally the presenting symptom in patients with primary lung cancer (Figure 8–5).

Invasion of the mediastinum may involve the

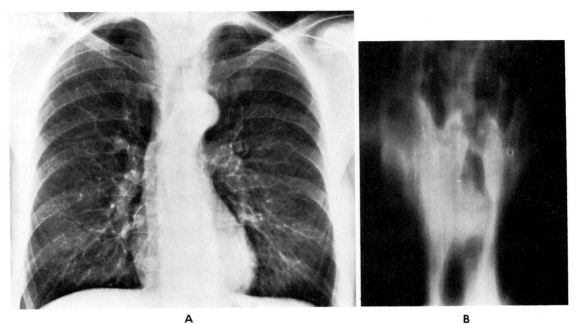

A   **B**

Figure 8–3. Primary Carcinoma of the Trachea. A posteroanterior roentgenogram *(A)* reveals increased volume of both lungs, attributable at least in part to emphysema. In addition, the air column of the cervical trachea approximately 2 cm distal to the larynx is markedly narrowed. A large mass can be identified arising from the right wall of the trachea and extending over a distance of at least 3 cm of its length. An anteroposterior tomogram *(B)* reveals the lesion to better advantage and shows the severe compromise of the tracheal air column. A sleeve resection was carried out with end-to-end anastomosis. Proved squamous-cell carcinoma. This 55-year-old man had complained of increasing dyspnea on effort during the past year.

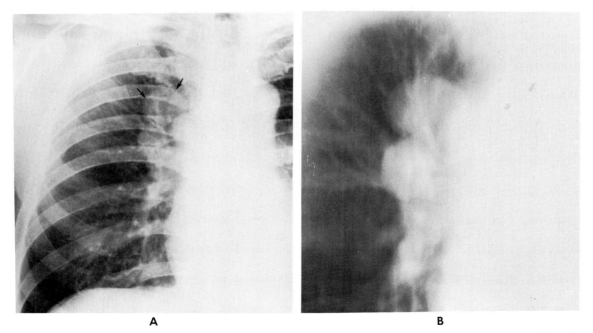

A   **B**

Figure 8–4. Anaplastic Bronchogenic Carcinoma with Hilar and Mediastinal Node Metastases. A view of the right hemithorax from a posteroanterior roentgenogram *(A)* reveals a large, smooth, sharply demarcated mass *(arrows)* situated immediately above an enlarged, nodular right hilum. There also appears to be a mass occupying the right tracheobronchial angle. An anteroposterior tomogram *(B)* shows the shadow to better advantage. This 61-year-old man had been told 5 years previously that he had an abnormality on his chest roentgenogram, although he had been asymptomatic until 3-and-a-half weeks prior to admission, when he had a brisk hemoptysis. At thoracotomy, the disease was felt to be unresectable because of the presence of both hilar and mediastinal lymph node metastases. Proved undifferentiated bronchogenic carcinoma.

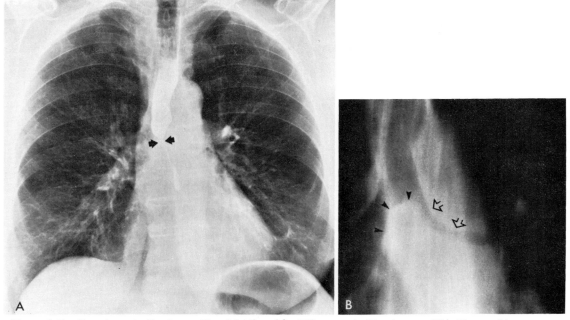

Figure 8–5. Bronchogenic Carcinoma First Manifested by Effects on the Esophagus. This 78-year-old woman was admitted to the hospital for investigation of increasing dysphagia over the past several weeks. The chest roentgenogram illustrated in *A* shows no abnormalities of the lungs or hila; however, the barium swallow reveals an annular constricting lesion of the esophagus at the level of the carina *(arrows)*. A tomogram in anteroposterior projection *(B)* confirms the presence of a lobulated soft tissue mass blunting the carinal angle and indenting the medial wall of the right main bronchus; in addition, it reveals a marked uniform narrowing of the left main bronchus throughout most of its length *(open arrows)*. Proved primary squamous-cell carcinoma of the left main bronchus with metastases to carinal and posterior mediastinal lymph nodes, the latter producing circumferential compression of the esophagus.

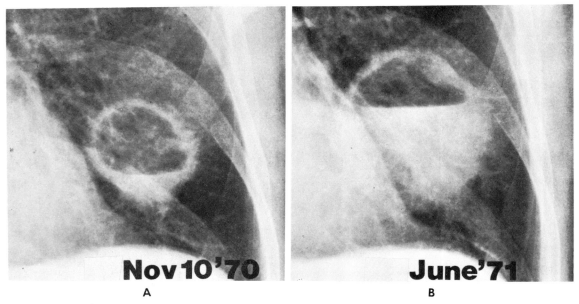

Figure 8–6. Cavitation in Primary Squamous-Cell Carcinoma. The original roentgenogram of this 64-year-old asymptomatic man *(A)* reveals a 4.5 cm cavity in the left lower lobe, possessing a wall thickness of about 3 mm, and a small accumulation of fluid within it. Seven months later *(B)*, the transverse diameter of the mass had increased to 6.5 cm, which represents a tripling in volume. Note that wall thickness is essentially unchanged from the original examination. Proved squamous-cell cancer.

phrenic nerve or recurrent laryngeal nerve, causing diaphragmatic paresis or hoarseness, respectively; compression or invasion of vascular channels may produce the superior vena cava syndrome.

CAVITATION. Cavitation in bronchogenic carcinoma is common, its reported incidence ranging from 2 to 16 per cent (*see* Table 8–2).[30, 67] It may occur in three ways:

1. *Central necrosis of the neoplasm:* This is undoubtedly the commonest form of cavitation. There is strong predilection for upper lung zones, the segments most frequently affected being the apicoposterior segment of the left upper lobe and the superior segment of the left lower lobe. The majority of cavitating neoplasms are squamous-cell, and over 60 per cent of these occur in the upper lobes. Most of these cavities are thick-walled, resembling acute lung abscess (Figure 8–6), but occasionally the wall may be extremely thin, resembling a bulla or bronchogenc cyst. The inner surface is usually irregular, bearing nodules or solid masses of neoplastic tissue. It is still not known why only some bronchial carcinomas undergo necrosis. The theory most often cited is that necrosis results from ischemia. However, for a variety of reasons it is necessary to invoke some mechanism in addition to simple ischemia—perhaps an immunologic mechanism such as type IV cell-mediated delayed hypersensitivity.

2. *Cavitary disease not restricted to the neoplasm:* A lung abscess distal to an obstructing neoplasm may communicate with the bronchial tree, especially after antibiotic or radiation therapy.

3. *Development of abscess elsewhere in the lung:* In the third variety of neoplastic cavitation, abscesses develop elsewhere in the lungs as a result of spill-over of purulent material from segmental obstructive pneumonitis and abscess formation.

MUCOID IMPACTION. Mucoid impaction of segmental and subsegmental bronchi is most commonly a manifestation of a hypersensitivity state usually seen in asthmatics and frequently associated ·with hypersensitivity bronchopulmonary aspergillosis (*see* page 386). Sometimes, however, impaction of inspissated secretions can occur within the bronchial tree, commonly at the segmental or subsegmental levels, behind an obstructing endobronchial lesion. Since the commonest roentgenographic manifestation of an endobronchial lesion is obstructive pneumonitis, the presence of mucoid impaction associated with distal air-containing parenchyma requires that there be no infection within the

bronchopulmonary segment at the time its airway is obstructed and that collateral air drift is functioning properly so that atelectasis does not occur. Since collateral air drift effectively reduces ventilation, local hypoxia leads to reflex vasoconstriction; the resultant oligemia can create a zone of radiolucency whose presence provides additional evidence of airway obstruction. This complex of roentgenographic signs is epitomized by bronchial atresia in which no communication exists between the major airways and peripheral parenchyma, commonly in the apicoposterior bronchus of the left upper lobe.

Mucoid impaction has been seen in a variety of lesions causing segmental bronchial occlusion, including primary and metastatic carcinoma, bronchial adenoma, bronchial atresia, and foreign body.[68] Three cases have been described in which a "bronchocele" was associated with primary oat-cell carcinoma of the lung;[69] in this series, neoplastic cells could be identified within the inspissated mucus.

The radiographic appearances of mucoid impaction are no different from those associated with a hypersensitivity state except that the impaction is localized to one specific segment (Figure 8–7). Depending on the extent of the impaction, the resultant opacity may be linear or branched in a V or Y configuration. The affected bronchi are almost invariably dilated, sometimes to a marked degree.

APICAL NEOPLASMS. The so-called superior pulmonary sulcus tumor or Pancoast tumor arises in lung parenchyma or contiguous pleura at the extreme apex of an upper lobe. The superior pulmonary sulcus is a groove in the lung formed by the subclavian artery as it crosses the lung apex in the cupola of the pleura. Most apical lung neoplasms arise in relationship to this sulcus; hence, their name. The superior inlet of the thorax is bounded laterally by the first rib, anteriorly by the first costal cartilage and manubrium, and posteriorly by the head of the first rib and body of the first thoracic vertebra. Most of the area is occupied by the apex of the lung. Neoplasms that arise from this location include all four cell types, with squamous-cell carcinoma predominating. These lesions may transgress the pleura and extend into contiguous thoracic wall, there causing bone destruction, Horner's syndrome, and other manifestations of the Pancoast syndrome.[70] In the absence of bone destruction on conventional roentgenograms, computed tomography can sometimes reveal abnormalities not otherwise suspected (Figure 8–8). Any

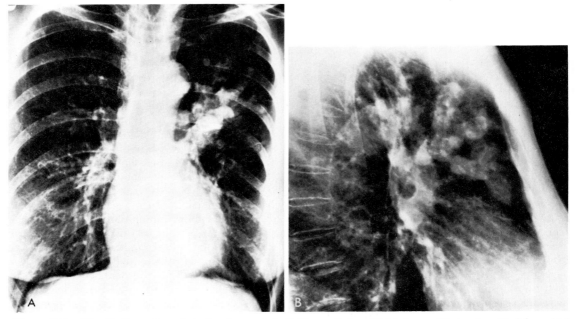

Figure 8–7. Mucoid Impaction, Anterior Segment Left Upper Lobe, Distal to an Obstructing Endobronchial Lesion. Posteroanterior *(A)* and lateral *(B)* roentgenograms of a middle-aged woman reveal several fingerlike opacities from the upper portion of the left hilum. The lungs are otherwise normal. Bronchoscopy revealed a squamous-cell carcinoma completely obstructing the orifice of the anterior segmental bronchus of the left upper lobe. Note that the parenchyma of this bronchopulmonary segment is air-containing as a result of collateral air drift from contiguous normally ventilated segments. (Courtesy of Dr. Kenneth Thomson, Flinders University Medical Center, Adelaide, Australia.)

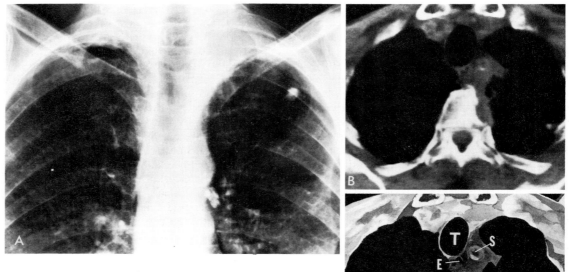

Figure 8–8. Superior Pulmonary Sulcus Neoplasm: Value of CT in Assessment. A posteroanterior roentgenogram *(A)* reveals a homogeneous opacity situated in the apical and paramediastinal zone of the left upper lobe. Roentgenograms of the left upper ribs and thoracic spine revealed no significant abnormality. However, a CT scan at the level of the body of T3 *(B)* and a diagrammatic representation of the scan *(C)* reveal a paravertebral mass associated with considerable destruction of the contiguous vertebral body *(arrows in C)*. In addition, there is no line of demarcation between the mass and retrotracheal soft tissues, indicating invasion of the mediastinum. T = trachea; S = left subclavian artery; E = esophagus. This is a 69-year-old man whose major complaint was pain in the left shoulder. Proven squamous-cell carcinoma.

asymmetry of presumed apical pleural thickening on the two sides should raise suspicion of such a neoplasm.

PLEURAL INVOLVEMENT. Pleural involvement in primary bronchogenic carcinoma is not uncommon, effusion having been observed in 8 per cent of patients in one large series[71] and in 15 per cent of another.[30] Pleural effusion does not invariably denote direct invasion by neoplastic cells (in one series[72] serous effusion resulted solely from lymphatic obstruction by involved mediastinal lymph nodes), but hemorrhagic effusion nearly always denotes direct tumor invasion. Regardless of the mechanism of its formation, effusion indicates a poor prognosis even when malignant cells are not discovered cytologically.

Spontaneous pneumothorax may occur as a result of direct transgression of the visceral pleural surface.

BONE INVOLVEMENT. The skeleton may be involved in bronchogenic carcinoma either by direct extension to the ribs or vertebrae (as in the Pancoast tumor) or by extension via the bloodstream to remote sites. Although metastases are predominantly osteolytic, purely osteoblastic lesions also occur. The bones most commonly involved are vertebrae (70 per cent), pelvic bones (40 per cent), and femora (25 per cent). Serum alkaline phosphatase values are almost invariably elevated.

DOUBLE PRIMARY CARCINOMAS OF THE LUNG. Double primary carcinomas of the lung are uncommon. A review of the literature in 1974[73] uncovered only 155 acceptable examples of multiple primary bronchogenic carcinomas, developing either simultaneously or asynchronously.

OTHER SIGNS. Other roentgenographic signs include unilateral diaphragmatic paralysis resulting from phrenic nerve involvement,[30] to be differentiated from hemidiaphragmatic elevation compensatory to atelectasis; bilateral parenchymal lesions resulting from contralateral hematogenous metastases;[30] and diffuse lymphangitic carcinomatosis, in which neoplasm spreads throughout the lungs (*see* page 445).[30]

Roentgenographic Techniques in Diagnosis

Special roentgenographic techniques often are indicated in the investigation of suspected bronchogenic carcinoma, for diagnostic purposes or for assessment of surgical resectability. *Roentgenograms of the chest at maximal expiration* may be of value when the lesion is largely endobronchial and is invisible on standard inspiratory roentgenograms. *Tomography* is invaluable in the study of the hila, particularly in the assessment of node enlargement; posterior oblique tomography at an angle of 55 degrees has been found by some to be superior to standard anteroposterior tomography for displaying a clearer outline of the anatomic components of the hila.[74] *Computed tomography* is of particular value in the determination of the presence and extent of mediastinal spread in patients with bronchogenic carcinoma, either by direct invasion (Figure 8–9) or by lymph node metastasis (Figure 8–10), and may be of value in the determination of pleural and chest wall involvement. In a prospective study of 54 patients suspected of having primary lung carcinoma, Hirleman and his colleagues[75] found CT to be the primary modality of choice in the investigation of central carcinomas, possessing a sensitivity of 95 per cent and a specificity of 80 per cent for predicting mediastinal metastases.

In our view, *bronchography* is seldom if ever indicated in the investigation of suspected bronchogenic carcinoma. The fiberoptic bronchoscope, because of the facility with which it can be used to study the airways as far as subsegmental divisions, has largely obviated the value of bronchography. With few exceptions, the diagnosis for pulmonary disease depends on microbiologic or morphologic examination, and many recently developed procedures provide adequate material for study, permitting precise diagnosis without recourse to bronchography.

Pulmonary and bronchial arteriography have been used to assess the resectability of proved cancer. Our attitude to these procedures is similar in many respects to our position regarding bronchography.

Lung scanning has limited potential in the study of the lungs and mediastinum of patients with bronchogenic carcinoma. Attempts to identify lung neoplasms by selective uptake of various isotopes have been disappointing, partly because not all neoplasms take up the isotope but mainly because certain infectious processes also result in positive scans. We consider that this procedure provides little information that cannot be obtained directly and more reliably with tomography, bronchoscopy, and mediastinoscopy. However, it is possible that radionuclide scanning may be useful in the identification of occult liver, brain, and bone metastases once the diagnosis of carcinoma of the lung has been established: more than half

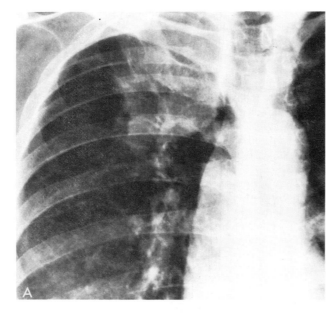

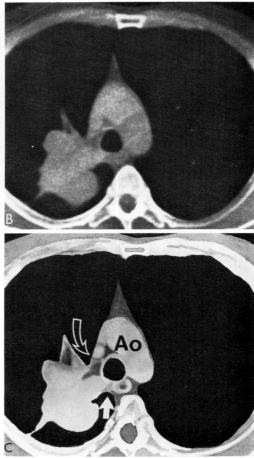

Figure 8–9. Squamous Cell Carcinoma, Right Upper Lobe: Value of CT in Assessment. A posteroanterior roentgenogram (A) reveals a large irregular homogeneous mass in the paramediastinal zone of the right upper lobe. The mass obscures the tracheal stripe. A CT scan through the midportion of the mass at the level of the aortic arch (B) and a diagrammatic representation of the scan (C) show the mass to excellent advantage but in addition reveal widening of the paratracheal soft tissues (*curved arrow* in C) and absence of demarcation between the mass and the retrotracheal soft tissues (*solid arrow* in C), both of which indicate mediastinal invasion and an inoperable lesion. Ao = transverse arch of the aorta.

(52.5 per cent) of 92 patients studied by Kelly and associates[76] had at least one abnormal scan of these three areas in the absence of significant symptoms referable to them.

Bone scanning is usually superior to roentgenographic surveys for the early detection of osseous metastases.[77] Until fairly recently strontium-85 was most often used. Now, however, the advantages of radioactive technetium (^{99m}Tc) and the facility with which it forms bone-seeking phosphato-anionic complexes offer new potential in skeletal scintiphotography.

Clinical Manifestations

Bronchopulmonary Manifestations

Bronchogenic carcinoma is commonest in men between the ages of 55 and 60 years; only 1 per cent of patients are under 40. About 10 per cent of patients are asymptomatic when first seen, the diagnosis being suspected initially from an abnormal chest roentgenogram or, very occasionally, from cytologic examination.[30] The commonest symptom by far is *cough*, usually mildly productive, occurring in 75 per cent of patients.[30] Since the majority of these patients are heavy smokers and have chronic bronchitis, cough may not be recognized as a new symptom. *Hemoptysis* occurs in about 50 per cent of cases[30] and may be the only clue in patients whose chest roentgenograms are normal. Initial symptoms may be the result of partial or complete obstruction of a bronchus, such as local wheeze, increased shortness of breath, or acute symptoms of obstructive pneumonitis. A local wheeze may be present when no abnormality is visible on a standard chest roentgenogram. Neoplasms in the lung periphery almost never cause local symptoms.

Extrapulmonary Intrathoracic Manifestations

The presenting symptoms and signs may result from extension of the disease beyond the lung to the mediastinum, pleura, diaphragm, chest wall, or thoracic inlet. Extension to the

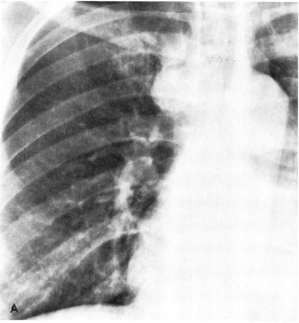

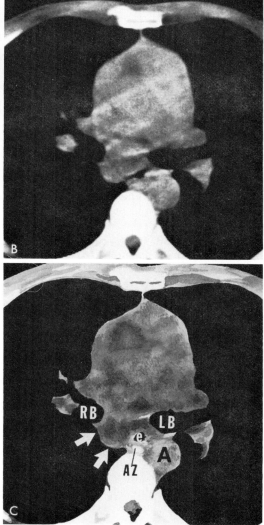

Figure 8–10. Value of CT in Assessment of Mediastinal Lymph Node Metastases. A posteroanterior roentgenogram (A) of a 43-year-old man reveals a somewhat irregular homogeneous mass in the paratracheal zone of the right upper lobe (*arrows*). On this somewhat underpenetrated roentgenogram, the carinal region is poorly seen. A CT scan 3 cm distal to the carina (B) and a diagrammatic representation of the scan (C) reveal a large soft tissue mass posteromedial to the right intermediate bronchus, protruding into and deforming the azygoesophageal recess (*arrows* in C). This mass represents enlarged carinal lymph nodes metastatic from what proved to be a squamous cell carcinoma of the right upper lobe. Compare with Figure 1–55, pages 82 and 83. RB = right intermediate bronchus; LB = left main bronchus; A = aorta; e = esophagus; AZ = azygos vein.

pleura may occasion pain on breathing, signs of pleural effusion, and friction rub. Effusion is more likely to be serous than grossly hemorrhagic and is not necessarily the result of direct invasion of the pleura by neoplastic cells. Spontaneous pneumothorax is very uncommon with bronchogenic carcinoma.

Mediastinal involvement is usually by metastatic spread to lymph node chains. Enlargement of hilar lymph nodes is by metastatic spread in most cases and seldom gives rise to symptoms. Compression or obstruction of the superior vena cava, usually by oat-cell carcinoma, results in the typical syndrome. Invasion of the recurrent laryngeal nerve may cause hoarseness, and invasion of the vagus nerve may cause dyspnea, particularly in patients with chronic bronchitis (as is so often the case).

Symptoms of *thoracic inlet* involvement al-most invariably indicate superior pulmonary sulcus tumor.[70] Important structures within the superior thoracic inlet are (from front to back) the subclavian and jugular veins, the phrenic and vagus nerves, the subclavian and common carotid arteries, the recurrent laryngeal nerve, the eighth cervical and first thoracic nerves, the sympathetic chain and stellate ganglion, and the first four ribs and upper vertebrae. A superior pulmonary sulcus tumor may involve one or several of these structures, so the signs and symptoms are highly variable and may include pain and weakness of the shoulder and arm, swelling of the arm, and Horner's syndrome.

Extrathoracic Metastatic Manifestations

Remote metastases develop from spread via the lymphatics and blood vessels and may be responsible for the initial clinical manifestations. Adenocarcinoma, in particular, tends to metastasize early and extensively via the bloodstream, although the prognosis is better with this tumor than with undifferentiated carcinoma. Bronchogenic carcinoma metastasizes beyond the thorax most commonly to lymph nodes, liver, adrenals, kidneys, bone, and brain.[30, 78] The incidence is highest with small cell and lowest with epidermoid carcinoma.

Lymph node extension is predominantly to the scalene group, and is chiefly ipsilateral from all parts of both lungs.

Metastatic involvement of *liver, adrenals,* and *kidneys* may produce symptoms and signs that confuse diagnosis. Symptoms due to *brain* metastases may antedate by some years those caused by the primary lung lesion.[79] Metastatic spread to *bone* occurs in up to 35 per cent[80] of cases. In roughly three-quarters of the patients, the lesions are osteolytic, predominantly from squamous-cell and anaplastic large cell primary lesions. Local bone pain is almost invariable.

Extrathoracic Nonmetastatic Manifestations

A small percentage of patients with bronchogenic carcinoma have multifarious symptoms and signs not directly related to neoplastic infiltration; in fact, such clinical manifestations may occur in the absence of bronchopulmonary symptoms. These manifestations can be divided into neuromuscular, metabolic, connective-tissue and osseous, and vascular and hematologic.[81] In addition to these symptoms of malfunction of specific tissues or organs, many patients with bronchogenic carcinoma complain of such nonspecific symptoms as malaise, weakness, lassitude, fever, or weight loss.

NEUROMUSCULAR MANIFESTATIONS. Carcinomatous neuropathies do occur with other neoplasms but principally with bronchogenic carcinoma. Their pathogenesis is unknown. Even when CNS metastases are absent, neurologic symptoms and signs are fairly common.[82] Neurologic symptoms precede those directly referable to the neoplasm in up to 85 per cent of cases; in fact, in about 3 per cent of bronchogenic carcinoma cases they antedate the diagnosis by as much as 3 years.[82] The neuromyopathy is usually progressive but may occur as a single episode or be recurrent. In some cases removal of the primary neoplasm has alleviated neurologic symptoms.[82] Oat-cell carcinoma is usually responsible. The syndrome includes myopathies, peripheral neuropathies, subacute cerebellar degeneration, encephalomyelopathy, and necrotizing myelopathy.

CONNECTIVE TISSUE AND OSSEOUS MANIFESTATIONS. Bronchogenic carcinoma is by far the commonest cause of hypertrophic pulmonary osteoarthropathy. It is much more frequently associated with squamous-cell lesions than with adenocarcinoma and occurs rarely if at all in association with oat-cell cancer. Its incidence is approximately 3 per cent of all patients with lung cancer.[83] High levels of human growth hormone (HGH), without clinical effects, have been reported in cases of lung cancer.[84] The main symptom is deep-seated burning pain in distal parts of the extremities; there is usually clubbing of the fingers and toes, and edema, warmth, and tenderness of the hands, wrists, feet, and lower end of the legs. Roentgenography reveals subperiosteal new bone formation, chiefly of the distal bones of the extremities. Since radionuclide bone scanning is a sensitive detector of new bone formation, it may offer a more complete description of the distribution of hypertrophic pulmonary osteoarthropathy than is possible by roentgenography alone.[85] Synovial effusions may develop. Both the roentgenologic and clinical changes in the digits may antedate roentgenographic visibility of the lung neoplasm by as much as two years. Relief of pain invariably follows resection of the primary neoplasm and usually after simple vagotomy without pulmonary resection.[86]

The association of bronchogenic carcinoma and scleroderma is fairly well recognized. Of four reported cases and one seen by us, three had bronchiolo-alveolar carcinoma and two adenocarcinoma. It is not known which disease predisposes to the other.

ENDOCRINE AND METABOLIC MANIFESTATIONS. Endocrinopathies associated with primary bronchogenic carcinoma include Cushing's syndrome; carcinoid syndrome; a hyperparathyroidlike picture, with hypercalcemia; inappropriate secretion of antidiuretic hormone, with hyponatremia; insulinlike secretion, with hypoglycemia; excess gonadotropin secretion, with gynecomastia; and excess secretion of melanocyte-stimulating hormone, with hyperpigmentation of the skin. These syndromes are described in considerable detail in our text *Diagnosis of Diseases of the Chest* 2nd ed. (pages 1043 to 1047), and the interested reader is directed to this source for further information.

VASCULAR AND HEMATOLOGIC MANIFESTATIONS. Migratory thrombophlebitis and various hematologic disorders, including purpura and anemia, are rare in cases of bronchogenic carcinoma but are considered more than coincidental.[81]

DIAGNOSTIC PROCEDURES

Diagnostic procedures used to investigate cases of bronchogenic carcinoma are described in detail elsewhere in this book; they include bronchoscopy (*see* page 134), mediastinoscopy (*see* page 135), cytologic examination of sputum, bronchial washings, and pleural fluid (*see* page 116), and biopsy techniques (*see* page 117). Particularly recommended is the section in Chapter 2, in which biopsy procedures are summarized and recommendations made as to our preferred techniques for investigating six basic patterns of disease (*see* page 118).

THE POSITIVE CYTOLOGY–NEGATIVE ROENTGENOGRAM PERPLEXITY

In a small but steadily increasing number of patients, serial sputum specimens are cytologically positive while the chest roentgenogram is normal. If bronchoscopy yields no diagnostic information, management of these patients is difficult. During the past few years the situation has changed somewhat as a result of the development of the fiberoptic bronchoscope. With this instrument one can study the bronchi down to subsegmental levels, including those in the upper lobes, and several groups of investigators have been able to locate almost every roentgenographically occult lung cancer later resected.[87-89] Several prolonged sessions of fiberoptic bronchoscopy under general anesthesia may be required before the tumor site is identified by direct vision and biopsy or by repeated brushing and cytologic examination. The abundant data accumulated by these writers indicate that prompt surgical treatment of *in situ* or early invasive bronchogenic carcinoma can prolong survival.[90, 91]

In patients with repeatedly positive sputum cytology and negative roentgenographic and bronchoscopic examination, we recommend a relatively simple, straightforward program: standard roentgenograms of the chest at *monthly* intervals, with posteroanterior studies at full inspiration and forced expiration (the latter is potentially more informative because it reveals expiratory air trapping), and bronchoscopy every 3 months at least. Obviously, the monthly examination should include detailed

auscultation to detect an expiratory wheeze. Since on the majority of bronchograms one can perceive minor deformities that could represent mucosal abnormalities, we consider bronchography to be positively contraindicated. At the time of writing, the precise role to be played by CT in the investigation of these patients has not been established.

THE SOLITARY PULMONARY NODULE

A great deal of attention has been devoted in recent years to the solitary circumscribed pulmonary nodule. This interest derives from the fact that many of these lesions are primary carcinomas, often discovered in asymptomatic patients in whom the diagnosis remains obscure until the nodule is removed. Greater interest is warranted by the current majority opinion that survival rates are much improved if the carcinoma is removed while still at the circumscribed nodular stage.[92]

A great variety of conditions may result in the development of solitary circumscribed pulmonary nodules. Using the criteria listed in Table 8–3, in a considerable percentage of cases one can distinguish benign from malignant lesions and thus decide whether thoracotomy is warranted. The percentage of cases of bronchogenic carcinoma varies considerably from series to series, depending not only upon how the solitary pulmonary nodule is defined but also upon whether the lesions were discovered by roentgenographic (photofluorographic) survey or by hospital screening roentgenograms and whether the series includes cases referred for resection. Solitary nodules discovered in roentgenographic surveys of the general population prove to be cancer in less than 5 per cent of cases, whether the nodule is surgically removed at the time[93] or the case is followed for five years.[94] Patients referred for tumor resection have a malignant nodule in approximately 40 per cent of cases, a granulomatous one in 40 per cent,[13] and benign lesions of various etiologies in the remainder. In any series of solitary lesions in which surgical resection is performed, malignant noncalcified lesions are found in approximately 50 per cent of males over the age of 50.[13, 95] The etiology of the granulomas depends at least partly upon the endemicity of fungal infections and the degree of control of pulmonary tuberculosis in the area, and its elucidation relates largely to the competence and patience of the pathologist in searching for a specific organism.[13]

TABLE 8–3. CLINICAL AND ROENTGENOGRAPHIC CRITERIA IN THE DIFFERENTIATION OF
BENIGN AND MALIGNANT SOLITARY PULMONARY NODULES

CLINICAL	BENIGN	MALIGNANT
Age	Below 40 years. Exception is hamartoma.	Over 45 years.
Sex	Female	Male
Symptoms	Absent	Present
Past history and functional enquiry	High incidence of granuloma in area. Exposure to tuberculosis. Mineral oil medication.	Diagnosis of primary lesion elsewhere.
Skin tests	Positive, usually with specific granulomas.	Negative or positive.
ROENTGENOGRAPHIC		
Size	Smaller (less than 2 cm in diameter).	Larger (more than 2 cm in diameter).
Location	No predilection except for tuberculosis (upper lobes).	Predominantly upper lobes except for lung metastases.
Definition and contour	Margins well-defined and smooth.	Margins ill-defined; lobulated; umbilicated.
Calcification	Almost pathognomonic of a benign lesion, particularly if of laminated, multiple punctate, or "popcorn" variety.	Very rare.
Satellite lesions	More common.	Less common.
Serial studies showing no change over 2 years	Almost diagnostic of benign lesion	Most unlikely

Comparison with previous chest roentgenograms is of fundamental importance in determining the benignity or malignancy of a solitary nodule. In many cases, a previous film may show an identical lesion, perhaps overlooked because of the roentgenographic technique employed or because it was obscured by a rib shadow. In such cases it is reasonable to withhold surgery and to follow up with periodic roentgenographic examination. In every case of enlargement of such a shadow in a patient over 35 years of age (Figure 8–11), thoracotomy is probably indicated, even though some benign conditions, such as hamartoma and histoplasmoma, also may enlarge.

Diagnostic procedures such as bronchoscopy and cytologic and bacteriologic examination of sputum usually are of little or no value in the investigation of a patient with a solitary nodule. Search for a primary neoplasm elsewhere on the assumption that a nodule might be metastatic is almost invariably unrewarding. Also, such a search is often superfluous; it is justifiable to remove a pulmonary metastasis reasonably established as solitary, and the lesion may reveal histologic characteristics indicative of a specific primary site.[12, 13]

Use of doubling time in estimating growth rate may be of value in differentiating benign and malignant nodules in individual patients. ("Doubling" refers to *volume*, not diameter.) In a study of 218 pulmonary nodules (177 malignant and 41 benign), Nathan and his colleagues[96] concluded that virtually all nodules whose doubling time is 7 days or less are benign; if metastatic choriocarcinoma, testicular neoplasms, and osteogenic sarcoma can be eliminated (usually relatively simple by the time pulmonary metastases appear), the doubling time for benign lesions can be increased to 11 days. Similarly, nodules whose volume doubles in 465 days or more are almost always benign. A pulmonary nodule whose rate of growth falls outside these "benign" limitations must be con-

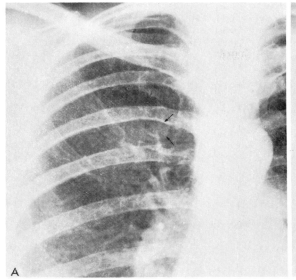

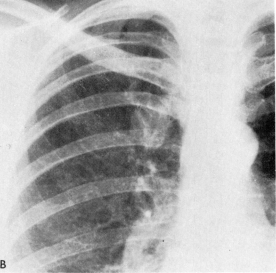

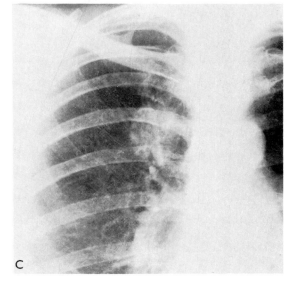

Figure 8–11. Enlarging Pulmonary Nodule: Broncho-genic Carcinoma. These are views of the upper half of the right lung from posteroanterior roentgenograms of a 52-year-old asymptomatic woman made as annual routine employee screening examinations. In 1965 *(A)*, the roentgenogram was interpreted as normal although in retrospect there is a rather poorly defined opacity measuring approximately 1 cm in diameter situated above the plane of the right hilum *(ar-rows)*. In 1967 *(B)*, the shadow measures slightly over 2 cm in diameter; such doubling of diameter means an eightfold increase in volume. In 1968 *(C)*, the lesion measures 3 cm in diameter. Such progression is virtually diagnostic of malig-nancy. At thoracotomy, the lobe was resected with ease; histologically the lesion was categorized as poorly differen-tiated carcinoma with mixed glandular and squamous fea-tures. Many lymph nodes submitted for examination showed no malignancy.

sidered malignant. Other investigators have quoted only slightly different figures—for ex-ample, a lesion that doubles in size in less than 1 month or more than 16 months is most unlikely to be malignant. Of the primary lung carcinomas, adenocarcinoma grows most slowly and undifferentiated and squamous-cell cancers most rapidly; giant cell carcinoma is character-ized by extremely rapid growth (Figure 8–12).

Roentgenographic signs often provide useful clues to diagnosis and may be pathognomonic. Undoubtedly the most important of these is calcification, the presence of which is almost certain evidence of benignity. Sometimes stand-ard roentgenograms reveal convincing evidence of calcification, particularly when laminated or

"target" in type, but perhaps just as often it is necessary to perform conventional tomography. Should the results of this procedure prove indeterminant, a CT study may be justified. The results obtained by Siegelman and his colleagues[97] in the differentiation of benign and malignant solitary pulmonary nodules are wor-thy of note: by assessing CT numbers from thin sections of 91 apparently noncalcified pulmo-nary nodules in 88 patients, these authors showed that benign lesions had relatively high CT numbers (164 H or greater), presumably because of diffuse calcification, and that malig-nant lesions had comparatively lower numbers (mean representative CT number was 92 H with a standard deviation of 18 H). While the

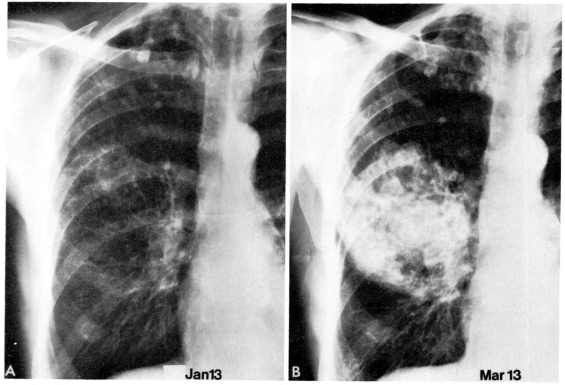

Figure 8–12. Giant Cell Carcinoma of the Right Lower Lobe. Views of the right lung from sequential roentgenograms of a 55-year-old asymptomatic man are illustrated, spanning a period of 2 months. The original examination (*A*) reveals a poorly defined opacity approximately 4 cm in diameter in the midportion of the right lung (situated in the superior segment of the lower lobe); there is obvious enlargement of the right hilum. By March 13 (*B*), only 2 months after the first examination, the volume of the mass had increased an estimated 20 times. Thoracotomy was performed and the lesion found to be unresectable. The extremely rapid growth observed roentgenologically is characteristic of giant cell carcinoma. (Courtesy of Dr. John Wrinch, Royal Inland Hospital, Kamloops, British Columbia.)

impressive results obtained by Siegelman and his colleagues have not been duplicated by all other investigators, they nevertheless have provided a stimulus to further research, which may in future years result in the development of a technique that will provide convincing evidence of the benign or malignant nature of these enigmatic lesions. At the time of this writing, digital radiography of the chest has just appeared on the horizon, and it appears entirely possible that this exciting new technique, particularly with dual-energy subtraction,[98] may prove successful in estimating the calcium content of nodules. Other techniques that hold promise include a dual-energy film subtraction technique[99] and a densitometric light-beam technique recently described by Revesz and his colleagues.[100]

The diagnosis and management of solitary pulmonary nodules have given rise to more discussion—and, possibly, more difference of opinion—than any other chest disease. Skin tests and complement-fixation tests may be of

value. History of exposure to known pathogens, notably *Histoplasma capsulatum* and *Coccidioides immitis*, may be highly significant. Previous chest roentgenograms may reveal no change in size over a lengthy period, or, if no previous studies are available, the patient may have been told in the past that he had a "shadow" on his lung. Finally, lung biopsy may provide definitive diagnostic information. Clinical and roentgenographic criteria of value in differentiating benign and malignant solitary pulmonary nodules are summarized in Table 8–3. Obviously, the management of each patient must be based on individual assessment. Young patients should be managed differently from those aged over 40 or 45 years. In patients under 35 years of age, less than 1 per cent of solitary nodules are malignant[101] and surgery is rarely indicated. We agree with Nathan[102] that, since the tumor has been growing for many years, in certain instances it is reasonable to follow the patient with serial roentgenograms, waiting for growth to occur, before operating.

Although it is difficult to establish strict criteria, we endorse Good's proposals,[103] as follows:

1. If no change is seen in the size of a nodule on roentgenograms made 2 or more years previously, the lesion may be assumed to be benign. In such circumstances, serial chest roentgenograms should be obtained at least every 6 months.

2. Calcification within a solitary nodule, particularly when of the central "target" or laminated type, is almost certain evidence of benignity.

3. If symptoms or signs direct attention to another body system, this should be investigated as a possible source of a primary neoplasm, of which the pulmonary nodule is metastatic. [We repeat that if no such symptoms or signs are present, a search for a primary site by roentgenologic or other techniques is so often unrewarding that it is seldom warranted.]

4. If none of the first three criteria is met *and the patient is over 35 to 40 years of age* [our italics], the lesion should be resected.

BRONCHIOLAR (ALVEOLAR CELL) CARCINOMA

Bronchiolar carcinoma (*synonyms:* alveolar cell and bronchiolo-alveolar carcinoma) accounts for 1 to 18 per cent of all pulmonary neoplasms. Its incidence appears to be increasing.[104] Although usually regarded as originating in bronchiolar epithelium, electron microscopic studies have shown that at least some of these lesions develop from type II alveolar epithelial cells.[105] The majority are detected in the middle-aged. In general, there is no predilection for either sex, except in association with scleroderma—which has a higher than expected incidence in both sexes but particularly in females.[106] Most series suggest an association with local parenchymal scarring or diffuse interstitial inflammation and fibrosis.[107]

It seems most likely that this neoplasm originates from a single primary focus, since many cases of bronchiolar carcinoma present as solitary peripheral masses in asymptomatic patients and, if they are resected when still local, the long-term prognosis is excellent.[108] If not resected, however, they invariably develop local and remote extensions. Growth may be very slow and insidious, over a period as long as 7 to 12 years.

It has been postulated that bronchiolar carcinoma may be of infectious origin. There is no convincing epidemiologic evidence that the tumor can be transmitted from one human to another, but there is a remarkable histologic similarity between bronchiolar carcinoma in man and jagziekte, a transmittable disease of sheep.

PATHOLOGIC CHARACTERISTICS

The gross appearance of these tumors is highly characteristic. Many are situated close to the pleura, with an area of atelectasis or scarring in between causing pleural dimpling. The tumors are grayish-white, mottled with black pigment, and poorly circumscribed. The distinctive histologic characteristics consist of sheets of well-differentiated tall columnar cells, with eosinophilic cytoplasm and nuclei at the bases lining the air spaces in a glandular pattern.[108] These cells produce mucus, abundant in some cases. The histologic picture may be identical to that of lung metastases from a primary adenocarcinoma elsewhere, particularly from the pancreas; the primary sites, in order of frequency, are pancreas, colon, breast, stomach, and kidney. Patients in whom a remote neoplasm is discovered should be excluded from any series of bronchiolar carcinoma.

Diffuse bilateral involvement in alveolar cell carcinoma occurs late and almost certainly results from spread via the bronchial tree. Tumor cells are found lying free in bronchial secretions in many cases and have been detected in the contralateral lung in association with proliferation of fibroblasts adherent to alveolar walls. Metastases occur in about 50 per cent of cases, in equal proportions in local lymph nodes, distant sites, and both locations. Contrary to common belief, lymphatic permeation is relatively common. Although bronchiolo-alveolar carcinoma is included in the WHO classification under adenocarcinoma, pathologic characteristics and clinical features support the concept that it is a distinct entity.[110]

ROENTGENOGRAPHIC MANIFESTATIONS

These may be local or widely disseminated, the former predominating in the great majority of cases. In either event, the basic roentgenographic pattern is one of air-space consolidation.

Local

The local variety shows no predilection for any lobe. The manifestation most commonly

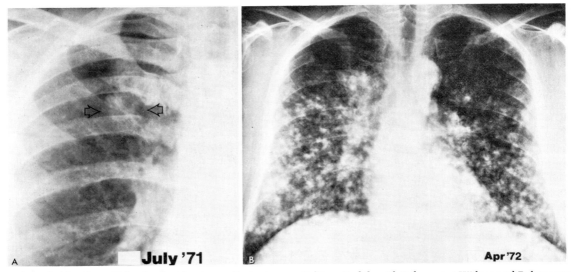

July '71   Apr '72

Figure 8–13. Bronchiolo-alveolar Carcinoma Beginning as a Solitary Nodule with Subsequent Widespread Pulmonary Involvement. A screening roentgenogram *(A)* of this 43-year-old asymptomatic man reveals a poorly defined solitary nodule 2 cm in diameter in the right upper lobe *(arrows)*. Nine months later *(B)*, there has occurred widespread involvement of both lungs by small discrete and confluent opacities characteristic of acinar shadows. The original right upper lobe mass has undergone considerable growth and there has developed evidence of right hilar lymph node enlargement. Proved bronchiolo-alveolar carcinoma.

seen is a rather well-circumscribed, peripheral, homogeneous mass, ranging in size from a small nodule no more than 1 cm in diameter to a large mass occupying most of a lobe. An air bronchogram or bronchiologram is a common roentgenographic feature and is of major importance in differential diagnosis. Air-containing airways in a peripheral mass may be visible in this neoplasm, in lymphoma, in pseudolymphoma, and in inflammatory pseudotumor, but rarely are seen in lesions of other etiologies. Another sign consists of linear strands extending from the nodule toward the pleura and in most cases reaching the pleural surface.[110] Although such linear streaks may occur in granulomatous disease, their association with a lesion containing an air bronchogram or bronchiologram is highly suggestive of bronchiolo-alveolar carcinoma. Many local masses grow very slowly, changing little for years.

Diffuse

The roentgenographic pattern of widely disseminated bronchiolar carcinoma may be fairly uniform throughout both lungs (Figure 8–13) or may vary regionally. The basic roentgenographic manifestation is the acinar shadow, indicating peripheral air-space consolidation. Acinar shadows may be discrete and readily identifiable as typical rosettes in one area of the lung or be more-or-less confluent—although seldom to the extent of homogeneous consoli-

dation—in other areas. In the latter circumstances, confluent disease was probably the source of disseminated spread, although diffuse bilateral disease develops from more localized lesions in some cases. Prominent line shadows extending along the bronchovascular bundles toward the hila usually represent lymphatic permeation.

Pleural effusion develops in 8 to 10 per cent of cases, always in association with pulmonary involvement. Uncommon roentgenographic manifestations include mediastinal lymph node enlargement, parenchymal atelectasis, spontaneous pneumothorax, and cavitation.

CLINICAL MANIFESTATIONS

The discovery rate of lesions during roentgenographic survey suggests that up to 50 per cent of these patients are asymptomatic.[111] The commonest symptom is cough, present in approximately 60 per cent of symptomatic patients. It may be dry or only slightly productive, but in 20 to 25 per cent of cases it gives rise to abundant mucoid expectoration; the latter feature is highly suggestive of the disease. Voluminous expectoration of lung liquid (bronchorrhea) — up to 4 l daily — usually indicates extensive lung involvement;[111] it may result in severe hypovolemia and electrolyte depletion. Other symptoms include weight loss, hemoptysis, fever, chest pain, thrombophlebitis and, as a late manifestation, dyspnea. Pulmonary signs are usually absent although widely scattered rales may be audible in advanced stages.

The discovery rate from cytologic examination of sputum varies widely in reported series. Cytologic study has been reported to be very unrewarding, positive only in far-advanced cases, and yielding positive results in only 20 to 50 per cent of cases.

As with the majority of bronchogenic carcinomas, prognosis depends largely on the extent of the disease when first detected. Survival times range from 4 to 15 years after resection in patients with local or unifocal disease to up to 3 years in those with multifocal lesions or metastases.

PROGNOSIS IN CASES OF BRONCHOGENIC CARCINOMA

The survival of patients with bronchogenic carcinoma depends upon many factors. These can be generally divided into factors inherent in the host and those attributable to the neoplasm itself. The latter include the influence of cell type and of morphologic extent of the neoplasm, growth rate, the size and location of the neoplasm, and whether there is regional or distant spread. Clinical considerations include the presence or absence of symptoms occasioned by the neoplasm, whether they are local or systemic, and their duration. Since treatment obviously affects survival rates, the influence of various forms of therapy must be taken into consideration. Many attempts have been made to correlate these many variables with survival rates in order to provide "staging," *i.e.*, grouping patients according to anatomic or clinical criteria, or both.

Although these factors are discussed individually, it must be borne in mind that the complexity of their interrelationships necessitates their overall consideration in relation to every patient.

INFLUENCE OF HOST FACTORS

Factors influencing survival that can be attributed to the "soil" in which the neoplasia develops include the patient's sex, age, immunocompetence, and certain ill-defined inherited components that affect not only the patient's innate susceptibility to malignant disease[52] but also his survival from it. The prognosis is poor for the young and the aged, because undifferentiated carcinoma is commoner in children and young adults and comorbidity is more prev-

alent in the aged. The major comorbid states in heavy smokers are chronic bronchitis and emphysema. In cigarette smokers, survival may be influenced by a decision to stop smoking, since continuance of the habit can lead to the development of second or third primary neoplasms.[112]

Finally, host resistance probably plays a major role in both preventing and combating neoplasia. Inherited qualities, in addition to immunocompetence, probably influence tumor growth rates and invasiveness.

PROGNOSIS BASED ON ANATOMIC STAGING

Influence of Cell Type

The cell type of bronchogenic carcinoma is a major factor in determining survival. Undifferentiated carcinomas, particularly oat-cell, carry a poor prognosis, since they grow rapidly and have a high metastatic potential. In contrast to squamous-cell carcinomas, which grow rapidly but show a low tendency to metastasize, adenocarcinomas grow slowly but have a high metastatic potential.

An exhaustive study of survival rates in lung cancer was published by Mountain and his colleagues in 1974.[113] Of 2155 histologically proved cases of bronchogenic carcinoma, 996 were of squamous-cell type, 521 adenocarcinoma, 195 undifferentiated large cell carcinoma, 368 undifferentiated small cell carcinoma, and 75 undifferentiated with cell type not specific. As shown in Figure 8–14, the overall prognosis of up to 90 months in cases of squamous-cell carcinoma is better than for other major cell types, regardless of any other factor. The relative survival rates for patients with adenocarcinoma and undifferentiated large cell carcinoma were intermediate and were almost identical. Survival with undifferentiated small cell (oat-cell) carcinoma was universally disastrous.

Influence of Morphologic Extent of the Neoplasm

Prognosis also relates very strongly to the stage of the disease at the time of detection, but here also there is a very strong interrelationship with cell type. Most attempts at staging bronchogenic carcinoma have been based on purely anatomic features as determined roentgenologically or at thoracotomy. Traditionally, patients have been grouped into three general categories: (1) those with a peripheral lesion

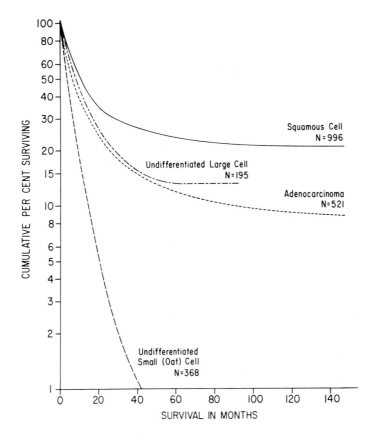

CUMULATIVE PER CENT SURVIVING

Squamous Cell
N = 996

Undifferentiated Large Cell
N = 195

Adenocarcinoma
N = 521

Undifferentiated
Small (Oat) Cell
N = 368

SURVIVAL IN MONTHS

Figure 8–14. Prognosis in Patients with Lung Cancer. Proportion of patients surviving lung cancer stratified by the histologic pattern of disease in 2080 cases. (Reprinted from Mountain, C. F., Carr, D. T., and Anderson, W. A. D.: Am. J. Roentgenol., *120*:130, 1974, with permission of the authors and editor.)

without evidence of involvement of regional lymph nodes or distant metastases; (2) those in whom the tumor has spread beyond the lung to regional lymph nodes; and (3) those who have distant metastases. Refinements of this form of staging include tumor size, mediastinal as distinct from hilar lymph node involvement, and, when thoracotomy is performed, whether all tumor tissue has been removed.[114] Patients with peripheral neoplasms have a much better prognosis than those with central ones, chiefly because most well-differentiated adenocarcinomas occur in peripheral lung parenchyma. Neoplasms that arise in main-stem bronchi carry an extremely poor prognosis. Survival rates fall off abruptly when regional lymph nodes become involved.

A tumor's size when first detected is a significant factor in survival.[114] A study of 392 men with asymptomatic pulmonary nodules recorded a 5-year survival rate of 48 per cent for tumors ≤ 2.5 cm in diameter but only 13 per cent for those 2.6 to 6 cm in diameter.

In general, about 15 per cent of patients with bronchogenic carcinoma survive 5 years or more. Five-year survival is virtually nil for patients whose neoplasms arise in a main-stem bronchus[115] and is about 40 per cent for those

with asymptomatic peripheral pulmonary nodules. In large series, operative mortality ranges from 10 to 12 per cent[116] and in older patients is as high as 20 per cent.

Perhaps the most convenient and simplest method of classifying lung cancer is the TNM classification.[117] This classification and its system for clinical staging have been described in detail by Mountain and his colleagues,[113] and much of the following is either abstracted or taken directly from their paper.

In the TNM system, "T" designates the primary tumor, with subscripts to denote increasing size or direct extension or both. "N" represents regional lymph node involvement, with subscripts to denote the absence of involvement or increasing involvement. "M" represents distant metastases, with subscripts to denote the absence of such involvement or increasing dissemination of the neoplasm. The categories of T, N, and M, as described by Mountain and his associates,[113] are as follows.

T—PRIMARY TUMORS

T_0 No evidence of primary tumor.
T_x Tumor proved by the finding of malignant cells in bronchopulmonary secretions but not visualized roentgenographically or bronchoscopically.

T_1 A tumor that is 3.0 cm or less in greatest diameter surrounded by lung or visceral pleura and without evidence of invasion proximal to a lobar bronchus at bronchoscopy.

T_2 A tumor more than 3.0 cm in greatest diameter, or a tumor of any size which, with associated atelectasis or obstructive pneumonitis, extends to the hilar region. At bronchoscopy the proximal extent of demonstrable tumor must be at least 2.0 cm distal to the carina. Associated atelectasis or obstructive pneumonitis must involve less than an entire lung, and there must be no pleural effusion.

T_3 A tumor of any size that extends directly into an adjacent structure such as the chest wall, diaphragm, or mediastinum, and its contents; or that at bronchoscopy is demonstrably less than 2.0 cm distal to the carina; or that is associated with atelectasis or obstructive pneumonitis of an entire lung or with pleural effusion.

Mountain and his associates[113] analyzed 2155 histologically proved bronchogenic carcinomas. Patients were included in the study only if their cancers had been diagnosed 4 or more years earlier and if follow-up information was available either up to the time of death or to survival for at least 4 years. Assessment of the T factor (Figure 8–15) revealed a direct relationship between the measurable clinical anatomic ex-

tent of the primary neoplasm and survival in cases of squamous-cell carcinoma, adenocarcinoma, and undifferentiated large cell carcinoma. Survival bore no relationship to the clinically recognized anatomic extent of disease in cases of undifferentiated small cell carcinoma. The most favorable variables were smallness of the primary neoplasm, a peripheral location, and absence of invasion of adjacent structures.

N—REGIONAL LYMPH NODES

N_0 No demonstrable metastasis to regional lymph nodes.

N_1 Metastasis to lymph nodes in the ipsilateral hilar region (including direct extension).

N_2 Metastasis to lymph nodes in the mediastinum.

Based on 1568 cases studied by Mountain and associates (excluding undifferentiated small cell carcinoma) (Figure 8–16), prognosis decreased sharply in proportion to the presence and extent of hilar and mediastinal node involvement.

M—DISTANT METASTASES

M_0 No distant metastasis.

M_1 Distant metastasis, as to scalene, cervical, or contralateral hilar lymph nodes, brain, bones, lung, or liver.

Figure 8–15. Prognosis in Patients with Lung Cancer: T Factor. Survival in lung cancer stratified by the anatomic extent of the primary tumor (T factor), excluding undifferentiated small cell carcinoma in 1678 cases. (Reprinted from Mountain, C. F., Carr, D. T., and Anderson, W. A. D.: Am. J. Roentgenol., 120:130, 1974, with permission of the authors and editor.)

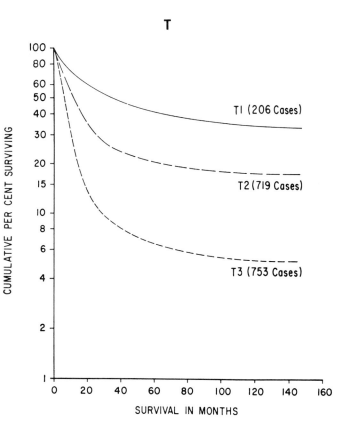

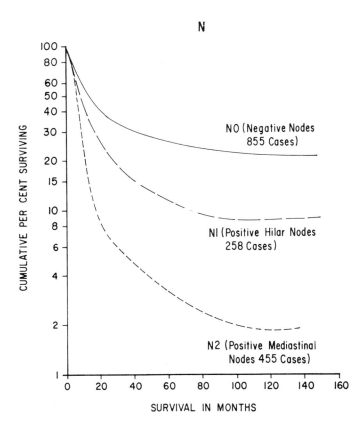

Figure 8–16. Prognosis in Patients with Lung Cancer: N Factor. Survival in lung cancer stratified by the extent of the regional lymph node involvement (N factor), excluding undifferentiated small cell carcinoma in 1568 cases. (Reprinted from Mountain, C. F., Carr, D. T., and Anderson, W. A. D.: Am. J. Roentgenol., *120*:130, 1974, with permission of the authors and editor.)

Figure 8–17. Prognosis in Patients with Lung Cancer: M Factor. Survival in lung cancer stratified by absence or presence of distant metastases (M factor), excluding undifferentiated small cell carcinoma in 1739 cases. (Reprinted from Mountain, C. F., Carr, D. T., and Anderson, W. A. D.: Am. J. Roentgenol., *120*:130, 1974, with permission of the authors and editor.)

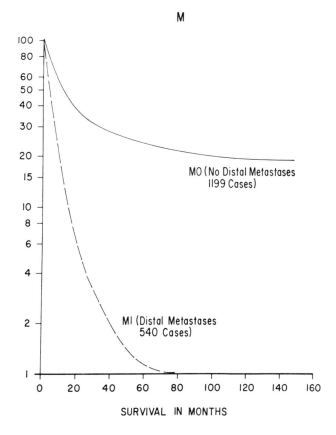

As expected (Figure 8–17), it was concluded that with current therapy lung cancer is incurable, regardless of cell type, once the disease has extended beyond the hemithorax of origin and beyond mediastinal lymph nodes.

Mountain and his colleagues later assigned the various TNM sets to stage groups, in order to minimize intragroup variation in survival and to create the greatest prognostic differences between stage groups. Their definitions of these stages are as follows.

Occult Carcinoma

$T_xN_0M_0$ An occult carcinoma with bronchopulmonary secretions containing malignant cells, but without other evidence of primary tumors, of metastasis to regional lymph nodes, or distant metastasis.

Invasive Carcinoma

Stage I

$T_1N_0M_0$ A tumor that can be classified T_1 without any metastasis or with metastasis to the lymph nodes in the ipsilateral hilar region only, or a tumor that can be classified T_2 without any metastasis to lymph nodes or distant metastasis. (Note that $T_xN_1M_0$ and $T_0T_1M_0$ also are theoretically possible, but clinically it would be difficult if not impossible to make such a diagnosis. If made, it should be included in stage I.)

Stage II

$T_2N_1M_0$ A tumor classified as T_2, with metastasis to the lymph nodes in the ipsilateral hilar region only.

Stage III

T_3 with any N or M

N_2 with any T or M

M_1 with any T or N

Any tumor more extensive than T_2 or any tumor with metastasis to the lymph nodes in the mediastinum or with distant metastasis.

Mountain and associates determined the survival relationships between the three stage groups, based on 2001 cases (Figure 8–18).

By using a common language for categorizing the extent of disease, the TNM system contributes to the attainment of several objectives: (1) the planning of treatment by the clinician; (2) the estimation of prognosis; (3) the validation of clinical evaluation and, thus, continuing self-assessment; and (4) perhaps most important,

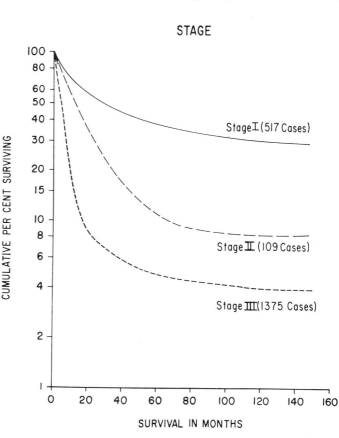

Figure 8–18. Prognosis in Patients with Lung Cancer: TNM Combinations. Survival in lung cancer stratified by stage (TNM combinations), with undifferentiated small cell carcinoma specified as stage III, in 2001 cases. (Reprinted from Mountain, C. F., Carr, D. T., and Anderson, W. A. D.: Am. J. Roentgenol., *120*:130, 1974, with permission of the authors and editor.)

STAGE

Stage I (517 Cases)

Stage II (109 Cases)

Stage III (1375 Cases)

CUMULATIVE PER CENT SURVIVING

SURVIVAL IN MONTHS

the facilitation of exchange of information among centers of study.

PROGNOSIS BASED ON COMBINED ANATOMIC AND CLINICAL STAGING

Feinstein, Carbone, and their colleagues[118, 119] have clearly demonstrated the importance of assessing tumor function (patient's symptoms) in determing survival rates and consider a combined anatomic and clinical classification a more valid starting point for assessing the results of therapy than staging by either method alone. They have proposed four clinicoanatomic stages. (1) Stage A, asymptomatic patients or those with "long primary" (6 months or more) symptoms, with anatomically local lesions. (2) Stage B, patients with no symptoms or with "long primary" symptoms associated with regional spread, or patients with "short primary" (less than 6 months) symptoms or systemic symptoms or both with anatomically local lesions. (3) Stage C, patients with "short primary" symptoms or systemic symptoms or both, associated with regional spread. (4) Stage D, patients with either anatomic or symptomatic evidence of metastases.

In an analysis of survival rates in 449 patients, these investigators[120] not only classified the neoplasms into six main histologic groups, but also correlated the tumor type with symptoms and anatomic stage. Epidermoid neoplasms were much more likely than the other groups to be detected in the biologically favorable stages A, B, or C; and within such stages the survival rates were highest for patients with epidermoid neoplasms, both operable and inoperable. For neoplasms detected in the unfavorable biologic stage D, however, inoperability rates and the outcome in operable or inoperable cases were not significantly affected by the histologic cell type. These results suggest that histologic typing adds a distinct prognostic gradient within the favorable symptom-anatomic stages of lung cancer but not within the unfavorable stages.

THERAPEUTIC CONSIDERATIONS IN PROGNOSIS

Surgical and, to a lesser extent, nonsurgical therapy (radiation therapy, chemotherapy, and immunotherapy) influence survival, since the great majority of patients who survive 5 years or longer after recognition of their disease have been treated. Few patients with lesions deemed inoperable or considered unresectable at thoracotomy live longer than 1 year, and most die within 6 months. In such patients life is probably not significantly prolonged with irradiation or chemotherapy or both. However, selected patients with bronchoscopically diagnosed oat-cell carcinoma considered to be potentially resectable may respond to radiotherapy, chemotherapy, or a combination of the two. In a study by the Medical Research Council of Great Britain,[121] three of 71 patients were alive 10 years after radical radiotherapy, whereas all 73 of a control group who underwent surgery were dead.

Although some authors believe that periodic chest roentgenograms of susceptible individuals have led to little[122] or no[123] improvement in survival, even when the lesions are solitary pulmonary nodules,[124] others[125] have found that roentgenologic and cytologic screening with fiberoptic bronchoscopy every four months may be of benefit in the "high-risk" group of middle-aged and older men who are chronic heavy smokers.

HODGKIN'S DISEASE

Hodgkin's disease is a malignant (though not necessarily neoplastic) affection of the lymphatic tissues and is usually classified as a lymphoma. Its major manifestation is lymph node enlargement, alone or concomitant with generalized disease of many organs, including the lungs. The clinical and histologic features of the disease vary in different parts of the world and in young and old patients.[126] MacMahon[127] described a bimodal incidence distribution, peaks occurring around the ages of 25 to 30 and around 70 years. There is a slight male predominance, and most patients are over the age of 20 years at time of diagnosis.

The etiology of Hodgkin's disease is unknown, but recent findings favor an environmental source to explain the uneven geographic distribution, the racial differences in incidence, the affinity for a high socioeconomic status population, and the alleged horizontal transmission.[128] The disease in young adults appears to differ somewhat from that in the older group, the former experiencing more nodular sclerosis and lymphocytic predominance.

In many mammalian species, lymphoid leukemias and lymphomas are caused by oncogenic viruses and can be induced experimentally by interfering with the animals' immune state. Although there have been reports of isolation of presumed causative organisms of lymphoproliferative disease in humans, the only viral etiology accepted at this time is that of the Epstein-Barr virus responsible for Burkitt's lymphoma.[129] Methods identical to those that have revealed viruses in other lymphoproliferative disease have failed to do so in Hodgkin's disease. Nevertheless, recent epidemiologic studies[130, 131] suggest that horizontal transmission may occur, predominantly from young patients to young or old persons.

The immune system is disrupted in patients with Hodgkin's disease, but it is not clear whether this reflects primary immunocompetence, is the result of the disease itself, or is both.

STAGING OF HODGKIN'S DISEASE

The purpose of staging is primarily to establish the type and amount of therapy required; it also aids in determining prognosis. A report of a Subcommittee at the Rye Conference in 1966[132] proposed the following classification.

STAGE I.   Disease limited to one anatomic region or two contiguous anatomic regions on the same side of the diaphragm.

STAGE II.   Disease in more than two anatomic regions or in two noncontiguous regions on the same side of the diaphragm.

STAGE III. Disease on both sides of the diaphragm, but not extending beyond the involvement of lymph nodes, spleen, and/or Waldeyer's ring.

STAGE IV.   Involvement of the bone marrow, lung parenchyma, pleura, liver, bone, skin, kidney, gastrointestinal tract, or any tissue or organ in addition to lymph nodes, spleen, or Waldeyer's ring.

All stages are subclassified as A or B, indicating the absence or presence of otherwise unexplained systemic symptoms: fever, night sweats, or pruritus. Staging can be based on physical findings alone, but many investigators include lymphography or computed tomography (CT) and some add exploratory laparotomy.

It has been shown that laparotomy alters the preoperative clinically determined staging in 25 to over 50 per cent of cases,[133] a finding of para-aortic lymph node or splenic involvement changing their status from stage I or II to III. In previous years, lymphangiography has proved a useful aid in determining the need for laparotomy, since an unequivocally positive lymphangiogram generally necessitates a change in therapeutic regimen. In recent years, however, it has been shown that CT yields more accurate information than lymphangiography and is the preferred method not only for the initial staging of patients with lymphoma but for follow-up studies after one year of therapy.[134]

The consensus in the management of Hodgkin's disease is total nodal irradiation (including the spleen) for patients with stages I and II disease above the diaphragm, and exploratory laparotomy (to assess whether liver or other nonlymphoid tissue is involved) for those with an abnormal CT scan or lymphangiogram or judged clinically to have stage III or IV disease.[133]

Intrathoracic involvement occurs in 90 per cent of patients at some stage in Hodgkin's disease, most commonly as mediastinal lymph node enlargement.

PATHOLOGIC CHARACTERISTICS

The pathologic classification of Hodgkin's disease includes four histologic types, as recommended by a Committee on Nomenclature of the American Cancer Society:[135] (1) lymphocyte predominance, (2) nodular sclerosis, (3) mixed cellularity, and (4) lymphocyte depletion.

The lymphocyte predominance type is as its name implies. Histiocytes are present in most cases and are numerous in about half. Reticulum cells and Reed-Sternberg cells are scanty. The histologic pattern may be nodular or diffuse.

The nodular sclerosis type is characterized by broad intersecting bands of doubly refractile collagenous fibrous tissue that partly or completely subdivides distinctively abnormal lymphoid tissue into isolated cellular nodules. The amount of collagen and the character of the cellular proliferation vary widely, even within the same specimen. The histologic pattern is predominantly cellular or sclerotic. A distinctive feature of the cellular proliferation is the extremely large size of the Reed-Sternberg cells. This binucleated or multinucleated cell with large nucleoli is a histologic requisite for the diagnosis of Hodgkin's disease of nodular sclerosing type. The cellular proliferation otherwise may be predominantly lymphocytic, or it may be mixed with numerous eosinophils or mature granulocytes or both. This form shows a predilection for local deposits in cervical and mediastinal node-bearing regions.

The mixed cellularity type is intermediate between lymphocyte predominance and lymphocyte depletion. The tumor contains lymphocytes, eosinophils, plasma cells, mature neutrophils, and histiocytes, as well as a proliferation of neoplastic reticulum and the characteristic giant cell, the Reed-Sternberg cell. Fibrosis may develop but birefringent collagen is absent. Growth is usually diffuse, but in some cases nodules are arranged in neoplastic pseudofollicles.

The lymphocyte-depletion type comprises several histologic expressions that have in common a scarcity of lymphocytes. This form of Hodgkin's disease is predominantly subdiaphragmatic, involving the liver, spleen, and retroperitoneal lymph nodes. All bone marrow sites are affected with severe marrow hyperplasia.

ROENTGENOGRAPHIC MANIFESTATIONS

Filly and his colleagues[136] have analyzed the incidence of various intrathoracic abnormalities identifiable on plain chest roentgenograms and tomograms in a series of 300 consecutive patients with untreated Hodgkin's disease and non-Hodgkin's lymphoma. The former condition was found to be associated with a higher incidence of intrathoracic disease at presentation (67 per cent compared with 43 per cent), manifested predominantly by bulky anterior mediastinal lymph node enlargement. Lung involvement was also more common in Hodgkin's disease (11.6 per cent compared with 3.7 per cent), and was always accompanied by mediastinal or hilar lymph node enlargement or both.

Mediastinal Lymph Node Enlargement

This is the most common roentgenographic finding in Hodgkin's disease and is seen on the initial chest roentgenogram of approximately 50 per cent of patients.[137]

In the majority, involvement is asymmetric but bilateral (Figure 8–19); unilateral node enlargement is unusual. The paratracheal and bifurcation groups are involved as often as or more often than the bronchopulmonary nodes. Involvement of anterior mediastinal and retrosternal nodes is common and may be associated with invasion of the sternum. This anatomic distribution is a major factor in the differential diagnosis from sarcoidosis, which seldom produces roentgenographically visible enlargement of nodes in the anterior compartment.

Enlargement of the posterior mediastinal

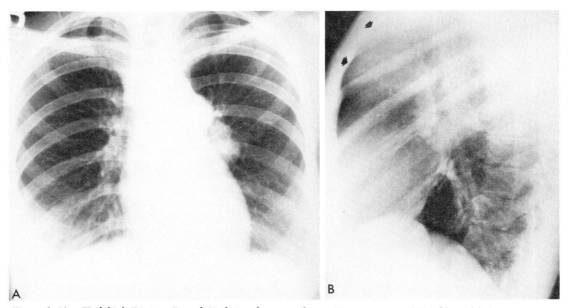

Figure 8–19. Hodgkin's Disease: Lymph Node Involvement Alone. Posteroanterior *(A)* and lateral *(B)* roentgenograms reveal marked enlargement of lymph nodes in the anterior and middle mediastinal compartments. Hilar node enlargement is left-sided and asymmetric; enlargement of the prevascular (anterior mediastinal) chain is best seen in lateral projection, where it is represented by a poorly defined increase in density anterosuperiorly *(arrows)*. The prominent bump on the left border of the mediastinum just above the left hilum represents enlargement of the lymph node of the ligamentum arteriosum. The combination of asymmetric hilar node enlargement and anterior mediastinal involvement constitutes strong evidence for the diagnosis of lymphoma. Support was obtained from an intravenous pyelogram, which revealed marked deformity of the left ureter caused by pressure from enlarged retroperitoneal nodes.

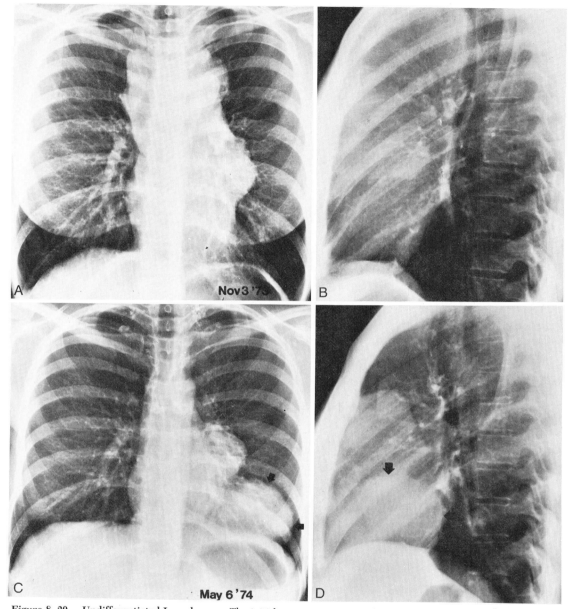

Figure 8–20. Undifferentiated Lymphoma. The initial roentgenograms on this 28-year-old woman (*A* and *B*) revealed markedly enlarged anterior mediastinal lymph nodes, biopsy of which showed undifferentiated lymphoma. A course of chemotherapy resulted in disappearance of all lymph node enlargement six weeks later. However, by four months (*C* and *D*), a large cardiophrenic mass had appeared (*arrows*) and a new group of prevascular nodes had developed in the anterior mediastinal compartment on the left. The cardiophrenic mass represents involvement of the diaphragmatic chain of parietal nodes.

nodes, which is rare, may be detected by extrinsic pressure defects in the barium-filled esophagus;[137] involvement of the posterior parietal chain may cause paravertebral masses and deform the posterior mediastinal line. The diaphragmatic group of parietal lymph nodes are not normally visible roentgenographically; when enlarged, they cause opacities that simulate pleuropericardial fat pads (Figure 8–20).[138]

Pleuropulmonary Involvement

Pulmonary involvement occurs in less than 30 per cent of patients, the great majority of whom have the nodular sclerosing type. With rare exception pulmonary involvement is accompanied by mediastinal lymph node enlargement.[139] Rarely if ever is Hodgkin's disease of the lung the sole manifestation of the dis-

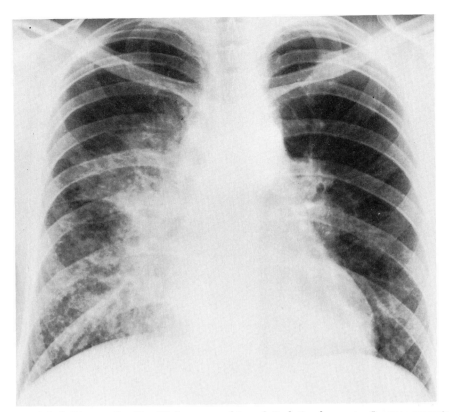

Figure 8–21. Hodgkin's Disease: Combined Pulmonary and Lymph Node Involvement. In posteroanterior projection, there is extensive disease of the right lung in the form of a coarse linear or reticular pattern extending outward along the bronchovascular bundles. In the right upper lobe, the shadows are largely confluent. Enlargement of hilar lymph nodes is masked by contiguous parenchymal disease, although there is definite evidence of paratracheal node enlargement (note the azygos node particularly). Kerley B lines are present above the costophrenic sulcus, probably owing to involvement of the interlobular septa by Hodgkin's tissue rather than to edema secondary to lymphatic obstruction. The patient is a 27-year-old man.

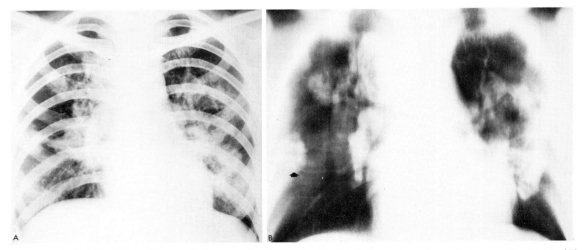

Figure 8–22. Hodgkin's Disease: Pulmonary Involvement with Cavitation. A posteroanterior roentgenogram *(A)* reveals extensive, bilateral parenchymal consolidation of a rather inhomogeneous nature occupying a "bat's wing" distribution. Hilar lymph node enlargement is present bilaterally but is partly obscured by contiguous parenchymal disease. In an anteroposterior tomogram *(B)*, an air bronchogram is clearly visualized in several areas, particularly the right upper lobe. Cavitation has occurred in a mass situated in the right axilla *(arrow)* and in the upper portion of the consolidation on the left. The predominantly right-sided hilar and paratracheal lymph node enlargement is readily apparent on the tomogram. (Courtesy of Dr. R. Lesperance.)

ease.[137, 139] In the exceptional cases in which pulmonary parenchymal lesions are present without mediastinal lymph node enlargement, either there is clinical or roentgenographic evidence of extrathoracic disease,[137] or the patient's disease has previously been treated and the present involvement represents recurrence.

Pulmonary parenchymal involvement usually occurs by direct extension from mediastinal nodes along the lymphatics of the bronchovascular sheaths (Figure 8–21). Consolidation of lung parenchyma remote from the mediastinum is not uncommon.[141] The size of such masses ranges widely and may vary with time; individual foci may coalesce to form a large homogeneous nonsegmental mass even involving a whole lobe.[141] This type of parenchymal consolidation is purely space-occupying, not causing loss of volume; its borders tend to be shaggy and ill defined. As the airways are not affected, an air bronchogram should be visible (Figure 8–22). Occasionally, parenchymal masses undergo cavitation.

Atelectasis occurs occasionally, but seldom if ever as a result of compression by enlarged lymph nodes.[142] Bronchial occlusion, almost always due to endobronchial disease invading the submucosal endobronchial lymphatic plexus,[137, 142] may give rise to lobar or segmental atelectasis or obstructive pneumonitis (Figure 8–23).

Pleural effusion occurs in approximately 30 per cent of cases, with other intrathoracic manifestations of the disease in most.[141] The fluid is serous, chylous, pseudochylous,[139] or (rarely) serosanguineous. Nonchylous pleural effusions result from lymphatic obstruction by enlarged mediastinal nodes;[143] in contrast to metastatic carcinoma, Hodgkin's disease seldom invades the pleura directly.

About 15 per cent of patients with Hodgkin's disease manifest bone involvement roentgenographically.[144] Vertebral involvement other than by direct extension is purely osteoblastic (ivory vertebrae) in some cases, although affection of nonthoracic bones (most commonly the spine and pelvis) usually results in mixed lytic and blastic lesions.[144]

CLINICAL MANIFESTATIONS

Most patients seek the advice of a physician as a result of noticing enlarged peripheral lymph nodes, an initial manifestation said to occur in 90 to 93 per cent of cases and localized to the cervical area in the great majority. Primary mediastinal involvement without superficial or retroperitoneal node enlargement occurs in about 6 to 11 per cent of cases.[145] The disease is usually most benign in cases in which the original presentation is enlarged nodes in the neck. Systemic symptoms such as fever, night sweats, pruritus, weight loss, weakness, and

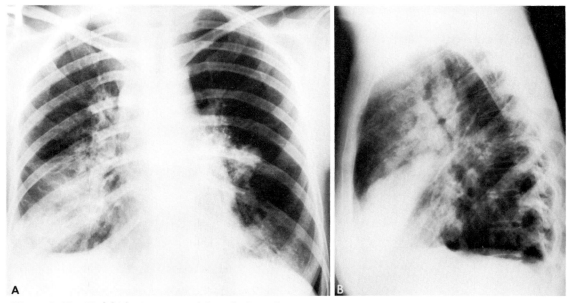

A   **B**

Figure 8–23. Hodgkin's Disease: Endobronchial Involvement. Posteroanterior (A) and lateral (B) roentgenograms demonstrate extensive bilateral parenchymal disease and paratracheal lymph node enlargement. On the left, the shadows are the result of parenchymal invasion by Hodgkin's disease. On the right, the middle lobe is airless and has lost considerable volume, the result of a combination of replacement of parenchyma by Hodgkin's disease and of bronchial obstruction resulting from endobronchial involvement. Proof obtained at necropsy.

fatigue are usually late manifestations. Although fever can be due to the primary disease, complicating infections should be excluded. Symptoms and signs usually depend upon the systems involved. In contrast to its occurrence in sarcoidosis, bilateral hilar node enlargement in Hodgkin's disease usually produces symptoms or detectable signs or both.[146] Pulmonary disease may be accompanied by cough, dyspnea, and pleural pain. The initial symptom may be retrosternal or abdominal pain due to enlargement of mediastinal or retroperitoneal lymph nodes. Involvement of bone commonly produces pain which, along with other symptoms, may be induced or worsened by the ingestion of alcohol. The spleen and liver are enlarged in about 50 per cent of cases.

In its later stages, especially when the patient is receiving corticosteroids or chemotherapeutic agents, Hodgkin's disease may be complicated by infection, usually opportunistic. The lungs may become infected, leading sometimes to serious difficulty in roentgenologic interpretation.

Major factors influencing *prognosis* are the histologic type and stage of disease at the time of diagnosis. The outlook is much better for patients with the lymphocyte predominance or nodular sclerosing type, particularly in stages I and II. At the University of Florida, Million[147] reported an overall 6-year survival of 53 per cent for treated patients, rising to 80 per cent for patients with stages IA, IIA, and IIIA disease. Diffuse disease of both lungs has a grave prognosis. As in bronchogenic carcinoma, symptoms, particularly systemic ones, carry a bad prognosis.[148] The presence of mediastinal lymph node enlargement as an initial manifestation of Hodgkin's disease has been found to be of prognostic importance: in a recent retrospective study of 189 patients, North[149] found that patients with stage I or II disease with mediastinal node enlargement at presentation had an 88 per cent five-year survival rate compared with a 98 per cent survival rate for those without mediastinal involvement. Disease-free survival was 66 per cent versus 78 per cent, respectively. Patients with Hodgkin's disease are at increased risk for leukemia or other malignancies, particularly acute leukemia.

NON-HODGKIN'S LYMPHOMAS

In addition to Hodgkin's disease (which is a specific entity identified histologically by the presence of Reed-Sternberg cells) are the lymphoproliferative diseases formerly known as the lymphosarcoma group but now usually referred to as non-Hodgkin's lymphomas; they originate from stem cells, reticulum cells, lymphoblasts, and lymphocytes. In contrast to Hodgkin's disease, which is a T cell disorder, most non-Hodgkin's lymphocytic lymphomas in adults appear to originate from B cells;[150] a few derive from stem cells or reticulum cells (histiocytes) of lymphoid tissue. Non-Hodgkin's lymphoma affects adults between the ages of 30 and 70 years and is slightly more common in females than males. A 1980 NIH Conference dealing with the non-Hodgkin's lymphomas reviewed the epidemiology, immunology, and pathology of this group of diseases.[151]

As with Hodgkin's disease, it seems likely that a transmissible agent is responsible for at least some cases of non-Hodgkin's lymphoma.[152] The Epstein-Barr virus has been implicated in the etiology of Burkitt's lymphoma. Non-Hodgkin's lymphomas, particularly the histiocytic variety (reticulum-cell sarcoma), occur with greater frequency than expected in immunosuppressed kidney transplant recipients, patients with primary immunologic deficiency syndromes, and in those with autoimmune diseases such as Sjögren's syndrome and scleroderma.[151, 152] Current concepts of the classification, diagnosis, and management of adult non-Hodgkin's lymphoma have recently been reviewed.[154]

PATHOLOGIC CHARACTERISTICS

The non-Hodgkin's lymphomas are subdivided on the basis of their histopathology; clinical and pathologic findings warrant a classification based on both cell type and architectural pattern. Bearing in mind that all types of non-Hodgkin's lymphoma (except Burkitt's lymphoma) can be either nodular or diffuse, the following classification, proposed by Rappaport[155] and slightly modified by Berard,[156] is most fitting.

Stem-Cell Lymphoma
1. Undifferentiated, Burkitt's type.
2. Undifferentiated, pleomorphic type.

Histiocytic Lymphoma
1. Histiocytic type (reticulum-cell sarcoma).
2. Histiocytic-lymphocytic (mixed cell) type.

Lymphocytic Lymphoma
1. Lymphocytic type, poorly differentiated.
2. Lymphocytic type, well differentiated.

Stem-Cell Lymphoma

Burkitt's lymphoma is characterized by cytologic uniformity of neoplastic cells, with no clear differentiation as to histiocytic or lymphocytic cell types despite moderate nuclear and cytoplasmic variations. Lymph node involvement is usually abdominal; peripheral and mediastinal nodes are affected in only a minority of cases.

The rare second form of stem-cell lymphoma—the undifferentiated pleomorphic type—occurs in older adults and its cellular pleomorphism readily distinguishes it from Burkitt's lymphoma. It may subsequently differentiate into either the histiocytic or the lymphocytic type.

Histiocytic Lymphoma

The *histiocytic type* (reticulum-cell sarcoma) can be subdivided according to histiocytic differentiation of neoplastic cells. It develops mostly in older adults and is characterized by either generalized enlargement of lymph nodes or limitation to a single lymph node group or extranodal site. The histologic pattern may be diffuse or nodular.

Mixed Cell Histiocytic-Lymphocytic Type

This type shows proliferation of roughly equal numbers of neoplastic histiocytes and lymphocytes. Later, histopathologic changes of the pure histiocytic type occur in about 90 per cent of cases.

Lymphocytic Lymphoma

Lymphocytic lymphoma includes poorly differentiated and well-differentiated types. The *poorly differentiated form* (lymphoblastic lymphoma), which accounts for about 90 per cent of cases, has a diverse cellular constitution. The nodular (follicular) variety is common in adults but rare in children. In adults, lymphoblastic cells vary greatly in size and configuration, but in children they are usually homogeneous. Acute leukemia develops in about 30 per cent of affected children. The *well-differentiated form* (lymphocytic lymphoma) accounts for the other 10 per cent of this group. Lymphocytes are small to medium-sized, mature, and with little intercellular variation. Compared with the poorly differentiated type, this form is usually much less nodular and occurs in older patients; it may represent a local manifestation of chronic lymphocytic leukemia.

Mycosis Fungoides

Mycosis fungoides is a lymphomatous process predominantly affecting the skin and clinically resembling eczema or psoriasis. The commonest presentation is as scaly cutaneous plaques or frank tumors, which may ulcerate; rarely, the disease begins with an exfoliative erythroderma. The viscera are invaded later, and necropsy may reveal lymphoma in almost every organ but chiefly in lymph nodes, spleen, liver, and lungs.[157] Histologically, the process may resemble any other lymphoma, consisting of lymphocytes, histiocytes, and atypical reticulum cells with large hyperchromatic nuclei. Mycosis fungoides appears to be a disorder of T lymphocytes. The prognosis is poor.

Pseudolymphoma

This term usually designates collections of apparently benign lymphocytes that lack the usual invasive characteristics of lymphoma. This disease is manifested in the lung by peripheral nodules, segmental parenchymal consolidation, or diffuse interstitial infiltration. In contrast to lymphocytic lymphomas (which have a uniform cellular infiltrate of mature or immature lymphocytes without germinal centers), pseudolymphoma has a mixed cellular infiltrate and lymphoid germinal centers. Another feature indicating benignity is lack of invasion of regional lymph nodes and extrapulmonary tissues.[158] In most cases in which diagnosis is based on these morphologic criteria, the clinical course supports the nonmalignant nature of the disease.[159]

ROENTGENOGRAPHIC MANIFESTATIONS

In a recently published retrospective review of 112 nonselected patients with histiocytic lymphoma, Burgener and Hamlin[160] found intrathoracic involvement in exactly 50 per cent: of these 56 cases, mediastinal node enlargement was present in 28 (50 per cent), hilar node enlargement in 19 (34 per cent), pulmonary involvement in 22 (40 per cent), and pleural involvement in 20 (36 per cent).

Mediastinal Lymph Node Involvement

Mediastinal or bronchopulmonary lymph node enlargement is the commonest intrathoracic manifestation of the disease.

Pleuropulmonary Involvement

Primary pulmonary non-Hodgkin's lymphoma is nearly always of the lymphocytic type and rarely histiocytic. In the lungs it usually presents as a homogeneous mass, in some cases occupying an entire lung.[161] In most cases the

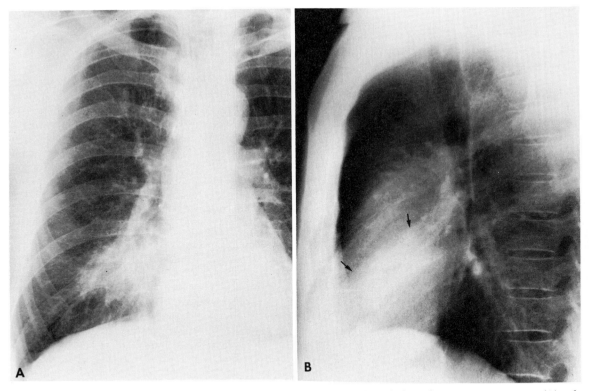

Figure 8–24. **Primary Pulmonary Lymphocytic Lymphoma.** Views of the right hemithorax in posteroanterior *(A)* and lateral *(B)* projection reveal a poorly defined shadow of homogeneous density in the right middle lobe (note the silhouette sign); the distribution does not conform to a bronchopulmonary segment *(arrows in B)*. Although an air bronchogram is not apparent on the plain roentgenogram, patency of the bronchial tree within the mass was demonstrated bronchographically. Note the absence of hilar or mediastinal lymph node enlargement. The resected right middle lobe showed well-circumscribed replacement of lung parenchyma by lymphosarcoma. This 48-year-old man had rather nonspecific complaints consisting of fatigue and frequent sweating. (Courtesy of Dr. George Genereux, University Hospital, Saskatoon.)

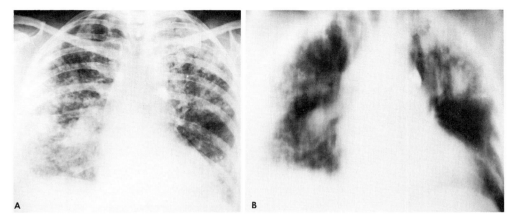

Figure 8–25. **Histiocytic Lymphoma (Secondary).** A posteroanterior roentgenogram *(A)* and anteroposterior tomogram *(B)* reveal extensive involvement of both lungs by a multitude of nodular and patchy shadows of homogeneous density. Individual shadows range from 2 to 10 mm in diameter and in some areas are confluent; in areas of confluence (such as the left midlung), an air bronchogram can be identified. Gross hilar and paratracheal lymph node enlargement is present. This 46-year-old woman also showed roentgenologic evidence of extensive involvement of her stomach and small bowel by histiocytic lymphoma. At necropsy, numerous firm, whitish-gray nodules measuring up to 1 cm in diameter were present throughout the lungs; the hilar and mediastinal lymph nodes were grossly enlarged.

mass has a rather smooth outline, with fairly sharply circumscribed margins, and is located centrally (Figure 8–24). A characteristic of this lesion is that it rarely obstructs the bronchial tree by either intraluminal invasion or extrabronchial compression; as a result, an air bronchogram almost invariably can be identified. When such consolidation involves most or all of a segment or a lobe, it may simulate acute air-space pneumonia.

In contrast to bronchogenic carcinoma, primary non-Hodgkin's lymphoma shows a propensity to transgress interlobar fissures and the pleura over the convexity of the lung.[162] A distinctive presentation of the histiocytic type of non-Hodgkin's lymphoma, seen in no other pulmonary neoplasm in our experience, is the rapid onset of extensive parenchymal disease early in the course of the illness. The extreme rapidity of roentgenographic progression of parenchymal consolidation invariably leads to a suspicion of acute infection, and lung biopsy is usually necessary to establish the true nature of the process.[163]

The typical roentgenographic pattern in *secondary* pulmonary non-Hodgkin's lymphoma is of solitary or multiple "nodular" lesions 3 mm to 7 cm in diameter (Figure 8–25).[161] Unlike primary pulmonary lymphoma, the secondary variety tends to be located endobronchially and thus results in atelectasis and obstructive pneumonitis.

Direct extension of the neoplasm from mediastinal nodes may cause pericardial effusion. Involvement of the skeleton in non-Hodgkin's lymphoma is fairly common; the lesions are characteristically osteolytic. Pleural effusion occurs in about one-third of all cases but, as in Hodgkin's disease, in only a few of those with primary disease.

CLINICAL MANIFESTATIONS

The extrathoracic manifestations of these processes often predominate, patients presenting with fever, anorexia, weight loss, and weakness. Involvement of the upper respiratory and gastrointestinal tracts, including the nasopharynx, tonsils, stomach, and bowel, is commoner than in Hodgkin's disease and may simulate carcinoma. The spleen usually enlarges as the disease progresses, and invasion of the spinal cord, cranial nerves, and meninges may produce pain, paresthesias, and paralyses.

About one-third of patients with primary pulmonary disease are asymptomatic; the remainder complain of cough, sometimes with hemoptysis, chest pain, and dyspnea.[162] Enlarged mediastinal lymph nodes may invade the recurrent laryngeal nerve, causing vocal cord paralysis, and may obstruct the superior vena cava.

PROGNOSIS

When extralymphatic lymphoma is confined to the lungs or elsewhere, the prognosis is more favorable than with either nodular or widespread nodal lymphomas.[153, 164] In the case of diffuse non-Hodgkin's lymphoma, the prognosis is determined by architectural pattern and cell type. Nodularity points to a better survival rate with all cell types except the histiocytic-lymphocytic (mixed cell) variety.[165] Within the nodular and diffuse groups the prognosis relates to cell type,[165] being better for the lymphocytic well-differentiated type than for the poorly differentiated type.

IMMUNOBLASTIC LYMPHADENOPATHY

Immunoblastic lymphadenopathy,[166] or angioimmunoblastic lymphadenopathy, is a hyperimmune disorder, most probably of B lymphocytes, which may closely resemble Hodgkin's disease. It is distinguishable morphologically from Hodgkin's disease, and although the clinical presentation may be similar it is associated with other immune phenomena, including autoimmune hemolytic anemia, polyclonal hyperglobulinemia, and in some cases initial hypersensitivity reactions to therapeutic agents. The disease is most commonly seen in patients over the age of 50, and, based on the limited data available, occurs more commonly in males than in females.[166]

Pathologic changes are found in lymph nodes, spleen, liver, bone marrow, and occasionally in other organs, including the lung.[166] The lymph nodes show a mixed cellular proliferation of immunologically reactive cells, including immunoblasts, plasmacytoid immunoblasts, and plasma cells. There is a striking proliferation of arborizing small vessels. Reed-Sternberg cells are not seen. The roentgenographic pattern is identical to that of Hodgkin's disease, with paratracheal and mediastinal lymph node enlargement.

Patients present with fever, sweats, weight loss, generalized lymphadenopathy, hepatosplenomegaly, and skin rashes. The course of the disease is usually progressive; many patients die from overwhelming infection.

LEUKEMIA

Leukemia may be granulocytic, lymphocytic, or monocytic, and acute or chronic. Lymphomas are solid tumors of blood-forming organs, and it may be impossible to determine whether a lymphoproliferative disorder represents lymphocytic leukemia or lymphocytic lymphoma. The acute leukemias are commonest in children; chronic lymphocytic leukemia has a predilection for middle-aged males. The main clinical manifestations of leukemia are excessive bleeding, enlargement of lymph nodes at various sites, and lack of resistance to infection.

Necropsy studies have confirmed that intrathoracic involvement is a common late development in leukemia. Mediastinal lymph node enlargement is found in about 50 per cent of cases[167] and pulmonary parenchymal disease in approximately 25 per cent.[168] Acute monocytic leukemia particulary tends to infiltrate the lungs. Of the chronic leukemias, the lymphocytic variety invades the lungs significantly more often than does the granulocytic types.[168]

In contrast to the relatively frequent finding of leukemic infiltration of the lungs at necropsy, *roentgenographic abnormalities* in the chest during life are much more likely to be due to infection or heart failure.[168] Some pulmonary opacities observed roentgenologically are due to hemorrhage.

The commonest roentgenographic sign of leukemia within the thorax is mediastinal and hilar lymph node enlargement; this occurs in about 25 per cent of patients[167] and is much commoner in the lymphocytic than the granulocytic form. (Note that this figure represents only half the incidence found at necropsy.)[167]

The usual pattern of pulmonary parenchymal involvement is diffuse bilateral reticulation resembling that of lymphangitic carcinoma and tending to occur only in the terminal stages (Figure 8–26).[168] Sometimes the pattern consists of extensive patchy air-space consolidation resembling acute pulmonary edema, an abnormality that can develop exceedingly rapidly.[169] Pleural effusion, usually unilateral, is second only to mediastinal node enlargement in frequency.

Typically, acute leukemia has an abrupt *clin-*

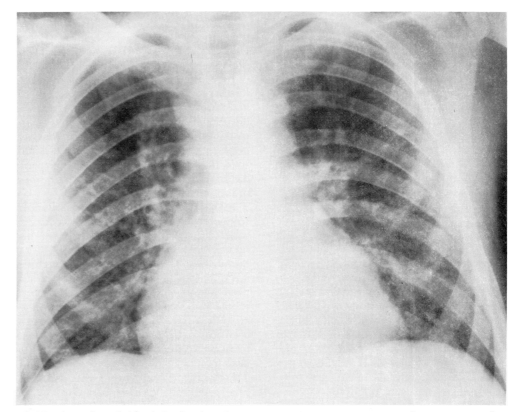

Figure 8–26. Acute Lymphoblastic Leukemia. An anteroposterior roentgenogram reveals a course reticular network throughout both lungs; there is no convincing evidence of hilar or mediastinal lymph node enlargement, although the spleen was markedly enlarged. This 17-year-old boy was in a terminal state with acute lymphoblastic leukemia. Necropsy showed extensive invasion of the interstitial tissues of the lungs by leukemic cells.

ical onset with major symptoms and signs related to bleeding or infection. Lymph nodes are enlarged at the onset in over one-third of cases, most frequently in lymphocytic leukemia. The spleen and liver are usually enlarged, and bleeding, oral infections, and retinal hemorrhages are frequent manifestations. Fever and pallor resulting from hemolysis or hemorrhage are almost invariable. Joint pain may simulate acute rheumatic fever.

Chronic leukemia usually develops insidiously, revealing itself by painless lymph node enlargement or hepatosplenomegaly. Lymph node enlargement and moderate enlargement of abdominal organs are usual in the lymphocytic form, whereas gross splenomegaly is characteristic of granulocytic leukemia. Generalized weakness and loss of weight and appetite develop as the disease progresses. In the chronic form, anemia and hemorrhage due to thrombocytopenia occur late.

Pulmonary symptoms, including cough, expectoration, and hemoptysis, usually are the result of infection rather than leukemic infiltration; in fact, leukemic infiltration of the lung parenchyma is seldom of clinical significance.

Leukemia is diagnosed on the finding of typical cells in the peripheral blood or bone marrow. The total leukocyte count is increased in nearly all cases, but may be normal or even reduced, with few immature cells in the peripheral blood. In the latter circumstances, examination of the bone marrow is required to establish the diagnosis.

THE PLASMA CELL DYSCRASIAS

These include multiple myeloma (plasma cell myeloma), Waldenström's macroglobulinemia, heavy-chain disease (IgG, IgA, or IgM), and amyloidosis. The first three are malignant proliferative diseases of plasma cells or plasmacytoid lymphocytes, justifying their inclusion in this chapter on neoplastic diseases. Amyloidosis sometimes develops in association with plasma cell myeloma, but more often it is secondary to chronic inflammatory disease. It is included here because it probably represents a *consequence* of plasma cell dyscrasia, chemical studies having shown that the major protein constituents of amyloid are fragments of immunoglobulin polypeptide chains.[170] The malignant plasma cell dyscrasias almost invariably show a monoclonal gammopathy. This anomalous immunoglobulin, which is detectable by serum or urine electrophoresis or immunoelectrophoresis, belongs to one of the five immunoglobu-

lins or to their heavy or light polypeptide chains. The term M peak (or M-type protein) designates these homogeneous immunoglobulin spikes. Monoclonal gammopathy does not necessarily indicate plasma cell dyscrasia, since M peaks (due to IgM, or less often to IgG) are present in some cases of chronic lymphocytic leukemia and lymphocytic lymphoma.

MULTIPLE MYELOMA (PLASMACYTOMA)

Thoracic involvement in multiple myeloma occurs in three forms: (1) direct extension from primary involvement of a rib, undoubtedly the commonest form;[171] (2) solitary plasmacytoma originating in the upper respiratory tract, including the trachea; and (3) solitary plasmacytoma originating in lung parenchyma.

Morphologically, these neoplasms are grossly firm, pale gray masses of various sizes, and histologically show the typical, uniform, monotonous pattern of abnormal plasma cells.

Primary plasmacytoma of the trachea is rare—as are all histologic types of primary tracheal neoplasms. Large lesions may obstruct either inspiration or expiration, depending upon their location in the cervical or thoracic trachea, respectively.

Secondary thoracic involvement from a primary lesion in the rib presents a rather typical roentgenographic appearance, a smooth homogeneous soft tissue mass protruding into the thorax, compressing the lung, and usually at an obtuse angle to contiguous chest wall (Figure 8–27). The association of an osteolytic lesion in a rib with a soft tissue mass protruding into the thorax should strongly suggest the possibility of myeloma,[171] although this combination may occur with other chest wall affections also (*e.g.,* osteomyelitis or rib metastases) and with lesions originating in the lung, including primary bronchogenic carcinoma and acute fungal infections.

Primary parenchymal myeloma presents as solitary or multiple masses, somewhat lobulated in contour and homogeneous in density, indistinguishable from peripheral bronchogenic carcinoma. Occasionally mediastinal lymph node enlargement will be evident.[172]

The great majority of patients with plasma-cell myeloma are symptomatic when first seen, by which time their disease is widely disseminated. In one large series,[173] initial findings included bone pain (68 per cent), anemia (62 per cent), renal insufficiency (55 per cent), hypercalcemia (30 per cent), palpable liver (21 per cent), and palpable spleen (5 per cent). Proteinuria was noted in 88 per cent, of Bence-

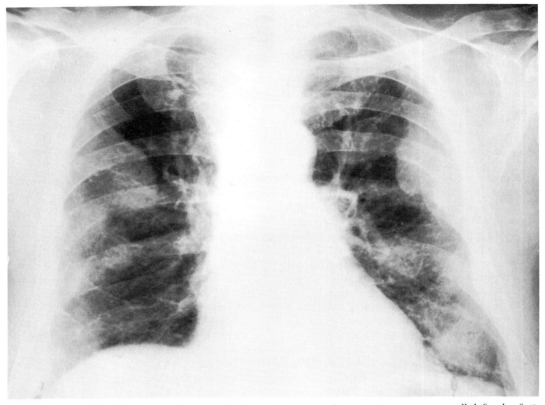

Figure 8–27. Multiple Myeloma. A posteroanterior roentgenogram demonstrates numerous, well-defined soft tissue masses of homogeneous density protruding into the thorax from the chest wall bilaterally. Each of the masses is related to a destructive lesion in an adjacent rib. Destructive lesions are present in both clavicles. This picture is highly suggestive if not diagnostic of multiple myeloma.

Jones type in 49 per cent. Approximately 60 per cent of symptomatic patients have monoclonal gammopathy of IgG type, and 20 per cent of IgA type; the remainder manifest Bence-Jones proteinuria or proteinemia, as determined by immunoelectrophoresis.[173]

The *prognosis* in plasma cell myeloma is considerably better in patients with one or two plasmacytomas than in those with generalized disease. Most patients with symptomatic multiple myeloma die from infection (usually bacterial) or renal insufficiency.[173]

WALDENSTRÖM'S MACROGLOBULINEMIA

This rare lymphoproliferative disorder is characterized by anemia, lymphocytic or plasmacytoid infiltration of the bone marrow, and monoclonal IgM gammopathy. An association with autoimmune disorders is frequent; a specific histocompatibility antigen has been detected in a family.[174] Hepatomegaly, splenomegaly, and palpable peripheral adenopathy are common. The lungs are seldom involved.

A review of the roentgenologic manifestations of primary macroglobulinemia[175] listed the following: the reticuloendothelial system (variable degrees of hepatosplenomegaly and lymphadenopathy); the osseous system (generalized osteopenia); the gastrointestinal tract (slight dilatation and thickening of the mucosal folds of the small bowel); the central nervous system (subarachnoid or subdural hemorrhage); miscellaneous areas (arthritis); and the chest. Characteristically, the chest roentgenogram shows a diffuse reticulonodular pattern or, less commonly, local homogeneous consolidation. Pleural effusion is present in about 50 per cent of cases.

HEAVY-CHAIN DISEASE

These plasma cell dyscrasias are associated with monoclonal gammopathies that result from Fc fragments of heavy chains from IgG, IgA, and IgM molecules. In *IgG heavy-chain disease*, enlargement of lymph nodes (including mediastinal ones) is common, and there is hepatosplenomegaly, anemia, and leukopenia. Most of these patients die from pneumonia within a year of diagnosis.[176] *IgA heavy-chain disease* is usually associated with an abdominal neoplasm and severe primary malabsorption syndrome.[177]

BRONCHOPULMONARY AMYLOIDOSIS

Amyloidosis is a disease of undetermined origin in which amyloid, a complex protein-polysaccharide, is deposited in various tissues. The major protein constituents are fragments of immunoglobulin polypeptide chains. Electrophoresis and immunoelectrophoresis have implicated plasma cell dyscrasia as the origin of the majority of cases of both "primary" and "secondary" amyloidosis.[170] In comparison with other organs, the lungs are seldom involved.

Amyloidosis occurs in three main forms, which differ in staining qualities, organs involved, and the degree of association with other diseases. Secondary amyloidosis, by far the commonest type, develops in rheumatoid arthritis, malignant neoplasms, and chronic suppurative disease. The amyloid, which characteristically is deposited in the spleen, liver, kidneys, and adrenals, readily absorbs Congo red, iodine, and methyl violet stains. The other two forms are primary amyloidosis (including an inherited subgroup), in which there is no clear-cut association with other diseases, and the amyloidosis that develops in some cases of multiple myeloma. In both these forms, amyloid deposition occurs in the heart, blood vessels, smooth and striated muscle, lymph nodes, spleen, gastrointestinal tract, and lungs, and the amyloid does not consistently stain by the usual histochemical methods. In primary amyloidosis, 35 to 70 per cent of cases show roentgenologic evidence of deposition in the lung; in fact, the disease may be confined to the lungs, apparently more often in men than in women.[178] By contrast, bronchopulmonary involvement is rare in secondary amyloidosis and can be appreciated only microscopically.

Pathologically, there are three main patterns of amyloid involvement in the chest, differing markedly in their anatomic sites and the effects they produce. (1) A *tracheobronchial form,* in which amyloid is deposited in the walls of the tracheobronchial tree, chiefly the submucosal muscle and adventitia. In this form the mucous membrane usually remains intact and the lung parenchyma is unaffected. (2) A *nodular parenchymal form,* in which solitary or, more often, multiple[178] masses of amyloid develop within the lung parenchyma. The pulmonary nodules, which are up to 9 cm in diameter, are very slow growing. Their histopathology frequently reveals calcification and ossification of the amyloid. (3) *A diffuse alveolar septal form,* histologically different from the nodular form, in which the amyloid infiltrates almost every alveolar septum diffusely and is deposited around capillaries and within the interstitial tissue.[178] It is usually associated with systemic amyloidosis or multiple myeloma.[178]

In the tracheobronchial form, *roentgenographic manifestations* range from general accentuation of bronchovascular markings associated with overinflation to the effects of bronchial obstruction by intramural masses of amyloid. The parenchymal form is evident as solitary or multiple masses, in some cases calcified or ossified and perhaps cavitated. The diffuse alveolar septal form has a nodular pattern simulating miliary tuberculosis, silicosis, or sarcoidosis.[179] Hilar and mediastinal lymph nodes may be enlarged, sometimes massively, and associated with dense calcification.[180] Occasionally, obstructive bronchial amyloidosis and peripheral parenchymal disease occur concomitantly.

In the variety with tracheobronchial involvement, the *clinical picture* may simulate bronchial asthma, with wheezing and dyspnea;[181] hemoptysis is common.[181] In the obstructive variety, symptoms and signs depend on the volume of lung involved and whether infection is present; hoarseness is common. The nodular parenchymal form usually provokes no symptoms,[178] whereas the diffuse alveolar septal amyloidosis often occasions severe dyspnea. Biopsy of rectal tissue or of subcutaneous abdominal fat may confirm the diagnosis, but transbronchial, needle, or open-lung biopsy may be required. Monoclonal gammopathy is absent in most cases.

The prognosis is much better for the nodular pulmonary parenchymal type than for the tracheobronchial, obstructive, or diffuse interstitial forms.[182] Diffuse septal involvement often leads to death from respiratory insufficiency.[178]

METASTATIC NEOPLASMS

Metastases to the lungs occur in approximately 30 per cent of all cases of malignant disease and are confined to the lungs in about half of these. Metastatic thoracic disease occurs most frequently after middle age, coincident with the increased incidence of neoplasia. There is no significant sex predominance.

Neoplasms originating elsewhere may spread to the lungs or pleura through the vascular or lymphatic systems or by direct extension. ("Direct extension of disease" may not be truly "metastatic," but the latter term is used here in its broadest sense.) *Direct extension* may occur from the chest wall, mediastinum, or below the diaphragm. This method of spread is relatively rare, and occurs mainly from carcinoma of the breast, liver, or pancreas. Encroachment on or invasion of the pulmonary parenchyma by mediastinal masses may simulate primary bronchogenic carcinoma arising in the paramediastinal lung areas and extending to mediastinal lymph nodes.

Vascular and Lymphatic Spread

Although over 80 per cent of lung metastases originate in the breast or skeletal or urogenital systems,[183] almost all primary neoplasms have a propensity to metastasize. Neoplasms with a rich vascular supply draining directly into the systemic venous system, such as renal cell carcinoma, sarcoma of bone, and trophoblastic tumors, have a very high incidence of pulmonary metastases.[184] The commonest pathway for metastases to the lungs is the systemic veins, either directly by invasion at the primary site or indirectly via the thoracic or right lymphatic duct and subclavian veins. Thoracic duct lymph is a common vehicle for dissemination of malignant cells in humans. Since remote spread of primary bronchogenic carcinoma will follow invasion of the pulmonary veins and dissemination by the systemic circulation, pulmonary hematogenous metastases from such neoplasms have a lower incidence than those arising elsewhere.

It is highly probable that the vast majority of neoplastic cells that reach the capillary sieve of the lungs do not find fertile ground for growth or are removed by macrophages. There is substantial evidence that metastases in the lungs are more likely to flourish when large numbers of cells reach the lung capillaries.[185]

Many malignancies, particularly carcinoma of the breast and stomach, characteristically disseminate through the lymphatic system of the lungs.[183] Spread to the pulmonary and pleural lymphatics is believed to occur in two ways: (1) hematogenous dissemination to the lung capillaries, followed by invasion of the peripheral lymphatics and spread along them toward the hila;[186] and (2) less commonly by retrograde lymphatic invasion, in which malignant cells first involve the anterior or posterior mediastinal chains of nodes (for example, from carcinoma of the breast or stomach), advance via anastomotic channels to the bronchomediastinal group of nodes, and finally spread retrogradely through the lung lymphatics. It has been suggested[186] that in the majority of cases the natural history of lymphangitic carcinomatosis is as follows. First, cancer cells reach the lungs by hematogenous spread, embolizing in small peripheral vessels; second, cells that are viable grow to form small parenchymal nodules; third, the neoplasm extends through blood vessel walls and invades adjacent interstitium and lymphatics; and finally, it spreads medially by permeation of the peribronchial-perivascular lymphatics. In this way, hilar lymph nodes may become the seat of metastatic neoplasms as a *result* of lymphangitic permeation.

Although the spontaneous disappearance of lung metastases is well documented, its mechanism is not fully understood. Renal or trophoblastic neoplasms are the primary lesions in most cases.

Pleural metastases from sites other than the lung are considered to represent tertiary spread from established hepatic secondaries; this is particularly true when pleural involvement is bilateral.[72] Of considerable importance is the fact that serous pleural effusions may result from lymphatic obstruction secondary to neoplastic infiltration of mediastinal lymph nodes; in such circumstances the effusion is not necessarily related to direct pleural invasion by neoplastic cells.[72] Effusions usually are hemorrhagic when caused by direct neoplastic involvement of pleural surfaces and serous when secondary to lymphatic obstruction.[72]

Pathologically, malignant cells that survive after reaching the lung via the bloodstream become encased in fibrin clinging to vascular endothelium; emboli tend to lodge at the bifurcation of capillaries and arterioles. Some traverse the vessel wall and lodge in the extravascular interstitial space, the lymphatics, or the alveoli. Massive intracapillary spread may develop, presumably as a result of the complete loss of defense mechanisms.[187] In such cases, and in those in which 70 to 75 per cent of the pulmonary vasculature is obstructed by tumor emboli, cor pulmonale results, with dilatation and hypertrophy of the right ventricle. Pathologically, lymphangitic carcinomatosis is distinctive, with features quite different from those of the usual hematogenous deposits. The neoplasm most likely to permeate the lymphatics is adenocarcinoma of the breast. Invasion of adjacent connective tissues varies: little fibrous stromal reaction is apparent with neoplasms entirely within the lymphatic vessels, but spread to contiguous connective tissue and parenchyma tends to provoke considerable desmoplasia, particularly in pleural and subpleural zones.

ROENTGENOGRAPHIC MANIFESTATIONS

The commonest roentgenographic evidence of metastatic disease consists of one or more well-defined nodular masses, from 3 mm to 6 cm in diameter or even larger. The lesions are multiple in 75 per cent of cases.[183]

Solitary Metastases

Solitary metastatic neoplasms represent a distinct group that must be differentiated from any other cause of a solitary nodule in the lungs. In the all-male Veterans' Administration series of 887 asymptomatic patients with solitary pulmonary nodules 6 cm or less in diameter, 3 per cent were solitary metastases.[13] Certain primary neoplasms are more likely than others to produce solitary metastases:. carcinoma of the colon, particularly the rectosigmoid area (which accounts for 30 to 40 per cent of all cases);[13] sarcomas, particularly those originating in bone; carcinoma of the kidney, testicle, and breast; and malignant melanoma.[13]

Most solitary metastatic lesions have smooth or slightly lobulated margins, occur predominantly in the lower lobes, and seldom if ever have satellite lesions. They tend to be well circumscribed, in contrast to the poor definition of primary bronchogenic carcinoma.

Identification of a primary neoplasm elsewhere, or even a history of resection of a primary neoplasm, does not *necessarily* indicate that a solitary mass in the lung is metastatic, and it may be exceedingly difficult to determine the most efficacious management of these patients.

Full lung tomography or CT scanning preoperatively may reveal small nodules not visible on standard roentgenograms whose presence would contraindicate surgery. (*See* page 106 for a discussion of this subject.)

When a solitary mass is identified in the lungs, some physicians feel obliged to put the patient through a battery of roentgenologic and other diagnostic procedures, searching for a primary malignancy. We decry this tendency, mainly because the great majority of such searches are fruitless, a conclusion supported

enthusiastically in two recent studies.[188, 189] In addition, we feel that nearly all patients with a solitary metastatic focus in the lung have symptoms or signs directing attention to the primary site. Further, if a resected lesion proves to be metastatic, there is a good possibility that its histologic appearance will be sufficiently specific to indicate the site of origin and lead to removal of the primary neoplasm.

Subepithelial endobronchial metastases are rare in comparison with parenchymal deposits. The most numerous extrathoracic neoplasms to metastasize to central airways are renal and colorectal carcinomas.[190] Other primary neoplasms reported include those of the breast, pancreas, adrenal glands, thyroid, and testicle, and malignant melanoma.

Disseminated Hematogenous Metastases

The pattern of widely disseminated metastatic disease varies from a normal roentgenogram (in the earliest stages, when deposits are too small to be visible), to diffuse micronodular shadows resembling miliary disease (Figure 8–28), to multiple large well-defined masses (the "cannonball" type of metastases; Figure 8–29).

A fine micronodular pattern is sometimes seen if the primary neoplasm is highly vascular, such as renal cell or thyroid carcinoma, sarcoma of bone, and trophoblastic disease (Figure 8–28). In such cases the many lesions may be of uniform size, indicating a simultaneous origin in one shower of emboli, or may differ, suggesting embolic inoculations of different ages; this latter pattern is rare in cases of benign diffuse pulmonary nodular disease.[184] In hematogenous spread, the mediastinal and hilar nodes are usually not enlarged.

Disseminated Lymphangitic Metastases

The most frequent origins of predominantly lymphangitic metastatic spread throughout the lungs are the breast, stomach, thyroid, pancreas, larynx, cervix, and lungs. The pathogenesis of this type of spread (discussed earlier in this section) almost certainly relates to the invasion of lymphatics from hematogenous metastases in the lung periphery, only a minority being caused by retrograde extension into the lungs from bronchopulmonary lymph nodes. The roentgenographic pattern consists of coarsened bronchovascular markings of irregular contour and sometimes indistinctly defined, simulating interstitial pulmonary edema. In most patients the pattern is uniform throughout

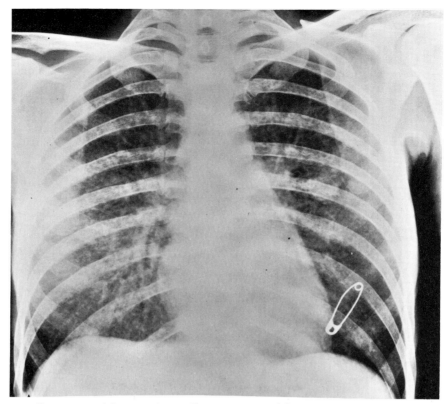

Figure 8–28. Diffuse Micronodular Metastases, Choriocarcinoma of the Uterus. An anteroposterior roentgenogram (*A*) of this 38-year-old woman reveals widespread nodular deposits distributed evenly throughout both lungs. In some areas the nodules are sharply circumscribed, but in others they are indistinct and partly coalescent, as revealed to better advantage in the magnified view of the right upper zone.

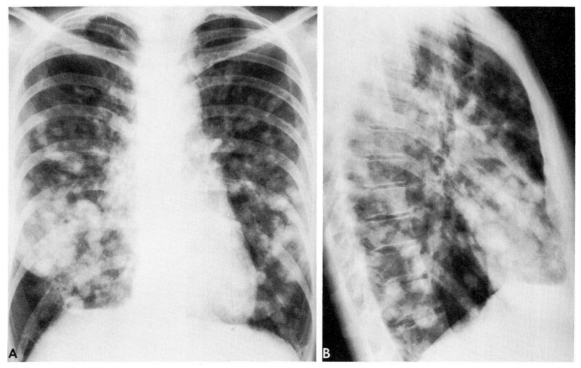

Figure 8–29. Nodular Metastases from Cylindroma of the Left Submaxillary Gland. Posteroanterior (*A*) and lateral (*B*) roentgenograms reveal multiple nodules of homogeneous density ranging in size from 5 mm to 2 cm, distributed widely through both lungs. The apices and bases are relatively less affected than the midzones. There is no evidence of cavitation.

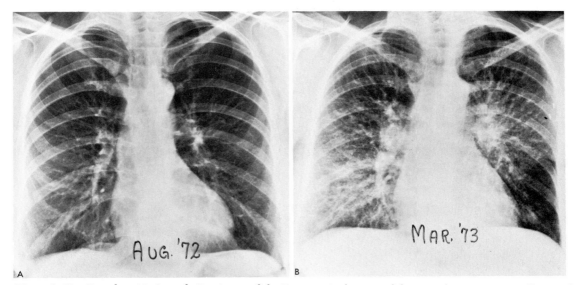

Figure 8–30. Lymphangitic Spread, Carcinoma of the Breast. At the time of the normal roentgenogram illustrated in *A*, this 50-year-old woman was discovered to have a carcinoma of the left breast and a modified radical mastectomy was carried out. Seven months later, at which time she was complaining of progressively increasing dyspnea, a roentgenogram *(B)* revealed extensive involvement of both lungs by a coarse linear and reticular pattern associated with bilateral hilar lymph node enlargement. Note the loss of lung volume that has occurred in this interval as a result of reduced compliance.

both lungs, but is more obvious in the lower zones because of their greater volume of tissue (Figure 8–30). This linear accentuation is sometimes associated with a nodular component, presumably resulting from hematogenous deposits, creating a very coarse reticulonodular pattern.[186]

In lymphangitic carcinoma, the onset of dyspnea may precede demonstrable roentgenographic change, and the patient may be severely incapacitated by this symptom by the time abnormality becomes visible.[191]

Cavitation

Excavation of metastatic lesions is not as common as with primary bronchogenic carcinoma. In one report it was identified in 4 per cent of metastatic deposits and 9 per cent of primary neoplasms.[192] As with primary bronchogenic carcinoma, cavitation is more likely in squamous-cell lesions; the site of the primary neoplasm most frequently is in the head and neck in men and in the genitalia in women.[192] Although not of absolute value in differential diagnosis, excavated small, thin-walled metastases usually indicate a primary site in the head or neck (Figure 8–31), whereas most larger thicker-walled secondaries arise from the genital tract. Cavitation may develop in only a small percentage of metastatic lung nodules; the characteristic variation in size of affected nodules may be diagnostic (Figure 8–31). As with pri-

mary neoplasms of the lung, cavitation occurs more frequently in the upper than the lower lobes.

CLINICAL MANIFESTATIONS

Symptoms may derive from two sources, the primary tumor and the lung metastases. The majority of patients (80 to 90 per cent) have symptoms or signs that direct attention to the primary site; in the others the first indication of disease is the roentgenographic demonstration of one or more pulmonary nodules.[13, 193] Metastases to the lungs seldom occasion symptoms, particularly if spread is hematogenous. Cough and hemoptysis are very uncommon, since metastatic lesions rarely erode the bronchial wall. Respiration may be painful when the pleura is involved.

The commonest symptom of metastatic lung disease is dyspnea, particularly in lymphangitic spread; it is typically insidious in onset but progresses rapidly and within a few weeks causes severe disability.

The great majority of patients with pulmonary metastases have normal pulmonary function in the early stages of the disease. Hematogenous metastases must be widespread before patients begin to note dyspnea, and at this stage function testing shows appropriate abnormalities. Diffusing capacity is uniformly reduced in all patients with lymphangitic spread, but is reduced in

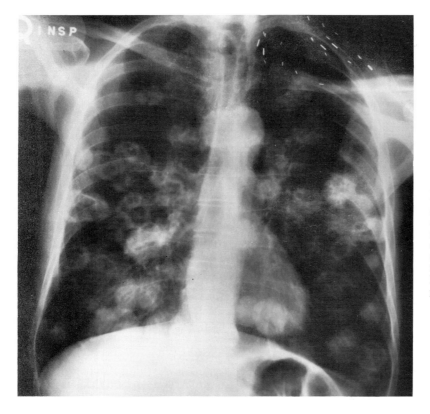

Figure 8–31. Cavitation in Metastatic Neoplasm. A posteroanterior roentgenogram reveals multiple nodules throughout both lungs ranging from 5 mm to 3 cm in diameter. The majority of the nodules are cavitated. For some unknown reason, such thin-walled cavities tend to occur in metastases from primary neoplasms arising in the head and neck. In this patient, the primary carcinoma was in the pharynx. Note the surgical clips over the left supraclavicular region from previous radical neck dissection.

those with hematogenous spread only if this is severe. Lung compliance is decreased in the lymphangitic group, but again only in the more extensively involved hematogenous cases.

REFERENCES

1. Pock-Steen, O. C.: Bronchial adenoma. Acta Radiol., 51:266, 1959.
2. Donahue, J. K., Weichert, R. F., and Ochsner, J. L.: Bronchial adenoma. Ann. Surg., 167:873, 1968.
3. Markel, S. F., Abell, M. R., Haight, C., and French, A. J.: Neoplasms of bronchus commonly designated as adenomas. Cancer, 17:590, 1964.
4. Good, C. A., and Harrington, S. W.: Asymptomatic bronchial adenoma. Proc. Mayo Clin., 28:577, 1953.
5. McGuinnis, E. J., and Lull, R. J.: Bronchial adenoma causing unilateral absence of pulmonary perfusion. Radiology, 120:367, 1976.
6. Allison, D. J., and Stanbrook, H. S.: A radiologic and physiologic investigation into hypoxic pulmonary vasoconstriction in the dog. Invest. Radiol., 15:178, 1980.
7. Giustra, P. E., and Stassa, G.: The multiple presentations of bronchial adenomas. Radiology, 93:1013, 1969.
8. Smith, R. A.: Bronchial carcinoid tumours. Thorax, 24:43, 1969.
9. Isawa, T., Okubo, K., Konno, K., Oshibe, M., Kidokoro, S., and Ouchi, A.: Cushing's syndrome caused by recurrent malignant bronchial carcinoid. Case report with 12 years' observation. Am. Rev. Resp. Dis., 108:1200, 1973.
10. Lawson, R. M., Ramanathan, L., Hurley, G., Hinson, K. W., and Lennox, S. C.: Bronchial adenoma: Review of an 18-year experience at the Brompton Hospital. Thorax, 31:245, 1976.
11. Bateson, E. M., and Abbott, E. K.: Mixed tumours of the lung, or hamartochondromas. A review of the radiological appearance of cases published in the literature and a report of fifteen new cases. Clin. Radiol., 11:232, 1960.
12. Bateson, E. M.: An analysis of 155 solitary lung lesions illustrating the differential diagnosis of mixed tumours of the lung. Clin. Radiol., 16:51, 1965.
13. Steele, J. D.: The solitary pulmonary nodule. Report of a cooperative study of resected asymptomatic solitary pulmonary nodules in males. J. Thorac. Cardiovasc. Surg., 46:21, 1963.
14. Sagel, S. S., and Ablow, R. C.: Hamartoma: On occasion a rapidly growing tumor of the lung. Radiology, 91:971, 1968.
15. Rosenbaum, H. D., Alavi, S. M., and Bryant, L. R.: Pulmonary parenchymal spread of juvenile laryngeal papillomatosis. Radiology, 90:654, 1968.
16. Singer, D. B., Greenberg, S. D., and Harrison, G. M.: Papillomatosis of the lung. Am. Rev. Resp. Dis., 94:777, 1966.
17. Greenfield, H., and Herman, P. G.: Papillomatosis of the trachea and bronchi. Am. J. Roentgenol., 89:45, 1963.
18. Agnos, J. W., and Starkey, G. W. B.: Primary leiomyosarcoma and leiomyoma of the lung. Review of the literature and report of two cases of leiomyosarcoma. N. Engl. J. Med., 258:12, 1958.

19. Bachman, D., and Wolff, M.: Pulmonary metastases from benign-appearing smooth muscle tumors of the uterus. Am. J. Roentgenol., *127*:441, 1976.

20. Kaplan, C., Katoh, A., Shamoto, M., Rogow, E., Scott, J. H., Cushing, W., and Cooper, J.: Multiple leiomyomas of the lung: Benign or malignant. Am. Rev. Resp. Dis., *108*:656, 1973.

21. Nair, S., Nair, K., and Weisbrot, I. M.: Fibrous histiocytoma of the lung (sclerosing hemangioma variant?). Chest, *65*:465, 1974.

23. Hutchinson, W. B., Friedenberg, M. J., and Saltzstein, S.: Primary pulmonary pseudolymphoma. Radiology, *82*:48, 1964.

22. Spencer, H.: Pulmonary blastomas. J. Pathol., *82*:161, 1961.

24. Julsrud, P. R., Brown, L. R., Li, C.-Y., Rosenow, E. C., III, and Crowe, J. K.: Pulmonry processes of mature-appearing lymphocytes: pseudolymphoma, well-differentiated lymphocytic lymphoma, and lymphocytic interstitial pneumonitis. Radiology, *127*:289, 1978.

25. Feigin, D. S., Siegelman, S. S., Theros, E. G., and King, F. M.: Nonmalignant lymphoid disorders of the chest. AJR, *129*:221, 1977.

26. Leading Article: Early diagnosis of lung cancer. Br. Med. J., 2:710, 1968.

27. Editorial: Bronchial adenoma. Radiology, *70*:588, 1958.

28. Miller, A. B.: Identification of adults at high risk of lung cancer. Can. Med. Assoc. J., *122*:985, 1980.

29. Miller, A. B.: Lung cancer. Can. Lung Assoc. Bull., 59:3, 1980.

30. Cohen, S., and Hossain, M. S.: Primary carcinoma of the lung. A review of 417 histologically proved cases. Dis. Chest, *49*:67, 1966.

31. Dorn, H. F.: Tobacco consumption and mortality from cancer and other diseases. Public Health Rep., 74:581, 1959.

32. Fletcher, C. M., and Horn, D.: Smoking and health. Presented at World Health Assembly Geneva, 17 May 1970. National Clearing House for Smoking and Health Bulletin, June, 1970.

33. Springett, V. H.: The beginning of the end of the increase in mortality from carcinoma of the lung. Thorax, *21*:132, 1966.

34. Wynder, E. L., Mabuchi, K., and Beattie, E. J., Jr.: The epidemiology of lung cancer. Recent trends. J.A.M.A., *213*:2221, 1970.

35. Belcher, J. R.: Adenocarcinoma and smoking. Chest, 67:622, 1975.

36. Berry, G., Newhouse, M. L., and Turok, M.: Combined effect of asbestos exposure and smoking on mortality from lung cancer in factory workers. Lancet, 2:476, 1972.

37. Selikoff, I. J., Bader, R. A., Bader, M. E., Churg, J., and Hammond, E. C.: Asbestosis and neoplasia. Am. J. Med., *42*:487, 1967.

38. Dutra, F., and Carney, J.: Asbestosis and pulmonary carcinoma. Arch. Environ. Health, *10*:416, 1965.

39. Selikoff, I. J., Churg, J., and Hammond, E. C.: Asbestos exposure and neoplasia. J.A.M.A., *188*:22, 1964.

40. Weiss, W., Moser, R. L., and Auerbach, O.: Lung cancer in chloromethyl ether workers. Am. Rev. Resp. Dis., *120*:1031, 1979.

41. Chovil, A. C., McCracken, W. J., Dowd, E. C., Stewart, C., Burton, D. F., and Dyer, D. W.: Occupational cancer: experience in Ontario. Can. Med. Assoc. J., *125*:1237, 1981.

42. Kotin, P.: Carcinogenesis of the lung: Environmental

and host factors. *In* Liebow, A. A., and Smith, D. E. (eds.): The Lung. Baltimore, Williams & Wilkins, 1968, p. 203.

43. Auerbach, O., Garfinkel, L., and Parks, V. R.: Scar cancer of the lung. Increase over a 21 year period. Cancer, *43*:636, 1979.

44. Lazo, B. G., Feiner, L. L., and Seriff, N. S.: A study of routine cytologic screening of sputum for cancer in 800 men consecutively admitted to a tuberculosis service. Chest, *65*:646, 1974.

45. Murasawa, K., and Altmann, V.: Primary lung cancer and pulmonary tuberculosis. A study based on 570 postmortem examinations. Sea View Hosp. Bull., *17*:37, 1958.

46. Greenberg, S. D., Jenkins, D. E., Bahar, D., Schweppe, H. I., Jr., and Block, H., Jr.: Coexistence of carcinoma and tuberculosis of the lung. Am. Rev. Resp. Dis., *90*:67, 1964.

47. Bariéty, M., and Rullière, R.: Carcinoma bronchique et tuberculose pulmonaire. (Bronchial carcinoma and pulmonary tuberculosis.) Rev. Tuberc., *27*:1, 1963.

48. Haddad, R., and Massaro, D.: Idiopathic diffuse interstitial pulmonary fibrosis (fibrosing alveolitis), atypical epithelial proliferation and lung cancer. Am. J. Med., *45*:211, 1968.

49. Genereux, G. P., and Merriman, J. E.: Desquamative interstitial pneumonia: Progression to the end-stage lung and the unusual complication of alveolar cell carcinoma. Case report. J. Can. Assoc. Radiol., *24*:144, 1973.

50. Twersky, J., Twersky, N., and Lehr, C.: Scleroderma and carcinoma of the lung. Clin. Radiol., *27*:203, 1976.

51. Tokuhata, G. K.: Familial factors in human lung cancer and smoking. Am. J. Public Health, *54*:24, 1964.

52. Kellermann, G., Shaw, C. R., and Luyten-Kellerman, M.: Aryl hydrocarbon hydroxylase inducibility and bronchogenic carcinoma. N. Engl. J. Med., *289*:934, 1973.

53. Waldmann, T. A., Strober, W., and Blaese, R. M.: Immunodeficiency disease and malignancy. Various immunologic deficiencies of man and the role of immune processes in the control of malignant disease. Ann. Intern. Med., *77*:605, 1972.

54. Brugarolas, A., and Takita, H.: Immunologic status in lung cancer. Chest, *64*:427, 1973.

55. Bolton, P. M., Mander, A. M., Davidson, J. M., James, S. L., Newcombe, R. G., and Hughes, L. E.: Cellular immunity in cancer: Comparison of delayed hypersensitivity skin tests in three common cancers. Br. Med. J., 3:18, 1975.

56. Kreyberg, L., in collaboration with Liebow, A. A., and Euhlinger, E. A.: Histological Typing of Lung Tumors. Geneva, World Health Organization, International Reference Center for the Histological Definition and Classification of Lung Tumors, 1967.

57. Auerbach, O., Garfinkel, L., and Parks, V. R.: Histologic type of lung cancer in relation to smoking habits, year of diagnosis and sites of metastases. Chest, *67*:382, 1975.

58. Galofré, M., Payne, W. S., Woolner, L. B., Clagett, O. T., and Gage, R. T.: Pathologic classification and surgical treatment of bronchogenic carcinoma. Surg. Gynecol. Obstet., *119*:51, 1964.

59. Bensch, K. G., Corrin, B., Pariente, R., and Spencer, H.: Oat-cell carcinoma of the lung. Its origin and relationship to bronchial carcinoid. Cancer, *22*:1163, 1968.

60. Jacques, J., Hill, D. P., Shier, K. J., Jindani, A., Miller, A. B.: Appraisal of the World Health Organization classification of lung tumors. Can. Med. Assoc. J., 122:897, 1980.

61. Lehar, T. J., Carr, D. T., Miller, W. E., Payne, W. S., and Woolner, L. B.: Roentgenographic appearance of bronchogenic adenocarcinoma. Am. Rev. Resp. Dis., 96:245, 1967.

62. Byrd, R. B., Miller, W. E., Carr, D. T., Payne, W. S., and Woolner, L. B.: The roentgenographic appearance of squamous cell carcinoma of the bronchus. Mayo Clin. Proc., 43:327, 1968.

63. Byrd, R. B., Miller, W. E., Carr, D. T., Payne, W. S., and Woolner, L. B.: The roentgenographic appearance of large cell carcinoma of the bronchus. Mayo Clin. Proc., 43:333, 1968.

64. Byrd, R. B., Miller, W. E., Carr, D. T., Payne, W. S., and Woolner, L. B.: The roentgenographic appearance of small cell carcinoma of the bronchus. Mayo Clin. Proc., 43:337, 1968.

65. Lisa, J. R., Trinidad, S., and Rosenblatt, M. B.: Site of origin, histogenesis, and cytostructure of bronchogenic carcinoma. Am. J. Clin. Pathol., 44:375, 1965.

66. Garland, L. H.: The rate of growth and natural duration of primary bronchial cancer. Am. J. Roentgenol., 96:604, 1966.

67. Chaudhuri, M. R.: Primary pulmonary cavitating carcinomas. Thorax, 28:354, 1973.

68. Felson, B.: Mucoid impaction (inspissated secretions) in segmental bronchial obstruction. Radiology, 133:9, 1979.

69. Aronberg, D. J., Sagel, S. S., Jost, R. G., and Levitt, R. G.: Oat cell carcinoma manifesting as a bronchocele. Am. J. Roentgenol., 132:23, 1979.

70. Pancoast, H. K.: Superior pulmonary sulcus tumor. Tumor characterized by pain, Horner's syndrome, destruction of bone and atrophy of hand muscles. J.A.M.A., 99:1391, 1932.

71. Emerson, G. L., Emerson, M. S., and Sherwood, C. E.: The natural history of carcinoma of the lung. J. Thorac. Cardiovasc. Surg., 37:291, 1959.

72. Meyer, P. C.: Metastatic carcinoma of the pleura. Thorax, 21:437, 1966.

73. Rohwedder, J. J., and Weatherbee, L.: Multiple primary bronchogenic carcinoma with a review of the literature. Am. Rev. Resp. Dis., 109:435, 1974.

74. Janower, M. L.: 55 posterior oblique tomography of the pulmonary hilum. J. Canad. Assoc. Radiol., 29:158, 1978.

75. Hirleman, M. T., Yiu-Chiu, V. S., Chiu, L. C., and Schapiro, R. L.: The resectability of primary lung carcinoma: A diagnostic staging review. CT, 4:146, 1980.

76. Kelly, R. J., Cowan, R. J., Ferree, C. B., Raben, M., and Maynard, C. D.: Efficacy of radionuclide scanning in patients with lung cancer. J.A.M.A., 242:2855, 1979.

77. Fletcher, J. W., Solaric-George, E., Henry, R. E., and Donati, R. M.: Radioisotopic detection of osseous metastases. Evaluation of ^{99m}Tc polyphosphate and ^{99m}Tc pyrophosphate. Arch. Intern. Med., 135:553, 1975.

78. Warren, S., and Gates, O.: Lung cancer and metastasis. Arch. Pathol., 78:467, 1964.

79. Brain, L.: The neurological complications of neoplasms. Lancet, 1:179, 1963.

80. Napoli, L. D., Hansen, H. H., Muggia, F. M., and Twigg, H. L.: The incidence of osseous involvement in lung cancer, with special reference to the development of osteoblastic changes. Radiology, 108:17, 1973.

81. Knowles, J. H., and Smith, L. H., Jr.: Extrapulmonary manifestations of bronchogenic carcinoma. N. Engl. J. Med., 262:505, 1960.

82. Morton, D. L., Itabashi, H. H., and Grimes, O. F.: Nonmetastatic neurological complications of bronchogenic carcinoma: The carcinomatous neuromyopathies. J. Thorac. Cardiovasc. Surg., 51:14, 1966.

83. Rassam, J. W., and Anderson, G.: Incidence of paramalignant disorders in bronchogenic carcinoma. Thorax, 30:86, 1975.

84. Beck, C., and Burger, H. G.: Evidence for the presence of immunoreactive growth hormone in cancers of the lung and stomach. Cancer, 30:75, 1972.

85. Ali, A., Tetalman, M. R., Fordham, E. W., Turner, D. A., Chiles, J. T., Patel, S. L., and Schmidt, K. D.: Distribution of hypertrophic pulmonary osteoarthropathy. Am. J. Roentgenol., 134:771, 1980.

86. Greenfield, G. B., Schorsch, H. A., and Shkolnik, A.: The various roentgen appearances of pulmonary hypertrophic osteoarthropathy. Am. J. Roentgenol., 101:927, 1967.

87. Marsh, B. R., Frost, J. K., Erozan, Y. S., Carter, D., and Proctor, D. F.: Flexible fiberoptic bronchoscopy. Its place in the search for lung cancer. Ann. Otol. Rhinol. Laryngol., 82:757, 1973.

88. Baker, R. R., Marsh, B. R., Frost, J. K., Stitik, F. P., Carter, D., and Lee, J. M.: The detection and treatment of early lung cancer. Ann. Surg., 179:813, 1974.

89. Fontana, R. S., Sanderson, D. R., Miller, W. E., Woolner, L. B., Taylor, W. F., and Uhlenhopp, M. A.: The Mayo lung project: Preliminary report of "early cancer detection" phase. Cancer, 30:1373, 1972.

90. Fontana, R. S., Sanderson, D. R., Woolner, L. B., Miller, W. E., Bernatz, P. E., Payne, W. S., and Taylor, W. F.: The Mayo lung project for early detection and localization of bronchogenic carcinoma: A status report. Chest, 67:511, 1975.

91. Woolner, L. B., David, E., Fontana, R. S., Andersen, H. A., and Bernatz, P. E.: In situ and early invasive bronchogenic carcinoma. Report of 28 cases with postoperative survival data. J. Thorac. Cardiovasc. Surg., 60:275, 1970.

92. Steele, J. D., Kleitsch, W. P., Dunn, J. E., Jr., and Buell, P.: Survival in males with bronchogenic carcinomas resected as asymptomatic solitary pulmonary nodules. Ann. Thorac. Surg., 2:368, 1966.

93. Oka, S., Konno, J., and Suzuki, S.: Differential diagnosis of solitary round shadow of the lung. Jap. J. Chest Dis., 22:361, 1963.

94. Holin, S. M., Dwork, R. E., Glaser, S., Rikli, A. E., and Stocklen, J. B.: Solitary pulmonary nodules found in a community-wide chest roentgenographic survey. A five-year follow-up study. Am. Rev. Tuberc. Pulm. Dis., 79:427, 1959.

95. Walske, B. R.: The solitary pulmonary nodule. A review of 217 cases. Dis. Chest, 49:302, 1966.

96. Nathan, M. H., Collins, V. P., and Adams, R. A.: Differentiation of benign and malignant pulmonary nodules by growth rate. Radiology, 79:221, 1962.

97. Siegelman, S. S., Zerhouni, E. A., Leo, F. P., Khouri, N. F., and Stitik, F. P.: CT of the solitary pulmonary nodule. Am. J. Roentgenol., 135:1, 1980.

98. Brody, W. R., Cassel, D. M., Sommer, F. G., Lehmann, L. A., Macovski, A., Alvarez, R. E., Pelc, N. J., Riederer, S. J., and Hall, A. L.: Dual-

energy projection radiography: Initial clinical experience. Am. J. Roentgenol., *137*:201, 1981.

99. Kruger, R. A., Armstrong, J. D., Sorenson, J. A., and Niklason, L. T.: Dual energy film subtraction technique for detecting calcification in solitary pulmonary nodules. Radiology, *140*:213, 1981.

100. Revesz, G., Kundel, H. L., and Toto, L. C.: Densitometric measurements of lung nodules on chest radiographs. Invest. Radiol., *16*:201, 1981.

101. Trunk, G., Gracey, D. R., and Byrd, R. B.: The management and evaluation of the solitary pulmonary nodule. Chest, *66*:236, 1974.

102. Nathan, M. H.: Management of solitary pulmonary nodules. An organized approach based on growth rate and statistics. J.A.M.A., *227*:1141, 1974.

103. Good, C. A.: Roentgenologic appraisal of solitary pulmonary nodules. Minn. Med., *45*:157, 1962.

104. Watson, W. L., and Farpour, A.: Terminal bronchiolar or "alveolar cell" cancer of the lung. Two hundred sixty-five cases. Cancer, *19*:776, 1966.

105. Coalson, J. J., Mohr, J. A., Pirtle, J. K., Dee, A. L., and Rhoades, E. R.: Electron microscopy of neoplasms in the lung with special emphasis on the alveolar cell carcinoma. Am. Rev. Resp. Dis., *101*:181, 1970.

106. Tomkin, G. H.: Systemic sclerosis associated with carcinoma of the lung. Br. J. Dermatol., *81*:213, 1969.

107. Beaver, D. L., and Shapiro, J. L.: A consideration of chronic pulmonary parenchymal inflammation and alveolar cell carcinoma with regard to a possible etiologic relationship. Am. J. Med., *21*:879, 1956.

108. Belgrad, R., Good, C. A., and Woolner, L. B.: Alveolar-cell carcinoma (terminal bronchiolar carcinoma). A study of surgically excised tumors with special emphasis on localized lesions. Radiology, *79*:789, 1962.

109. Rosenblatt, M. B,. Lisa, J. R., and Collier, F.: Primary and metastatic bronchiolo-alveolar carcinoma. Dis. Chest, *52*:147, 1967.

110. Schraufnagel, D., Peloquin, A., Paré, J. A. P., and Wang, N.-S.: Differentiating bronchiolo-alveolar carcinoma from adenocarcinoma. Am. Rev. Resp. Dis., *125*:74, 1982.

111. Marcq, M., and Galy, P.: Bronchioloalveolar carcinoma. Clinicopathologic relationships, natural history, and prognosis in 29 cases. Am. Rev. Resp. Dis., *107*:621, 1973.

112. Salerno, T. A., Munro, D. D., Blundell, P. E., and Chiu, R. C. J.: Second primary bronchogenic carcinoma: Life-table analysis of surgical treatment. Ann. Thorac. Surg., *27*:3, 1979.

113. Mountain, C. F., Carr, D. T., and Anderson, W. A. D.: A system for the clinical staging of lung cancer. Am. J. Roentgenol., *120*:130, 1974.

114. Slack, N. H., Chamberlain, A., and Bross, I. D. J.: Predicting survival following surgery for bronchogenic carcinoma. Chest, *62*:433, 1972.

115. Stoloff, I. L.: The prognostic value of bronchoscopy in primary lung cancer. A new perspective for an old procedure. J.A.M.A., *227*:299, 1974.

116. Editorial: Operability of lung cancer. Br. Med. J., *2*:299, 1975.

117. TNM Classification of Malignant Tumors. Joint Publication of International Union Against Cancer and American Joint Committee on Cancer Staging and End Results Reporting. Geneva, 1972.

118. Feinstein, A. R.: A new staging system for cancer and reappraisal of "early" treatment and "cure" by radical surgery. N. Engl. J. Med., *279*:747, 1968.

119. Carbone, P. P., Frost, J. K., Feinstein, A. R., Higgins, G. A., Jr., and Selawry, O. S.: Lung cancer: Perspective and prospects. Ann. Intern. Med., *73*:1003, 1970.

120. Feinstein, A. R., Gelfman, N. A., and Yesner, R.: The diverse effects of histopathology on manifestations and outcome of lung cancer. Chest, *66*:225, 1974.

121. Fox, W., and Scadding, J. G.: Medical Research Council comparative trial of surgery and radiotherapy for primary treatment of small-celled or oat-celled carcinoma of bronchus. Ten-year follow-up. Lancet, *2*:63, 1973.

122. Brett, G. Z.: Earlier diagnosis and survival in lung cancer. Br. Med. J., *4*:260, 1969.

123. Boucot, K. R., Cooper, D. A., and Weiss, W.: The Philadelphia pulmonary neoplasm research project. Med. Clin. North Am., *54*:549, 1970.

124. Weiss, W., and Boucot, K. R.: The prognosis of lung cancer originating as a round lesion. Am. Rev. Resp. Dis., *116*:827, 1977.

125. Fontana, R.: Early diagnosis of lung cancer. Am. Rev. Resp. Dis., *116*:399, 1977.

126. Editorial: Epidemiology of Hodgkin's disease. Lancet, *2*:647, 1973.

127. MacMahon, B.: Epidemiological evidence on the nature of Hodgkin's disease. Cancer, *10*:1045, 1957.

128. Editorial: Hodgkin's disease: A clue or a fluke? Br. Med. J., *4*:564, 1972.

129. MacMahon, B.: Is Hodgkin's disease contagious? N. Engl. J. Med., *289*:532, 1973.

130. Vianna, N. J., and Polan, A. K.: Epidemiologic evidence for transmission of Hodgkin's disease. N. Engl. J. Med., *289*:499, 1973.

131. Vianna, N. J., Davies, J. N. P., Polan, A. K., and Wolfgang, P.: Familial Hodgkin's disease: An environmental and genetic disorder. Lancet, *2*:854, 1974.

132. Rosenberg, S. A.: Report of the committee on the staging of Hodgkin's disease. Cancer Res., *26*:1310, 1966.

133. O'Connell, M. J., Wiernik, P. H., Sklansky, B. D., Greene, W. H., Abt, A. B., Kirschner, R. H., Ramsey, H. E., and Murphy, W. L.: Staging laparotomy in Hodgkin's disease. Further evidence in support of its clinical utility. Am. J. Med., *57*:86, 1974.

134. Lee, J. K. T., Stanley, R. J., Sagel, S. S., Melson, G. L., and Koehler, R. E.: Limitations of the post-lymphangiogram plain abdominal radiograph as an indicator of recurrent lymphoma: Comparison to computed tomography. Radiology, *134*:155, 1980.

135. Lukes, R. J., Craver, L. F., Hall, T. C., Rappaport, H., and Ruben, P.: Report of the nomenclature committee. Cancer Res., *26*:1311, 1966.

136. Filly, R., Blank, N., and Castellino, R. A.: Radiographic distribution of intrathoracic disease in previously untreated patients with Hodgkin's disease and non-Hodgkin's lymphoma. Radiology, *120*:277, 1976.

137. Martin, J. J.: The Nisbet Symposium: Hodgkin's disease. Radiological aspects of the disease. Australas. Radiol., *11*:206, 1967.

138. Castellino, R. A., and Blank, N.: Adenopathy of the cardiophrenic angle (diaphragmatic) lymph nodes. Am. J. Roentgenol., *114*:509, 1972.

139. Strickland, B.: Intra-thoracic Hodgkin's disease. Part II. Peripheral manifestations of Hodgkin's disease in the chest. Br. J. Radiol., *40*:930, 1967.

140. Costello, P., and Mauch, P.: Radiographic features of

recurrent intrathoracic Hodgkin's disease following radiation therapy. Am. J. Roentgenol., *133*:201, 1979.

141. Fisher, A. M. H., Kendall, B., and Van Leuven, B. D.: Hodgkin's disease. A radiological survey. Clin. Radiol., *13*:115, 1962.

142. Stolberg, H. O., Patt, N. L., MacEwen, K. F., Warwick, O. H., and Brown, T. C.: Hodgkin's disease of the lung: Roentgenologic-pathologic correlation. Am. J. Roentgenol., *92*:96, 1964.

143. Weick, J. K., Kiely, J. M., Harrison, E. G., Jr., Carr, D. T., and Scanlon, P. W.: Pleural effusion in lymphoma. Cancer, *31*:848, 1973.

144. Beachley, M. C., Lau, B. P., and King, E. R.: Bone involvement in Hodgkin's disease. Am. J. Roentgenol., *114*:559, 1972.

145. Ultmann, J. E., and Moran, E. M.: Clinical course and complications in Hodgkin's disease. Arch. Intern. Med., *131*:332, 1973.

146. Winterbauer, R. H., Belic, N., and Moores, K. D.: A clinical interpretation of bilateral hilar adenopathy. Ann. Intern. Med., *78*:65, 1973.

147. Million, R. R.: Hodgkin disease in 1974. J.A.M.A., *229*:328, 1974.

148. Korst, D. R., Meyer, O. O., and Jaeschke, W. H.: Survival in Hodgkin disease. A study of patients with at least ten-year survival. Arch. Intern. Med., *134*:1043, 1974.

149. North, L. B., Fuller, L. M., Hagemeister, F. B., Rodgers, R. W., Butler, J. J., and Shullenberger, C. C.: Importance of initial mediastinal adenopathy in Hodgkin disease. Am. J. Roentgenol., *138*:229, 1982.

150. Jaffe, E. S., Shevach, E. M., Frank, M. M., Berard, C. W., and Green, I.: Nodular lymphoma—evidence for origin from follicular B lymphocytes. N. Engl. J. Med., *290*:813, 1974.

151. Berard, C. W., Greene, M. H., Jaffe, E. S., Magrath, I., and Ziegler, J.: A multidisciplinary approach to non-Hodgkin's lymphomas. Ann. Intern. Med., *94*:218, 1981.

152. Schimpff, S. C., Schimpff, C. R., Brager, D. M., and Wiernik, P. H.: Leukaemia and lymphoma patients interlinked by prior social contact. Lancet, *1*:124, 1975.

153. Aisenberg, A. C.: Malignant lymphoma (first of two parts). N. Engl. J. Med., *288*:883, 1973.

154. Rassiga, A. L.: Advances in adult non-Hodgkin's lymphoma. Current concepts of classification, diagnosis, and management. Arch. Intern. Med., *140*:1647, 1980.

155. Rappaport, H.: Tumors of the Hemopoietic System. Atlas of Tumor Pathology, Section III, Fasc. 8: Armed Forces Institute of Pathology, Washington, D.C., 1966.

156. Berard, C. W.: Histopathology of the lymphomas. *In* Williams, W. J., Beutler, E., Ersley, A. J., and Rundles, R. W. (eds.): Hematology. New York, McGraw-Hill, 1972.

157. Marglin, S. I., Soulen, R. L., Blank, N., and Castellino, R. A.: Mycosis fungoides. Radiology, *130*:35, 1979.

158. Al-Saleem, T., and Peale, A. R.: Lymphocytic tumors and pseudotumors of the lung. Report of five cases with special emphasis on pathology. Am. Rev. Resp. Dis., *99*:767, 1969.

159. Reich, N. E., McCormack, L. J., and Van Ordstrand, H. S.: Pseudolymphoma of the lung. Chest, *65*:424, 1974.

160. Burgener, F. A., and Hamlin, D. J.: Intrathoracic histiocytic lymphoma. Am. J. Roentgenol., *136*:499, 1981.

161. Robbins, L. L.: The roentgenological appearance of parenchymal involvement of the lung by malignant lymphoma. Cancer, *6*:80, 1953.

162. Rees, G. M.: Primary lymphosarcoma of the lung. Thorax, *28*:429, 1973.

163. Cathcart-Rake, W., Bone, R. C., Sobonya, R. E., and Stephens, R. L.: Rapid development of diffuse pulmonary infiltrates in histiocytic lymphoma. Am. Rev. Resp. Dis., *117*:587, 1978.

164. Kim, H., and Dorfman, R. F.: Morphological studies of 84 untreated patients subjected to laparotomy for the staging of non-Hodgkin's lymphomas. Cancer, *33*:657, 1974.

165. Patchefsky, A. S., Brodovsky, H. S., Menduke, H., Southard, M., Brooks, J., Nicklas, D., and Hoch, W. S.: Non-Hodgkin's lymphomas: A clinicopathologic study of 293 cases. Cancer, *34*:1173, 1974.

166. Lukes, R. J., and Tindle, B. H.: Immunoblastic lymphadenopathy: A hyperimmune entity resembling Hodgkin's disease. N. Engl. J. Med., *292*:1, 1975.

167. Klatte, E. C., Yardley, J., Smith, E. B., Rohn, R., and Campbell, J. A.: The pulmonary manifestations and complications of leukemia. Am. J. Roentgenol., *89*:598, 1963.

168. Green, R. A., and Nichols, N. J.: Pulmonary involvement in leukemia. Am. Rev. Resp. Dis., *80*:833, 1959.

169. Armstrong, P., Dyer, R., Alford, B. A., and O'Hara, M.: Leukemic pulmonary infiltrates: Rapid development mimicking pulmonary edema. Am. J. Roentgenol., *135*:373, 1980.

170. Glenner, G. G., Ein, D., and Terry, W. D.: The immunoglobulin origin of amyloid. Am. J. Med., *52*:141, 1972.

171. Wolfel, D. A., and Dennis, J. M.: Multiple myeloma of the chest wall. Am. J. Roentgenol., *89*:1241, 1963.

172. Kaplan, J. O., Morillo, G., Weinfeld, A., and Ostrov, S. G.: Mediastinal adenopathy in myeloma. J. Canad. Assoc. Radiol., *31*:48, 1980.

173. Kyle, R. A.: Multiple myeloma. Review of 869 cases. Mayo Clin. Proc., *50*:29, 1975.

174. Blattner, W. A., Garber, J. E., Mann, D. L., McKeen, E. A., Henson, R., McGuire, D. B., Fisher, W. B., Bauman, A. W., Goldin, L. R., and Fraumeni, J. F., Jr.: Waldenström's macroglobulinemia and autoimmune disease in a family. Ann. Intern. Med., *93*:830, 1980.

175. Renner, R. R., Nelson, D. A., and Lozner, E. L.: Roentgenologic manifestations of primary macroglobulinemia (Waldenström). Am. J. Roentgenol., *113*:499, 1971.

176. Bloch, K. J., Lee, L., Mills, J. A., and Haber, E.: Gamma heavy chain disease—an expanding clinical and laboratory spectrum. Am. J. Med., *55*:61, 1973.

177. Pittman, F. E., Tripathy, K., Isobe, T., Bolanos, O. M., Osserman, E. F., Pittman, J. C., Lotero, H. R., and Duque, E. E.: IgA heavy-chain disease. A case detected in the Western hemisphere. Am. J. Med., *58*:424, 1975.

178. Lee, S.-C., and Johnson, H. A.: Multiple nodular pulmonary amyloidosis. A case report and comparison with diffuse alveolar-septal pulmonary amyloidosis. Thorax, *30*:178, 1975.

179. Wang, C. C., and Robbins, L. L.: Amyloid disease. Its roentgen manifestations. Radiology, *66*:489, 1956.

180. Gross, B. H.: Radiographic manifestations of lymph node involvement in amyloidosis. Radiology, *138*:11, 1981.
181. Prowse, C. B., and Elliott, R. I. K.: Diffuse tracheobronchial amyloidosis: A rare variant of a protein disease. Thorax, *18*:326, 1963.
182. Schraufnagel, D. E., Knight, L., Ying, W. L., and Wang, N. S.: Favourable outcome in a case of endobronchial amyloidosis. Can. Med. Assoc. J., *122*:559, 1980.
183. Paglicci, A.: Metastatic tumours of the lung: A study of 152 cases. Radiol. Med. (Torino), *42/2*:184, 1956.
184. Willis, R. A.: The Spread of Tumours in the Human Body. London, Butterworth, 1952, pp. 169–177.
185. Burn, J. I., Watne, A. L., and Moore, G. E.: The role of the thoracic duct lymph in cancer dissemination. Br. J. Cancer, *16*:608, 1962.
186. Janower, M. L., and Blennerhassett, J. B.: Lymphangitic spread of metastatic cancer to the lung: A radiologic-pathologic classification. Radiology, *101*:267, 1971.
187. Spencer, H.: Pathology of the Lung, 2nd ed. Oxford, Pergamon, 1968.
188. Nystrom, J. S., Weiner, J. M., Wolf, R. M., Bateman, J. R., and Viola, M. V.: Identifying the primary site in metastatic cancer of unknown origin. Inadequacy of roentgenographic procedures. J.A.M.A. *241*:381, 1979.
189. Steckel, R. J., and Kagan, A. R.: Diagnostic persistence in working up metastatic cancer with an unknown primary site. Radiology, *134*:367, 1980.
190. Braman, S. S., and Whitcomb, M. E.: Endobronchial metastasis. Arch. Intern. Med., *135*:543, 1975.
191. Goldsmith, H. S., Bailey, H. D., Callahan, E. L., and Beattie, E. J., Jr.: Pulmonary lymphangitic metastases from breast carcinoma. Arch. Surg., *94*:483, 1967.
192. Dodd, G. D., and Boyle, J. J.: Excavating pulmonary metastases. Am. J. Roentgenol., *85*:277, 1961.
193. Bateson, E. M.: An analysis of 155 solitary lung lesions illustrating the differential diagnosis of mixed tumors of the lung. Clin. Radiol., *16*:51, 1965.

9

Embolic and Thrombotic Diseases of the Lungs

PULMONARY THROMBOEMBOLISM

DEFINITION

The term "pulmonary thromboembolic disease" implies the clinical and pathologic state that results when the blood supply to a part of the lungs is interrupted by obstruction of its feeding vessel by a clot originating from a thrombus. Thromboembolic disease does not imply pulmonary infarction, which occurs in only a small proportion—probably not more than 10 to 15 per cent—of embolic episodes.[1] The precise meaning of infarction requires clarification: as defined in *The Shorter Oxford English Dictionary*, an infarct is a portion of tissue stuffed with extravasated blood or serum. Despite this clear definition, the term still denotes different things to different observers, even among pathologists; for example, Spencer[2] considers necrosis of lung parenchyma necessary to the diagnosis, whereas some other pathologists do not. Roentgenologically, since opacification of pulmonary parenchyma distal to an occluded vessel is often the result of hemorrhage rather than of tissue death, and these two conditions can be differentiated roentgenologically only by their time of resolution (as shown later), we feel it proper *to use the word "infarct" in all situations in which a parenchymal opacity develops distal to an occluded pulmonary artery*. Should follow-up examinations show rapid clearing, it would be reasonable to term the lesion hemorrhagic. Should the shadow clear more slowly, over several weeks, the reasonable inference can be made that the vascular insult resulted in tissue death.

INCIDENCE

It is estimated that about 80 per cent of pulmonary thromboembolic episodes go unrecognized, since the great majority do not cause symptoms. The exact incidence is unknown, but it seems to be increasing,[3] particularly in previously healthy young adults. Some of this increase can be attributed to a higher index of clinical suspicion and improved, readily accessible diagnostic facilities,[3] but, in addition, there appears to be a real increase for which not all the causal factors are known, although the increasing complexity of surgical procedures and the vast increase in the use of oral contraceptives (*see* further on) are partly responsible. The frequency of pulmonary embolism directly parallels that of peripheral venous thrombosis.

In summary, there are two major points that should be emphasized: (1) Thromboembolism is by far the commonest pathologic process involving the lungs of patients in general hospitals.[1] (2) Of even greater importance perhaps is the fact that, although the majority of these patients are asymptomatic, pulmonary embolism is one of the most lethal diseases and probably the most often misdiagnosed.[4]

PATHOGENESIS

The great majority of pulmonary thromboemboli originate from intravascular thrombi in the legs or pelvis. In some cases of heart disease, the thrombus causing a pulmonary embolism may originate in the right atrium or right ventricle. Necropsy of 78 patients known to have had pulmonary embolism[4] showed peripheral thrombi in 62, at multiple sites in more than

454

one-third; the leg veins were involved in 46 per cent, the right atrium in 23 per cent, the inferior vena cava in 19 per cent, and the pelvic veins in 16 per cent. It is important to realize that the site of thrombosis is not found during life in up to 50 per cent of cases of fatal embolism[5] and may not be found even at necropsy.[5]

Slowing of the circulation is a major factor in the high incidence of peripheral venous thrombosis in patients with cardiorespiratory disease, in otherwise healthy persons whose lower limbs are immobilized for a long while, and in association with pregnancy, obesity, or varicose veins. Most patients have predisposing factors leading to intravascular clotting, such as slowing of the peripheral venous circulation by leg casts applied for fractures, sitting for long periods in a cramped position while traveling, or standing for long periods at work in occupations such as nursing. In addition to the effects of endothelial trauma and slowing of the venous circulation, patients with increased clotting tendencies may have elevated levels of one or more components of the clotting mechanism or deficient fibrinolysis.

In the late 1960's, three studies in the United Kingdom showed increased morbidity and mortality from thromboembolism in women taking oral contraceptives.[6-8] Although these drugs may be a risk factor, however, they are of relatively little consequence compared with other causes of thrombosis, such as obesity and pregnancy. Thus, to take an obese young woman off the pill and not put her on a diet is to miss the forest for the trees!

Increases in factors accelerating the clotting mechanism and platelet aggregation, and decreases in fibrinolysis and the protective component, antithrombin III (heparin cofactor), have been reported in women taking oral contraceptives.[9, 10] The culpable ingredient in the hormonal pill is thought to be estrogen, which augments clotting but impairs fibrinolysis. The risk of thromboembolism is dose-related. Both synthetic and natural equine estrogen, but not progestogen, raise the levels of extrinsic clotting factors VII and X and accelerate prothrombin time. Therefore, one would expect that patients in whom thrombosis develops while taking the pill would be less subject to recurrence after its cessation, and this has been confirmed.[11] It is estimated that healthy married women between the ages of 20 and 34 taking oral contraceptives run a risk of death from pulmonary or cerebral embolism that is seven to eight times that in nonusers.[7] Since thromboembolism is an un-

common cause of death in healthy women in this age group, these figures are statistically equivalent to eight deaths per half-million users of the contraceptive pill compared with one death per half-million nonusers.

Most patients in whom venous thrombosis develops have obvious reasons for slowing of the peripheral circulation, including immobilization of the legs, inflammation adjacent to a peripheral vein (*e.g.*, with a fracture), and interference with venous return to the right side of the heart (as in heart failure, varicose veins, and pregnancy, particularly postpartum and in association with eclampsia). Whether coagulation on the venous side is caused solely by sequential conversion of certain blood protein coenzymes to enzymes and, finally, to fibrin formation from fibrinogen is now in question,[12] it having been suggested that clotting in both veins and arteries may be initiated by the formation of a small platelet nidus. If so, rational therapy would include not only anticoagulants, such as heparin and the coumarin drugs, but also those substances (*e.g.*, acetylsalicylic acid) that prevent platelet aggregation and adhesiveness by inhibiting the release of platelet adenosine diphosphate.[12]

In about 30 to 50 per cent of patients who die postoperatively, necropsy reveals deep vein thrombosis, with or without pulmonary emboli.[13] Similarly, deep vein thrombosis is detected in about 30 per cent of patients postoperatively, almost always in the calf, by scanning the legs with ^{125}I-labeled fibrinogen.[13]

The chief medical conditions leading to thromboembolic disease are those associated with prolonged immobilization and venostasis, such as myocardial infarction and heart failure,[3] strokes, obesity,[3] and varicose veins. Isotopic scanning techniques and radiographic phlebography have shown deep vein thrombosis in from 30 per cent to over 50 per cent of patients with these risk factors. In addition, there are some disease entities that predispose to clotting because of an associated hypercoagulable state; these include hypertension, hyperlipidemia, multiple myeloma, sickle-cell anemia, and cancer. Certain neoplasms—notably carcinoma of the lung, gastrointestinal tract, or genitourinary tract[14]—show a strong predisposition to venous thrombosis.

In addition to increasing venous pressure in the legs and the risk of varicosities in the pelvic and leg veins, pregnancy increases the concentration of several components of the clotting mechanism. Thromboembolic disease occurs particularly in the postpartum period, most often after difficult or traumatic delivery and especially if there is hemorrhage.[15] Pulmonary embolism during pregnancy poses a special problem in therapy, since coumarin drugs, unlike heparin, cross the placental barrier and are reported to have caused fetal death in 19 per cent of cases.[16]

It is emphasized that few peripheral thromboses detected by modern techniques in high-risk patients are clinically apparent. Most of the clots are in the deep veins of the calf and rarely embolize to the lungs. In fact, if a thrombosis remains confined to the calf, major pulmonary embolism is unlikely. Dangerous thrombi are those in the thighs and the femoral and iliac veins, few of which are in continuity with calf thrombi.[13, 17]

The clinical manifestations and roentgenographic signs in pulmonary thromboembolic disease depend on several factors which, individually or in combination, influence the effect of vascular occlusion on the lung parenchyma: the presence or absence of cardiopulmonary disease; the size, number, and location of emboli; whether vessel occlusion is complete or partial; and the time interval between embolic episodes. Although supposedly normal persons may die suddenly as a result of pulmonary embolism, even a large embolus obstructing a major vessel may give rise to only minor disturbance in circulatory dynamics and minimal clinical and roentgenographic findings. In such cases, serial angiograms show disappearance of the clot within a few days as a result of lysis, or fragmentation and dispersal to smaller vessels, or a combination of both. In a patient with cardiovascular disease, however, a similar episode usually leads to infarction, cardiac arrhythmia, systemic hypotension, and death. Prior embolic episodes are evident in the clinical history or at necropsy in most cases of death due to massive pulmonary embolism.

Multiple small pulmonary emboli rarely cause sudden death and do so only when there is severe underlying lung disease.[18] These patients may have no symptoms indicative of an embolic episode, but occlusion of the major portion of the pulmonary vascular tree almost inevitably results in acute pulmonary hypertension, cor pulmonale, and right-sided heart failure. Even if there are multiple pulmonary emboli, pulmonary hypertension is not sustained until at least 50 per cent (probably closer to 70 per cent) of the pulmonary vascular tree is occluded.[18] However, transient pulmonary hypertension may result from vasoconstriction, particularly when smaller vessels are occluded.[19]

PATHOLOGIC CHARACTERISTICS

The morphologic consequences of embolic occlusion of the pulmonary arteries depend on the size of the embolic mass (and thus the order of artery affected) and the general state of the circulation. Three distinctive effects may be observed:

1. With occlusion of a large central, segmental, or subsegmental vessel in younger persons with good cardiovascular function, there may be no significant alteration in the peripheral lung parenchyma. It is not known why sudden occlusion of a pulmonary artery does not necessarily result in infarction; the bronchial circulation may be adequate to maintain the integrity of the involved parenchyma, or, as has been shown by postmortem angiography, emboli lodged in vessels may not completely occlude them. In such circumstances, surfactant deficit may reduce lung volume but the lung parenchyma remains air containing and structurally intact.

2. Arterial occlusion results in consolidation of distal lung parenchyma caused by hemorrhage and edema unassociated with lung necrosis. Although lung structure may be obscured by suffusion of blood and edema fluid, this type of infarct is distinguished by the preservation of lung architecture. The consolidative process may resolve in 3 to 10 days. Lung parenchyma does not undergo necrosis, and organization of the hemorrhage rarely leaves fibrous scarring.[20] These hemorrhagic infarcts are 1 to 10 cm in diameter, depending upon the size of the occluded vessel; some very small ones may occur in a single secondary pulmonary lobule.[21] When bronchopulmonary vascular anastomoses develop, extravasated blood is removed and the involved area again becomes air containing.

3. In patients with cardiovascular disease or serious debilitating illness such as advanced malignancy, pulmonary vascular occlusion results in infarction with necrosis. About three-quarters of all such infarcts affect the lower lobes, and in over half the cases they are multiple. Characteristically, but not invariably, they extend to a visceral pleural surface and are roughly conical, with the apex pointing toward the lung hilum. Grossly, the infarct is classically hemorrhagic and, in its early stages, appears as a raised, blue-red area.[22] The adjacent pleural surface usually is covered by a fibrinous exudate. The occluded vessel may be identified near the apex of the infarcted zone. Within 48 hours, the red cells begin to lyse, and the cyanotic blue-red appearance begins to fade. In time, fibrous replacement begins at the margins

of the infarct, appearing as a gray-white peripheral zone. It eventually converts the entire infarct into a scar, which contracts below the level of the surrounding lung tissue, drawing the pleura with it.[22] Histologically, the characteristic feature of this form of pulmonary infarction is ischemic necrosis of lung substance, affecting not only alveolar walls but also interstitial tissue, bronchioles, and pulmonary vessels. Consolidation in such infarcts is composed of (a) a central zone, which undergoes necrosis and eventual fibrous replacement, and (b) a peripheral zone, which is purely hemorrhagic and resolves completely in a few days. It is the latter zone that gives rise to the poor definition of infarcts roentgenographically.

The fact that only a few lobules in a poorly perfused area may undergo infarction explains the frequent discrepancy between lung scans and roentgenographic changes in thromboembolism.[21] The perfusion deficit seen on a lung scan is often much larger than the opacity observed roentgenographically, implying that the opacity represents involvement of only a few secondary lobules within a larger subsegmental zone of lung whose vessel has been occluded.

Diffuse pulmonary edema sometimes develops after pulmonary embolism. Many of these patients are in heart failure at the time of the embolic episode, in which case the edema is readily explained on this basis alone. Another possible pathogenesis of pulmonary edema, applicable only in patients suffering massive embolism, is the pulmonary arterial hypertension that accompanies obstruction of a large cross section of the pulmonary vascular bed. Since right ventricular output must pass through a markedly reduced vascular bed, the pulmonary hypertension that inevitably ensues can conceivably cause high capillary hydrostatic pressures with resultant edema.

As discussed later, both angiographic[23] and perfusion scanning[24] studies have established that perfusion through initially obstructed arteries tends to return relatively rapidly in the first few days after embolization and then more slowly over the next several weeks, presumably by a process of lysis and fragmentation.

PATHOPHYSIOLOGIC MANIFESTATIONS

Pathophysiologic consequences of sudden occlusion of a pulmonary vessel include local decrease in compliance and in ventilation, caused at least partly by bronchoconstriction of small bronchi, bronchioles, or alveolar ducts[26]

resulting from decreased PCO_2 within the bronchus supplying the occluded segment.[25] The effects on the pulmonary vasculature are somewhat similar to those on the airways. Minor pulmonary emboli increase pulmonary arterial pressure and arterial hypoxemia, the pressure rise depending on both mechanical blockage and vasoconstriction. Clinical and physiologic studies in humans and in experimental animals have indicated that pulmonary emboli induce the release of vasoactive substances such as serotonin, prostaglandins, and histamine, leading to bronchoconstriction, vasoconstriction, and perhaps altered pulmonary microcirculatory permeability.[27] Physiologic evidence of bronchoconstriction was found in 61 of 72 patients with pulmonary emboli.

ROENTGENOGRAPHIC MANIFESTATIONS

Consideration of the manifestations of pulmonary thromboembolic disease should be prefaced by a further reminder that most episodes are asymptomatic and produce no detectable changes on plain chest roentgenograms. Even if the diagnosis is suspected clinically and confirmed angiographically, in many cases no abnormalities are seen on plain films. Roentgenologically apparent changes occur only when a fairly large segmental artery is occluded or when obstruction of many small vessels has impaired pulmonary hemodynamics.[28]

Anatomic Distribution

Most embolic occlusions occur in the lower lobes, probably as a result of hemodynamic flow patterns. The right lung is involved more frequently than the left, especially the posterior basal segment.[28] The roentgenographic manifestations of thromboembolism can be divided into those with and those without increase in roentgenographic density—that is, with and without infarction.

Thromboembolism Without Infarction

When changes relating to thromboembolism without infarction are visible on plain roentgenograms of the chest, they may be distinctive and should strongly suggest the diagnosis. There are four changes: oligemia, change in vessel size, alteration in size and configuration of the heart, and loss of lung volume.

OLIGEMIA. Peripheral oligemia may be local, caused by occlusion of a fairly large lobar

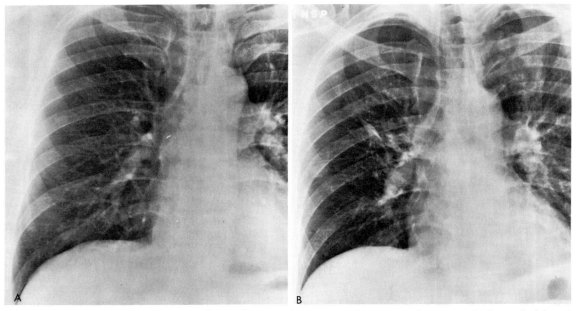

Figure 9–1. Pulmonary Embolism Without Infarction: The Westermark Sign. On admission to the hospital of this 52-year-old man a posteroanterior roentgenogram (A) revealed no significant abnormalities. Several days following abdominal surgery, he experienced abrupt onset of right chest pain and dyspnea. A roentgenogram at this time (B) showed an obvious increase in diameter and a change in configuration of the right interlobar artery; also, the distal end of this artery appeared "knuckled" and the vessels peripheral to it diminutive. The overall density of the right lower zone was considerably less than that of the left, indicating diminished perfusion (the Westermark sign). A lung scan revealed absence of perfusion of the lower half of the right lung.

or segmental pulmonary artery (Figure 9–1), or general, the result of widespread small vessel thromboembolism. The first description of local oligemia resulting from embolism was by Westermark in 1938,[29] and this valuable sign now bears his name. In a study of 25 patients with massive pulmonary embolism in whom plain film and angiographic abnormalities were correlated,[30] local oligemia was observed in *all*—in fact, 79 per cent of such zones apparent on the arteriogram were recognizable on the plain roentgenogram. It was concluded that changes in vascularity were the principal diagnostic changes on the plain roentgenogram. It is entertaining to conjecture whether CT might be able to identify local areas of oligemia with a greater degree of confidence than standard roentgenography; in fact, a recent experimental study on 17 dogs positively identified oligemia distal to acute pulmonary arterial occlusion in all animals;[31] interestingly, oligemia was found to be identified conclusively only when animals were examined in the prone position.

General pulmonary oligemia in thromboembolic disease is almost invariably the result of widespread occlusion of smaller arteries. The diffuse oligemia is nearly always accompanied by signs of pulmonary artery hypertension—enlargement of the central pulmonary arteries, cor pulmonale, cardiac decompensation, and dilation of the superior vena cava and the azygos vein.[32]

CHANGES IN THE PULMONARY ARTERY. Enlargement of a major hilar pulmonary artery is a leading sign of pulmonary embolism (Figures 9–1 and 9–2)[20, 33] and is of particular value when serial roentgenograms reveal progressive enlargement of the affected vessel.[33] The increase in size is the result of distention of the vessel by bulk thrombus—*not* of increased vascular resistance in the lung involved. In the right hilum, the presence of a thrombus can be assessed by measurement of the diameter of the descending branch of the pulmonary artery where it relates to the intermediate stem bronchus. The normal maximal diameter of this artery at total lung capacity (TLC) is 16 mm in adult men and 15 mm in adult women; when values are exceeded it may be reasonably concluded that the vessel is enlarged.[34] Perhaps more reliable than this absolute measurement, however, is increase in size of the affected vessel in serial examinations, which is strong evidence of thromboembolism, especially if peripheral oligemia is present (Figure 9–1). Widening of the pulmonary artery usually dimin-

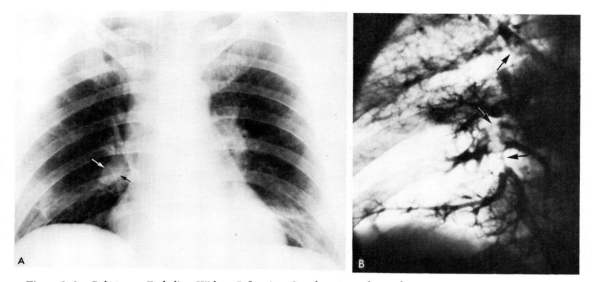

Figure 9–2. Pulmonary Embolism Without Infarction. On admission to hospital, a posteroanterior roentgenogram of a 40-year-old man revealed a normal appearance of the pulmonary vasculature and lung parenchyma. Six weeks later, shortly after the abrupt onset of dyspnea and severe pain in the right chest, an anteroposterior roentgenogram exposed in the supine position *(A)* reveals a slight but definite asymmetry in the density of the two lungs, the lower two-thirds of the right lung being more translucent than the left (Westermark's sign). In addition, there had been a change in the diameter and configuration of the descending branch of the right pulmonary artery, this vessel showing a distinct bulge both medially and laterally *(arrows)*. The diagnosis of pulmonary embolism without infarction was confirmed by a selective right pulmonary angiogram *(B)*; several large defects can be identified within the major branches of the right pulmonary artery *(arrows)*. At thoracotomy, several wormlike thrombi were extracted from the right pulmonary artery. Recovery was uneventful.

ishes rapidly and the artery reverts to normal size within a few days as a result of lysis and fragmentation of the clot.[35]

Of equal importance to increase in size is the abrupt tapering of an occluded vessel distally; the vessel may terminate suddenly, creating the so-called "knuckle sign" (Figures 9–1 and 9–2).

CARDIAC CHANGES (COR PULMONALE). Acute cor pulmonale is not a common roentgenologic accompaniment of thromboembolism, being observed in only about 10 per cent of patients. It occurs more often with widespread multiple peripheral emboli and sometimes—when a large enough area of the arterial system is occluded—with massive central embolization. The signs are those of cardiac enlargement due to dilation of the right ventricle, increase in size of the main pulmonary artery, and usually, increase in size and rapidity of tapering of the hilar pulmonary vessels.[33] Dilation of the azygos vein and superior vena cava may be apparent, reflecting right-sided cardiac decompensation.

LOSS OF LUNG VOLUME. Loss of volume of a lower lobe in pulmonary embolism without infarction may be manifested roentgenographically by elevation of the hemidiaphragm, or downward displacement of the major fissure, or both. The mechanism probably relates to a deficit of surfactant resulting from loss of pulmonary artery perfusion. Loss of lung volume is a more frequent finding when infarction is present.

Thromboembolism With Infarction

Thromboembolism may increase roentgenographic density by consolidating lung parenchyma, regardless of whether the infarction is associated with tissue necrosis or with simple hemorrhage and edema. The roentgenologic changes in embolism with and without infarction are basically the same, except that in the former instance the oligemia is replaced by parenchymal consolidation. Increased size and abrupt tapering of the feeder artery are common to both conditions, but loss of lung volume occurs most often and is more severe with infarction. In a retrospective study of 66 necropsy-proved cases of pulmonary embolism with infarction, Talbot and associates[36] found elevation of the hemidiaphragm in 26 (40 per cent) and regarded this as the single most useful roentgenographic sign of infarction.

The roentgenographic patterns of pulmonary infarction are specific only insofar as the shadows are segmental in distribution and homoge-

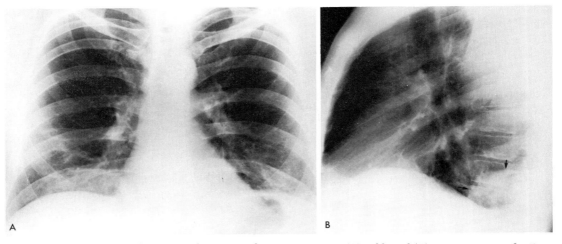

Figure 9–3. Pulmonary Infarction, Right Lower Lobe. Posteroanterior *(A)* and lateral *(B)* roentgenograms of a 40-year-old man reveal a fairly well-circumscribed shadow of homogeneous density occupying the posterior basal segment of the right lower lobe. In lateral projection, the shadow has the shape of a truncated cone with its apex directed toward the hilum (Hampton's hump) *(arrows)*. A small effusion can be identified in lateral projection. This combination of changes is highly suggestive of pulmonary infarction; the history and biochemical findings were compatible with the diagnosis.

neous in density. In the early stages particularly, any increase in density is ill-defined; it is most common in the base of the right lower lobe, often nestled in the costophrenic sinus (Figure 9–3). The majority of cases of pulmonary infarction involve one or perhaps two bronchopulmonary segments, thus affecting a relatively small volume of lung parenchyma. The oft-repeated observation that infarction invariably relates to a visceral pleural surface[28] is of little value in differential diagnosis, since the majority of pneumonias do also. The interval between the embolic episode and any increase in roentgenographic density ranges from 10 to 12 hours to 1 week after occlusion, although the shorter period is much more frequent.[37]

The classic configuration of an infarction as a "truncated cone" is not uncommon in our experience. This "typical" configuration consists of homogeneous wedge-shaped consolidation in the lung periphery, with its base contiguous to a visceral pleural surface and its rounded, convex apex toward the hilum (Figure 9–3).[28, 37] Originally described by Hampton and Castleman[38] in 1940, this configuration has come to bear the euphonious eponym "Hampton's hump"; it is highly suggestive of pulmonary infarction. The size of the consolidated area varies from patient to patient and, in the case of multiple infarctions, from one area to another. They are usually 3 to 5 cm in diameter,[37] in a range extending from bare visibility up to 10 cm. An air bronchogram is rarely seen in a pulmonary infarct; this absence, combined with peripheral homogeneous consolidation,

should strongly suggest infarction rather than acute air-space pneumonia. However, an air bronchogram does not completely rule out infarction: in three of our patients with pulmonary embolism, an air bronchogram was apparent within 24 hours of appearance of a pulmonary opacity, presumably reflecting delayed filling of the airways with blood and edema fluid. Cavitation in pulmonary infarction is rare.

The time of resolution of infarction varies widely and is a reliable indicator of the nature of the consolidative process. If embolism results only in parenchymal hemorrhage and edema (as is common), clearing may occur within 4 to 7 days,[39] often without residua. When infarction leads to necrosis, however, resolution averages 20 days[35] and may take as long as 5 weeks.[40] Serial roentgenography usually shows pattern changes, most often "line shadows," culminating in permanent linear streaking representing residual fibrosis, but in some cases the lungs eventually appear normal. In a follow-up study of 58 angiographically proven pulmonary infarcts in 32 patients, McGoldrick and his colleagues[41] found complete roentgenographic resolution in 29 (50 per cent). Residual abnormalities that were observed in the remaining 29 infarcts included linear scars (in 14), pleural diaphragmatic adhesions (in 9), and localized pleural thickening (in 6). These abnormalities were regarded as minimal in extent. It is noteworthy that the age of the patient seemed to have no effect on the frequency of residual abnormalities.

A valuable sign differentiating pulmonary infarction from acute pneumonia is the pattern of resolution.[42] The shadow of acute pneumonia appears to break up, rendering an originally homogeneous opacity inhomogeneous as scattered areas of radiolucency appear within it, whereas the shadow of a pulmonary infarct gradually diminishes but maintains its homogeneity and roughly its original shape. Woesner and associates[42] likened a resolving infarct to a melting ice cube; thus the term "the melting sign."

LINE SHADOWS. These probably constitute one of the most frequent roentgenographic manifestations of pulmonary embolism and infarction. Four types may occur: "platelike atelectasis," parenchymal scarring, thrombosed arteries and veins, and line shadows of pleural origin.

"Platelike Atelectasis." These linear opacities, almost always in the lung bases 1 to 3 cm above the hemidiaphragm, are usually roughly horizontal. They are 1 to 3 mm thick and usually several centimeters long; at least one extremity abuts against the pleural surface. In thromboembolic disease, the pathogenesis probably relates to a combination of (a) mucous plugging of small bronchi and bronchioles caused by decreased ventilation as a result of diminished diaphragmatic activity, and (b) altered alveolar surface tension resulting from decreased surfactant production. We are still not convinced that these linear opacities are in fact the result of atelectasis.

Parenchymal Scarring. As with "platelike atelectasis," linear shadows caused by scarring secondary to lung necrosis extend to a pleural surface. They lie in any plane and run in almost any direction, apparently without regard to segmental distribution. They may be up to 10 cm long. The long line shadows of healed infarction may have a sizable pleural component. In pathologic studies Reid found that, as the necrotic tissue of infarction shrinks through scarring, it causes inward retraction of contiguous visceral pleura, and she suggested that this infolded pleura may contribute to the formation of line shadows (*see* Figure 4-53, page 210).[43]

Thrombosed Arteries and Veins. Simon[44] described line shadows, usually horizontal in the lung bases, in middle-aged and elderly subjects who had no abnormalities that might suggest a cause for "platelike atelectasis." Although the pathologic basis of many of these lines is elusive, some have been shown to represent a thrombosed artery or vein, with or without fibrosis in contiguous lung parenchyma.

More recently, it has been suggested[45] that horizontal or obliquely oriented long line shadows represent thrombosed veins more often than arteries. Evidence was both inferential and direct: inferential in that the direction of the line shadow was identical to that followed by a pulmonary vein, particularly the relationship of its medial extremity to the left atrium; and direct in that the position of the line shadow was related to that of the vein in subsequent angiography. We have seen many cases in which the distribution of line shadows was similar to that described by Simon.[45] The major clues to their nature lie in their orientation (not conforming to bronchovascular distribution) and the relationship of their medial extremity to the left atrium. The shadows are 2 to 10 mm thick, and in our cases followed the distribution of a major upper lobe vein just as frequently as veins draining the middle and lower zones. These opacities cannot be caused purely by blood clot within the vein itself: the density of clot is identical to that of blood and thus should not produce a different roentgenographic shadow. Until pathologic confirmation is possible—and this appears singularly difficult—it seems reasonable to assume that the opacity is created by a combination of edema and hemorrhage in lung parenchyma surrounding the vein, with or without atelectasis and fibrosis.

Despite the lack of more precise pathologic confirmation, the evidence that has accumulated over the past few years lends considerable support to the thesis that these opacities represent thrombosed veins (or occasionally arteries) associated with edema and hemorrhage in the surrounding parenchyma. Current knowledge dictates that visualization of such shadows on a chest roentgenogram, particularly if the clinical setting is such that a thromboembolic episode might be anticipated, should alert physicians to the possibility of thromboembolism.

Line Shadows of Pleural Origin. These line shadows are seen frequently and are caused either by thickening of an interlobar fissure or by fibrous pleural thickening over the anterior or posterior lung surfaces, resulting from the serosanguineous effusion that frequently accompanies pulmonary infarction. These rather stringy shadows are usually horizontal or oblique, not unlike scars of old pulmonary infarction.

PLEURAL EFFUSIONS. As a roentgenographic manifestation of thromboembolic disease, pleural effusion is as common as, if not commoner than, parenchymal consolidation: it nearly always indicates infarction. The parenchymal shadow may be diminutive or hidden by the fluid,[20, 28] so confusing the diagnostic possibilities that an embolic episode will be suggested only if there is a high index of suspicion. The amount of pleural fluid is frequently small but may be abundant. It is more often unilateral.[33, 37] When predominantly infrapulmonary, it may be mistaken for hemidiaphragmatic elevation.[37] Pleural fluid usually develops and absorbs synchronously with the infarction, but sometimes appears later and clears sooner.[35]

PULMONARY ANGIOGRAPHY

Pulmonary arteriography is the single most definitive technique for investigating suspected pulmonary thromboembolic disease,[46] and even extremely ill patients usually tolerate the procedure well.[35] However, it carries a risk of morbidity and mortality.

Technique

Best results are obtained if the contrast medium is injected through a catheter whose tip is in the undivided pulmonary artery (Figure 9–2). This permits not only clear visualization of the entire pulmonary arterial tree but also the measurement of right ventricular and pulmonary artery pressures. The study may reveal partial or complete occlusion of lobar or segmental vessels, but is seldom useful when the obstructed vessels are subsegmental or smaller; in such cases, it may be necessary to perform segmental arteriography in an anteroposterior or oblique plane.[47]

Angiographic Abnormalities

The multifarious angiographic criteria reported for the diagnosis of pulmonary embolism are listed in the Table 9–1. Although the importance of secondary signs has been stressed, these signs reflect nothing more than diminished pulmonary arterial perfusion, a common manifestation of several pulmonary and cardiac diseases from which pulmonary embolism must be differentiated.[48] In fact, there is only one established angiographic criterion for the definitive diagnosis of pulmonary embolism—direct observation of an intraluminal filling defect (Figure 9–2).[49, 50] However, the secondary signs listed in Table 9–1 may be useful by directing attention to areas in which manifestations of embolism may be subtle; in such cases, segmental or wedge arteriography, especially with

TABLE 9–1. ANGIOGRAPHIC CRITERIA REPORTED FOR THE DIAGNOSIS OF PULMONARY EMBOLISM*

PRIMARY SIGN
A. Filling defect
1. Persistent intraluminal radiolucency, central or marginal, without complete obstruction of blood flow
2. Trailing edge of an intraluminal radiolucency when there is complete obstruction of distal blood flow
SECONDARY SIGNS
A. Abrupt occlusion ("cutoff") of a pulmonary artery without visualization of an intraluminal filling defect
B. Perfusion defect (asymmetric filling)
1. Areas of oligemia or avascularity
2. Focal areas in which the arterial phase is prolonged (especially when localized to the lower lung fields); this is usually accompanied by slow filling and emptying of the pulmonary veins
3. Tortuous, abruptly tapering peripheral vessels, with a paucity of branching vessels ("pruning")

*Reprinted from Sagel, S. S., and Greenspan, R. H.: Radiology, 99:541, 1971, with permission of the authors and editor.

magnification, should reveal intraluminal defects in smaller vessels.

In patients in whom pulmonary angiography is contraindicated for one reason or another, *computed tomography* can provide a noninvasive alternative in selected circumstances. Although experience is rather limited to date, Godwin and his colleagues[51] effectively employed CT to demonstrate emboli and thrombi in central pulmonary arteries in three patients; the technique established the diagnosis in one patient and in another served as a follow-up of central thromboembolism, thus avoiding repeat angiography. More recent experimental evidence[52] suggests that CT scanning with contrast enhancement may be capable of identifying emboli in lobar and segmental arteries.

PHLEBOGRAPHY (VENOGRAPHY)

This procedure is used to outline the deep veins extending from the calf to the inferior vena cava, to determine the site of thrombus formation. Usually the veins are opacified by injecting contrast medium into a foot vein; the iliac veins can be displayed by femoral vein or intraosseous injection.[53] The procedure is recommended in patients with recurrent pulmonary embolism for whom thrombectomy and venous ligation are being contemplated, particularly if anticoagulant therapy has apparently been unsuccessful.[54]

PULMONARY ARTERY PRESSURES

Measurement of the right ventricular and pulmonary arterial pressures is often very helpful in the evaluation of patients with thromboembolic disease,[55] and these pressures should always be carefully recorded before pulmonary angiography. Even if the angiogram reveals no evidence of major vessel occlusion, the pulmonary arterial pressure may be raised, indicating multiple microemboli throughout the lungs. The pulmonary arterial pressure probably is raised in most patients with positive angiographic findings, and those with a mean right ventricular pressure exceeding 22 mm Hg (30 cm saline) are likely to die. When the main pulmonary arterial pressure is raised and the differential diagnosis is between acute pulmonary embolism and myocardial infarction with shock, capillary wedge pressure can be obtained with much less risk than an angiogram and usually distinguishes the two conditions, being normal in embolism and raised in myocardial infarction.[56]

RADIOISOTOPIC SCANNING

Radioisotopic scanning in the diagnosis and assessment of pulmonary embolism consists of the injection of macroaggregates of albumin tagged with ^{131}I, ^{51}Cr, ^{99m}Tc, or ^{113m}In. The aggregates, which are two to five times the size of human red blood cells, are loosely bound and easily fragmented. Aggregates larger than 10 to 15 μ are trapped in the arteriolar-capillary pulmonary bed. False positive scans may be recorded in lung zones that are poorly perfused because of impaired ventilation, even if no vascular obstructive lesions are present.[57] The scanning technique measures blood flow, and this may be diminished for reasons other than organic intraluminal obstruction.[57] For instance, local decrease in ventilation, reducing blood flow, is particularly characteristic of bronchitis, with or without emphysema, and of asthma even in remission.[58] Fairly distinctive perfusion patterns have been described[59] for pulmonary embolism, congestive heart failure, and emphysema. Perhaps the clearest distinguishing feature was the nature of the perfusion defects, which were focal, segmental, or lobar in pulmonary emboli and irregular and nonsegmental in congestive heart failure and emphysema. Gilday and his colleagues[60] emphasized that the patterns do not provide an absolute differential diagnosis, but rather probabilities. Based on the type of perfusion abnormality and its loca-

TABLE 9–2. PROBABILITY OF PULMONARY EMBOLISM: SCAN CLASSIFICATION

SCAN FINDING	PROBABILITY OF PULMONARY EMBOLISM
Focal:	
Segmental-subsegmental	High
Lobar	High
Entire lung	Indeterminate*
Nonanatomic	Low
Diffuse	
Patchy	Low
Normal	None

*Becomes a high probability if there is a focal defect in the opposite lung. (Reprinted from Gilday, D. L., Poulose, K. P., and Deland, F. H.: Am. J. Roentgenol., *115*:739, 1972, with permission of the authors and editor.)

tion, they judged that the probability of pulmonary embolism was high if a focal perfusion abnormality corresponded to an anatomic division of the lung (Table 9–2), was low if any other perfusion abnormality was observed, and was zero if the scan was normal.

Both lateral and posterior oblique views are useful aids in the assessment of lung scans in pulmonary embolism. As with the plain chest roentgenogram, a lateral view is necessary to establish the segmental nature of a defect and hence define the probability of embolism. If the chest roentgenogram shows no opacity, a segmental lung scan pattern can help distinguish pulmonary embolism from congestive heart failure and emphysema. However, segmental defects are common in pneumonia, and in many cases this is the diagnosis that must be excluded.

Another method for differentiating pulmonary embolism from chronic obstructive pulmonary disease (COPD) when lung scan reveals perfusion defects is aerosol inhalation lung imaging. The inhalation scan should show defects corresponding to zones of underperfusion in cases of COPD but should be relatively normal in pulmonary embolism.[61] Hypoperfusion due to embolic arterial occlusion is unaccompanied by regional hypoventilation, thus resulting in increased dead space ventilation and a high $\dot{V}/\dot{Q}$ ratio.[62] Using the same ^{133}Xe method to study patients with COPD, it has been shown[62] that regional hypoventilation was accompanied by regional hypoperfusion; however, the decrease in ventilation was greater than that in perfusion, resulting in venous admixture and a low $\dot{V}/\dot{Q}$ ratio. Several studies[63-65] have confirmed these findings and have established the value of combined ventilation and perfusion scanning.

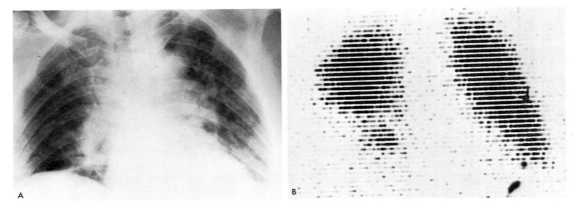

Figure 9–4. Right Lower Lobe Pulmonary Embolism; Value of Radioisotope Scanning. An anteroposterior roentgenogram *(A)* reveals signs that are virtually pathognomonic of embolism of the right lower lobe without infarction. The lower half of the right lung is relatively radiolucent compared with the left lung (Westermark's sign), and the descending branch of the right pulmonary artery is enlarged and bulging (note the "knuckle sign"). On the same day, an anterior scan *(B)* of the lungs following the intravenous injection of macroaggregates of radioiodinated serum albumin shows a large triangular defect in the lower portion of the right lung, indicating absence of blood flow.

The necessity for correlation of scan patterns with chest roentgenograms is obvious. The chief value of scanning lies in the detection of areas of absent radioactivity when the chest roentgenogram is normal or shows a suspicious area of oligemia (Figure 9–4). In patients with clinically suspected pulmonary thromboembolism in whom roentgenographic opacities are present (parenchymal or pleural or both), evaluation of the significance of perfusion defects can be difficult, although the studies of Biello and his colleagues[66] have thrown some light on this issue. In a scintigraphic study of 111 patients who had matching perfusion defects and roentgenographic abnormalities, of the 14 patients in whom the perfusion defects were substantially smaller than the roentgenographic opacity, only 1 (7 per cent) had pulmonary embolism; of 77 patients in whom the opacities and perfusion defects were of similar size, embolism was established in 20 (26 per cent); when perfusion defects were substantially larger than the roentgenographic opacities (18 patients), pulmonary embolism was present in 16 (89 per cent). Clearly, the larger the size of the perfusion defect in relation to the roentgenographic opacity, the greater the likelihood of pulmonary embolism.

FIBRINOGEN SCANNING FOR DEEP VEIN THROMBOSIS

The intravenous injection of ^{125}I-labeled fibrinogen (along with daily doses of oral iodine), followed by scanning of the legs, can aid in the detection of thrombosis and thus the prevention of **pulmonary embolism.** Fibrinogen scanning is inaccurate in the veins of the upper thigh and pelvis where methods for flow detection may provide more information (*see* further on). A ^{125}I-labeled fibrinogen uptake study can be used to monitor deep vein thrombosis postoperatively, to detect extension of thrombosis from the leg into the thigh, and to decide whether anticoagulant therapy is needed. In recent years this technique has been combined with Doppler ultrasonic detection or impedance plethysmography as a noninvasive means of diagnosing deep vein thrombosis.[67, 68]

ULTRASONIC DETECTIONS OF DEEP VEIN THROMBOSIS

The Doppler ultrasound flow detection method[69] records the cyclic nature of venous sound coincident with the respiratory cycle, and its modification with the Valsalva and Mueller maneuvers. Thrombosis in the iliofemoral veins is recognizable by alteration in audible sounds or flow-velocity patterns recorded over the common femoral vein. This method of assessing flow variation has largely been replaced by impedance plethysmography.

IMPEDANCE PLETHYSMOGRAPHY

This technique, originally described by Mullick and Wheeler and their colleagues in the 1970's,[70, 71] is based on variations in blood flow measured by a change in electrical resistance between electrodes fastened to the calf. Since blood is an excellent conductor of electricity, the change in limb venous blood volume when a thigh cuff is inflated normally results in decreased resistance; when the cuff pressure is released, there follows a prompt increase in resistance. Constant dilatation of the deep venous system caused by thrombotic occlusion results in little or no change in resistance with this maneuver.

Since lower limb venography can induce deep venous thrombosis in 3 to 4 per cent of patients,[68] a safe and reliable noninvasive method for determining deep vein patency is highly desirable, and there is an increasing body of evidence that impedance plethysmography is the method of choice, especially when combined with fibrinogen scanning.[73] Some authors[17, 73] advocate radiofibrinogen leg scanning and impedance plethysmography as screening procedures in all patients suspected of having pulmonary embolism.

Comparison of Angiography and Isotopic Scanning

In several studies, pulmonary photoscans and angiograms have been correlated in the evaluation of patients with pulmonary embolism. By and large, all studies agree on two basic principles: (1) pulmonary perfusion scans and angiograms are complementary—not competitive—techniques in the evaluation of pulmonary embolic disease; and (2) each method has diagnostic limitations. A study of 14 patients with pulmonary embolism established by both lung scanning and selective pulmonary angiography, and in whom other cardiopulmonary disease had been excluded, showed that the lung scan better depicted capillary flow and the angiogram better detected embolic material in large vessels, but that the findings with both correlated reasonably well overall in the assessment of embolic involvement. When embolization involved less than 40 per cent of the lung, it was better demonstrated by the perfusion scan, whereas more extensive involvement was more reliably recorded by angiogram. Agreement was closest when a massive clot completely obstructed either a part of the main pulmonary artery or a junction of the main and lobar pulmonary arteries. It was concluded that although overall correlation was good, either technique could significantly underestimate the extent of embolism and both might be necessary to determine this reasonably accurately.

In a study of 71 patients with clinical findings indicative of pulmonary embolism who underwent lung scanning and then pulmonary angiography, the scan predicted specific arteriographic evidence of pulmonary embolism in 75 per cent of those in whom the scan defects were characteristic of embolism (*i.e.*, the perfusion defects corresponded to specific anatomic segments and the chest roentgenograms were normal or suggested pulmonary embolism). This study confirmed previous observations that in patients with COPD, congestive cardiac failure, or bronchial asthma, only pulmonary arteriography can establish the diagnosis of embolism with certainty. A remarkably high degree of correlation of results of scanning and arteriography was found in a study of 48 patients in whom these were performed because of the clinical possibility of pulmonary embolism. There was 94 per cent agreement between the scan and both arteriogram and plain roentgenogram, and in all cases a negative scan correlated with a negative arteriogram. All correlative studies have shown that although scanning is not as reliable as angiography in assessing oligemia at the lung bases, it has the theoretic advantage of depicting the circulation in the lung periphery, an area poorly visualized by angiography. The volume of lung parenchyma is 20 to 30 times the size of a supply vessel 1 to 2 mm in diameter and is easily visualized by scanning when the vessel is occluded; by contrast, vessels of this size are seldom well depicted angiographically.

Finally, Gilday and associates' study of 101 patients thought clinically to have pulmonary embolism who were subjected to both lung scanning and angiography sums up the current position of these two procedures in the investigation of a suspected embolic episode. All 44 patients with pulmonary emboli shown by angiography had abnormal scans, and none of the 21 with normal lung scans had emboli on angiography. Correlation between scan and angiogram was good (85 per cent) when the distribution of focal scan defects was lobar but was less (64 per cent) when this was segmental. Seventy-seven per cent of the 53 patients judged on pulmonary scanning to have a high probability of pulmonary embolism had angiographically demonstrated emboli.

The conclusions reached by Gilday and his colleagues[60] have been supported by other workers[65, 74] and include an initial screening procedure by lung scan followed by pulmonary angiography in those instances when the scan findings are abnormal or inconclusive (lack of focal lobar or segmental defects or a corresponding roentgenographic opacity). Angiography is also recommended to confirm the scan diagnosis before pulmonary embolectomy, inferior vena caval interruption, or thrombolytic therapy. We are in general agreement with these guidelines with perhaps one qualification: we believe that there is little indication for a lung scan in a patient whose chest roentgenogram reveals an abnormality consistent with acute pulmonary embolism or infarction when there is convincing clinical evidence of phlebitis.

CLINICAL MANIFESTATIONS

Symptoms

Most pulmonary emboli produce no symptoms or occasion such minimal distress that they are recognized only in retrospect.

The major clue to the diagnosis of pulmonary embolism is a well-defined predisposing condition.[75] The onset of dyspnea or pain is usually *abrupt*, which aids in differentiation from pneumonia, whose onset usually is more gradual and accompanied by cough productive of purulent material. In perhaps 50 per cent of cases, questioning elicits a history of one or more transitory episodes of dyspnea, harbingers of the more distressing acute embolism and infarction.[76] The three commonest symptoms of angiographically proved emboli are dyspnea (in over 80 per cent of patients), cough (70 per cent), and pleural pain (58 to 70 per cent). Hemoptysis is comparatively uncommon (20 to 33 per cent of cases).[20, 75, 76] Two types of chest pain occur: retrosternal, characteristic of angina pectoris, and pleuritic, a consequence of pulmonary infarction.

Neurologic signs include restlessness, anxiety, syncope, convulsions, irrational behavior, hemiparesis or monoparesis, confusion, and coma. They appear mainly in elderly bedridden or cardiac patients and almost certainly are caused by a combination of previous cerebrovascular disease, hypoxemia, and acute cerebral vasospasm resulting from hypocarbia. The commonest physical findings are nonspecific—tachypnea, rales, tachycardia (with or without arrhythmias), and manifestations of pulmonary hypertension. Fever occurs with infarction.

In general, pulmonary thromboembolic disease consists of the following three fairly well-defined syndromes that reflect the size and numbers of clots:

1. *Massive pulmonary embolism*, when a thrombus lodges in the bifurcation of main branches of the pulmonary artery, obstructing at least 50 per cent of the pulmonary vascular bed. As a result of acute cor pulmonale, central venous pressure rises and cardiac output falls. Peripheral venous vasoconstriction may prevent systemic hypotension, but with very high resistance in the lesser circulation the blood pressure falls, and the clinical presentation is that of circulatory collapse or shock.[56] Patients complain of severe dyspnea and retrosternal pain, and tachycardia, tachypnea, and—in some—cyanosis develop. Auscultation reveals only *increased* air entry, and rarely rales or a friction rub. The jugular veins are distended, and gallop rhythm is invariably audible. There may be a diffuse systolic lift at the left sternal edge, with accentuation of the second pulmonic sound.

2. *Pulmonary infarction*, when a lobar or segmental artery is occluded by a medium-sized embolus. Usually, the patient complains of dyspnea of acute onset, pain on breathing, and possibly hemoptysis. Tachycardia and fever are often present; the latter is usually low grade (37.2 to 37.7° C), but temperature may go as high as 39.5° C. Fever occurs in up to 50 per cent of cases.[77] Findings include locally decreased breath sounds, rales, rhonchi, friction rub, and signs of pleural effusion.[20] The differential diagnosis includes pneumonia, atelectasis, and primary pleural effusion. However, pneumonia usually causes higher fever and purulent expectoration and has a more insidious onset. It may be difficult to rule out atelectasis, since both complications are common postoperatively. The pleural effusion of pulmonary infarction is usually grossly bloody.

3. *Multiple pulmonary microthromboemboli*, when a multitude of small clots impact in small arteries and arterioles and do not cause infarction. If only a small cross section of the vascular bed is occluded, most patients are asymptomatic. If more than 50 per cent of the vascular bed is affected, progressive dyspnea on exertion develops, and, in some patients, right ventricular failure occurs. Some complain of episodic transient dyspnea, presumably a result of intermittent microembolism. Recurrent attacks of cardiac arrhythmia, particularly atrial flutter, may occur.[78]

Diagnostic laboratory tests are concerned mainly with levels of serum enzymes and of fibrin and fibrinogen degradation products, and experience over the years has indicated that these are of limited value. The leukocyte count seldom exceeds 15,000 per cu mm. Any increase in neutrophils is usually associated with fever and symptoms and signs of pulmonary infarction.

Sanguineous pleural fluid strongly suggests

pulmonary infarction, particularly if malignancy has been excluded. Serous effusion is probably caused by cardiac failure.

Pulmonary function studies reveal restrictive disease. The resting lung volume is decreased and airway resistance is increased, and lung compliance and diffusing capacity are reduced. Most of the patients hyperventilate. Arterial blood gas analysis reveals low PO_2 values and respiratory alkalosis. However, the urokinase study group reported arterial PO_2 values of 80 mm Hg or greater in 13 of 113 patients, including three of 70 mm Hg with massive pulmonary embolism.[75, 79] Furthermore, pulmonary embolism is commoner in older patients, in whom PaO_2 is normally 80 mm Hg or less. The value of blood gas studies in this disorder is limited by the occurrence of similar changes in heart failure, atelectasis, and pneumonia, the main conditions to be differentiated. This hypoxemia cannot always be corrected by the patient's breathing 100 per cent oxygen, suggesting intrapulmonary venous shunting that may be due to pulmonary edema.[77] Some authors[80] stress the value of determining the difference between end tidal and arterial PCO_2 as a measurement of large areas of ventilated but unperfused lung. It is estimated that at least 20 to 30 per cent of lung parenchyma must be unperfused before the PCO_2 difference exceeds 6 mm Hg, and compensatory measures that restrict ventilation of the unperfused lung develop rapidly after embolism and render this test almost valueless by 48 hours after the event.[77]

Electrocardiographic Changes

These appear early and are often transient; they are caused by acute pulmonary hypertension and hypoxemia and therefore are commonest after massive pulmonary embolism.[81] Certain ECG patterns are considered diagnostic of acute pulmonary embolism; these include an S wave in lead I and an inverted Q wave or T wave or both in lead III, with inversion of the T waves recorded over the right side of the heart. Other less reliable changes are those of right axis deviation and a pattern of right bundle branch block or right ventricular hypertrophy. Atrial arrhythmias are frequent, particularly in patients with established heart disease.[81]

PROGNOSIS

It is very likely that most people suffer thromboembolic episodes which, because of the very efficient fibrinolytic system, are unrecognized clinically. Careful search of the pulmonary vascular tree at necropsy has revealed organized thrombi in over 50 per cent of patients, most of whom had neither a clinical history suggestive of thromboembolic episodes nor pathologic evidence that the emboli had caused morbidity or mortality.[1] Probably the majority of patients with massive pulmonary embolism die within 30 minutes to 2 hours. Follow-up studies of 15 patients who survived major or massive embolism[82] showed earliest complete resolution at 14 days, and in two others at 15 and 34 days. Serial photoscanning of 69 patients[83] revealed that most of them had complete or nearly complete return of pulmonary blood flow by 4 months. Similarly, follow-up of 33 patients at 30 months[84] showed residual angiographic abnormalities in four and chronic cor pulmonale in none.

The prognosis is improved by anticoagulant and thrombolytic therapy, and by surgical procedures such as thrombectomy and inferior vena cava ligation. The indications for and effectiveness of pulmonary embolectomy remain obscure.

Summary

Pulmonary thromboembolism, with or without infarction, is a common disease that is often undiagnosed or misdiagnosed. It is the commonest cause of death as determined by postmortem examination. Because of the difficulty in establishing a definitive diagnosis and the anxiety that develops over the possibility of a sudden catastrophic event, there has emerged in recent years a tendency to overdiagnosis, with resultant potentially serious therapeutic consequences.[85]

Diagnosis frequently depends upon the physician's alertness to complaints of the sudden onset of dyspnea or pleuritic pain, particularly if this is followed by hemoptysis. Suspicion should be heightened if there are predisposing conditions such as recent fracture, surgical procedures, heart disease, obesity, pregnancy, or estrogen therapy.

The diagnosis is virtually certain if the pulmonary symptoms develop in patients with evidence of peripheral venous thrombosis, although the latter is apparent in less than 50 per cent of cases.

If there is even the slightest clinical evidence of pulmonary embolus, a chest roentgenogram, ECG, arterial blood gas analysis, fibrinogen scanning, and impedance plethysmography should be carried out promptly. If these studies indicate the presence of deep venous thrombosis in the thigh and the likelihood of pulmonary embolism, radioisotopic lung scanning should be followed in a minority of patients by pulmonary angiography.

A normal chest roentgenogram does not exclude the diagnosis. Positive findings include local oligemia (Westermark's sign), increased caliber and abrupt tapering of the descending branch of the pulmonary artery, hemidiaphragmatic elevation, basal line shadows, and parenchymal consolidation. Parenchymal consolidation varies widely but is nearly always basal and abutting against a visceral pleural surface and often is associated with a small pleural effusion.

Local "cold" zones on a radioisotopic scan without corresponding roentgenographic opacities are virtually pathognomonic of thromboembolism if the scan defect is segmental and the ventilation scan is normal (ventilation/perfusion mismatch).

Pulmonary angiography is the most definitive technique for diagnosing thromboembolism, although indications for its use are in dispute. Whereas it is generally agreed that pulmonary angiography must be performed to confirm a scan diagnosis before pulmonary embolectomy, inferior vena cava interruption, or thrombolytic therapy, some dispute its requirement before starting anticoagulant therapy. While recognizing the views of those who insist upon angiographic proof before instituting this therapy, we subscribe to the position that if a pulmonary scan is positive in a patient with strong clinical evidence of an acute embolic episode, and the chest roentgenogram is normal or reveals abnormalities compatible with the diagnosis, angiography should be avoided and anticoagulant therapy started at once. Possible exceptions are patients with chronic obstructive pulmonary disease, in whom matching ventilation/perfusion scans are likely without embolism. Although the diagnosis sometimes cannot be established short of pulmonary angiography, the administration of anticoagulant therapy on suspicion alone is preferable to confirmation of the diagnosis at necropsy.

PULMONARY EMBOLIC DISEASE OF VARIED ETIOLOGY

SEPTIC EMBOLISM

The pulmonary manifestations of septic emboli may be the only indication of serious underlying infection, and since the roentgenographic changes are often distinctive, their recognition early in the disease should permit diagnosis and prompt institution of therapy.[86]

ETIOLOGY AND PATHOGENESIS

Septic pulmonary embolism occurs most often in younger people, the majority of the 17 patients described by Jaffe and Koschmann being under 40 years of age.[87] Emboli originate from two major sites—the heart (in association with bacterial endocarditis of the tricuspid valve or a ventricular septal defect) and the peripheral veins (septic thrombophlebitis). The tricuspid valve may have been normal before infection, or may have been congenitally malformed or the site of rheumatic endocarditis. Staphylococcal osteomyelitis may also be the primary site of origin of septic embolic disease.

In 13 of Jaffe and Koschmann's 17 cases, the emboli were thought to arise from lesions in the right side of the heart (two of the 13 had septic thrombophlebitis also). A predisposing factor is nearly always present, most often drug addiction, alcoholism, general infections in patients with immunologic deficiencies (particularly lymphoma), congenital heart disease, and dermal infections.[88]

Sites of septic thrombophlebitis include arm veins in patients with a history of intravenous drug abuse, tonsillar and internal jugular veins in those with acute pharyngeal infection, pelvic veins in association with pelvic infection,[86] and veins near infected indwelling catheters and arteriovenous shunts, such as those used for hemodialysis.

In Jaffe and Koschmann's series, the organism most often grown on blood cultures was coagulase-positive Staphylococcus aureus and secondly streptococci.

ROENTGENOGRAPHIC MANIFESTATIONS

Septic pulmonary emboli, which are nearly always multiple, are usually visualized as rather ill-defined, round or wedge-shaped opacities in the periphery of the lungs (Figure 9–5). They may be uniform in size or vary widely, reflecting recurrent showers of emboli. Cavitation is frequent (Figure 9–5) and may occur rapidly; the cavities are usually thin-walled and many have no fluid level. Occasionally there develops within one or more cavities a central loose body simulating a fungus ball;[89] we suspect that this situation is analogous to the loose bodies that develop in the presence of acute lung gangrene. Hilar and mediastinal lymph node enlargement may occur and may be massive.[90] Pleural effusion, in the form of empyema, is an infrequent complication. With appropriate therapy, in most cases the lesions resolve rapidly and completely.

CLINICAL MANIFESTATIONS

Dominant clinical findings are shaking chills, high fever, and severe sinus tachycardia.[86] If the infection originates from a right heart valve it may give rise to a murmur, but in many cases this is soft and atypically located and its significance may be overlooked.[88] The source of infection must be identified, since antibiotic therapy alone may not control the infection.

FAT EMBOLISM

Nearly all pulmonary fat emboli result from trauma, usually leg fractures. Less frequent conditions are pancreatitis, severe burns, acute fatty liver in alcoholics, and extracorporeal circulation. Fat embolism to the lungs after fracture is probably common. Necropsy series on patients who have died after injury have shown incidences ranging from 67 to 97 per cent.[91] In a clinical study in which the diagnosis was based on fat in the urine, 52 per cent of the emboli followed moderate or severe trauma.[92] By contrast, in a review of 670 patients with fractures of the femur or tibia,[91] only eight (1.2 per cent) had clinical evidence of fat embolism.

Fat is believed to enter the circulation via torn veins near a fracture. It almost certainly originates in the marrow, a conclusion supported by instances of the complication after intraosseous phlebography and the finding of other bone-marrow particles in pulmonary vessels.[91] Fat appears to be transported to the lungs in the form of neutral triglycerides. Within the lungs, lipase converts the triglycerides into unsaturated fatty acids, leading to congestion, edema, and intra-alveolar hemorrhage. Intravascular coagulation also occurs, probably initiated by the release of thromboplastin from the fat; whether fibrin is present depends on the degree of fibrinolytic response to the clotting. There is also evidence that severe trauma increases the serum catecholamines, inducing lipolysis of depot fat. The normally small blood chylomicrons coalesce into larger fat droplets that are carried to the lungs and there are hydrolyzed by pulmonary lipase into chemically active fatty acids.[91]

Typically, the full clinical syndrome develops 1 to 3 days after trauma.[93] This delay can be explained by (1) continuing embolization from the site of injury, (2) the conversion of neutral triglycerides to unsaturated fatty acids, and (3) imbalance between coagulation and fibrinolysis, leading to deposition of fibrin in pulmonary vessels.[91] From the pulmonary circulation, small fat droplets pass into the general systemic circulation and form emboli in many organs, notably the brain, kidneys, and skin.

PATHOLOGIC CHARACTERISTICS

Radiologic-pathologic studies of three patients with pulmonary fat embolism[94] showed identical pathologic findings: the lungs weighed 1¼ to 3 times normal and were reddish-purple; there were sanguineous secretions in the tracheobronchial tree; and microscopically, the most striking finding was extensive intra-alveolar hemorrhage and lesser amounts of edema fluid. In addition, alveolar capillaries and alveoli contained fatty vacuoles. None of the patients had pleural effusion.

Histologic evidence of fat embolism is rare if the interval between injury and death is more than 4 weeks. Some patients survive the acute toxic pneumonitis but have residual severe brain damage due to cerebral infarction and hemorrhage induced by fat emboli.[91]

The commonest cause of death is respiratory failure, usually within 2 weeks of the trauma.

ROENTGENOGRAPHIC MANIFESTATIONS

Pulmonary fat embolism goes unrecognized in many cases if not severe, partly because symptoms are mild but more especially because the chest roentgenogram may be normal—as, for example, in 87.5 per cent of patients in whom the diagnosis of fat embolism was based on the presence of lipiduria.[92] Roentgenographic appearances in the lungs are distinctive, consisting of widespread air-space consolidation due to alveolar hemorrhage and edema, often with discrete acinar shadows. The distribution is predominantly peripheral rather than central,[94] usually involving the basal regions to a greater degree than does pulmonary edema of cardiac origin. The time lapse between trauma and both symptoms and roentgenographic signs is usually 1 to 2 days, although symptoms may develop immediately after trauma.[94] This delay in the appearance of signs differentiates oil embolism from traumatic lung contusion: in the latter, roentgenographic opacity invariably ap-

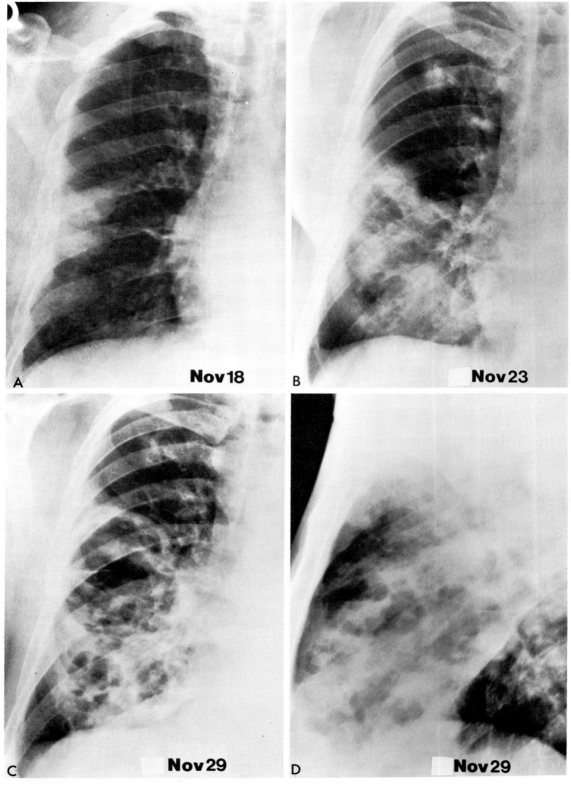

Figure 9–5
See legend on opposite page

pears immediately after injury, and whereas the opacity usually clears rapidly (in 24 to 48 hours), the roentgenographic resolution of traumatic fat embolism commonly takes 7 to 10 days or even longer.

CLINICAL MANIFESTATIONS

Fat embolism is most common in young people with leg fractures sustained in vehicular accidents[91] and elderly people with hip fractures or after arthroplasty. Symptoms usually appear 1 to 2 days after injury. The clinical manifestations can be divided into those arising from the lungs and those originating in other viscera. Symptoms from involvement of the lungs are cough, dyspnea, hemoptysis, and pleural pain; signs include pyrexia, tachypnea, tachycardia, rales, rhonchi, and friction rub.[91, 95] Acute cor pulmonale with cardiac failure, cyanosis, and circulatory shock may occur.[95] Manifestations of fat embolism elsewhere chiefly affect the central nervous system and skin; they include confusion, restlessness, stupor, delirium, and coma,[95] the last-named signifying a poor prognosis. Petechiae are common,[95] particularly along the anterior axillary folds and in the conjunctiva and retina. Hypocalcemia usually develops because of the affinity of calcium ions for free fatty acids released by the hydrolysis of fat emboli; the serum calcium level may be of prognostic value.[95] The triad of petechial rash, cerebral manifestations, and typical pulmonary changes 1 to 2 days after trauma is virtually pathognomonic of fat embolism. Fat droplets may be detected in the urine or sputum,[95] but the latter particularly is not a reliable indication of the diagnosis;[96] fat droplets are found rarely in cerebrospinal fluid.

Pulmonary function tests reveal stiffness of the lungs, a diffusion defect, increase in the A-a O_2 gradient and $\dot{V}/\dot{Q}$ inequality.[95] Severe hypoxemia may persist despite inhalation of 100 per cent oxygen.

AMNIOTIC FLUID EMBOLISM

Amniotic fluid with its contained fetal squames, mucin, fat, bile pigments, lanugo hairs, and amorphous debris from the pregnant uterus can enter the maternal circulation and embolize to the lungs. The entity was not clearly defined until the publication in 1941 of Steiner and Lushbaugh's review,[97] and their description still stands:

Profound shock coming on suddenly and unexpectedly in a woman who is in unusually severe labor or has just finished such a labor, especially if she is an elderly multipara with an excessively large, perhaps dead, fetus and with meconium in the amniotic fluid, should lead to a suspicion of this possibility. If, also, the shock is introduced by a chill which is followed by dyspnea, cyanosis, vomiting, restlessness and the like and is accompanied by a pronounced fall in blood pressure and a rapid, weak pulse, the picture is more complete. If pulmonary edema now develops quickly in the known absence of previously existing heart disease the diagnosis is reasonably certain.

In 1967 it was estimated that about 10 per cent of the 1400 maternal deaths in the United States were attributable to amniotic fluid embolism.[98] Courtney's review[99] stated that this condition accounts for 4 to 6 per cent of all maternal deaths. Perhaps a more realistic index of the significance of amniotic fluid embolism is the statement in the 1961 report from the Sloan Hospital for Women[100] that it was the commonest cause of maternal death during labor or immediately postpartum.

PATHOGENESIS

Virtually no amniotic fluid escapes into the maternal circulation during normal pregnancy, labor, and delivery. Experiments in which filtered amniotic fluid was injected into the peripheral circulation showed no significant harmful effects.[101] The fullblown syndrome develops

---

Figure 9–5. Massive Septic Embolism. This 31-year-old man suffered a massive right pulmonary embolism originating in severe thrombophlebitis of one leg. A lung scan revealed a total lack of perfusion of the right lung and a segmental defect in the midportion of the left lung. Five days after the acute episode (A), a poorly defined opacity appeared in the axillary portion of the right lung in a configuration compatible with a pulmonary infarct; there was a small right pleural effusion. Five days later (B), much of the lower half of the right lung became consolidated, with several areas of radiolucency scattered throughout the consolidated lobe suggesting cavitation. After another 5 days (C and D), numerous shaggy cavities appeared in the consolidation, representing multiple abscesses as a result of septic infarction. The disease is situated predominantly in the right middle and upper lobes.

only if the amniotic fluid contains certain fetal products, principally squames and meconium.[102]

There appear to be three major routes by which amniotic fluid infuses into the maternal circulation: (1) the endocervical veins, which are lacerated even during normal labor and are probably the commonest route of entry; (2) the placental site, usually in cases of uterine rupture, placenta previa, premature separation, and cesarean section, when the incision involves the placental implantation site; and (3) in other types of uterine trauma, such as a split in the myometrium.[99]

The pathogenesis derives from three factors: overwhelming embolic obstruction of the pulmonary vasculature, anaphylactoid reaction to particulate matter in the amniotic fluid, and coagulation failure.

VASCULAR EMBOLIZATION. Once the amniotic fluid enters the maternal circulation, particulate matter is quickly filtered out in the pulmonary vascular bed, causing mechanical obstruction. Pulmonary artery pressure rises abruptly (probably caused at least partly by reflex vasoconstriction), blood flow to the left side of the heart decreases and cardiac output falls, systemic hypotension develops, and peripheral vascular collapse occurs; pulmonary edema rapidly develops. The severe pulmonary hypertension induces acute cor pulmonale and right ventricular failure, and the hypoxemia causes cerebral manifestations including restlessness, convulsions, and coma.

ANAPHYLACTOID REACTION. This has been proposed[97] as the cause of death in rapidly fatal cases. Meigs[103] surmised that intense phagocytic activity directly implicates particulate meconium as the cause of fatal anaphylactic shock.

COAGULATION FAILURE. Amniotic fluid, which is a powerful coagulant, constitutes a quarter of total blood volume at term; thus it is the body's largest reservoir of active coagulant. Disturbances in blood coagulation, which may occur in up to 40 per cent of patients who survive the first hour after the catastrophe,[104] probably relate chiefly to a decrease in circulating fibrinogen. Whatever the mechanism, the result is severe fibrin depletion and disseminated intravascular coagulation (DIC). Since 1 ml of a thrombokinase-like constituent of amniotic fluid can coagulate 10 liters of blood,[105] this substance may contribute to the hemorrhage secondary to hypofibrinogenemia. Prompt treatment with heparin[106] may combat the impairment of the microcirculation caused by DIC.

Predisposing factors to amniotic fluid embolism include tumultuous labor, uterine stimulants, meconium in the amniotic fluid, intrauterine fetal death, older age of the mother, and multiparity. In all reported series, patients were in the thirty-fifth to forty-second week of pregnancy at the time of embolization. The high correlation with intrauterine death and fetal distress suggests that conditions resulting in contamination of amniotic fluid, particularly with meconium, render the effects of amniotic fluid infusion unusually lethal.

PATHOLOGIC CHARACTERISTICS

The most complete description of the lungs at necropsy has been provided by Peterson and Taylor,[107] who analyzed 40 cases at the U.S. Armed Forces Institute of Pathology. The findings are diagnostic: grossly, most lungs evidenced pulmonary edema, the combined weight of the lungs averaging 748 g; minimal to moderate pulmonary edema was seen histologically in 24 cases, severe in four. Amniotic fluid debris was not visible grossly in pulmonary vessels but was readily identified histologically. Intravascular mucin was found in all cases, chiefly within small pulmonary arteries (this substance is derived almost entirely from the infant's intestinal tract and is a major constituent of meconium); mucin was the chief particulate matter identified in pulmonary vessels in 80 per cent of lungs examined. Squames from the fetus' skin (present in normal amniotic fluid) were identified by special keratin stains in 32 cases and were the major embolic constituent in eight; they were chiefly in arterioles and capillaries, usually mixed with mucin. Other recognizable elements were lanugo hair, fat from the vernix caseosa, and amorphous debris.

ROENTGENOGRAPHIC MANIFESTATIONS

In line with the pathologic characteristics, the major roentgenologic sign is air-space pulmonary edema indistinguishable from acute pulmonary edema of other cause. Whether cardiac enlargement accompanies the edema depends on the severity of pulmonary arterial hypertension and consequent cor pulmonale, but almost certainly vascular occlusion severe enough to cause roentgenographically demonstrable cardiomegaly will be fatal.

Since the predominant roentgenographic manifestation is widespread air-space consolidation, the chief differential diagnoses are massive pulmonary hemorrhage and Mendelson's syndrome (*see* page 505).

CLINICAL MANIFESTATIONS

All of Peterson and Taylor's 40 cases[107] manifested abrupt onset of signs and symptoms of pulmonary embolism. The embolization was heralded by dyspnea and cyanosis in 20 patients, sudden profound shock disproportionate to blood loss in 12, and signs of CNS irritability (convulsions, hyper-reflexia, and other signs) in eight. Thirty patients died as a direct result of the embolic episode, 29 within 6 hours of the clinical onset and one after 31 hours; excessive bleeding was a contributory cause in eight. In the other 10 cases, death was attributed to uncontrollable uterine hemorrhage. Fibrinogen levels were low in all four patients in whom they were measured.

EMBOLIC MANIFESTATIONS OF PARASITIC INFESTATION

Of the two major groups of parasitic infestations (protozoan and metazoan) of the lung, only the latter can cause embolic manifestations. The parasites chiefly responsible are blood flukes, the cause of schistosomiasis. Although the protozoan larvae—*Ascaris lumbricoides, Strongyloides stercoralis, Ancylostoma duodenale, Necator americanus, Trichinella spiralis, Dirofilaria immitis,* and *Toxocara*—must pass through the lung capillaries in order to reach the airways, they obstruct the vessels only slightly or not at all. Of the numerous flatworm infestations, *Schistosoma* are the only organisms that can cause pulmonary vascular occlusion. These diseases are described fully in Chapter 6 (*see* page 339).

EMBOLIC MANIFESTATIONS OF METASTATIC CANCER

Malignant disease metastasizes to the lungs in about 30 per cent of all cases, and only to that site in about half of these.[108] The usual route is the systemic veins, directly by invasion at the primary site or indirectly via the thoracic or right lymphatic duct and subclavian veins. Despite this high incidence of a vascular origin for metastatic disease, the incidence of recognizable embolic phenomena is very low indeed. Metastatic neoplasms are discussed in Chapter

8 (*see* page 443); only the implications for vascular occlusion are considered here.

Pathologically, malignant cells that survive after reaching the lung via the bloodstream are found encased in fibrin clinging to the vascular endothelium; emboli tend to lodge at the bifurcation of capillaries and arterioles. Some traverse the vessel wall and lodge in the interstitial space, lymphatics, or alveoli. Massive intracapillary spread develops in some cases, presumably as the result of total loss of defense mechanisms.[2] In such cases, and in those with 70 to 75 per cent of the pulmonary vasculature obstructed by tumor emboli, cor pulmonale results, with right ventricular dilation and hypertrophy. Histologic examination reveals blockage of vessels by tumor, alone or mixed with thrombus, or by fibro-obliterative endarteritis.[109]

Roentgenographically, changes in the cardiac silhouette and pulmonary vasculature are indistinguishable from other causes of pulmonary arterial hypertension: the main pulmonary artery is prominent and the hilar arteries are enlarged and taper rapidly distally. Micronodular opacities may be present throughout both lungs, but often without a background to suggest metastatic disease. The chest roentgenogram may be normal, since enlargement of the main pulmonary arteries and right ventricle (reflecting the diffuse vascular obstruction) is not invariable.[109] In cases of acute cor pulmonale resulting from extensive embolic occlusion by metastatic trophoblastic neoplasms, therapy may reverse the roentgenographic changes.

AIR EMBOLISM

Air may enter (1) the systemic venous circulation and pass to the right side of the heart and thence to the lungs (*venous air embolism*), or (2) the pulmonary venous circulation, the left side of the heart, and the systemic arterial network (*arterial air embolism*). In venous air embolism, the effects derive from obstruction of the pulmonary circulation and thus are felt *by* the lungs, whereas in arterial air embolism the effects derive from an abnormality *within* the lung and are felt chiefly by the two vital organs, the heart and the brain.

PATHOGENESIS

ARTERIAL AIR EMBOLISM. Air can enter a pulmonary vein (the most common but not the only cause of arterial air embolism) only when

(1) there is an opening in a vessel exposed to air, and (2) the pressure of the air exceeds the pressure in the vessel. These two criteria are met in various situations, the easiest to comprehend (and possibly the commonest) being the insertion of a needle into the thoracic cavity for thoracentesis, therapeutic pneumothorax, or needle biopsy. In view of the frequency of these procedures and the apparent rarity of the occurrence of air embolism, it is clear that special circumstances must exist for air to enter the pulmonary venous system. Three such situations are possible:[110] (1) when a needle, accidentally inserted into the lung during attempted induction of pneumothorax, enters a pulmonary vein, injection of air will obviously result in embolism; (2) when a needle containing no stylet or stopcock is introduced into the lung for biopsy and enters a pulmonary vein, air may enter the vein if atmospheric pressure exceeds venous pressure, as during deep inspiration (atmosphere to pulmonary vein fistula); and (3) when a needle introduced into the lung for biopsy pierces a bronchus or pulmonary cyst and a contiguous vein, air may enter the vein if the bronchial or cyst pressure exceeds venous pressure, as during a cough. It is apparent that such episodes can be prevented by ensuring that suction on a syringe does not produce blood, that the needle hole is occluded by a stylet or stopcock, and that patients undergoing lung biopsy are cautioned against coughing or straining after the needle point has entered the lung.

With the thorax intact (*i.e.*, if no needle has entered the lung), arterial air embolism can occur in several clinical situations. Probably the common denominator is a bulla or bleb that is poorly ventilated because of partial or complete obstruction of its feeding airway. Perhaps air embolism occurs most frequently during scuba diving. Smith[111] calculated that the volume of air in a space distal to a partly or completely occluded bronchus doubles every 33 ft of a diver's ascent, producing sufficient distention to explode the air space. This excess pulmonary pressure and volume force air into the pulmonary circulation, sending a stream of bubbles to the left side of the heart. Such episodes can be prevented by exhaling during ascent, so that poorly ventilated spaces do not overdistend as pressure within them diminishes. Similar circumstances are possible during assisted positive pressure breathing, perhaps particularly in neonates: Kogutt[112] has reported six cases of systemic air embolism as a complication of respiratory therapy in neonates; in the only infant who survived, there was no clinical symptomatology, the diagnosis being made by roentgenographic findings alone. A similar pathophysiologic process undoubtedly underlies the arterial air embolism that occurs in status asthmaticus[113] and hyaline membrane disease of the newborn.[114] Arterial air embolism also results from direct injection into the systemic arterial system, usually via intra-arterial catheters or cannulas.

VENOUS AIR EMBOLISM. Venous air embolism occurs as a result of air entering the systemic venous circulation and passing to the right side of the heart and the lungs. Although fatalities from venous air embolism have been reported, small amounts of air on the right side of the heart and pulmonary arterial tree have little deleterious effect and, in fact, even large amounts may be well tolerated. The embolism can occur if air enters the circulation through an intravenous infusion apparatus, during surgery of the head and neck, or (occasionally) during operative obstetrics. In the case of infusion catheters, the usual mode of entry is direct injection.

PATHOLOGIC CHARACTERISTICS

The gross morphologic changes in patients who die from venous air embolism are well documented.[115] Bloody froth formed by the whipping action of the right atrium and ventricle fills these chambers and extends into the central and peripheral branches of the pulmonary artery and sometimes the superior and inferior vena cavae. The pulmonary veins are virtually empty of blood; so also are the left atrium and left ventricle, which are contracted upon themselves and contain only a very small quantity of black blood. The systemic arterial system contains no air bubbles. Thus it might be assumed that the cause of death would be formation of an air block in the outflow tract of the right ventricle and pulmonary arteries, preventing peripheral pulmonary blood flow. However, experimental studies[116] have clearly shown that the ill effects of air embolism cannot be attributed solely to vascular obstruction by air bubbles; a highly complex series of events is involved, chief of which is probably the formation of fibrin plugs and their impaction in terminal branches of the pulmonary arteries.

ROENTGENOGRAPHIC MANIFESTATIONS

The roentgenologic manifestations of air embolism in living patients have been fairly well documented in the small number of reports that have appeared in the literature.[112, 117-119] As expected, the only sign is the presence of visible gas in cardiac chambers, major pulmonary arteries, or systemic arteries in many sites throughout the body. In venous air embolism, gas is present in the right heart chambers and central pulmonary arteries; in arterial or systemic air embolism, gas will be identified in the left heart chambers, aorta, or more peripheral branches of the systemic arterial tree such as in the neck, shoulder girdles, or upper abdomen.

CLINICAL MANIFESTATIONS

Air embolism, whether arterial or venous, is so often rapidly fatal—at least in cases in which the diagnosis has been proved—that the clinical manifestations are of little consequence. Clinically, there is abrupt onset of hypotension, bradycardia, shock, and early asystole; convulsions may occur.

EMBOLISM IN DRUG ADDICTS

Reference has been made to septic thromboembolism in intravenous drug abusers. This section describes a different form of embolic disease in drug addicts, resulting from the intravenous injection of oral medications. Over the past decade, heroin addicts have acquired the habit of injecting themselves intravenously ("mainlining") with a variety of medications intended solely for oral use. Oral medications misused in this way include amphetamines and closely related drugs such as methylphenidate hydrochloride (Ritalin) and tripelennamine, methadone hydrochloride, meperidine, propylhexedrine (Benzedrine), and hydromorphone hydrochloride (Dilaudid).[120] These oral medications have in common an insoluble filler, talc (magnesium silicate), added for its lubricant effect in preventing the tablets from sticking to punches and dies during manufacture. The talc particles elicit a granulomatous reaction in and around the pulmonary vessels. Heroin addicts given methadone as replacement therapy and those who inject stimulants to counteract the sedative effect of narcotic drugs crush the pills in a spoon or bottle top and add water; they heat the mixture and draw it into a syringe, sometimes using absorbent cotton as a filter.

In a study of ex-addicts who had injected methadone,[120] we found impaired pulmonary function and roentgenographic evidence of granulomata in heavy users (10 to 20 tablets daily for 5 to 7 years) and retinal granulomas but normal chest roentgenograms in "more moderate" users.

PATHOLOGIC CHARACTERISTICS

The talc crystals impact in pulmonary vessels and elicit an endovascular and perivascular foreign body granulomatous reaction. Smaller particles traverse the lesser circulation and become embedded in other viscera, including the retina.[121] Histologically, there is extensive replacement of lung parenchyma by confluent foreign body granulomas, chiefly interstitial and sometimes involving the walls of small arteries. Intravascular thrombi may contain talc crystals. Foreign body giant cells are numerous and contain doubly refractile crystals that are identifiable as talc by x-ray diffraction and are optically refractive when viewed with polarized light. In advanced cases there is extensive interstitial pulmonary fibrosis and a remarkable loss of pulmonary vascular bed.[120, 122]

ROENTGENOGRAPHIC MANIFESTATIONS

Of the 15 chronic "mainline" methadone users described by Paré and his coworkers,[120] six had unequivocally abnormal chest roentgenograms. Two distinct patterns of disease emerged, one with widespread micronodulation without any loss of lung volume (four patients) and the other with both general and local loss of volume (two patients). The nodular pattern consisted of a multitude of discrete opacities whose diameter ranged from bare visibility to about 1 mm (Figure 9–6). There was no suggestion of a reticular component, the opacities being remarkably distinct and "pinpoint" in character, simulating alveolar microlithiasis. In contrast to the midzonal predominance described by others[122] the distribution in our first four patients was symmetric and uniform throughout both lungs, slightly greater profusion in lower zones reflecting the greater volume of lung.

In one of the two patients with reduced lung volume, diffuse cicatrization progressed over a period of four years to a point where roentgenography revealed very little air in either lung (Figure 9–7). In the second patient, not only was lung volume reduced generally but also there was coalescence of opacities in both upper zones, much greater on the left. Changes in the upper zones resembled the progressive massive fibrosis of coal-worker's pneumoconiosis except

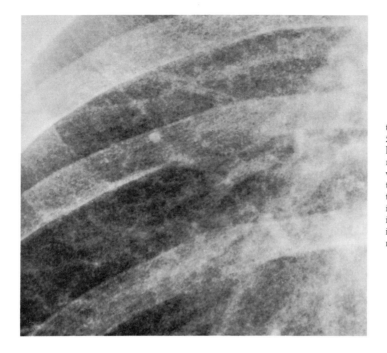

Figure 9–6. Pulmonary Talcosis in Intravenous Drug Abuse. This asymptomatic 22-year-old white male had been "shooting" heroin and methadone for 4 years when this roentgenogram was obtained. There is widespread involvement of both lungs by tiny micronodular opacities seen to advantage on a roentgenographically magnified image (2:1) of the right lower zone. There is no anatomic predominance. The pattern is similar to the discrete opacities of alveolar microlithiasis.

that the borders of the opacity were less well defined and a prominent air bronchogram was visible. Identical changes of conglomerate pulmonary disease have been described more recently by Sieniewicz and Nidecker.[123]

The granulomatous lesions of talcosis are so strategically placed in and around arterioles and capillaries that a slowly progressive obliteration of the microvascular circulation might be anticipated, resulting in diffuse vascular obstruction and angiothrombotic pulmonary hypertension.[124]

CLINICAL MANIFESTATIONS

Probably most addicts who inject oral medications containing talc are asymptomatic, granulomas being found incidentally at necropsy in those who die from other causes. Many heavy users experience dyspnea and some complain

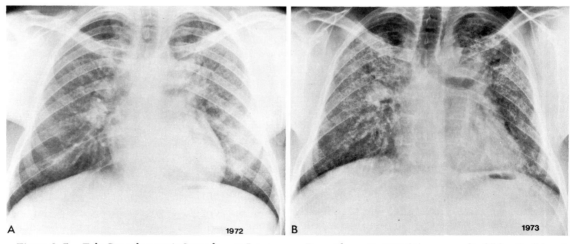

Figure 9–7. Talc Granulomatosis Secondary to Intravenous Drug Abuse. In 1972 (A), as a result of "shooting" heroin and methadone for a period of about 2 years, this 21-year-old white male demonstrated in both lungs a multitude of tiny nodular opacities that created almost a ground-glass appearance. Considerable loss of lung volume was present. Hilar lymph nodes were enlarged as a result of sarcoidosis, previously diagnosed. One year later (B), the micronodules had increased in both size and number and, in the upper lung zones, particularly, were becoming confluent. Lung volume was still further reduced.

of persistent cough.[120, 122] Extensive vascular and perivascular disease may lead to cor pulmonale.

Organized thrombi and scars are visible in the forearms of nearly all addicts who "mainline," and accumulations of glistening particles can be seen in the fundi, principally at the posterior pole surrounding the foveal area; these may be the earliest clue to illicit use of such drugs, since they have been detected in addicts whose chest roentgenograms and pulmonary function were normal.[120] Although fundal deposits of talc generally result in only a mild reduction in visual acuity, a case recently has been reported in which there was severe bilateral visual loss as a result of retinal detachment and vitreous hemorrhage.[125] Farber and associates[126] have recently described six young men with intravenous talc granulomatosis who manifested increased levels of serum angiotensin-converting enzyme, positive gallium lung scans, and increased lymphocyte counts: birefringent particles could be identified in broncho-alveolar lavage.

As in the pneumoconioses resulting from inhalation of silicon dioxide and silicates, intravenous talc granulomatosis progresses and disability increases, even after cessation of exposure.[120] Follow-up studies (unpublished) of drug abusers reported in 1979 by Paré and his colleagues[120] have revealed the development of progressive lower lobe emphysema in several cases; one of these has had repeated pneumothoraces.

PULMONARY FUNCTION TESTS. Function abnormalities are common in heavy users and may be present in those who admit to lesser abuse. The pattern is unusual and should suggest the diagnosis. There is a combination of "restrictive" and "obstructive" dysfunction, reducing bronchial air flow well below that expected in heavy cigarette smokers of this age. Hyperinflation and air trapping are not evident at the outset but in some patients the full pattern of advanced emphysema, including increased compliance, occurs as a late development; in many cases diffusing capacities are significantly decreased. Hypoxemia is present in advanced stages of the disease.

IODIZED OIL EMBOLISM

Iatrogenic pulmonary oil embolism is almost invariably a complication of lymphangiography with ethiodized oil (Ethiodol) and only occasionally after procedures such as hystero-salpingography, urethrography, and myelography. In one study, lung biopsy performed within 12 hours after the lymphatic injection of ethiodized oil[127] showed lipid droplets widely distributed throughout the pulmonary capillary bed, corresponding to fine granular stippling observed throughout both lungs roentgenologically. Biopsy specimens obtained the next day revealed less lipid in the parenchymal interstitial space; and it was no longer exclusively in the capillary bed, much having passed into the extravascular interstitial tissue and some into the alveoli. At this stage, roentgenography usually shows a fine reticular pattern.[128] Roentgenographic evidence of oil embolism was found in 44 of 80 patients,[128] most of whom had pelvic or abdominal lymphatic obstruction. The small peripheral vessels may be so filled with lipid contrast material as to present an arborizing pattern similar to that seen on pulmonary arteriography.

Few patients have symptoms. Mild fever may develop within 48 hours after lymphangiography. Very rarely, cough, chills, dyspnea, cyanosis, or hypotension may develop, and the ECG shows evidence of right ventricular strain.[128] Several investigators have documented decreased diffusing capacity after lymphangiography.[127, 129] Decrease is maximal at 24 to 48 hours, an early fall in gas transfer being attributed to reduced pulmonary capillary blood flow and a later drop to interference with the membrane component of diffusion when the oil moves into the interstitial tissue.[129] There is also reduction in lung compliance and in arterial PO_2, particularly after a high dose of a contrast agent.[127]

METALLIC MERCURY EMBOLISM

Like air, mercury may be introduced into either the arterial or the venous circulation. In the former case, since it is the peripheral arterial circulation that is involved, the thorax is not affected.

Venous embolization may be accidental, from injury from a broken thermometer or venous blood sampling with a mercury-sealed syringe, or intentional, from injection by drug abusers or patients attempting suicide. The metal reaches the right ventricle and is disseminated throughout the pulmonary arterial tree: the result is a distinctive, almost alarming, roentgenographic appearance (Figure 9–8).

Pathologically, the inflammatory reaction in the lungs is relatively mild.[130] The mercury may

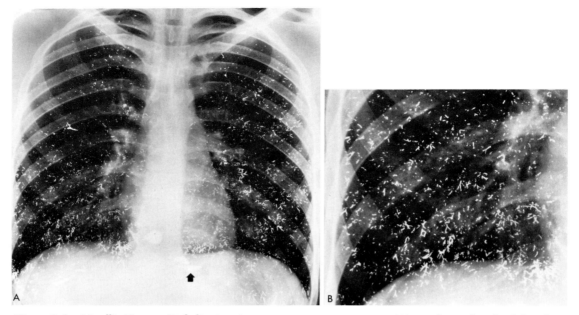

Figure 9–8. **Metallic Mercury Embolization.** A posteroanterior roentgenogram *(A)* reveals a multitude of short linear and branching opacities of metallic density distributed widely throughout both lungs, seen to better advantage in a magnified view of the lower portion of the right lung *(B)*. It would be difficult to be certain whether this metallic mercury was within the vascular or airway system of the lungs if it were not for the presence of a pool of mercury lying in the inferior aspect of the right ventricular chamber, seen in posteroanterior projection *(arrow)*. This young male drug addict injected metallic mercury into an antecubital vein for a special "kick." (Courtesy of Dr. William Beamish, University Hospital, Edmonton, Alberta.)

remain within the pulmonary arteries, eventually becoming encased in thrombus; it may also get into the interstitium and alveoli, presumably from rupture of capillaries, and in these locations may give rise to a granulomatous foreign body reaction surrounding each droplet.

Roentgenographically, the appearance is distinctive because of the very high density of the intravascular material. The presentation may be in the form of spherules or of short tubular structures resembling mercury-filled arterial segments. The distribution is usually bilateral and fairly symmetric. Being denser than plasma, mercury flows to the dependent portions of the lung, so that the predominant distribution depends on the body position at the moment of injection. A local collection of mercury may be apparent in the heart, usually near the apex of the right ventricle, distinguishing it from aspirated mercury in the bronchi (Figure 9–8). Roentgenograms of the abdomen may reveal scattered mercury deposits in the liver, spleen, or kidney as a result of passage through the pulmonary capillary bed and into the systemic circulation. In patients in whom the mercury has been self-administered, roentgenograms of the forearms may reveal aggregations of mercury droplets within the soft tissues at the site of injection.[72]

Clinically, the body's reaction to metallic mercury varies but appears to be predominantly systemic. Mercurialism occurs when sufficient metallic mercury is oxidized to the soluble mercuric ion Hg^{++}, whose toxicity derives from its selective affinity for sulfhydryl groups and its inhibition of enzymes containing such groups.[130] Toxicity is manifested by a metallic taste, excessive salivation, gingivitis, stomatitis, diarrhea, nephrosis, tremor (hatter's shakes), and erethism.[130] Excretion is chiefly via the kidneys.

REFERENCES

1. Freiman, D. G., Suyemoto, J., and Wessler, S.: Frequency of pulmonary thromboembolism in man. N. Engl. J. Med., *272*:1278, 1965.
2. Spencer, H.: Pathology of the Lung. 2nd ed. Oxford, Pergamon, 1968.
3. Silver, D., Helfrich, L. R., and Woodard, W. T.: Management of pulmonary embolism. Med. Clin. North Am., *54*:361, 1970.
4. Smith, G. T., Dexter, L., and Dammin, G. J.: Postmortem quantitative studies in pulmonary embolism. *In* Sasahara, A. A., and Stein, M. (eds.): Pulmonary Embolic Disease. New York, Grune & Stratton, 1965, pp. 120–130.
5. Greenberg, H.: Refractory dyspnea and orthopnea. Evidence of recurrent pulmonary embolism and infarction. Am. Rev. Resp. Dis., *92*:215, 1965.

6. Royal College of General Practitioners Report by Records Unit and Research Advisory Service of R.C.G.P.: Oral contraception and thrombo-embolic disease. J. Coll. Gen. Pract., 13:267, 1967.

7. Inman, W. H. W., and Vessey, M. P.: Investigation of deaths from pulmonary, coronary, and cerebral thrombosis and embolism in women of child-bearing age. Br. Med. J., 2:193, 1968.

8. Vessey, M. P., and Doll, R.: Investigation of relation between use of oral contraceptives and thromboembolic disease. Br. Med. J., 2:199, 1968.

9. Editorial: Predisposition to thrombosis. Lancet, 2:1430, 1974.

10. Coope, J., Thomson, J. M., and Poller, L.: Effects of "natural oestrogen" replacement therapy on menopausal symptoms and blood clotting. Br. Med. J., 4:139, 1975.

11. Badaracco, M. A., and Vessey, M. P.: Recurrence of venous thromboembolic disease and use of oral contraceptives. Br. Med. J., 1:215, 1974.

12. Salzman, E. W., Harris, W. H., and DeSanctis, R. W.: Reduction in venous thromboembolism by agents affecting platelet function. N. Engl. J. Med., 284:1287, 1971.

13. Le Quesne, L. P.: Relation between deep vein thrombosis and pulmonary embolism in surgical patients. N. Engl. J. Med., 291:1292, 1974.

14. Greenspan, R. H., and Steiner, R. E.: The radiologic diagnosis of pulmonary thromboembolism. In Simon, M., Potchen, E. J., and LeMay, M. (eds.): Frontiers of Pulmonary Radiology. New York, Grune & Stratton, 1969, pp. 222–245.

15. Aaro, L. A., and Juergens, J. L.: Thrombophlebitis and pulmonary embolism as complications of pregnancy. Med. Clin. North Am., 58:829, 1974.

16. Villasanta, U.: Thromboembolic disease in pregnancy. Am. J. Obstet. Gynecol., 93:142, 1965.

17. Moser, K. M., and LeMoine, J. R.: Is embolic risk conditioned by location of deep venous thrombosis? Ann. Intern. Med., 94(Part 1):439, 1981.

18. Gorham, L. W.: A study of pulmonary embolism: Part II. The mechanism of death; based on a clinicopathological investigation of 100 cases of massive and 285 cases of minor embolism of the pulmonary artery. Arch. Intern. Med., 108:189, 1961.

19. Dexter, L.: Cardiovascular responses to experimental pulmonary embolism. In Sasahara, A. A., and Stein, M. (eds.): Pulmonary Embolic Disease. New York, Grune & Stratton, 1965, pp. 101–109.

20. Fleischner, F. G.: Pulmonary embolism. Can. Med. Assoc. J., 78:653, 1958.

21. Heitzman, E. R., Markarian, B., and Dailey, E. T.: Pulmonary thromboembolic disease: A lobular concept. Radiology, 103:529, 1972.

22. Robbins, S. L.: Pathology, 3rd ed., vol. II. Philadelphia, W. B. Saunders Co., 1967.

23. Dalen, J. E., Banas, J. S., Jr., Brooks, H. L., Evans, G. L., Paraskos, J. A., and Dexter, L.: Resolution rate of acute pulmonary embolism in man. N. Engl. J. Med., 280:1194, 1969.

24. Secker-Walker, R. H., Jackson, J. A., and Goodwin, J.: Resolution of pulmonary embolism. Br. Med. J., 4:135, 1970.

25. Comroe, J. H., Jr.: Pulmonary arterial blood flow: Effects of brief and permanent arrest. Am. Rev. Resp. Dis., 85:179, 1962.

26. Nadel, J. A., Colebatch, H. J. H., and Olsen, C. R.: Location and mechanism of airway constriction after barium sulfate microembolism. J. Appl. Physiol., 19:387, 1964.

27. Meth, R. F., Tashkin, D. P., Hansen, K. S., and Simmons, D. H.: Pulmonary edema and wheezing after pulmonary embolism. Am. Rev. Resp. Dis., 111:693, 1975.

28. Torrance, D. J., Jr.: Roentgenographic signs of pulmonary artery occlusion. Am. J. Med. Sci., 237:651, 1959.

29. Westermark, N.: On the roentgen diagnosis of lung embolism. Acta Radiol., 19:357, 1938.

30. Kerr, I. H., Simon, G., and Sutton, G. C.: The value of the plain radiograph in acute massive pulmonary embolism. Br. J. Radiol., 44:751, 1971.

31. Grossman, Z. D., Ritter, C. A., Tarner, R. J., Somogyi, J. W., Johnson, A. C., Lyons, B., Fernandes, P., Thomas, F. D., Gagne, G. M., Bassano, D., and Zens, A.: Successful identification of oligemic lung by transmission computed tomography after experimentally produced acute pulmonary arterial occlusion in the dog. Invest. Radiol., 16:275, 1981.

32. Fleischner, F. G.: Recurrent pulmonary embolism and cor pulmonale. N. Engl. J. Med., 276:1213, 1967.

33. Fleischner, F. G.: Pulmonary embolism. Clin. Radiol., 13:169, 1962.

34. Chang, C. H. (J.), and Davis, W. C.: A roentgen sign of pulmonary infarction. Clin. Radiol., 16:141, 1965.

35. Figley, M. M., Gerdes, A. J., and Ricketts, H. J.: Radiographic aspects of pulmonary embolism. Semin. Roentgenol., 2:389, 1967.

36. Talbot, S., Worthington, B. S., and Roebuck, E. J.: Radiographic signs of pulmonary embolism and pulmonary infarction. Thorax, 28:198, 1973.

37. Fleischner, F. G.: Roentgenology of the pulmonary infarct. Semin. Roentgenol., 2:61, 1967.

38. Hampton, A. O., and Castleman, B.: Correlation of postmortem chest teleroentgenograms with autopsy findings. With special reference to pulmonary embolism and infarction. Am. J. Roentgenol., 43:305, 1940.

39. Castleman, B.: Pathologic observations on pulmonary infarction in man. In Sasahara, A. A., and Stein, M. (eds.): Pulmonary Embolic Disease. New York, Grune & Stratton, 1965, pp. 86–92.

40. Fleischner, F. G.: Observations on the radiologic changes in pulmonary embolism. In Sasahara, A. A., and Stein, M. (eds.): Pulmonary Embolic Disease. New York, Grune & Stratton, 1965, pp. 206–213.

41. McGoldrick, P. J., Rudd, T. G., Figley, M. M., and Wilhelm, J. P.: What becomes of pulmonary infarcts? Am. J. Roentgenol., 133:1039, 1979.

42. Woesner, M. E., Sanders, I., and White, G. W.: The melting sign in resolving transient pulmonary infarction. Am. J. Roentgenol., 111:782, 1971.

43. Reid, L.: Quoted by Simon, G., as a personal communication. Br. J. Radiol., 43:327, 1970.

44. Simon, G.: The cause and significance of some long line shadows in the chest radiograph. Proc. R. Soc. Med., 58:861, 1965.

45. Simon, G.: Further observations on the long line shadow across a lower zone of the lung. Br. J. Radiol., 43:327, 1970.

46. Dalen, J. E., Brooks, H. L., Johnson, L. W., Meister, S. G., Szucs, M. M., Jr., and Dexter, L.: Pulmonary angiography in acute pulmonary embolism: Indications, techniques, and results in 367 patients. Am. Heart J., 81:175, 1971.

47. Johnson, B. A., James, A. E., Jr., and White, R. I., Jr.: Oblique and selective pulmonary angiography in diagnosis of pulmonary embolism. Am. J. Roentgenol., 118:801, 1973.

48. Sagel, S. S., and Greenspan, R. H.: Nonuniform

pulmonary arterial perfusion: Pulmonary embolism? Radiology, 99:541, 1971.

49. Simon, M., and Sasahara, A. A.: Observations on the angiographic changes in pulmonary thromboembolism. In Sasahara, A. A., and Stein, M. (eds.): Pulmonary Embolic Disease. New York, Grune & Stratton, 1965, pp. 214–224.

50. Alexander, J. K., Gonzalez, D. A., and Fred, H. L.: Angiographic studies in cardiorespiratory diseases. Special reference to thromboembolism. J.A.M.A., 198:575, 1966.

51. Godwin, J. D., Webb, W. R., Gamsu, G., and Ovenfors, C.-O.: Computed tomography of pulmonary embolism. Am. J. Roentgenol., 135:691, 1980.

52. Ovenfors, C.-O., Godwin, J. D., and Brito, A. C.: Diagnosis of peripheral pulmonary emboli by computed tomography in the living dog. Radiology, 141:519, 1981.

53. Leading Article: Management of pulmonary embolism. Br. Med. J., 4:133, 1968.

54. Mavor, G. E., and Galloway, J. M. D.: The iliofemoral venous segment as a source of pulmonary emboli. Lancet, 1:871, 1967.

55. MacLean, L. D., Shibata, H. R., McLean, A. P. H., Skinner, G. B., and Gutelius, J. R.: Pulmonary embolism: The value of bedside scanning, angiography and pulmonary embolectomy. Can. Med. Assoc. J., 97:991, 1967.

56. Oakley, C. M.: Diagnosis of pulmonary embolism. Br. Med. J., 2:773, 1970.

57. Fred, H. L., Burdine, J. A., Jr., Gonzalez, D. A., Lockhart, R. W., Peabody, C. A., and Alexander, J. K.: Arteriographic assessment of lung scanning in the diagnosis of pulmonary thromboembolism. N. Engl. J. Med., 275:1025, 1966.

58. Secker-Walker, R. H.: Scintillation scanning of lungs in diagnosis of pulmonary embolism. Br. Med. J., 2:206, 1968.

59. Gilday, D. L., and James, A. E., Jr.: Lung scan patterns in pulmonary embolism versus those in congestive heart failure and emphysema. Am. J. Roentgenol., 115:739, 1972.

60. Gilday, D. L., Poulose, K. P., and DeLand, F. H.: Accuracy of detection of pulmonary embolism by lung scanning correlated with pulmonary angiography. Am. J. Roentgenol., 115:732, 1972.

61. Isawa, T., Hayes, M., and Taplin, G. V.: Radioaerosol inhalation lung scanning: Its role in suspected pulmonary embolism. J. Nucl. Med., 12:606, 1971.

62. Bass, H., Heckscher, T., and Anthonisen, N. R.: Regional pulmonary gas exchange in patients with pulmonary embolism. Clin. Sci., 33:355, 1967.

63. McNeil, B. J., Holman, B. L., and Adelstein, S. J.: The scintigraphic definition of pulmonary embolism. J.A.M.A., 227:753, 1974.

64. Farmelant, M. H., and Trainor, J. C.: Evaluation of a ¹³³Xe ventilation technique for diagnosis of pulmonary disorders. J. Nucl. Med., 12:586, 1971.

65. Cheely, R., McCartney, W. H., Perry, J. R., Delany, D. J., Bustad, L., Wynia, V. H., and Griggs, T. R.: The role of noninvasive tests versus pulmonary angiography in the diagnosis of pulmonary embolism. Am. J. Med., 70:17, 1981.

66. Biello, D. R., Mattar, A. G., Osei-Wusu, A., Alderson, P. O., McNeil, B. J., and Siegel, B. A.: Interpretation of indeterminate lung scintigrams. Radiology, 133:189, 1979.

67. Moser, K. M., Brach, B. B., and Dolan, G. F.: Clinically suspected deep venous thrombosis of the lower extremities. A comparison of venography, impedance plethysmography, and radiolabeled fibrinogen. J.A.M.A., 237:2195, 1977.

68. Hull, R., Hirsh, J., Sackett, D. L., Taylor, D. W., Carter, C., Turpie, A. G. G., Zielinsky, A., Powers, P., and Gent, M.: Replacement of venography in suspected venous thrombosis by impedance plethysmography and ¹²⁵I-fibrinogen leg scanning. A less invasive approach. Ann. Intern. Med., 94:12, 1981.

69. Little, J. M., and Binns, M.: Spontaneous change in frequency of deep-vein thrombosis detected by ultrasound. Lancet, 2:1229, 1972.

70. Mullick, S. C., Wheeler, H. B., and Songster, G. F.: Diagnosis of deep venous thrombosis by measurement of electrical impedance. Am. J. Surg., 119:417, 1970.

71. Wheeler, H. B., Mullick, S. C., Anderson, J. N., and Pearson, D.: Diagnosis of occult deep vein thrombosis by a noninvasive bedside technique. Surgery, 70:20, 1971.

72. Vas, W., Tuttle, R. J., and Zylak, C. J.: Intravenous self-administration of metallic mercury. Radiology, 137:313, 1980.

73. Sasahara, A. A., Sharma, G. V. R. K., and Paris, A. F.: New developments in the detection and prevention of venous thromboembolism. Am. J. Cardiol., 43:1214, 1979.

74. Moses, D. C., Silver, T. M., and Bookstein, J. J.: The complementary roles of chest radiography, lung scanning, and selective pulmonary angiography in the diagnosis of pulmonary embolism. Circulation, 49:179, 1974.

75. Wenger, N. K., Stein, P. D., and Willis, P. W., III: Massive acute pulmonary embolism. The deceivingly nonspecific manifestations. J.A.M.A., 220:843, 1972.

76. Goodwin, J. F.: The clinical diagnosis of pulmonary thromboembolism. In Sasahara, A. A., and Stein, M. (eds.): Pulmonary Embolic Disease. New York, Grune & Stratton, 1965, pp. 239–255.

77. Sasahara, A. A.: Clinical studies in pulmonary thromboembolism. In Sasahara, A. A., and Stein, M. (eds.): Pulmonary Embolic Disease. New York, Grune & Stratton, 1965, pp. 256–264.

78. Johnson, J. C., Flowers, N. C., and Horan, L. G.: Unexplained atrial flutter: A frequent herald of pulmonary embolism. Chest, 60:29, 1971.

79. Urokinase pulmonary embolism trial: Phase I results. A cooperative study. J.A.M.A., 214:2163, 1970.

80. Robin, E. D., Julian, D. G., Travis, D. M., and Crump, C. H.: A physiologic approach to the diagnosis of acute pulmonary embolism. N. Engl. J. Med., 260:586, 1959.

81. Szucs, M. M., Jr., Brooks, H. L., Grossman, W., Banas, J. S., Jr., Meister, S. G., Dexter, L., and Dalen, J. E.: Diagnostic sensitivity of laboratory findings in acute pulmonary embolism. Ann. Intern. Med., 74:161, 1971.

82. Dalen, J. E., Banas, J. S., Jr., Brooks, H. L., Evans, G. L., Paraskos, J. A., and Dexter, L.: Resolution rate of acute pulmonary embolism in man. N. Engl. J. Med., 280:1194, 1969.

83. Tow, D. E., and Wagner, H. N., Jr.: Recovery of pulmonary arterial blood flow in patients with pulmonary embolism. N. Engl. J. Med., 276:1053, 1967.

84. Paraskos, J. A., Adelstein, S. J., Smith, R. E., Rickman, F. D., Grossman, W., Dexter, L., and Dalen, J. E.: Late prognosis of acute pulmonary embolism. N. Engl. J. Med., 289:55, 1973.

85. Robin, E. D.: Overdiagnosis and overtreatment of pulmonary embolism: The emperor may have no clothes. Ann. Intern. Med., 87:775, 1977.

86. Fred, H. L., and Harle, T. S.: Septic pulmonary embolism. Dis. Chest, 55:483, 1969.

87. Jaffe, R. B., and Koschmann, E. B.: Septic pulmonary emboli. Radiology, 96:527, 1970.

88. Roberts, W. C., and Buchbinder, N. A.: Right-sided valvular infective endocarditis. A clinicopathologic study of twelve necropsy patients. Am. J. Med., 53:7, 1972.

89. Silingardi, V., Canossi, G. C., Torelli, G., and Russo, G. L.: The radiologic 'target sign' of septic pulmonary embolism in a case of acute myelogenous leukemia. Respiration, 42:61, 1981.

90. Gumbs, R. V., and McCauley, D. I.: Hilar and mediastinal adenopathy in septic pulmonary embolic disease. Radiology, 142:313, 1982.

91. Benatar, S. R., Ferguson, A. D., and Goldschmidt, R. B.: Fat embolism—some clinical observations and a review of controversial aspects. Q. J. Med., 41:85, 1972.

92. Glas, W. W., Grekin, T. D., and Musselman, M. M.: Fat embolism. Am. J. Surg., 85:363. 1953.

93. Feldman, F., Ellis, K., and Green, W. M.: The fat embolism syndrome. Radiology, 114:535, 1975.

94. Heitzman, E. R.: The Lung: Radiologic-Pathologic Correlations. St. Louis, The C. V. Mosby Co., 1973, pp. 127, 137.

95. Burgher, L. W., Dines, D. E., Linscheid, R. L., and Didier, E. P.: Fat embolism and the adult respiratory distress syndrome. Mayo Clin. Proc., 49:107, 1974.

96. Editorial: Fat embolism. Lancet, 1:672, 1972.

97. Steiner, P. E., and Lushbaugh, C. C.: Maternal pulmonary embolism by amniotic fluid as a cause of obstetric shock and unexpected deaths in obstetrics. J.A.M.A., 117:1245, 1941.

98. Philip, R. S.: Amniotic fluid embolism. N.Y. State J Med., 67:2085, 1967.

99. Courtney, L. D.: Amniotic fluid embolism. Obstet. Gynecol. Surv., 29:169, 1974.

100. Shnider, S. M., and Moya, F.: Amniotic fluid embolism. Review article. Anesthesiology, 22:108, 1961.

101. Attwood, H. D., and Downing, S. E.: Experimental amniotic fluid and meconium embolism. Surg. Gynecol. Obstet., 120:255, 1965.

102. Willocks, J., Mone, J. G., and Thomson, W. J.: Amniotic fluid embolism: Case with biochemical findings. Br. Med. J., 2:1181, 1966.

103. Meigs, L. C.: Amniotic fluid embolism. Pulmonary histopathologic findings in a rapidly fatal occurrence of amniotic fluid embolism. Am. J. Obstet. Gynecol., 111:1069, 1971.

104. Aguillon, A., Andjus, T., Grayson, A., and Race, G. J.: Amniotic fluid embolism: A review. Obstet. Gynecol. Surv., 17:619, 1962.

105. Weiner, A. E., Reid, D. E., and Roby, C. C.: The hemostatic activity of amniotic fluid. Science, 110:190, 1949.

106. Chung, A. F., and Merkatz, I. R.: Survival following amniotic fluid embolism with early heparinization. Obstet. Gynecol., 42:809, 1973.

107. Peterson, E. P., and Taylor, H. B.: Amniotic fluid embolism: An analysis of 40 cases. Obstet. Gynecol., 35:787, 1970.

108. Johnson, R. M., and Lindskog, G. E.: 100 cases of tumor metastatic to the lung and mediastinum. J.A.M.A., 202:94, 1967.

109. Altemus, L. R., and Lee, R. E.: Carcinomatosis of the lung with pulmonary hypertension. Pathoradiologic spectrum. Arch. Intern. Med., 119:32, 1967.

110. Westcott, J. L.: Air embolism complicating percutaneous needle biopsy of the lung. Chest, 63:108, 1973.

111. Smith, F. R.: Air embolism as a cause of death in scuba diving in the Pacific Northwest. Dis. Chest, 52:15, 1967.

112. Kogutt, M. S.: Systemic air embolism secondary to respiratory therapy in the neonate: Six cases including one survivor. Am. J. Roentgenol., 131:425, 1978.

113. Segal, A. J., and Wasserman, M.: Arterial air embolism: A cause of sudden death in status asthmaticus. Radiology, 99:271, 1971.

114. Siegle, R. L., Eyal, F. G., and Rabinowitz, J. G.: Air embolus following pulmonary interstitial emphysema in hyaline membrane disease. Clin. Radiol., 27:77, 1976.

115. Gottlieb, J. D., Ericsson, J. A., and Sweet, R. B.: Venous air embolism: A review. Anesth. Analg., 44:773, 1965.

116. Warren, B. A., Philp, R. B., and Inwood, M. J.: The ultrastructural morphology of air embolism: Platelet adhesion to the interface and endothelial damage. Br. J. Exp. Pathol., 54:163, 1973.

117. Tuddenham, W. J., and Paskin, D. L.: Radiographic demonstration of air embolism. Med. Radiogr. Photogr., 50:16, 1974.

118. Faer, M. J., and Messerschmidt, G. L.: Nonfatal pulmonary air embolism: Radiographic demonstration. Am. J. Roentgenol., 131:705, 1978.

119. Cholankeril, J. V., Joshi, R. R., Cenizal, J. S., Ketyer, S., and O'Connor, W. T.: Massive air embolism from the pulmonary artery. Radiology, 142:33, 1982.

120. Paré, J. A. P., Fraser, R. G., Hogg, J. C., Howlett, J. G., and Murphy, S. B.: Pulmonary "mainline" granulomatosis: Talcosis of intravenous methadone abuse. Medicine, 58:229, 1979.

121. Atlee, W. E., Jr.: Talc and cornstarch emboli in eyes of drug abusers. J.A.M.A., 219:49, 1972.

122. Douglas, F. G., Kafilmout, K. J., and Patt, N. L.: Foreign particle embolism in drug addicts: Respiratory pathophysiology. Ann. Intern. Med., 75:865, 1971.

123. Sieniewicz, D. J., and Nidecker, A. C.: Conglomerate pulmonary disease: A form of talcosis in intravenous methadone abusers. Am. J. Roentgenol., 135:697, 1980.

124. Genereux, G. P., and Emson, H. E.: Talc granulomatosis and angiothrombotic pulmonary hypertension in drug addicts. J. Can. Assoc. Radiol., 25:87, 1974.

125. Bluth, L. L., and Hanscom, T. A.: Retinal detachment and vitreous hemorrhage due to talc emboli. J.A.M.A., 246:980, 1981.

126. Farber, H. W., Fairman, R. P., and Glauser, F. L.: Talc granulomatosis: Laboratory findings similar to sarcoidosis. Am. Rev. Resp. Dis., 125:258, 1982.

127. Fraimow, W., Wallace, S., Lewis P., Greening, R. R., and Cathcart, R. T.: Changes in pulmonary function due to lymphangiography. Radiology, 85:231, 1965.

128. Bron, K. M., Baum, S., and Abrams, H. L.: Oil embolism in lymphangiography: Incidence, manifestations, and mechanism. Radiology, 80:194, 1963.

129. White, R. J., Webb, J. A. W., Tucker, A. K., and Foster, K. M.: Pulmonary function after lymphography. Br. Med. J., 4:775, 1973.

130. Naidich, T. P., Bartelt, D., Wheeler, P. S., and Stern, W. Z.: Metallic mercury emboli. Am. J. Roentgenol., 117:886, 1973.

10

Pulmonary Hypertension and Edema

GENERAL CONSIDERATIONS OF PULMONARY BLOOD FLOW AND PRESSURE

The major roentgenologic effects of many intrathoracic diseases are reflected in changes in the pulmonary vascular tree. Some of these diseases are local (*e.g.*, unilateral or lobar emphysema) and usually produce changes in roentgenographic density that can be appreciated by comparison with zones of normal lung. However, the majority, whether pulmonary or cardiac in origin, are of general distribution. Since assessment of *change in lung density* owing to generalized increase or decrease in blood flow may be grossly inaccurate, in this group of diseases density change must be of less importance than *alterations in vascular pattern*. The present section deals with the pulmonary vasculature and the variations in size and pattern of linear markings that may provide information concerning underlying hemodynamic change.

The principles that govern hemodynamic flow through the pulmonary vascular tree are discussed in some detail in Chapter 1 (*see* page 42). In summary, in the pulmonary circuit, pressure is dependent upon flow and upon the cross-sectional area of perfused vascular bed. The pulmonary vascular circuit is a low-pressure system, amounting to about one-sixth the systemic arterial pressure, and has a remarkable capacity to compensate for a large physiologic increase in flow without a corresponding increase in pressure. This apparent reduction in vascular resistance is achieved mainly by "recruiting" pulmonary vessels that are not perfused at rest. When increased flow is maintained for long periods (as in cases of intracardiac left-to-right shunts), vascular distention occurs and the increased vascular vol-

ume is recognizable roentgenologically. Pulmonary hypertension occurs only when the cross-sectional area of the pulmonary vascular bed is severely reduced.

In the roentgenologic assessment of diseases of the pulmonary vascular system, signs are related to a relative change in the caliber of hilar pulmonary arteries and of peripheral pulmonary arteries as they proceed distally in the lung tissue. Attention must be directed not only to the pulmonary vessels themselves but also to the size and contour of the heart, the size of the main pulmonary artery, and the pulmonary veins, since each is important to the overall evaluation of any abnormality in hemodynamics.

PULMONARY HYPERTENSION

With several exceptions, abnormalities of the pulmonary vascular tree are related to the presence of pulmonary hypertension, which may be defined as prolonged increase to above normally accepted values for pressure in the main pulmonary artery at rest or during exercise, as measured by a catheter. Generally accepted values for these pressures are 30 mm Hg systolic and 18 mm Hg mean pulmonary arterial pressure, above which pulmonary hypertension may be said to be present.

In the fetus, the muscular arteries have relatively thick media and small lumina that restrict pulmonary blood flow during intrauterine life and divert the blood through the ductus arteriosus into the aorta. After birth, with the first breath, blood flows into the low-resistance pulmonary arteries, and the arterioles undergo progressive decrease in wall thickness and increase in luminal diameter.

The *pathologic changes* seen in the pulmonary vessels in pulmonary hypertension are most striking in arterioles and in small pulmonary arteries less than 500 μ in diameter. Changes in the arterioles consist of muscular thickening and intimal proliferation. Arterioles normally have no media; in grades I to III of pulmonary hypertension a distinct muscular media develops that may form up to 25 per cent of the external diameter of the vessel and is separated by internal and external elastic laminae.[1] Intimal proliferation usually occurs as a later manifestation; at first it is cellular but subsequently it becomes fibrous; finally, elastic tissue may develop and intimal proliferation may progress to complete obliteration of the lumen. The intima of the pulmonary trunk and large elastic vessels becomes atherosclerotic, and the vessels' media may be thickened by muscular hyperplasia.

The *pathogenesis* of pulmonary hypertension varies from case to case, and multiple factors are responsible in many. In some instances, there is reason to believe that the rise in pulmonary arterial pressure is due to vasoconstriction and, therefore, is reversible. In other cases, obstruction of the pulmonary vascular tree appears to be largely morphologic and thus irreversible, but even in these circumstances some degree of reversibility may be demonstrated.[2] The early stages of primary pulmonary hypertension are considered to be the result of vasoconstriction of undetermined cause, on the evidence that vasodilator drugs may produce pressure decreases. Vasoconstriction may be produced by hypoxia and acidosis, high altitude, the secretion of either serotonin or histamine, and postcapillary hypertension. An "epidemic" of pulmonary hypertension in Europe during the late 1960's that was attributed to an anorectic drug (aminorex fumarate)[3, 4] and the production of pulmonary hypertension in animals given pyrrolizidine alkaloids[5-8] have raised the possibility that substances taken by mouth may be responsible for some cases of primary pulmonary hypertension.[9] This concept of dietary pulmonary hypertension and the occasional association of portal hypertension with the development of pulmonary hypertension[10] has led to the interesting hypothesis of a "gut-liver-lung axis," in which the liver fails to deal appropriately with the products of digestion, resulting in pulmonary vasospasm and eventually morphologic vascular abnormality.[11] Additional factors contributing to pulmonary arterial hypertension in some cases include increase in pulmonary blood flow, increase in pulmonary blood volume, and increase in blood viscosity such as is seen in polycythemia.

It is useful conceptually to divide the causes of pulmonary hypertension into three general groups, each of which shows somewhat different clinical, physiologic, and roentgenologic characteristics (Table 10–1): those in which the major mechanisms of production are *precapillary* in location, those in which the significant physiologic disturbance arises from disease in the *postcapillary* vessels, and those in which the hypertension reflects a disturbance in ves-

TABLE 10–1. CLASSIFICATION OF PULMONARY HYPERTENSION

PRECAPILLARY PULMONARY HYPERTENSION
  Primary Vascular Disease
    1. *Increased flow (large left-to-right shunts)*
    2. *Decreased flow (tetralogy of Fallot)*
    3. *Primary pulmonary hypertension*
    4. *Pulmonary thromboembolic disease:*
      Thrombotic
      Metastatic neoplastic
      Parasitic
      Trophoblastic
      Foreign bodies; fat embolism; talc
        granulomatosis
    5. *Pulmonary arteritides*
  Primary Pleuropulmonary Disease
    1. *Emphysema*
    2. *Diffuse interstitial or air-space disease of the
        lungs:*
      Granulomatous
      Fibrotic
      Neoplastic: metastatic, bronchiolo-alveolar
      Miscellaneous: alveolar microlithiasis, idiopathic hemosiderosis, alveolar proteinosis, mucoviscidosis, bronchiectasis
      Postresection changes
    3. *Pleural disease (fibrothorax)*
    4. *Chest deformity:*
      Thoracoplasty
      Kyphoscoliosis
    5. *Alveolar hypoventilation:*
      Neuromuscular
      Obesity
      Idiopathic
      Chronic upper airway obstruction in children
    6. *High altitude pulmonary hypertension*
POSTCAPILLARY HYPERTENSION
  Cardiac
    1. *Left ventricular failure*
    2. *Mitral valvular disease*
    3. *Myxoma (or thrombus) of the left atrium*
    4. *Cor triatriatum*
  Pulmonary Venous
    1. *Congenital stenosis of the origin of the pulmonary
        veins*
    2. *Mediastinal granulomas and neoplasms*
    3. *Idiopathic veno-occlusive disease*
    4. *Anomalous pulmonary venous return*
COMBINED PRECAPILLARY AND POSTCAPILLARY
  HYPERTENSION

---

sels on both sides of the capillary bed—*combined precapillary and postcapillary hypertension.* In each of these groups, the capillaries may be involved to some extent and may contribute considerably to the increase in vascular resistance.

PRECAPILLARY PULMONARY HYPERTENSION

PRIMARY VASCULAR DISEASE

Increased Flow

Included in this category are the congenital cardiovascular defects with left-to-right shunt—atrial septal defect, ventricular septal defect, patent ductus arteriosus, aorticopulmonary window, and partial anomalous pulmonary venous connection. Pulmonary artery flow may be greatly increased for a long time before increased peripheral resistance results in hypertension. It is assumed that the increase in peripheral resistance is caused by an increase in vasomotor tone and that, subsequently, the morphologic changes of increased flow hypertension develop. The elastic and large muscular arteries (larger than 500 μ in diameter) are uniformly dilated throughout the lungs. More striking changes in the hypertrophied small arteries and arterioles consist of local mural dilatations that occur in relation to occluded or markedly narrowed arteries and arterioles, evidencing attempts to re-establish flow around affected vessels.

The main roentgenographic sign in these conditions is an increase in caliber of all of the pulmonary vessels throughout the lungs (Figure 10–1). Since the hemodynamic change is one of increased flow, the degree of enlargement of the main and hilar pulmonary arteries usually is proportional to the degree of distention of the intrapulmonary vessels. Thus, when peripheral resistance is normal, the arteries taper gradually and proportionately distally.

When pulmonary hypertension is long-standing and severe, usually in association with an Eisenmenger reaction, the pulmonary arteries may develop calcification, presumably on an atherosclerotic basis. This calcification usually is located in the main pulmonary artery and its major hilar branches.

It may be extremely difficult roentgenologically to recognize the presence of pulmonary arterial hypertension in cases of left-to-right

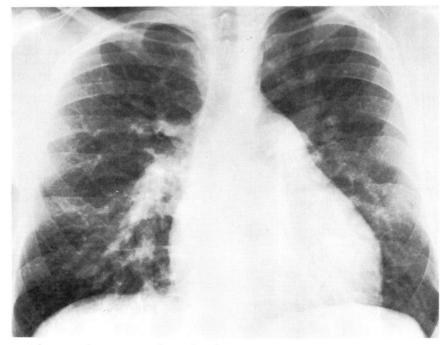

Figure 10–1. Pulmonary Pleonemia: Atrial Septal Defect. A posteroanterior roentgenogram of an asymptomatic 19-year-old male reveals a marked increase in the caliber of the pulmonary arteries and veins throughout both lungs; the vessels taper normally. The heart is moderately enlarged, possessing a contour consistent with enlargement of the right atrium and right ventricle. The electrocardiogram showed a right bundle branch block. An atrial septal defect was satisfactorily corrected surgically.

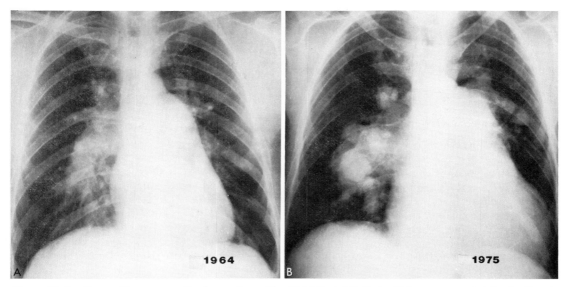

Figure 10–2. Severe Eisenmenger Syndrome Caused by Atrial Septal Defect. This man presented for the first time at the age of 32 with a history of increasing shortness of breath on exertion. A roentgenogram *(A)* revealed marked enlargement of the hilar pulmonary arteries which tapered rapidly as they proceeded distally. The peripheral vasculature was clearly diminished, and the size and configuration of the heart were consistent with cor pulmonale. Cardiac catheterization revealed a secundum-type atrial septal defect. Pressures in the main pulmonary artery were 113/42 mm Hg and those in the ascending aorta 99/56 mm Hg. There was a right-to-left shunt of approximately 21%; pulmonary vascular resistance was equivalent to systemic levels at approximately 17 units. Eleven years later *(B)*, the main pulmonary arteries and the heart had undergone remarkable enlargement; the peripheral oligemia was much more evident. The patient showed severe cyanosis and polycythemia. Despite supportive therapy, he died shortly after this examination. At necropsy, the lumen of the main pulmonary artery was considerably larger than that of the ascending aorta. Mural thrombi were present in the major pulmonary arteries and there was severe muscular hypertrophy and calcification of the walls of these vessels. (Courtesy of Dr. Murray Mazer, St. Boniface Hospital, Manitoba.)

shunt, mainly owing to the fact that although the small branches of the pulmonary arterial tree are narrowed in some instances, usually they are beyond the range of visibility on plain roentgenography or angiography. The difficulty is compounded by the fact that other signs of pulmonary arterial hypertension, such as enlargement of the main and hilar pulmonary arteries, are unreliable, since these structures may be greatly enlarged when resistance is normal. However, the rapidity of tapering of the pulmonary vessels as they proceed distally may be a useful sign in assessing the development of hypertension, particularly in atrial septal defect (ASD) (Figure 10–2).

As might be anticipated, the ratio of blood flow to upper and lower lung zones is altered in left-to-right shunts. In a radioisotopic study of regional pulmonary blood flow in erect normal subjects and in patients with congenital heart disease, it was found that in the former upper-lower blood flow ratios averaged 0.43, whereas in patients with left-to-right shunting this ratio was slightly but significantly raised, more so in the presence of pulmonary arterial hypertension. However, upper-lower ratios never exceeded 1.00 unless pulmonary venous hypertension was present, regardless of pulmonary arterial pressure.

The diagnosis of left-to-right shunts may be facilitated by fluoroscopic observation of increased amplitude of pulsation of the enlarged pulmonary arteries (which tends to be of greatest magnitude in atrial septal defect and least in patent ductus arteriosus) and enlargement of individual cardiac chambers.

Clinically, the character of the cardiac murmur may be distinctive, and specific findings may indicate strongly one particular anomaly (for example, incomplete right bundle branch block in atrial septal defect). In many cases, however, cardiac catheterization, with or without angiocardiography, is requisite to thorough assessment.

Most symptoms and signs of pulmonary hypertension are due to cor pulmonale. Retrosternal pain, identical to angina pectoris, accompanies the very high pulmonary arterial pressures that develop in primary pulmonary hypertension and in severe hypertension with mitral stenosis. Pulmonary hypertension also causes accentuation of the second pulmonic sound and an early diastolic murmur along the left sternal border as a result of pulmonary valvular insufficiency. The parasternal thrust, tricuspid insufficiency, and liver and neck pulsations are caused by failure of the right ventricle.

Primary Pulmonary Hypertension

This is an uncommon condition[12] whose authenticity has been questioned by some on the basis of demonstration at necropsy of multiple pulmonary emboli in patients considered to have had the disease during life.[13, 14] However, the dramatic response to the intravenous injection of acetylcholine in some cases, the tendency to familial occurrence, its preponderance in young women, and clinical and experimental evidence that it may be drug- or food-induced strongly support the existence of this disease as a distinct entity with a multifactorial pathogenicity.[9] Primary pulmonary hypertension has been reported in twins, in five members in three generations of one family, and in a father and his two children. Recent data suggest an autosomal dominant mode of genetic transmission.[15]

Roentgenographically, the lungs show evidence of diffuse oligemia, the peripheral pulmonary arteries being narrow and inconspicuous.[16] The hilar pulmonary arteries are enlarged and taper rapidly distally; the main pulmonary artery usually is prominent and often shows increased amplitude of pulsation fluoroscopically. There may be roentgenologic evidence of right ventricular enlargement. Overinflation does not occur, permitting ready differentiation from the diffuse pulmonary oligemia associated with emphysema.

In one series of 23 cases,[16] there was a female predominance of 5 to 1, and the median age at the time of death was 34 years. Symptoms consisted of dyspnea (in 22 patients), Raynaud's phemonenon (in seven), and syncope (in six). In a more recent report of 38 patients with primary pulmonary hypertension seen at the Cleveland Clinic,[17] the commonest symptoms in order of frequency were dyspnea on exertion (in 97 per cent), easy fatigability, chest pain, cough, dizziness, and syncope. Signs of cor pulmonale and cardiac failure may be present, including giant jugular A waves, right atrial gallop, a loud pulmonary ejection click, an accentuated pulmonic sound, a palpable lift along the left sternal border, and, in some cases, murmurs caused by pulmonic and tricuspid insufficiency.[16] Catheterization of the right side of the heart reveals pulmonary arterial hyper-

tension, a normal pulmonary capillary wedge pressure, high pulmonary vascular resistance, and, in cases of right ventricular failure, a low cardiac output.[16] Pulmonary function may be completely normal, although more severe cases may have decreased arterial oxygen saturation and moderately decreased diffusing capacity. The ECG typically shows evidence of right ventricular hypertrophy and tall peaked P waves.

Patients with primary pulmonary hypertension do not always show a progressive downhill course and some regression may occur; in fact, repeated catheterizations may even reveal improvement.[18] This considerable variation in survival makes assessment of any form of therapy most difficult. Nevertheless, the fact that vessel muscle hypertrophy can be reversible warrants biopsy[19] and, if appropriate, the institution of vasodilator therapy.[20] Of note is the fact that these patients are at particular risk for cardiac arrest following surgery, lung scanning,[21] cardiac catheterization, or angiography.[22]

Pulmonary Thromboembolic Disease

The majority of cases of pulmonary arterial hypertension of vascular origin probably are attributable to multiple pulmonary embolic episodes occurring over a period of many years. However, patients with thromboembolic pulmonary hypertension usually do not give a history suggesting major pulmonary embolism or infarction.[23] Microemboli originate from thromboses in the systemic veins of the legs or pelvis and occasionally in the heart from myocardial or valvular disease. Webs and bands found in smaller pulmonary arteries at necropsy are considered to represent old organized emboli and are accepted by most pathologists as confirmatory evidence for this cause of the hypertension. Identical lesions, presumably representing organized thrombi, have been described in pelvic and leg veins. In addition to thrombi, many other materials can embolize to the lungs and cause pulmonary hypertension, including metastatic neoplasm, schistosomal parasites, and talc, the base in oral preparations injected intravenously by drug addicts.

In contrast to thrombi that form in the systemic circulation and embolize to the lung, primary thrombosis sometimes develops in the pulmonary arterial circulation itself. Slowing of the circulation and the increased blood viscosity typical of polycythemia probably contribute to such thromboses, as do pulmonary vascular changes resulting from increased vasomotor tone, inflammation of the vessel wall, and sickling due to hemoglobin SC and hemoglobin SS disease. When either thrombosis or embolism occurs in the major hilar pulmonary arteries, the combination of bulging hilar pulmonary arteries, severe peripheral oligemia, and cor pulmonale constitutes a virtually pathognomonic roentgenologic triad.

Pulmonary Veno-Occlusive Disease

As a cause of pulmonary arterial hypertension, this unusual condition of unknown etiology is very uncommon, only 34 cases having been recognized by 1981.[24-27] It is a disease with no sex predilection; age at recognition has ranged from infancy to 48 years, approximately half the patients being 16 years of age or younger.[26]

Pathologically, there is narrowing and obliteration of the lumina of small pulmonary veins and venules by intimal fibrous tissue proliferation, usually widespread throughout both lungs. Larger pulmonary veins are usually spared. It is probable that the venous occlusions are thrombotic in origin although the cause of the thrombosis is unknown. The presence of fever in some cases has suggested the possibility of a viral etiology.[27]

Roentgenographically, signs of pulmonary arterial hypertension are no different from those associated with primary or thromboembolic disease but with the important addition of signs of postcapillary hypertension, chiefly pulmonary edema. The left atrium is not enlarged and there is no evidence of redistribution of blood flow to upper lung zones, both important signs in distinguishing this condition from mitral stenosis.

Cardiac catheterization reveals the expected elevation of pulmonary artery pressures but normal pulmonary wedge pressures. This latter finding is vital to the diagnosis. The triad of normal wedge pressure, pulmonary arterial hypertension, and pulmonary edema is virtually diagnostic. It is important to recognize that pulmonary wedge pressure is also normal in other causes of precapillary pulmonary hypertension, so that the recognition of pulmonary edema is cardinal to the triad.

Clinically, the picture closely resembles that of primary pulmonary hypertension, the first symptoms being fatigue and dyspnea on exertion. Most patients die within two years of the onset of symptoms.[26]

Pulmonary Arteritides

Arteritis associated with scleroderma and occasionally with rheumatoid arthritis and isolated Raynaud's disease is a rare cause of pulmonary hypertension. This subject is considered further in the section on collagen diseases (*see* Chapter 7). Even rarer forms of primary pulmonary vascular disease resulting in pulmonary hypertension are those associated with Takayasu's arteritis[28] and multiple pulmonary artery stenoses or coarctations.[29]

Compression of the Main Pulmonary Artery or its Branches

Occasionally, an acquired disease of the mediastinum results in diffuse pulmonary oligemia of "central" origin. For example, a mediastinal mass lying contiguous to the main pulmonary artery may compress this vessel to a degree sufficient to compromise pulmonary arterial flow. In one of our patients an aneurysm of the ascending arch of the aorta compressed the pulmonary outflow tract so severely that cor pulmonale ensued; there was clear-cut roentgenographic evidence of pulmonary oligemia.

Vasoconstrictive (Vasospastic) Vascular Disease

This includes chronic vasoconstriction due to direct chemical-induced effects on the small arteries and arterioles. Chronic hypoxia, metabolic or respiratory acidosis, and excessive amounts of catecholamines are reputed to produce this change and give rise to pulmonary hypertension.[30] Prolonged vasospasm is believed to be the first stage of idiopathic (primary) pulmonary arterial hypertension, successive events thereafter being hypertrophy, "muscularization" of arterioles, and subsequently marked luminal occlusions caused by severe fibrosis of the intima.

PRIMARY PLEUROPULMONARY DISEASE

A wide variety of primary diseases of the lungs, pleura, chest wall, and respiratory control center (*see* Table 10–1) may cause a rise in pulmonary arterial pressure without significant change in pulmonary venous pressure. Pulmonary arterial pressures seldom reach the levels attained in cases of primary vascular disease. It is probable that the main cause of pulmonary arterial hypertension in this group of conditions is hypoxemia, with or without respiratory acidosis. The reduction in arterial oxygen saturation may be due to ventilation-perfusion inequality or to generalized alveolar hypoventilation. Other probable contributory factors include hypervolemia and polycythemia, and pulmonary capillary destruction.

Emphysema and Chronic Bronchitis

Pulmonary hypertension in chronic bronchitis and emphysema appears to be caused primarily by a combination of hypoxemia and destruction of the microvasculature. Physiologic studies have shown a close correlation between pulmonary vascular resistance, oxygen saturation, and diffusing capacity during exercise.[31] The roentgenographic manifestations of pulmonary hypertension in emphysema are identical to those of primary vascular disease; however, the invariable presence of overinflation permits ready differentiation. A recent study[32] has shown excellent correlation between the diameters of the right and left descending pulmonary arteries and the presence and severity of pulmonary arterial hypertension in patients with chronic obstructive pulmonary disease; a combined increase in the diameter of the right descending pulmonary artery (>16 mm) and of the left descending pulmonary artery (>18 mm) permitted the correct diagnosis of pulmonary arterial hypertension in 45 of 46 patients. Even in the presence of cor pulmonale, the ECG usually does not show the characteristic pattern of right ventricular hypertrophy that is associated with primary pulmonary vascular disease.

Diffuse Interstitial or Air-Space Disease of the Lungs

In these diseases, elevation of pulmonary artery pressure probably is related to the limited distensibility of the pulmonary vascular tree, and, therefore, hypertension becomes particularly manifest during exercise-induced increases in cardiac output. The roentgenologic changes are almost invariably dominated by the underlying pulmonary disease, and in many cases the peripheral vascular markings are obscured. However, in a study of 29 patients with chronic diffuse interstitial pulmonary disease (20 with progressive systemic sclerosis, 6 with sarcoidosis, and 3 miscellaneous), Austin and his colleagues[33] showed that pulmonary arterial pressure was significantly related to the severity of parenchymal disease and to the size of central pulmonary arteries. The symptoms usually are attributable to the underlying disease, and the presence of pulmonary hypertension may not be clinically detectable until cor pulmonale and cardiac failure develop.

Surgical Resection

Although pneumonectomy does not appear to cause a rise in pressure in a remaining normal lung in the immediate postoperative period, pathologic and physiologic evidence of hypertension can be found in patients living for 4 or more years and presumably results from small vessel sclerosis secondary to increased blood flow.

Chest Deformity

Severe degrees of kyphoscoliosis and thoracoplasty may lead to pulmonary arterial hypertension and cor pulmonale, again on the basis of a poorly ventilated but relatively well-perfused lung.

Alveolar Hypoventilation Syndromes

Underventilation of normal lungs, with consequent decreased arterial blood Po_2 and increased Pco_2, may result in pulmonary hypertension. This syndrome may be primary in origin (Ondine's curse—Figure 10–3) or due to obesity, upper airway obstruction, loss of altitude acclimatization, or continuous depression of the respiratory center by drugs. There is increasing evidence that patients who chronically hypoventilate from these various causes have in common a decreased sensitivity of their respiratory center to carbon dioxide. A more complete account of the many diseases leading to hypoventilation may be found in Chapters 11 and 18.

POSTCAPILLARY PULMONARY HYPERTENSION

Postcapillary pulmonary hypertension results from any condition that increases pulmonary venous pressure above a critical level. Undoubtedly the most common of these is mitral stenosis, but also included are left ventricular failure, cor triatriatum, left atrial myxoma, primary pulmonary venous obstruction from any cause, and total anomalous pulmonary venous drainage (either with connection below the diaphragm or with atresia of the common pulmonary vein).

Morphologically, the earliest lesions of pulmonary venous hypertension (as in mitral stenosis) are tortuosity and dilatation of capillaries in alveolar walls. Hemorrhage occurs early and probably originates in small pulmonary veins. It results in the accumulation of

Figure 10–3. Severe Pulmonary Arterial Hypertension in Primary Alveolar Hypoventilation (Ondine's Curse). A posteroanterior roentgenogram of a 55-year-old white man reveals marked dilatation of the main pulmonary artery and its hilar branches, with rapid diminution in caliber of pulmonary arteries as they proceed distally. The heart is moderately enlarged in a configuration compatible with cor pulmonale. The lungs are not overinflated nor do they show evidence of primary disease. This is a case of Ondine's curse, an abnormality characterized by a failure to "remember" to breathe, with resultant alveolar hypoventilation (particularly during sleep), hypoxemia, hypercarbia, pulmonary vasoconstriction, arterial hypertension, and cor pulmonale. The pacemaker projected over the base of the left lung was pacing the left phrenic nerve in order to achieve repeated diaphragmatic contraction. (Courtesy of Dr. Richard Greenspan, Yale University, New Haven.)

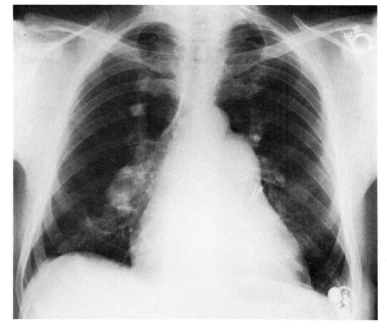

hemosiderin in macrophages in alveoli and around respiratory and terminal bronchioles. Fibrosis of the alveolar septa develops gradually. Dilatation of lymphatics and edema of lobular septa are prominent features. Venous intimal proliferation is an outstanding feature, as may be hypertrophy of venous muscle. Dilatation occurs in the central pulmonary arteries in about one-third of cases and in the conducting arteries to the upper zones (greater than 1 mm in diameter) in about the same proportion. By contrast, the lower zone conducting vessels—particularly from the level of segmental arteries to those 1 mm in diameter—often are narrowed owing to muscular hypertrophy.[34] Perivascular edema occurs in this region. Anastomoses develop between pulmonary and bronchial veins in many cases, with bronchial vein varicosities that give rise to the bright red hemoptysis seen in this form of pulmonary hypertension. As the pressure rises in the pulmonary venous system, the pulmonary arteries undergo reflex constriction which lightens the pressure on the capillaries by restricting flow (combined precapillary and postcapillary hypertension; *see* further on).

Roentgenologically, the changes in the pulmonary vasculature are characteristic. When pulmonary vascular resistance is increased in part of the lungs and unaffected elsewhere, blood flow is redistributed from zones of high resistance to those of normal resistance. When areas of lung thus affected are sufficiently large,

the discrepancy in size between normal and abnormal lung markings is readily apparent roentgenographically. This effect is observed in several primary pulmonary diseases (*e.g.*, local obstructive emphysema), as well as in some affections of the cardiovascular system; we are concerned with the latter group here. In 1958, Simon[35] observed that in mitral stenosis or left ventricular failure the lower lobe pulmonary vessels are narrowed and the upper lobe vessels distended, and he postulated that increase in pulmonary venous pressure above a critical level results in venous vasoconstriction. In erect humans, pulmonary venous pressure is higher in the lower than in the upper lobes because of a difference in hydrostatic pressure (averaging approximately 12 to 15 mm Hg in adult subjects). Therefore, the critical level is reached first in lower lung zones and resultant vasoconstriction occurs in the same order, so that peripheral vascular resistance rises in the lower zones. Since resistance in the upper lobes is unchanged initially, blood is diverted to those areas, giving a roentgenographic picture of upper lobe pleonemia and lower lobe oligemia (Figure 10–4). This is in striking contrast to the normal situation, in which pulmonary perfusion increases from apex to base. With continued increase in venous pressure, the reduction in venous caliber progresses upward from the lung bases and eventually involves the upper lobes, constricting the engorged upper lobe veins and producing a pattern of diffuse alteration in the

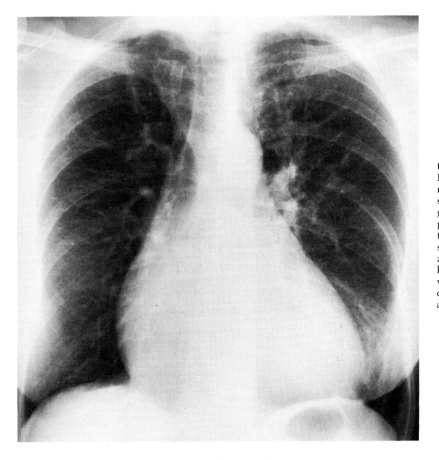

Figure 10–4. Redistribution of Blood Flow to Upper Lung Zones Caused by Pulmonary Venous Hypertension. A posteroanterior roentgenogram reveals unusually prominent vascular markings in the upper zones and rather sparse markings in the lower zones. This 42-year-old woman had recurrent episodes of left ventricular decompensation consequent upon cardiomyopathy.

pulmonary vasculature. The inevitable result is generalized elevation of peripheral vascular resistance and pulmonary arterial hypertension.

West and associates[36] used radioactive xenon to measure the distribution of blood flow in an isolated dog lung and found greatly increased vascular resistance in the dependent lung zone when the pulmonary venous pressure was raised. Rapidly frozen sections showed accumulations of edema fluid around small arteries and veins, suggesting that resistance increases when there is interference with the tethering effect of the lung parenchyma that normally holds these vessels open.

Although more recent studies[37, 38] have cast some doubt on this hypothesis, there is no doubt that a disparity between the caliber of upper and lower lobe vessels represents one of the most useful roentgenographic signs of pulmonary venous hypertension. All too frequently, there exists an unfortunate semantic inaccuracy regarding this sign. It is common to hear the term "upper lobe venous engorgement" used to describe redistribution of blood flow from lower to upper zones; in fact, however, the redistribution of blood flow is *arterial*

rather than venous as the result of increased resistance to blood flow through lower zones. Thus, *both* arteries and veins show distention, and it is conceptually preferable to employ the phrase "upper zone vascular distention" to indicate redistribution of blood flow.

It is important to recognize that "recruitment" of upper zonal vessels such that their caliber is increased occurs in circumstances other than those associated with pulmonary venous hypertension. As previously noted, this disappearance of the normal apex-to-base gradient is characteristic of large left-to-right shunts. Upper zonal vessel recruitment is also characteristic of pulmonary arterial hypertension[39] and of parenchymal diseases, such as emphysema, which tend to affect lower lung zones more than upper. An excellent review of the whole subject of pulmonary blood flow distribution has been published by Milne.[40]

The alteration in pulmonary vascular pattern seen in mitral stenosis may be observed in mild left ventricular failure also but then is transient. In fact, however, the changes in the vascular pattern may be similar in all respects, including the signs of pulmonary arterial hypertension. It is of interest that signs of left ventricular failure may be apparent roentgenographically without clinical evidence of decompensation. Of 94 patients who had chest roentgenograms obtained on admission to a coronary care unit,[41] 31 (33 per cent) were found to have roentgenographic evidence of pulmonary venous hypertension (manifested most commonly by distention of upper zone vessels) without associated clinical signs. In 23 of these, however, clinically evident failure developed subsequently. In a study of 30 patients with acute myocardial infarction,[42] the severity of roentgenographic abnormality generally correlated well with levels of pulmonary capillary wedge pressure. It was found that redistribution of blood flow was the earliest manifestation of elevated wedge pressure, followed sequentially by loss of the normal sharp margins of the pulmonary vessels, the development of perihilar haze, and finally rosette formation.

In addition to the typical alteration in vascular pattern observed in pulmonary venous hypertension, particularly in mitral stenosis, other pulmonary changes occur that are worthy of note. Signs of *interstitial pulmonary edema* frequently are visible, including septal edema (Kerley A and B lines) and perivascular edema (manifested by loss of definition of pulmonary vascular markings). *Hemosiderosis*, although often visible pathologically, is not readily identifiable roentgenographically unless severe, probably because of the low density of the deposits; it is manifested by tiny punctate shadows situated mainly in the mid- and lower lung zones. Morphologically, these deposits consist of focal areas of fibrosis situated around phagocytic cells containing hemosiderin, undoubtedly the result of previous alveolar hemorrhage.

Bone formation occurs in some cases of mitral stenosis and is virtually pathognomonic of this entity, although it has been described in pulmonary veno-occlusive disease as well. Roentgenographically, these deposits appear as densely calcified nodules, 2 to 5 mm in diameter, mainly in the midlung zones and sometimes containing demonstrable trabeculae.

Finally, *pulmonary fibrosis* may be apparent as a rather coarse, poorly defined reticulation, again predominantly in the mid- and lower lung zones, and probably related to recurrent episodes of interstitial and alveolar edema and hemorrhage.

Clinically, the symptoms associated with postcapillary hypertension usually are readily differentiated from those of precapillary origin. Patients typically are dyspneic and orthopneic and may be subject to paroxysmal nocturnal dyspnea, manifestations of interstitial and air-space edema. In left ventricular failure, which perhaps is the most common cause of pulmonary venous hypertension, symptoms and signs are predominantly those arising from acute pulmonary edema. In mitral stenosis, in addition to the pink frothy expectoration typical of acute pulmonary edema, bright red blood from hemorrhaging varicosities of the bronchial veins may be expectorated. The pulmonary vascular pressure does not increase until the size of the mitral valve orifice is less than 50 per cent of normal. When the orifice is very tight, a severe degree of pulmonary arterial hypertension may develop that can be differentiated from primary pulmonary hypertension only by the symptoms and signs of pulmonary edema, by the loud opening snap of the first heart sound, and by the rumbling diastolic murmur associated with this valvular abnormality. Pulmonary function studies in patients with mitral valve disease show a progressive decrease in vital capacity and diffusing capacity and, with advancing disease, in midexpiratory flow rates. Mitral valvotomy in patients with severe disease does not result in an improvement in diffusing capacity.

COMBINED PRECAPILLARY AND POSTCAPILLARY HYPERTENSION

When postcapillary hypertension is severe and long standing, it induces changes within the pulmonary arterial circulation that are indistinguishable from those seen in precapillary hypertension (apart from the changes in cardiac contour, which almost always permit differentiation). Simon[43] suggests that this condition be referred to as combined precapillary and postcapillary hypertension. The roentgenographically demonstrable changes evidence superimposition of the two patterns of hypertension.

CHRONIC COR PULMONALE

Although the presence of pulmonary hypertension does not necessarily imply cor pulmonale, it does indicate that there is a strain on the right ventricle which, if prolonged, will inevitably lead to right ventricular hypertrophy. Strictly speaking, the term "cor pulmonale" should be restricted to those instances in which abnormality of lung structure or function results in right ventricular hypertrophy. Although disease of the left side of the heart and congenital cardiac disease may closely mimic true cor pulmonale, they are not generally accepted under this definition. Approximately 80 per cent of cases of chronic cor pulmonale result from chronic bronchitis and emphysema.

Roentgenologically, cardiac enlargement is not always apparent, even when right ventricular hypertrophy is evident postmortem. This failure to appreciate cardiac enlargement is particularly notable in the presence of pulmonary emphysema, when only serial roentgenography may reveal the increase.

Clinically, right ventricular thrust, usually felt along the left sternal border, may be similarly obscured by pulmonary overinflation in emphysema. A systolic thrust, sometimes a diastolic shock, and a systolic thrill may be felt over the pulmonary area. A loud P_2 sound with a pulmonary systolic ejection click, and in some cases harsh systolic and diastolic murmurs, may be heard over the same area. As right-sided heart failure develops, a systolic murmur becomes audible along the left sternal border, which is louder during inspiration. It may be associated with a palpable pulse in the (enlarged) liver, a systolic venous pulse in the neck and, in many cases, with peripheral edema and ascites, all attributable to insufficiency of the tricuspid valve. The electrocardiogram may be normal even in cases of known severe right ventricular hypertrophy.

PULMONARY EDEMA

Normally, anatomic and physiologic mechanisms within the lungs keep the alveoli dry, or, perhaps more correctly, ideally moist. As in other body tissues, two physiologic factors are chiefly responsible: (1) a balance between capillary pressure and plasma osmotic pressure, the latter always exceeding the former; and (2) maintenance of normal capillary wall permeability. A disturbance of sufficient magnitude in one or both of these factors will result in the exudation of fluid from the capillaries into the interstitial tissues and air spaces of the lungs—pulmonary edema. These statements might imply that, in normal circumstances, the balance of hydrostatic and osmotic forces across capillary walls is so precise that escape of water or protein into the interstitial tissue of the alveolar septa is prevented, but this is not strictly true. Some water and protein does escape in small quantities but is removed promptly and continuously by the intricate network of pulmonary lymphatics that absorb the excess and dump it into the systemic circulation. The net effect of all these forces is to keep the quantity of extravascular water and proteins in the normal lung stable from day to day, such that alveolar surfaces are maintained in a moist but unflooded condition.

The commonest cause of pulmonary edema is elevation of pulmonary microvascular* pressure secondary to elevated pulmonary venous pressure, usually produced by mitral stenosis or left ventricular decompensation. This might conveniently be called *hemodynamic* or *elevated microvascular pressure* pulmonary edema. A less common but nevertheless significant pathogenetic mechanism consists of increased permeability of the alveolar-capillary barrier as a result of toxic injury or other influence. In its pure form, this mechanism results in accumulation of excess water and protein in the lungs in the absence of elevated microvascular pressure and may thus be termed *permeability* or *normal microvascular pressure* pulmonary edema. Still a third pathogenesis of pulmonary edema exists in which the relative roles played by hemodynamic and permeability factors are unclear, although both are probably operative to a greater or lesser degree. This type, an example of which is the pulmonary edema of heroin intoxication, can be designated *mixed* pulmonary edema.

Before beginning a discussion of each of these three varieties of pulmonary edema and the diseases with which they are associated, it is desirable to review certain anatomic and physiologic considerations relating to the alveolar-capillary apparatus. Much of the following material has been gleaned from the excellent reviews of the subject by Fishman,[44] Robin and his colleagues,[45][46] Staub,[47-49] Butler,[50][51] and Snashall.[52]

ANATOMIC CONSIDERATIONS

The Interstitium

There are two major compartments of the lung in which excess fluid may accumulate—the interstitial space and the air space. Their distinction is important, since the pathophysiologic and clinical manifestations of edema of these compartments differ. The interstitial space can be further subdivided, not altogether arbitrarily, into an alveolar wall component and a bronchovascular component. The latter con-

---

*The term "microvascular" is more accurate than "capillary," since liquid exchange occurs from small pulmonary arterioles and venules as well as from capillaries.

ists of an extensive and continuous network of loose connective tissue forming a cuff around the pulmonary arteries and bronchi (the bronchovascular bundle) and the pulmonary veins and situated within the interlobular septa and subpleural space. While there are no qualitative differences in the connective tissue in these two "compartments," their distinction is important, since, as shown by Staub and his coworkers,[53] not only does an interstitial phase of edema exist for a variable period before alveolar flooding occurs, but edema develops in the loose interstitial space before it appears in the alveolar septa.

The Alveolar Wall

It will be recalled from the description of the morphology of the alveolus in Chapter 1 that the alveolar membrane consists of a continuous epithelium composed of thin cytoplasmic extensions of type I alveolar epithelial cells, with type II cells being interposed at irregular intervals. Deep to these cells is a continuous, well-defined basement membrane. The intercellular junctions of the alveolar epithelium are of the tight variety (zonulae occludentes), so that the membrane exhibits low permeability to all lipid-insoluble substances other than water itself.[54]

In contrast to the tight junctions of cells composing the alveolar membrane, the endothelial cells of the pulmonary capillaries are separated by clefts approximately 200 Å wide which are narrowed at irregular distances from the capillary ostia to form "pores" or "junctions" 40 to 50 Å wide (maculae occludentes).[54] Although the entire endothelial surface is available for the movement of water and lipid-soluble substances, lipid-insoluble substances appear to traverse the endothelial wall via these clefts and junctions.[44] It is clear that in normal circumstances, permeability of the capillary wall will depend in large measure on molecular dimensions. Large molecules (mol wt > 90,000) are arrested by the junctions, whereas smaller molecules (mol wt approximately 10,000) pass through. However, as emphasized by Fishman,[44] the dimensions of the junctions are not fixed and appear to be strongly influenced by hydrostatic pressures. At pulmonary capillary pressures > 50 mm Hg inert tracers measuring approximately 30 Å are arrested, whereas at higher intraluminal pressure the pores stretch, permitting the tracer to pour into the interstitial space.

A facet of alveolar wall structure that is of considerable importance in a discussion of pulmonary edema is the concept of the "thick side–thin side." As pointed out by Fishman,[44] an alveolar septum viewed on edge through the electron microscope (not evident on light microscopy) reveals two distinct functional zones, a thin side for gas exchange and a thick side that serves for both support and water exchange (see Figure 1-8, page 9). The difference between the two sides depends upon the amount of interstitial tissue separating the endothelial and epithelial aspects. On the thin side, the alveolar-capillary membrane measures no more than 300 to 500 Å and consists of three anatomic layers: the alveolar epithelium, the capillary endothelium, and fused basement membranes in between. This arrangement provides the lungs with an enormous expanse for gas exchange without the encumbrance of excessive mass. In contrast, between the basement membranes on the thick side there is a wide interstitium consisting of collagen and elastic fibers, fibroblasts, macrophages, and ground substance—the interstitial connective tissue. Five discrete layers separate alveolar air from capillary blood in this region: alveolar epithelium, basement membrane, interstitial space, basement membrane, and capillary endothelium. This thick side not only provides support for the capillary network, but constitutes an essential component of the water-exchanging apparatus of the lung, operating to expedite the removal of water and protein from the septal interstitial space toward lymphatic capillaries.[44] When excess water and protein accumulate in the alveolar septa (interstitial pulmonary edema) they do so exclusively or predominantly on the thick side (Figure 10–5).

The Lymphatics

Pulmonary lymphatic capillaries are similar to those in other organs, possessing a larger lumen than blood capillaries, a discontinuous or absent basement membrane, and attenuated, irregular endothelial lining cells with many loose intercellular junctions.[56] It is generally agreed that lymphatic capillaries begin in the region of the alveolar ducts and respiratory bronchioles, there being none within the alveolar septa. The absence of lymphatic channels within the alveolar walls is easily understandable functionally. As pointed out by Staub,[47] the three-dimensional structure of the alveolar wall junctions forms an interconnecting pathway through which interstitial fluid can drain proximally to a point where it can be picked up by lymphatic capillaries. Numerous valves, 1 to 2

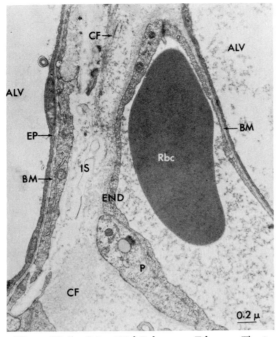

Figure 10–5. Interstitial Pulmonary Edema. The interstitial space *(IS)* of the thick portion of the alveolar septum has been considerably widened by edema fluid during hemodynamic pulmonary edema, whereas the opposite thin part, containing the fused basement membranes *(BM)*, remains unchanged in thickness. Compare with Figure 1–8, page 9. *ALV* = alveolar space; *EP* = alveolar epithelium; *BM* = basement membrane; *IS* = interstitial space; *CF* = collagen fibers; *END* = capillary endothelium; *Rbc* = red blood cell. TEM section stained with uranil acetate and lead citrate, × 12,000. (Reprinted from Fishman, A. P.: Pulmonary edema: The water-exchanging function of the lung. Circulation, *46*:389, 1972, with permission of the author and editor.)

mm apart, direct the flow of lymph in both pleural and intrapulmonary lymphatics toward the hilum.

PHYSIOLOGIC CONSIDERATIONS

Four factors require discussion with respect to forces that govern the formation and removal of extravascular fluid within the lungs, in both normal conditions and pathologic states: (1) intravascular forces; (2) extravascular forces; (3) changes in the characteristics of the alveolar-capillary membrane; and (4) mechanisms for removal of fluid.

Intravascular Forces

In all organs, under normal conditions there is a continual net outward flow of fluid and protein from the vascular bed to the interstitium and back to the bloodstream via the lymphatics. Two basic equations describe the movement of water and solutes across a membrane—the fluid transport equation (the Starling equation) and the solute transport equation. The Starling forces are illustrated schematically in Figure 10–6.

As already pointed out, the commonest cause of pulmonary edema is elevation of pulmonary microvascular pressure secondary to pulmonary venous hypertension. The differential between the two pressures (microvascular hydrostatic pressure and plasma colloid osmotic pressure) is greater in the lung than anywhere else in the body. The relatively low pulmonary capillary pressure of approximately 8 mm Hg, compared with an osmotic pressure of plasma proteins of about 25 mm Hg, creates a difference of such magnitude that quite severe hemodynamic changes can occur before fluid is lost from the capillaries (Figure 10–6). Edema may develop when the microvascular pressure is raised, or the plasma osmotic pressure is lowered, or both. Although hypoproteinemia as a cause of decreased intravascular osmotic pressure undoubtedly plays a significant role in the edema seen in severe liver disease or nutritional deficiency, it is seldom if ever the *sole* precipitating factor in any disease process. In fact, a decrease in plasma protein concentration, even to low levels, should not produce pulmonary edema because it would be accompanied by similar decreases in protein concentration in the perimicrovascular space. Even in the presence of increased microvascular pressure, forces within the vessels may be so balanced that edema can occur only when the capillary blood volume is increased by overloading the circulation with intravenous fluid, by increasing cardiac output (*e.g.*, during exercise), or by increasing the blood flow to the lungs (which occurs when the patient is lying down—paroxysmal nocturnal dyspnea).

Extravascular Forces

Referring again to Figure 10–6, it can be seen that the hydrostatic pressure of the interstitial space and the osmotic pressure contributed by solutes in this space are intimately concerned with net transvascular fluid flow; similarly, the latter is involved in net protein flow. In fact, both these pressures together (10 mm Hg + 17 mm Hg) exert a force (favoring edema formation) greater than colloid osmotic pressure of the plasma (25 mm Hg), which

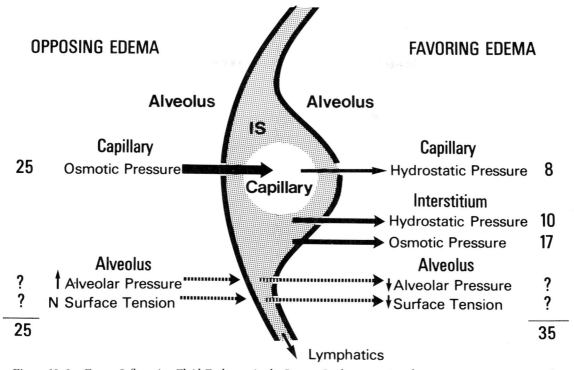

OPPOSING EDEMA

FAVORING EDEMA

Alveolus

Alveolus

IS

Capillary

Capillary

25 Osmotic Pressure

Capillary

Hydrostatic Pressure 8

Interstitium

Hydrostatic Pressure 10

Osmotic Pressure 17

Alveolus

Alveolus

? ↑ Alveolar Pressure

↓ Alveolar Pressure ?

? N Surface Tension

↓ Surface Tension ?

25

35

Lymphatics

Figure 10–6. Forces Influencing Fluid Exchange in the Lung. In the center is a diagrammatic representation of an alveolar septum containing a single capillary and surrounding interstitium (*IS*). On the left are indicated the forces opposing flow of fluid out of the capillary and on the right forces favoring it. The balance of forces clearly favors constant flow of water and protein from capillary to interstitium. The influence of alveolar pressure and surface tension has not been quantified.

opposes edema formation. Disregarding for the moment the effect of forces exerted by alveolar pressure and surfactant, it can be seen (Figure 10–6) that forces within the lung that oppose edema formation (colloid osmotic pressure of plasma = 25 mm Hg) are considerably exceeded by forces that favor edema (intravascular hydrostatic pressure + extravascular hydrostatic pressure + extravascular colloid osmotic pressure = 35 mm Hg). Thus, under normal conditions the combination of forces is such that there is a constant flow of water and protein from the capillaries into the interstitial space, an excess that can be handled adequately by the lymphatics and dumped back into the systemic circulation. When fluid transudation into the interstitium increases as a result of a rise in capillary hydrostatic pressure, the perivascular (interstitial) hydrostatic pressure also rises and tissue colloid pressure falls as a result of protein dilution.[49, 51] Along with increased lymph flow, these homeostatic mechanisms protect the lung against alveolar filling.

As pointed out by Staub,[47] the role of changes in interstitial fluid hydrostatic pressure is complicated because of related changes in lung

volume, pleural pressure, and intravascular pressure. For example, when sheep were subjected to continuous positive airway pressure breathing, there was observed a slight but definite *decrease* in lung lymph flow, thus actually increasing the extravascular water content of the lungs. Fishman[44] suggests that the success of positive pressure breathing in decreasing pulmonary edema is perhaps more attributable to its effect on reducing systemic venous return to the lungs than to its direct effect on the pulmonary capillaries.

Changes in the Characteristics of the Alveolar-Capillary Membrane

Since edema fluid may accumulate in the interstitial space (alteration in the microvascular component) and in the alveoli (alteration in the alveolar epithelium), both components of the membrane must be considered. Alveolar edema fluid always contains substantial quantities of protein, indicating a marked change in the apparent alveolar membrane permeability to macromolecules.[47] Staub states that this protein content must indicate a large change in the equivalent pore structure of the alveolar membrane, probably due to opening of the intercellular junctions. The reasons why the junctions open are unknown.

Precisely the same mechanism must exist in the capillary endothelium. Changes in membrane characteristics leading to pulmonary edema mean an increase in equivalent size of pores or an increase in their number. The physiologic correlate of these changes is increased fluid filtration at a given hydrostatic pressure and normal or even increased lymph-plasma protein ratios. This represents "permeability" or normal microvascular pressure pulmonary edema.

The composition of lung fluid is different in cardiogenic and noncardiogenic pulmonary edema. When pulmonary edema is caused by high filtration pressure, the protein concentration of tracheal fluid is usually less than half that of plasma; in contrast, alveolar fluid protein composition in permeability edema is much higher and similar to that in circulating plasma.[47]

Mechanisms for Removal of Fluid

In normal circumstances, water and protein are moved from the perimicrovascular space toward the lymphatic capillaries by gradients of subatmospheric pressure. Once in the larger lymphatics, water and protein are advanced toward the hilum primarily by ventilatory movements. Warren and Drinker[57] showed in anesthetized dogs that cessation of ventilation results in abrupt diminution of flow in mediastinal lymphatics draining lung lymph. It has been suggested that flow of lymph through pulmonary lymphatic channels depends on a "pumping" action of ventilation.[57]

Although the rate of lung lymph flow in pulmonary edema is unknown in man, Staub[47] has predicted that steady state lung lymph flows up to 200 ml per hour may be achieved in adult humans. It has been suggested[58] that the ceiling for lymphatic drainage is set by the relatively small caliber of the thoracic and right lymphatic ducts. In chronic left ventricular failure, the entire lymphatic system proliferates and the exit lymphatics increase in caliber. For example, Uhley, Leeds, and their colleagues[59-61] produced acute pulmonary edema in dogs by partial obstruction of the left atrium by a balloon and observed only a very small absolute increase in lymph flow through the right lymphatic duct. In contrast, dogs in which chronic heart failure was induced by creation of an aortocaval anastomosis showed gross increases in pulmonary lymph flow ranging from 300 to 2800 per cent over the normal flow of 4 ml per hour. Thus, in these experiments at least, although the lymphatics were unable to function significantly to relieve *acute* accumulation of lung water, they underwent important functional expansion over a period of time, thus acting as a compensatory mechanism for the prevention of overt alveolar edema. These latter experiments were felt to be analogous to the clinical state of chronic mitral stenosis, in which the lymphatics might be expected to aid in the

TABLE 10–2. CLASSIFICATION OF PULMONARY EDEMA

ELEVATED MICROVASCULAR PRESSURE (EMP)
  Cardiogenic:
    Left ventricular failure
    Mitral valvular disease
    Left atrial myxoma
    Cor triatriatum
  Affection of the pulmonary veins:
    Primary (idiopathic) veno-occlusive disease
    Secondary to mediastinal fibrosis or granuloma
  Neurogenic:
    Head trauma
    Increased intracranial pressure
    Postictal
NORMAL MICROVASCULAR PRESSURE (NMP)
(INCREASED CAPILLARY PERMEABILITY)
  Inhalation of noxious fumes and soluble aerosols:
    Nitrogen dioxide (silo-filler's disease)
    Sulfur dioxide
    Carbon monoxide
    Oxygen
    Ozone
    Smoke (burns)
    Ammonia
    Chlorine
    Phosgene
    Organophosphates
  Inhalation (aspiration) of noxious fluids:
    Liquid gastric contents (Mendelson's syndrome)
    Near-drowning
    Hypertonic contrast media
    Ethyl alcohol
  High altitude
  Transient tachypnea of the newborn
  Rapid re-expansion of lung in thoracentesis
  Other causes of NMP pulmonary edema:
    Traumatic fat embolism
    Post-traumatic (contused lung)
    Acute radiation reaction
    Circulating toxins (alloxan, snake venom)
    Circulating vasoactive substances (histamine, kinins, prostaglandins, serotonin)
    Decreased capillary oncotic pressure
    Lymphatic insufficiency
COMBINED ELEVATION OF MICROVASCULAR
PRESSURE AND INCREASED CAPILLARY PERMEABILITY
  Overdose of narcotic agents
  Acute pulmonary insufficiency due to a variety of causes (ARDS; shock lung)

removal of interstitial edema and thus effectively reduce the hazard of acute air-space edema.

CLASSIFICATION OF PULMONARY EDEMA

Table 10–2 divides the multiple etiologies of pulmonary edema into the major groups previously described: those associated with *elevated microvascular pressure,* those associated with *normal microvascular pressure,* and those in which a combination of these two factors is operative *(mixed).* In the following pages, the pathologic and roentgenologic characteristics of pulmonary edema secondary to cardiac disease will be described in detail. The other etiologies will be discussed in general terms, but their pathologic and roentgenologic manifestations will be referred to only insofar as they deviate from the pattern observed in cardiogenic edema.

PULMONARY EDEMA ASSOCIATED WITH ELEVATED MICROVASCULAR PRESSURE

CARDIOGENIC PULMONARY EDEMA

Undoubtedly the most common cause of interstitial and air-space edema of the lungs is a rise in pulmonary venous pressure, secondary to disease of the left side of the heart. Increased pressure within the left atrium may be transmitted to pulmonary veins as a result of back pressure from the left ventricle—which itself is secondary to long-standing systemic hypertension, aortic valvular disease, cardiomyopathy, coronary artery disease, myocardial infarction—or as a result of obstruction proximal to the left ventricle, such as mitral valvular disease, left atrial myxoma, or cor triatriatum. Rarely, pulmonary edema may follow electroconversion of arrhythmias, a complication believed to be caused by restoration of sinus rhythm in the presence of ineffective contraction of the left atrium.

PATHOLOGIC CHARACTERISTICS

In a study of the sequence of fluid accumulation in the lungs of dogs in which pulmonary edema was induced by elevation of microvascular pressure and by alteration of microvascular permeability, Staub and his colleagues[53] found a definite sequence of accumulation in both hydrostatic and permeability situations—an interstitial phase, an alveolar wall phase, and an alveolar air-space phase.

Interstitial Phase

As observed through the light microscope, the earliest manifestation of pulmonary edema was the appearance of fluid in the loose connective tissue around extra-alveolar conducting vessels and airways. Excess fluid was evidenced by widening of the perivascular and peribronchial interstitial space and by distention of lymphatics. The appearance of fluid in this compartment occurred before there was evidence of alveolar filling and when measurements of alveolar wall thickness were virtually normal. Once fluid accumulation filled the interstitial compartment and exceeded lymphatic transport capacity, additional fluid leakage was necessarily at the alveolar level.

Alveolar Wall Phase

As the quantity of edema fluid increased, there was observed a progressive increase in total alveolar wall thickness, by about 2 μ at most. A transition between this phase and overt alveolar edema was observed in which small accumulations of fluid were confined to the alveolar corners.

Alveolar Air-Space Phase

In some regions, all alveoli were filled with edema fluid, while in others they were either completely filled or were normal (air-filled). The lack of intermediate grades of filling in the latter areas suggested to Staub and his coworkers that edema formation was rapid and quantal in nature—*i.e.,* that individual alveoli filled essentially independently of their neighbors. The walls of the fluid-filled alveoli showed moderate to marked folding, indicating loss of volume.

On the basis of necropsy findings in 16 patients, Heard and his associates[62] concluded that most of the pathologic changes in pulmonary edema were visible roentgenologically, the notable exception being the pulmonary fibrosis that developed consequent upon organization of intra-alveolar fibrin. It was emphasized that the fibrosis which occurs in chronic left ventricular failure is *intra-alveolar* and is caused by organization of fibrinous edema.

ROENTGENOGRAPHIC MANIFESTATIONS

The sequence of fluid accumulation in the lungs of dogs subjected to elevated microvascular pressure[53] is also observed in humans roentgenologically, there being two major patterns related to whether edema fluid remains relatively localized in the interstitial space or whether it occupies the air spaces of the lung also. Whether or not it is possible for "interstitial" edema to be "pure" in the human lung has not been established to the best of our knowledge, but the distinction between predominantly interstitial and predominantly air-space edema serves the useful purpose of describing two situations whose clinical and functional characteristics are different.

Predominantly Interstitial Edema

Transudation of fluid into the interstitial spaces of the lung inevitably constitutes the first stage of pulmonary edema, since the capillaries are situated in this compartment. Using a double-indicator dilution technique and external counting over the chest to measure intravenously injected gamma-emitting radioisotopes, Fazio and associates[63] showed that roentgenographic abnormality becomes apparent with increases in lung water ranging from 30 to 80 per cent; similarly, in experimental studies in dogs, Snashall[52] demonstrated a "diffuse increase in hazy shadowing" when gravimetrically measured extravascular lung water increased by more than 30 per cent. When pulmonary venous hypertension is moderate in degree or transient, fluid transudation occurs into the interstitial space and is deposited within the perivascular sheath and interlobular septa. It is this anatomic localization that produces the typical roentgenographic pattern of loss of the normal sharp definition of pulmonary vascular markings and thickening of the interlobular septa (A and B lines of Kerley—Figure 10–7). The roentgenologic characteristics of Kerley A and B lines are discussed in detail in Chapter 4 (see page 206). Several studies have indicated that Kerley B lines due to interstitial pulmonary edema may develop when pulmonary venous pressure (wedge pressure) is 17 to 20 mm Hg or higher.[43, 64] Disappearance of the lines generally parallels that of other signs of the edema, and their persistence after adequate therapy (such as mitral commissurotomy for mitral stenosis) usually indicates that chronic congestion and edema of the septa have led to irreversible fibrosis and hemosiderosis.

We have not been impressed with the value of so-called perihilar haze as a sign of interstitial edema. Although it is frequently cited as a reliable sign of interstitial edema, in our experience the definition of hilar pulmonary arteries is seldom lost in cases of "pure" interstitial pulmonary edema, and for good reason. Since the major bronchi and arteries situated within the hila do not enter the lung until after they have divided into lobar branches, they do not possess the peribronchial and perivascular interstitium that is characteristic of intrapulmonary bronchovascular bundles. Thus, there is no reason for them to lose their definition until alveolar edema affects contiguous parenchyma and obscures their margin by a silhouetting effect. Loss of demarcation of hilar shadows should therefore be considered a sign of air-space rather than interstitial edema.

If evidence for interstitial pulmonary edema is equivocal as judged from the signs described, confirmatory evidence may be provided in some cases by appreciating an increased thickness of the wall of bronchi commonly visualized end-on in the parahilar zones. These bronchial walls, which we have visualized in 80 per cent of a large number of normal subjects, are normally hairline in thickness (in the absence of severe chronic bronchitis). When fluid accumulates in the loose interstitial tissue surrounding them, their shadow thickens and loses its sharp definition. In this regard, Don and Johnson[65] have suggested that peribronchial cuffing may be caused not only by an accumulation of edema fluid in the peribronchial interstitium but also by edema of the bronchial wall itself secondary to transudation from capillaries in the bronchial circulation. This should conceivably result in a narrowing of the lumen of bronchi viewed end-on, and we agree that narrowing is apparent in some cases. However, an alternative explanation for lumen narrowing is loss of pulmonary compliance: the accumulation of excess water makes the lungs stiffer than normal and reduces compliance; it is inevitable that the reduction in lung volume achieved on inspiration will be associated with a reduction in bronchial cross section. It is possible that both mechanisms are operative; clearly, further work is necessary to clarify these issues.

Another sign of interstitial edema, but one that usually becomes evident only when the accumulation of excess water is severe, is thickening of the interlobar fissure lines by fluid accumulation in the subpleural space (Figure 10–7), an abnormality that is sometimes confused with pleural effusion. The subpleural con-

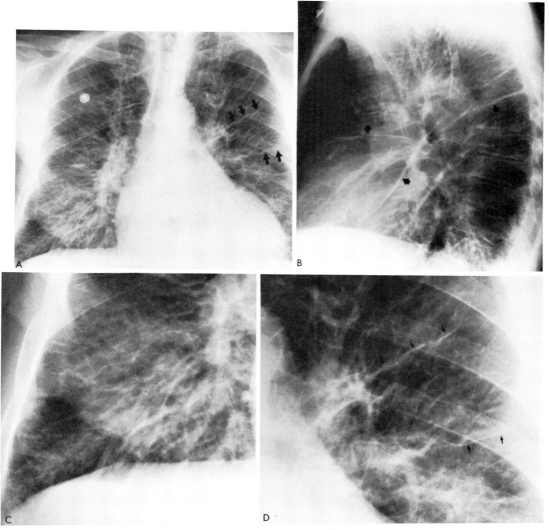

Figure 10–7.   Interstitial Pulmonary Edema.   Posteroanterior *(A)* and lateral *(B)* roentgenograms reveal multiple linear opacities throughout both lungs, seen to better advantage in magnified views of the right lower *(C)* and left upper *(D)* lungs. These lines consist of a combination of long septal lines (Kerley A), predominantly in the midlung zones *(arrows in B and D)*, and shorter peripheral septal lines (Kerley B). In lateral projection *(B)*, the interlobar fissures are very prominent *(arrows)*, representing subpleural edema. Twenty-four hours later, the edema had cleared completely.

nective tissue layer is in continuity with the interlobular septa and it is reasonable to assume that when edema fluid accumulates in the latter sites (creating Kerley B lines), it might also collect in the subpleural space.

Clinically, the findings in interstitial edema vary widely. Since the increased fluid remains relatively localized in the interstitial space, auscultation may reveal no signs. Even when patients complain of dyspnea and orthopnea and have a dry cough, there may be no abnormal physical findings, particularly when the interstitial edema results from mild left ventricular decompensation.

Pulmonary function is affected by interstitial edema in the development of hypoxemia caused partly by an increased pathway for diffusion but more importantly by a ventilation-perfusion inequality.[51, 66] Fluid in this compartment would not be expected to interfere appreciably with diffusion but can affect airway and vascular resistance.[36] In fact, the interstitial phase of edema may exert a beneficial function in that it represents preferential accumulation of fluid before the alveolar walls are affected, thereby protecting the gas exchange function of the lungs.

The chest roentgenogram usually is more

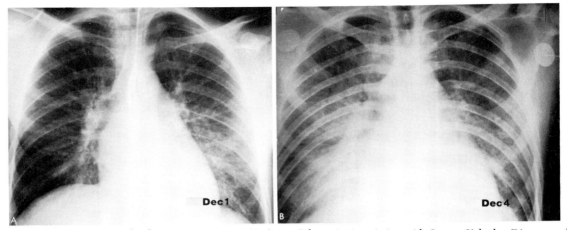

Figure 10–8. Interstitial Edema Progressing to Air-Space Edema in Association with Severe Valvular Disease and Subacute Bacterial Endocarditis. The initial posteroanterior roentgenogram of this 22-year-old man *(A)* reveals diffuse interstitial edema manifested by loss of definition of vessel markings throughout both lungs and by septal lines in both costophrenic recesses. Three days later *(B)*, the lungs had become massively consolidated by air-space edema. Heart size had increased considerably in this interval. Proved aortic insufficiency, mitral insufficiency, and subacute bacterial endocarditis.

accurate than is the physical examination in identifying interstitial pulmonary edema. In a hemodynamic, electrocardiographic, and roentgenographic assessment of 36 acutely ill patients with myocardial infarction or serious angina, Heikkilä and associates found a very good correlation between pulmonary capillary wedge pressure and evidence of pulmonary venous hypertension as assessed from bedside chest

roentgenograms. They found that a normal chest roentgenogram was an exceptional feature of the early stages of acute myocardial infarction, since evidence for pulmonary venous hypertension presented itself immediately after mean left ventricular filling pressure rose above 10 mm Hg. However, McHugh and coworkers found that serious roentgenologic misinterpretation of left ventricular failure occurred occa-

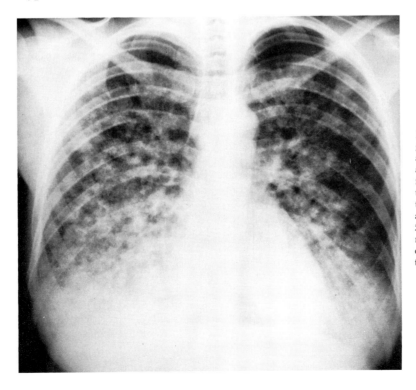

Figure 10–9. Acute Pulmonary Edema. A posteroanterior roentgenogram reveals widespread patchy airspace consolidation. Individual acinar shadows can be visualized in some areas, although generally these are coalescent, particularly in the lower lung zones. Cardiac size and configuration are normal. This 28-year-old woman had severe, periodic systemic arterial hypertension caused by a pheochromocytoma of the adrenal gland.

sionally in the presence of severe hypoxemia. They also observed considerable phase lags; *i.e.*, pulmonary capillary wedge pressure rose before roentgenographic signs became apparent and pulmonary edema persisted following successful therapy and lowering of wedge pressure to normal.

Air-Space Edema

Interstitial edema invariably precedes alveolar edema (Figure 10–8), and in some patients the chest roentgenogram shows evidence of both simultaneously. The sheet anchor in the roentgenologic diagnosis of air-space edema is the acinar shadow (Figure 10–9). In the majority of cases these shadows are confluent, creating irregular, rather poorly defined, patchy shadows of unit density scattered randomly throughout the lungs; in the medial third of the lungs particularly, coalescence of acinar consolidation is common and permits visualization of an air bronchogram. The distribution varies from patient to patient but may be surprisingly similar during different episodes in one patient. In acute pulmonary edema resulting from left ventricular failure, which commonly follows myocardial infarction, patchy air-space consolidation sometimes extends to the subpleural zone or "cortex" of the lung—although the

cortex may be completely spared, thus creating the "bat's-wing" or "butterfly" pattern of edema (*see* further on).

Edema caused by cardiac disease usually is bilateral and fairly symmetric, although it may be predominantly unilateral or in other respects "inappropriate"—that is, occupying zones of one or both lungs out of keeping with the "expected" distribution of disease arising from a central influence (Figure 10–10).

The mechanisms underlying the development of unilateral pulmonary edema are not known for certain. In patients with cardiac decompensation, it is probably related primarily to dependency.[67] In a thorough review of the subject, Calenoff and associates[68] enumerated 18 conditions associated with unilateral pulmonary edema. These they divided into two equal groups: one, which they termed "ipsilateral," consisting of an alteration in the alveolocapillary apparatus of one lung only that favored accumulation of excess water (*e.g.*, unilateral veno-occlusive disease or prolonged lateral decubitus position); and the other, which they termed "contralateral," comprising a group of disorders in which edema developed on the side opposite a lung with impaired perfusion (*e.g.*, Swyer-James syndrome or massive unilateral pulmonary thromboembolism).

When edema is predominantly unilateral or

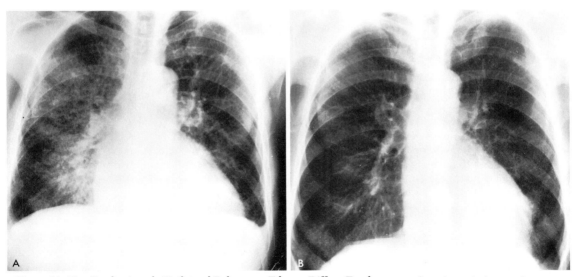

Figure 10–10. Predominantly Unilateral Pulmonary Edema. Diffuse Emphysema. A posteroanterior roentgenogram (*A*) of this 70-year-old man admitted with acute myocardial infarction reveals patchy air-space consolidation occupying the medial two-thirds of the right lung characteristic of acute pulmonary edema. The left lung is much less severely affected. The heart is moderately enlarged. A visit to the patient's bedside revealed the fact that he lay on his right side most of the time, since other positions seemed to intensify his shortness of breath. A roentgenogram following resolution of the edema (*B*) shows a marked increase in volume of both lungs characteristic of diffuse pulmonary emphysema. The unilaterality of the edema was clearly related to the influence of gravity. The reduction in lung volume associated with the edema was the result of reduced compliance (increased stiffness), an important and frequent concomitant of pulmonary edema.

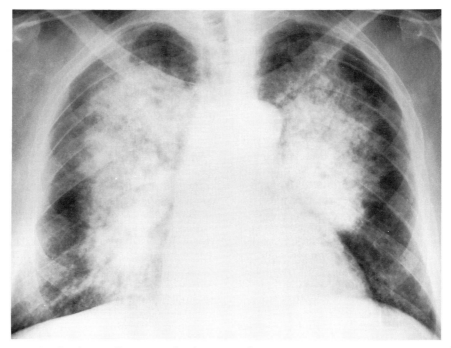

Figure 10–11. The "Bat's Wing" Pattern of Pulmonary Edema. A posteroanterior roentgenogram demonstrates consolidation of the parahilar and "medullary" portions of both lungs, creating a "bat's wing" or "butterfly" appearance; the "cortex" of both lungs is relatively unaffected. The margins of the edematous lung are rather sharply defined. The consolidation is fairly homogeneous and is associated with a well-defined air bronchogram on both sides. This 59-year-old man had suffered a massive myocardial infarction 48 hours previously; he had a cough productive of pinkish sputum but was able to lie flat in bed.

in other ways "inappropriate," the differential diagnosis from pneumonia may be difficult but may be facilitated by roentgenologic visualization of changes typical of interstitial edema.

The "bat's-wing" or "butterfly" pattern of edema describes an anatomic distribution of air-space edema in which the hilum and "medulla" of the lungs are fairly uniformly consolidated and the peripheral 2 to 3 cm of lung parenchyma—the "cortex"—is relatively uninvolved (Figure 10–11). Nessa and Rigler[69] recorded an incidence of 5 per cent in 110 cases of moderate to severe edema of varying etiology. Although it has been said that this pattern of edema is seen commonly in association with uremia, Hodson[70] states that there is convincing evidence that the lesion is the result of acute left ventricular failure and that it bears no specific relationship to uremia. He further states that its association with uremia is caused by concomitant left-sided heart failure.

Definition of the margin of consolidated parenchyma often is rather indistinct but may be remarkably sharp. Resolution of the edema generally begins in the periphery and spreads medially. Many theories have been propounded to explain the mechanism of this unusual anatomic distribution of pulmonary edema. The most

recent of these, put forward by Fleischner,[71] is based on Mayerson's observation: "Pulmonary edema arises when capillary filtration exceeds the point where the lymphatic drainage is adequate to maintain the relatively 'dry' state of pulmonary tissue."[72] Fleischner proposed that the accumulation of fluid is dependent upon the efficiency with which the lymphatics can remove an excess. He postulated that during respiration the peripheral portion of the lungs undergoes greater volumetric change than does the medulla, and that this increased movement operates in much the same way as does muscular exercise in the extremities to stimulate increased lymphatic flow. This theory is plausible, but further experimental work is required to determine its validity.

Like interstitial pulmonary edema, air-space pulmonary edema usually clears fairly rapidly in response to adequate treatment of the underlying condition, and resolution appears complete roentgenographically in not more than 3 days in most cases. It is likely that the degree of efficiency of the lymphatic system plays a major role in clearance time.

Clinically, the classic symptoms of acute pulmonary edema are severe dyspnea and orthopnea, usually associated with cough which may be dry or may be productive of copious frothy sputum. Expectorated material may be pink or, as in mitral stenosis, frankly bloody. In mitral stenosis or in left ventricular failure secondary to systemic hypertension or aortic valvular disease, the episode of acute pulmonary edema may develop only following exertion or may be consequent upon the increase in pulmonary blood volume associated with the change in position when the patient lies flat. Most of these patients appear apprehensive and evidence tachypnea and cyanosis; almost invariably crepitations are audible over the lung bases and in the more severe cases extend up to the apices. Other signs of congestive failure, such as elevated systemic venous pressure, hepatosplenomegaly, and peripheral edema may be present.

The effects of edema on pulmonary function consist of a decrease in compliance and an increase in resistance. Some degree of hypoxemia is present in virtually all patients with clinically evident pulmonary edema and in approximately half of patients with acute myocardial infarction. The hypoxemia usually is more severe in overt air-space edema than in predominantly interstitial edema and its pathogenesis is related more to vascular shunt; it often develops in severe degree in the presence of alveolar hypoventilation due to widespread air-space edema or respiratory muscle fatigue. In this situation, hypercapnia and acute tissue hypoxia may result in a mixed acidemia.

The clinical manifestations of "butterfly" edema may be almost as unimpressive as the roentgenographic appearance is dramatic. Even when there is roentgenographic evidence of massive consolidation of the medial two-thirds of the lungs, the clinical presentation may be unremarkable, and even those patients who complain of dyspnea and orthopnea may have minimal or nonexistent physical signs—much the same as in diffuse interstitial edema. This dissociation of clinical and roentgenologic findings probably is attributable to the fact that the lack of involvement of the parenchymal compartment of the lungs (whose prime function is gas exchange) minimizes the effect on function and physical signs.

PULMONARY EDEMA ASSOCIATED WITH RENAL DISEASE, HYPERVOLEMIA, OR HYPOPROTEINEMIA

Both acute glomerulonephritis and chronic renal disease—with or without uremia—may be associated with acute pulmonary edema or pulmonary edema of "butterfly" distribution. In acute glomerulonephritis, children may die so abruptly from this consequence of cardiac failure that the diagnosis may be made postmortem. In fact, the incidence of pulmonary edema in acute glomerulonephritis of infants and children is so high that Macpherson and Banerjee[73] suggested that the diagnosis can be made with a high degree of accuracy from the plain chest roentgenogram.

It is very likely that the major contributing cause to the development of pulmonary edema in renal disease is left ventricular failure, although it is probable that decreased oncotic pressure and hypervolemia also play a part, as may increased capillary permeability.

Patients with chronic renal failure may also develop "metastatic" calcification, particularly in the kidneys, stomach, and lungs. These organs are believed to be particularly susceptible because they secrete acid, thus encouraging calcium deposition because of a higher tissue pH.

Overloading of the circulation by intravenous infusion, with resultant rise in microvascular pressure, is a common cause of pulmonary edema, particularly during the postoperative period and in elderly patients. A decrease in plasma protein levels leading to reduction in the plasma osmotic pressure may play a role in some patients, but probably only as a contributory factor in those who are on the verge of cardiac decompensation from some other cause.

It is worthy of emphasis that pulmonary edema developing in association with blood transfusion need not always be the result of overloading of the circulation; in some instances it probably is caused by increased capillary permeability resulting from leukoagglutinins[74] demonstrable in the donors, who generally are multiparous. The antibodies develop because of incompatibility with fetal leukocytes, much in the same manner as Rhesus antibodies develop.

PULMONARY EDEMA SECONDARY TO AFFECTION OF THE PULMONARY VEINS

Obstructive disease of the pulmonary veins is a relatively rare cause of pulmonary venous hypertension. Five different etiologies may be seen: (1) congenital heart disease of both high and low flow types; (2) congenital stenosis of the origin of the pulmonary veins; (3) idiopathic veno-occlusive disease involving the small and medium-sized veins (*see* page 487); (4) chronic mediastinitis, in which the pulmonary veins are involved in the cicatricial process; and (5) anomalous pulmonary venous return, above or below the diaphragm, in which venous compression, stenosis, or increased resistance of the hepatic sinusoids leads to a rise in pulmonary venous pressure.

The *roentgenographic manifestations* usually are indistinguishable from those of pulmonary venous hypertension from cardiac causes, except that in most cases the heart is of normal size. The edema may be predominantly interstitial in location, although associated periodically with acute air-space edema. The chronic elevation of venous pressure leads to pulmonary arterial hypertension indistinguishable from that due to chronic mitral stenosis.

Clinically, these patients typically have slowly progressive dyspnea and orthopnea punctuated by attacks of acute pulmonary edema; hemoptysis may occur.

NEUROGENIC AND POSTICTAL PULMONARY EDEMA

Acute pulmonary edema in association with raised intracranial pressure, head trauma, and seizures is a well known but infrequent phenomenon. Its mechanism is poorly understood, although experimental work in recent years has pointed to elevated microvascular pressure as the likeliest mechanism. Probably the most logical pathophysiologic mechanism for neurogenic edema is related to massive sympathetic discharge from hypothalamic centers. Since one of the major effects of sympathetic discharge on the cardiovascular system is venous constriction, it is logical to invoke this mechanism to explain elevation of pulmonary venous pressure and subsequent pulmonary edema, even in the absence of overt cardiac decompensation. However, the persistence or worsening of edema following the return to normal of capillary hydrostatic pressure suggests that there may be a component of increased capillary permeability, perhaps caused by the high microvascular pressure itself.[52]

Of the various causes of neurogenic edema head trauma is one of the most frequent, and though often severe it may be relatively mild and nonfatal.[75] In nontraumatized patients in whom edema develops as a consequence of raised intracranial pressure, the rise in pressure may or may not be abrupt. The mechanism of development of postictal pulmonary edema is undoubtedly the same as that with trauma and increased intracranial pressure. It may develop immediately after an epileptic seizure or be delayed for several hours.

Characteristically, the edema disappears within several days following surgical relief of increased intracranial pressure. Most patients are comatose and have frequent periods of apnea when pulmonary edema develops. Thus they are likely to aspirate acid gastric juice and suffer prolonged hypoxemia. It is possible that these mechanisms can be invoked as the pathogenesis in some cases.

PULMONARY EDEMA ASSOCIATED WITH NORMAL MICROVASCULAR PRESSURE

Of the many different etiologies of permeability pulmonary edema, the majority are associated with inhalation of noxious substances (*e.g.*, nitrogen dioxide or liquid gastric contents) that must traverse the tracheobronchial tree to reach the terminal units of the lung (*see* Table 10–2, page 496). Several gases and soluble aerosols, notably nitrogen dioxide, sulfur dioxide, phosgene, chlorine, carbon monoxide, and hydrocarbon compounds, induce within the lungs acute pulmonary edema whose severity depends chiefly upon intensity and duration of exposure. However, in the majority of cases, the pulmonary edema is transient and is no more than a part of the lung's reaction to the insult, a much more ominous and long-lasting reaction being an acute, severe fibrinous bronchiolitis and peribronchiolitis. The result in many cases is extensive bronchiolitis fibrosa obliterans, generalized bronchiectasis, and severe obstructive airway disease. Thus, although edema is the usual initial manifestation of these insults—and occasionally is severe enough to cause death—the long-term effects are generally more significant. Therefore we have included this group of diseases with the inhalation diseases of the lung (*see* Chapter 12).

INHALATION (ASPIRATION) OF NOXIOUS FLUIDS

Liquids that may induce acute pulmonary edema when inhaled include fresh and sea water (near-drowning), hypertonic contrast media, and—by far the most common—acid gastric juice. Ethyl alcohol has also been reported to induce acute pulmonary edema but will not be discussed here. Kerosene and other hydrocarbons also induce pulmonary edema, although the pathogenesis of the acute pulmonary disease is controversial. There is good experimental evidence that these materials cause toxic capillary damage through the pulmonary circulation following their absorption from the gastrointestinal tract rather than by aspiration; therefore this condition is considered in the chapter on inhalation diseases (*see* Chapter 12).

MENDELSON'S SYNDROME (ASPIRATION OF ACID GASTRIC CONTENTS)

This might more properly be designated "acute inhalational pulmonary edema" because, in fact, the lung changes are predominantly those of edema.

The history is usually that the patient vomited while under anesthesia (or, perhaps more commonly, while coming out of anesthesia) or while in a coma produced by alcohol, barbiturate poisoning, cerebrovascular accident, or epileptic seizure. Liquid gastric contents are aspirated in varying amounts and, because of their highly irritative character, usually are distributed widely and diffusely throughout both lungs in an explosive fashion as a result of violent coughing and the deep inspirations that such coughing usually engenders. Since the aspirate is fluid, it typically passes out to the most peripheral air spaces. The hydrochloric acid of the gastric juice is the chief offending agent and causes direct damage to the capillary wall, with resultant increase in capillary permeability. Experimental work suggests that pulmonary edema develops when the pH of the aspirate is less than 2.5. However, it seems logical that aspiration of large amounts of fluid whose pH is greater than 2.5 should have the same effect as near-drowning in water. In a study of the ultrastructure of pulmonary alveolar capillaries in Mendelson's syndrome, Alexander[76] examined the lungs of experimental animals into which solutions of varying pH and tonicity had been instilled. Pulmonary edema was present in all specimens, including those in which distilled water was the aspirated fluid. Electron microscopy revealed fluid in the alveoli, as well as separation of the vascular endothelium from the alveolar epithelium by interstitial fluid. The pH and tonicity increased the reaction only in terms of degree and time, suggesting that the pathologic process produced by fresh water aspiration is similar to that produced by acid aspiration and that the major mechanism must be increased capillary permeability.

Although the major response of the lungs to the presence of large quantities of acid gastric juice is massive edema, descriptions of the *pathologic characteristics* usually reflect the presence of superimposed bacterial infection.[77]

The *chest roentgenogram* reveals general involvement of both lungs by typical air-space consolidation similar in many ways to the pulmonary edema of cardiac origin (Figure 10–12).

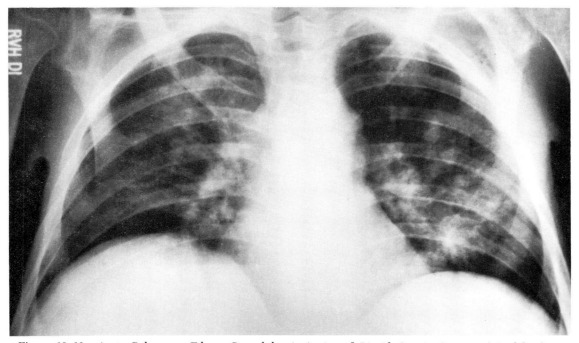

Figure 10–12. Acute Pulmonary Edema Caused by Aspiration of Liquid Gastric Contents (Mendelson's Syndrome). An anteroposterior roentgenogram of the chest in the supine position reveals widespread, patchy air-space consolidation typical of acute pulmonary edema of any etiology. Heart size and configuration are normal. This 19-year-old male aspirated liquid gastric contents postoperatively.

In a review of the roentgenographic manifestations of aspiration of gastric contents in 60 patients, Landay and his colleagues[78] observed three basic patterns of disease: (1) extensive bilateral air-space consolidation (confluent acinar opacities); (2) fairly discrete acinar shadows; and (3) irregular opacities whose pattern did not fit into either of the other two categories (this last named was the most frequent pattern, comprising slightly over 40 per cent).

It is to be emphasized that this form of aspiration "pneumonia" may not show an anatomic distribution reflecting the influence of gravity. If the patient was lying in the prone or supine position when he aspirated, the highly irritative nature of the aspirate will result in widespread dissemination throughout the lungs, although *predominant* changes may be unilateral if the patient was lying on his side or in the upper zones if he was lying on his back. In most cases, resolution is relatively rapid, averaging 7 to 10 days in our experience.

Clinical manifestations vary with the material aspirated. Aspiration of vomitus may occur after emergency surgery or obstetric delivery[79] when the patient has eaten recently. In these circumstances the toxic pulmonary edema produced by hydrochloric acid is complicated to some extent by the obstructive influence of solid food particles. Endotracheal intubation with cuff inflation during anesthesia does not necessarily prevent this complication, since vomited material may accumulate proximal to the inflated bag and be aspirated only when the cuff is deflated and the endotracheal tube removed.

The main symptom is shortness of breath, which may be noted before roentgenographic changes become manifest in the chest. Cough, which is initially dry, eventually produces copious purulent sputum if the patient survives the stage of acute pulmonary edema; a variety of aerobic and anaerobic pathogens and commensals may be cultured from this material.

NEAR-DROWNING

In the experimental animal, the effects of inhaling sea water (which has about three times the tonicity of human extracellular fluid) differ from the effects of inhaling fresh water (which has a negligible solute content), but in humans the life-threatening consequences are hypoxemia and acidosis, there being no convincing evidence that other factors such as hemodilution result in a significant rise in microvascular pressure.

Near-drowning may be subdivided into three types, depending on whether water enters the lung and whether the inhaled water contains contaminants.

Dry Drowning

In a fit individual whose laryngeal reflexes are brisk, spasm may prevent inhalation of water. If this is maintained until the resulting cerebral anoxia causes paralysis of the respiratory center, the individual can lose consciousness without water entering the lungs. It has been estimated that between 20 and 40 per cent of all near-drownings fall into this category. Clinically, patients present a picture of simple asphyxia.

Near-Drowning in Fresh or Sea Water

In near-drowning in either sea or fresh water, there is usually a period of apnea and struggling, which may be followed by violent inspiratory effort. Water enters the mouth and at first is swallowed in large quantities and then inhaled. Pulmonary edema is almost invariable, being observed roentgenographically in 27 of 32 patients studied by Hasan and colleagues.[80] In this group, serum electrolyte changes were minimal and included slight hypokalemia in 17 patients; minimal elevation of serum sodium was found in approximately 25 per cent of sea water victims. In both fresh and salt water drowning, there is considerable loss of protein from the blood, manifested pathologically in fatal cases by hyaline membrane formation in the alveoli and clinically by the characteristic foam found in the airways.

As pointed out by Miles,[81] the theoretical and experimental differences between the effects of inhalation of salt and fresh water have tended to confuse the issue as far as humans are concerned, since complete investigations are seldom made during recovery. Where it has been possible to carry out such examinations, *no evidence of significant electrolyte transfer, hemoconcentration, or hemodilution has been found.*[82] Similarly, no difference is seen between fresh water and salt water victims clinically.[83] It is clear that water entering the alveoli must act as an irritant, whatever its tonicity and whichever way electrolytes flow, and it is quite possible that such irritation may lead to increased permeability of pulmonary capillaries.

Secondary Near-Drowning

In most cases, the water inhaled contains debris such as small marine growths, sand,

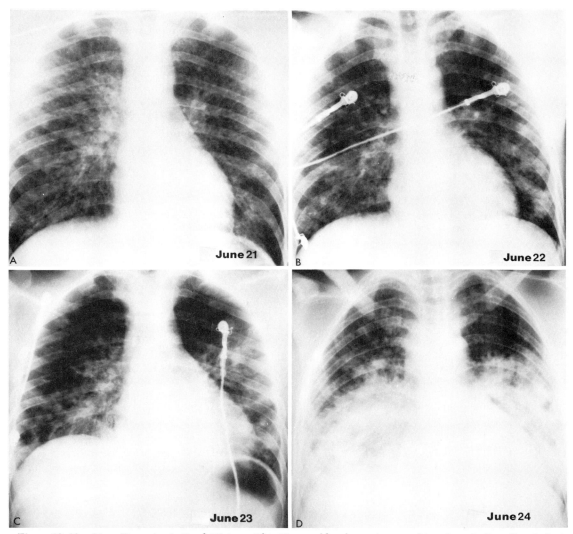

Figure 10–13. Near-Drowning in Fresh Water. This 19-year-old male was immersed in a dirty, badly polluted, fresh-water lake for a period of about 4 minutes before being rescued; he was under the influence of drugs at the time. The roentgenogram obtained shortly after his arrival in the emergency department *(A)* reveals widespread patchy air-space consolidation evenly distributed throughout both lungs. Heart size and configuration are normal. Twenty-four hours later *(B)*, the upper zones of both lungs had cleared considerably, although moderate edema persists in the lower zones. Forty-eight hours later *(C)*, the edema appeared to have worsened somewhat in the lower zones, suggesting the possibility of secondary near-drowning. Three days after the acute episode *(D)*, massive air-space consolidation had developed throughout the lower two-thirds of both lungs, and the patient's clinical status had deteriorated markedly. This represents the characteristic sequence of events following near-drowning in badly polluted water and the development of acute pneumonia caused by chemicals and debris—secondary near-drowning.

mud, fuel oil, sewage, and other pollution, all of which increase the hazard to the lungs. These substances may result in a deterioration in clinical status following initial improvement. For example, a patient who has recovered consciousness and seems to be progressing favorably may, within a few hours, show increasing respiratory distress with progressive restlessness, breathlessness, pain in the chest, cyanosis, and cough. It is probable that the major cause of this deterioration is progressive pul-

monary edema and pneumonia resulting from toxic debris (Figure 10–13*D*).

Roentgenographic Manifestations

The report of 36 patients by Hasan and colleagues[80] revealed no significant differences in the roentgenographic picture between fresh and sea water aspiration. The basic roentgenographic finding is one of pulmonary edema (Figure 10–13), the severity presumably depending upon the amount of water inhaled; in the most severe cases there is almost complete opacification of both lungs. Air-space edema is generally bilateral and symmetric and in less severe cases may be predominantly parahilar and midzonal. Most patients show marked clearing of their lungs within 3 to 5 days and complete resolution in 7 to 10 days.

Clinical Manifestations

According to Miles,[81] the period between the onset of respiratory failure and cardiac arrest rarely exceeds 3 to 4 minutes, and the longer cardiac arrest continues the less likely is resuscitation to be effective. The resulting cerebral hypoxia results in cerebral edema, which may have prolonged aftereffects.

Hasan and colleagues[80] reviewed in detail the clinical manifestations in 36 patients with near-drowning, 32 in salt water and 4 in chlorinated pools. Severe hypoxia was a constant finding, mean PO_2 being 55 mm Hg (SD $\pm$ 24) with patients breathing supplemental oxygen. Significant metabolic acidosis was present in 19 patients, mean values of pH for the entire group being 7.23 (SD $\pm$ 17) and base excess -10 mEq/L (SD $\pm$ 9). The metabolic acidosis is presumably caused by the formation of lactic acid in the hypoxic tissues of a person struggling to survive. Respiratory acidosis is usually not observed in near-drowning patients, probably because victims are artificially ventilated before initial arterial blood gas samples are drawn in the hospital.[80]

The prognosis in patients with near-drowning has been reviewed by Modell and associates on the basis of a retrospective study of 91 victims, of whom 81 survived.[84] Patients who were alert on arrival in the emergency room survived, but those who were comatose and whose pupils were fixed and dilated invariably died. All patients with normal chest roentgenograms survived, but it is notable that several of these had significant hypoxemia. Only two of the survivors manifested residual neurologic damage.

It is apparent that prolonged submersion in cold water improves chances of survival,[85] possibly because the hypothermia serves to protect the brain from hypoxic injury.

HYPERTONIC CONTRAST MEDIA

A number of reports have appeared in the literature describing the development of acute pulmonary edema following aspiration of water-soluble contrast media,[86] commonly in patients with chronic pulmonary disease, and for unknown reasons usually unassociated with overt clinical signs of aspiration. Although case reports of deaths from such causes have been infrequent,[86] it is clear that extreme caution must be exercised in the use of these oral agents in patients in whom there is a danger of aspiration, especially in the presence of known pre-existing pulmonary disease.

SALICYLATE-INDUCED PULMONARY EDEMA

Noncardiogenic pulmonary edema is a known complication of salicylate intoxication.[55, 87] It is usually nonfatal and is seen most commonly in older individuals who ingest salicylates chronically and who have a history of smoking.[87] Serum salicylate levels usually are greater than 40 mg/ml; the pulmonary edema characteristically responds to measures that lower serum salicylate levels.

PULMONARY EDEMA OCCURRING AT HIGH ALTITUDE

Many patients develop a variety of symptoms while becoming acclimatized to high altitudes. This symptom complex, known as mountain or altitude sickness, may become manifest on both acute[88] and prolonged exposure[89] at 3500 to 4000 m (11,500 to 13,000 feet). Symptoms include headache, giddiness, dizziness, tiredness, weakness, body aches, anorexia, nausea, vomiting, abdominal pain, insomnia, restlessness, cough, dyspnea on exertion, and occasionally fever. All symptoms and signs characteristically disappear on descent to sea level or on administration of oxygen. A small percentage of persons arriving at high altitudes develop overt pulmonary edema which occasionally proves fatal.[90] This is a relatively rare occurrence, as illustrated by one study in which edema developed in only one of 200 persons.[91] Usually the move from sea level to high altitude is abrupt, commonly by airplane. It is rare for edema to develop at altitudes of less than 3350 m (11,000 feet), but reports have originated in the United States of cases developing at 2750 m (9000 feet). Characteristically, the patients are young and healthy; some have arrived at high altitudes for the first time but the condition appears to show a predilection for former residents who are returning after being at sea level for a few days to several weeks.[90, 91] Edema usually develops within 2 to 3 days and almost always within the first month after arrival at high altitude. Physical exertion and cold weather are considered precipitating factors in some cases.

The pathogenetic sequence presumably starts with a constitutionally predisposed individual who develops an inordinate degree of pulmonary arterial hypertension when exposed to tolerable levels of hypoxia.[44] It has been suggested that the cause of high altitude pulmonary edema is intense vasoconstriction of a large fraction of the pulmonary arterial vessels, forcing blood flow at high pressures through the remaining patent vessels. This explanation requires the presence of regional inhomogeneities in pulmonary capillary pressures owing to non-uniform populations of precapillary resistances, so that the extraordinary pulmonary arterial hypertension affects some pulmonary capillary pressures more than others. Just how or why this occurs is not known, although a combination of mechanisms has been proposed including increased capillary permeability, luminal occlusions distal to spastic arterioles, and severe contraction of nonmuscular arterioles resulting in wider opening of perpendicular muscular arterioles. This severe constriction of muscular pulmonary arterioles is believed to be caused by hypoxia; the nonmuscular arterioles would thus take the brunt of the increased cardiac output, also resulting from the hypoxia. Visscher[92] suggested that obstruction of 75 per cent of the pulmonary vascular bed in dogs resulted in pulmonary edema because of the high pressures necessary to produce adequate flow through the remaining microvascular bed.

Catheterization studies in humans have revealed raised pulmonary arterial pressure, and in at least two patients, normal pulmonary wedge pressures.[93] Thus, while high altitude pulmonary edema is not caused by generalized elevation of microvascular pressure, it can be considered a form of high pressure pulmonary edema, the high pressure being on the arterial rather than the venous side. Probably of the same pathogenesis is the localized pulmonary edema that follows surgically created left-to-right shunts and that which occurs sometimes in association with massive pulmonary embolism.

The roentgenographic appearances are typical of acute pulmonary edema although the distribution tends to be rather irregular and patchy, reflecting the pathogenesis of inhomogeneous distribution of precapillary resistances.

Symptoms develop within 12 hours to 3 days after arrival at high altitude[91] and consist of cough, dyspnea, weakness, and hemoptysis, often associated with substernal discomfort. Common findings include cyanosis and tachy-cardia. Patients respond rapidly to the administration of oxygen or to a return to sea level. The chest roentgenogram clears within 24 to 48 hours.

RAPID RE-EXPANSION OF LUNG IN THORACENTESIS

Unilateral pulmonary edema may develop following rapid removal of air or fluid from the pleural space in the presence of pneumothorax or hydrothorax.[94] Three features are common to almost all cases: (1) the pneumothorax or hydrothorax is moderate or large in size (amounting to at least 50 per cent); (2) the pulmonary edema is strictly localized to the ipsilateral lung; and (3) the pneumothorax or hydrothorax has been present for a considerable period of time, usually several days, prior to rapid re-expansion (Figure 10–14). Typically, the edema resolves spontaneously within a few days.

The pathogenesis of this form of edema is not understood, but normal microvascular pressure is common to the four current theories: (1) the sudden increase in negative intrapleural pressure; (2) a delay in venous or lymphatic return caused by stasis in the pulmonary venules and lymphatics during prolonged collapse; (3) the alteration in alveolar surface tension that may accompany prolonged relaxation atelectasis; and (4) an anoxic effect on pulmonary capillaries during the period of lung collapse. Whether or not the edema is secondary to anoxia, increased capillary permeability would appear to be at least one factor in pathogenesis as judged by the protein content of the edema fluid that has been shown to be at a level usually associated with permeability rather than hydrostatic influences.[95]

It is almost certain that pulmonary edema from this cause occurs much more commonly than reports indicate; in fact we have personally seen several cases within recent years. It is important to be aware of this potential complication of rapid thoracentesis in pneumothorax or hydrothorax, since it may be prevented by slow withdrawal of gas or fluid by underwater drainage.

OTHER CAUSES OF PERMEABILITY PULMONARY EDEMA

A number of causes of permeability edema are best considered in relationship to the etiology of the underlying disease, although in

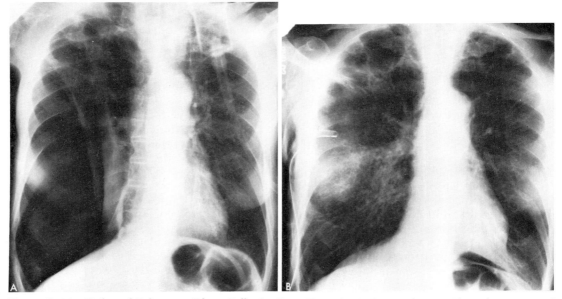

Figure 10–14. **Unilateral Pulmonary Edema Following Lung Expansion in Pneumothorax.** Three days prior to the roentgenogram illustrated in *A*, this 74-year-old man had experienced the abrupt onset of severe right-sided pleural pain and dyspnea. The chest pain subsided but shortness of breath persisted, and he presented himself to the emergency department. The admission roentgenogram reveals a large right pneumothorax, the upper portion of the lung being unaffected because of obliterative pleuritis. An intercostal drainage tube was inserted and negative pressure applied. A roentgenogram obtained shortly thereafter *(B)* reveals patchy air-space edema in the mid and lower portions of the right lung. Note that the upper zone is unaffected by edema because of the presence of multiple bullae. There is evidence of diffuse emphysema.

each, edema forms a significant part of their pathologic characteristics—*e.g., traumatic fat embolism, post-traumatic edema* (contused lung), and *acute radiation pneumonitis.* Of a somewhat different nature (in terms of the requirement for a slight to moderate rise in microvascular pressure) is the pulmonary edema accompanying *decreased pulmonary capillary oncotic pressure* and *lymphatic insufficiency.* It has been shown in experiments on dogs that acute reduction of plasma oncotic pressure from 25 to 15 mm Hg produces demonstrable pulmonary edema when pulmonary capillary hydrostatic pressures are only modestly elevated to 15 mm Hg.[96] Therefore, it is reasonable to assume that patients whose plasma protein concentrations are reduced may develop pulmonary edema with only moderate fluid overload in the absence of overt left ventricular decompensation.[46, 51] The importance of the lymphatics in maintaining the lungs in a "dry" state has been emphasized previously, and it has been shown experimentally that impairment of lymphatic drainage by partial ligation of the right lymphatic channels results in pulmonary edema in association with hemodynamically inconsequential elevation of left atrial pressure to 15 mm Hg.[97] The clinical equivalent of these experimental studies is rep-

resented by the occurrence of pulmonary edema in disorders characterized by abnormalities of lymphatic drainage—*e.g.,* silicosis and lymphangitic carcinomatosis—in which pulmonary edema may develop in the presence of only modestly elevated pulmonary venous pressure, and in cirrhosis of the liver, in which the quantity of lymph flow from below the diaphragm overloads the thoracic duct (*see* Chapter 18).

PULMONARY EDEMA ASSOCIATED WITH COMBINED ELEVATION OF MICROVASCULAR PRESSURE AND INCREASED CAPILLARY PERMEABILITY

In cases of severe pulmonary edema, both elevated capillary pressure and increased capillary permeability contribute to the accumulation of excess extravascular fluid. It is believed that profound hypoxemia and acidosis, whether of respiratory or metabolic origin, not only damage the microvasculature but also impair myocardial function. Frequently, overloading of the circulation with intravenous fluids in such patients is an additional contributory and often irreversible factor. Such combined mechanisms of edema formation are operative in two major conditions: narcotic overdose, chiefly from heroin, and a miscellaneous group of disorders generally lumped under the term "adult respiratory distress syndrome" (ARDS).

PULMONARY EDEMA ASSOCIATED WITH NARCOTIC ABUSE

Although the complications of drug abuse are many, including aspiration and bacterial pneumonia, septic pulmonary emboli, angiothrombotic pulmonary hypertension, bacterial endocarditis, mycotic aneurysms, arterial occlusion, arterial laceration, osteomyelitis, and hepatitis, one of the most important and dramatic is acute pulmonary edema. As a major complication of heroin overdose, the incidence of pulmonary edema ranges from 48 per cent to 75 per cent.[98] Addicts are predominantly males aged between 20 and 35 years. In one series of 149 cases of heroin overdose reported from New York City,[98] 71 developed pulmonary edema and six died. In the institutions serving this low income population, heroin overdose has become the commonest cause of pulmonary edema in patients under 40 years of age and accounts for up to six admissions per week. Most patients who die following heroin overdose show severe pulmonary edema at necropsy.[99] There are several settings in which overdose may occur, the most frequent being a lack of awareness of the potency of the heroin packet, which can vary considerably from "bag" to "bag" purchased on the streets.[100] Casual heroin users and addicts returning to heroin after a period of abstinence constitute a large percentage of victims of overdose.[98]

In virtually all cases, pulmonary edema develops within a few hours of the overdose and invariably in patients who fulfill the criteria of the "acute intoxication syndrome," consisting of the clinical triad: (1) an acutely ill patient in a stuporous or comatose state; (2) depressed respiration; and (3) constricted pupils.

The *pathogenesis* of the pulmonary edema is not thoroughly understood but is probably related to increased capillary permeability, with an element of elevated microvascular pressure in some cases. The hallmark of increased permeability edema[47]—a substantial increase in lymphatic protein flow (the product of lymph flow and lymph protein concentration)—was well illustrated in a study of 10 patients with acute pulmonary edema, in five resulting from

heroin overdose and in the other five from ischemic cardiac decompensation.[101] In the latter group the concentration of protein in edema fluid averaged 40.0 per cent (± 7.8) of serum protein compared with a level of 98.3 per cent (± 10) in the heroin group; all 10 patients were severely hypoxemic. It is probable that the increased permeability results chiefly from hypoxemia and acidosis, there being no convincing evidence that the drug itself exerts a toxic effect on pulmonary capillaries. Elevated microvascular pressure may be contributory in some cases as a result of left ventricular decompensation, an effect which is to be expected if hypoxemia and acidosis are severe enough to compromise myocardial performance.[44] A third pathogenetic mechanism acting in concert with elevated microvascular pressure and increased capillary permeability is impaired lymphatic drainage resulting from inadequate ventilatory excursions. An additional factor[44] may be nonuniform transmission to the pulmonary capillaries of pulmonary arterial hypertension elicited by hypoxemia and acidosis.

The *roentgenographic manifestations* of pulmonary edema following heroin and methadone overdose are similar to those from other causes. The pattern is bilateral and symmetric and usually rather patchy (Figure 10–15); massive confluent consolidation occurs in the most severe cases. Roentgenographic resolution characteristically occurs in as brief a time as 24 to 48 hours. If a roentgenogram obtained 24 to 48 hours after admission shows persisting opacities, aspiration or superimposed bacterial pneumonia should be suspected.

Clinically, heroin pulmonary edema usually follows intravenous injection, although occasional cases have been reported after nasal inhalation or "snorting" of the drug.[98] Methadone may be taken orally or by injection.[102] Pulmonary edema has also been reported in association with overdose of other respiratory depressant drugs such as propoxyphene, chlordiazepoxide (Librium), and ethchlorvynol (Placidyl).

The drug abuser with pulmonary edema is usually admitted in coma, often with frothy, pink edema fluid oozing from nostrils and mouth. Hypoxemia is severe and the patient is acidotic, usually of mixed respiratory and metabolic origin. By the time the first arterial blood gas is drawn, hypoxemia is probably the result of a combination of alveolar hypoventilation from depression of the respiratory center and ventilation-perfusion inequality from air-space edema. Patients who manifest hypocapnia have presumably recovered from central nervous sys-

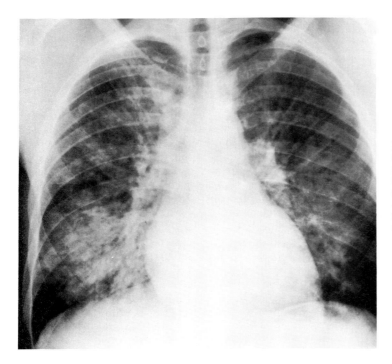

Figure 10–15. Acute Pulmonary Edema Caused by Drug Abuse. A posteroanterior roentgenogram reveals widespread, patchy air-space consolidation typical of acute pulmonary edema of any etiology. Several hours previously, this 19-year-old man had injected intravenously a high dose of Demerol and methadone. Uneventful recovery.

tem depression; persisting hypoxemia and acidosis then reflect the severe pulmonary edema and hypoperfusion of tissues.

ADULT RESPIRATORY DISTRESS SYNDROME (ARDS)

The appellation "adult respiratory distress syndrome" was coined by Petty and Ashbaugh in 1971[103] to describe a clinical picture of severe, unexpected, and life-threatening acute respiratory distress occurring after a widely diverse group of clinical insults. Although its pathogenesis is incompletely understood and its multiple predisposing conditions are of widely differing natures, it presents a characteristic clinical and roentgenologic picture that justifies its recognition as a distinct syndrome, i.e., the abrupt onset of marked dyspnea, increased respiratory effort, and severe hypoxemia associated with roentgenographic evidence of widespread air-space consolidation. Not only are the clinical and roentgenographic manifestations of the syndrome identical regardless of the predisposing condition, but the pathologic changes observed at necropsy are constant. Depending on the duration of pulmonary insufficiency prior to death, the lungs are found to be heavy, airless, and grossly hemorrhagic and show microscopic evidence of capillary congestion, interstitial edema, intra-alveolar edema and hemorrhage, hyaline membrane formation, hypertrophy and

hyperplasia of alveolar lining cells, interstitial and alveolar fibroblastic proliferation, and, as a final phase, extensive collagen deposition and fibrosis.

The wide diversity of predisposing conditions has led to a multitude of synonyms for ARDS, the most frequently employed of which are shock lung, post-traumatic pulmonary insufficiency, hemorrhagic lung syndrome, Da Nang lung, stiff lung syndrome, respirator lung, pump lung, congestive atelectasis, oxygen toxicity, catastrophic pulmonary failure, and acute respiratory distress in adults. The designation ARDS will be employed throughout the present discussion.

PREDISPOSING CONDITIONS

As has been indicated, a widely diverse group of conditions predispose to ARDS, including hemorrhagic or septic shock, massive pulmonary or general body trauma, acute pancreatitis, and a number of conditions whose etiology can be more precisely identified, including aspiration of liquid gastric contents (Mendelson's syndrome), heroin and methadone intoxication, massive viral pneumonia, traumatic fat embolism, near-drowning and, in fact, virtually all the conditions considered previously in this chapter under the heading of permeability pulmonary edema (see classification on page 496). It is to be emphasized that regardless of the etiology or predisposing condition, the clinical, roentgenologic, functional, and morphologic features of the syndrome are identical.

PATHOGENESIS

Despite the variety of precipitating events, the pathologic characteristics common to all cases of ARDS would suggest that either there is one common activating factor or the lung is capable of reacting to injury in only a limited manner. As will be seen in the discussion of pathology to follow, there occurs a complete breakdown in the integrity of the lung resulting in a marked increase in permeability of the microvascular bed and alveolar epithelium. Although hypovolemic shock is often present, it is difficult to produce lung damage by shock alone,[104] and other factors must be involved. These factors, each of which is carried by the blood, include endotoxins from sepsis, the products of disseminated intravascular coagulation, and a wide variety of vasoactive agents. Of potential importance in contributing to the pathologic changes are surfactant deficit, oxygen toxicity, prolonged respirator use, cardiopulmonary bypass, and left ventricular decompensation.

Sepsis. Experimental studies in unanesthetized sheep in which *Pseudomonas aeruginosa* bacteremia was induced[105] have shown a marked increase in lymph flow from the lungs: protein flow (product of lymph flow and lymph protein concentration) was greatly increased— the hallmark of increased permeability edema. Similar studies in man have confirmed the value of protein measurement in pulmonary edema as an indicator of pathogenesis.[106, 107] MacLean and his coworkers[108] have shown that pulmonary edema can occur in endotoxin shock in the presence of normal pulmonary capillary pressures.

Disseminated Intravascular Coagulation (DIC). This acquired hemorrhagic syndrome (*synonyms:* consumption coagulopathy, diffuse intravascular thrombosis, defibrination syndrome) has been observed in a wide variety of clinical disorders and has been implicated as a major pathogenetic feature of ARDS.[104, 109, 110] In fact, coagulation changes, which in most instances do not fulfill the criteria for DIC, are a hallmark of capillary permeability edema.[126] DIC includes a tetrad of laboratory findings:[109] (1) deficiency of clotting factors, primarily of fibrinogen; (2) thrombocytopenia; (3) the presence of circulating anticoagulants; and (4) excessive fibrinolysis. The abnormality occurs primarily in the microcirculation and it is important that it should be distinguished from thromboembolic disease affecting major vessels. It has been suggested[111] that DIC involves two major factors. The first is *slowing of capillary flow* caused by arterial hypotension; arterial or venous constriction; opening of all capillaries simultaneously; or opening of arteriovenous shunts. The second factor comprises *hypercoagulability and stimuli to clotting of blood,* including acidosis; hemolysis; high levels of clotting factors; bacterial toxins; surface factor activation as in extracorporeal circulation by glass, air, or metal surfaces; cancer or necrotic tissue; particulate matter introduced into the blood such as amniotic fluid; snake venom; and thrombin. It has been proposed that extensive obstruction of the pulmonary microcirculation initiates a complex series of events that ultimately result in interstitial edema, alveolar hemorrhage caused by altered capillary permeability, atelectasis, and hyaline membrane formation. Depletion of clotting factors by the diffuse coagulopathy paradoxically results in a bleeding diathesis which may be occult or massive.

Vasoactive Agents. In addition to the endotoxins that may cause direct damage to the alveolar-capillary membrane in cases of sepsis, a variety of vasoactive agents that modify pulmonary vascular permeability, or cause platelet aggregation, or both, may be released from damaged organs and tissues remote from the lungs, either from traumatized tissue or from blood constituents. These include *histamine, serotonin, adenosine triphosphate* (ATP) and its product *adenosine diphosphate* (ADP), and *catecholamines.*

Surfactant Deficit. It has been shown[112] that appreciable depletion of surfactant may occur following nonthoracic trauma, usually most evident after 18 to 36 hours. Such depletion results from defective production caused either by direct damage to type II alveolar epithelial cells or by a break in the chemical chain of production, such as occurs with the increase in phospholipase A activity in acute pancreatitis. In either event, the result is alveolar instability and progressive microatelectasis. Although atelectasis results in an increase in venoarterial shunting in the lung, a prominent pathophysiologic consequence of ARDS, it is unlikely that its role in the production of the basic lung lesion is primary.[104]

Left Ventricular Decompensation. Although the pulmonary edema of ARDS is characteristically associated with normal microvascular pressure and is due to altered permeability of the pulmonary microvascular bed, cardiogenic edema may show identical clinical and physiologic features and may be confused with or superimposed upon ARDS. For example, of 14 patients with adult respiratory distress syndrome admitted to a medical intensive care unit,[113] four were found to have left ventricular failure (defined as a pulmonary arterial wedge pressure greater than 12 mm Hg). All patients were studied with a balloon-tipped, flow-directed Swan-Ganz catheter. In this series, analysis of the standard clinical and laboratory data demonstrated no criteria that could differentiate those patients with left ventricular decompensation from those without. Left ventricular decompensation in such patients may be primary or may be secondary to the pathophysiologic consequences of ARDS itself, including severe hypoxemia, tissue hypoxia, endotoxemia, or DIC. The detection of pulmonary venous hypertension in patients with ARDS is of more than academic interest, since it can substantially influence therapy. For example, digitalis would be used in the presence of left ventricular failure, whereas this drug is contraindicated in patients without cardiac decompensation, partly because it possesses no therapeutic value but more importantly because it is actually hazardous (digitalis possesses a substantial potential for promoting cardiac arrhythmia in the presence of hypoxemia and electrolyte imbalance).

Stevens[114] has formulated a useful flow diagram (Figure 10–16) which aids in the assessment of the patient with acute respiratory failure and in establishing the pathogenesis of the pulmonary edema. However, it should be emphasized that mechanical ventilation and respiratory disease impose both theoretical and practical limitations on the interpretation of hemodynamic measurements.[115]

Oxygen Alveolopathy. Oxygen toxicity is a well-documented cause of lung damage, particularly when the oxygen is delivered for prolonged periods in high concentrations or partial pressures.[116] In many cases, it must be exceedingly difficult to distinguish the pathogenetic influences described earlier (*e.g.*, DIC, endotoxemia, and vasoactive agents) from those resulting from oxygen therapy. In fact, studies in human patients with normal lungs who have been placed on ventilators suggest that even after 4 or 5 days of administration of 100 per cent oxygen pathologic changes are minimal, even though abnormalities may be observed in pulmonary function. Thus, it appears likely that whereas the administration of oxygen in high concentration over long periods of time can conceivably damage normal lungs, oxygen therapy cannot reasonably be implicated in the

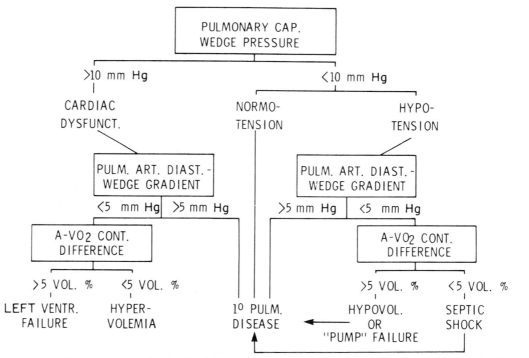

Figure 10–16. Flow Diagram Indicating Probable Pathogenesis of Pulmonary Edema on the Basis of Pulmonary Capillary Wedge Pressure in Patients with Acute Respiratory Failure. (Reprinted from Stevens, P. M.: Assessment of acute respiratory failure: Cardiac versus pulmonary causes. Chest, 67:1, 1975, with permission of the author and editor.)

initial pulmonary changes of ARDS, especially when used in concentrations of less than 50 per cent.

Prolonged Respirator Care. Patients with ARDS require artificial ventilation with either intermittent positive pressure breathing (IPPB) or positive end-expiratory pressure (PEEP), and although it is difficult to establish the role played by this form of therapy in the production of pathologic changes, there is little doubt that in some instances it is significant.[117] Alveolar edema caused by IPPB at high levels for prolonged periods may result from surfactant depletion caused by large excursions of alveolar surface area and an increase in surface tension at end expiration.

Cardiopulmonary Bypass. ARDS sometimes occurs after cardiopulmonary bypass. In a comparison of 14 patients who developed ARDS following cardiopulmonary bypass with a control group of 10 patients who had an uneventful postoperative recovery,[118] it was concluded that initiating factors of ARDS included a prolonged cardiopulmonary bypass time, a history of heavy cigarette smoking, and a tendency to develop cardiocirculatory failure postoperatively. The mechanism for capillary leak following cardiopulmonary bypass is not known, although surfactant deficiency may play a role in conjunction with the commonly associated left ventricular failure and hypotension. An increase in pulmonary artery pressure has been recorded in some cases and has been recognized as a potential cause.[119]

PATHOLOGIC CHARACTERISTICS

There are few differences in the observed morphologic changes in the lungs reported by different observers,[104, 111, 120, 121] the severity of changes depending in large measure on the duration of the pulmonary insufficiency prior to death. Without exception, all changes affect the lungs uniformly without significant anatomic predilection.

Up to 12 hours: Three groups of observers[103, 120, 121] described fibrin and platelet microemboli in arterioles 50 to 100 mμ in diameter, unassociated with macroscopic or other microscopic evidence of disease.

Twelve to 24 hours: Interstitial edema has appeared, affecting both the perivascular interstitium and the alveolar walls.

Twenty-four to 48 hours: Grossly, the lungs are hemorrhagic, heavy, and airless, and appear beefy or liverlike. Fluid is not easily expressed from the cut surface. Microscopically, there is evidence of capillary congestion, extensive interstitial and intra-alveolar proteinaceous edema and hemorrhage, and widespread microatelectasis. During this acute exudative phase, there is evidence of widespread destruction of type I alveolar epithelial cells, probably the major mechanism for the massive alveolar edema.[122] It is of considerable interest that this destruction of alveolar epithelial cells affects type I cells almost exclusively; during the reparative phase, it is the type II cells that undergo proliferation, resulting not only in an increase in their own cell numbers but in a relining of alveolar surfaces by type I cells formed by differentiation from proliferated type II cells.[122]

Five to 7 days: Grossly, the lungs are still heavy and airless, although the previously hemorrhagic appearance has been replaced by a grayish discoloration. Microscopically, the highly proteinaceous edema fluid within the alveoli is less evident, but there has occurred extensive hyaline membrane formation lining the alveoli, alveolar ducts, and sacs. Type II alveolar lining cells are undergoing hypertrophy and hyperplasia. There may be early fibroblastic proliferation and deposition of collagen. Scattered areas of bronchopneumonia may be observed.

Seven to 14 days: Grossly, the lungs are still heavy and almost airless. The previous histologic changes have largely been replaced by extensive fibroblastic proliferation in both interstitial and alveolar compartments, associated with rapidly progressing collagen deposition and fibrosis. By this stage pneumonia is almost invariable, and in view of the propensity for these patients to develop infection with gram-negative organisms, there is often tissue necrosis and microabscesses.

ROENTGENOGRAPHIC MANIFESTATIONS

Remarkably good correlation has been reported between the roentgenographic patterns observed during life and the pathologic changes observed at necropsy (Figure 10–17).[120, 121]

Up to 12 hours: All observers report a characteristic delay of up to 12 hours from the clinical onset of respiratory failure to the appearance of abnormalities on the chest roentgenogram.

Twelve to 24 hours: Patchy, ill-defined opacities appear throughout both lungs. The appearance is the same as patchy air-space edema of cardiac origin, except that heart size is usually normal and there is no convincing evidence of redistribution of blood flow to upper zones.

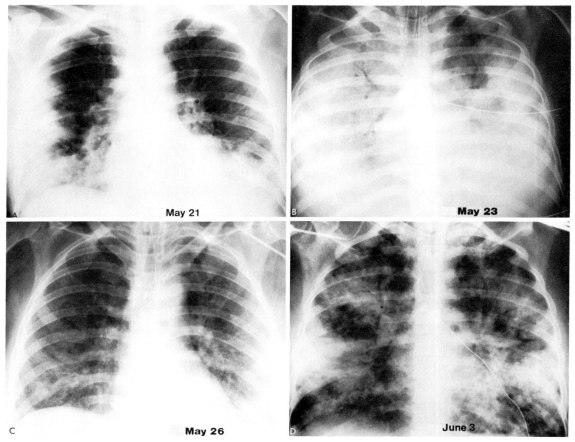

Figure 10–17. Acute Posttraumatic Respiratory Insufficiency ("Shock Lung," ARDS). This 18-year-old girl was admitted to the intensive care unit in severe shock following a motor vehicle accident. A roentgenogram the day after admission (*A*) revealed homogeneous consolidation of the left lower lobe and the axillary portion of the right lung. Two days later (*B*), both lungs were massively consolidated by pulmonary edema; note the prominent air bronchogram. It is predicted that at this time, histologic sections of the lung would have shown the interstitium and alveoli to be filled with highly proteinaceous edema fluid, associated with extensive necrosis of alveolar lining cells. Three days later, following vigorous supportive therapy and positive end-expiratory pressure (PEEP) ventilation, the patient's condition improved slightly and a roentgenogram (*C*) revealed considerable clearing of the diffuse air-space edema. At this time, it is predicted that the edema fluid would have largely disappeared from the alveoli but that thick hyaline membranes would have been present on alveolar walls. Eight days later (*D*), both lungs had become massively consolidated in a pattern compatible with combined edema and acute air-space pneumonia. The patient died shortly thereafter. At necropsy, both lungs were found to be massively consolidated and very heavy. Histologically, there was extensive fibroblastic proliferation and collagen deposition, not only within the interstitium but within alveoli.

Twenty-four to 48 hours: The patchy zones of consolidation rapidly coalesce to a point of massive air-space consolidation of both lungs (Figure 10–17B). Pleural effusion is characteristically absent; its presence should strongly suggest a complicating acute pneumonia or pulmonary infarction.

Five to 7 days: Characteristically, there occurs improvement in the roentgenographic picture, the homogeneous consolidation becoming inhomogeneous, suggesting diminution of the amount of alveolar edema (Figure 10–17C). It is during this period that acute pneumonia frequently becomes evident in the form of local areas of consolidation. Continuous positive

pressure ventilation can lead to diffuse interstitial emphysema, which may be readily visible against the background of extensive parenchymal consolidation. It is important to recognize this development because of the frequency of impending pneumomediastinum and pneumothorax.

Over 7 days: The lungs remain diffusely abnormal but the pattern tends to become reticular[120] or "bubbly."[123] It is likely that this pattern represents diffuse interstitial and patchy air-space fibrosis so characteristic of the end-stage picture observed pathologically.

Probably the most important differential diagnostic possibility in the early stages of the disease is massive thromboembolism. The clinical manifestations may be identical, and although there may be roentgenographic evidence of pulmonary oligemia and a bulging of central pulmonary arteries, such signs may be absent and only clinical awareness and a lung scan will permit diagnosis.

CLINICAL MANIFESTATIONS

The symptoms and signs of ARDS vary from patient to patient, depending upon the exciting cause. Although precipitating causes are multitudinous,[124] reports in the literature and our own experience suggest that the most frequent are gram-negative septicemia, severe body trauma, major surgery, particularly cardiovascular, viral pneumonia due to influenza or adenovirus types 4 and 7, and narcotic overdose.

The clinical presentation varies widely and may represent either end of a broad spectrum. For example, patients may present with clinical features of septic shock including peripheral vasodilatation and high fever, or with peripheral vasoconstriction, hypopyrexia, and hypotension. Hypotension is by no means invariable. Tissue hypoxia is manifested by confusion and anxiety; metabolic acidosis is evident on blood gas analysis. Shock is associated with hyperventilation and hypocapnia. As edema fluid accumulates in the lungs, cyanosis usually becomes evident and may be accentuated by fluid replacement for hypovolemia. Cough is initially dry but may become productive of viscous mucoid material and eventually, if the patient lives long enough, may become purulent as a result of superimposed bacterial pneumonia. Physical findings vary with the precipitating cause; rales and signs of consolidation are usually detected on examination of the chest.

Blood gas analysis reveals a severe degree of hypoxemia, which often persists and even worsens despite IPPB; the institution of PEEP may be crucial to survival. The hypoxemia frequently is accompanied by acidemia, which is initially due to accumulation of lactic acid but later reflects both metabolic and respiratory components as gas exchange deteriorates. The establishment of a diagnosis is facilitated very little by other laboratory tests, although a greater sensitivity and specificity in measurement of lung water holds some hope for the future.[50]

Patients who recover may show remarkably few abnormalities of pulmonary function;[125] however, despite apparent good health, most patients manifest some decrease in lung volume and flow rate and particularly in diffusing capacity.

PULMONARY EDEMA ASSOCIATED WITH NORMAL HEART SIZE

As discussed previously, the most common cause of pulmonary edema is a rise in pulmonary venous pressure secondary to disease of the left side of the heart, either from chronic states such as mitral stenosis, or, more commonly, from acute myocardial ischemia or infarction affecting the left ventricle. In both these circumstances the heart is usually enlarged, but sometimes acute myocardial infarction results in interstitial or air-space pulmonary edema in the absence of roentgenographic evidence of cardiomegaly. Of all other causes of edema unassociated with cardiac enlargement, the two most common are also usually associated with elevated microvascular pressure—heroin intoxication and some forms of adult respiratory distress syndrome. Of the remaining causes—left atrial myxoma, cor triatriatum, pulmonary veno-occlusive disease, neurogenic edema, inhalation of noxious fumes, aspiration of liquids (Mendelson's syndrome or near-drowning), high altitude, post-traumatic lung contusion, fat embolism, and rapid thoracentesis—only the first four are associated with elevated microvascular pressure. The differential diagnosis of these many causes of pulmonary edema associated with a normal heart size can usually be established without difficulty on the basis of history, although there are few if any distinguishing roentgenographic features.

REFERENCES

1. Harris, P., and Heath, D.: The Human Pulmonary Circulation: Its Form and Function in Health and Disease. Baltimore, Williams & Wilkins, 1962.
2. Dantzker, D. R., and Bower, J. S.: Partial reversibility of chronic pulmonary hypertension caused by pulmonary thromboembolic disease. Am. Rev. Resp. Dis., 124:129, 1981.
3. Follath, F., Burkart, F., and Schweizer, W.: Drug-induced pulmonary hypertension? Br. Med. J., 1:265, 1971.
4. Guertner, H. P., Gertsch, M., Salzmann, C., Scherrer, M., Stucki, P., and Wyss, F.: Häufen sich die primär vasculären Formen des chronischen Cor pulmonale? Schweiz. Med. Wochenschr., 98:1579, 1968.
5. Kay, J. M., Heath, D., Smith, P., Bras, G., and Summerell, J.: Fulvine and the pulmonary circulation. Thorax, 26:249, 1971.
6. Kay, J. M., Smith, P., and Heath, D.: Electron microscopy of *Crotalaria* pulmonary hypertension. Thorax, 24:511, 1969.
7. Wagenvoort, C. A., Wagenvoort, N., and Dijk, H. J.: Effect of fulvine on pulmonary arteries and veins of the rat. Thorax, 29:522, 1974.
8. Heath, D., Shaba, J., Williams, A., Smith, P., and

Kombe, A.: A pulmonary hypertension-producing plant from Tanzania. Thorax, *30*:399, 1975.

9. Fishman, A. P., and Pietra, G. G.: Primary pulmonary hypertension. Ann. Rev. Med., *31*:421, 1980.

10. Senior R. M., Britton, R. C., Turino, G. M., Wood, J. A., Langer, G. A., and Fishman, A. P.: Pulmonary hypertension associated with cirrhosis of the liver and with portacaval shunts. Circulation, *37*:88, 1968.

11. Fishman, A. P.: Primary pulmonary hypertension: More light or more tunnel? Ann. Intern. Med., *94*:815, 1981.

12. Evans, W.: The less common forms of pulmonary hypertension. Br. Heart J., *21*:197, 1959.

13. Shinnick, J. P., Cudkowicz, L., Blanco, G., Calderon, C., Haskin, M., Johnston, R., Kauffman, L., Najmi, M., Oslick, T., Segal, B., and Shirley, D.: A problem in pulmonary hypertension. Part 1: The clinical course. Chest, *65*:69, 1974.

14. Shinnick, J. P., Cudkowicz, L., Saldana, M., and Brodsky, I.: A problem in pulmonary hypertension. Part 2: The final course and autopsy findings. Chest, *65*:192, 1974.

15. Thompson, P., and McRae, C.: Familial pulmonary hypertension. Evidence of autosomal dominant inheritance. Br. Heart J., *32*:758, 1970.

16. Walcott, G., Burchell, H. B., and Brown, A. L., Jr.: Primary pulmonary hypertension. Am. J. Med., *49*:70, 1970.

17. Gupta, B. D., Moodie, D. S., and Hodgman, J. R.: Primary pulmonary hypertension in adults. Clinical features, catheterization findings and long-term follow-up. Cleve. Clin. Q., *47*:275, 1980.

18. Yu, P. N.: Primary pulmonary hypertension: Report of six cases and review of literature. Ann. Intern. Med., *49*:1138, 1958.

19. Wagenvoort, C. A.: Lung biopsy specimens in the evaluation of pulmonary vascular disease. Chest, *77*:614, 1980.

20. Reeves, J. T.: Hope in primary pulmonary hypertension? N. Engl. J. Med., *302*:112, 1981.

21. Williams, J. O.: Death following injection of lung scanning agent in a case of pulmonary hypertension. Br. J. Radiol., *47*:61, 1974.

22. Caldini, P., Gensini, G. G., and Hoffman, M. S.: Primary pulmonary hypertension with death during right heart catheterization: A case report and a survery of reported fatalities. Am. J. Cardiol., *4*:519, 1959.

23. Riedel, M., Stanek, V., Widimsky, J., and Prerovsky, I.: Longterm follow-up of patients with pulmonary thromboembolism. Late prognosis and evolution of hemodynamic and respiratory data. Chest, *81*:151, 1982.

24. Wagenvoort, C. A., and Wagenvoort, N.: Pulmonary veno-occlusive disease. *In* Wagenvoort, C. A., and Wagenvoort, N. (eds.): Pathology of Pulmonary Hypotension. New York, John Wiley and Sons, 1977, p. 217.

25. Rambihar, V. S., Fallen, E. L., and Cairns, J. A.: Pulmonary veno-occlusive disease: Antemortem diagnosis from roentgenographic and hemodynamic findings. C.M.A. Journal, *120*:1519, 1979.

26. Shackelford, G. D., Sacks, E. J., Mullins, J. D., and McAlister, W. H.: Pulmonary venoocclusive disease: Case report and review of the literature. Am. J. Roentgenol., *128*:643, 1977.

27. McDonnell, P. J., Summer, W. R., and Hutchins, G. M.: Pulmonary veno-occlusive disease. Morphological changes suggesting a viral cause. J.A.M.A., *246*:667, 1981.

28. Lupi, H. E., Sanchez, T. G., Horwitz, S., and Gutierrez, F. E.: Pulmonary artery involvement in Takayasu's arteritis. Chest, *67*:69, 1967.

29. Gay, B. B., Jr., Franch, R. H., Shuford, W. H., and Rogers, J. V., Jr.: The roentgenologic features of single and multiple coarctations of the pulmonary artery and branches. Am. J. Roentgenol., *90*:599, 1963.

30. Steiner, R. E.: Radiology of pulmonary circulation. Chamberlain lecture—1963. Am. J. Roentgenol., *91*:249, 1964.

31. Emirgil, C., Sobol, B. J., Herbert, W. H., and Trout, K. W.: Routine pulmonary function studies as a key to the status of the lesser circulation in chronic obstructive pulmonary disease. Am. J. Med., *50*:191, 1971.

32. Matthay, R. A., Schwarz, M. I., Ellis, J. H., Jr., Steele, P. P., Siebert, P. E., Durrance, J. R., and Levin, D. C.: Pulmonary artery hypertension in chronic obstructive pulmonary disease: Determination by chest radiography. Invest. Radiol., *16*:95, 1981.

33. Austin, J. H. M., Yount, B. G., Jr., Thomas, H. M., III, and Enson, Y.: Radiologic assessment of pulmonary arterial pressure and blood volume in chronic, diffuse, interstitial pulmonary diseases. Invest. Radiol., *14*:9, 1979.

34. Harrison, C. V.: Pulmonary hypertension. A symposium. IV. The pathology of the pulmonary vessels in pulmonary hypertension. Br. J. Radiol., *31*:217, 1958.

35. Simon, M.: The pulmonary veins in mitral stenosis. J. Fac. Radiol., *9*:25, 1958.

36. West, J. B., Dollery, C. T., and Heard, B. E.: Increased pulmonary vascular resistance in the dependent zone of the isolated dog lung caused by perivascular edema. Circ. Res., *17*:191, 1965.

37. Muir, A. L., Hall, D. L., Despas, P., and Hogg, J. C.: Distribution of blood flow in the lungs in acute pulmonary edema in dogs. J. Appl. Physiol., *33*:763, 1972.

38. Surette, G. D., Muir, A. L., Hogg, J. C., and Fraser, R. G.: Roentgenographic study of blood flow redistribution in acute pulmonary edema in dogs. Invest. Radiol., *10*:109, 1975.

39. Ravin, C. E., Greenspan, R H., McLoud, T. C., Lange, R. C., Langou, R. A., and Putman, C. E.: Redistribution of pulmonary blood flow secondary to pulmonary arterial hypertension. Invest. Radiol., *15*:29, 1980.

40. Milne, E. N. C.: Pulmonary blood flow distribution. Invest. Radiol., *12*:479, 1977.

41. Chait, A., Cohen, H. E., Meltzer, L. E., and VanDurme, J.-P.: The bedside chest radiograph in the evaluation of incipient heart failure. Radiology, *105*:563, 1972.

42. McHugh, T. J., Forrester, J. S., Adler, L., Zion, D., and Swan, H. J. C.: Pulmonary vascular congestion in acute myocardial infarction: Hemodynamic and radiologic correlations. Ann. Intern. Med., *76*:29, 1972.

43. Simon, M.: The pulmonary vessels: Their hemodynamic evaluation using routine radiographs. Radiol. Clin. North Am., *1*:363, 1963.

44. Fishman, A. P.: Pulmonary edema: The water-exchanging function of the lung. Circulation, *46*:390, 1972.

45. Robin, E. D., Cross, C. E., and Zelis, R.: Pulmonary edema (first of two parts). N. Engl. J. Med., *288*:239, 1973.

46. Robin, E. D., Cross, C. E., and Zelis, R.: Pulmonary

edema (second of two parts). N. Engl. J. Med., *288*:292, 1973.

47. Staub, N. C.: 'State of the art' review. Pathogenesis of pulmonary edema. Am. Rev. Resp. Dis., *109*:358, 1974.
48. Staub, N. C.: Pulmonary edema. Physiol. Rev., *54*:678, 1974.
49. Staub, N. C.: Pulmonary edema. Physiologic approaches to management. Chest, *74*:559, 1978.
50. Butler, J.: Pulmonary oedema. Clin. Sci., *60*:1, 1981.
51. Noble, W. H.: Pulmonary oedema: A review. Canad. Anaesth. Soc. J., *27*:286, 1980.
52. Snashall, P. D.: Pulmonary oedema. Br. J. Dis. Chest, *74*:2, 1980.
53. Staub, N. C., Nagano, H., and Pearce, M. L.: Pulmonary edema in dogs, especially the sequence of fluid accumulation in lungs. J. Appl. Physiol., *22*:227, 1967.
54. Schneeberger-Keeley, E. E., and Karnovsky, M. J.: The ultrastructural basis of alveolar-capillary membrane permeability to peroxidase used as a tracer. J. Cell Biol., *37*:781, 1968.
55. Anderson, R. J., Potts, D. E., Gabow, P. A., Rumack, B. H., and Schrier, R. W.: Unrecognized adult salicylate intoxication. Ann. Intern. Med., *85*:745, 1976.
56. Lauweryns, J. M., and Boussauw, L.: The ultrastructure of pulmonary lymphatic capillaries of newborn rabbits and of human infants. Lymphology, *2*:108, 1969.
57. Warren, M. F., and Drinker, C. K.: The flow of lymph from the lungs of the dog. Am. J. Physiol., *136*:207, 1942.
58. Dumont, A. E., Clauss, R. H., Reed, G. E., and Tice, D. A.: Lymph drainage in patients with congestive heart failure. Comparison with findings in hepatic cirrhosis. N. Engl. J. Med., *269*:949, 1963.
59. Uhley, H. N., Leeds, S. E., Sampson, J. J., and Friedman, M.: Some observations on the role of the lymphatics in experimental acute pulmonary edema. Circ. Res., *9*:688, 1961.
60. Uhley, H. N., Leeds, S. E., Sampson, J. J., and Friedman, M.: Role of pulmonary lymphatics in chronic pulmonary edema. Circ. Res., *11*:966, 1962.
61. Leeds, S. E., Uhley, H. N., Sampson, J. J., and Friedman, M.: Significance of changes in the pulmonary lymph flow in acute and chronic experimental pulmonary edema. Am. J. Surg., *114*:254, 1967.
62. Heard, B. E., Steiner, R. E., Herdan, A., and Gleason, D.: Oedema and fibrosis of the lungs in left ventricular failure. Br. J. Radiol., *41*:161, 1968.
63. Fazio, F., Jones, T., MacArthur, C. G. C., Rhodes, C. G., Steiner, R. E., and Hughes, J. M. B.: Measurement of regional pulmonary oedema in man using radioactive water ($H_2^{15}O$). Br. J. Radiol., *49*:393, 1976.
64. Milne, E. N. C.: Physiological interpretation of the plain radiograph in mitral stenosis, including a review of criteria for the radiological estimation of pulmonary arterial and venous pressures. Br. J. Radiol., *36*:902, 1963.
65. Don, C., and Johnson, R.: The nature and significance of peribronchial cuffing in pulmonary edema. Radiology, *125*:577, 1977.
66. Hogg, J. C., Agarawal, J. B., Gardiner, A. J. S., Palmer, W. H., and Macklem, P. T.: Distribution of airway resistance with developing pulmonary edema in dogs. J. Appl. Physiol., *32*:20, 1972.

67. Leeming, B. W. A.: Gravitational edema of the lungs observed during assisted respiration. Chest, *64*:719, 1973.
68. Calenoff, L., Kruglik, G. D., and Woodruff, A.: Unilateral pulmonary edema. Radiology, *126*:19, 1978.
69. Nessa, C. G., and Rigler, L. G.: The roentgenological manifestations of pulmonary edema. Radiology, *37*:35, 1941.
70. Hodson, C. J.: Pulmonary oedema and the "batswing" shadow. J. Fac. Radiol., *1*:176, 1950.
71. Fleischner, F. G.: The butterfly pattern of acute pulmonary edema. Am. J. Cardiol., *20*:39, 1967.
72. Mayerson, H. S.: The physiologic importance of lymph. *In* Hamilton, W. F. (ed.): Handbook of Physiology, sect. 2, vol. II. Washington, D.C., American Physiological Society, 1963, p. 1035.
73. Macpherson, R. I., and Banerjee, A. K.: Acute glomerulonephritis: A chest film diagnosis? J. Can. Assoc. Radiol., *25*:58, 1974.
74. Thompson, J. S., Severson, C. D., Parmely, M. J., Marmorstein, L., and Simmons, A.: Pulmonary "hypersensitivity" reactions induced by transfusion of non–HL-A leukoagglutinins. N. Engl. J. Med., *284*:1120, 1971.
75. Felman, A. H.: Neurogenic pulmonary edema: Observations in 6 patients. Am. J. Roentgenol., *112*:393, 1971.
76. Alexander, I. G. S.: The ultrastructure of the pulmonary alveolar vessels in Mendelson's (acid pulmonary aspiration) syndrome. Br. J. Anaesth., *40*:408, 1968.
77. Ribaudo, C. A., and Grace, W. J.: Pulmonary aspiration. Am. J. Med., *50*:510, 1971.
78. Landay, M. J., Christensen, E. E., and Bynum, L. J.: Pulmonary manifestations of acute aspiration of gastric contents. Am. J. Roentgenol., *131*:587, 1978.
79. Berris, B., and Kasler, D.: Pulmonary aspiration of gastric acid—Mendelson's syndrome. Can. Med. Assoc. J., *92*:905, 1965.
80. Hasan, S., Avery, W. G., Fabian, C., and Sackner, M. A.: Near drowning in humans: A report of 36 patients. Chest, *59*:191, 1971.
81. Miles, S.: Drowning. Br. Med. J., *3*:597, 1968.
82. Fuller, R. H.: The 1962 Wellcome Prize Essay: "Drowning and the postimmersion syndrome. A clinicopathologic study." Milit. Med., *128*:22, 1963.
83. Bradley, M. E.: Near-drowning: CPR is just the beginning. J. Resp. Dis., *2*:37, 1981.
84. Modell, J. H., Graves, S. A., and Ketover, A.: Clinical course of 91 consecutive near-drowning victims. Chest, *70*:231, 1976.
85. Sekar, T. S., MacDonnell, K. F., Namsirikul, P., and Herman, R. S.: Survival after prolonged submersion in cold water without neurologic sequelae. Report of two cases. Arch. Intern. Med., *140*:775, 1980.
86. Ansell, G.: A national survey of radiological complications: Interim report. Clin. Radiol., *19*:175, 1968.
87. Heffner, J. E., and Sahn, S. A.: Salicylate-induced pulmonary edema. Clinical features and prognosis. Ann. Intern. Med., *95*:405, 1981.
88. Kamat, S. R., and Banerji, B. C.: Study of cardiopulmonary function on exposure to high altitude. I. Acute acclimatization to an altitude of 3500 to 4000 meters in relation to altitude sickness and cardiopulmonary function. Am. Rev. Resp. Dis., *106*:404, 1972.
89. Kamat, S. R., Rao, T. L., Sarma, B. S., Venkataraman, C., and Raju, V. R. K.: Study of cardiopul-

monary function on exposure to high altitude. II. Effects of prolonged stay at 3500 to 4000 meters and reversal on return to sea level. Am. Rev. Resp. Dis., *106*:414, 1972.

90. Viswanathan, R., Jain, S. K., Subramanian, S., Subramanian, T. A. V., Dua, G. L., and Giri, J.: Pulmonary edema of high altitude. II. Clinical, aerohemodynamic, and biochemical studies in a group with history of pulmonary edema of high altitude. Am. Rev. Resp. Dis., *100*:334, 1969.

91. Menon, N. D.: High-altitude pulmonary edema. A clinical study. N. Engl. J. Med., *273*:66, 1965.

92. Visscher, M. B.: The pathophysiology of lung edema: A physical and physicochemical problem. Lancet, *82*:43, 1962.

93. Hultgren, H. N., Lopez, C. E., Lundberg, E., and Miller, H.: Physiologic studies of pulmonary edema at high altitude. Circulation, *29*:393, 1964.

94. Waqaruddin, M., and Bernstein, A.: Re-expansion pulmonary oedema. Thorax, *30*:54, 1975.

95. Buczko, G. B., Grossman, R. F., and Goldberg, M.: Re-expansion pulmonary edema: Evidence for increased capillary permeability. C.M.A. Journal, *125*:460, 1981.

96. Guyton, A. C., and Lindsey, A. W.: Effect of elevated left atrial pressure and decreased plasma protein concentration on the development of pulmonary edema. Circ. Res., *7*:649, 1959.

97. Rusznyák, I., Földi, M., and Szabó, G.: Lymphatics and Lymph Circulation: Physiology and Pathology, 2nd English ed. Oxford, Pergamon Press, 1967.

98. Duberstein, J. L., and Kaufman, D. M.: A clinical study of an epidemic of heroin intoxication and heroin-induced pulmonary edema. Am. J. Med., *51*:704, 1971.

99. Helpern, M., and Rho, Y.-M.: Deaths from narcotism in New York City. Incidence, circumstances, and postmortem findings. N.Y. State J. Med., *66*:2391, 1966.

100. Helpern, M.: Interim report on narcotic program, August 12, 1963. Summarized in National Association for the Prevention of Addiction to Narcotics Newsletter, *2*, No. 2, 1964.

101. Katz, S., Aberman, A., Frand, U. I., Stein, I. M., and Fulop, M.: Heroin pulmonary edema. Evidence for increased pulmonary capillary permeability. Am. Rev. Resp. Dis., *106*:472, 1972.

102. Presant, S., Knight, L., and Klassen, G.: Methadone-induced pulmonary edema. Can. Med. Assoc. J., *113*:966, 1975.

103. Petty, T. L., and Ashbaugh, D. G.: The adult respiratory distress syndrome. Clinical features, factors influencing prognosis and principles of management. Chest, *60*:233, 1971.

104. Blaisdell, F. W., and Schlobohm, R. M.: The respiratory distress syndrome: A review. Surgery, *74*:251, 1973.

105. Brigham, K. L., Woolverton, W. C., and Staub, N. C.: Increased pulmonary vascular permeability after *Pseudomonas aeruginosa* (Ps.) bacteremia in unanesthetized sheep. Fed. Proc., *32*:440, 1973.

106. Fein, A., Grossman, R. F., Jones, J. G., Overland, E., Pitts, L., Murray, J. F., and Staub, N. C.: The value of edema fluid protein measurement in patients with pulmonary edema. Am. J. Med., *67*:32, 1979.

107. Sprung, C. L., Rackow, E. C., Fein, I. A., Jacob, A. I., and Isikoff, S. K.: The spectrum of pulmonary edema: differentiation of cardiogenic, intermediate, and noncardiogenic forms of pulmonary edema. Am. Rev. Resp. Dis., *124*:718, 1981.

108. MacLean, L. D., Duff, J. H., Scott, H. M., and Peretz, D. I.: Treatment of shock in man based on hemodynamic diagnosis. Surg. Gynecol. Obstet., *120*:1, 1965.

109. Kwaan, H. C.: Disseminated intravascular coagulation. Med. Clin. North Am., *56*:177, 1972.

110. Connell, R. S., Swank, R. L., and Webb, M. C.: The development of pulmonary ultrastructural lesions during hemorrhagic shock. J. Trauma, *15*:116, 1975.

111. Webb, W. R.: Pulmonary complications of nonthoracic trauma: Summary of the National Research Council Conference. J. Trauma, *9*:700, 1969.

112. Greenfield, L. J., Barkett, V. M., and Coalson, J. J.: The role of surfactant in the pulmonary response to trauma. J. Trauma, *8*:735, 1968.

113. Unger, K. M., Shibel, E. M., and Moser, K. M.: Detection of left ventricular failure in patients with adult respiratory distress syndrome. Chest, *67*:8, 1975.

114. Stevens, P. M.: Assessment of acute respiratory failure: Cardiac versus pulmonary causes. Chest, *67*:1, 1975.

115. King, E. G.: Influence of mechanical ventilation and pulmonary disease on pulmonary artery pressure monitoring. C.M.A. Journal, *121*:901, 1979.

116. Burrows, F. G. O., and Edwards, J. M.: A pulmonary disease in patients ventilated with high oxygen concentrations. Br. J. Radiol., *43*:848, 1970.

117. Barsch, J., Birbara, C., Eggers, G. W. N., Jr., Krumlofsky, F., Sanit, Y. W., Smith, W., Smith, R., and Webster, J.: Positive pressure as a cause of respirator-induced lung disease. Ann. Intern. Med., *72*:810, 1970.

118. Llamas, R., and Forthman, H. J.: Respiratory distress syndrome in the adult after cardiopulmonary bypass. A successful therapeutic approach. J.A.M.A., *225*:1183, 1973.

119. Byrick, R. J., Finlayson, D. C., and Noble, W. H.: Pulmonary arterial pressure increases during cardiopulmonary bypass, a potential cause of pulmonary edema. Anesthesiology, *46*:433, 1977.

120. Ostendorf, P., Birzle, H., Vogel, W., and Mittermayer, C.: Pulmonary radiographic abnormalities in shock. Roentgen-clinical-pathological correlation. Radiology, *115*:257, 1975.

121. Putman, C. E., Minagi, H., and Blaisdell, F. W.: The roentgen appearance of disseminated intravascular coagulation (DIC). Radiology, *109*:13, 1973.

122. Weibel, E. R.: Looking into the lung: What can it tell us? Am. J. Roentgenol., *133*:1021, 1979.

123. Dyck, D. R., and Zylak, C. J.: Acute respiratory distress in adults. Radiology, *106*:497, 1973.

124. Sutton, F. D., Hudson, L. D., and Petty, T. L.: Recognition and management of the adult respiratory distress syndrome. Chest, *66*:(Suppl.):34s, 1974.

125. Klein, J. J., van Haeringen, J. R., Sluiter, H. J., Holloway, R., and Peset, R.: Pulmonary function after recovery from the adult respiratory distress syndrome. Chest, *69*(Suppl.):350, 1976.

126. Carlson, R. W., Schaeffer, R. C., Jr., Carpio, M., and Weil, M. H.: Edema fluid and coagulation changes during fulminant pulmonary edema. Chest, *79*:43, 1981.

11

Diseases of the Airways

OBSTRUCTIVE AIRWAY DISEASE

This chapter is concerned with several lung diseases that are grouped together because of their common characteristics of hypersecretion from and obstruction of the airways. Obstruction can occur in either the upper or the lower airways, and in the latter site may be local or diffuse. Although the clinical manifestations of obstruction of the upper airways (defined as that portion of the conducting system from the mouth to the tracheal carina) are usually sufficiently distinctive to permit prompt recognition, a significant number of cases of chronic upper airway obstruction are misdiagnosed as asthma or chronic bronchitis. Lower airway obstruction results from a large number of entities of varying etiology and pathogenesis whose clinical manifestations may overlap.

In recent years, as a result of correlative clinical, pathologic, roentgenologic, and physiologic studies, our knowledge of diseases characterized by chronic lower airway obstruction has been greatly extended, but with the better understanding has come the realization that precise differentiation of the individual diseases often is difficult. The majority of patients with "chronic obstructive pulmonary disease," or COPD, have chronic bronchitis, intractable asthma, obstructive emphysema, bronchiectasis, or a combination of these conditions. However, the term is not restricted to these four disorders. Other diseases can give rise to similar clinical and physiologic manifestations.

The recognition of diseases within the broad category of "chronic obstructive pulmonary disease" implies identification of increased resistance to air flow in the conducting system. In the later stages of these diseases or in acute exacerbations, airway obstruction is judged to be present on the basis of rhonchi or continuous wheezing, prolonged expiration, and poor air entry. Dyspnea is a frequent complaint, although diffuse rhonchi may be present in pa-

tients who are asymptomatic. In this latter group the chest roentgenogram almost invariably is normal, and in these patients as well as those who manifest neither physical signs nor roentgenologic evidence of airway obstruction the diagnosis must be based on tests of pulmonary function. Chronic obstructive pulmonary disease can be assessed fairly accurately roentgenologically when the disease is advanced; by contrast, roentgenograms may sometimes present convincing evidence of abnormality when there is little or no clinical evidence of obstructive pulmonary disease. In many of these latter cases the roentgenographic examination is part of a screening procedure and subsequent direct questioning reveals evidence of deteriorating exercise tolerance or cough.

In no other area of pulmonary disease is a close correlation of the clinical, roentgenologic, and pulmonary function parameters so vital in the overall assessment of the patient as in chronic obstructive airway disease.

This chapter is divided into two major sections: affections of the upper airways (pharynx, larynx, and trachea) and the much larger group of diseases that affect the lower airways.

OBSTRUCTIVE DISEASE OF THE UPPER AIRWAYS

ACUTE UPPER AIRWAY OBSTRUCTION

This disorder occurs most commonly in infants and young children because of the small intraluminal caliber of their upper airways. Regardless of etiology, the cardinal symptom is a sudden onset of dyspnea or even suffocation, sometimes requiring emergency tracheostomy. The cause of respiratory distress usually is readily apparent from the history. For example, patients with angioneurotic edema may give a history of allergy, with or without familial occurrence, and have usually experienced pre-

521

vious episodes dating back to childhood. Stridor is common, and its presence warrants immediate direct or indirect visualization of the larynx.

Roentgenographic manifestations vary somewhat according to the specific etiology. Whereas chronic obstruction of the intrathoracic trachea or of the lower airways characteristically results in pulmonary overinflation, acute obstruction of the upper airways may be associated with lungs of normal or even small volume; at the same time, the airway *proximal* to the site of obstruction will be unusually distended during inspiration. This combination of changes should be readily apparent on lateral views of the soft tissues of the neck and thorax and constitutes highly suggestive evidence of acute upper airway obstruction.

The causes of acute upper airway obstruction include infection, edema, hemorrhage, and foreign bodies.

Infection

Infection may cause severe narrowing of the upper airways in infants and young children. Acute pharyngitis and tonsillitis most commonly are caused by β-hemolytic streptococci. Acute laryngotracheitis (croup) is caused by parainfluenza or respiratory syncytial viruses and results in a characteristic narrowing of the subglottic trachea. A variant of this usual picture is seen in so-called membranous croup in which the inflammatory narrowing of the upper trachea is associated with the presence of adherent or semiadherent mucopurulent membranes resulting in marked irregularity of contour of the proximal tracheal mucosa.[1] Acute epiglottitis usually is caused by *Haemophilus influenzae* and occasionally by *Staphylococcus aureus* or *Streptococcus pneumoniae*.[2] Although acute epiglottitis most commonly affects infants and young children, it also occurs in adults, in whom it often is unrecognized.[3, 4] Roentgenographic findings include swelling of the epiglottis, aryepiglottic folds, arytenoids, uvula, and prevertebral soft tissues; the hypopharynx and oropharynx tend to be ballooned and the valleculae obliterated. Narrowing of the subglottic trachea, simulating croup, occurs in roughly a quarter of affected children.[5] The presenting symptoms are severe sore throat and difficulty in breathing.

Acute retropharyngeal abscess can result in severe upper airway obstruction in both infants and adults (Figure 11–1) and may extend into the mediastinum, where it sets up an acute mediastinal abscess.

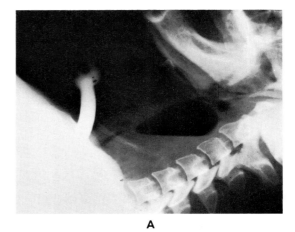

A

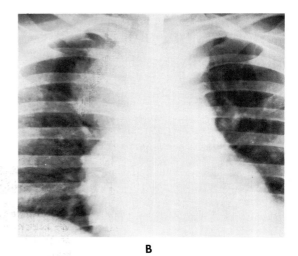

B

Figure 11–1. Acute Retropharyngeal and Mediastinal Abscess. This 29-year-old woman was admitted to the hospital with an 8-day history of increasing dyspnea, difficulty in swallowing, and loss of voice. An emergency tracheostomy was performed. Lateral roentgenography of the soft tissues of the neck with a horizontal x-ray beam (A) revealed a large accumulation of gas and fluid in the retropharyngeal space associated with complete obliteration of the air space of the hypopharynx and anterior displacement of the cervical trachea. An anteroposterior roentgenogram of the chest (B) showed a large mediastinal mass projecting predominantly to the right of the midline. The retropharyngeal and mediastinal abscesses were evacuated and drained surgically; 3 weeks later the mediastinal silhouette was almost normal.

Edema

As a cause of acute upper airway obstruction, edema of noninfective origin characteristically affects the larynx. Underlying causes include trauma, the inhalation of irritant noxious gases, and "angioneurotic edema." The last named is perhaps the commonest cause of acute upper airway obstruction and includes a variety of subgroups, some with an allergic or anaphylactic etiology, some inherited, and others of idiopathic origin.[6] Although many patients are atopic, with or without a familial history, the precise mechanism for the development of angioedema is identified in less than one-fifth of cases. In a minority, acute episodes characteristic of a type I reaction are provoked by certain foods, inhalants, bee stings, or drugs. Type III reactions of a less acute nature may be caused by antiserum, certain drugs such as penicillin, and some radiographic contrast media. Certain drugs such as aspirin may cause nonimmunologic histamine release, particularly in adults with nasal polyps.

The hereditary form of angioneurotic edema usually begins in childhood and is characterized by recurrent attacks, often in association with abdominal cramps. These attacks are not precipitated by allergens, but may follow local trauma such as tonsillectomy or tooth extraction or may be associated with emotional upsets. Simultaneously with laryngeal obstruction, the skin may show angioedema or urticaria. The prognosis in the hereditary form of angioneurotic edema is very grave, approximately one-third of affected family members dying from suffocation.[6]

Retropharyngeal Hemorrhage

Acute upper airway obstruction may result from hemorrhage into the retropharyngeal space from a variety of causes, including neck surgery, external trauma, carotid angiography, transbrachial retrograde catheterization, and erosion of an artery secondary to infection. Hemorrhage may occur spontaneously in hemophiliacs or in patients with acute leukemia or receiving anticoagulant therapy.[7]

Foreign Bodies

Obstruction of the air and food passages by foreign bodies occurs most frequently in infants and young children and tends to affect the esophagus and major bronchi much more commonly than the upper airway.[8]

CHRONIC UPPER AIRWAY OBSTRUCTION

GENERAL CONSIDERATIONS

In contrast to acute upper airway obstruction, whose cause is generally apparent, chronic obstructive disease of the pharynx, larynx, and trachea frequently is misdiagnosed as asthma or bronchitis. Dyspnea is the usual presenting complaint, often first noted on exertion and sometimes exacerbated when the patient assumes a recumbent position. In a minority of patients obstruction results in serious impairment of gas exchange, cor pulmonale, and sleep disturbance.

Etiology

A wide variety of conditions affecting all levels of the upper airway, from the nasopharynx to the tracheal carina, can cause chronic upper airway obstruction. The following list is by no means comprehensive: hypertrophy of the tonsils and adenoids, tracheal stenosis following tracheostomy or prolonged tracheal intubation, primary neoplasms, and a number of rare primary diseases of the trachea such as relapsing polychondritis, "saber-sheath" trachea, and tracheobronchomegaly. Disturbance in the dynamic activity of the trachea as a result of increased compliance of its walls—tracheomalacia—may occur as a part of some of these conditions. Each of these possesses fairly characteristic roentgenographic manifestations that permit their differentiation, and each is discussed in some detail further on. However, certain physiologic, roentgenologic, and clinical manifestations are common to all, regardless of their precise nature, and these will be described first.

Physiologic Manifestations

An excellent method of portraying how physiologic determinants of flow can be affected by various obstructing lesions of the conducting system is the flow-volume loop, which combines maximum expiratory and inspiratory curves from TLC and RV, respectively (Figure 11–2). The flow-volume loop is altered by having normal subjects breathe through fixed external resistances.[9] Miller and Hyatt[9] found that the most sensitive test under these circumstances was peak expiratory flow, which did not decrease significantly until the orifice was 10 mm in size; this finding correlates well with the clinical observation that dyspnea on exertion occurs only when the caliber of the tracheal air column is reduced to half normal. Breathing through an external orifice of 6 mm reduces peak flows and produces plateaus on both inspiration and expiration (Figure 11–2), a loop pattern closely resembling that of fixed airway obstruction.

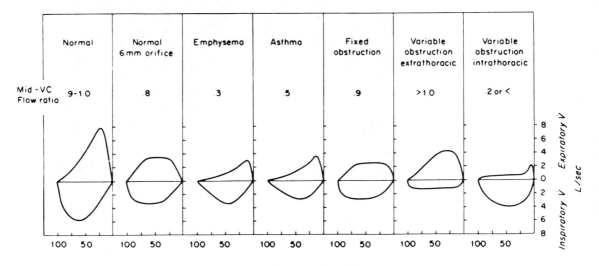

Figure 11–2. Flow-Volume Loops of Various Obstructive Conditions Compared with Normal. Volume is given as a percentage of vital capacity exhaled from total lung capacity. Representative mid-vital capacity flow ratios are given. (Reproduced from Miller, R. D., and Hyatt, R. E., Mayo Clin. Proc., 44:145, 1969, with permission of the authors and editor.)

The dynamic effects of lesions of the upper airway depend in part on the extent to which the obstruction is "fixed" (the airway is unable to change cross-sectional area in response to transmural pressure differences—usually produced by circumferential benign strictures or bilateral vocal cord paralysis) or "variable" (the airway responds to transmural stress—most often resulting from neoplasms that arise from the wall of the airway and create a crescentic lumen, thus permitting a variable cross-sectional diameter throughout the forced ventilatory cycle). Characteristic flow-volume loop patterns are produced by fixed and variable lesions (Figure 11–2). Since fixed upper airway obstructions, either intrathoracic or extrathoracic, are not influenced by transmural pressure gradients, both inspiratory and expiratory flow are proportionately slowed. When a lesion is variable, however, its location (intrathoracic or extrathoracic) becomes important because the airway responds to transmural pressure. During inspiration the extrathoracic airway has a transmural pressure favoring narrowing because intraluminal pressure is subatmospheric while extraluminal pressure is approximately atmospheric. Intraluminal pressure below the lesion becomes subatmospheric to the extent that the lesion produces turbulence; as a result of airway narrowing, a further pressure drop occurs because of acceleration of gas flow (the Bernoulli effect), and the overall effect is to reduce flow on inspiration. In contrast to the dynamic

events that occur during inspiration in variable extrathoracic lesions, during expiration intraluminal pressure is positive relative to extraluminal pressure, thus tending to dilate the airway and obscure the presence of the lesion. Thus, *a variable extrathoracic lesion tends to cause predominant decrease in maximum inspiratory flow and relatively little effect on maximum expiratory flow.*[9]

This situation is reversed when a variable lesion is intrathoracic in location. During inspiration, extraluminal pressure (equivalent to pleural pressure) is negative relative to intraluminal pressure so that transmural pressure favors airway dilatation. By contrast, during expiration extraluminal pressure is positive relative to intraluminal pressure so that airway narrowing occurs. Thus, *a variable intrathoracic lesion results in a predominant reduction in maximum expiratory flow with relative preservation of maximum inspiratory flow* (Figure 11–2).[9]

Since the clinical and roentgenologic diagnosis of upper airway obstruction may be exceedingly difficult, it is of vital importance to recognize the basic physiologic changes caused by lesions in this area and to know how they are reflected in pulmonary function tests. Since in some laboratories flow-volume loops are not routine procedures, it is pertinent to compare the results of tests that measure effort-dependent expiratory flow with those that reflect the effort-independent flow contribution. This is done by determining the ratio FEV_1-MMF, the former measuring both effort-dependent and effort-independent flow and the latter effort-independent flow only.

The breathing of helium-oxygen mixtures can differentiate between upper and lower airway obstruction.[10] The resistance caused by turbulent flow in the larger bronchi is reduced by the breathing of this less dense gas mixture, whereas laminar flow in peripheral airways remains unchanged (see Figure 3–7, page 155).

Roentgenographic Manifestations

As in acute upper airway obstruction, these vary somewhat according to the specific etiology, although there are certain unusual manifestations, particularly in infants and children, which should alert the radiologist to the possibility of upper airway obstruction.

Unequivocal evidence of pulmonary overinflation, particularly in a young patient, should immediately raise the suspicion of intrathoracic upper airway obstruction, especially since overinflation is such a surprisingly infrequent manifestation of spasmodic asthma. Obviously of much greater importance than this indirect sign of obstructive airway disease is the narrowing of the airway, and it is in this area that the roentgenologist can play a very useful—and sometimes vital—role. Once the presence of a lesion has been discovered on standard PA and lateral roentgenograms, its more precise anatomic nature can be established by tomography. Other roentgenographic techniques that may be of value in selected cases include lateral roentgenograms of the soft tissues of the neck (particularly in infants and young children, in whom such abnormalities as hypertrophied tonsils and adenoids may be responsible for upper airway obstruction) and studies of the dynamic activity of the trachea with either cineradiographic or videotape recording to assess the fixed or variable nature of an obstruction (e.g., tracheomalacia). Powdered tantalum has been strongly recommended as the contrast medium of choice for these studies,[11] although at the time of writing this substance has not been approved by the FDA for clinical use.

Two unusual roentgenographic manifestations of chronic upper airway obstruction relate to the heart. The first is cardiac enlargement (cor pulmonale) that results from pulmonary arterial hypertension secondary to chronic hypoxemia and acidosis.[12] The second unusual manifestation consists of a paradoxical change in heart size between inspiration and expiration.

Normally, cardiac diameter is greater on expiration than inspiration; in the presence of chronic (and sometimes acute) upper airway obstruction, the heart is smaller on expiration than inspiration, a paradox that also occasionally occurs in association with chronic lower airway obstruction such as emphysema.

Clinical Manifestations

Obviously, the symptoms and signs of chronic upper airway obstruction will vary with the nature of the underlying lesion and, to some extent, with the age of the patient. As might be expected, the major complaint is dyspnea, either during exercise or at rest, depending on the severity of obstruction. Stridor also may be noted either at rest or during exercise, and its timing may be inspiratory, expiratory, or both. Nonproductive cough is common.

In some patients partial occlusion of the upper airways is associated with an insidious form of hypoventilation that results in hypoxemia, hypercarbia, and pulmonary hypertension and cor pulmonale, with or without cardiac failure. The airway tends to become obstructed periodically during sleep, resulting in periods of apnea lasting from 60 to 90 seconds; hypoxemia and hypercarbia result. These patients complain of an inability to stay awake during the day that results from the poor quality of nocturnal sleep, constituting the syndrome of hypersomnia and periodic breathing. The disturbance usually results from a combination of obesity[10] and periodic obstruction of the upper airway by the tongue or lax pharyngeal muscles. In a study of nine children with sleep-related upper airway obstruction, Felman and his colleagues[13] performed cinefluorography of the upper airways while the children were asleep and found that during inspiration the tongue and hypopharyngeal soft tissues approximated, obliterating the hypopharyngeal air space and causing intermittent and almost complete obstruction to air flow. There is evidence that a number of muscles of the upper airway, including the genioglossus, are activated physically during inspiration. Contraction of these muscles serves to stabilize the airway and prevent its collapse by the negative intra-airway pressure generated during diaphragmatic contraction. Any reduction in intensity or delay in contraction of upper airway muscles could result in airway occlusion.[14] Other causes include enlarged tonsils and adenoids, congenital or acquired defects of the mandible (micrognathia), and occasionally granulomas or neoplasms. When observed during sleep, these patients have repeated episodes of apnea lasting up to 90 seconds, terminating in a loud snore, a return of ventilation, and often arousal. The apnea is associated with prolonged periods of hypoxemia, hypercapnia, and acidosis, resulting eventually in pulmonary hypertension.[15]

Although airway obstruction undoubtedly plays the primary role in many cases of hypersomnia with periodic breathing, there is evidence that in most the pathogenesis is complicated and multifactorial. The whole subject of alveolar hypoventilation is discussed in detail in Chapter 18.

HYPERTROPHY OF TONSILS AND ADENOIDS

Hypertrophy of the palatine tonsils results in a characteristic roentgenographic appearance of a smooth, well-defined, elliptical mass of unit density extending downward from the soft palate into the hypopharynx (Figure 11–3); hypertrophy of the nasopharyngeal adenoids is a commonly associated condition. Both should be readily apparent on lateral roentgenograms of the soft tissues of the neck. The major effect of the chronic upper airway obstruction is alveolar hypoventilation, with resultant hypoxemia, hy-

percapnia, and pulmonary arterial hypertension and cor pulmonale.[16]

A similar picture is seen in obese subjects as a result of obstruction of the pharynx by the tongue when the patient is recumbent,[10] and in patients with micrognathia, a congenital or acquired condition characterized by a small mandible (Pierre Robin syndrome).[17]

TRACHEAL STENOSIS FOLLOWING INTUBATION

One of the commonest causes of chronic upper airway obstruction is tracheal stenosis occurring as a complication of intubation or tracheostomy, a reflection of the ever-increasing tendency to support ventilation in seriously ill patients.

Post-tracheostomy tracheal stenosis may occur at the level of the stoma, at the level of the inflatable cuff, or, rarely, where the tip of the tracheostomy tube impinges on the tracheal mucosa. When the inflatable cuff is involved, the most susceptible portion of the trachea is where the mucosa overlies rigid cartilaginous rings, and it is here that pressure necrosis occurs most often.[19] The lesion begins as a superficial tracheitis and progresses to shallow mucosal ulcerations, usually 2 or more days

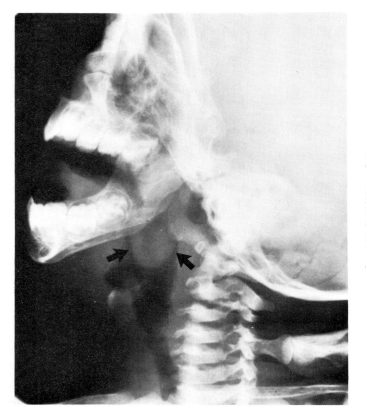

Figure 11–3. Hypertrophied Tonsils Resulting in Upper Airway Obstruction. A view of the soft tissues of the neck in lateral projection reveals a large soft tissue mass (*arrows*) protruding downward into the hypopharynx from the oropharynx. This represents huge hypertrophied tonsils. There is in addition evidence of moderate enlargement of the nasopharyngeal adenoids. This 3-month-old girl was experiencing severe respiratory distress. (Courtesy of Dr. Bernard Epstein, University of Texas, San Antonio.)

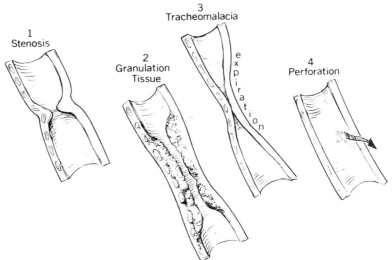

Figure 11–4. Diagrammatic Representation of Distal Post-tracheostomy Lesions that Occur in the Area of the Balloon Cuff. (Reproduced from MacMillan, A. S., Jr., James, A. E., Jr., Stitik, F. P., and Grillo, H. C., Thorax, 26:696, 1971, with permission of the authors and editor.)

following the inflation of the cuff. As the tracheal mucosa becomes eroded, the cartilaginous rings are exposed and become softened, split, fragmented, and eventually completely destroyed. Following deflation of the cuff and removal of the tracheostomy tube, fibrosis occurs in the damaged tracheal wall, resulting in cicatricial stenosis (Figure 11–4).

Roentgenologically, the narrowing of the tracheal lumen typically begins 1 to 1.5 cm distal to the inferior margin of the tracheostomy stoma and involves 1.5 to 2.5 cm of tracheal wall (including 2 to 4 cartilaginous rings).[19] James and his colleagues described three different roentgenographic appearances: (1) the tracheal lumen is circumferentially narrowed over a distance of approximately 2 cm; (2) a thin membrane or diaphragm (caused by fresh granulation tissue rather than mature cicatrization) may project almost at right angles from the tracheal wall; and (3) a long, thickened, eccentric opacity of soft tissue density compromises the tracheal lumen. Adequate roentgenographic assessment can usually be made by standard films of the chest, along with tomography in anteroposterior and lateral projections. Occasionally, precise delineation of the length of stenosis may require opacification.

Occasionally, thinning of the trachea results in tracheomalacia rather than cicatricial stenosis, usually as a result of excessive removal of cartilage at the time of tracheostomy or destruction of cartilage by pressure necrosis and infection.[20] In such circumstances, the increased compliance of the affected tracheal segment can be appreciated by fluoroscopic examination or cinefluorography.[11]

Clinically, most patients are symptom-free

for a variable period following removal of the tracheostomy tube, although edema of the tracheal wall may be present. Eventually, they experience increasing difficulty in raising secretions and note shortness of breath on exertion; these symptoms may progress to stridor and marked dyspnea on minimal exertion.[19] Symptoms and signs of upper airway obstruction may not become apparent for several weeks, during which time the edema subsides and progressive cicatrization occurs.

Resection of the stenotic segment with primary end-to-end anastomosis appears to be the definitive treatment of choice. As pointed out by Grillo,[21] more than half of the trachea may be resected and primary anastomosis performed.

TRACHEAL NEOPLASMS

Compared with the larynx and bronchi, the trachea is a rare site of primary cancer. The commonest primary cancer of the trachea is squamous-cell carcinoma, constituting 50 per cent or more of cases in various series and being approximately four times as common in men as in women.[22] Adenoid cystic carcinoma (cylindroma) is slightly less common and shows no sex predilection. Patients with tracheal neoplasms often are treated for asthma for considerable periods of time before the correct diagnosis is made. Although initially dyspnea may be noted only on exertion, eventually its paroxysmal occurrence at night may suggest the diagnosis of asthma. Hoarseness, cough, and wheeze are common and, when associated with hemoptysis, virtually eliminate the possibility of spasmodic bronchospasm. A characteristic wheeze (stridor) may be heard with or without a stethoscope placed over the trachea. The timing of the wheeze is characteristically inspiratory with extrathoracic lesions and expiratory with intrathoracic lesions.

"SABER-SHEATH" TRACHEA

In cross section the resting trachea is roughly horseshoe-shaped, the open end of the cartilage rings being closed by the compliant posterior sheath. Very occasionally, the coronal diameter is markedly reduced and the sagittal diameter correspondingly increased, a condition called "saber-sheath" trachea by Greene and Lechner.[23] These authors reported 13 patients with this condition, the only criterion for selection being an internal coronal diameter of the intrathoracic trachea one-half or less the corresponding sagittal diameter. All patients were men ranging in age from 52 to 75 years. Generally, the narrow coronal diameter extended the entire length of the intrathoracic trachea from carina to thoracic outlet.

Since this original report,[23] Greene[24] has reported a very high incidence of chronic obstructive pulmonary disease in patients with the "saber-sheath" trachea: of 60 men so affected, 57 (95 per cent) had clinical evidence of obstructive airway disease compared to only 18 per cent in a group of 60 control subjects. Of perhaps greater diagnostic importance, 26 of the 57 patients with COPD (45 per cent) lacked conventional roentgenographic evidence of obstructive airway disease; thus, the "saber-sheath" deformity provided a clue to the presence of COPD when other signs were absent.

RELAPSING POLYCHONDRITIS

This collagen or connective tissue disease (see page 363) affects cartilage in many anatomic sites throughout the body, including the ribs, tracheobronchial tree, ear lobes, nose, and central or peripheral joints. A poor prognostic feature is said to be involvement of the cartilages of the upper airways, and respiratory complications have accounted for most of the reported deaths.[25] Inflammation is localized to tissues with high glycosoaminoglycan concentrations. The mechanism of cartilage destruction appears to be the release or activation of lysosomal enzymes that destroy connective tissue and release chondroitin sulfate from the cartilage matrix.

Histologically, affected cartilage shows fragmentation, round cell infiltration, loss of normal basophilic staining, and replacement of destroyed cartilage by fibrous connective tissue. Electron microscopic examination of synovium and articular cartilage[26] has been reported to show changes identical to those of rheumatoid arthritis.

The *roentgenographic manifestations* of relapsing polychondritis include articular cartilage destruction, calcification of the ear lobes, and narrowing of the tracheal and major bronchial airway columns. In one patient we observed, the major involvement was of the left mainstem bronchus, bronchography revealing marked irregular narrowing of its air column (Figure 11–5). The left lung showed severe air trapping on expiration and was diffusely oligemic, presumably reflecting reflex vasoconstriction as a result of hypoventilation and hypoxia.

The diagnosis is made on the basis of recurrent inflammation of two or more cartilaginous sites, most commonly the ears and nose. Chondrolysis of the joints may lead to severe arthritis.

TRACHEOBRONCHOMEGALY

This condition consists of a dilatation of the tracheobronchial tree that may extend all the way from the larynx to the periphery of the lung.[27] Originally described by Mounier-Kuhn, it is reported to have a familial incidence.[27] The disease occurs predominantly in males, the majority of whom are in their third and fourth decades of life.

The mean coronal diameter of the trachea is 17.5 mm (range 11 to 26 mm) and the mean sagittal diameter 19.5 mm (range 11 to 30 mm) (see page 20). We have adopted the arbitrary figure of 30 mm as the upper limit of normal in any subject; a measurement at or above this extreme is considered to represent tracheobronchomegaly (the figure 30 is perhaps somewhat conservative and we now feel that 25 mm may be more realistic). In this condition the increased compliance of the tracheal and bronchial walls results in abnormal flaccidity and easy collapsibility during forced expiration and cough. *Pathologically*, both the cartilaginous and membranous portions of the trachea and bronchi are affected, having thin, atrophied muscular and elastic tissue.

Roentgenologically, the diagnosis of tracheobronchomegaly may be apparent at a

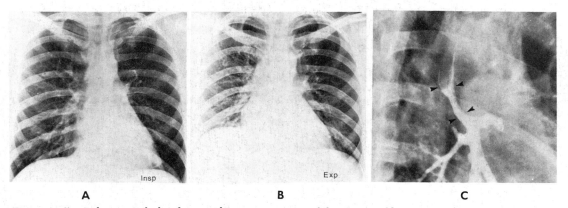

Figure 11–5.   Relapsing Polychondritis.   The major symptom of this 25-year-old man was polyarthralgia. In addition, he manifested a saddle deformity of his nose and an ulcer on the pinna of one ear. He had no symptoms referable to his chest. Posteroanterior roentgenograms at inspiration (*A*) and expiration (*B*) reveal a moderate degree of oligemia of the whole of the left lung, although the left hilum is only slightly smaller than the right. The volume of the left lung on inspiration is roughly normal, although it shows a severe degree of air trapping on expiration (*B*). These plain roentgenographic findings are consistent with a diagnosis of Swyer-James' syndrome, and the patient might have been given that diagnosis had it not been for a high index of suspicion of a possible lesion affecting the left main bronchus. A left bronchogram was performed (*C*) and demonstrated a severe degree of narrowing of the whole length of the left main bronchus (*arrowheads*); the lower lobe bronchi were otherwise normal. This bronchial narrowing resulted from chondritis affecting the cartilage rings of this airway. Some years later, the patient died in respiratory insufficiency when a similar process affected the major bronchi of the right lung. (Courtesy of Dr. John Henderson, Ottawa General Hospital.)

glance. The caliber of the trachea and major bronchi generally is increased and the air columns have an irregular corrugated appearance caused by the protrusion of redundant musculomembranous tissue between the cartilaginous rings (sometimes called tracheal diverticulosis). This appearance is often best visualized in lateral projection.[27] The inefficient cough mechanism leads to retention of mucus with resultant recurrent pneumonia, emphysema, bronchiectasis, and parenchymal scarring. The bronchoscopic appearance may simulate multiple diverticula.

Clinically, symptoms are usually indistinguishable from those caused by chronic bronchitis or bronchiectasis. The presence of prolonged cough and a loud, harsh, rasping sound on auscultation in a patient who complains of inability to expectorate secretions should arouse suspicion of the diagnosis. Pulmonary function tests typically show decrease in bronchial flow rates,[27] an enlarged dead space, and increased tidal volume.

OBSTRUCTIVE DISEASE OF THE LOWER AIRWAYS

The concepts involved and the practical application of the many methods of pulmonary function testing were described in detail in Chapter 3 (*see* page 148). Since a knowledge of these measurements is necessary to a thorough understanding of the pathophysiology of obstructive diseases of the lower airways, a review of this material is recommended before proceeding.

ASTHMA

Asthma is a disease of the airways, characterized by hyper-reactivity of the trachea and bronchi to a variety of stimuli. It is usually intermittent and variable in severity; remission between attacks is generally complete, either spontaneously or as a result of therapy. During attacks, widespread narrowing of the bronchi results in diffuse wheezing often associated with dyspnea, even at rest. A major characteristic of the airway obstruction in asthma is its reversibility.

The term "asthma" frequently is misused and applied to "bronchospasm" or "wheezing," despite the recognition of other clinical entities that can produce intermittent airway obstruction. "Asthma" should be restricted to a state characterized by reversible bronchial obstruction in patients with a clear-cut history of allergy, in patients in whom bronchospasm is precipitated by infection, and in those in whom no obvious cause is discoverable.

INCIDENCE

Asthma is a common disease, estimates of prevalence in children ranging from less than 1 per cent to up to 12 per cent.[28] The first attack may appear at any age, although the onset of extrinsic (atopic) asthma is almost invariably before the age of 30 years while the intrinsic (nonatopic) variety occurs more commonly in middle age. Onset is as frequent after as before the age of 15 years.

ETIOLOGY

Despite the intensive investigation that has resulted in important discoveries in recent years, the factors that provoke asthmatic attacks and their mechanisms of action are still incompletely understood. It is now well accepted that asthmatics have in common a basic hyper-reactivity of the airways that makes them unusually susceptible to a great variety of inhaled substances that induce bronchospasm. Asthmatics may be somewhat arbitrarily categorized as either extrinsic (atopic) or intrinsic (nonatopic). The extrinsic group is subject to attacks from environmental allergens to which they are sensitive, whereas the intrinsic group, although showing some features of allergy, often develops bronchospasm for undetermined reasons. In a relatively small number of asthmatics, episodes of dyspnea are precipitated by analgesics, exercise, or emotion.

HOST PREDISPOSITION

Inhaled particles or gases are believed to act on irritant (rapidly adapting stretch) receptors, which, in the human and in many experimental animals, have been demonstrated to lie just below the epithelium.

The airway hyperirritability so characteristic of the asthmatic state occurs not only in response to nonspecific irritants but also to specific allergens,[29] *e.g.*, histamine, methacholine, and prostaglandins. In addition to its direct and reflex bronchoconstricting effect, histamine produces vagally-induced hyperpnea and hyperventilation when administered in aerosol form.[30] There is evidence that some atopic individuals are lacking or deficient in IgA, thus altering host defense and facilitating allergen invasion.

A predisposition to allergy and positive skin tests has been found in both homozygotes and heterozygotes for the cystic fibrosis gene.[31]

It is generally assumed that there is a genetic basis for asthma, at least for the extrinsic variety, and the major criteria for the diagnosis of atopy are a positive family history along with positive skin and aerosol challenge tests. Current studies of the genetics of IgE-mediated immune response in humans[32] indicate that such nongenetic factors as age of initial exposure to allergen, breast feeding experience, occurrence of infectious diseases early in childhood, and localized changes in airborne pollutants must be controlled before hereditary predisposition can be implicated.

PROVOKING FACTORS

Susceptible individuals are prone to develop episodic bronchospasm, which can be precipitated by a variety of mechanisms. The most thoroughly studied and accepted of these provoking factors is the inhalation, ingestion, or parenteral injection of antigenic material in a sensitized person, resulting in extrinsic asthma. Infection also may initiate either atopic or nonatopic attacks in predisposed individuals. Exercise frequently induces bronchospasm in patients with either extrinsic or intrinsic asthma, and in some it is the only provoking factor. In a few susceptible patients, notably nonatopic middle-aged females with nasal polyps, certain analgesics, particularly acetylsalicylic acid (ASA), can produce severe, even fatal, bronchoconstriction. Psychophysiologic factors are probably responsible for some attacks. A growing number of substances encountered in industry are being accepted as initiators of bronchospasm.[33, 34]

Allergens

Specific antigens provoke asthmatic attacks in sensitized persons who frequently suffer from other allergic manifestations such as hay fever and eczema (as do members of their families) and who usually manifest positive prick or intradermal skin tests to a variety of allergens. However, despite such indications for a state of hypersensitivity, the antigen responsible for a specific attack of bronchospasm frequently is not identified. In a minority of patients with extrinsic asthma, the timing of attacks coincident with exposure to certain antigens leaves little doubt as to the cause of the bronchospasm, particularly with antigens such as pollens, animal dander, some foods, and substances inhaled in the working environment.[34, 35] More frequently, incrimination of a suspected allergen requires confirmation by more reliable means such as inhalation challenge tests,[36] the radioallergosorbent test (RAST),[37] or the demonstration of passive cutaneous anaphylaxis (the Prausnitz-Küstner or PK reaction).

Potential antigens in our environment are innumerable. Surveys of the population at large with immediate skin-test reactivity to a variety of antigens indicate that approximately 30 per cent have a positive prick test response to at least one allergen. Many of these sensitive individuals are asymptomatic, and those with allergies usually suffer from only seasonal or perennial rhinitis. A number of surveys of atmospheric pollens and fungal spores (and skin-test reactions to them) reveal geographical variation. Grass and tree pollens appear to be universal and are the commonest cause of hay fever. These antigens cause positive skin reactions and inhalation challenge in many atopic asthmatics but are not thought to be common causes of asthmatic attacks. In fact, seasonal asthma caused by pollens usually is not severe. A variety of foods, especially eggs, fish, shellfish, nuts, spices, and chocolate, tend to cause immediate wheal and erythematous skin reactions to intracutaneous skin testing, particularly in children. Evidence of hypersensitivity to the specific food may be corroborated by the occurrence of an asthmatic attack following ingestion of the food in question and sometimes by the absence of attacks when the specific allergens are avoided. By contrast, some young people who manifest positive skin test reactions to specific food allergens can consume these foods repeatedly with apparent impunity.

Support for the theory that insects can act as allergens has been provided in recent years by evidence incriminating house mites as a responsible allergen in house dust. Many asthmatics show positive skin test reactions to house dusts, and although such dusts contain many substances, including potentially allergenic molds and disintegrating fibers, a number of studies have shown that various house mites are present in large numbers, particularly in dust from mattresses.[38, 39]

A particularly serious and sometimes fatal manifestation of anaphylaxis in humans can occur following administration of drugs.[40] The reaction usually occurs when the drug is administered intravenously or intramuscularly, although oral, percutaneous, or even respiratory exposure may produce a response in highly sensitive individuals. The commonest drug implicated in this reaction is penicillin. Another cause of potentially fatal anaphylaxis is a sting from one of the insects of the Hymenoptera order, including bees, wasps, hornets, and yellow jackets.

Occupational asthma may be allergen-induced. Allergic mechanisms have been reported following exposure to animal danders, *Bacillus subtilis* enzymes, castor and green coffee beans, papaya, platinum, nickel, chemical fumes from epoxy resins, paints, polyvinylchloride, soldering flux, isocyanates, plicatic acid, and trimellitic and phthalic anhydrides.[33, 34]

In contrast to patients with extrinsic asthma in whom sensitization is due to specific antigens, those with a typical clinical picture of intrinsic asthma (*i.e.*, negative skin tests, negative allergic histories, some eosinophilia, and long-term severe bronchospasm requiring steroid therapy) have lymphocytes that are sensitive *in vitro* to a large variety of nonspecific antigens, as judged by the production of macrophage inhibitory factor.[41]

Infections

Nonatopic patients with episodic bronchospasm usually are referred to as "intrinsic" asthmatics. The major provoking factor in the production of attacks in this group is believed to be infection. The commonest association is upper respiratory infection, including sinusitis.[42] Exacerbations of asthma are likely to be related to viral infections, particularly in families with children. In contrast to respiratory infections of bacterial origin, which seldom appear to precipitate asthma, a good correlation is found between the severity of viral respiratory infections and the likelihood of an asthmatic attack.[43] The mechanism by which respiratory infection precipitates attacks of asthma in either atopic or nonatopic patients is by no means clear. There is very little evidence to implicate an immunologic mechanism and it is likely that virus particles exert a nonspecific effect on the irritant receptors in the large bronchi, resulting in vagally mediated bronchospasm.

In some asthmatics, particularly adults, bronchoconstriction never remits, and such patients are considered to have "chronic intractable" asthma. Frequently the clinical presentation suggests the combination of both infective asthma and chronic bronchitis with intermittent exacerbations of bronchospasm (asthmatic bronchitis).

Analgesics

Acetylsalicylic acid (ASA) and several other unrelated analgesics are capable of provoking attacks in a significant percentage of asthmatics. The ASA-sensitive asthmatic typically is a non-atopic female over the age of 20 with a long history of perennial rhinitis and nasal polyps. The incidence of intolerance increases with age, being six times more common after the age of 50 than before 20.[44] Peripheral eosinophilia and a family history of atopy are observed in over 50 per cent of patients. Symptoms and signs develop within two hours of taking the drug and include angioedema, bronchospasm, and cyanosis; asphyxia, coma, and death may follow. Although ASA may occasionally act as an antigen and stimulate antibody production, there is abundant evidence that ASA-induced bronchospasm is not allergic in nature.[45] It has been postulated that patients with ASA-sensitive asthma produce large amounts of the bronchodilator prostaglandin (PGE_2) in partial compensation for the continuing bronchoconstrictor stimulus; when ASA or other analgesics are ingested, a drop in PGE_2 synthesis precipitates an acute asthmatic attack.[45]

Exercise

Most asthmatics become increasingly dyspneic following exertion and many show an increase in airway resistance of 25 per cent or more over pre-exercise values.[46] At rest, some of these patients are completely free of symptoms and have normal pulmonary function tests. As in normal subjects, an initial period of bronchodilation occurs in asthmatics during the first 2 to 4 minutes of exercise, followed by severe bronchoconstriction, which reaches a peak approximately 3 to 5 minutes after cessation of exercise and gradually decreases in intensity until resistance returns to normal about 20 minutes later.[46] To be effective in producing bronchospasm the exercise must be of moderate duration; maximal response appears to occur after 6 minutes. Exercise-induced asthma (EIA) occurs less with longer[46] or repeated[47] periods of exercise during the same day.

Recent studies clearly show that EIA can be virtually abolished by breathing moist air at 37° C.[48, 49] The degree of bronchospasm induced by exercise is directly proportional to the magnitude of airway cooling.[48] The reduction in the severity of obstruction with repeated exercise testing and the protection accorded by cromolyn sodium suggests a mediator release from mast cells; however, this hypothesis is not compatible with the finding that a minority of asthmatics with EIA do not become refractory to exercise after an initial test episode breathing warm, humid air.[49]

Emotion

It is difficult to evaluate the influence of psychologic factors in the etiology of asthma and the provocation of individual attacks. Asthmatics tend to be emotionally unstable and dependent, and it has been found that both bronchospasm and bronchodilation may be induced by suggestion, presumably acting through the vagus nerve.[50] There is little evidence that emotional distress is ever the sole etiologic factor, although it may trigger an attack in a predisposed person. Children with asthma appear to manifest different psychologic patterns. Those whose symptoms remit rapidly on admission to the hospital tend to be rather neurotic, whereas those whose asthma is steroid-dependent tend to manifest less psychopathologic behavior.

Environment

The role played by air pollution in the production of asthmatic attacks is not known. Since patients with bronchial asthma have a low threshold for nonspecific irritants, one might expect a close correlation between atmospheric pollution and exacerbations of asthma. Studies in the New Orleans area showed a sharp increase in the incidence of asthmatic attacks during June and July and October and November, periods during which atmospheric pollution increased.[51] In an investigation of the relationship between air pollution and asthmatic attacks in the Los Angeles area, it was found that a significantly greater number of persons had attacks on days when oxidant levels were high enough to cause eye irritation and damage to plants. The increased incidence of asthmatic attacks at night is well recognized, and it is postulated that this may relate to the presence of mites in mattresses.

PATHOGENESIS

The pathophysiology is one of airway obstruction resulting from spasm of bronchial smooth muscle, edema of the mucosa and submucosa, and excessive secretion of viscous mucus. Major advances have been made in our understanding of the mechanisms provoking bronchoconstriction, but the factors responsible for persistence of obstruction and the development of mucous plugging remain poorly understood. Recent observations stress the importance of vagal reflex action in the initiation of bronchospasm. Chemical mediators liberated from mast cells appear to play a lesser role and perhaps are more responsible for prolonging airway resistance.

Irritant receptors within the bronchial mucosa are stimulated either directly or indirectly by nonspecific irritants, antigens, and a variety of substances known to produce smooth muscle spasm, such as histamine. The result is vagally mediated reflex bronchoconstriction. However, studies of asthma in both experimental animals and humans indicate that the stimuli producing bronchoconstriction are only partly blocked by vagotomy or the administration of atropine. Direct stimulation of smooth muscle is particularly evident in extrinsic asthma, resulting from either the allergen itself or a release of chemical mediators from mast cells. The latter cells are plentiful in the vicinity of blood vessels, and their abundance appears to correlate with the connective tissue content of organ or tissue.[53]

Studies in humans and in various species of animals have shown that chemical mediators can be released from certain tissues and cells; the two cells generally accepted as the sources of these materials are the mast cell and the circulating basophil. In humans, there exist a number of chemical mediators including histamine, SRS-A, eosinophil-chemotactic factor of anaphylaxis (ECF-A), platelet activating factor (PAF), serotonin, bradykinin, and prostaglandins.[54] Histamine, SRS-A, ECF-A, and PAF are considered to be primary mediators. Histamine and ECF-A are stored preformed, whereas SRS-A and PAF are generated immediately before release. The prostaglandins and bradykinin are considered to be secondary mediators. Slow-reacting substance of anaphylaxis (SRS-A) is composed of prostaglandin-like substances (leokotrienes), which are derived from the metabolism of arachidonic acid. Besides being potent contractors of bronchial smooth muscle,[55] they interfere with mucociliary transport[56] and may cause airway edema as a result of an increase in endothelial permeability.

The mode of action of the chemical mediators is described in considerable detail in our book *Diagnosis of Diseases of the Chest* (page 1339), and the interested reader is directed there for further information.

PATHOLOGIC CHARACTERISTICS

Since the bulk of our knowledge of the morphologic characteristics of asthma derives from studies at necropsy, it is probable that the changes described represent the effects of prolonged, severe bronchial asthma. However, evidence provided from bronchial biopsies suggests that morphologic changes may disappear between acute attacks.[57]

The lungs of patients dying of asthma are very distended. The bronchi and bronchioles are plugged with large amounts of viscid, tenacious mucus,[58, 59] which, in some cases, extends into and even fills the alveoli. In one case observed by us, mucous plugging extended into the trachea and main bronchi. On histologic examination, the mucus contains eosinophils, bronchial epithelial cells, and Charcot-Leyden crystals. The walls of the bronchi, particularly those smaller than 10 mm in diameter, are thickened and edematous and contain many eosinophils and plasma cells. The thickening is largely the result of hypertrophy of mucous glands, thickening and hyalinization of the basement membrane, and hypertrophy of smooth muscle. Goblet cells are increased in number, and the columnar epithelial cells of the mucosa may be partly replaced by cuboidal cells. The destructive changes in the alveoli characteristic of chronic bronchitis and emphysema are lacking, although focal areas of collapse and congestion are common. Approximately 25 per cent of patients show evidence of local bronchiectasis.

ROENTGENOGRAPHIC MANIFESTATIONS

In many patients with bronchial asthma the chest roentgenogram is normal. As discussed further on, the incidence of abnormality is influenced to a considerable extent by age of onset of the asthma, its severity, and its constancy. In the presence of status asthmaticus or during prolonged, intractable asthmatic attacks, the characteristic roentgenographic signs are those of severe overinflation and air trapping. Roentgenograms exposed at full expiration show diminution in diaphragmàtic excursion caused by air trapping. In contrast to the findings in emphysema, the vascular markings throughout the lungs are of normal caliber. The hilar shadows usually are normal; sometimes, however, the hilar pulmonary arteries appear to be slightly enlarged, a finding attributable to reversible pulmonary arterial hypertension.

The influence of age of onset of asthma on the presence or absence of roentgenographic changes was illustrated graphically in a study by Hodson and associates[60] of 117 asthmatic patients over 15 years of age. In this adult group, roentgenographic abnormalities were identified in 31 per cent of the patients whose asthma had its onset before the age of 15 years but in none of those in whom it occurred after

30 years of age. The incidence of roentgenographic abnormalities is also affected by severity. In a study of 58 patients ranging in age from 10 to 69 years (mean age 32.7) in whom the asthma was categorized as "severe," evidence of pulmonary overinflation was detected in 42 (73 per cent).[61] The incidence of roentgenographic abnormalities also bears a relationship to the constancy or intermittent nature of symptoms. In a study of 218 children with asthma and a control group of 162 normal children, Simon and his colleagues[62] found that the asthmatics with the most marked roentgenographic abnormalities were, without exception, suffering from severe or moderately severe *constant* asthma; those with *intermittent* symptoms usually had roentgenograms that appeared normal, even during asthmatic episodes. Overall, 73 per cent of the asthmatics were roentgenographically normal. In some patients with chronic asthma—usually those with a history of repeated episodes of infection—the bronchial walls are thickened, an abnormality sometimes detectable roentgenographically.

The primary importance of chest roentgenography in patients with bronchial asthma is its usefulness in excluding other conditions associated with diffuse wheezing throughout the chest—emphysema, bronchiectasis, and obstructions of the trachea or major bronchi.

CLINICAL MANIFESTATIONS

The diagnosis of asthma is based largely on a history of periodic paroxysms of dyspnea, usually at rest as well as on exertion, with intervals of complete or nearly complete remission. Meticulous inquiry into circumstances initiating attacks, although time-consuming, undoubtedly constitutes the most important diagnostic procedure leading to rational therapy. If the patient is a child, questioning should be directed toward the possible association of food with the onset of attacks. Seasonal occurrence is of importance in suggesting either pollen sensitivity or an allergic asthma precipitated by insects. Careful inquiry should be made into possible antigens in the home, especially domestic pets and feather pillows. The patient may have recognized an association between the onset of symptoms and exposure to a dusty environment at his or her place of work. A history of drug intake should be looked for. Analgesic drugs, particularly acetylsalicylic acid, may initiate bronchospasm, rhinorrhea, flushing, pruritus, urticaria, hypotension, loss of consciousness,

and, rarely, death. Asthmatics usually manifest an increase in airway resistance after exercise that is exaggerated in contrast to the mild bronchospasm occurring in normal subjects. Rarely, exercise is the *only* provoking factor; in such circumstances the presence of the disease may go unrecognized if clinical examination and pulmonary function tests are not performed at appropriate times.[46]

The patient should be questioned as to whether there is an association between the onset of asthmatic attacks and infections of the upper or lower respiratory tract, with particular emphasis on the occurrence of postnasal drip and facial pain. An attempt should be made to correlate the onset of attacks with emotional disturbance; if the patient is a child, this should include interview of the parents. Finally, the patient should be questioned as to the relationship between onset of attacks and exposure to irritating dusts, fumes, or odors, and the effects of changing temperature and humidity.

In the majority of patients the onset of an attack of asthma is heralded by an unproductive cough and wheeze, and only subsequently do the sensations of suffocation and tightness in the chest develop. The onset of dyspnea seldom is abrupt. These paroxysms occur most commonly at night. Nocturnal breathlessness is a common symptom in asthma and probably results from the formation of mucous plugs in the airways during sleep.

Physical findings in asthma include hyperventilation, hyper-resonance on percussion, and auscultatory evidence of inspiratory and expiratory sonorous and sibilant rhonchi, diminished air entry, and prolonged expiration. An abnormal degree of pulsus paradoxus has been correlated with severity of asthma.[63]

An attack of asthma usually lasts for 30 to 60 minutes and may abate spontaneously after the expectoration of mucous plugs. Asthmatic attacks seldom last for less than half an hour and may persist for several hours or even days or weeks. When an attack persists beyond 12 hours and there is no therapeutic response to inhaled bronchodilators or subcutaneous injections of adrenalin, the patient can be considered to be in status asthmaticus and to require immediate hospitalization.[64]

LABORATORY FINDINGS

The sputum expectorated by patients with uncomplicated bronchial asthma is characteristic, containing spiral casts (Curschmann's spirals) up to several centimeters long, eosinophils, and in some cases colorless, elongated, octahedral crystals, 20 to 40 μ in diameter (Charcot-Leyden crystals). When infection is superimposed, as is so often the case, the sputum becomes mucopurulent and rarely, blood-streaked. The white cell count usually is normal or slightly elevated, with slight eosinophilia in the majority of cases. In adult asthmatics, peripheral blood eosinophilia is almost invariably present, and absolute counts are recommended to monitor therapeutic effect.[65] A decrease in eosinophilia correlates well with improvement of pulmonary function; it has been recommended that a count of 85 cells or less per cu mm be achieved in subjects treated with steroids.[65]

Skin tests for various foods and inhalants are discussed in Chapter 3. They are particularly useful in confirming the responsibility of a specific allergen suspected by the patient. A positive reaction does not necessarily indicate that the specific allergen will cause bronchoconstriction, nor does a negative result exclude the specific substance as a causal agent in any individual case. Generally, however, a positive history shows a highly significant correlation with a positive prick test. A very reliable method of identifying suspected antigens is bronchial (inhalational) provocation testing.[36] When the history suggests a specific allergen and skin testing is negative, a nebulized extract may be administered by aerosol with relative impunity. However, when skin testing is positive, the inhaled allergen should be well diluted and initially administered in small amounts. This method of testing may elicit immediate or delayed reactions that should be documented objectively by spirographic recordings made before and at intervals after the administration of the extract. Bronchial provocation tests are most valuable in determining immunologic reactions to substances, both organic and inorganic, suspected of being causative agents in occupational asthma.[34, 66]

PULMONARY FUNCTION ABNORMALITIES

As might be expected, aberrations in pulmonary function in asthma vary, depending largely upon whether the condition is in remission or exacerbation and, if the latter, upon the severity of the attack. Many patients whose asthma is in remission have normal pulmonary function, values being normal even when auscultation reveals wheezing.

An asthmatic attack is associated with bronchospasm, edema of bronchial mucous membranes, and increased secretion of mucus. These pathologic changes cause airway obstruction, the bronchoconstriction resulting from smooth muscle contraction in large or small airways or both, and the accumulation of mucus exerting its influence largely in the smaller airways. Since considerable obstruction may be present in small airways without increasing total pulmonary resistance, patients who manifest predominantly peripheral bronchiolar constriction may show no abnormality on routine pulmonary function testing, at least during mild to moderate attacks. However, if the obstruction is severe or if it is the result of large airway spasm, the increased expiratory resistance can be detected by body plethysmographic measurements or by a decrease in FEV_1. The latter determination and the FEV_1-VC ratio are useful in the assessment of changes in airway resistance from day to day.[67]

One effect of increased airway resistance is air trapping, which results partly from obstruction of airways during expiration and partly from collateral air drift distal to totally obstructed bronchioles or bronchi. Air trapping causes an increase in residual volume and upward movement of the end-expiratory level; the usual result is a decrease in vital capacity. The FRC (RV plus ERV) almost invariably is increased,[67] and TLC (VC plus RV) usually increases, particularly in children.[68] Such pulmonary hyperinflation is advantageous to the asthmatic with acute airway obstruction, since the increase in elastic recoil tends to keep the airways open by increasing traction on bronchial walls.

In the presence of bronchospasm, airway obstruction varies in degree regionally within the lungs, resulting in nonuniformity of both distribution of inspired air and lung perfusion. The regional distribution of bronchial obstruction in asthma results in abnormal ventilation-perfusion ratios ($\dot{V}/\dot{Q}$) which persist even during periods of remission. This mismatching of ventilation and perfusion can be detected by the use of radioactive xenon or by scanning with macroaggregates of labeled serum albumin.[69] In our experience and that of others,[67] the majority of asthmatics have a normal steady state diffusing capacity in contrast to patients with emphysema, in whom diffusion is reduced.

Most patients with asthma have some degree of hypoxemia, even when asymptomatic, whereas hypocapnia develops early in the attack. Hypoxemia is largely the result of regional $\dot{V}/\dot{Q}$ inequality. As airway obstruction worsens and the lungs become progressively more hyperinflated, hypoxemia increases in severity. By the time the clinical picture suggests status asthmaticus, the PaO_2 generally has dropped to below 60 mm Hg and often close to 40 mm Hg,[70] and the peak expiratory flow rate will be less than 60 liters/min.[70] As the severity of the obstruction increases and the patient becomes exhausted, values for PCO_2 gradually rise to normal and hypercapnia eventually develops.

COMPLICATIONS

Complications of asthma are much more common in children than in adults and consist of pneumonia, atelectasis, mucoid impaction and mucous plugging, pneumomediastinum and, rarely, arterial air embolism.

Lower respiratory tract infection has a distinctly higher incidence among patients with asthma than in the population at large, an observation that applies generally to all forms of obstructive airway disease.

Atelectasis occurs predominantly in children and is the result of mucous plugging or mucoid impaction. Although roentgenographically demonstrable atelectasis occurs very uncommonly in adult asthmatics, it is probable that mucous plugging of smaller bronchi and bronchioles occurs much more frequently than is recognized. In such circumstances, it is assumed that pulmonary collapse distal to the obstructed airway is prevented by collateral air drift.

Pneumomediastinum is an uncommon complication of asthma. It occurs predominantly in children and occasionally in young adults. The presumed mechanism is alveolar rupture consequent upon the trapping of air beyond mucous plugs in the bronchioles, with subsequent dissection of air through the perivascular sheath to the hilum and mediastinum.[71] In infants, particularly, there is a tendency for the additional development of pneumothorax, the release of air into the pleural space relieving the pressure within the mediastinum.[71]

PROGNOSIS

Studies in children[72] have shown that a number of factors are associated with a poor prognosis—early onset, high frequency of attacks in the initial year, clinical and physiologic evidence of persisting airway obstruction, pulmonary hyperinflation, chest deformity, and impairment of growth. Prognosis is considerably

better in both children and adults whose asthmatic attacks are intermittent and who show evidence of lability than in patients whose symptoms are continuous and whose obstruction is relatively fixed. Follow-up studies in children indicate that maximal flow at 50 per cent of FVC may deteriorate with serial measurements.[73]

A recent study by Chan-Yeung and her colleagues[74] of occupational asthma caused by western red cedar (*Thuja plicata*) has shown that the disease may persist in 50 per cent of workers after removal from the source of air pollution. Previous work by these same authors[75] indicated that bronchial hyper-reactivity may be the consequence rather than the predisposing factor in occupational asthma.

Deaths caused by asthma occur predominantly in adults aged 40 to 60 years, in children under the age of 2 years, in teenagers,[76] and in pregnant women.[77] Deaths resulting from asthma outside the hospital often occur suddenly and before a physician can be summoned.[58] When patients are seen by general practitioners during an asthmatic attack, hospitalization frequently is not advised; even if it is, the patient may die in the ambulance.[58] Both patients and physicians should be made more aware of the seriousness of the disease; patients who are considered at risk of developing fatal asthma should be admitted to the hospital promptly when clinical and physiologic findings indicate a severe attack.

CHRONIC BRONCHITIS AND EMPHYSEMA

Chronic bronchitis and emphysema are the commonest forms of chronic obstructive pulmonary disease (COPD) (*synonyms:* chronic obstructive lung disease, obstructive airway disease, chronic air flow obstruction). Recently,[78] Thurlbeck advocated the term "chronic air flow limitation," giving emphasis to the fact that flow is limited rather than that airways are obstructed. In the lung, the pressure that is applied to air flow is the elastic recoil of the lung, the loss of which is thought to be the most characteristic feature of emphysema. Thus, flow can be limited in the presence of perfectly normal airways.

Although our knowledge of the chronic obstructive pulmonary diseases has been greatly extended in recent years, with this better understanding has come the realization that in many cases the precise differentiation of individual diseases is difficult. As Macklem stated,[79] "In the syndrome of chronic obstructive lung disease, the abnormalities that result from chronic bronchitis have proved enormously difficult to dissect from those which result from emphysema and those which result from a combination of both. Indeed, it was because of this difficulty that the term chronic obstructive lung disease was coined. Although this term successfully masks our ignorance, it hardly advances our knowledge of emphysema *per se* or chronic bronchitis *per se—both specific disease entities in their own right"* (italics ours).

In the following pages, the incidence, etiology, pathogenesis, pathologic characteristics, and roentgenographic manifestations are described separately for chronic bronchitis and emphysema, and the clinical and physiologic manifestations of the two diseases are considered together subsequently.

CHRONIC BRONCHITIS

In its simplest form, the definition of chronic bronchitis is a chronic productive cough without a demonstrable cause, either local or general. Since this definition is purely clinical, some standardization was necessary so that studies of population groups could be compared. For this purpose, quantitative (and somewhat arbitrary) terms were introduced. For example, expectoration must occur on most days during at least 3 consecutive months for not less than 2 successive years.[80]

The definition requires that all other causes of chronic cough and expectoration be eliminated before a diagnosis of chronic bronchitis is accepted. In some cases it may be difficult to differentiate chronic bronchitis from asthma; however, the definition of asthma as a disease characterized by widespread reversible narrowing of the bronchial airways, changing rapidly in severity either spontaneously or with treatment, is of differential value in the majority. Some patients cough and expectorate sufficiently to qualify for the diagnosis of chronic bronchitis as just defined, but also experience episodes of airway obstruction that are rapidly reversible. There may be nothing in their history or test results to suggest an allergic background, and many such patients are considered to have "asthmatic bronchitis." Others give a history of allergy, or of spasmodic asthma for a number of years before the onset of daily expectoration, suggesting that in those patients the two diseases coexist.

ETIOLOGY AND PATHOGENESIS

There is abundant evidence to incriminate several etiologic factors as acting singly or in concert to produce chronic bronchitis. The majority of clinical and experimental investigations to determine the causes have been concerned with five factors—tobacco smoking, air pollution (either occupational or urban), infection, heredity, and social class; each is considered in the following pages. It is stressed that in any individual case a combination of these factors may be responsible and they may have synergistic relationships.[81]

Influence of Smoking

In 1968, the American Advisory Committee for Research on Tobacco and Health reiterated conclusions reached in its 1964 report, which documented convincing evidence that tobacco smoking is a significant cause of lung disease. Clinical studies of the incidence of respiratory disease in nonsmokers have shown that chronic obstructive pulmonary disease is very rare in these people,[82] and studies of adolescent male and female smokers and nonsmokers have shown a significantly greater frequency of infection in both the lower and upper respiratory tracts in smokers of both sexes. Comparative studies on the prevalence of cough and expectoration in adult smokers and nonsmokers have shown a remarkable predominance among cigarette smokers.[82, 83] Data obtained by standard questionnaire and pulmonary function tests of an East Boston population[84] showed that 82 per cent of the observed prevalence of chronic bronchitis could be attributed to cigarette smoking, both men and women showing a linear increase in incidence with increased smoking. Men appear to be at greater risk than women for the development of chronic bronchitis but less clearly so for the development of obstructive airway disease.

Comparisons of expiratory flow rates of smokers and nonsmokers have revealed a significant increase in airway obstruction in smokers, particularly obvious in the maximal midexpiratory and three-quarter fractions; in addition, a statistically significant relationship has been observed between the degree of impairment of flow and the number of cigarettes smoked.[85] Cessation of smoking has resulted in significant reduction of air flow limitation.[82, 86, 87] Pathologically, cigarette smoking has been related to hyperplasia of the bronchial mucous glands—

as evidenced by an increase in the Reid index[88]—and to the development of squamous metaplasia of the respiratory tract epithelium.

Influence of Air Pollution

There seems no doubt that certain chemicals in dusts, if present in sufficient concentrations, can cause acute and probably chronic bronchial damage, although the consequences of this form of pollution are minor compared to those of cigarette smoking. Urban air pollution can be divided into two major categories according to the chemicals involved: (1) reducing agents, consisting mainly of carbonaceous particulate matter and sulfur dioxide; and (2) oxidizing substances, including the hydrocarbons, oxides of nitrogen, and photochemical reaction pollutants such as ozone, aldehydes, and organic nitrates. There seems little doubt that a sudden increase in the amount of air pollution, such as occurs with smog, can result in increased morbidity and mortality in patients with established chronic airway obstruction (CAO).[89] Recent studies in which other variables have been controlled have incriminated air pollution as a cause of both chronic bronchitis and air flow limitation when urban and rural population groups are compared.[90] Urban air pollution appears to play an additive role in smokers and may be partly responsible for progression of disability in patients with CAO.

Many epidemiologic studies have been made to try to correlate chronic obstructive pulmonary disease with occupations linked with air pollution.[91] However, evidence is conflicting and it is clear that more long-term studies are indicated.

It has been suggested that smoking habits of individuals in a family may exert an effect on the health of other family members, particularly children, because of environmental exposure to tobacco smoke.[92] Similarly, a recent study has produced convincing evidence of small airways dysfunction in nonsmokers who are chronically exposed to tobacco smoke in the work environment.[93]

Influence of Infection

Although pulmonary infection probably plays an etiologic role in only a minority of cases, it is a recognized cause of acute exacerbations of already established disease and is possibly a factor in the progression of disability. It is almost certain that the lower respiratory tract in healthy patients is sterile. Infection results

in acute episodes in which there is symptomatic and physiologic deterioration. The sputum often becomes purulent, cultures usually growing *Haemophilus influenzae* and sometimes *Streptococcus pneumoniae*.[94] Although bacteria may play a role in acute exacerbations of the disease, it is more likely that they act as a secondary invader following an acute viral infection of the lower respiratory tract. Viral infection is almost certainly responsible for the majority of clinical exacerbations in patients with chronic bronchitis. The rhinoviruses and myxoviruses—the latter particularly during epidemics—appear to be the commonest etiologic agents,[95, 96] but other respiratory viruses and nonbacterial organisms such as *Mycoplasma pneumoniae*[95] have been isolated in a small percentage of cases. Identification of these organisms in conjunction with acute clinical exacerbations has clearly established their role as primary pathogens.

Influence of Heredity

An inherited susceptibility may be as important a factor as smoking in the pathogenesis of chronic bronchitis and CAO. Larson and associates[97] compared the pulmonary function of 156 relatives of 61 chronically obstructed patients with that of a control group of relatives of the patients' spouses and found an increased familial incidence that was not attributable to alpha$_1$-antitrypsin (A_1AT) deficiency. In this group females and males were affected equally, there was a tendency to early onset of disease, and dyspnea rather than cough was the major symptom. Studies of monozygotic twins[98] have demonstrated a significant concordance in the occurrence of chronic cough, a correlation that was clearly independent of cigarette smoking. Additional support for the influence of heredity is provided by the observation that chronic bronchitis and CAO tend to occur in households.[99]

Influence of Social Status

The mortality from chronic bronchitis has been shown to increase with descending socioeconomic class, an increase applying to both men and their wives.[100] This presumed pathogenetic factor is closely linked with and difficult to dissociate from such influences as the increased incidence of respiratory infections among underprivileged citizens and the crowding and regional pollution of poorer districts, all of which are capable of producing a harmful environment.

PATHOLOGIC CHARACTERISTICS

In chronic bronchitis, not only is there hypertrophy and hyperplasia of mucus-secreting glands, but the secretions become more viscous, resulting in interference with mucociliary transport[101] and plugging of small airways. In patients with an unusually high degree of bronchospasm, airway smooth muscle may be increased in amount and peribronchiolar fibrosis may contribute to airway obstruction.[102]

Secretions into the bronchial lumen originate in branched tubular glands and in goblet cells of the surface epithelium. The branched tubular glands are found in the trachea and in all cartilage-containing bronchi and possess an acinar appearance in cross section. The majority lie beneath the surface epithelium between the basement membrane and the cartilage plates, a few extending between plates of cartilage and even lying external to them. They open into the lumen through a duct. Goblet cells exist mainly in the large airways, where they may represent one in perhaps 30 epithelial cells. In normal subjects the volume of mucous glands is approximately 100 times that of goblet cells, so that the former are considered the main source of secretions.[103, 104]

The yardstick devised by Reid[104] for the assessment of the presence and severity of chronic bronchitis consists of the measurement from histologic sections of the width of the mucous glands and the width of the bronchial wall, from the basement membrane of the epithelium to the inner edge of the perichondrium at a point at which the epithelium is roughly parallel to the inner edge of the cartilage. The ratio of the width of the gland to the width of the wall is known as the Reid index; it is usually determined by averaging measurements of three to five transverse sections from main, lobar, or segmental bronchi. In her original description, Reid[104] found a gland-wall mean ratio of 0.26 in seven normal subjects and 0.59 in 20 patients with bronchitis. A relationship has been reported between chronic productive cough during life and the size of bronchial mucous glands at necropsy.[104] Similarly, Reid[104] found a close correlation between the amount of sputum produced during life and the gland-wall ratio at necropsy. Patients who expectorated 1 ounce of sputum per day had a mean Reid index of 0.53, whereas those producing 6 ounces per day had a ratio of 0.76. In addition to mucous gland hypertrophy and increase in goblet cells, some cases of chronic bronchitis show evidence of chronic inflammation of the bronchial and bronchiolar walls, although any cellular infiltration is usually of minor degree.[103, 104]

Controversy still exists as to the mechanism or mechanisms responsible for airway obstruction in uncomplicated chronic bronchitis. In patients who die from CAO, by far the most important morphologic correlate of the clinical state is destructive emphysema.[105] It is very likely that it is small airway obstruction that results in disability in patients with chronic bronchitis and plays a role in the development of emphysema.[103] The pathologic correlate of physiologically detected disease of the small airways is almost certainly mucous plugging of bronchioles, identifiable even in the absence of emphysema.[106]

Mucus Production in Chronic Bronchitis

The production and expectoration of bronchial secretions depend upon several factors. In bronchitis, not only is the quantity of mucus increased in proportion to the degree of hyperplasia and hypertrophy of mucous glands and the increase in goblet cells, but it is likely that the composition of the mucus is abnormal. Such change in composition results in an alteration in consistency of the sputum, rendering expectoration more difficult. Other factors that influence expectoration of sputum include the ciliary activity of the bronchial mucosa, patency of the airways, and the action of gravity and cough in ridding the bronchial tree of its secretions.

Volume of sputum in chronic bronchitics varies considerably from day to day.[107] The bulk of expectorated material is coughed up during the first hour after rising, although it has been found[107] that as the total quantity of sputum production increases, the first hour volume decreases from two-thirds to approximately one-third of the total 24-hour expectorated material.

ROENTGENOGRAPHIC MANIFESTATIONS

The roentgenographic appearances in uncomplicated chronic bronchitis are inadequately documented, mainly because no large series has been reported of an assessment of premortem roentgenograms of known bronchitics who have been shown to have no emphysema at necropsy. As in spasmodic asthma, the main roentgenologic requirement is to exclude other conditions, such as bronchiectasis, that may mimic the disease clinically. We wish to emphasize at the outset that *chronic bronchitis cannot be diagnosed roentgenologically.*

Changes may be observed in the lungs that *suggest* that bronchitis may be present, but on the basis of plain roentgenograms it is never appropriate to do more than indicate that the findings are compatible with or suggestive of that diagnosis. If one were to obtain chest roentgenograms of a number of cigarette smokers picked at random from passers-by on the street, each of whom satisfied the clinical criteria for the diagnosis of chronic bronchitis, it is very likely that the great majority would show no changes suggesting that diagnosis.

Roentgenographic abnormalities include prominence of lung markings (the "dirty chest") and tubular shadows.[107] *Increased lung markings* consist of a general accentuation of linear markings throughout the lungs. In a recently reported radiologic-pathologic correlative study of lungs obtained from consecutive autopsies, Feigin and Abraham[108] found good correlation between the roentgenographic appearance of increased pulmonary markings and histologic evidence of edema, chronic inflammatory cell infiltration, and mild fibrosis in the perivenous interstitium. Although this roentgenographic sign is admittedly a very subjective finding, we consider it useful evidence in support of a diagnosis of chronic bronchitis. The appearance is similar to the "increased marking" pattern of emphysema (*see* page 546), the major difference being the absence of pulmonary arterial hypertension and cor pulmonale in the uncomplicated chronic bronchitic.

Tubular shadows, consisting of parallel or slightly tapering line shadows outside the boundary of the pulmonary hila, are probably always abnormal and are thought with good reason to represent thickened bronchial walls. Unfortunately, there exists considerable intra- and interobserver variation in the frequency with which they are identified, the main reason probably relating to the physical nature of a tubular structure. Since a "tramline" represents a bronchus viewed longitudinally, roentgenographic visibility of this air-containing tube depends upon the absorptive power of its tissue in tangent. Therefore, because the image of the tangential wall thickness fades off at the margins, causing loss of definition, the *total* wall thickness cannot be accurately appreciated. However, when the bronchus is visualized end-on, in cross section, a substantially greater amount of tissue is traversed by the x-ray beam, particularly at the periphery, thus producing a sharp air-tissue interface and a well-defined margin. These end-on bronchi range in diameter from approximately 3 to 7 mm and thus represent different stages in bronchial subdivision. Their accompanying arteries are nearly always identifiable, but because of slight angulation may not be sharply defined. Thickening of these bronchial shadows visualized end-on can usually be easily identified. In a study by Fraser and his coworkers,[238] step-wise discriminant analysis of six variables showed that the median estimate of bronchial wall thickness was of some value in discriminating normal subjects from chronic bronchitics, but that the presence of thickening could not be used as an absolute criterion for the presence of chronic bronchitis, nor could its absence be construed as evidence against that diagnosis.

Overinflation at TLC occurs when there is diminished elastic recoil of the lungs as in emphysema, and in fact an increase in TLC is usual in this disease. However, since both TLC and elastic recoil are normal in chronic bronchitics, logically there should be no evidence of overinflation on standard roentgenograms exposed at full inspiration.

PULMONARY EMPHYSEMA

It is generally agreed that emphysema can be accurately defined in morphologic terms only. Two such definitions are available, one drawn up at a Ciba symposium[109] in 1958 and reported in 1959, and the other composed by the American Thoracic Society[80] in 1962 and the World Health Organization[110] in 1961. The former group defined emphysema as a condition of the lung characterized by increase beyond normal in the size of air spaces distal to the terminal bronchiole, either from dilatation or from destruction of their walls. Both the American Thoracic Society and the W.H.O. limited the use of the term "emphysema" to enlargement of these air spaces *accompanied by destruction*. We prefer to adopt the latter definition and to employ the term "overinflation" to describe the state of the lungs as defined in the Ciba symposium.

PATHOLOGIC CHARACTERISTICS

Examination of macroscopic sections of inflated lung reveals a varied degree and distribution of destruction of the acinar unit. The likelihood that such destruction has produced symptoms during life depends not only upon its severity but also upon its location within the acinus and its distribution through the parenchymal tissue. Selective involvement of the acinus at the level of the first and second generations of respiratory bronchioles results in a proportionately greater degree of function loss than of structural damage. If destruction takes place predominantly in the alveolar sacs and alveoli, extensive involvement of the lung parenchyma may be present without accompanying disability.

Morphologically, emphysema has been divided into "selective" and "nonselective" on the basis of the distribution of destruction within the acinus or the secondary lobule.[111] The selective emphysemas include those in which destruction occurs in specific areas of the acinus or secondary lobule—*centrilobular emphysema, focal-dust emphysema,* and *alveolar duct emphysema.* Unselective distribution of emphysema refers to general destruction of the acinus or lobule, without favoring any specific region; in this category is *panlobular* or *panacinar emphysema.*

Panlobular Emphysema (PLE)

Macroscopically, panlobular (panacinar) disease is manifested by a change in the normal architecture of the lobule, consisting of loss of contrast between the larger, rounded alveolar ducts and the smaller, multifaceted alveoli. The alveoli are enlarged, lose their angles, and become indistinguishable from the alveolar ducts. Examination of thick sections of lung reveals abnormal fenestrations approximately 20μ in diameter in the walls of the dilated alveoli. In the end stages of the disease, affected parenchyma may consist of no more than thin strands of tissue surrounding blood vessels— the so-called cotton-candy lung. Panlobular emphysema occurs in more or less random distribution throughout the lungs, with some predilection for the lower lobes and anterior zones.[103, 112] It may be associated with centrilobular emphysema, in which circumstance chronic bronchitis is almost invariable, usually in patients with a history of heavy cigarette smoking. PLE occurs in aged patients more commonly than does CLE, being identified occasionally in the eighth and ninth decades, occurring with equal frequency in males and females.[103] Although it is clear that both types of emphysema are more common in men than in women, panlobular disease appears to be more common than centrilobular in females. In some instances panlobular emphysema is associated with a family history of the disease and with a deficiency of alpha$_1$-antitrypsin. Gough[113] considers this type of emphysema to be distinguished by absence of inflammation.

Centrilobular Emphysema (CLE)

In centrilobular (centriacinar) emphysema, the earliest change is dilatation of respiratory bronchioles, usually those of the two distal orders; the periphery of the lobule—alveolar ducts, alveolar sacs, and alveoli—is spared (Figure 11–6). As destruction progresses, a number of respiratory bronchioles become confluent both in series and in parallel, creating a common pool supplied by a terminal bronchiole proximally and leading to relatively normal alveolar tissue distally.[103, 114] Fenestrations appear in the thinned-out bronchiolar walls and open into the outer intact lobular parenchyma. Both the terminal and the respiratory bronchioles often show evidence of inflammation and may be completely obstructed by mucous plugs. Lymphocytes, plasma cells, and sometimes polymorphonuclear leukocytes and dust-containing macrophages are present.

Obstruction of bronchioles in CLE, either by inflammation or by mucous plugging, implies that ventilation of the "pools" and of the alveoli distal to them must occur through fenestrations and alveolar pores connecting with contiguous ventilated parenchyma. The air that enters these obstructed zones has been in contact with capillaries containing venous blood; thus the capillaries in the obstructed areas are exposed to a relatively low Po_2 and a high Pco_2. Even when the bronchioles supplying a zone of CLE are patent, the size of the centrilobular "pool" may be such that the interface between inspired gas and gas already present within the acinus occurs within the "pool" rather than more peripherally in the alveolar ducts. Either of these effects (or both) results in a greater distance for gas diffusion and can lead to ineffective alveolar ventilation with consequent reduction in arterial Po_2 and elevation of arterial Pco_2.[115]

In its early stages, CLE occurs predominantly in the upper two-thirds of the lungs, particularly in the apical and posterior segments of the upper lobes and the superior segments of the lower lobes.[103, 112] Considerable amounts of carbon pigment are commonly found in areas of destruction in the middle of the lobules.

A large proportion of patients with CLE are heavy cigarette smokers and consequently usually show morphologic evidence of chronic bronchitis.[103]

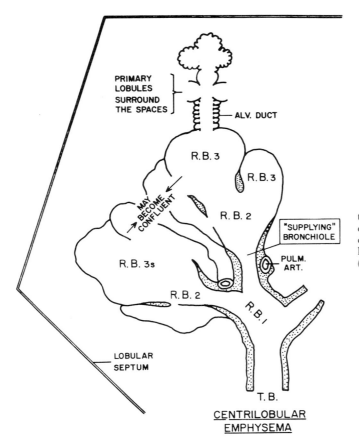

**PRIMARY
LOBULES
SURROUND
THE SPACES**

ALV. DUCT

R.B. 3

R.B. 3

MAY
BECOME
CONFLUENT

R.B. 2

"SUPPLYING"
BRONCHIOLE

R.B. 3s

PULM.
ART.

R.B. 2

R.B. I

LOBULAR
SEPTUM

T.B.

**CENTRILOBULAR
EMPHYSEMA**

Figure 11–6. Diagram of the Acinus in Centrilobular Emphysema. The second and third order respiratory bronchioles (RB) are severely dilated while the periphery of the lobule—alveolar ducts, alveolar sacs, and alveoli—are spared. (Courtesy of Professor J. Gough.)

Other Forms of Emphysema

Focal-Dust Emphysema (FDE). Gough[113] reviewed his findings in cases showing the accumulation of coal dust in terminal and respiratory bronchioles and its association with bronchiolar dilatation in later life. Atrophy of smooth muscle occurs in the walls of the bronchioles in advanced cases. The distention of terminal and respiratory bronchioles causes little or no disturbance of respiratory function and may be differentiated from early CLE by the lack of bronchiolitis.[113] FDE closely resembles CLE and is not universally recognized as a separate entity. However, there does appear to be an excess of emphysema affecting the respiratory bronchioles of coal workers who do not appear to be excessive cigarette smokers.

Alveolar Duct Emphysema (ADE). Increase in the diameter of alveolar ducts is a common finding in elderly persons and seldom is associated with clinical or functional evidence of disease.

Paraseptal Emphysema. This form selectively involves the periphery of the lung deep to the pleura and along interlobar septa. Bullae may develop from coalescence of distended, destroyed alveoli and commonly are multiple; in fact, paraseptal emphysema is thought to represent the basic lesion of bullous lung disease. In the majority of cases this form of emphysema gives rise to no symptoms and is well localized. It is thought that this is the abnormality that often leads to spontaneous pneumothorax.

Small areas of alveolar distention and destruction commonly occur in the vicinity of pulmonary scars. "Paracicatricial" or "scar" emphysema may occur anywhere in the lungs and, like paraseptal disease, is of no clinical consequence unless confluence of lesions results in the formation of a bulla.

INCIDENCE

Since emphysema must be defined in morphologic terms, the only meaningful data on incidence are obtained from necropsy series. In a random necropsy series of 138 patients, Thurlbeck[116] found some degree of emphysema in 50 per cent, but lung destruction was severe enough to cause death or disability in only 6.5 per cent of these. The incidence of CLE is slightly higher than that of PLE and the former occurs over a wider age range, being more common in the younger age groups. CLE is much more common in males than in females and in fact, all observers are agreed on the higher frequency of more severe grades of emphysema of all types in men compared with women of similar ages.

ETIOLOGY AND PATHOGENESIS

The etiology and pathogenesis of emphysema are incompletely understood. It is very likely that several factors act not only in initiating changes that lead to the disease but also in contributing to its progress once it is established. These factors are discussed in detail in our text *Diagnosis of Diseases of the Chest* (page 1375), and the interested reader is directed there for further information. In the following paragraphs, the essential features of etiology and pathogenesis are summarized.

Although many unanswered questions still remain, a considerable body of knowledge has accumulated that permits speculation as to the etiology and pathogenesis of human emphysema. The major pieces in this jigsaw puzzle have been identified, and it remains for us to attempt to fit them together to see whether an image is created that explains the end result of dilatation and destruction of alveolar membranes. Two of the largest pieces in the puzzle bear the labels bronchitis and small airway inflammation. Our primary concern here is to summarize the effects of elastolysis and to describe the body defense mechanisms against this enzymatic process. Any acceptable hypothesis must incorporate at least five important and incontrovertible advances in the field.

1. *The discovery that animal and human phagocytes contain elastolytic enzymes.* Human polymorphonuclear leukocytes contain proteolytic enzymes that can digest lung proteins both *in vitro*[117] and *in vivo*.[118] Proteases are also present in purulent sputum.[119] An elastase-like esterase and protease activity also has been identified in human alveolar macrophages.[120] When grown in a culture medium, alveolar macrophages from rats are also capable of synthesizing and secreting alpha$_1$-proteinase inhibitor.[121] The elastase in human granulocytes is inhibited by serum alpha$_1$-antitrypsin,[122] whereas macrophage elastase is less effectively inhibited by the same substance.[123] In a study of nine alpha$_1$-antitrypsin–deficient (Pi^{ZZ}) individuals, the severity of pulmonary dysfunction appeared to correlate with the concentration of elastolytic protease in the granules of polymorphonuclear leukocytes rather than with the amount of cigarette smoking.[124] This observation may explain why nonsmoking children with severe alpha$_1$-antitrypsin deficiency sometimes have severe panlobular emphysema.

2. *Patients with severe alpha$_1$-antitrypsin deficiency have an increased susceptibility to emphysema.* The emphysema of alpha$_1$-antitrypsin deficiency characteristically possesses a striking lower lobe anatomic distribution, a fact that has been attributed to the tendency for leukocytes to become sequestered in lower lobe pulmonary capillaries.[125] It is believed that in the absence of antiproteolytic enzymes, this potential source of elastase permits uninhibited action of proteolytic enzymes in basal segments of the lungs.

3. *Experimentally, proteolytic enzymes induce elastin destruction.* It has been suggested[126] that experimental emphysema produced by aerosolized proteases may not be attributable solely to the elastase-like effect of these enzymes but may also involve macrophage injury and production of chemotactic factor resulting in invasion by neutrophils and a cascade-type cellular destructive reaction. In fact, papain-induced emphysema can be prevented by intratracheal installation of alpha$_1$-antitrypsin, even though this substance does not inhibit papain *in vitro*.[127] On the other hand, a single elastolytic enzyme has been purified from dog neutrophils that produces a dose-related degree of canine emphysema.[128]

4. *There is a highly significant correlation between the prevalence and amount of cigarette smoking and the development of emphysema.* A statistical association between cigarette smoking and emphysema has been firmly established[129] and it has been shown that the extent of alveolar destruction increases with the amount smoked in both men and women. Cigarette smoke causes immobilization of leukocytes[130] and degradation of intracellular membranous structures. The number of circulating leukocytes has been reported to be increased in cigarette smokers compared with nonsmokers, and it is possible that they are attracted to the lungs because cigarette smoke stimulates alveolar macrophages to produce neutrophil chemotactic factor.[131] Similarly, increased numbers of alveolar macrophages[120] possessing a greatly reduced half-life have been obtained in the bronchial lavage of smokers. In addition to their greater number, the alveolar macrophages of cigarette

smokers demonstrate relatively greater elastolytic activity than those of nonsmokers[120]; in addition, lavage fluids from smokers show a 50 per cent reduction in functional alpha$_1$-antiproteinase compared with nonsmokers.[132]

5. *Some patients tend to develop centriacinar (centrilobular) emphysema while others acquire panacinar (panlobular) disease.* Although the proteolytic-antiproteolytic explanation for destruction or protection, respectively, of the alveolar septa is convincing, it is somewhat more difficult to understand why there should be two fundamentally different forms of emphysema, centrilobular and panlobular. The former involves the upper lobes predominantly and shows its major pathologic effects in the respiratory bronchioles. This form of the disease characteristically is found in heavy smokers, a finding that correlates with the observed destruction of the more proximal portions of the acinus resulting from inhaled noxious substances. By contrast, panlobular emphysema is a disease of the lower lobes, an anatomic bias that may be explained by the fact that polymorphonuclear leukocytes tend to sequester in vessels at the base of the lungs and elastase-like enzymes from this source (with or without the aid of alveolar macrophages activated by cigarette smoke) induce the characteristic destruction of more peripheral portions of the acinus. Two groups of investigators[134, 135] have described an animal model in which neutrophil sequestration has been observed in pulmonary capillaries, induced by repeated injections of endotoxin, with resulting emphysema. There is also reason to believe that sequestered platelets may stimulate human leukocytic elastase against lung elastin by releasing factor 4.[132]

ROENTGENOGRAPHIC MANIFESTATIONS

In a 1970 correlative study of 61 patients with morphologically proved emphysema,[136] two different roentgenographic patterns were recognized and were designated "arterial deficiency" (AD) and "increased markings" (IM). AD represented peripheral vascular deficiency (oligemia), in most cases associated with severe overinflation, and IM indicated increased prominence of the vascular markings, almost invariably with milder overinflation. In the latter group, pulmonary arterial hypertension was ev-

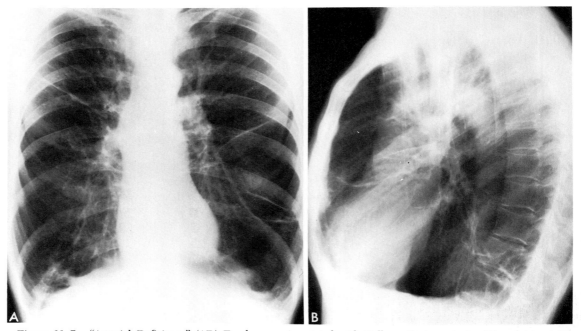

Figure 11–7. "Arterial Deficiency" (AD) Emphysema Associated with Bullae. Posteroanterior (*A*) and lateral (*B*) roentgenograms of a 43-year-old woman reveal severe overinflation of both lungs. The diaphragm is low and its superior surface concave. Note the prominent costophrenic muscle slips. The retrosternal air space is deepened. The peripheral vasculature of the lungs is severely diminished, but there is no evidence of pulmonary arterial hypertension. (It is probable that the upper lung zones are less severely involved than the lower, permitting redistribution of blood flow and a lack of any tendency for the development of hypertension.) Numerous bullae are present in both lower lung zones, particularly the left.

ident in the great majority and cor pulmonale in many.

THE "ARTERIAL DEFICIENCY" (AD PATTERN) OF EMPHYSEMA

The roentgenologic signs of this pattern of emphysema include pulmonary overinflation and oligemia. Bullae may or may not be visible.

Overinflation

Characteristically, overinflation is of severe degree, usually 4+ and never less than 3+ (assessed on a scale of 0 to 4+). Probably the most dependable single piece of evidence of pulmonary overinflation is flattening of the diaphragmatic domes (Figure 11–7). In the careful roentgenologic-pathologic correlative study by Nicklaus and his colleagues,[137] of the five roentgenologic criteria employed, diaphragmatic flattening was the most accurate indicator of the presence of morphologic emphysema and gave rise to the least intra- and interobserver variation. We find that if the configuration of the diaphragm is concave superiorly, the presence of emphysema is virtually certain, at least in adults (Figure 11–7). "Tenting" of the diaphragm sometimes results from the invagination of thickened visceral pleura attached to septa between basal bullae. Other traditional signs of overinflation include increase in the width of the retrosternal air space, anterior bowing of the sternum, accentuation of the thoracic kyphosis, and horizontally inclined, widely spaced ribs; however, none of these signs is as valuable as diaphragmatic flattening.

In addition to these static changes observed on standard posteroanterior and lateral roentgenograms exposed at TLC, air trapping constitutes an important sign in the assessment of patients with emphysema. Limitation of diaphragmatic excursion provides convincing evidence for the presence of air trapping, but is only an indirect indication of overinflation.

The development of left-sided heart failure in emphysematous patients with roentgenographic evidence of overinflation gives rise to a curious change in the chest roentgenogram. In addition to the usual evidence of interstitial pulmonary edema, the signs of overinflation may diminish or disappear altogether.[138] Milne and Bass[138] also found that left-sided heart failure has a marked effect on lung function by concealing evidence of overinflation and, in some cases, by improving diffusing capacity and flow rates.

Alteration in Pulmonary Vasculature (Oligemia)

Diminution in the caliber of the pulmonary vessels, with increased rapidity of tapering distally, is regarded by several investigators[136, 139] as the most reliable roentgenologic sign of emphysema. In our experience, diminution of the peripheral vasculature is a sign of great value in differentiating emphysema from other diseases in which hyperinflation is an integral part, notably spasmodic asthma. This differentiation is particularly accurate if full lung tomography is employed in addition to standard roentgenograms of the chest.[140] Simon[141] has emphasized the value of the "marker vessel" in the assessment of vascular loss in emphysema. It is common for blood to be diverted from more severely affected zones to those least affected, producing dilatation of segmental vessels in either upper or lower zones.

In a 1973 roentgenologic-physiologic study of 101 patients with chronic air flow obstruction, Simon and his colleagues[142] found that when the roentgenogram showed widespread vascular attenuation as well as overinflation, the impairment in FEV_1 and other tests of pulmonary function was considerably more severe than when there was evidence of overinflation alone. We are in general agreement with this observation. However, if the presence of overinflation can be regarded as convincing evidence of loss of elastic recoil *in the absence of clinical evidence of asthma*, then this sign by itself should permit a confident diagnosis of emphysema. The *additional* finding of oligemia, either local or general, might then be construed as evidence of *severity* of the disease rather than simply of its presence.

In our experience, emphysema occurs more often in local form than is usually recognized. In one series, fully half of the 26 cases had oligemia localized to one or more areas of both lungs, the vasculature in the remaining portions being normal or of increased caliber.[140] In this series the lower lung zones were most predominantly involved. The type of emphysema associated with alpha$_1$-antitrypsin deficiency usually involves the lower lobes predominantly, with relatively normal or distended vasculature to upper lung zones.[143] However, such anatomic predilection also is found in a significant percentage of patients with normal alpha$_1$-antitrypsin values. Xenon-133 studies of patients with pulmonary emphysema have confirmed the observation that destructive lung disease frequently is local rather than general.[144]

Pulmonary arterial hypertension secondary

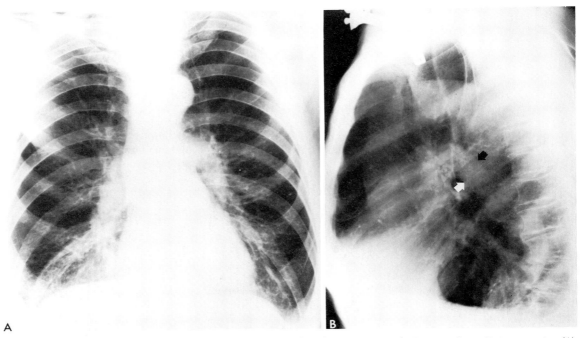

A   B

Figure 11–8. "Arterial Deficiency" (AD) Emphysema with Pulmonary Arterial Hypertension. Posteroanterior (A) and lateral (B) roentgenograms reveal severe overinflation of both lungs as evidenced by marked flattening of the diaphragm (seen to best advantage in lateral projection) and increase in the depth of the retrosternal air space. The lungs generally are oligemic, arterial deficiency being more apparent in the upper two-thirds than in the bases. The hilar pulmonary arteries are moderately enlarged and taper rapidly distally. In lateral projection, note the shadow of the dilated descending branch of the left pulmonary artery (*arrows*). Despite the evidence of severe pulmonary arterial hypertension, the heart is only slightly enlarged. The patient is a 71-year-old man severely incapacitated by longstanding emphysema.

to emphysema usually is easily recognizable, not by a deficiency in the peripheral vasculature alone but with the additional finding of dilatation of hilar pulmonary arteries (Figure 11–8). Tapering of arteries distally may be so striking as to constitute sufficient evidence of cor pulmonale despite a small cardiac size. It is well recognized that cor pulmonale cannot be appreciated in the majority of cases of emphysema unless cardiac failure has developed, since the heart shadow typically is long and narrow.

Bullae

Bullae are local, air-containing cystic spaces within the lung, ranging from 1 to 2 cm in diameter up to the volume of a whole hemithorax. They may be single or multiple. Their walls are usually of no more than hairline thickness, so that it may be difficult to distinguish them from uninvolved parenchyma. In fact, Laws and Heard[145] showed that frequently large bullae may be observed pathologically that are quite invisible roentgenologically, even in retrospect. When bullae occur as part of general panlobular emphysema, the diagnosis of bullous emphysema is only semantic; as pointed out by

Bates and Christie,[146] cystic spaces up to 1 cm in diameter are common in severe panlobular emphysema and whether they should be regarded as bullae or merely as large emphysematous spaces is a matter of preference.

THE "INCREASED MARKINGS" (IM) PATTERN OF EMPHYSEMA

The roentgenographic appearance of "IM emphysema" is the antithesis of the AD pattern (Figure 11–9). Instead of the vascular markings being attenuated and diminished in caliber, they are more prominent than normal and tend to be irregular in contour and indistinct in definition.[136] Thus, in contrast to the exceptionally clear lungs characteristic of "AD emphysema," the appearance is that of the "dirty chest" suggestive of some cases of severe chronic bronchitis. Overinflation seldom is present to the degree seen in AD disease and, in the majority of cases, is no more than slight or moderate. Pulmonary arterial hypertension (as evidenced by enlargement of the hilar pulmonary arteries) is invariable and in many cases is associated with cardiac enlargement (cor pulmonale); in fact, cardiac enlargement is a much more frequent feature of IM than of AD disease. Bullae seldom are seen.

THE SIGNIFICANCE OF THE AD AND IM PATTERNS AND THEIR RELATIONSHIP TO PLE AND CLE

Although the relationships are by no means definitive, and the designations represent the two ends of a wide spectrum, there is some indication that *patients who manifest the arterial deficiency pattern roentgenographically have panlobular emphysema morphologically and that those who show the increased markings pattern have centrilobular emphysema.* Extending this relationship to the clinical presentation and employing the euphemistic terms coined by Dornhorst,[147] patients with the AD pattern present as "pink puffers" and those with the IM pattern as "blue bloaters." Supporting the re-

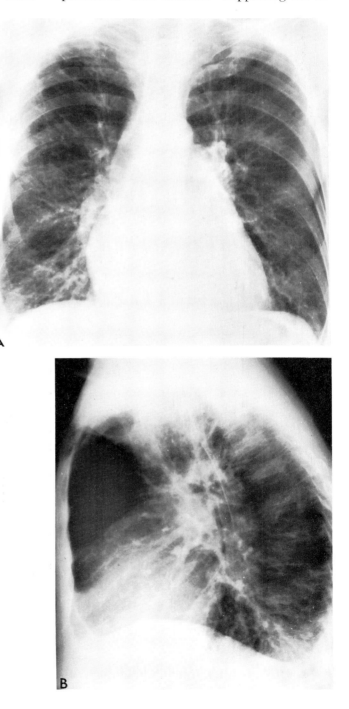

Figure 11–9. "Increased Markings" (IM) **Emphysema.** Roentgenograms of the chest in posteroanterior (A) and lateral (B) projection reveal only slightly increased volume (note the deep retrosternal air space). The vascular markings throughout the lungs are prominent except in the subapical zones, where there appears to be local vascular deficiency. The heart is moderately enlarged (consistent with right ventricular enlargement) and the hilar pulmonary arteries dilated, indicating the presence of pulmonary arterial hypertension. At necropsy, the lungs were found to be extensively involved by emphysema, which was almost purely centrilobular in type.

lationship between the AD pattern and PLE is the observation that patients with either Swyer-James' syndrome or alpha₁-antitrypsin deficiency manifest an arterial deficiency pattern roentgenographically and have panlobular emphysema morphologically.[148]

It is conceivable that the IM pattern is due, at least in part, to the "inflammatory changes" described by Burrows and associates[149] or the "recurrent bronchopneumonitis" reported by Milne and Bass.[150] Their roentgenologic criteria for the diagnosis of "recurrent bronchopneumonitis" include tortuosity, marginal blurring and segmentation of the vasculature, enlargement of the central arteries, patchy interstitial fibrosis, and loss of vascular lability. The irregularity and slight tortuosity of the peripheral pulmonary vessels are stated to be affected by contiguous areas of fibrosis and by arteriolar endarteritis obliterans.

Other possibilities have been suggested as the morphologic basis for this pattern. In a review of the roentgenographic features of chronic obstructive pulmonary disease, Heitzman and his colleagues[151, 152] describe and illustrate a patient who showed a typical IM roentgenographic pattern during life and whose lung at necropsy revealed gross bronchial dilatation and a pulmonary arterial tree whose branches were of large caliber out to the periphery of the lung. They speculate that one or both of these abnormalities could have contributed to the prominence of lung markings, and this explanation appears perfectly valid in this patient. However, since bronchiectasis was not a prominent feature of most of the cases with the IM pattern described by Thurlbeck and associates,[136] it might be concluded that the vascular nature of the shadows would be the more likely explanation in that group. In fact, Scarrow[153] has documented dilatation of intrapulmonary branches of the pulmonary artery in some cases of chronic obstructive pulmonary disease.

ACCURACY OF THE ROENTGENOLOGIC DIAGNOSIS OF EMPHYSEMA

Perhaps the definitive study on the accuracy of the roentgenologic diagnosis of emphysema was carried out by Thurlbeck and Simon,[154] who performed a roentgenologic-pathologic correlative study of 696 patients from whose lungs paper-mounted, whole-lung sections were available. Only occasionally were patients without emphysema or with mild emphysema thought to have the disease based on roentgenologic evidence. Of the patients with moderately se-

vere and severe emphysema, 41 per cent were diagnosed as having the disease, as were two-thirds of those with the most severe grade of emphysema. Centrilobular disease was usually present when emphysema was diagnosed roentgenologically in upper lung zones, as was panacinar disease when emphysema was diagnosed in lower zones. No combination of roentgenologic variables, including those generally accepted as indicating overinflation, was found that recognized emphysema better than the subjective diagnosis of the disease based on arterial deficiency.

Finally, we regard the roentgenologic signs of morphologically proved emphysema to consist of two distinctly different patterns, "arterial deficiency" (AD) and "increased markings" (IM). Provided that both patterns are recognized, the roentgenologic diagnosis of emphysema is highly accurate in cases of severe disease and reasonably precise in those of less severity. If only the traditional roentgenologic criteria of emphysema are recognized—general pulmonary overinflation and pulmonary oligemia—many patients with severe emphysema will not be recognized, including those with clear-cut evidence of pulmonary hypertension and cor pulmonale.

The terms "emphysema" and "chronic bronchitis" mean different things to different people. For example, Fletcher and his colleagues[155] found an almost identical spectrum of diseases in an "emphysema clinic" in Chicago and a "chronic bronchitic" clinic in London. The euphemistic terms "pink puffer" and "blue bloater" applied by Dornhorst[147] to patients who manifest predominantly emphysematous and chronic bronchitic characteristics, respectively, describe two ends of a spectrum between which are the majority of patients who manifest elements of both. If the selection of a therapeutic regime depends in part on the categorization of a patient into one or the other of these two types, as has been suggested, the radiologist should recognize changes appropriate to each type and describe them in a manner clearly understood not only by the referring physician but by his radiologist-colleagues.

The confusion existing in the radiologic literature derives not from the "classic" picture of emphysema—marked pulmonary overinflation and oligemia—but from the picture designated as the "IM pattern" of disease. Whether or not the pathophysiology of this disease is related to the presence of emphysema is disputable. Reid[156] has stated that CLE is not associated with roentgenologic abnormality, whereas others, including ourselves, have found the contrary,[103, 136] *a discrepancy due to differences in morphologic rather than roentgenologic interpretation.* It is almost certain that patients categorized by us as having the IM pattern are similar or identical to the British "chronic bronchitic with cardiac decompensation." Which label one wishes to place on this roentgenographic pattern of disease is probably more of semantic than of practical importance, although logically it must be differentiated from the classic AD pattern.

CLINICAL AND PHYSIOLOGIC MANIFESTATIONS OF CHRONIC BRONCHITIS AND EMPHYSEMA

Although the morphologic and roentgenologic manifestations of chronic bronchitis can be described separately from those of emphysema, it is extremely difficult to separate their clinical manifestations. Therefore, the clinical features and physiologic manifestations of the two diseases are described together under the general heading of chronic obstructive pulmonary disease.

SYMPTOMS OF CHRONIC OBSTRUCTIVE PULMONARY DISEASE

Patients with chronic obstructive pulmonary disease caused by chronic bronchitis, with or without emphysema, complain of cough and expectoration. In over 75 per cent of cases, cough either antedates the onset of dyspnea or the two symptoms appear simultaneously. The 10 to 15 per cent of patients with established chronic obstructive pulmonary disease who do not have a productive cough and complain only of exertional dyspnea are presumed to have primary emphysema.[157]

The majority of patients who complain of cough and expectoration have mucoid sputum, only periodically yellow or green. Hemoptysis is very uncommon in chronic bronchitis, and its presence should stimulate careful search for other causes. Most patients attest to an increased frequency of respiratory infections during the winter, and such episodes may increase the severity of dyspnea. Most patients are heavy smokers.[157]

A number of studies have shown that the great majority of working people with chronic bronchitis do not develop progressive chronic airway obstruction. Approximately 10 per cent—almost invariably heavy smokers—experience increasing dyspnea and subsequently develop respiratory insufficiency. When ventilatory impairment becomes sufficiently severe to result in dyspnea, progression to severe disability can be expected within 6 to 10 years.[158] Although a gradual decline to respiratory failure and death seems virtually inevitable once the patient with COPD seeks medical aid because of dyspnea, the life span of these patients has been greatly prolonged with modern therapy. In one study,[159] 64 patients with hypercapnia survived for a period of 2 to 15 years. When disease is this far advanced, repeated episodes of acute respiratory failure may occur. Seventy to 75 per cent of such patients survive such crises,[160, 161] although approximately 50 per cent die within 1 year[160] and 70 per cent within 2 years of the initial episode.[161] When cor pulmonale develops, most observers judge the prognosis to be extremely bad, although in our experience some patients survive for 5 years or more. Certainly, the outlook seems to have improved in recent years.

It is probable that despite the elimination of cigarette smoking, progression of COPD results from repeated infections of the lower respiratory tract, largely of viral etiology and from chemical irritation of the distal airways and air spaces by atmospheric pollution. Microorganisms and inert particles have the dual effect of increasing mucous secretion (which obstructs small airways) and attracting phagocytes (with resultant elastolysis). In most patients with cor pulmonale the blood gas values are markedly abnormal, including decreased PO_2 and arterial oxygen saturation and increased PCO_2. Clinically, such patients have cyanosis, peripheral edema, liver enlargement, and sometimes ascites as well as jugular venous distention; they may be most comfortable in a sitting position. Examination reveals faint heart sounds and a right ventricular heave, usually of lesser degree than in other types of cor pulmonale.[162] The presence of a pansystolic murmur accentuated on inspiration and heard close to the lower left sternal border or in the epigastrium indicates tricuspid insufficiency.

The electrocardiogram may be perfectly normal in patients with CAO despite the development of increased pulmonary vascular resistance on exercise. However, as airway obstruction becomes more severe, signs of right axis deviation develop, with large S waves and diphasic T waves over the left precordium beyond the V_2 position. These changes correlate best with total pulmonary vascular resistance.[163]

Neurologic symptoms and signs are common

in patients with advanced chronic obstructive pulmonary disease and in some cases are severe enough to divert attention from the underlying condition. Symptoms include somnolence, headaches, and mental confusion, sometimes associated with a tremor or twitch of the extremities. Coma, depressed tendon reflexes, extensor plantar responses, and occasionally papilledema may suggest the presence of a brain tumor. The precise mechanism by which these symptoms and signs develop is not completely understood. They appear to relate to the presence of hypoxemia and particularly hypercapnia.[164]

The increased incidence of peptic ulcer in patients with chronic obstructive pulmonary disease is well documented, ranging from 10 to over 35 per cent compared with 3 per cent in control groups.[165] Often it is not associated with pain, being suspected only because of gastrointestinal hemorrhage. This increased incidence may be explained, at least partly, by gastric hypersecretion stimulated by increased arterial PCO_2 and decreased arterial PO_2.

Pulmonary hypertension, cor pulmonale, and heart failure may be the major causes of symptoms in chronic obstructive pulmonary disease. Right ventricular hypertrophy occurs most often in patients with severe CAO or advanced emphysema,[136] but it is occasionally seen with little or no morphologic emphysema and with only moderate airway obstruction. In the latter circumstances the right heart strain probably is the result of ventilation-perfusion inequality caused by disease in the small airways. Right ventricular hypertrophy occurs in response to pulmonary hypertension, which may be episodic and associated with acute attacks of respiratory failure.

When both hypoxemia and hypercarbia coexist with cor pulmonale caused by emphysema, secondary polycythemia is prone to develop. Although both hemoglobin and hematocrit values are low in many hypoxic emphysema patients at sea level compared with normal high altitude dwellers with similar degrees of hypoxemia, in some patients an increased red cell volume is masked by a proportional increase in plasma volume. In such circumstances, demonstration of the absolute polycythemia requires direct measurements of blood volume.

Although spontaneous pneumothorax is a rare complication of emphysema, it may have serious consequences since it tends to occur in patients with little respiratory reserve.

The treatment of respiratory failure in emphysema patients with hypoxemia and hyper-capnia may result in serious complications. Uncontrolled oxygen therapy increases $\dot{V}/\dot{Q}$ mismatching resulting in hypoventilation, an abrupt and sometimes catastrophic rise in PCO_2, coma, and death.[165a] Hypoventilation may also occur following attempts to restore the acid-base balance to normal by the administration of bicarbonate.

Patients with COPD manifest impaired water handling and electrolyte exchange.[166] Renal excretion is impaired during respiratory failure and usually improves during recovery. Potassium depletion can be a major complication of both acute and chronic respiratory failure. Potassium tends to move from tissue cells to plasma, and although serum potassium values may be normal, total exchangeable potassium may be greatly reduced.[167]

PHYSICAL SIGNS IN CHRONIC OBSTRUCTIVE PULMONARY DISEASE

In many patients with chronic cough and expectoration, physical examination of the chest reveals no abnormalities, at least during quiet breathing. At maximal expiration or during rapid, deep breathing, however, expiratory rhonchi are audible in most cases. The presence of rhonchi in a patient who does not have dyspnea but who otherwise fulfills the criteria for the diagnosis of chronic bronchitis probably represents the earliest objective sign of airway obstruction and presumably reflects the presence of increased secretions within the bronchi. Rhonchi usually are more numerous in the patient with chronic bronchitis who complains of shortness of breath on exertion, and commonly they are present during both inspiration and expiration. When high-pitched sibilant rhonchi and crepitations are heard in addition to sonorous rhonchi, it can be assumed that the disease has affected the smaller bronchi and bronchioles also.

When emphysema becomes widespread it gives rise to physical signs attributable to the combination of airway obstruction, destruction of alveolar septa, formation of bullae, loss of parenchymal elasticity, and pulmonary overinflation. The most characteristic of these additional signs is decreased intensity of breath sounds, usually described as a reduction in "air entry." Expiration becomes prolonged. Loss of parenchymal elasticity results in wide fluctuations in intrapleural pressure that may be manifested clinically by intercostal and supraclavicular indrawing during inspiration and jugular venous filling during expiration. When lung volumes are markedly increased and the thoracic cage is fixed in an inspiratory position, the physical signs are characteristic: the chest becomes barrel-shaped, and the thoracic kyphosis may be considerably increased; the shoulders are raised, and the chest tends to move *en bloc*, often with contraction of the accessory muscles of respiration in the neck. Pulmonary overinflation may be evidenced by increased resonance of the percussion note, although this may be difficult to evaluate in obese or muscular patients. Separation of the heart from the anterior chest wall by overinflated lung results in varying degrees of faintness of heart sounds; in some cases, auscultation of the heart can be performed satisfactorily only when the stethoscope is placed over the epigastrium.

PULMONARY FUNCTION STUDIES IN CHRONIC OBSTRUCTIVE PULMONARY DISEASE

The lesions responsible for airway obstruction in primary emphysema and in simple bronchitis are distinctly different, and yet the functional abnormalities are surprisingly similar. The major pathophysiologic result of alveolar destruction is loss of elastic recoil, whereas that of bronchitis is an increase in airway resistance.[79] Elastic recoil is usually expressed as the maximum intrapleural pressure attained at TLC[168]; airway resistance is measured either directly in a body plethysmograph or indirectly by flowtime or flow-volume curves. Early in the course of both chronic bronchitis and emphysema, the pathophysiology may not be reflected in these measurements but may be identified by abnormalities caused by bronchiolar obstruction,[169] or elastolytic disease detected in tests of smaller lung units. Although it would appear feasible to be able to distinguish bronchial from extrabronchial factors in the pathophysiology of CAO, at least in its early stages, this is not so in the majority of cases of advanced COPD when chronic bronchitis and emphysema coexist.

Assessment of Airway Obstruction

Although the designation "chronic obstructive pulmonary disease" implies resistance to the flow of air in the conducting system, some patients with chronic productive cough and expiratory rhonchi throughout their lungs on physical examination reveal no objective evidence of airway obstruction during routine pulmonary function testing. It is probable that in such patients the small airways are chiefly affected. Since these are responsible for only a small percentage of the total resistance of the conducting system,[171] the degree of their obstruction must be considerable before it gives rise to abnormal routine direct or indirect measurements of flow resistance However, by the time most patients seek medical aid they not only have cough and expectoration but some degree of dyspnea also, and their routine pulmonary function tests reveal significant abnormalities of bronchial air flow and resistance.

Routine indirect methods for detecting airway obstruction include forced expiratory volume (FEV) measured against time, and flow rates plotted against lung volume from TLC to RV. Various flow rates can be calculated from the FEV curve, but it is generally accepted that measurements in the lower 75 per cent of vital capacity are earlier indicators of COPD since they are independent of effort and measure flow through smaller airways.[172, 173] As a screening procedure for large numbers of patients, the most practical test is the FEV_1,[173] which is averaged from three to five tracings of a forced expiration recorded on a rapidly revolving kymograph. Some investigators have found the midexpiratory area of this curve (MMFR) and the maximum expiratory flow volume (MEFV) to be abnormal in subjects with normal closing volumes, a test whose sensitivity has been stressed.[174] Good correlation has been shown between the MMFR, $FEV_{1.0}$, and MBC and the extent of emphysema found at necropsy. A particularly useful and often used index of the degree of airway obstruction is the ratio of FEV_1 to FVC.[175] Most patients with severe airway obstruction as evidenced by indirect methods of measurement have blood gas abnormalities, although this association is not invariable.

The precise mechanism of airway obstruction in chronic obstructive pulmonary disease is incompletely understood. Since small airways are responsible for less than 25 per cent of the total resistance in the conducting system, their deterioration cannot explain the severe degree of expiratory obstruction common to many patients with chronic bronchitis and emphysema. Expiratory obstruction almost certainly is caused by collapse of bronchi (the result of loss of elasticity), atrophy of bronchial walls, and the marked increase in transmural pressure that characteristically occurs in emphysema.

Clinical-pathologic correlation of patients with COPD at the Royal Victoria Hospital in Montreal[136] suggested that the degree of airway obstruction in chronic obstructive pulmonary disease relates more to the morphologic extent of emphysema than to the presence or severity of chronic bronchitis. This observation may explain the lack of response to bronchodilators (as judged by flow rates) in the great majority of cases of chronic obstructive pulmonary disease.

It has been shown[158, 176] that patients with COPD manifest an average decrease in FEV_1 of 50 to 75 ml per year in contrast to the decline of 25 ml found in normal individuals. This suggests that a 20- to 30-year history of disease is required before ventilatory impairment becomes severe enough to produce dyspnea, and it is conceivable that simultaneous slowly progressive alveolar destruction may cause this gradual decrease in flow rates. In contrast to the findings in one much quoted study,[177] it has been shown by others[178] that patients who manifest a low FEV_1 on initial testing do not show an accelerated decrease in FEV_1 over time. In fact, Burrows[179] has found so much variability in FEV_1 in patients with COPD over a four- to five-year period that meaningful individual regression slopes cannot be calculated.

Disturbances in Lung Volumes

The finding of severe emphysema at necropsy denotes disturbances in lung volumes during life that are largely predictable: an increase in TLC and FRC of approximately 50 per cent over predicted normal values, approximate doubling of the RV, and a decrease in VC of about 50 per cent. The RV-TLC ratio is about 40 per cent greater than the generally accepted normal value of 35 per cent in late middle age.[136] The initial increase in FRC in patients with chronic obstructive pulmonary disease undoubtedly results from air trapping distal to obstructed bronchioles in acinar units ventilated by collateral air drift. With progressive lung destruction and the formation of larger "air pools," the tethering effect of elastic fibers in the alveolar septa is diminished, permitting the bronchioles to collapse during expiration and thereby leading to further air trapping and a greater increase in FRC.

It is the loss of elastic recoil and perhaps collagen destruction that causes the thorax to assume a more "inspiratory" position and leads to a reduction in the maximal negative intrapleural pressure at full inspiration.[168] In contrast to patients with pulmonary fibrosis (who have "stiff" lungs), most patients with emphysema have increased static compliance; as previously discussed, however, the dynamic compliance is

in large measure frequency-dependent, probably reflecting obstruction in the small bronchi and bronchioles.

Disturbances in Arterial Blood Gases

Arterial blood gas values are commonly disturbed in patients with chronic obstructive lung disease, hypoxemia and hypercapnia being present more frequently in those with more severe grades of emphysema. Although decrease in Po_2, with or without increase in Pco_2, may result from a combination of factors including ventilation-perfusion inequality, alveolar hypoventilation, and venoarterial shunting, it is probable that the major role is played by nonuniform distribution of alveolar ventilation and capillary perfusion. When a sufficient number of acinar units are poorly ventilated but well perfused, the Po_2 is decreased and Pco_2 is increased; this tends to lead to hyperventilation, which readily compensates for any carbon dioxide retention that might develop from perfusion of underventilated units. With more severe grades of obstructive pulmonary disease, retention of carbon dioxide occurs eventually, either because of the lack of sufficient normally functioning lung tissue to compensate for retention through hyperventilation or because hyperventilation has been replaced by hypoventilation. Patients so affected may show further impairment of gas exchange while sleeping, without evidence of upper airway obstruction.[180, 181]

Some patients with chronic obstructive pulmonary disease who can hyperventilate (and thus reduce carbon dioxide levels to within normal range) tend rather to underventilate. This tendency is perhaps best explained on the basis of the increased work of breathing in emphysema—the patient hypoventilates and thus settles for a new level of Pco_2 rather than occasion the unpleasant sensation of dyspnea. The strong correlation between decreased Po_2 and increased Pco_2 in patients with bronchitis suggests that widespread alveolar hypoventilation contributes significantly to the development of these blood gas abnormalities.

Other arterial blood determinations may provide information important to the assessment of patients with chronic obstructive pulmonary disease, including pH or hydrogen ion concentration and bicarbonate levels. When an excess of carbon dioxide is compensated for by an increase in bicarbonate, to the extent that the hydrogen ion concentration is within normal range, there is clear indication that the respiratory failure is not of "acute" onset. Such patients show a greater efficiency in buffering acute changes in carbon dioxide levels. On the other hand, elevated PCO_2 associated with normal bicarbonate levels indicates that the respiratory failure leading to hypoventilation and respiratory acidosis is of recent onset. However, the latter conclusion is not justified if there is coexisting metabolic acidosis (which tends to depress bicarbonate levels). When metabolic acidosis occurs in patients with COPD, it reflects tissue hypoperfusion rather than hypoxemia *per se*.

In any assessment of arterial blood gas abnormalities and their relationship to neurologic symptoms and signs, it must be remembered that gas tensions and acid-base balance in the cerebrospinal fluid are different from those in arterial blood and perhaps more correctly reflect the environment of the respiratory center.

The breathing of high concentrations of oxygen by patients who have an elevated arterial PCO_2 results in physiologic effects of utmost importance in proper management. These effects include decrease in the work of breathing and reduction in regional vasoconstriction. Although the reduction in work of breathing implies decrease in carbon dioxide production by the tissues, the reduction in vasoconstriction in poorly ventilated areas has the opposite effect— the PCO_2 rises and may reach levels that promote neurologic signs and symptoms.[182]

Disturbances in Diffusion

The diffusing capacity measured by both the single-breath and the steady-state carbon monoxide methods is commonly reduced in chronic obstructive pulmonary disease. There is close correlation between severely reduced diffusing capacity during life and the finding of extensive morphologic emphysema at necropsy.[136] Some authors consider the diffusing capacity to be of differential diagnostic value in cases of obstructive pulmonary disease, reduction indicating emphysema and normal values indicating chronic bronchitis.[149] It should be appreciated, however, that anatomic emphysema of mild to moderate degree may be observed at necropsy in patients who had normal diffusing capacity.[136] The reduction in diffusing capacity in chronic obstructive pulmonary disease is generally considered to be due to decrease in the membrane component, the result of ventilation-perfusion inequality. It is probable, however, that there are other contributing factors, including reduction in capillary bed, widespread alveolar hypoventilation, and perhaps even limitation of diffusion in the gas phase occasioned by the large "air pools" typical of emphysema.

Studies in asymptomatic and mildly disabled individuals with severe alpha$_1$-antitrypsin deficiency reveal a pattern of disturbed function that is believed to represent early emphysema. The two major findings are a loss of elastic recoil and a redistribution of blood flow with loss of the normal perfusion gradient from apex to base. These alpha$_1$-antitrypsin–deficient patients may manifest pulmonary hyperinflation but need not show evidence of airway obstruction, at least as measured by routine methods. When symptoms develop in patients with phenotype Pi^{zz}, routine pulmonary function testing reveals a number of abnormalities, including a reduction of FEV_1; there is a trend toward increased impairment close to the fourth decade of life.[183] In advanced homozygous alpha$_1$-antitrypsin deficiency the disturbances of pulmonary function are similar to those seen in ordinary emphysema.

BULLOUS DISEASE OF THE LUNGS

Considerable semantic confusion surrounds this diagnosis, chiefly because the words "bulla," "cyst," and "bleb" tend to be used interchangeably; it is debatable whether their distinction serves a useful purpose. The word "cyst" mostly is used to describe the congenital variety of bronchial or bronchogenic cyst. The word "bleb" usually connotes a collection of air within the layers of visceral pleura; this lesion is often associated with the development of spontaneous pneumothorax. A "bulla" is an air-filled, thin-walled space within the lung usually considered to result from destruction of alveolar tissue. The walls of bullae are formed by pleura, connective tissue septa, or compressed lung parenchyma; the character of the wall depends on the site of the bulla. The Ciba symposium report[109] of 1959 recommended the definition of a bulla as an air-containing space within the lung greater than 1 cm in diameter in the distended state.

PATHOLOGIC CHARACTERISTICS

A bulla represents a local, sharply demarcated area of emphysema, an air-containing space that may contain overdistended and ruptured alveolar septa and blood vessels. Bullae occur both singly and in multiples, either in otherwise normal lung or as part of generalized obstructive emphysema. Reid[184] divided bullae into three types.

Type 1 bullae originate in a subpleural location or in the vicinity of parenchymal scars ("linear emphysema"). Such a bulla commonly is located in the apex of an upper lobe or along the costophrenic rim of the middle lobe and lingula. It characteristically has a narrow neck and usually contains only gas, without evidence of alveolar remnants or blood vessels. This type of air sac may rupture, permitting air to escape into the pleural cavity and causing spontaneous pneumothorax. These also are the bullae that may become enormous, initiating passive collapse of normal lung tissue, extending across the mediastinum into the contralateral hemithorax, and interfering with the function of the opposite lung.

Type 2 bullae also are superficial in location but have a very broad neck. They may occur anywhere over the lung surface, but most commonly develop over the anterior edge of the upper and middle lobes and over the diaphragmatic surface. In contrast to type 1 bullae, this variety characteristically contains strands of emphysematous lung, and blood vessels course through it. It may arise in association with any type of emphysema.

Type 3 bullae lie deep within the lung substance and have a broad base. Contained strands of emphysematous lung and intact blood vessels commonly are identifiable. They appear to affect both upper and lower lobes equally. Although a type 3 bulla represents a large area of overinflated, destroyed lung, it may develop in the absence of generalized emphysema.

ROENTGENOGRAPHIC MANIFESTATIONS

The diagnosis of bullous disease of the lungs depends upon roentgenologic identification of local, thin-walled, sharply demarcated areas of avascularity (Figure 11–10). The walls are characteristically apparent as hairline shadows, but since the air cysts are most often at or near the lung surface, usually only a portion of the wall is visible. Location within the substance of the lung renders identification much more difficult, and even peripheral bullae may be extremely difficult to identify. Since the bullae trap air during expiration, they may be identified on roentgenograms exposed at RV and yet be barely or not at all visible on those exposed at TLC.

Tomography may provide greatly improved visibility of a bulla already identified and may reveal bullae not even suspected on plain roentgenograms. Similarly, tomography may be useful in the assessment of the vasculature throughout the lungs, particularly in establishing whether the bullae are part of general obstructive emphysema or merely local abnormalities in otherwise normal lungs (Figure 11–10).

Rarely, bullae disappear as a result of secondary infection.[185] In the majority of cases, however, they enlarge progressively. Some increase slowly and continuously, whereas others remain

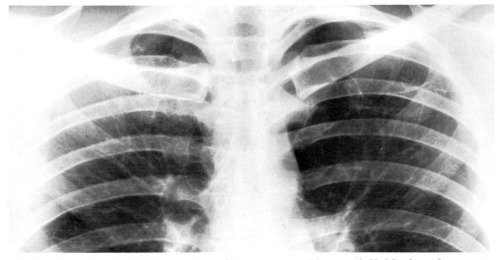

Figure 11–10. Multiple Bullae in Otherwise Normal Lung.   A view of the upper half of the thorax from a posteroanterior roentgenogram reveals numerous curved hairline shadows in the upper portion of the left lung representing the walls of multiple large bullae. A single bulla is present in the right paramediastinal area.

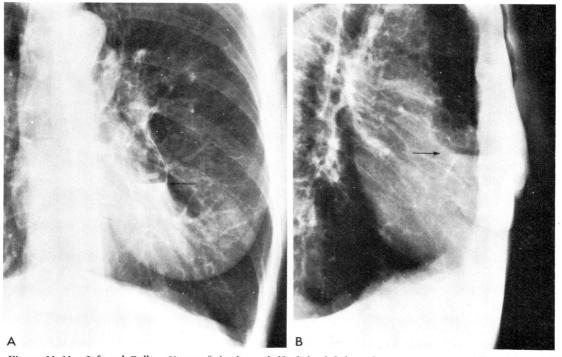

Figure 11–11. Infected Bulla. Views of the lower half of the left lung from posteroanterior (A) and lateral (B) roentgenograms reveal a cystic space in the anterior portion of the lingula. Its wall is of hairline thickness and it contains a prominent fluid level (*arrow*). This 60-year-old white female with severe emphysema had low-grade fever but no symptoms attributable to chest infection. Three weeks later the infection had cleared, leaving only a thin-walled bulla.

constant in size for several years and then, for no obvious reason, enlarge.

Infection of a bulla usually is manifested roentgenographically by a fluid level within the air sac, with or without some degree of pneumonitis in the surrounding lung parenchyma (Figure 11–11). In such circumstances, the roentgenographic appearance may be misinterpreted as a lung cavity secondary to abscess formation, but differentiation is aided by the fact that most patients with infected bullae are much less ill than those with acute lung abscess. Also, most infected bullae have much thinner walls, are surrounded by lesser degrees of pneumonitis, and usually contain much less fluid than cavitated lung abscesses. Complete clearing of fluid from infected bullae may be protracted, averaging about six weeks.[186]

CLINICAL MANIFESTATIONS

Since the majority of bullae occasion no symptoms or physical signs, their recognition depends upon adequate roentgenography. The roentgenologic identification of a single bulla in a patient who is severely dyspneic is a clear indication that the bulla is part of diffuse obstructive emphysema.

It is essential to divide patients with bullous disease of the lungs into two groups—those with chronic obstructive pulmonary disease and those judged to have normal pulmonary parenchyma between the bullae and who thus are free of airway obstruction.[185]

Primary bullous disease (paraseptal emphysema) characteristically occasions no symptoms or signs. A familial occurrence has been reported.[187] Usually there is minimal abnormality in pulmonary function. Bullae rarely contribute significantly to dead space ventilation because they are so poorly ventilated.[188] However, they permit relaxation of surrounding normal lung and thus reduce elastic recoil pressure. The rationale for bullectomy lies in the potential for healthy lung to expand and fill the space occupied by the bullae and in the expected increase in elastic recoil pressure that reduces the tendency for airways to collapse on expiration.[189] In the great majority of patients with primary bullous disease, there is no clinical disability and hence surgery is not indicated. However, when bullae are large, their surgical removal may become necessary; in such cases, pulmonary function studies carried out before and after surgery have revealed significant improvement.[189, 190]

Bullae associated with chronic obstructive pulmonary disease show little difference clinically or functionally from chronic obstructive pulmonary disease without bullae. In this group, surgical intervention is not nearly as successful as in patients with primary bullous disease, although some patients improve clinically and show better gas exchange and lung elastic recoil postoperatively,[188, 189] particularly when the bullae are large.

LOCAL EMPHYSEMA

As already discussed, the emphysema that forms part of chronic obstructive pulmonary disease is just as often local as it is general, at least in its roentgenographic manifestations. For example, predominant involvement of both lower lung zones with comparatively little involvement of the upper zones results in a typical roentgenographic appearance of oligemic lower lungs containing thin attenuated vessels and upper zones whose vessels are larger than normal as a result of redistribution of blood from the zones of higher resistance. Clinically and functionally these cases represent variations on the theme of chronic obstructive pulmonary disease. However, this section is concerned with one type of disease that may be categorized as "emphysema" but whose etiology and pathogenesis, roentgenographic manifestations, and clinical presentations differ somewhat from those of classic emphysema—unilateral hyperlucent lung (Swyer-James' or Macleod's syndrome).

UNILATERAL OR LOBAR EMPHYSEMA (SWYER-JAMES' OR MACLEOD'S SYNDROME)

Unilateral hyperlucent lung is one of the very few "diseases" whose name derives entirely from the manifestations it produces roentgenographically—a state in which the density of one lung is markedly less than the density of the other. Morphologically, there is bronchitis, bronchiolitis, bronchiolitis obliterans, and dilatation and destruction of lung parenchyma.[191–193] These changes are virtually indistinguishable from those of obstructive emphysema except that dust accumulation is generally absent. The condition does not always affect just one lung to the total exclusion of the other. It may occur in various anatomic distributions, including one lobe, two lobes in the right lung, and the lower lobe of one lung and the upper lobe of the other. In addition, undoubtedly some patients who present in adulthood with chronic obstructive pulmonary disease, shown roentgenologically and physiologically to be local emphysema (for example, disease localized to both upper lobes), clearly represent examples of this disease pathogenetically.

In many cases this disease is recognized (or at least suspected) in childhood when chest roentgenography is carried out in the investigation of repeated respiratory infections. However, the condition may not become apparent until adulthood, on the basis of a screening chest roentgenogram in a completely asymptomatic patient. Inquiry often reveals a history of acute lower respiratory tract infection, generally during childhood. The character of the morphologic abnormality—bronchiolitis obliterans, bronchiectasis, and distal airspace distention and destruction—lends support to the impression that the basic cause in the majority of cases is infection, probably of viral origin. Furthermore, a report by MacPherson and Gold[194] of six children with unilateral or lobar emphysema whose previous history showed definite or highly suggestive evidence of adenoviral pneumonia suggests that this organism may be the responsible agent in the majority of cases. It is probable that the pathogenesis follows a predictable pattern: acute bronchiolitis leads to obliteration of small airways, peripheral parenchyma being ventilated by collateral air drift; air trapping and overdistention develop in the peripheral parenchyma; and ultimately the destructive changes characteristic of emphysema occur. It is also conceivable that infection could persist for some time after the acute viral infection, with consequent elastolysis from phagocytic proteases.

The roentgenographic manifestations usually are easily recognized and are virtually pathognomonic. A posteroanterior roentgenogram of the chest exposed at TLC reveals a remarkable difference in the radiolucency of the two lungs, caused *not* by a relative increase in air in the affected lung but by decreased perfusion (Figure 11–12). The peripheral pulmonary markings are diminutive, indicating severe narrowing and attenuation of the vessels. The ipsilateral hilum also is diminutive but is *present*, a feature of great value in the differentiation from proximal interruption of a pulmonary artery (pulmonary artery agenesis). In roentgenograms exposed at

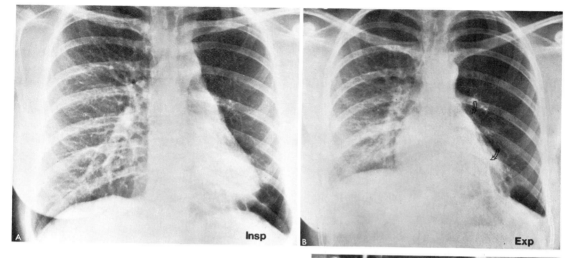

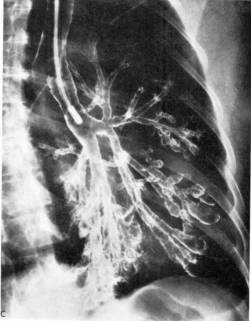

Figure 11–12. Swyer-James' Syndrome Associated with Absence of the Ipsilateral Breast. Posteroanterior roentgenograms at inspiration (*A*) and expiration (*B*) reveal marked oligemia of the left lung and severe air trapping on expiration. A left breast shadow is not visualized nor was breast tissue apparent on physical examination. The left lower lobe shows a severe degree of loss of volume (*open arrows* in *B*) and the left hilum is diminutive. A left bronchogram (*C*) reveals bronchiectasis of all segments, those in the lower lobe being the most severely involved and thus accounting for the loss of volume. All bronchial segments terminate abruptly in a configuration characteristic of obliterative bronchiolitis. Whether a relationship exists between the left-sided emphysema and congenital absence of the left breast is not known. This young woman complained of chronic cough productive of mucopurulent sputum. (Courtesy of The Montreal Chest Hospital Center.)

TLC, the volume of the affected lung (or lobe) either is comparable to that of the normal contralateral lung or is reduced (Figure 11–12); volume is seldom increased. The volume of the affected lung depends almost entirely on the age of the patient at the time of the infectious insult. The younger the patient at the time of the pneumonia, the smaller the fully developed lung, since the insult prevents further maturation.[192]

One of the characteristic roentgenologic features of unilateral or lobar emphysema—in fact, a *sine qua non* for diagnosis—is the presence of air trapping during expiration (Figure 11–12). This indicates the presence of airway obstruction and is of absolute value in differentiation from other conditions that may give rise to unilateral or lobar translucency. Since the contralateral lung is normal, expiration causes the mediastinum to swing abruptly toward the normal lung, and excursion of the hemidiaphragms is markedly asymmetric, being severely diminished on the affected side.

Pulmonary arteriography is seldom indicated in the investigation of these patients, but a perfusion lung scan may provide useful information in selected cases and is less hazardous. In the majority of patients, bronchography reveals a characteristic deformity of the bronchial tree. The segmental bronchi are irregularly dilated and end abruptly in squared or club-shaped terminations in the vicinity of the fifth- or sixth-stage divisions, a pattern typical of obliterative bronchiolitis. Filling of peripheral bronchiolar radicals is notable by its absence, even with repeated deep respirations (Figure 11–12).

Clinically, the presentation is highly variable. Some patients are completely asymptomatic, some complain of dyspnea on exertion, and others present with a history of repeated lower respiratory tract infection.[191] Physical examination reveals restriction of chest expansion on the affected side, associated with diminished air entry, relative hyperresonance, and sometimes scattered rales. Pulmonary function test values are as might be anticipated with destruction of virtually half the functioning parenchyma of both lungs. There is reduction in VC and to a lesser extent in expiratory flow. Diffusing capacity measured by the steady-state method usually is reduced but may be normal with the single-breath method, since breath-holding permits time for more uniform gas distribution. Blood gas concentrations usually are normal but may fall during exercise.

Differential diagnosis is rarely a problem. Other conditions that give rise to unilateral or lobar radiolucency, such as proximal interruption of a pulmonary artery, hypogenetic lung syndrome, and obstruction of a pulmonary artery or one of its branches from thromboembolic disease are readily differentiated by the absence of air trapping during expiration and by other roentgenologic signs that characterize these conditions.

BRONCHIECTASIS

Bronchiectasis may be defined as irreversible dilatation of the bronchial tree. Formerly a relatively common affliction, bronchiectasis has decreased considerably in incidence since the advent of antibiotic therapy. Its precise incidence in the population as a whole or even in a general hospital population is not known, but its frequency as a disease requiring surgical resection has greatly decreased, at least in developed countries.[195] Bronchiectasis is bilateral in approximately 50 per cent of cases and in the great majority involves the basal segments of the lower lobes. In only about 10 per cent of cases is the middle lobe or lingula affected without concomitant involvement of the ipsilateral lower lobe.

PATHOGENESIS

Bronchiectasis is predominantly a pediatric disease, the history commonly dating from early childhood. In a majority of cases one can elicit a history of pneumonia developing as a complication of measles, whooping cough, or some other contagious disease of childhood, and it is thought that the bacterial pneumonia and associated atelectasis are responsible for the destruction and dilatation of the bronchial walls.

A small percentage of cases are associated with other diseases, deficiencies, or structural abnormalities that contribute directly or indirectly to the development of bronchial dilatation and destruction. These can be divided into three groups. (1) *Congenital defects of a "structural" nature*, including cystic fibrosis, Kartagener's syndrome, and bronchial cartilage deficiency (Williams-Campbell syndrome). Pathologic studies suggest that defects of the structures that support the bronchi, abnormal secretions, or abnormal ciliary action may play a part, singly or in combination. (2) *Congenital or acquired deficiencies in host defense* are usually immunologic in nature and the result of a deficiency of gamma globulin.[196] However, they may result from a defect in cell-mediated immunity, phagocytic deficiency, or even alpha$_1$-antitrypsin deficiency.[197] It is quite possible that a developmental defect of cilia may be an important feature in the pathogenesis of bronchiectasis. Originally described in patients with Kartagener's syndrome (*see* further on), immotile cilia have since been identified in other groups of patients. Electronmicroscopy reveals structural deficiencies in the dynein arms[197] or the radial spokes.[198] In patients with bronchiectasis, a variety of ciliary abnormalities may be present.[199] (3) In addition to these "congenital" defects, bronchiectasis may occur as a complication of several primary lung diseases. These include the "central" bronchiectasis associated with mucoid impaction, the bronchiectasis that almost invariably results from chronic bronchial obstruction by neoplasms or an aspirated foreign body, and that occurring as a result of chronic granulomatous or acute viral infections or following aspiration of liquid gastric contents or inhalation of toxic fumes.

PATHOLOGIC CHARACTERISTICS

The definitive description of the pathologic findings and the pathologic-roentgenographic correlation of bronchiectasis was reported by Lynne Reid in 1950. By correlating the pathologic and bronchographic findings in 45 lobes removed because of bronchiectasis, this author classified the disease into three groups, using the criteria of severity of bronchial dilatation and degree of bronchial and bronchiolar obliteration.

GROUP I: CYLINDRICAL BRONCHIECTASIS. The bronchi were of regular outline and not greatly increased in diameter distally; their lumens ended squarely and abruptly (Figure 11–13A and B). Although patent anatomically, the smaller bronchi and bronchioles were plugged with thick, yellow, purulent material and did not fill with bronchographic contrast medium. Cellular infiltration and swelling of the bronchial walls were common. The number of subdivisions of the bronchial tree from the main bronchus to the periphery was considered to be within normal limits (16 subdivisions compared with 17 to 20 normally).

GROUP II: VARICOSE BRONCHIECTASIS. The degree of dilatation was somewhat greater than in group I. Local constrictions caused an irregularity of outline that resembled varicose veins (Figure 11–13C and D). This irregularity and bulbous termination of bronchi were the cardinal features in this group, in contrast to the regular outline and abrupt termination seen in group I. There was much more obliteration of peripheral bronchial lumens than in group I, some bronchi terminating abruptly in a bed of fibrous tissue that continued as a discrete cord of tissue toward the periphery of the lung. The average number of patent bronchial subdivisions was 4 bronchographically, 6.5 macroscopically, and 8 microscopically (compared with 17 to 20 normally).

GROUP III: SACCULAR (CYSTIC) BRONCHIECTASIS. Bronchial dilatation increased progressively toward the periphery. The bronchi had a ballooned outline (Figure 11–13E and F), and the maximum number of subdivisions that could be counted by any technique was five. No remnants of the peripheral bronchial tree could be shown to be directly continuous with the dilated bronchi. Despite the fact that only five subdivisions of the bronchial tree could be counted, the cysts or saccules were situated immediately deep to the pleura.

ROENTGENOGRAPHIC MANIFESTATIONS

We have found Reid's classification[200] eminently satisfactory for roentgenologic descrip-

tion. Not only does it permit accurate description of the degree of bronchial deformity, but it has the added advantage of supplying fairly precise information on the amount of parenchymal destruction encountered in each group.

The plain roentgenogram reveals changes highly suggestive of bronchiectasis in the great majority of patients. The typical changes on plain roentgenograms consist of the following: (a) Increase in size and loss of definition of the markings in specific segmental areas of the lungs. (b) Markings are crowded, indicating the almost invariable associated loss of volume. (c) In more advanced disease, particularly groups II, and III, cystic spaces, up to 2 cm in diameter and sometimes containing fluid levels, may be identified. (d) In advanced disease, atelectasis may be complete and associated with total airlessness of a lobe. Signs of compensatory overinflation of the remainder of lung parenchyma are present in most cases.

Although the plain roentgenogram may strongly suggest the diagnosis of bronchiectasis, bronchography is mandatory to establish its presence beyond question and to determine its precise extent, particularly if surgery is contemplated. Bronchography should be performed only after adequate postural drainage and antibiotic therapy have rendered the bronchial tree as free as possible of retained secretions. The bronchographic findings in the three types of bronchiectasis are as described in the section on pathology (Figure 11–13).

Reversible bronchiectasis designates the form of bronchial dilatation that usually is a manifestation of acute pneumonia.[201] Dilatation develops as a result of retained secretions and of the atelectasis that is an invariable accompaniment of resolving pneumonia. With complete resolution of the pneumonia the dilatation gradually disappears, although it may be as long as 3 to 4 months before the integrity of the bronchial tree is restored. Consequently, to be on the safe side, it is advisable to allow 4 to 6 months to elapse after acute pneumonia before performing bronchography for the assessment of bronchiectasis.

CLINICAL MANIFESTATIONS

The main symptoms are cough and the expectoration of purulent sputum. The quantity of sputum varies with the severity of the disease, but mose patients expectorate daily. Some patients become aware of purulent expectoration only after respiratory infections (which tend

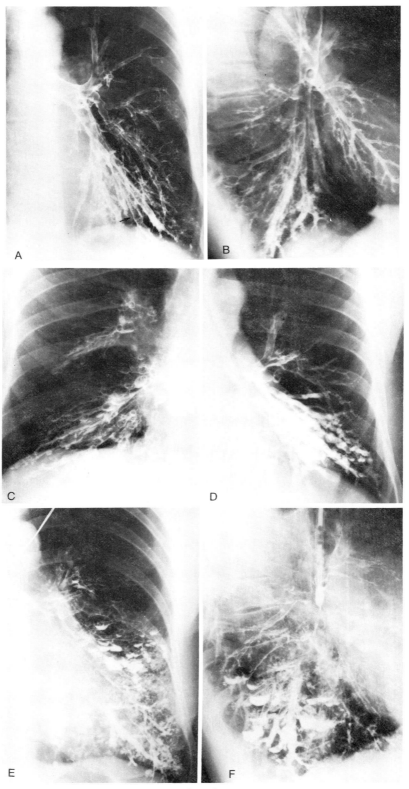

Figure 11–13. *See legend on opposite page.*

to be frequent). Hemoptysis occurs in about 50 per cent of older patients but is relatively rare in children. If the disease is widespread, the patient may complain of shortness of breath. In almost every case there are persistent rales localized to the area of major involvement. Extrathoracic manifestations include finger clubbing, seen in about one-third of cases, and rarely brain abscess and amyloidosis.

In our experience there is no specific pattern of pulmonary function in bronchiectasis. Patients with well-localized disease unassociated with chronic bronchitis suffer little or no functional impairment. However, with appropriate testing, such patients may show generalized disease of small airways,[202] a well-recognized pathologic finding in this disease. In diffuse disease, the pattern is that of obstructive disease, with decrease in the timed VC and, in many cases, impairment of mixing, increase in the FRC, and reduction of diffusing capacity.

KARTAGENER'S SYNDROME

Kartagener's syndrome consists of situs inversus, paranasal sinusitis, and bronchiectasis.[203] Other associated congenital anomalies include transposition of the great vessels, trilocular or bilocular heart, pyloric stenosis, urethral meatus on the ventral ridge of the glans penis, and postcricoid web (Paterson-Brown-Kelly syndrome). Congenital cardiac anomalies occur less frequently when bronchiectasis is present than when dextrocardia is an isolated anomaly. The incidence of Kartagener's syndrome in the total Caucasian population is estimated to be one in 40,000.[204] The complete syndrome has a high familial incidence, although transmission does not appear to occur in successive generations.[205]

It has been thought for some time that the pathophysiology of the syndrome must relate to abnormalities of ciliary action or abnormal mucus production.[205, 206] It is noteworthy that although the bronchiectasis may be acquired, the incidence of bronchiectasis in patients with situs inversus (12 to 25 per cent) is much higher than in the general population (0.2 to 0.5 per cent).[205] It has now been shown that the axoneme (central core) of the cilia of epithelial cells and of sperm tails is functionally inefficient. This abnormality explains both the sterility seen in male patients with this syndrome and the dextrocardia that is believed to be caused by deficient embryonic cilia.[207]

Roentgenologically, the bronchiectasis is indistinguishable from the usual form unassociated with sinusitis and situs inversus.

CHRONIC OBSTRUCTIVE DISEASE OF SMALL AIRWAYS

In 1971, Macklem and his colleagues[208] described seven cases of chronic obstructive pulmonary disease characterized by inflammatory narrowing, mucous plugging, and fibrous obliteration of the small airways of the lungs. In all cases, pathologic specimens obtained at necropsy or biopsy showed no evidence of significant emphysema, and chest roentgenograms

Figure 11–13. **A and B, Cylindrical Bronchiectasis.**   A left bronchogram in posteroanterior (*A*) and lateral (*B*) projections reveals uniform dilatation of all basal bronchi of the left lower lobe; prominent transverse striations are present in the lateral basal bronchus (*arrow*). All bronchiectatic segments end abruptly, and there is little or no peripheral filling. The remainder of the bronchial tree is normal. In lateral projection, note the crowding of the bronchiectatic segments and the elevation of the posterior portion of the hemidiaphragm, both findings indicating moderate loss of volume. Cinefluorographic studies revealed normal bronchial dynamics. This 31-year-old man had a history of productive cough dating from an attack of whooping cough and bronchopneumonia as a child. Pulmonary function studies were normal. **C and D, Varicose Bronchiectasis.**   Right (*C*) and left (*D*) bronchograms reveal extensive dilatation of all basal bronchi of the lower lobes and of the right middle lobe; the dilatation is not uniform, as in *A* and *B*, but is characterized by numerous local constrictions that give the bronchi a configuration resembling varicose veins. There is a notable absence of peripheral filling. It is unusual for such extensive bronchiectasis to be associated with the inconspicuous plain roentgenographic changes depicted; it is assumed that the alteration in vascular pattern resulted from a redistribution of blood flow from the lower lobes as a result of bronchial artery hypertrophy and systemic pulmonary arterial anastomoses. This patient gave a history of the accidental ingestion of camphorated oil 1 year previously and had had cough productive of "dirty" sputum ever since; it seems reasonable to postulate a cause and effect relationship between this episode and the severe bronchiectasis. **E and F, Cystic (Saccular) Bronchiectasis.**   Posteroanterior (*E*) and lateral (*F*) projections of a left bronchogram reveal numerous cystic spaces containing contrast material in many areas presenting as fluid levels. There is somewhat less loss of volume than one might anticipate from the extensive bronchial destruction, an observation that undoubtedly reflects the presence of considerable emphysema. A right bronchogram was normal. The patient was a 46-year-old woman.

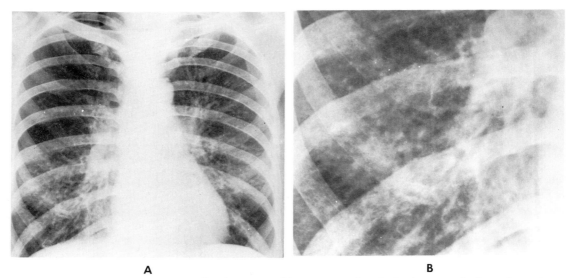

A   **B**

Figure 11–14. "Small Airway Disease." This 34-year-old woman complained of a chronic smoker's cough, productive of thick sputum, for many years. She had noted vague shortness of breath on exercise during the previous 3 months. She was cyanotic. A posteroanterior roentgenogram (A) revealed diffuse involvement of both lungs by a coarse reticular pattern, seen to advantage in a magnified view of the lower portion of the right lung (B). There are no associated findings, such as hilar lymph node enlargement, pleural effusion, or cardiomegaly. Several months later she developed a spontaneous pneumothorax followed by a chronic bronchopleural fistula and a progressive downhill course characterized by uncontrollable respiratory failure. At necropsy, there was evidence of extensive bronchiolar obstruction caused by mucous plugs and by peribronchiolar inflammation and fibrosis.

revealed the widespread involvement of both lungs by medium-to-coarse reticulation suggestive of a restrictive type of disease such as sarcoidosis (Figure 11–14). Roentgenologic evidence of pulmonary arterial hypertension and cor pulmonale was present in one patient. Pulmonary function tests were of considerable interest. Despite moderate impairment of expiratory flow rates the FRC was consistently normal, although values for RV were slightly increased and diffusing capacity tended to be moderately reduced. Elastic recoil was normal, although values for dynamic compliance diminished with increasing frequency of respiration (frequency-dependent small airway disease). Hypoxemia and hypercapnia were present in six of the seven patients.

Like bronchiolitis obliterans, this disease does not fit easily into the spectrum of diseases characterized by obliteration of small airways. It appears to be a distinct entity in that the roentgenographic pattern suggests restrictive lung disease, and yet the functional impairment is chiefly obstructive in nature. Although local bronchiectasis was demonstrated in one patient at necropsy and may have been present in others (although not investigated), the morphologic picture was characterized by a relative absence of emphysema.

CYSTIC FIBROSIS

This hereditary disease of Mendelian recessive transmission is also known as cystic fibrosis of the pancreas, or simple CF. Although the fundamental abnormality consists of the secretion of thick tenacious mucus from the exocrine glands, there are other pathophysiologic phenomena such as abnormalities of sweat and salivary gland secretions. The major manifestations are chronic obstructive pulmonary disease (found in varying degrees of severity in almost all cases) and pancreatic insufficiency (absent in 10 to 20 per cent of patients).[209] Although a family history may suggest the diagnosis, confirmation requires the demonstration of elevated levels of sodium and chloride in sweat.

Cystic fibrosis is the commonest lethal genetically transmitted syndrome among white children. The estimated incidence is approximately one case per 2000 to 3500 live births.[210-212] There is no sex predominance, but the disease is almost completely restricted to Caucasians. It is chiefly a disease of infants and children, although adult cases are being recognized with greater frequency. As a result of improved medical care, chiefly through antibiotic therapy, life expectancy has been greatly increased. Undoubtedly this improved prognosis can be explained at least partly by earlier recognition of the disease and by the detection of milder cases. Infants with severe pancreatic insufficiency usually die from meconium ileus and children and young adults from progressive lung disease.

Cystic fibrosis is believed to be transmitted as an autosomal recessive trait. In the Caucasian population, approximately one in 20 individuals is heterozygous for cystic fibrosis. No clinical characteristics have been demonstrated that identify heterozygotes, since they do not express the disease and generally are unaware that they are carriers until they have children with cystic fibrosis.[213] If a carrier of the gene marries another person who is heterozygous with the same gene, each pregnancy has a 25 per cent risk of resulting in a child with the disease. If one parent has no history of cystic fibrosis and the other parent has the disease, there is a one in 40 chance of the child's being affected.[213] Since at the present time there are no means of identifying heterozygotes and no test for the detection of an affected homozygous fetus *in utero*, genetic counseling has its limitations.

PATHOGENESIS

Despite intensive investigation, the pathogenesis and pathophysiology of the many manifestations of cystic fibrosis are not completely understood. The morphologic changes in affected organs are the result of plugging of the tubes into which the secretions of exocrine glands are poured. In the tracheobronchial tree, in addition to an abnormality of mucous secretion, there is considerable evidence to implicate disturbances of autonomic control of bronchial mucous glands and of mucociliary transport.

The water content of bronchopulmonary secretions is diminished, either because of an increased solid content or hyperpermeability of mucus.[214] A primary biologic function of mucus is to protect cell membranes from hydrostatic, osmotic, and concentration gradients. Hyperpermeability would permit the passage of water more easily through the mucous lining barrier. It has been postulated that an increased calcium content in bronchial mucoproteins is responsible for this hyperpermeable state.[214] Tracheobronchial mucous secretions contain lower than normal amounts of sodium and chloride.[209] A number of organic substances present in exocrine secretions could play a role in the formation of the thick, tenacious material that obstructs conducting systems. In the lung, most

interest has centered around mucous glycoproteins, which are secreted in increased amounts and are capable of forming viscoelastic gels. A recent study has shown that the lipid content of airway secretions is increased and that this may be responsible in part for the tenacity and insolubility of the secretions and for the concomitant airway obstruction.[215]

Limited studies of mucociliary transport have yielded conflicting results. It is unclear whether disordered mucociliary transport is a nonspecific feature of chronic inflammatory airway disease or whether it represents a primary pathogenetic factor in the development of pulmonary disease. A disturbance in mucociliary transport could result from one or more of three factors: (1) the physicochemical properties of the mucous blanket, (2) overproduction of mucus, or (3) defective ciliary function. Evidence for ciliary dysfunction in cystic fibrosis rests largely on the discovery by Spock and associates[216] of a cilio-inhibitory factor in the euglobulin fraction of the serum of patients with the disease and of the "carrier" parent. These workers observed that serum from patients with cystic fibrosis disorganized the ciliary rhythm in explants of the respiratory epithelium of rabbits. Some investigators[217] have been able to confirm these original observations, but others have been unable to reproduce ciliary dyskinesia.[218]

The abnormal secretion of electrolytes varies from one exocrine gland to another. The concentration of sodium and chloride is slightly diminished in tracheobronchial and cervical mucus. Pancreatic secretions are severely deficient in electrolytes, particularly bicarbonate. Saliva from parotid, submaxillary, and sublingual glands contains normal amounts of sodium and chloride, but the minor salivary gland secretion, like that from sweat glands, shows an excess of these electrolytes.[209, 219] Submaxillary saliva has a high concentration of calcium. The sweat of patients with cystic fibrosis contains elevated concentrations of sodium and chloride and, to a lesser extent, of potassium. The primary secretions in sweat glands are normally isotonic, but become hypotonic in the duct system as a result of the reabsorption of sodium in excess of water.[209] The determination of sodium and chloride concentrations in sweat is a basic requirement for the diagnosis of cystic fibrosis (*see* further on).

Patients with cystic fibrosis have an increased susceptibility to infection and possibly to asthma. Both these manifestations are probably secondary to lung destruction and to increased permeability of the epithelial barrier. Progressive pulmonary involvement is almost invariably associated with repeated or persistent infections with *Staphylococcus aureus* or *Pseudomonas aeruginosa* or both. Immunologic host defense mechanisms are not impaired, and in fact, immunoglobulin levels are often increased, at least in adults. A recent study[220] has revealed hypogammaglobulin-G in a number of patients under the age of ten years with relatively mild cystic fibrosis, leading to the conclusion that progression of lung dysfunction may be due in part to a hyperimmune response.

Local defenses are defective because of reduced mucociliary transport and perhaps because of interference with alveolar macrophage phagocytosis of *Pseudomonas* organisms by a serum inhibitory factor.[221]

PATHOLOGIC CHARACTERISTICS

Exocrine glands that secrete mucus are most plentiful in the pancreas, the tracheobronchial tree, and, to a lesser extent, in the liver and cervix. In the pancreas, the abnormally tenacious mucus obstructs the ducts, resulting in acinar atrophy and fibrotic and cystic changes throughout the organ. The lungs are involved to some extent in virtually all patients with the disease. Mucus plugs the bronchial tree, partly or completely obstructing air passages and giving rise to a wide variety of pathologic changes, including focal atelectasis, pneumonitis, bronchiolar obstruction and dilatation,[222] cylindrical and cystic bronchiectasis, abscesses, and focal areas of overinflation distal to obstructed segmental bronchi, chiefly through the mechanism of collateral air drift.[210–212] Appreciable emphysema rarely develops, except in patients who reach adulthood. The bronchial mucosa may undergo squamous metaplasia.

ROENTGENOGRAPHIC MANIFESTATIONS

Plain roentgenography reveals a pattern typical of extensive obstruction of medium-sized and small airways of the lungs; hyperinflation is almost invariable. The earliest change perhaps is accentuation of the linear markings, usually generalized throughout the lungs (Figure 11–15). Atelectasis may be subsegmental, segmental, or lobar (the last having been reported in 10 per cent of cases), most frequently in the right upper lobe. Curiously, lobar collapse seldom occurs in the left lung. Recurrent local pneumonitis occurs in most cases. Cylindrical and even cystic bronchiectasis and multiple small bronchiolar abscesses may be present. A pattern of nodular, finger-like shadows along the distribution of the bronchovascular bundles indicates the presence of mucoid impaction.[223] Focal areas of parenchymal overinflation are

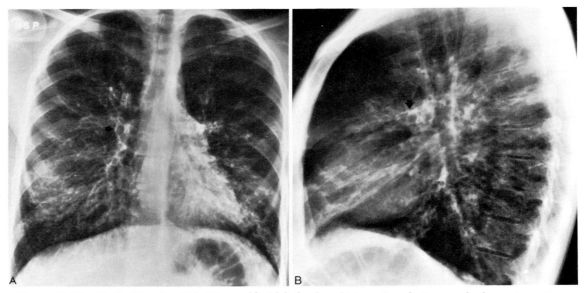

Figure 11–15. Cystic Fibrosis. This 16-year-old girl had a long history of productive cough, frequent respiratory infections, and bulky, fatty stools. Posteroanterior (A) and lateral (B) roentgenograms showed unusual prominence and irregularity of lung markings bilaterally. Tubular shadows can be visualized, particularly in the lower lobes, and are strongly suggestive of bronchiectasis. One markedly dilated bronchus is present in the anterior segment of the right upper lobe, indicated by an *arrow* in both projections. The sweat test was positive.

probably largely compensatory in nature, but true bullous emphysema has been reported, particularly in adults.

CLINICAL AND BIOCHEMICAL FINDINGS

The lack of pancreatic enzymes results in poor digestion, particularly of fat, in the small bowel, so that patients characteristically have bulky fatty stools. Approximately 10 to 20 per cent of neonates with cystic fibrosis develop intestinal obstruction as a result of meconium ileus; surgical therapy is usually required.

Involvement of the lungs usually is manifested clinically by recurrent chest infections associated with wheezing, dyspnea, productive cough, and occasionally hemoptysis. Such cases may present clinically as simple bronchiectasis. Occasionally, hemoptysis may be massive; it usually occurs as a result of bronchiectasis but sometimes may be associated with bronchial artery–pulmonary artery anastomoses.[224] Although bronchoscopy is the definitive method of identifying the bleeding site in such cases, in circumstances in which bronchoscopy cannot be performed because of continuous hemorrhage or because the severity of the lung disease precludes the use of general anesthesia, bronchial arteriography may effectively demonstrate the bleeding site.

Physical findings in adult patients with cystic fibrosis are typical of bronchiectasis and obstructive airway disease. Coarse rales may be localized but are often diffuse; generalized wheezing may suggest asthma. Finger clubbing is a frequent sign in patients with advanced disease.

Complications include spontaneous pneumothorax, respiratory insufficiency, cor pulmonale, infertility in the male, maldigestion and malabsorption, liver and pancreatic cirrhosis, and rectal prolapse. Pneumothorax is common and frequently recurrent.

Respiratory insufficiency and cor pulmonale develop frequently in the later stages of the disease. Ventilation-perfusion inequality is worsened by acute infectious episodes and may lead to cardiac decompensation. Hypoxemia may be corrected by breathing a high concentration of oxygen (which frequently results in a fall in pulmonary arterial pressure to normal levels[210–212]) or by treatment of the infection. Eventually, however, some degree of persistent pulmonary arterial hypertension develops as a result of intimal thickening of the medium-sized arteries.

Reproductive failure in males was first described by Kaplan and his associates in 1968.[225]

A review of 25 patients over 17 years of age revealed aspermia that was shown in surgical and autopsy specimens to result from absence of the vas deferens. In a 1972 survey of 105 cystic fibrosis centers,[226] normal fertility was found in only 2 to 3 per cent of affected males.

Maldigestion and occasionally malabsorption may be present, particularly in children. Hepatic involvement includes a fatty liver and focal biliary cirrhosis. Pancreatic involvement is reflected in recurrent attacks of acute pancreatitis. A curious unexplained abnormality found in a significant percentage of cases is rectal prolapse, observed in 87 (22.6 per cent) in one series of 386 patients.[227]

Although the diagnosis of cystic fibrosis may be suggested by family history, persistent respiratory disease, or clinical evidence of pancreatic insufficiency, confirmation requires a positive sweat test. The most generally accepted method is the pilocarpine iontophoresis sweat collection, with chemical analysis of ionic composition. Employing this method, a Mayo Clinic group[228] showed a clear differentiation of normal subjects from patients with the disease, although a few (generally adults in the 40-to-70-year-old range) fell into a gray area. The amount of sweat collected should never weigh less than 50 mg and ideally should be over 100 mg. Sweat electrolyte testing is not reliable in newborn infants. In children a chloride concentration of 60 mEq/L or higher indicates the presence of cystic fibrosis; a value of 50 mEq/L requires repeating. Since normal adults may have values above 60 mEq/L, a diagnosis of cystic fibrosis should not be made at this level in the absence of an appropriate clinical history and unless repeated values of sodium and chloride are at or above this level.[213]

Screening for pancreatic insufficiency is generally carried out by measuring the trypsin and chymotrypsin content of stool, but a more reliable method is the determination of bicarbonate and enzyme content of duodenal secretions obtained by intubation following stimulation with secretin and pancreozymin.[209]

Most investigators[229] have found that the various tests that measure small airway function are the most sensitive means of detecting pulmonary involvement in patients with cystic fibrosis. As the disease progresses, vital capacity diminishes and residual volume increases, the latter sometimes to four or five times predicted normal, with a resultant increase in total thoracic gas volume.[229, 230] FEV_1 values fall and carbon monoxide diffusing capacity also may decrease. The major factor reducing expiratory flow appears to be airway obstruction. Hypoxemia is present in some cases, with hypercapnia present in a minority of cases. The impairment in gas exchange has been shown to be due equally to shunt and $\dot{V}/\dot{Q}$ inequality.[231] Elaborate studies of respiratory center control and of the mechanics of ventilation have been reported in children.[232] Overall, correlation between abnormalities in pulmonary function and roentgenologically detectable pulmonary disease is excellent.[233]

FAMILIAL DYSAUTONOMIA (RILEY-DAY SYNDROME)

This disease, which is probably the result of a biochemical, perhaps enzymatic, anomaly, is manifested by malfunction of the autonomic nervous system with consequent hypersecretion of mucous glands and obstruction of the bronchial tree.[234] It is transmitted as an autosomal recessive trait and occurs almost exclusively in Jewish infants.

Clinical manifestations suggest a widespread neural disturbance, better explained on a metabolic than on a primary structural basis.[235] Much of the pathophysiology appears to result from an inability to release catecholamines. More recent interest has centered around nerve growth factor (NGF), a protein that causes a striking increase in sensory and sympathetic ganglions when injected into chick embryos. A bioassay method has been described that can measure the blood level of this substance.[236] Using a radioimmunoassay of three subunits of this substance called alpha, beta, and gamma, Siggers and associates[236] found a threefold increase in serum antigen levels of the biologically active subunit beta NGF in patients with dysautonomia as compared with normal subjects.

The disease usually becomes manifest in infancy and the prognosis is extremely poor. A small number of patients live into adulthood, although it appears that none has had children.[235] Recurrent respiratory infections are common and are the most frequent direct cause of death. Some of these episodes may be caused by aspiration, since a large percentage of patients manifest swallowing difficulties.

The roentgenographic picture is one of diffuse interstitial disease associated with patchy areas of pneumonia, atelectasis, and emphysema that may undergo remission and exacerbation. It is not surprising that the roentgenographic pattern resembles that of cystic fibrosis, since the basic cause of pulmonary abnormality in both diseases is increased secretions in the tracheo-bronchial tree. Atelectasis occurs predominantly in the right upper lobe and with less frequency in the right middle and left lower lobes. It has been emphasized that standard barium studies in the erect position may not reveal the primary esophageal disturbance, a delay in coordinated relaxation of the upper esophageal sphincter. This abnormality accounts for tracheal aspiration and can only be demonstrated satisfactorily by cineroentgenography.[235]

Clinically, the picture is characterized by episodes of acute respiratory difficulty with fever, cough, and shortness of breath associated with typical signs of bronchopneumonia, usually over both lungs. In their series of 210 patients, Brunt and McKusick[235] described the following clinical features in addition to the pulmonary manifestations: absence of fungiform papillae on the tongue (100 per cent of patients), absence of overflow tears (100 per cent), vasomotor disturbances exemplified by blotching of the skin (98 per cent), abnormal sweating (97 per cent), episodic fever (92 per cent), incoordination and unsteadiness (90 per cent), swallowing difficulty, particularly in infants (85 per cent), physical retardation (78 per cent), episodic vomiting (67 per cent), breathholding attacks (66 per cent), marked emotional instability (65 per cent), scoliosis (55 per cent), and bowel disturbances (49 per cent). Intellect is unimpaired.[235]

Although the clinical and roentgenographic findings usually suggest the diagnosis, the lack of a flare reaction to scratch or intradermal histamine is considered by Riley and Moore[237] to be a requirement for confirmation.

REFERENCES

1. Han, B. K., Dunbar, J. S, and Striker, T. W.: Membranous laryngotracheobronchitis (membranous croup). Am. J. Roentgenol., *133*:53, 1979.
2. Bass, J. W., Steele, R. W., and Wiebe, R. A.: Acute epiglottitis. A surgical emergency. J.A.M.A., *229*:671, 1974.
3. Schabel, S. I., Katzberg, R. W., and Burgener, F. A.: Acute inflammation of epiglottitis and supraglottic structures in adults. Radiology, *122*:601, 1977.
4. Ossoff, R. H., and Wolff, A. P.: Acute epiglottitis in adults. J.A.M.A., *244*:2639, 1980.
5. Shackelford, G. D., Siegel, M. J., and McAlister, W. H.: Subglottic edema in acute epiglottitis in children. Am. J. Roentgenol., *131*:603, 1978.
6. Michel, R. G., Hudson, W. R., and Pope, T. H.: Angioneurotic edema. A review of modern concepts. Arch. Otolaryngol., *101*:544, 1975.
7. Genovesi, M. G., and Simmons, D. H.: Airway

obstruction due to spontaneous retropharyngeal hemorrhage. Chest, 68:840, 1975.

8. Brooks, J. W.: Foreign bodies in the air and food passages. Ann. Surg., 175:720, 1972.

9. Miller, R. D., and Hyatt, R. E.: Obstructing lesions of the larynx and trachea: Clinical and physiologic characteristics. Mayo Clin. Proc., 44:145, 1969.

10. Kryger, M., Bode, F., Antic, R., and Anthonisen, N.: Diagnosis of obstruction of the upper and central airways. Am. J. Med., 61:85, 1976.

11. Stitik, F. P., Bartelt, D., James, A. E., Jr., and Proctor, D. F.: Tantalum tracheography in upper airway obstruction: 100 experiences in adults. Am. J. Roentgenol., 130:35, 1978.

12. Capitanio, M. A., and Kirkpatrick, J. A.: Obstructions of the upper airway in children as reflected on the chest radiograph. Radiology, 107:159, 1973.

13. Felman, A. H., Loughlin, G. M., Leftridge, C. A., Jr., and Cassisi, N. J.: Upper airway obstruction during sleep in children. Am. J. Roentgenol., 133:213, 1979.

14. Hyland, R. H., Hutcheon, M. A., Perl, A., Bowes, G., Anthonisen, N. R., Zamel, N., and Phillipson, E. A.: Upper airway occlusion induced by diaphragm pacing for primary alveolar hypoventilation: Implications for the pathogenesis of obstructive sleep apnea. Am. Rev. Respir. Dis., 124:180, 1981.

15. Tilkian, A. G., Guilleminault, C., Schroeder, J. S., Lehrman, K. L., Simmons, F. B., and Dement, W. C.: Hemodynamics in sleep-induced apnea. Studies during wakefulness and sleep. Ann. Intern. Med., 85:714, 1976.

16. Djalilian, M., Kern, E. B., Brown, H. A., Facer, G. W., Stickler, G. B., Weidman, W. H., and O'Connell, E. J.: Hypoventilation secondary to chronic upper airway obstruction in childhood. Mayo Clin. Proc., 50:11, 1975.

17. Tammeling, G. J., Blokzijl, E. J., Boonstra, S., and Sluiter, H. J.: Micrognathia, hypersomnia and periodic breathing. Bull. Physiopathol. Respir. (Nancy), 8:1229, 1972.

18. Pearson, F. G., Goldberg, M., and da Silva, A. J.: Tracheal stenosis complicating tracheostomy with cuffed tubes. Clinical experience and observations from a prospective study. Arch. Surg., 97:380, 1968.

19. James, A. E., Jr., MacMillan, A. S., Jr., Eaton, S., B., and Grillo, H. C.: Roentgenology of tracheal stenosis resulting from cuffed tracheostomy tubes. Am. J. Roentgenol., 109:455, 1970.

20. Harley, H. R. S.: Laryngotracheal obstruction complicating tracheostomy or endotracheal intubation with assisted respiration: A critical review. Thorax, 26:493, 1971.

21. Grillo, H. C.: Surgical approaches to the trachea. Surg. Gynecol. Obstet., 129:347, 1969.

22. Hajdu, S. I., Huvos, A. G., Goodner, J. T., Foote, F. W., Jr., and Beattie, E. J., Jr.: Carcinoma of the trachea. Clinicopathologic study of 41 cases. Cancer, 25:1448, 1970.

23. Greene, R., and Lechner, G. L.: "Saber-sheath" trachea: A clinical and functional study of marked coronal narrowing of the intrathoracic trachea. Radiology, 115:265, 1975.

24. Greene, R.: "Saber-sheath" trachea: Relation to chronic obstruction pulmonary disease. Am. J. Roentgenol., 130:441, 1978.

25. Gibson, G. J., and Davis, P.: Respiratory complications of relapsing polychondritis. Thorax, 29:726, 1974.

26. Mitchell, N., and Shepard, N.: Relapsing polychon-

dritis: An electron microscopic study of synovium and articular cartilage. J. Bone Joint Surg., 54A:1235, 1972.

27. Johnston, R. F., and Green, R. A.: Tracheobronchiomegaly. Report of five cases and demonstration of familial occurrence. Am. Rev. Respir. Dis., 91:35, 1965.

28. Williams, H., and McNicol, K. N.: Prevalence, natural history, and relationship of wheezy bronchitis and asthma in children. An epidemiological study. Br. Med. J., 4:321, 1969.

29. Yu, D. Y. C., Galant, S. P., and Gold, W. M.: Inhibition of antigen-induced bronchoconstriction by atropine in asthmatic patients. J. Appl. Physiol., 32:823, 1972.

30. Guz, A.: Control of ventilation in man with special reference to abnormalities in asthma. In Austen, K. F., and Lichtenstein, L. M. (eds.), Asthma—Physiology, Immunopharmacology and Treatment, Vol. II. New York, Academic Press, 1977.

31. Warner, J. O., Norman, A. P., and Soothill, J. F.: Cystic fibrosis heterozygosity in the pathogenesis of allergy. Lancet, 1:988, 1976.

32. Bias, W. B., and Marsh, D. G.: The genetic basis of asthma. Current studies of the genetics of IgE-mediated immune response in man. In Austen, K. F., and Lichtenstein, L. M. (eds.), Asthma—Physiology, Immunopharmacology and Treatment, Vol. II. New York, Academic Press, 1977.

33. Chan-Yeung, M.: Occupational asthma. Med. North Am., 22:2187, 1982.

34. Pepys, J.: Occupational asthma: Review of present clinical and immunologic status. J. Allergy Clin. Immunol., 66:179, 1980.

35. Jones, R. N., Hughes, J. M., Lehrer, S. B., Butcher, B. T., Glindmeyer, H. W., Diem, J. E., Hammad, Y. Y., Salvaggio, J., and Weill, H.: Lung function consequences of exposure and hypersensitivity in workers who process green coffee beans. Am. Rev. Respir. Dis., 125:199, 1982.

36. Pepys, J.: New tests to assess lung function: Inhalation challenge tests in asthma. N. Engl. J. Med., 293:758, 1975.

37. Freedman, S. O.: New perspectives in allergic asthma. Can. Med. Assoc. J., 114:346, 1976.

38. Blythe, M. E., Ubaydi, F. A., Williams, J. D., and Smith, M. J.: Study of dust mites in three Birmingham hospitals. Br. Med. J., 1:62, 1975.

39. Tovey, E. R., Chapman, M. D., Wells, C. W., and Platts-Mills, T. A. E.: The distribution of dust mite allergen in the houses of patients with asthma. Am. Rev. Respir. Dis., 124:630, 1981.

40. Parker, C. W.: Drug therapy: Drug allergy (third of three parts). N. Engl. J. Med., 292:957, 1975.

41. Caspary, E. A., Feinmann, E. L., and Field, E. J.: Lymphocyte sensitization in asthma with special reference to nature and identity of intrinsic form. Br. Med. J., 1:15, 1973.

42. Stevenson, D. D., Mathison, D. A., Tan, E. M., and Vaughan, J. H.: Provoking factors in bronchial asthma. Arch. Intern. Med., 135:777, 1975.

43. Minor, T. E., Dick, E. C., DeMeo, A. N., Ouellette, J. J., Cohen, M., and Reed, C. E.: Viruses as precipitants of asthmatic attacks in children. J.A.M.A., 227:292, 1974.

44. Settipane, G. A., Chafee, F. H., and Klein, D. E.: Aspirin intolerance. II. A prospective study in an atopic and normal population. J. Allergy Clin. Immunol., 53:200, 1974.

45. Parker, C. W.: Aspirin-sensitive asthma. In Lichten-

stein, L. M., and Austen, K. F. (eds.), Asthma—Physiology, Immunopharmacology and Treatment, Vol. II. New York, Academic Press, 1977.

46. Fitch, K. D., and Godfrey, S.: Asthma and athletic performance. J.A.M.A., 236:152, 1976.

47. Jones, R. S., Buston, M. H., and Wharton, M. J.: The effect of exercise on ventilatory function in the child with asthma. Br. J. Dis. Chest, 56:78, 1962.

48. Deal, E. C., Jr., McFadden, E. R., Jr., Ingram, R. H., Jr., Strauss, R. H., and Jaeger, J. J.: Role of respiratory heat exchange in production of exercise-induced asthma. J. Appl. Physiol., 46:467, 1979.

49. Ben-Dov, I., Bar-Yishay, E., and Godfrey, S.: Refractory period after exercise-induced asthma unexplained by respiratory heat loss. Am. Rev. Respir. Dis., 125:530, 1982.

50. Spector, S., Luparello, T. J., Kopetzky, M. T., Souhrada, J., and Kinsman, R. A.: Response of asthmatics to methacholine and suggestion. Am. Rev. Respir. Dis., 113:43, 1976.

51. Weill, H., Ziskind, M. M., Dickerson, R. C., and Derbes, V. J.: Epidemic asthma in New Orleans, J.A.M.A., 190:811, 1964.

52. Schoettlin, C. E., and Landau, E.: Air pollution and asthmatic attacks in the Los Angeles area. Public Health Rep., 76:545, 1961.

53. Guz, E., and Orange, R. P.: Mast cells and endocrine (APUD) cells of the lung. *In* Austen, K. F., and Lichtenstein, L. M. (eds.), Asthma—Physiology, Immunopharmacology and Treatment, Vol. II. New York, Academic Press, 1977.

54. Foreman, J. C., and Garland, L. G.: Cromoglycate and other antiallergic drugs: A possible mechanism of action. Br. Med. J., 1:820, 1976.

55. Drazen, J. M., Venugopalan, C. S., Austen, K. F., Brion, F., and Corey, E. J.: Effects of leukotriene E on pulmonary mechanics in the guinea pig. Am. Rev. Respir. Dis., 125:290, 1982.

56. Ahmed, T., Greenblatt, D. W., Birch, S., Marchette, B., and Wanner, A.: Abnormal mucociliary transport in allergic patients with antigen-induced bronchospasm: Role of slow reacting substance of anaphylaxis. Am. Rev. Respir. Dis., 124:110, 1981.

57. Glynn, A. A., and Michaels, L.: Bronchial biopsy in chronic bronchitis and asthma. Thorax, 15:142, 1960.

58. MacDonald, J. B., Seaton, A., and Williams, D. A.: Asthma deaths in Cardiff 1963–74: 90 deaths outside hospital. Br. Med. J., 1:1493, 1976.

59. MacDonald, J. B., MacDonald, E. T., Seaton, A., and Williams, D. A.: Asthma deaths in Cardiff 1963–1974: 53 deaths in hospital. Br. Med. J., 2:721, 1976.

60. Hodson, M. E., Simon, G., and Batten, J. C.: Radiology of uncomplicated asthma. Thorax, 29:296, 1974.

61. Rebuck, A. S.: Radiological aspects of severe asthma. Australas. Radiol., 14:264, 1970.

62. Simon, G., Connolly, N., Littlejohns, D. W., and McAllen, M.: Radiological abnormalities in children with asthma and their relation to the clinical findings and some respiratory function tests. Thorax, 28:115, 1973.

63. Rebuck, A. S., and Pengelly, L. D.: Development of pulsus paradoxus in the presence of airways obstruction. N. Engl. J. Med., 288:66, 1973.

64. Banner, A. S., Shah, R. S., and Addington, W. W.: Rapid prediction of need for hospitalization in acute asthma. J.A.M.A., 235:1337, 1976.

65. Horn, B. R., Robin, E. D., Theodore, J., and Van

Kessel, A.: Total eosinophil counts in the management of bronchial asthma. N. Engl. J. Med., 292:1152, 1975.

66. Hendrick, D. J., Davies, R. J., and Pepys, J.: Baker's asthma. Clin. Allergy, 6:241, 1976.

67. Meisner, P., and Hugh-Jones, P.: Pulmonary function in bronchial asthma. Br. Med. J., 1:470, 1968.

68. Blackhall, M. I., and Jones, R. S.: Lung volume and its subdivisions in normal and asthmatic males. Thorax, 28:89, 1973.

69. Wilson, A. F., Surprenant, E. L., Beall, G. N., Siegel, S. C., Simmons, D. H., and Bennett, L. R.: The significance of regional pulmonary function changes in bronchial asthma. Am. J. Med., 48:416, 1970.

70. Senior, R. M., Lefrak, S. S., and Korenblat, P. E.: Status asthmaticus. J.A.M.A., 231:1277, 1975.

71. Macklin, C. C.: Pnemothorax with massive collapse from experimental local over-inflation of the lung substance. Can. Med. Assoc. J., 36:414, 1937.

72. McNicol, K. N., and Williams, H. B.: Spectrum of asthma in children. I. Clinical and physiological components. Br. Med. J., 4:7, 1973.

73. Woolcock, A., Leeder, S., Peat, J., and Blackburn, C.: The influence of bronchitis and asthma in infancy and childhood on lung function in schoolchildren. Chest, 77(Suppl.):251, 1980.

74. Chan-Yeung, M., Lam, S., and Koerner, S.: Clinical features and natural history of occupational asthma due to western red cedar *(Thuja plicata)*. Am. J. Med., 72:411, 1982.

75. Lam, S., Wong, R., and Yeung, M.: Nonspecific bronchial reactivity in occupational asthma. J. Allergy Clin. Immunol., 63:28, 1979.

76. Collins-Williams, C., Zalesky, C., Battu, K., and Chambers, M. T.: Death from asthma. CMA Journal, 125:341, 1981.

77. Turner, E. S., Greenberger, P. A., and Patterson, R.: Management of the pregnant asthmatic patient. Ann. Intern. Med., 6:905, 1980.

78. Macklem, P. T., and Permutt, S. (eds.): The Lung in Transition Between Health and Disease. New York, Dekker, 1979, p. 389.

79. Macklem, P. T.: The pathophysiology of chronic bronchitis and emphysema. Med. Clin. North Am., 57:669, 1973.

80. American Thoracic Society (Statement by Committee on Diagnostic Standards for Nontuberculous Respiratory Diseases): Definitions and classification of chronic bronchitis, asthma, and pulmonary emphysema. Am. Rev. Respir. Dis., 85:762, 1962.

81. Cohen, B. H., Menkes, H. A., Bias, W. B., Chase, G. A., Diamond, E. L., Graves, C. G., Levy, D. A., Meyer, M. B., Permutt, S., and Tockman, M. S.: Multiple factors in airways obstruction. Chest, 77(Suppl.):257, 1980.

82. Higgins, M. W., Keller, J. B., Becker, M., Howatt, W., Landis, J. R., Rotman, H., Weg, J. G., and Higgins, I.: An index of risk for obstructive airways disease. Am. Rev. Respir. Dis., 125:144, 1982.

83. Thurlbeck, W. M.: Chronic Airflow Obstruction in Lung Disease, Major Problems in Pathology, Vol. 5. Philadelphia, W. B. Saunders Co., 1976.

84. Tager, I. B., and Speizer, F. E.: Risk estimates for chronic bronchitis in smokers: A study of male-female differences. Am. Rev. Respir. Dis., 113:619, 1976.

85. Weiss, William, Boucot, K. R., Cooper, D. A., and Carnahan, W. J.: Smoking and the health of older men. II. Smoking and ventilatory function. Arch. Environ. Health, 7:538, 1963.

86. Nemery, B., Moavero, N. E., Brasseur, L., and

Stănescu, D. C.: Changes in lung function after smoking cessation: An assessment from a cross-sectional survey. Am. Rev. Respir. Dis., 125:122, 1982.

87. Beck, G. J., Doyle, C. A., and Schachter, E. N.: Smoking and lung function. Am. Rev. Respir. Dis., 123:149, 1981.

88. Mitchell, Roger S., Ryan, S. F., Petty, T. L., and Filley, G. F.: The significance of morphologic chronic hyperplastic bronchitis. Am. Rev. Respir. Dis., 93:720, 1966.

89. Bates, D. V.: Air pollutants and the human lung. The James Waring memorial lecture. Am. Rev. Respir. Dis., 105:1, 1972.

90. Detels, R., Sayre, J. W., Coulson, A. H., Rokaw, S. N., Massey, F. J., Jr., Tashkin, D. P., and Wu, M.-M.: The UCLA population studies of chronic obstructive respiratory disease. Am. Rev. Respir. Dis., 124:673, 1981.

91. Chan-Yeung, M., Schulzer, M., Maclean, L., Dorken, E., Tan, F., Lam, S., Enarson, D., Grzybowski, S.: A follow-up study of the grain elevator workers in the port of Vancouver. Arch. Environ. Health, 36:75, 1981.

92. Tager, I. B., Weiss, S. T., Rosner, B., and Speizer, F. E.: Effect of parental cigarette smoking on the pulmonary function of children. Am. J. Epidemiol., 110:15, 1979.

93. White, J. R., and Froeb, H. F.: Small-airways dysfunction in nonsmokers chronically exposed to tobacco smoke. N. Engl. J. Med., 302:720, 1980.

94. May, J. R., and May, D. S.: Bacteriology of sputum in chronic bronchitis. Tubercle, 44:162, 1963.

95. McNamara, M. J., Phillips, I. A., and Williams, O. B.: Viral and Mycoplasma pneumoniae infections in exacerbations of chronic lung disease. Am. Rev. Respir. Dis., 100:19, 1969.

96. Gump, D. W., Phillips, C. A., Forsyth, B. R., McIntosh, K., Lamborn, K. R., and Stouch, W. H.: Role of infection in chronic bronchitis. Am. Rev. Respir. Dis., 113:465, 1976.

97. Larson, R. K., Barman, M. L., Kueppers, F., and Fudenberg, H. H.: Genetic and environmental determinants of chronic obstructive pulmonary disease. Ann. Intern. Med., 72:627, 1970.

98. Cederlöf, R., Edfors, M.-L., Friberg, L., and Jonsson, E.: Hereditary factors, "spontaneous cough" and "smoker's cough." A study on 7,800 twin-pairs with the aid of mailed questionnaires. Arch. Environ. Health, 14:401, 1967.

99. Higgins, M., and Keller, J.: Familial occurrence of chronic respiratory disease and familial resemblance in ventilatory capacity. J. Chronic Dis., 28:239, 1975.

100. Leading article: Beginnings of bronchitis. Br. Med. J., 2:190, 1970.

101. Mossberg, B., and Camner, P.: Impaired mucociliary transport as a pathogenetic factor in obstructive pulmonary disease. Chest, 77(Suppl.):265, 1980.

102. Dunnill, M. S.: The contribution of morphology to the study of chronic obstructive lung disease. Am. J. Med., 57:506, 1974.

103. Thurlbeck, W. M.: Chronic obstructive lung disease. Pathol. Ann., 3:367, 1968.

104. Reid, L.: Measurement of the bronchial mucous gland layer: A diagnostic yardstick in chronic bronchitis. Thorax, 15:132, 1960.

105. Mitchell, R. S., Stanford, R. E., Johnson, J. M., Silvers, G. W., Dart, G., and George, M. S.: The morphologic features of the bronchi, bronchioles, and alveoli in chronic airway obstruction: A clinicopathologic study. Am. Rev. Respir. Dis., 114:137, 1976.

106. Matsuba, K., and Thurlbeck, W. M.: Disease of the small airways in chronic bronchitis. Am. Rev. Respir. Dis., 107:552, 1973.

107. Miller, D. L., Tinker, C. M., and Fletcher, C. M.: Measurement of sputum volume in factory and office workers. Br. Med. J., 1:291, 1965.

108. Feigin, D. S., and Abraham, J. L.: "Increased pulmonary markings"—A radiologic-pathologic correlation study (abstract). Invest. Radiol., 15:425, 1980.

109. A report of the conclusions of a Ciba Guest Symposium: Terminology, definitions and classification of chronic pulmonary emphysema and related conditions. Thorax, 14:286, 1959.

110. World Health Organization, Report of an Expert Committee: Definition and diagnosis of pulmonary diseases with special reference to chronic bronchitis and emphysema. In Chronic Cor Pulmonale, WHO Technical Report Series #213, 1961, pp. 14–19.

111. Thurlbeck, W. M.: Chronic Airflow Obstruction in Lung Disease. Philadelphia, W. B. Saunders Co., 1976, p. 220.

112. Anderson, A. E., Jr., and Foraker, A. G.: Centrilobular emphysema and panlobular emphysema: Two different diseases. Thorax, 28:547, 1973.

113. Gough, J.: The pathogenesis of emphysema. In Liebow, A. A., and Smith, D. E. (eds.), International Academy of Pathology, Monographs in Pathology, Vol. 8, The Lung. Baltimore, Williams & Wilkins Co., 1968, pp. 109–133.

114. McLean, K. H.: The histology of generalized pulmonary emphysema. I. The genesis of the early centrolobular lesion: Focal emphysema. Australas. Ann. Med., 6:124, 1957.

115. Horsfield, K., Cumming, G., and Hicken, P.: A morphologic study of airway disease using bronchial casts. Am. Rev. Respir. Dis., 93:900, 1966.

116. Thurlbeck, W. M.: Pulmonary emphysema. Am. J. Med. Sci., 246:332, 1963.

117. Loeven, W. A.: Elastolytic activity in blood. In Mittman, C. (ed.): Pulmonary Emphysema and Proteolysis. New York, Academic Press, 1972, p. 269.

118. Janoff, A., Sloan, B., Weinbaum, G., Damiano, V., Sandhaus, R. A., Elias, J., and Kimbel, P.: Experimental emphysema induced with purified human neutrophil elastase: Tissue localization of the instilled protease. Am. Rev. Respir. Dis., 115:461, 1977.

119. Lieberman, J.: Digestion of antitrypsin-deficient lung by leukoproteases. In Mittman, C. (ed.): Pulmonary Emphysema and Proteolysis. New York, Academic Press, 1972, p. 189.

120. Harris, J. O., Olsen, G. N., Castle, J. R., and Maloney, A. S.: Comparison of proteolytic enzyme activity in pulmonary alveolar macrophages and blood leukocytes in smokers and nonsmokers. Am. Rev. Respir. Dis., 111:579, 1975.

121. White, R., Lee, D., Habicht, G. S., and Janoff, A.: Secretion of alpha$_1$-proteinase inhibitor by cultured rat alveolar macrophages. Am. Rev. Respir. Dis., 123:447, 1981.

122. Janoff, A.: Inhibition of human granulocyte elastase by serum alpha$_1$-antitrypsin. Am. Rev. Respir. Dis., 105:121, 1972.

123. Kuhn, C., III, and Senior, R. M.: The role of elastases in the development of emphysema. Lung, 155:185, 1978.

124. Kidokoro, Y., Kravis, T. C., Moser, K. M., Taylor, J. C., and Crawford, I. P.: Relationship of leukocyte elastase concentration to severity of emphysema in

homozygous alpha$_1$-antitrypsin-deficient persons. Am. Rev. Respir. Dis., 115:793, 1977.

125. Robin, E. D.: Symposium on pulmonary emphysema and proteolysis. In Mittman, C. (ed.): Pulmonary Emphysema and Proteolysis. New York, Academic Press, 1972, p. 527.

126. Mustafa, M. G., Lê, C. T., Harris, N. E., and Cross, C. E.: Effects of proteases and lipases on membrane-associated biochemical reactions of alveolar macrophage and lung tissue. In Mittman, C. (ed.): Pulmonary Emphysema and Proteolysis. New York, Academic Press, 1972, p. 281.

127. Morse, J. O.: Alpha$_1$-antitrypsin deficiency. (Second of two parts.) N. Engl. J. Med., 299:1099, 1978.

128. Sloan, B., Abrams, W. R., Meranze, D. R., Kimbel, P., and Weinbaum, G.: Emphysema induced in vitro and in vivo in dogs by a purified elastase from homologous leukocytes. Am. Rev. Respir. Dis., 124:295, 1981.

129. Thurlbeck, W. M.: Chronic Airflow Obstruction in Lung Disease. Philadelphia, W. B. Saunders Co., 1976, p. 297.

130. Eichel, B., And Shahrik, H. A.: Tobacco smoke toxicity: Loss of human oral leukocyte function and fluid-cell metabolism. Science, 166:1424, 1969.

131. Hunninghake, G., Gadek, J., and Crystal, R.: Mechanism by which cigarette smoke attracts polymorphonuclear leukocytes to lung. Chest, 77(Suppl.):273, 1980.

132. Snider, G. L.: The pathogenesis of emphysema—twenty years of progress. Am. Rev. Respir. Dis., 124:321, 1981.

133. Janoff, A., White, R., Carp, H., Harel, S., Dearing, R., Lee, D.: Lung injury induced by leukocytic proteases. Am. J. Pathol., 97:111, 1979.

134. Wittels, E. H., Coalson, J. J., Welch, M. H., and Guenter, C. A.: Pulmonary intravascular leukocyte sequestration. A potential mechanism of lung injury. Am. Respir. Dis., 109:502, 1974.

135. Guenter, C. A., Coalson, J. J., and Jacques, J.: Emphysema associated with intravascular leukocyte sequestration. Comparison with papain-induced emphysema. Am. Rev. Respir. Dis., 123:79, 1981.

136. Thurlbeck, W. M., Henderson, J. A., Fraser, R. G., and Bates, D. V.: Chronic obstructive lung disease. A comparison between clinical, roentgenologic, functional and morphological criteria in chronic bronchitis, emphysema, asthma and bronchiectasis. Medicine, 49:81, 1970.

137. Nicklaus, T. M., Stowell, D. W., Christiansen, W. R., and Renzetti, A. D., Jr.: The accuracy of the roentgenologic diagnosis of chronic pulmonary emphysema. Am. Rev. Respir. Dis., 93:889, 1966.

138. Milne, Eric, N. C., and Bass, H.: Roentgenologic and functional analysis of combined chronic obstructive pulmonary disease and congestive cardiac failure. Invest. Radiol., 4:129, 1969.

139. Simon, G.: Principles of Chest X-Ray Diagnosis, 3rd ed. London, Butterworth, 1971.

140. Fraser, R. G., and Bates, D. V.: Body section roentgenography in the evaluation and differentiation of chronic hypertrophic emphysema and asthma. Am. J. Roentgenol., 82:39, 1959.

141. Simon, G.: Complexities of emphysema. In Simon, M., Potchen, E. J., and LeMay, M. (eds.): Frontiers of Pulmonary Radiology. New York, Grune & Stratton, Inc., 1969, pp. 142–153.

142. Simon, G., Pride, N. B., Jones, N. L., and Raimondi, A. C.: Relation between abnormalities in the chest radiograph and changes in pulmonary function in chronic bronchitis and emphysema. Thorax, 28:15, 1973.

143. Rosen, R. A., Dalinka, M. K., Gralino, B. J., Jr., Goldenberg, D. B., and Walsh, R. E.: The roentgenographic findings in alpha-1 antitrypsin deficiency (AAD). Radiology, 95:25, 1970.

144. Bentivoglio, L. G., Beerel, F., Stewart, P. B., Bryan, A. C., Ball, W. C., Jr., and Bates, D. V.: Studies of regional ventilation and perfusion in pulmonary emphysema using xenon^{133}. Am. Rev. Respir. Dis., 88:315, 1963.

145. Laws, J. W., and Heard, B. E.: Emphysema and the chest film: A retrospective radiological and pathological study. Br. J. Radiol., 35:750, 1962.

146. Bates, D. V., Macklem, P. T., and Christie, R. V.: Respiratory Function in Disease; An Introduction to the Integrated Study of the Lung, 2nd ed. Philadelphia, W. B. Saunders Co., 1971.

147. Dornhorst, A. D.: Respiratory insufficiency. Lancet, 1:1185, 1955.

148. Lieberman, J.: Alpha$_1$-antitrypsin deficiency. Med. Clin. North Am., 57:691, 1973.

149. Burrows, B., Fletcher, C. M., Heard, B. E., Jones, N. L., and Wootliff, J. S.: The emphysematous and bronchial types of chronic airways obstruction: A clinicopathological study of patients in London and Chicago, Lancet, 1:830, 1966.

150. Milne, E. N. C., and Bass, H.: Roentgenologic diagnosis of early chronic obstructive pulmonary disease. J. Can. Assoc. Radiol., 30:3, 1969.

151. Heitzman, E. R.: The Lung. Radiologic-Pathologic Correlations. St. Louis, C. V. Mosby Co., 1973, p. 350.

152. Heitzman, E. R., Markarian, B., and Soloman, J.: Chronic obstructive pulmonary disease: A review, emphasizing roentgen pathologic correlations. Radiol. Clin. North Am., 11:49, 1973.

153. Scarrow, G. D.: The pulmonary angiogram in chronic bronchitis and emphysema. Clin. Radiol., 17:54, 1966.

154. Thurlbeck, W. M., and Simon, G.: Radiographic appearance of the chest in emphysema. Am. J. Roentgenol., 130:429, 1978.

155. Fletcher, C. M., Jones, N. L., Burrows, B., and Niden, A. H.: American emphysema and British bronchitis. A standardized comparative study. Am. Rev. Respir. Dis., 90:1, 1964.

156. Reid, L. M.: The Pathology of Emphysema. London, Lloyd-Luke, 1967.

157. Kass, I., O'Brien, L. E., Zamel, N., and Dyksterhuis, J. E.: Lack of correlation between clinical background and pulmonary function tests in patients with chronic obstructive pulmonary diseases. A retrospective study of 140 cases. Am. Rev. Respir. Dis., 107:64, 1973.

158. Burrows, B., and Earle, R. H.: Course and prognosis of chronic obstructive lung disease. A prospective study of 200 patients. N. Engl. J. Med. 280:397, 1969.

159. Vandenberg, E., Clement, J., and van de Woestijne, K. P.: Course and prognosis of patients with advanced chronic obstructive pulmonary disease. Evaluation by means of functional indices. Am. J. Med., 55:736, 1973.

160. Burke, R. H., and George, R. B.: Acute respiratory failure in chronic obstructive pulmonary disease. Arch. Intern. Med., 132:865, 1973.

161. Moser, K. M., Shibel, E. M., and Beamon, A. J.: Acute respiratory failure in obstructive lung disease: Long-term survival after treatment in an intensive care unit. J.A.M.A., 225:705, 1973.

162. Bishop, J. M.: Cardiovascular complications of chronic bronchitis and emphysema. Med. Clin. North Am., 57:771, 1973.

163. Taha, R. A., Boushy, S. F., Thompson, H. K., Jr., North, L. B., and Aboumrad, M. H.: The electrocardiogram in chronic obstructive pulmonary disease. Am. Rev. Respir. Dis., 107:1067, 1973.

164. Dulfano, M. J., and Ishikawa, S.: Hypercapnia: Mental changes and extrapulmonary complications. An expanded concept of the "CO₂ intoxication" syndrome. Ann. Intern. Med., 63:829, 1965.

165. Zasly, L., Baum, G. L., and Rumball, J. M.: The incidence of peptic ulceration in chronic obstructive pulmonary emphysema. A statistical study. Dis. Chest, 37:400, 1960.

165a. Filley, G. F.: Acid regulation and CO₂ retention. Chest, 58:417, 1970.

166. White, R. J., and Woodings, D. F.: Impaired water handling in chronic obstructive airways disease. Br. Med. J., 2:561, 1971.

167. Schloerb, P. K., King, C. R., Kerby, G., and Ruth, W. E.: Potassium depletion in patients with chronic respiratory failure. Am. Rev. Respir. Dis., 102:53, 1970.

168. Macklem, P. T., and Becklake, M. R.: The relationship between the mechanical and diffusing properties of the lung in health and disease. Am. Rev. Respir. Dis., 87:47, 1963.

169. Cosio, M., Ghezzo, H., Hogg, J. C., Corbin, R., Loveland, M., Dosman, J., and Macklem, P. T.: The relations between structural changes in small airways and pulmonary-function tests. N. Engl. J. Med., 298:1277, 1977.

170. Petty, T. L., Silvers, G. W., and Stanford, R. E.: Functional correlations with mild and moderate emphysema in excised human lungs. Am. Rev. Respir. Dis., 124:700, 1981.

171. Macklem, P. T., Hogg, J. C., and Thurlbeck, W. M.: The flow resistance of central and peripheral airways in human lungs. In Cumming, G., and Hunt, L. B. (eds.): Form and Function in the Human Lung. Edinburgh, E. & S. Livingstone, Ltd., 1968, pp. 76–88.

172. McFadden, E. R., Jr., and Linden, D. A.: A reduction in maximum mid-expiratory flow rate. A spirographic manifestation of small airway disease. Am. J. Med., 52:725, 1972.

173. Burrows, B.: Early detection of airways obstruction. Chest, 65:239, 1974.

174. Abboud, R. T., and Morton, J. W.: Comparison of maximal mid-expiratory flow, flow volume curves, and nitrogen closing volumes in patients with mild airway obstruction. Am. Rev. Respir. Dis., 111:405, 1975.

175. Higgins, M. W., and Keller, J. B.: Seven measures of ventilatory lung function. Population values and a comparison of their ability to discriminate between persons with and without chronic respiratory symptoms and disease. Tecumseh, Michigan. Am. Rev. Respir. Dis., 108:258, 1973.

176. Knudson, R. J., and Burrows, B.: Early detection of obstructive lung diseases. Med. Clin. North Am., 57:681, 1973.

177. Fletcher, C. M., Peto, R., Tinker, C. M., and Speizer, F. E.: The Natural History of Chronic Bronchitis and Emphysema. Oxford, Oxford University Press, 1976.

178. Knudson, R. J., Armet, D. B., and Lebowitz, M. D.: Reevaluation of tests of small airways function. Chest, 77(Suppl.):284, 1980.

179. Burrows, B.: Course and prognosis of patients with chronic airways obstruction. Chest, 77(Suppl.):250, 1980.

180. Koo, K. W., Sax, D. S., and Snider, G. L.: Arterial blood gases and pH during sleep in chronic obstructive pulmonary disease. Am. J. Med., 58:663, 1975.

181. Flenley, D. C., Calverly, P. M. A., Douglas, N. J., Catterall, J. R., Lamb, D., and Brezinova, V.: Nocturnal hypoxemia and long-term domiciliary oxygen therapy in "blue and bloated" bronchitics. Physiopathologic correlations. Chest, 77(Suppl): 305, 1980.

182. Pain, M. C. F., Read, D. J. C., and Read, J.: Changes of arterial carbon-dioxide tension in patients with chronic lung disease breathing oxygen. Aust. Ann. Med., 14:195, 1965.

183. Rawlings, W., Jr., Kreiss, P., Levy, D., Cohen, B., Menkes, H., Brashears, S., and Permutt, S.: Clinical, epidemiologic, and pulmonary function studies in alpha₁-antitrypsin–deficient subjects of PiZ type. Am. Rev. Respir. Dis., 114:945, 1976.

184. Reid, L.: The Pathology of Emphysema. London, Lloyd-Luke, Ltd., 1967.

185. Boushy, S. F., Kohen, R., Billig, D. M., and Heiman, M. J.: Bullous emphysema: Clinical, roentgenologic and physiologic study of 49 patients. Dis. Chest, 54:327, 1968.

186. Stark, P., Gadziala, N., and Greene, R.: Fluid accumulation in preexisting pulmonary air spaces. Am. J. Roentgenol., 134:701, 1980.

187. Gibson, G. J.: Familial pneumothoraces and bullae. Thorax, 32:88, 1977.

188. Pride, N. B., Barter, C. E., and Hugh-Jones, P.: The ventilation of bullae and the effect of their removal on thoracic gas volumes and tests of overall pulmonary function. Am. Rev. Respir. Dis., 107:83, 1973.

189. Pride, N. B., Hugh-Jones, P., O'Brien, E. N., and Smith, L. A.: Changes in lung function following the surgical treatment of bullous emphysema. Q. J. Med., 39:49, 1970.

190. Foreman, S., Weill, H., Duke, R., George, R., and Ziskind, M.: Bullous disease of the lung. Physiologic improvement after surgery. Ann. Intern. Med., 69:757, 1968.

191. Swyer, P. R., and James, G. C. W.: A case of unilateral pulmonary emphysema. Thorax, 8:133, 1953.

192. Reid, L., and Simon, G.: Unilateral lung transradiancy. Thorax, 17:230, 1962.

193. MacLeod, W. M.: Abnormal transradiancy of one lung. Thorax, 9:147, 1954.

194. Gold, R., Wilt, J. C., Adhikari, T. K., Chernick, V., and MacPherson, R. I.: Adenoviral pneumonia and its complications in infancy and childhood. J. Can. Assoc. Radiol., 20:218, 1969.

195. Sanderson, J. M., Kennedy, M. C. S., Johnson, M. F., and Manley, D. C. E.: Bronchiectasis: Results of surgical and conservative management. A review of 393 cases. Thorax, 29:407, 1974.

196. Longstreth, G. F., Weitzman, S. A., Browning, R. J., and Lieberman, J.: Bronchiectasis and homozygous alpha₁-antitrypsin deficiency. Chest, 67:233, 1975.

197. Rossman, C. M., Forrest, J. B., Ruffin, R. E., and Newhouse, M. T.: Immotile cilia syndrome in persons with and without Kartagener's syndrome. Am. Rev. Respir. Dis., 121:1011, 1980.

198. Sturgess, J. M., Chao, J., Wong, J., Aspin, N., and Turner, J. A. P.: Cilia with defective radial spokes. A cause of human respiratory disease. N. Engl. J. Med., 300:53, 1979.

199. Wakefield, S., and Waite, D.: Abnormal cilia in

Polynesians with bronchiectasis. Am. Rev. Respir. Dis., *121*:1003, 1980.

200. Reid, L., McA.: Reduction in bronchial subdivision in bronchiectasis. Thorax, 5:233, 1950.
201. Nelson, S. W., and Christoforidis, A.: Reversible bronchiectasis. Radiology, *71*:375, 1958.
202. Landau, L. I., Phelan, P. D., and Williams, H. E.: Ventilatory mechanics in patients with bronchiectasis starting in childhood. Thorax, *29*:304, 1974.
203. Kartagener, M., and Stucki, P.: Bronchiectasis with situs inversus. Arch. Pediatr., *79*:193, 1962.
204. Holmes, L. B., Blennerhassett, J. B., and Austen, K. F.: A reappraisal of Kartagener's syndrome. Am. J. Med. Sci., *255*:13, 1968.
205. Katsuhara, K., Kawamoto, S., Wakabayashi, T., and Belsky, J. L.: Situs inversus totalis and Kartagener's syndrome in a Japanese population. Chest, *61*:56, 1972.
206. Wolfe, R. R.: Kartagener's syndrome: A pediatic responsibility. Chest, *69*:573, 1976.
207. Afzelius, B. A.: "Immotile-cilia" syndrome and ciliary abnormalities induced by infection and injury. Am. Rev. Respir. Dis., *124*:107, 1981.
208. Macklem, P. T., Thurlbeck, W. M., and Fraser, R. G.: Chronic obstructive disease of small airways. Ann. Intern. Med., *74*:167, 1971.
209. Wood, R. E., Boat, T. F., and Doershuk, C. F.: Cystic fibrosis. Am. Rev. Respir. Dis., *113*:833, 1976.
210. di Sant'Agnese, P. A., and Talamo, R. C.: Pathogenesis and physiopathology of cystic fibrosis of the pancreas. Fibrocytic disease of the pancreas (mucoviscidosis). N. Engl. J. Med., *277*:1287, 1967.
211. di Sant'Agnese, P. A., and Talamo, R. C.: Pathogenesis and physiopathology of cystic fibrosis of the pancreas. Fibrocystic disease of the pancreas (mucoviscidosis). (Continued.) N. Engl. J. Med., *277*:1344, 1967.
212. di Sant'Agnese, P. A., and Talamo, R. C.: Pathogenesis and physiopathology of cystic fibrosis of the pancreas. Fibrocystic disease of the pancreas (mucoviscidosis) (Concluded.) N. Engl. J. Med., *277*:1399, 1967.
213. Bowman, B. H., and Mangos, J. A.: Current concepts in genetics: Cystic fibrosis. N. Engl. J. Med., *294*:937, 1976.
214. Gibson, L. E., Matthews, W. J., Jr., and Minihan, P. T.: Hyperpermeable mucus in cystic fibrosis. Lancet, 2:189, 1970.
215. Sahu, S., and Lynn, W. S.: Lipid composition of airway secretions from patients with asthma and patients with cystic fibrosis. Am. Rev. Respir. Dis., *115*:233, 1977.
216. Spock, A., Heick, H. M., Cress, H., and Logan, W. S.: Abnormal serum factor in patients with cystic fibrosis of the pancreas. Pediatr. Res., *1*:173, 1967.
217. Wanner, A.: Clinical aspect of mucociliary transport. Am. Rev. Respir. Dis., *116*:73, 1977.
218. Wood, R. E., and di Sant'Agnese, P. A.: Bioassays of cystic-fibrosis factor. Lancet, 2:1452, 1973.
219. di Sant'Agnese, P. A., and Davis, P. B.: Research in cystic fibrosis (third of three parts). N. Engl. J. Med., *295*:597, 1976.
220. Matthews, W. J., Jr., Williams, M., Oliphint, B., Geha, R., and Colten, H. R.: Hypogammaglobulinemia in patients with cystic fibrosis. N. Engl. J. Med., *302*:245, 1980.
221. Boxerbaum, B., Kagumba, M., and Matthews, L. W.: Selective inhibition of phagocytic activity of rabbit alveolar macrophages by cystic fibrosis serum. Am. Rev. Respir. Dis., *108*:777, 1973.

222. Esterly, J. R., and Oppenheimer, E. H.: Cystic fibrosis of the pancreas: Structural changes in peripheral airways. Thorax, *23*:670, 1968.
223. Waring, W. W., Brunt, C. H., and Hilman, B. C.: Mucoid impaction of the bronchi in cystic fibrosis. Pediatrics, *39*:166, 1967.
224. Holsclaw, D. S., Grand, R. J., and Shwachman, H.: Massive hemoptysis in cystic fibrosis. J. Pediatr., *76*:829, 1970.
225. Kaplan, E., Shwachman, H., Perlmutter, A. D., Rule, A., Khaw, K.-T., and Holsclaw, D. S.: Reproductive failure in males with cystic fibrosis. N. Engl. J. Med., *279*:65, 1968.
226. Taussig, L. M., Lobeck, C. C., di Sant'Agnese, P. A., Ackerman, D. R., and Kattwinkel, J.: Fertility in males with cystic fibrosis. N. Engl. J. Med., *287*:586, 1972.
227. Kulczycki, L. L., and Shwachman, H.: Studies in cystic fibrosis of the pancreas. Occurrence of rectal prolapse. N. Engl. J. Med., *259*:409, 1958.
228. Jones, J. D., Steige, H., and Logan, G. B.: Variations of sweat sodium values in children and adults with cystic fibrosis and other diseases. Mayo Clin. Proc., *45*:768, 1970.
229. Landau, L. I., and Phelan, P. D.: The spectrum of cystic fibrosis. A study of pulmonary mechanics in 46 patients. Am. Rev. Respir. Dis., *108*:593, 1973.
230. Tomashefski, J. F., Christoforidis, A. J., and Abdullah, A. K.: Cystic fibrosis in young adults. An overlooked diagnosis, with emphasis on pulmonary function and radiological patterns. Chest, *57*:28, 1970.
231. Dantzker, D. R., Patten, G. A., and Bower, J. S.: Gas exchange at rest and during exercise in adults with cystic fibrosis. Am. Rev. Respir. Dis., *125*:400, 1982.
232. Coates, A. L., Desmond, K. J., Milic-Emili, J., and Beaudry, P. H.: Ventilation, respiratory center output, and contribution of the rib cage and abdominal components to ventilation during CO_2 rebreathing in children with cystic fibrosis. Am. Rev. Respir. Dis., *124*:526, 1981.
233. Reilly, B. J., Featherby, E. A., Weng, T.-R., Crozier, D. N., Duic, A., and Levison, H.: The correlation of radiological changes with pulmonary function in cystic fibrosis. Radiology, 98:281, 1971.
234. Riley, C. M., Day, R. L., Greeley, D. McL., and Langford, W. S.: Central autonomic dysfunction with defective lacrimation. I. Report of five cases. Pediatrics, *3*:468, 1949.
235. Brunt, P. W., and McKusick, V. A.: Familial dysautonomia: A report of genetic and clinical studies, with a review of the literature. Medicine, 49:343, 1970.
236. Siggers, D. C., Rogers, J. G., Boyer, S. H., Margolet, L., Dorkin, H., Banerjee, S. P., and Shooter, E. M.: Increased nerve-growth-factor β-chain cross-reacting material in familial dysautonomia. N. Engl. J. Med., *295*:629, 1976.
237. Riley, C. M., and Moore, R. H.: Familial dysautonomia differentiated from related disorders. Case reports and discussions of current concepts. Pediatrics, *37*:435, 1966.
238. Fraser, R. G., Fraser, R. S., Renner, J. W., Bernard, C., and Fitzgerald, P. J.: The roentgenologic diagnosis of chronic bronchitis: A reassessment with emphasis on parahilar bronchi seen end-on. Radiology, *120*:1, 1976.

12

The Pneumoconioses and Chemically-Induced Lung Diseases

The inorganic dust diseases, often termed the "pneumoconioses," are in large measure occupational diseases. In recent years, however, it has become increasingly apparent that these diseases may develop, as a result of atmospheric pollution, in persons who live in the vicinity of industrial plants (particularly those handling asbestos and beryllium) but do not work there.

The region of the respiratory tract affected and the pathologic changes produced depend not only on the chemical composition and density of particles in the atmosphere but also on particle size and shape. The great majority of particles that penetrate to the alveoli measure 5μ or less in diameter, larger particles being deposited on contact with the upper respiratory tract, trachea, and larger bronchi. The notable exception is the asbestos fiber, which may penetrate deep into the parenchyma of the lung despite a length of 30μ or more.

Pneumoconiosis can be defined as "the accumulation of dust in the lungs and the tissue reactions to its presence." Dust is regarded as an aerosol composed of solid inanimate particles, and the tissues react to it in two different ways: (1) a desmoplastic reaction resulting in permanent scarring—the collagenous pneumoconioses such as silicosis and asbestosis; and (2) a minimal stromal reaction consisting mainly of reticulin fibers—the noncollagenous pneumoconioses such as iron, tin, and barium. This definition excludes occupational diseases such as byssinosis, berylliosis, and the hypersensitivity pneumonitides in which particles do not accumulate in the lungs. Partly for this reason and partly because of the strong evidence for

their immunopathogenesis, the *organic dust* pneumoconioses are discussed in the chapter on immunologic lung disease. However, since beryllium poisoning has been traditionally included among the inorganic pneumoconioses, we have included it in the present chapter.

INHALATION DISEASES CAUSED BY INORGANIC DUST (INORGANIC DUST PNEUMOCONIOSES)

FACTORS INFLUENCING LUNG REACTION

The reaction of the lung to inhaled dust depends on seven factors, each of which is important in itself but all of which must be considered in combination, since they are to a certain extent interdependent.

1. *The chemical nature of the dust.* The majority of inorganic dusts, if inhaled in sufficient quantity over a long time, result in pulmonary fibrosis. Even though a few dusts are "inert" and are not fibrinogenic (for example, tin, iron, and barium), they can produce some degree of function impairment if inhaled in sufficient quantity over a sufficient period of time. It is unreasonable to expect the lung to act as a "physiologic dust trap" without its function being impaired to some extent.

The reaction of the lungs to inhaled particulate matter depends largely upon the particles' solubility. Soluble particles that reach the alveoli may give rise to an acute reaction, such as edema, or a more subacute granuloma formation. Insoluble particles may provoke a slowly progressive fibrogenic reaction if they reach the air spaces.

2. *The size of dust particles.* Three main physical processes determine particle deposition in the lungs: inertial impaction, sedimentation, and diffusion.

Nearly all particles 20 μ or more in diameter are deposited out on the walls of the nasopharynx, trachea, and bronchi as a result of inertial impaction and, to a lesser extent, sedimentation. The majority of particles less than 3 μ in diameter are deposited in the respiratory bronchioles or alveoli, chiefly by the mechanism of diffusion but partly by sedimentation. The three major physical processes that determine particle deposition in the lungs are influenced by transient changes in air flow and residence times at each level of the respiratory tract.[1]

3. *The distribution of inhaled dust particles.* There has been very little experimental work to determine the distribution of inert particles in normal lungs, but since ventilation in the erect position is relatively greater in lower than in upper lung regions, the former should be slightly more susceptible to lung damage. That this is not always the case in practice, however, is illustrated by the fact that silicosis commonly shows an *upper* zonal predominance.

4. *Concentration of dust particles.* It has been shown that the ability of the healthy lung to cope with the introduction of dust particles into the alveoli appears to relate roughly to the concentration of air-borne dust inhaled. Less than ten particles of 5 μ or less per ml can be completely eliminated, whereas only about 90 per cent of a concentration of approximately 1000 such particles per ml will be eliminated, and the retained 10 per cent can produce a slowly developing pneumoconiosis. With concentrations as high as 1,000,000 particles per ml, a very high proportion is retained and lung disease can develop rapidly.

5. *Duration of exposure.* The great majority of cases of pneumoconiosis develop only after many years of dust exposure. Occasionally, however, severe progressive lung disease develops after only relatively brief exposure—a few months for example. In these instances, it is probable that two factors are chiefly responsible: a very high concentration of dust and an individual susceptibility.

6. *Individual susceptibility.* This is a difficult factor to assess, but there is no doubt that different individuals with identical dust exposure may have different reactions: one may be free of disease while another may show advanced progressive massive fibrosis.

7. *Clearance of dust particles.* This is accomplished by one or both of two mechanisms—transport up the mucociliary escalator and lymphatic drainage. It is probable that variation in the efficiency of these mechanisms may account for individual susceptibility to the development of pneumoconiosis. Particles deposited on the tracheobronchial tree are rapidly transported on the mucociliary apparatus and reach the pharynx in 1 to 2 hours, where they are either expectorated or swallowed along with mucus. Smaller particles that reach the alveoli are thought to be deposited through random motion on the surface of alveolar macrophages, which engulf them. It is probable that these dust-containing macrophages are carried along by passive transport in fluid movement, either within the conducting airways or via the lymphatics.[3] Dust particles, either free or within macrophages, may enter the interstitial tissues and be carried either centripetally to centrilobar lymphatics or centrifugally to perilobar lymphatics.

The diagnosis of a pneumoconiosis usually is based on a specific exposure history, an abnormal chest roentgenogram, and the results of pulmonary function studies. During the last decade, newer methods of analyzing material obtained by lung biopsy have proven to be very useful in establishing an unequivocal diagnosis. These techniques complement the use of light and polarized light microscopy and include scanning and transmission electronmicroscopy, back-scattered electron imaging, x-ray energy spectrometry, x-ray diffractometry, and selected area electron diffraction.[4, 5]

The evaluation of potential hazards in the work place is of utmost importance in uncovering occupationally-induced disease.[6] A detailed occupational history is essential for the establishment of a causal relationship between an inhaled dust and an adverse biologic effect, since certain jobs not usually regarded as hazardous may become so if carried out in proximity to other workers involved in hazardous occupations such as welding or sandblasting.[7] The chest roentgenogram is an important epidemiologic tool that is useful not only in detecting the effects of dust particle deposition in the lungs but also in measuring progression.[8] In order for the roentgenogram to be useful in epidemiologic studies, however, it is essential that an international classification of extent of involvement be followed and an acceptable nomenclature be employed.

INTERNATIONAL CLASSIFICATION OF RADIOGRAPHS OF THE PNEUMOCONIOSES AND RECOMMENDED TERMINOLOGY

In response to a growing need for an internationally acceptable system for coding the changes seen on chest roentgenograms of individuals exposed to asbestos, a committee of l'Union Internationale Contre le Cancer (the International Union Against Cancer, UICC), together with other groups, met in Cincinnati in 1967 for the purpose of developing a new classification. This was subsequently adopted and became known as the UICC/Cincinnati (UC) classification.[9] Shortly thereafter, the ILO 1958 classification was revised (based in part on the U/C 1968 classification) and became known as the ILO 1968 classification. Following a period of experience with these two classifications, a meeting was convened in 1971 and it was recommended that the ILO 1968 and U/C classifications, including standard reference roentgenograms, be combined. The obvious benefits to be derived from such a combination were the establishment of uniform international standards and the ability to compare results around the world. These recommendations were approved in 1971 and subsequently modified once again in 1980, thus giving official recognition to the classification now widely used throughout the world, the ILO 1980 international classification of radiographs of the pneumoconioses (Table 12–1).

The object of the classification is to codify the roentgenographic changes of the pneumoconioses in a simple, reproducible manner. It does not define pathologic entities but possesses the considerable advantage of providing a uniform method of reporting the type and extent of pneumoconiosis, thus leading to international comparability of pneumoconiosis statistics. The classification (Table 12–1) is intended primarily for a comprehensive and semiquantitative description of the roentgenographic changes of all the principal features, including those of the pleura; it is likely to be particularly useful for epidemiologic studies.

GLOSSARY OF TERMS IN DESCRIBING ROENTGENOGRAPHIC CHANGES IN THE PNEUMOCONIOSES

Small Rounded Opacities

These are well-circumscribed opacities or nodules ranging in diameter from barely visible up to 10 mm. The qualifiers p, q, and r subdivide the predominant opacities into three diameter ranges—up to 1.5 mm, 1.5 to 3 mm, and 3 mm to 10 mm.

Small Irregular Opacities

This term is employed to describe a pattern which, elsewhere in this book, has been designated "linear" or "reticular"—in other words, a netlike pattern. Although the nature of these opacities is such that the establishment of quantitative dimensions is considerably more difficult than with rounded opacities, the ILO has seen fit to establish three categories—s (width up to about 1.5 mm), t (width exceeding 1.5 mm and up to about 3 mm), and u (width exceeding 3 mm and up to about 10 mm).

To record shape and size, two letters must be used. Thus, if the reader considers that all or virtually all opacities are of one shape and size, this should be noted by recording the symbol twice, separated by an oblique stroke (for example, q/q). If, however, another shape or size is seen, this should be recorded as the second letter (for example, q/t). The designation q/t would mean that the predominant small opacity is round and of size q, but that there are, in addition, significant numbers of small irregular opacities of size t. In this way, any combination of small opacities may be recorded.

Profusion

This term denotes the number of small rounded or small irregular opacities per unit area or zone of lung. There are four basic categories:

Category 0: small opacities absent or less profuse than in category 1.

Category 1: small opacities definitely present but few in number. The normal markings are usually visible.

Category 2: numerous small opacities. The normal lung markings are usually partly obscured.

Category 3: very numerous small opacities. The normal lung markings are usually totally obscured.

These categories can be further subdivided by employing a 12-point scale by which the classification recognizes the existence of a continuum of changes from complete normality to the most advanced category or grade. The 12-point scale is listed as follows:

0/ –	0/0	0/1
1/0	1/1	1/2
2/1	2/2	2/3
3/2	3/3	3/ +

Employing this scale, profusion of opacities is categorized as follows: the roentgenogram is

TABLE 12–1. ILO 1980 INTERNATIONAL CLASSIFICATION OF RADIOGRAPHS OF THE PNEUMOCONIOSES

FEATURE	CODE			DEFINITION
Small Opacities				
Shape and Size				
Rounded				The nodules are classified according to the approximate diameter of the predominant opacities.
	p	q	r	p = rounded opacities up to about 1.5 mm in diameter. q = rounded opacities exceeding about 1.5 mm and up to about 3 mm in diameter. r = rounded opacities exceeding about 3 mm and up to about 10 mm in diameter.
Irregular	s	t	u	s = width up to about 1.5 mm. t = width exceeding 1.5 mm and up to about 3 mm. u = width exceeding 3 mm and up to about 10 mm.
				To record shape and size, two letters must be used. Thus if the reader considers that all or virtually all opacities are of one shape and size, then this should be noted by recording the symbol twice, separated by an oblique stroke (for example, q/q). If, however, another shape or size is seen, then this should be recorded as the second letter (for example, q/t). The recording q/t would mean that the predominant small opacity is round and of size q, but that there are significant numbers of small irregular opacities of size t. In this way any combination of small opacities may be recorded.
Profusion				The category of profusion is based on assessment of the concentration (profusion) of opacities in the affected zones. The standard radiographs define the midcategories (1/1, 2/2, 3/3).
	0/−	0/0	0/1	Category 0 = small opacities absent or less profuse than in category 1.
	1/0	1/1	1/2	Category 1 = small opacities definitely present, but few in number. The normal lung markings are usually visible.
	2/1	2/2	2/3	Category 2 = small opacities, numerous. The normal lung markings are usually partly obscured.
	3/2	3/3	3/4	Category 3 = small opacities, very numerous. The normal lung markings are usually totally obscured.
Extent	RU LU	RM LM	RL LL	The zones in which the opacities are seen are recorded. Each lung is divided into three zones—upper, middle, and lower.
Large Opacities				
Size	A	B	C	Category A = an opacity having a greatest diameter exceeding about 1 cm and up to and including about 5 cm, or several opacities each greater than about 1 cm the sum of whose greatest diameters does not exceed about 5 cm.
				Category B = one or more opacities larger or more numerous than in category A whose combined areas do not exceed the equivalent of the right upper zone.
				Category C = one or more opacities whose combined areas exceed the equivalent of the right upper zone.
Pleural Thickening				
Costophrenic angle	R	L		Obliteration of the costophrenic angle is recorded separately from thickening over other sites. A lower limit standard radiograph is provided.

TABLE 12–1. ILO 1980 IINTERNATIONAL CLASSIFICATION OF RADIOGRAPHS OF THE PNEUMOCONIOSES *(Continued)*

FEATURE	CODE				DEFINITION
Chest wall					
Types					Circumscribed (plaques) and/or diffuse
Site		R		L	
Width	a	b		c	Grade a = up to about 5 mm thick at the widest part of any pleural shadow.
					Grade b = over about 5 mm and up to about 10 mm thick at the widest part of any pleural shadow.
					Grade c = over about 10 mm at the widest part of any pleural shadow.
Extent	1	2		3	Grade 1 = definite pleural thickening in one or more places such that the total length does not exceed one quarter of the projection of one lateral wall. The standard radiograph defines the lower limit of grade 1.
					Grade 2 = pleural thickening whose total length exceeds one quater but not one half of the projection of the lateral chest wall.
					Grade 3 = pleural thickening whose total length exceeds one half of the projection of the lateral chest wall.
Diaphragm		R		L	A plaque involving the diaphragmatic pleura is recorded separately as present or absent, right or left. This is illustrated by an example in the standard radiographs.
Pleural Calcification					
Site	Chest Wall	Diaphragm R		Other L	
Extent	1	2		3	Grade 1 = one or more areas of pleural calcification the sum of whose greatest diameters does not exceed about 2 cm.
					Grade 2 = one or more areas of pleural calcification the sum of whose greatest diameters exceeds about 2 cm but not above about 10 cm.
					Grade 3 = one or more areas of pleural calcification the sum of whose greatest diameters exceeds about 10 cm.
Additional Symbols					ax = coalescence of small pneumoconiotic opacities bu = bulla(e) ca = cancer of lung or pleura cn = calcification in small pneumoconiotic opacities co = abnormality of cardiac size or shape cp = cor pulmonale cv = cavity di = marked distortion of intrathoracic organs ef = effusion em = definite emphysema ex = eggshell calcification of hilar or mediastinal lymph nodes fr = fractured rib(s) hi = enlargement of hilar or mediastinal lymph nodes ho = honeycomb lung id = ill-defined diaphragm ih = ill-defined heart outline kl = septal (Kerley) lines od = other significant abnormality pi = pleural thickening in an interlobar fissure or along the mediastinum px = pneumothorax rp = rheumatoid pneumoconiosis tb = tuberculosis

classified in the usual way into one of the four categories, 0, 1, 2, or 3. If during the process the category above or below is considered as a serious alternative, this is recorded, *e.g.*, a roentgenogram in which profusion is considered to be category 2 but for which category 1 was seriously considered as an alternative would be graded category 2/1. If no alternative was considered—*i.e.*, the profusion was definitely category 2—it would be classified 2/2.

Large Opacities

This includes opacities that are larger than the maximum permitted for small rounded opacities, *i.e.*, greater than 10 mm. Three categories are recognized:

Category A: an opacity having a greatest diameter exceeding 1 cm and up to and including 5 cm, or several opacities each greater than 1 cm, the sum of whose greatest diameters does not exceed 5 cm.
Category B: one or more opacities larger or more numerous than in category A whose combined areas do not exceed the equivalent of the right upper zone.
Category C: one or more opacities whose combined areas exceed the equivalent of the right upper zone.

Extent

Each lung is divided into three zones—upper, middle, and lower—by horizontal lines drawn at one-third and two-thirds of the vertical distance between the apex of the lung and the dome of the diaphragm.

All other terms used in the classification are self-explanatory and are identical in context to the same terms used elsewhere in this book.

Standard reference roentgenograms* have been selected to illustrate the ILO 1980 classification.

SILICOSIS

EPIDEMIOLOGY

Silicon dioxide exists in two forms, amorphous and crystalline. Sandstone is almost pure silica, granite between 20 and 70 per cent silica,

*In North America, a set of the ILO 1980 Standard Reference Radiographs can be purchased from the regional center of the International Labor Office, 1750 New York Avenue N.W., Washington, D.C. 20006. In other parts of the world, it can be purchased from the International Labor Office, Geneva, Switzerland.

and slate about 40 per cent. Tunneling, mining, or quarrying inevitably leads to exposure to silica dust unless it is into pure limestone or marble.[10] Exposure to high concentrations of silica or silicon dioxide (SiO_2), resulting in the characteristic roentgenographic and pathologic picture of silicosis, may occur in many occupations.[11] In North America, exposure is most commonly to quartz in the mining of gold, but some cases of silicosis are seen in foundry workers, sandblasters, in persons exposed to potter's clay in the ceramics industry and in the manufacture of artificial grinding wheels, in ocher workers, granite workers, and in persons exposed to high concentrations of enamel.

Silica particles 0.5 to 5 μ in diameter are those likely to produce the disease. Most of the coarser particles, 5 to 10 μ or larger in diameter, are removed in the upper respiratory tract. The free silica content of dust varies considerably with particle size. In foundry dust, larger particles (5 to 10 μ or more in diameter) usually have a high free silica content, but smaller particles (less than 5 μ in diameter), those largely responsible for the disease, contain a relatively low free silica percentage.[12] The U.S. Public Health Service statements of *concentration* of dust particles in the atmosphere describe primary and secondary thresholds. *The primary threshold* consists of 5×10^6 particles less than 10 μ in size per cubic foot; exposure to concentrations below this level does not result in silicosis. *The secondary threshold* consists of 100×10^6 particles of the same size per cubic foot; all those exposed at or above this level will acquire silicosis.

PATHOGENESIS

The small particles that are deposited in alveoli are engulfed by alveolar macrophages, where they are acted upon by lysosomal enzymes that liberate the dust and allow it to enter the cytoplasm, resulting in cell death. *In vitro* studies have shown that nonlipid material released by macrophage destruction stimulates fibroblasts to form collagen, which subsequently becomes hyalinized.[13] This process takes place not only within alveoli and respiratory bronchioles but also within lymphatics and lymphoid tissue to which macrophages are carried.

Although the mechanism by which silicon dioxide produces its reaction in the lungs is not fully understood, it is believed that adsorption of protein onto the silica particle enables the protein to act as a nonspecific antigen. It is postulated that the presence of this antigen over a long period of time slowly results in the production of antibody. Such a mechanism would explain why the disease may progress for long periods after the patient is no longer exposed to silica.

PATHOLOGIC CHARACTERISTICS

The characteristic pulmonary lesions of silicosis are nodules consisting of layers of laminated connective tissue arranged in onion-skin fashion. These nodules measure 2 to 3 mm in diameter. They are scattered diffusely throughout the lungs and are most numerous in the upper lobes and parahilar regions.[11] Dust particles have a tendency to accumulate in alveoli in the vicinity of bronchovascular bundles, pulmonary veins, and pleural surfaces. For this reason, silicotic nodules commonly occur in these anatomic regions, particularly around the smaller vessels. This relationship may result in the gradual obliteration of perivascular lymphatic channels and may even lead to destruction of the arterial wall itself.

Silica particles can be readily identified histologically by the use of polarized light, not only in the lung nodules but also in hilar or prescalene lymph nodes.

The reaction of the lungs to overwhelming exposure to particles 1 to 3 μ in diameter, usually in sandblasters, is somewhat different from the usual chronic reaction, both pathologically and clinically.[14] At necropsy, the lungs of these patients show diffuse interstitial cellular infiltration and some fibrosis but only rare silicotic nodules. The striking feature is an accumulation within alveolar spaces of proteinaceous material that stains with periodic–acid Schiff (PAS) reagent. The clinical course tends to be much more acute than in ordinary silicosis, leading to the designation of this disease as acute silicoproteinosis.[14] Superimposed mycobacterial, nocardial, and mycotic infections are common.

The large irregular lesions characteristic of conglomerate silicosis are found usually in the upper lobes; they occur not only in silicosis, but also in some silicatoses and in mixed dust diseases. Conglomerate lesions may cavitate as a result of either central ischemic necrosis or tuberculous caseation.

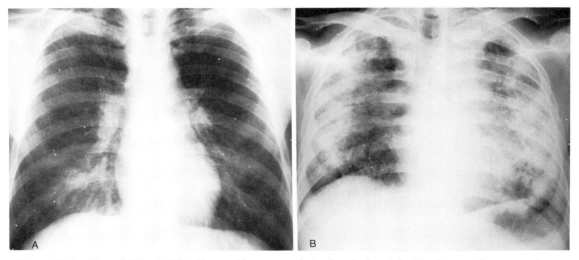

Figure 12–1. "Acute" Silicosis. This 29-year-old man was admitted to the hospital with a history of increasing dyspnea for 6 months and cough productive of thick yellow sputum for 1 week. During the previous 3 years, he was employed full time as a sandblaster inside huge nonventilated metal tanks. He was provided with a loosely-fitting face mask with a continuous flow of supposedly sand-free air (although the air flow was not filtered). He frequently worked without the air hose connected. On admission, a posteroanterior roentgenogram (A) revealed multiple fairly well-circumscribed nodules scattered diffusely throughout both lungs but more numerous in the upper and mid zones. The nodules ranged in size from bare visibility to 3 mm in diameter. Bilateral hilar lymph node enlargement was present. Pulmonary function studies showed lung volumes, mixing efficiency, and flow rates to be normal; the diffusing capacity at rest was low and did not rise with exercise. Blood gases and mechanical properties of the lung were within the normal range. Lung biopsy revealed gross disorganization of much of the pulmonary parenchyma suggestive of silicosis. Ashing of the lung biopsy specimen showed a residuum of 20 per cent of silicon dioxide. The patient's subsequent course was progressively and rapidly downhill, leading to severe respiratory failure. A roentgenogram 2 years after the initial study (B) reveals marked loss of lung volume, much of the lung parenchyma being replaced by a very coarse reticular pattern which in many areas is confluent as a result of conglomeration (large opacities).

Roentgenographic Manifestations

The diagnosis of silicosis requires the combination of a history of exposure to dust containing high concentrations of silicon dioxide and the roentgenographic appearance of changes compatible with the disease. Ten to 20 years' exposure usually is necessary before the appearance of roentgenographic abnormality, although the onset of silicosis sometimes is acute, particularly in patients exposed to high concentrations of dust in a relatively confined area (Figure 12–1).[15]

The classic roentgenographic pattern of silicosis consists of multiple nodular shadows from 1 to 10 mm in diameter (Figure 12–1A). The nodules tend to be fairly well circumscribed and of uniform density. Calcification of pulmonary nodules occurs more frequently than is realized (Figure 12–2). In one series of 724 miners who showed roentgenographic evidence of pneumoconiosis, calcification of nodules was present in 20 per cent.[16]

The nodular pattern may be preceded by or associated with a reticular pattern—the small irregular opacities of the ILO classification—which sometimes is the earliest roentgenographic abnormality. Seldom during either stage is there evidence of pleural abnormality.

The roentgenographic pattern of small round or irregular opacities is commonly referred to as "simple" silicosis in contrast to "complicated" silicosis, which is characterized by large opacities or conglomerate shadows. Large opacities represent homogeneous areas of consolidation of nonsegmental distribution usually affecting the upper lobes and measuring more than 1 cm in diameter; they may become very large (Figure 12–3), some even exceeding the volume of an upper lobe. The shadows' margins usually

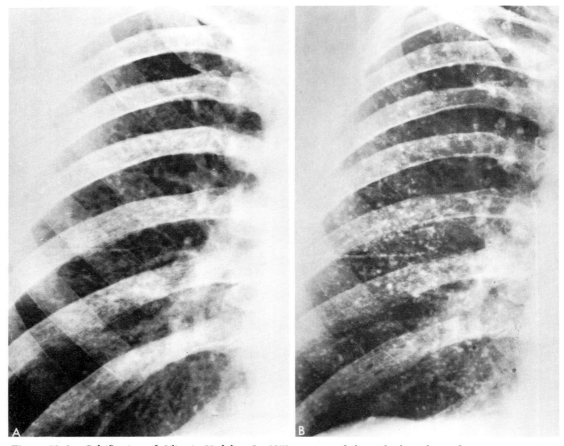

Figure 12–2. Calcification of Silicotic Nodules. In 1953, a view of the right hemithorax from a posteroanterior roentgenogram of a 32-year-old South African black male reveals involvement of all lung zones by small irregular opacities of unit density. By 1971, 18 years later, multiple punctate calcifications had developed throughout the right lung representing calcification of silicotic nodules. The patient had a history of 26 years in South African gold mines. (Courtesy of Dr. Raymond Glynn-Thomas, Medical Bureau for Occupational Diseases, Johannesburg, South Africa.)

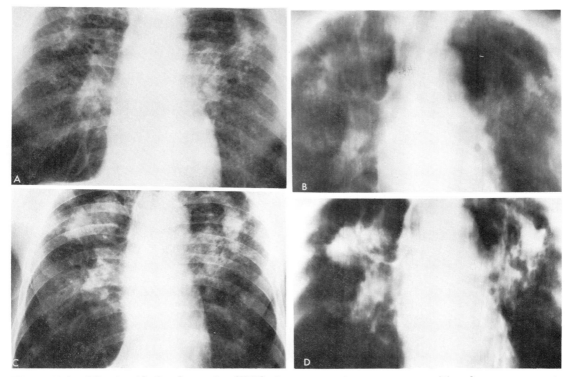

Figure 12–3. Silicosis with Conglomeration (PMF). A posteroanterior roentgenogram (A) and an anteroposterior tomogram (B) of this 54-year-old foundry worker reveal extensive irregular opacities involving predominantly the upper and mid lung zones. In the subapical regions bilaterally, poorly defined shadows of homogeneous density represent large opacities (category B). Four years later similar roentgenographic studies (C and D) show considerable enlargement of the large opacities, which are now category C. Most of the enlargement appears to have occurred hilarward, suggesting "migration" of the lesions medially. The lung peripheral to the zones of PMF has shown a loss of markings suggesting the development of emphysema; the lower lung zones also have shown signs of progressive emphysema.

are irregular and somewhat ill-defined, with multiple "pseudopodia" extending outward from their edges.[17] These shadows represent confluence of individual silicotic nodules, sometimes associated with superimposed tuberculous infection. They commonly develop in the midzone or periphery of the lung and tend to migrate later toward the hilum, leaving overinflated emphysematous lung tissue between the consolidation and the pleural surface (Figure 12–3).[18] The more extensive the progressive massive fibrosis, the less the apparent nodularity in the remainder of the lungs.[18] This unique characteristic presumably is owing to gradual incorporation of nodular lesions into the massive consolidation in the upper lungs, leaving behind overinflated and emphysematous parenchymal tissue. The conglomerate lesions may cavitate.

Hilar lymph node enlargement is a common roentgenographic finding and may occur at any stage of silicosis.[18] So-called egg-shell calcification is caused by the deposition of calcium salts in the periphery of enlarged lymph nodes and

is almost pathognomonic of silicosis (Figure 12–4), although seen occasionally in sarcoidosis. Of 1905 cases of silicosis reported by Bellini, it was identified in 4.7 per cent.[19] Egg-shell calcification involves not only the hilar lymph nodes but also (rarely) those in the anterior and posterior mediastinum, the thoracic wall, and the intraperitoneal and retroperitoneal areas.

Two other variants of the classic roentgenographic changes of the disease are the acute silicosis of sandblasters and the nodular lesions of Caplan's syndrome. Acute silicoproteinosis is associated with a pattern of diffuse air space disease, similar if not identical to that of alveolar proteinosis.[14] In addition to the typical interstitial silicotic nodules, histologic examination in these cases shows the alveoli to be filled with granular, PAS-positive material containing cell ghosts and needle-shaped clefts.[20] Caplan's syndrome (*see* page 371) consists of the presence of large necrobiotic nodules superimposed on a background of simple silicosis (Figure 12–5). It is a manifestation of rheumatoid lung disease

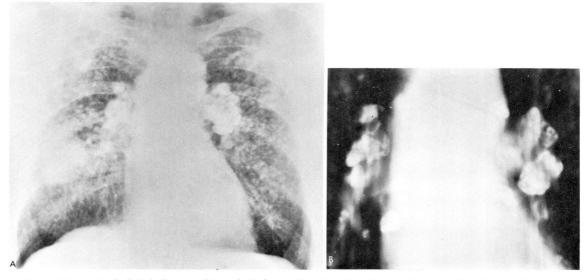

Figure 12–4. Eggshell Calcification of Lymph Nodes in Silicosis. This 62-year-old man had worked in a foundry for 30 years. A posteroanterior roentgenogram (*A*) reveals general involvement of both lungs by small rounded opacities with conglomeration in the upper lobes bilaterally and in the right lower zone. Extensive calcification of hilar lymph nodes is readily apparent. An anteroposterior tomogram of the hilar region (*B*) reveals dense calcification of the nodes bilaterally, the distribution being largely peripheral. (Courtesy of Dr. J. F. Meakins, Royal Victoria Hospital. Montreal.)

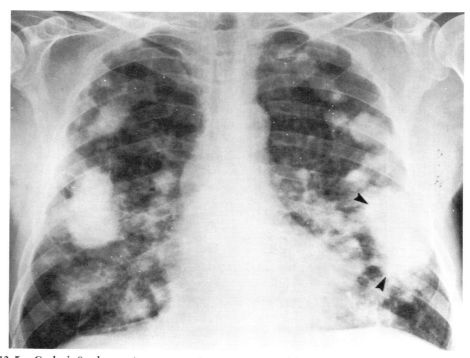

Figure 12–5. Caplan's Syndrome. A posteroanterior roentgenogram (*A*) reveals a multitude of fairly well-circumscribed nodules ranging in diameter from 1 to 5 cm, scattered randomly throughout both lungs with no notable anatomic predilection. No cavitation is apparent, nor is there evidence of calcification. This 56-year-old man had been a coal miner for many years and in recent years had developed arthralgia, which proved to be due to rheumatoid arthritis. As a means of establishing the nature of the pulmonary nodules, a percutaneous needle aspiration was carried out on the large mass situated in the lower portion of the left lung (*arrowheads*): several milliliters of inky black fluid were aspirated. The necrotic nature of this mass was thus established, as was the presence of large quantities of coal dust within it. (Courtesy of Dr. Michael O'Donavan, Montreal General Hospital.)

and is seen more commonly in coal-worker's pneumoconiosis than in silicosis.

CLINICAL MANIFESTATIONS

The diagnosis of silicosis usually is based on the identification of a diffuse nodular or irregular pattern on the chest roentgenogram of patients with an occupational history compatible with exposure to dust containing high concentrations of silicon dioxide. Many patients are totally asymptomatic when first seen. Some may complain of shortness of breath, first noted on exertion only but becoming progressively more severe as the roentgenographic changes worsen. With progressive destruction of functioning pulmonary tissue, pulmonary hypertension develops, resulting in cor pulmonale and, eventually, right-sided heart failure.

It is not uncommon for these patients to present with symptoms many years after leaving the occupation responsible for the dust exposure. This is an important point to remember, since only a complete occupational history, ranging over a patient's entire working life, may provide a clue to the diagnosis. Unlike many other inhalation diseases caused by inorganic and organic dusts, the fibrosis and associated disability in silicosis frequently are progressive, even after removal of the patient from the dusty environment.

Although the combination of a positive history and typical roentgenographic changes usually suffices to permit confident diagnosis in most cases, often it is necessary to prove *clinical disability*, and for this purpose pulmonary function tests are essential. Function may be normal in the early stages of the disease.[21] When dyspnea is present, impairment of function may be obstructive or restrictive, or a combination of both. Diffusing capacity may be decreased, and the combination of this with hyperinflation and decrease in flow rates constitutes a pattern of function impairment identical to that of uncomplicated pulmonary emphysema. Although arterial oxygen saturation may be normal at rest, exercise often gives rise to hypoxemia, at least in patients with progressive massive fibrosis.[22] In the late stages of the disease, carbon dioxide retention may develop.[15]

RELATIONSHIP TO PULMONARY TUBERCULOSIS

There appears to be little question that silicosis predisposes to tuberculosis. It is customary to suspect this complication with the development of progressive massive fibrosis, although sputum cultures of acid-fast bacilli are positive in as many patients with nodular opacities alone as in those with conglomerate shadows.[23] Even progressive massive fibrosis does not necessarily indicate the presence of tuberculous infection, since such shadows may develop in patients in whom the response to repeated Mantoux testing is negative. It may be extremely difficult to isolate tubercle bacilli during life in patients with progressive massive fibrosis, despite subsequent postmortem demonstration of active tuberculous infection.[23]

SILICATE PNEUMOCONIOSES

The silicatoses are a group of pneumoconioses in which salts of silicic acid are the exciting agents. Silicates occur in both fibrous and nonfibrous forms, the former being the most important and including asbestos and talc. The nonfibrous silicates—mica, kaolin, Fuller's earth, nepheline, and cement—are relatively rare causes of disease.

ASBESTOSIS

Asbestosis is a general term given to a group of minerals that are fibrous in nature and resistant to high temperatures. These minerals represent combinations of silicic acid with magnesium, calcium, sodium, and iron, and their importance lies not only in the hazard they present to those involved in their mining but also, and perhaps more importantly, in their extensive use in a wide variety of occupations. The monograph by Preger[24] and the more recent articles by Craighead and Mossman[25] and by Becklake[26] are recommended to those readers wishing to delve more deeply into this fascinating disease.

EPIDEMIOLOGY

The use of asbestos in industry has increased enormously during this century—world production jumped from 500 tons in 1900 to an estimated 5 million tons in 1974.[27]

The prevalence of this mineral throughout the world is indicated by the frequency with which "asbestos bodies" are found in routine necropsies, the incidence ranging from 1 per cent in rural Italy[28] to 60 per cent in New York City.[29] "Asbestos bodies" are yellow-brown in color, approximately 20 to 150 μ in length and 2 to 5 μ in width, and are usually found in patients with asbestosis. These bodies are best designated as ferruginous,[30] since definitive identification of the asbestos nature of the core is difficult and not feasible in most epidemiologic studies. In routine necropsies ferruginous bodies are found more often in the lungs of males than females and of urban than rural residents. When many such bodies are present there may be a minimal degree of fibrosis, but usually there is no tissue reaction. Patients with asbestosis generally show a much larger number of asbestos bodies than those without the disease.

There are two major sources of exposure to asbestos dust: (1) primary occupations of asbestos mining and its processing in a mill; and (2) secondary occupations such as insulation, textile manufacturing, construction, and ship building. The major producers of asbestos are the Soviet Union, Canada, South Africa, and the United States.[27] There are four major types of asbestos that cause pleuropulmonary disease—crocidolite, amosite, chrysotile, and anthophyllite. Amosite is produced largely in the Transvaal, crocidolite in Cape Town, chrysotile in the Soviet Union and Quebec, and anthophyllite in Finland. Crocidolite, amosite, and anthophyllite belong to the amphibole group of fibers, whereas the chrysotile fiber is serpentine. The amphiboles, particularly crocidolite and amosite, have greater pathogenic potential than chrysotile, notably with respect to the development of mesothelioma and bronchogenic carcinoma.[25, 26] The differences in oncogenicity are believed to be related to both the physical and chemical properties of the fibers.[26] Exposure to only one type of fiber occurs largely in mining and milling, whereas mixtures of fibers are commonly employed in construction and in the manufacture of textiles. Because they are long and pliable chrysotile fibers are particularly suitable for textile manufacture, whereas crocidolite and amosite are of greater value for marine insulation since they are more acid-resistant.

Insulation or lagging of pipes in factories, homes, and ships has been shown to be associated with both pulmonary fibrosis and mesothelioma. Naval dockyard workers, particularly laggers and sprayers, also are prone to develop fibrosis and mesothelioma, the incidence varying directly with the degree of exposure. Selikoff and his colleagues[31] found roentgenographically evident asbestosis in almost half of 1117 insulation workers, prevalence again being re-

lated directly to duration of exposure. It is during the process of manufacturing and even more so during repair and demolition that asbestos fibers are released. Once incorporated into manufactured products the fiber is well bound and unlikely to cause harm.

Although the finding of ferruginous bodies in routine necropsies indicates a worldwide exposure to asbestos dust, there is no evidence to date that this degree of exposure represents a risk.[27] However, there is irrefutable evidence that individuals living in the vicinity of a mine, mill, or factory associated with heavy asbestos dust pollution develop pleural plaques and mesotheliomas.[32] In fact, the disease can develop in persons who repeatedly handle the clothes of asbestos workers.[33]

PATHOGENESIS

The inhaled asbestos fiber, which may be 100 μ or more in length, exerts its deleterious effects in the respiratory bronchioles and alveoli. The exact mechanism by which asbestos induces pleuropulmonary fibrosis, mesotheliomas, and increased susceptibility to bronchogenic carcinoma is unknown. Three major theories have been proposed to explain its fibrogenic property: (1) direct physical irritation; (2) a response to released silicic acid and metallic ions; and (3) an autoimmune reaction resulting from antigens liberated through the interaction of macrophages and asbestos fibers. Like the silica particles, the asbestos fiber becomes coated with protein and is engulfed by macrophages. It is relatively soluble compared with quartz dust, which may explain the diffuse nature of the fibrosis and the relative paucity of asbestos bodies in some cases of advanced asbestosis.[25] Evidence for autoimmunity lies chiefly in the finding of circulating rheumatoid and antinuclear factors, reported to be present in 28 per cent and 27 per cent, respectively, of asbestos workers with positive chest roentgenograms.[34] In this study by Turner-Warwick and Parkes,[34] the autoantibodies were of the IgM type and were present in titers considerably lower than those usually identified in connective tissue diseases.

PATHOLOGIC CHARACTERISTICS

In experimental asbestosis, the fibers are found first in bronchioles and respiratory bronchioles and within a few hours in alveoli. Peribronchiolar edema and intra-alveolar hemorrhage result. Botham and Holt[35] have beautifully illustrated the formation of asbestos bodies. These are formed by the deposition of ferritin on the asbestos fibers within macrophages, first as a smooth coating and then in the form of beading as the macrophages shrink and rupture. Fibrosis first occurs in the peribronchiolar region and then in the interstitium. Varying degrees of fibrosis and distortion result, ranging from relative preservation of lung architecture to gross distortion with formation of microcysts and honeycombing (bronchiolectasis). Asbestos fibers lie both in the interstitium and free in air spaces. Striking pleural thickening is usually present.

Lower lobes tend to be affected first, then midlung zones, and eventually upper lobes.[27] Conglomerate lesions of massive fibrosis, comparable to the progressive massive fibrosis of silicosis and coal-worker's pneumoconiosis, are uncommon in asbestosis and when present tend to be situated in lower rather than upper lobes. Necrobiotic nodules of the type described by Caplan in coal miners are occasionally seen in patients with combined asbestosis and rheumatoid disease.

Pleural involvement consists of effusion, pleural plaques (which may be calcified), and mesotheliomas (*see* further on). Pleural effusion is associated with cellular infiltration, fibrosis, and the presence of asbestos fibers and bodies in the pulmonary interstitium. Generalized pleural thickening is an almost invariable accompaniment of asbestosis. Isolated pleural plaques occur with or without generalized pleural fibrosis; they are discrete, gray-white lesions that develop on the parietal pleura over the convexity of the lung and on the diaphragm. The latter structure is usually involved in the area of the central tendon; the pericardium also may be affected. Histologically, plaques consist of cell-poor collagenous connective tissue that does not contain asbestos bodies.

ROENTGENOGRAPHIC MANIFESTATIONS

The roentgenographic changes in the chest in asbestosis may be both pleural and parenchymal, but in most reported series the former are far more striking than the latter.[36, 37]

Pleural Manifestations

Four types of roentgenographic changes occur in the pleura—plaque formation, diffuse pleural thickening, calcification, and pleural effusion—each of which may occur alone or in combination with the others. These pleural manifestations dominate the picture roentgenographically in the majority of series.[36] Of 56 cases described by Freundlich and Greening,[36] 48 per cent showed pleural thickening alone, 41 per cent showed combined pleural and parenchymal manifestations, and only 11 per cent showed parenchymal changes alone. The shaggy heart sign, a partial obscuration of the heart border caused by a combination of parenchymal and pleural changes, was observed in 20 per cent. *Pleural thickening* or *pleural plaques* usually are bilateral, more prominent in the middle third of the thorax, and tend to follow the rib contours.[38, 38a] Pleural plaques are fibrotic processes that begin in the deepest part of the parietal pleura and morphologically are ivory white in color. They may be smooth or nodular in contour and may measure up to 1 cm in thickness, although they are usually thinner. They occur most commonly on the aponeurotic portion of the diaphragm, on the posterolateral chest wall between the seventh and tenth ribs, and on the lateral chest wall between the sixth and ninth ribs (Figure 12–6).[37] Their origin in the parietal pleura is in contrast to the visceral pleural involvement that characterizes previous hemothorax or empyema. They may be very difficult to visualize, particularly when viewed *en face*, and tangential roentgenograms may be necessary (Figure 12–7). In fact, the frequency with which plaques occur along the posterolateral or anterolateral portion of the thorax suggested to Fletcher and Edge[37] that oblique projections of the thorax should be standard in the roentgenographic investigation of patients suspected of having asbestos-related disease. Although pleural thickening posteriorly may be difficult to recognize roentgenographically, its presence may be detected by CT or ultrasonic examination. The greatest problem in the roentgenologic diagnosis of early plaque formation lies in distinguishing them from normal companion shadows of the chest wall, and, in fact, distinction sometimes is impossible with conviction. Despite these difficulties, it is clear that noncalcified plaques occur often enough to be regarded as virtually diagnostic of asbestos-related disease.

Although uncalcified pleural plaque formation is probably the commonest roentgenographic manifestation of asbestos-related disease, the most striking abnormality is calcification of pleural plaques. The frequency of pleural calcification is variable. Anton[39] re-

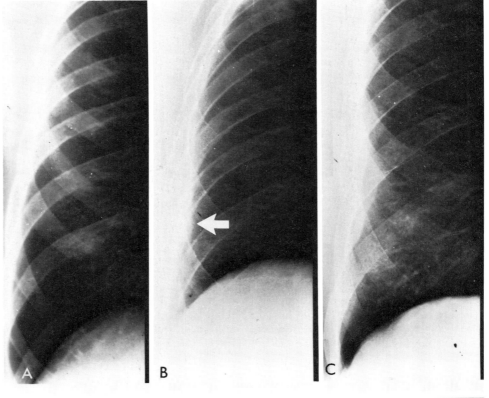

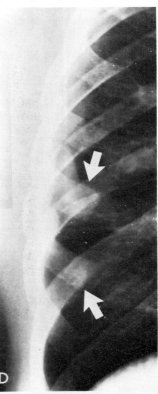

Figure 12–6. Pleural Plaques as Manifestations of Asbestos-related Disease. Views of the axillary lung region from PA roentgenograms of four different patients, revealing variations in pleural plaque formation. *A* is a normal subject for control. In *B*, there is uniform thickening of the pleura over the right lung with a local elevation inferiorly *(arrow)*, indicating plaque formation. In *C*, numerous plaques measuring almost 1 cm in diameter are clearly identifiable. In *D*, the plaques are still larger, some measuring 12 to 15 mm in thickness; vague opacities projected more medially *(arrows)* represent plaques *en face*. (Courtesy of Dr. Charles Ochs, Cooper Green Hospital, Birmingham, Alabama, and the American College of Radiology.)

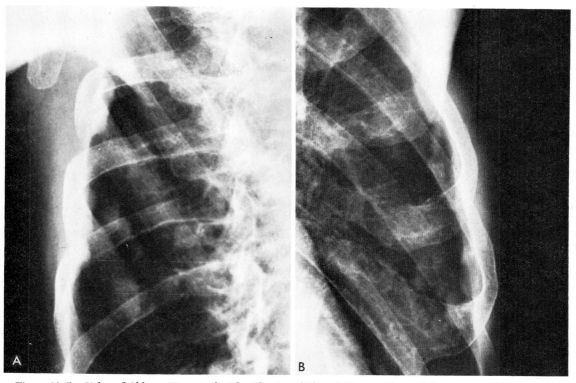

Figure 12–7. Value of Oblique Views in the Identification of Pleural Plaques. Views of the posterolateral aspect of the right hemithorax (A) and the anterolateral aspect of the left hemithorax (B) reveal multiple pleural plaques of typical configuration. These plaques were difficult to appreciate on a standard posteroanterior roentgenogram. (Courtesy of Dr. Charles Ochs, Cooper Green Hospital, Birmingham, Alabama, and the American College of Radiology.)

ported finding calcified and noncalcified plaques in roughly equal numbers of his 40 cases, whereas Freundlich and Greening[36] observed calcification in only 21 per cent of their 56 cases. Calcified plaques vary from small linear or circular shadows commonly situated over the diaphragmatic domes to complete encirclement of the lower portion of the lungs. When calcification is minimal, a roentgenogram overexposed at maximal inspiration facilitates visibility. No portion of the pleura is immune to calcification, although the most common site is the diaphragm.[40]

The third pleural manifestation of asbestos-related disease, which often is not appreciated, is pleural effusion.[41-43] The most comprehensive report of the prevalence and incidence of pleural effusion in an asbestos-exposed population was by Epler and his colleagues,[43] who studied 1135 exposed workers and 717 control subjects. Benign asbestos effusion was defined by (1) exposure to asbestos, (2) confirmation by roentgenograms or thoracentesis, (3) no other disease related to pleural effusion, and (4) no

malignant tumor within three years. These authors found 34 benign effusions among the exposed workers (3 per cent), compared with no otherwise unexplained effusions among the control subjects. Prevalence was dose related. The latency period was shorter than for other asbestos-related disorders, benign effusion being the most common abnormality during the first 20 years after exposure. Most effusions were small, 28 per cent recurred, and 66 per cent were asymptomatic. Chest pain is the most common symptom.[41] In most if not all cases, the fluid is a sterile, serous or blood-tinged exudate. The differential diagnoses must include tuberculosis and mesothelioma.

Pulmonary Manifestations

The roentgenographic changes in the lungs occur in two forms, small and large opacities.

SMALL OPACITIES. These opacities may be round or irregular or a combination of the two. Changes caused by small opacities may be divided into three stages: (1) a fine reticulation

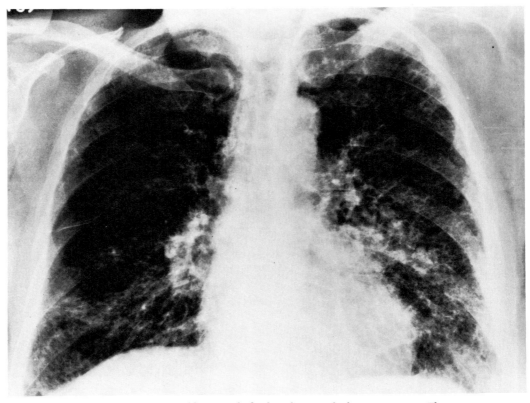

Figure 12–8. Asbestosis. This 64-year-old woman had a long history of asbestos exposure. There is a coarse reticular pattern throughout both lungs with some basal predominance. This pattern of small irregular opacities is characteristic but not diagnostic of asbestosis. This patient also had primary squamous cell carcinomas arising in both lower lobes.

predominantly occupying the lower lung zones and associated with "ground-glass" appearance that is probably the result of combined pleural thickening[39] and early interstitial pneumonitis or fibrosis; (2) a stage in which irregular small opacities become more marked, creating a prominent interstitial reticulation (Figure 12–8) (a combination of parenchymal and pleural changes leads to partial obscuration of the heart border—the so-called shaggy heart sign—and of the diaphragm); and (3) a late stage in which reticulation becomes visible in the midlung and upper lung zones and the cardiac and diaphragmatic contours become more obscured.[18] Hilar lymph node enlargement is seldom if ever notable.

LARGE OPACITIES. These opacities measure 1 cm or more in diameter and are an uncommon manifestation of asbestosis. They are invariably associated with widespread interstitial fibrosis[44] and usually with calcified or uncalcified pleural plaques. Although a tuberculous etiology of the large opacities, as in the massive fibrosis of silicotics, cannot be positively denied, no acid-fast bacilli could be identified pathologically in the four cases studied at necropsy by Solomon and colleagues.[44] Roentgenographically, the large opacities may be well- or ill-defined, are nonsegmental in distribution, may be multiple, and may become very large in size. Although they may occur in both upper and lower lung zones, they tend to show a lower zonal predominance in contrast to the upper lobe predominance of the large opacities of silicosis.[44] Unlike the large opacities of silicosis or coal-worker's pneumoconiosis, the massive fibrosis of asbestosis does not appear to "migrate" toward the center of the lung. Further, the opacities have not been known to undergo roentgenographically demonstrable cavitation.

So-called rounded atelectasis (*see* page 175), an unusual form of peripheral lung collapse, has been reported to be associated fairly frequently with asbestos-induced pleural disease.[45] Such an opacity could conceivably be mistaken for primary bronchogenic carcinoma or mesothelioma although the roentgenographic appearances of rounded atelectasis are usually sufficiently characteristic that little difficulty should be encountered in differential diagnosis.

CLINICAL MANIFESTATIONS

The great majority of patients with pleuropulmonary asbestosis have no symptoms. Occasionally, an acute pleural effusion is precipitated by asbestos fibers, in which circumstance the patient may experience pleural pain.[41] Breathlessness is almost invariably associated with interstitial fibrosis, although thickened pleura may be partly responsible for this symptom in some patients. Dyspnea is usually progressive, despite removal of the patient from asbestos exposure. Symptoms seldom develop before at least 20 to 30 years' exposure[46] and in addition to shortness of breath on exertion include cough, sometimes with mucopurulent sputum.

Basal crepitations may be present on physical examination and finger clubbing occurs in many cases.[46] Asbestos bodies are almost invariably found in the sputum of patients with roentgenographic evidence of the disease, even in the absence of symptoms. If the patient lives long enough and survives complicating mesothelioma or bronchogenic carcinoma, signs of cor pulmonale may develop. In chrysotile mining, excess mortality, has been observed in patients who had been exposed to the heaviest dust concentrations over periods of 20 years or longer, the response to increasing dose being effectively linear for lung cancer and for pneumoconiosis.[47]

Patients with interstitial fibrosis caused by asbestos exposure usually show a restrictive pattern of pulmonary function, with decreased vital capacity, residual volume, and diffusion capacity, and preservation of relatively good ventilatory function. Hypoxemia may be observed on exercise but the PCO_2 is normal or low. Pulmonary compliance characteristically is greatly reduced.[22, 48, 46] Cigarette smokers sometimes manifest an obstructive pulmonary function pattern. This finding may be analogous to the greater prevalence of pulmonary fibrosis in asbestos workers who smoke and to the additive or synergistic carcinogenic effect of cigarette smoking and asbestos exposure reported by Selikoff and his colleagues.

RELATIONSHIP TO NEOPLASIA

Of all non-neoplastic pulmonary diseases, asbestosis undoubtedly has the highest incidence of associated neoplasia, including bronchogenic carcinoma and mesothelioma.[49] Epidemiologic observations, particularly regarding time since first exposure and intensity of exposure, aid in attributing bronchogenic carcinoma to asbestos exposure.[50] Fibrosis of pulmonary interstitium appears to be invariably present pathologically when cancer develops in association with asbestos exposure; however, this fibrosis may not be detectable roentgenologically or by pulmonary function studies.[51] Asbestos-associated lung cancer is most frequently adenocarcinoma,[51, 173] although squamous-cell carcinoma is also seen (Figure 12–8). It has been stated[51] that asbestos-related carcinoma occurs more commonly in lower than in upper lobes.

Of the two most common asbestos-induced cancers, bronchogenic carcinoma is almost invariably related to cigarette smoking, whereas mesothelioma is not. This dichotomy has been observed for other asbestos-associated neoplasms as well: cancers of the esophagus, larynx, and oropharynx are of increased incidence in asbestos workers who have a history of cigarette smoking, whereas the incidence of colorectal and renal cancers is increased whether or not the workers have smoked.[52]

As pointed out by Selikoff and Hammond,[52] the burden of asbestos–lung cancer is borne by asbestos workers who smoke. These investigators reported on a ten-year follow-up study of 8220 asbestos insulation workers who had volunteered their histories of smoking at the outset of the study in 1967; 6841 had a history of cigarette smoking, 1379 did not. For comparison, a group of 73,763 men in the American Cancer Society's prospective cancer prevention study was analyzed as controls; these men had the same distribution of smoking habits and were alike in most other respects except that they had not been exposed to asbestos. Death rates for lung cancer (per 100,000 man-years, standardized for age) were as follows: 11.3 for men who neither worked with asbestos nor smoked cigarettes; 58.4 for men who worked with asbestos but did not smoke; 122.6 for cigarette smokers who had not worked with asbestos; and 601.6 for men who had been exposed to both cigarettes and asbestos. The bottom line is ominous indeed: among asbestos workers who smoke, one in every five deaths is due to lung cancer. Equally ominous is the mortality rate for bronchogenic carcinoma and mesothelioma in asbestos workers in whom the presence of asbestosis had been established: in one study,[53] almost 50 per cent died from these malignancies.

A latent period of at least 20 years' exposure is characteristic of those asbestos workers in whom pleuropulmonary malignancy develops. Even when fibrosis is only of minimal degree, asbestos bodies are present in the lung parenchyma and in some cases in the neoplasm also.

The incidence of associated neoplasia appears to relate to the type of asbestos involved. This is particularly true for mesothelioma, in which the most commonly implicated dust is crocidolite. It is generally agreed that the risk of developing mesothelioma is somewhat less for individuals working with amosite and considerably less for those involved with chrysotile than with crocidolite. Despite thorough search, mesothelioma has not been found to be associated with anthophyllite asbestos production in Finland.

The incidence of peritoneal mesotheliomas also is greater in patients with asbestosis. Enticknap and Smither[54] described 11 patients with peritoneal neoplasms, who had all worked in the same asbestos factory.

In a comparative study of mesothelioma and asbestosis using computed tomography and conventional chest roentgenography, Rabinowitz and his colleagues[55] found that the major pathologic features of both asbestosis and mesothelioma were well demonstrated by both modalities, although CT demonstrated the findings more frequently and in greater detail. Of interest was the observation that no distinguishing features between pleural plaques and mesothelioma could be established based on configuration and size of the lesion; many pleural plaques associated with advanced asbestosis were large and irregular and resembled those associated with mesothelioma. Features that predominated in mesothelioma included nodular involvement of the pleural fissures, pleural effusion, and ipsilateral volume loss with a fixed mediastinum.

TALCOSIS

This relatively uncommon variety of *silicatosis* results from many years' exposure to high concentrations of fibrous or tremolite talc (magnesium silicate). Talc is chemically closely related to chrysotile, anthophyllite, and tremolite, and deposits usually contain varying proportions of asbestos fibers and silica. Most reported cases of talcosis result from exposure of individuals in mining and milling, but also at risk are soapstone workers, persons engaged in handling milled material in manufacturing, and those who coat rubber goods with talc for storage. Pulmonary talcosis may also result from intravenous misuse of oral medications containing talc as a filler, a form of microembolization (*see* page 000).

Pathologically, in several cases necropsy has revealed diffuse and nodular fibrosis with scattered ferruginous bodies and numerous birefringent particles, resembling short needles, within the nodules. Irregular areas of fibrosis surround bronchioles and small vessels, resulting in dilatation of the bronchioles.

The hallmark in the *roentgenologic diagnosis* of talcosis is pleural plaque formation. These are often diaphragmatic in position and may be massive, often bizarre in shape and extending over much of the surface of both lungs[56] and sometimes involving the pericardium. The incidence of pleural abnormality in talcosis is similar to that in asbestosis. Parenchymal involvement is said to be similar to that in asbestosis.[56]

Clinical manifestations are similar to those of any other disabling pneumoconiosis, symptoms including dyspnea and productive cough. Decreased breath sounds (presumably due to pleural thickening), rales at the lung bases, limited chest expansion, and finger clubbing are found on physical examination.[56] An increased incidence of bronchogenic and pleural neoplasms has been reported.[57]

OTHER SILICATOSES

Mica, Fuller's earth, kaolin (china clay), cement dust, and nepheline rock dust are all silicates that are capable of producing pneumoconiosis, although the incidence of disease is very low.[11, 58, 59] Roentgenographic and clinical manifestations may be indistinguishable from those of asbestosis (as in exposure to mica), but more commonly consist of no more than general accentuation of lung markings in patients who have no clinical disability.

COAL-WORKER'S PNEUMOCONIOSIS

Coal miners are susceptible to a variety of respiratory diseases, including coal-worker's pneumoconiosis (CWP), silicosis, chronic bronchitis, emphysema, and tuberculosis.[60] In this section we will discuss the coal macule and its relation to progressive massive fibrosis, and the somewhat controversial clinical and physiologic significance of these well-accepted pathologic entities. This subject has recently been reviewed, with emphasis on pathogenesis and pathology.[61]

EPIDEMIOLOGY

Whereas in a small percentage of coal miners silicosis develops as a result of the high quartz content of certain coal seams,[62, 63] in the majority a pneumoconiosis develops that is entirely different and is characterized by the absence of symptoms in the early stages, a roentgenographic pattern that lacks the well-defined nodularity of silicosis, and a morphologic picture quite distinct from that of pure silicosis. Although a small amount of free silica is present in all coal dust and can be found in the ash of coal-workers' lungs at necropsy, it seems that the morphologic changes are caused chiefly by the deposition in the lungs of large quantities of carbon. The finding of pathologic changes identical to those of coal-worker's pneumoconiosis in carbon electrode workers, in whom the inhaled dust consists of coke and anthracite and almost no quartz, and in graphite workers, supports the contention that free silica plays little part in the lung disease of coal workers.[64] The disease is much more common in miners working at the coal face and in transportation workers than in maintenance and surface workers.

Pathogenesis

Inhaled particles of coal dust larger than 5 μ in diameter are deposited out in the conducting system and removed by mucociliary clearance. It has been estimated that geometric mean size of particles in airborne coal mine dust is slightly less than 1 μ and many of these particles penetrate to the peripheral air spaces. When in relatively small numbers, particles that are deposited on the alveoli or respiratory bronchioles are engulfed by phagocytic macrophages and become caught up in the mucous transport system to be expectorated or swallowed. It is only when this clearance mechanism is overwhelmed by an excessive load that coal dust is retained in the respiratory bronchioles and alveoli. An additional factor predisposing to the development of CWP may be the coal rank, anthracite being associated with a higher prevalence of disease than bituminous coal.[65] When the coal dust is relatively pure—*i.e.*, there is little or no associated silica—collagen does not form and the primary lesion consists of an admixture of coal dust, macrophages, and fibroblasts enmeshed in a reticulin network, the *coal macule*.[60] If the coal dust contains significant quantities of silicon dioxide, reaction within the macrophages results in liberation of a fibrogenic substance and the formation of collagen.

The factors responsible for the development of progressive massive fibrosis (PMF) in coal-worker's pneumoconiosis remain uncertain. In contrast to the conglomerate lesions of silicosis, which consist of a confluence of many silicotic nodules, the massive lesions of coal-worker's pneumoconiosis are amorphous accumulations of protein, mineral dust, and calcium phosphate.[60] Although mycobacterial infection may play a role in the development of PMF in some cases, additional unrecognized pathogenic factors exist in most. The presence of rheumatoid, antinuclear, and antilung autoantibodies, particularly in the more advanced cases of coal-worker's PMF, suggest an immunologic mechanism.[66, 67] Positive tests for rheumatoid factor have been found in 30 to 40 per cent[68] of patients with PMF. In one study of 109 coal workers with pneumoconiosis, circulating antinuclear antibody and rheumatoid factor were found in 13 per cent of the miners with simple pneumoconiosis and in 45 per cent of those with category C PMF.[66] However, in a more recent study,[69] an increased incidence of ANA was not observed in patients with PMF, nor was there seen to exist an increased incidence of serologic differences between miners with simple pneumoconiosis and those with complicated disease.

Pathologic Characteristics

Anthracotic pigment deposition and accompanying reticulin fiber formation and fibrosis, equal in extent to that found in some coal miners, has been described in city dwellers;[70] presumptive evidence of coal-worker's pneumoconiosis requires sufficient coal dust accumulation to form a "macule." On gross examination of full lung sections, coal macules are seen as evenly distributed black dots, with some predilection for the upper lobes. They measure up to 5 mm in diameter and relate to dilated respiratory bronchioles, a morphologic change known as focal emphysema.[60] This peribronchiolar deposition of dust associated with focal emphysema is usually referred to as "simple" pneumoconiosis of coal workers. If exposure to the dusty atmosphere continues, the pneumoconiosis may become "complicated" by the development of PMF.[71] The lesion of PMF is restricted almost exclusively to the posterior segment of an upper lobe or the superior segment of a lower lobe.[72, 73] In contrast to the PMF of silicosis, ill-defined bundles of coarse hyalinized collagen are confined to the capsule of the lesion, the center being composed of insoluble proteins stabilized by some form of cross-linking. Remnants of obliterated vessels and bronchi can be identified within the central amorphous mass. Cavitation may occur as a result of either superimposed tuberculosis or ischemic necrosis, the latter almost certainly being the more common mechanism. Pathologic evidence of cor pulmonale is frequently found at necropsy in patients with complicated coal-worker's pneumoconiosis.

The incidence of emphysema in patients with coal-worker's pneumoconiosis compared with control groups of nonminers is disputatious: in one survey,[74] it was found that emphysema was much more common in both simple and complicated pneumoconiosis than in the control group, whereas in another study[70] no significant differences concerning incidence or types of emphysema or frequency of chronic cor pulmonale were encountered between the two populations. In any event, the precise nature of the emphysema and its relation to the pneumoconiosis cannot always be determined, even at necropsy, particularly if the changes are advanced.[75]

ROENTGENOGRAPHIC MANIFESTATIONS

The roentgenographic pattern of "simple pneumoconiosis" is typically one of small, round opacities, but may be composed predominantly of small, irregular opacities, particularly in the early stages. The nodules range from 1 to 5 mm in diameter, tend to be somewhat less well defined than those of silicosis, and are of a "granular" density unlike the homogeneous density of silicotic nodules. Roentgenologic-pathologic correlative studies suggest that the opacity of individual nodules is caused almost entirely by tissue reaction, with little contribution from the coal dust, whose density is only slightly greater than unity.[71] Calcification occurs in at least a few of the nodules in up to 10 per cent of older coal miners. Eggshell calcification of lymph nodes is uncommon.

The appearance of large opacities (larger than 1 cm in diameter) indicates the development of "complicated" pneumoconiosis—PMF. These lesions range from a minimum of 1 cm in diameter to the volume of a whole lobe and are almost always restricted to the upper half of the lungs. They usually develop on a background pattern of simple pneumoconiosis but have been observed in miners whose initial chest roentgenograms four to five years earlier were considered to be within normal limits.[76] PMF is said to develop in about 30 per cent of patients with diffuse bilateral opacities.[77] PMF typically starts near the periphery of the lung and presents as a mass with a smooth, well-defined lateral border that parallels the rib cage

and is projected 1 to 3 cm from it. The medial margin of the mass is often ill-defined in contrast to its sharp lateral border. Such masses tend to be thicker in one dimension than the other; for example, they tend to produce a broad face on a posteroanterior roentgenogram and a thin shape on a lateral roentgenogram, frequently paralleling the major fissure. As might be expected, this spindle-shaped configuration creates a roentgenographic opacity that is considerably less dense in one projection than in the other. Both the smooth, sharply defined lateral border and the somewhat flattened configuration characteristic of these lesions can be employed to considerable advantage in differentiation from bronchogenic carcinoma, whose borders tend to be less well defined and whose configuration is typically spherical. PMF is usually homogeneous in density unless cavitation has developed. Cavitation occurs occasionally and is caused by ischemic necrosis or superimposed tuberculosis. As with the conglomerate shadows of silicosis, PMF usually originates in the lung periphery and gradually migrates toward the hilum, leaving a zone of overinflated emphysematous lung between it and the chest wall. Coal-worker's PMF may develop after exposure to coal dust has ceased and, unlike simple pneumoconiosis, may progress in the absence of further exposure.[77]

CLINICAL MANIFESTATIONS

Unlike patients with silicosis, coal workers with simple pneumoconiosis suffer little clinical disability and seldom show progress of their disease[78, 79] if removed from their dust-ridden environment. Symptoms usually develop only when the disease becomes complicated with PMF. Symptoms include cough, mucoid expectoration, dyspnea on exertion, hemoptysis, frequent attacks of acute purulent bronchitis, and the expectoration of jet-black fluid.[80] The production of copious amounts of black sputum occurs when an ischemic lesion of progressive massive fibrosis liquefies and ruptures into a bronchus, in which circumstance a cavity should be visible roentgenographically.[80] With progression of the disease, dyspnea usually worsens; cor pulmonale and right-sided heart failure may ensue. The degree of breathlessness appears to be directly related to the stage of the disease. In simple pneumoconiosis, there is usually no breathlessness on exertion, despite increasing roentgenographic abnormality. By contrast, in complicated pneumoconiosis, breathlessness is nearly always severe and increases with progression of roentgenographic changes.

An often cited study of pulmonary function of patients with simple pneumoconiosis compared with a control group of the same age, published in 1955, showed no significant differences apart from minor disturbances in gas distribution.[81] In patients with simple CWP, a decrease in ventilatory capacity, as measured by FEV_1 and FVC, can be explained largely on the basis of smoking, whereas patients with PMF show larger defects than appropriate normal controls.[60] By contrast, an increase in residual volume has been found in miners with or without airway obstruction, the degree of air trapping increasing with radiographic categories.[82] Diffusing capacity may be reduced in miners who smoke, but is usually normal in nonsmokers with simple CWP. In contrast to simple pneumoconiosis, PMF is frequently associated with physiologic evidence of airway obstruction, reduced diffusing capacity, abnormal blood gases, and increased pulmonary arterial pressures.[60, 83] In a study in which pathology and function were correlated, Lyons and Campbell[84] concluded that PMF and the extent of emphysema were not sufficient to explain impairment of ventilation, and that small airway disease and interstitial fibrosis must be invoked as additional factors.

MIXED DUST PNEUMOCONIOSES

In certain occupations workers are exposed to a combination of dusts, including silicon dioxide, silicates, and nonfibrogenic minerals such as iron. The clinical, roentgenologic, and pathologic findings depend upon the relative content of individual dusts. In these occupations, free silica usually presents less than 10 per cent of the inhaled dust, and although this substance is responsible for most of the lung damage, its low concentration requires heavy prolonged exposure to produce pathologic changes.

SILICOSIDEROSIS

This mixed dust pneumoconiosis (synonyms: siderosilicosis; hematite foundry worker's lung; hematite pneumoconiosis) develps when silica is mixed in varying proportions with iron oxide in the inhaled dust. Iron is radiopaque and nonfibrogenic, and in the absence of silica causes siderosis (see further on in the section on radiopaque dusts). Silicosiderosis usually oc-

curs in iron ore or foundry workers, boiler scalers, or others whose work is associated with the steel and iron industry.

When the content of free silica in the atmosphere is relatively small—for example, less than 10 per cent—the roentgenographic and pathologic picture is very similar to that of coalworker's pneumoconiosis. When the free silica content is high, the roentgenographic picture is identical to that of silicosis, with the addition of iron oxide deposits.[85] The severity of the fibrosis varies with the amount of free silica, there being no correlation between the degree of fibrosis and the amount of iron found in the lung.[85] The incidence of bronchogenic carcinoma is significantly higher in patients with siderosis or silicosiderosis than in the general population.[86]

ARGYROSIDEROSIS

A rather characteristic roentgenographic pattern may be seen in the pneumoconiosis of silver polishers, quite different from that of siderosis (see further on). Argyrosiderosis presumably results from the inhalation of very fine particles of silver in addition to iron oxide. The chest roentgenogram reveals a fine, stippled pattern in contrast to the widely disseminated reticulonodular pattern of siderosis. Pathologic examination in such cases reveals staining of the elastic tissue by the inhaled silver, in addition to the usual nonfibrogenic deposits of iron oxide.[85]

PNEUMOCONIOSIS CAUSED BY RADIOPAQUE DUST

The clinically significant radiopaque dusts include iron, tin, barium, emery, and antimony, the density of the roentgenographic shadows varying with the atomic weight of the element.[85] Characteristically, these substances are not fibrogenic and thus cause little clinical disability; their major importance lies in the dramatic changes they produce in the chest roentgenogram.

SIDEROSIS

Workers in many industries are exposed to iron dust, which may be mixed with various percentages of free silica and thereby give rise to silicosiderosis. The iron is usually in the form of hematite and ferric oxide (Fe_2O_3), which produce opacities whose density is greater than unity.

The majority of patients with siderosis are electric arc welders; the remainder include silver polishers, iron ore miners, ocher miners, foundry workers, and boiler scalers. It is believed that when iron oxide is inhaled in relatively pure form—that is, free from significant amounts of silicon dioxide—little or no pulmonary fibrosis develops. In fact, persons exposed to iron oxide in high concentrations for many years usually are not disabled and show little evidence of fibrosis at necropsy.[85]

Pathologically, deposits of iron oxide are seen predominantly within phagocytes in the peribronchial and perivascular lymphatics. There is no evidence of fibrotic reaction to this inert dust.[87]

The roentgenographic pattern is reticulonodular and widely disseminated. In contrast to the majority of pneumoconioses, the roentgenographic abnormality may disappear partly or completely when patients are removed from dust exposure.[87]

Clinically, patients with siderosis have no symptoms of chest disease, and pulmonary function studies of welders have shown values considered to be within normal limits.

STANNOSIS

Stannosis is a pneumoconiosis caused by the inhalation of tin oxide. The hazard exists for tin ore miners and hearth tinners and for workers in industries in which tin oxide fumes form. *Pathologically*, the findings closely simulate the bronchiolar lesions of coal-worker's pneumoconiosis, including focal emphysema.[88] Histologic staining shows only dust without associated fibrosis. The *roentgenographic pattern* consists of multiple tiny shadows of high density, about 1 mm in diameter, distributed evenly throughout the lungs.

BARYTOSIS

Barytosis is a "benign" pneumoconiosis that results from the inhalation of particulate barium sulfate. Owing to the high radiopacity of barium, the discrete shadows in the chest roentgenogram are extremely dense, creating an awesome appearance. The apices and bases usually are spared, and massive shadows do not occur. Roentgenographic abnormalities may develop after only relatively brief exposure. The lesions characteristically regress roentgenographically after the patient is removed from the dust-filled environment.[85]

ANTIMONY PNEUMOCONIOSIS

Antimony is present in cosmetics and is used in the manufacture of paints and lacquers, in the compounding of rubber, and in flameproofing. The metal is heated in a rotating kiln and is inhaled as a fine white powder. The chest roentgenogram reveals minute dense opacities scattered widely throughout both lungs. There is no evidence that the dust is fibrogenic or causes disturbances in lung function.[89]

RARE-EARTH PNEUMOCONIOSIS

Rare-earth pneumoconiosis is an uncommon inorganic dust disease that occurs with exposure over a period of several years to the smoke of carbon arc lamps.[90] The rare-earth elements are used in reactor control rods, in manufacturing and polishing of colored glass, in the manufacture of flints, and as part of the alloy in cast iron, light metals, and heating conductors. Industrial exposure occurs chiefly in workers in the graphic arts and in the factories producing cored carbon for arc lamps.

The typical roentgenographic pattern is one of widely disseminated punctate shadows of great density. The disease produces no symptoms and is associated with only minor degrees of pulmonary dysfunction.[90]

BERYLLIOSIS (BERYLLIUM PNEUMOCONIOSIS)

EPIDEMIOLOGY

The major commercial source of beryllium is beryl, a beryllium aluminum silicate. Its industrial use is related to three commodities—beryllium alloys, beryllium oxides, and metallic beryllium. Cases of berylliosis that have been reported most recently have been associated with the processing and handling of beryllium compounds in the aerospace industry and in the manufacture of gyroscopes and nuclear reactors.[91]

Although the pathogenesis of berylliosis is incompletely understood, there is good reason to believe that it represents a delayed hypersensitivity reaction. Cutaneous granulomas develop in approximately 70 per cent of patients on skin testing, and an equal number show blast transformation and macrophage inhibition factor production when their lymphocytes are cultured in the presence of beryllium.[92] In contrast to other dusts that cause true pneumoconiosis, beryllium is largely removed from the lungs and excreted in the urine and may be stored in bones and liver for many years.

Beryllium poisoning may occur in an acute or chronic form, the latter being much more common.

ACUTE BERYLLIOSIS

The majority of patients are exposed to the dust while working in beryllium refineries. Depending on the intensity of exposure, the clinical presentation may be either fulminating or insidious.

The fulminating variety of acute berylliosis develops rapidly following an overwhelming exposure. Its clinical and roentgenographic manifestations are those of acute pulmonary edema, which may be rapidly fatal.[93]

The insidious variety of acute berylliosis produces symptoms weeks or even months after the initial exposure. The onset is heralded by a dry cough, substernal pain, shortness of breath on exertion, anorexia, weakness, and weight loss. Pathologically, the insidious form of acute disease may show a severe organizing pneumonitis. Hyaline membranes line the alveoli and are similar in appearances to that found in viral or "uremic" pneumonitis. The chest roentgenogram usually does not become abnormal until 1 to 4 weeks after the onset of symptoms. Diffuse, symmetric, bilateral "haziness" is seen in the earliest stage of the disease, with subsequent development of irregular patchy opacities scattered rather widely throughout the lungs. Complete roentgenographic clearing may take 2 to 3 months.[94]

Pulmonary function studies in the insidious form of acute disease have shown greatly decreased arterial oxygen saturation during exercise and even at rest, with an increase in the alveolar-arterial gradient for oxygen. Removal from exposure to the dust results in gradual return to normal function.

CHRONIC BERYLLIOSIS

The chronic variety of berylliosis is much commoner and more serious than acute beryl-

lium poisoning. In the majority of patients in the earlier reports, the disease resulted from exposure in the fluorescent phosphor industry or from working with beryllium alloys.[94] In some patients, however, the only known source of exposure was contaminated work clothes at home or atmospheric contamination from neighborhood beryllium plants.

Pathologically, chronic berylliosis is a widespread systemic disease, producing lesions in the lungs, lymph nodes, liver, spleen, kidney, myocardium, skin, skeletal muscle, and pleura.[95] In the lungs, the earliest lesion apparent histologically is a focal, noncaseating granuloma that gradually undergoes transition to fibrous tissue, with associated interstitial fibrosis. It has been stated that the histologic picture of chronic berylliosis is entirely nonspecific and that differentiation from sarcoidosis cannot be made with certainty.[95]

The *roentgenographic pattern* is neither specific nor diagnostic.[96] When the degree of involvement is relatively minor, the pattern is described as a diffuse, finely granular "haziness" with a tendency to sparing of the apices and bases. With more severe involvement, ill-defined nodules of moderate size are scattered diffusely throughout the lungs, sometimes with associated lymph node enlargement. Calcification of nodules occurs and when present permits differentiation from sarcoidosis. In advanced cases, the pattern may be chiefly reticular and may be associated with great decrease in volume and will some conglomeration of nodular shadows. Spontaneous pneumothorax occurs in slightly more than 10 per cent of cases.

Clinically, symptoms usually develop insidiously after a latent period that may be as long as 15 years following the last exposure to dust.[94] Early symptoms include minimal cough, fatigue, weight loss, increasing dyspnea on exertion, and sometimes migratory arthralgia. With progression of the disease, cyanosis may become obvious, and in approximately 30 per cent of patients, clubbing of the fingers and toes develops; cor pulmonale is frequent. Hypergammaglobulinemia, hypercalciuria, and polycythemia are not uncommon findings.[94]

Results of pulmonary function studies may be normal or may indicate some degree of restrictive insufficiency.[97] In many cases the arterial oxygen tension is decreased, even at rest. Diffusing capacity may be reduced.

The diagnosis of chronic beryllium disease may be suspected from a history of exposure to the dust and a chest roentgenogram showing

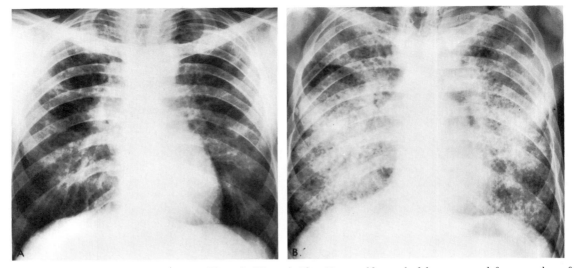

Figure 12–9. Bauxite Pneumoconiosis (Shaver's Disease). This 29-year-old man had been exposed for a number of years to bauxite in the manufacture of corundum. The first posteroanterior roentgenogram (A) reveals a coarse reticulonodular pattern throughout both lungs involving predominantly the upper and midlung zones. Slightly over 1 year later (B), the disease has extended to a remarkable degree, the reticulonodular shadows being confluent in many areas. (Courtesy of the Herbert Reddy Hospital, Montreal, and the Montreal Chest Hospital Center.)

diffuse nodular disease. Confirmation may be obtained by a patch test showing hypersensitivity to beryllium.[98] Confusion in diagnosis may arise with sarcoidosis, a disease that is much more frequent asymptomatic and carries a better prognosis.

ALUMINUM PNEUMOCONIOSIS (ALUMINOSIS)

There are two types of pneumoconiosis associated with aluminum, that related to the inhalation of minute particles of metallic aluminum, and that related to the mining and processing of bauxite, a complex hydrous aluminum oxide that constitutes the principal source of metallic aluminum used in industry. In both, pathologic changes are thought to consist initially of edema of the alveolar walls, followed by interstitial pneumonitis and subsequently fibrosis. The end result is diffuse interstitial fibrosis, without nodule formation. Emphysematous bullae may develop and rupture.

Roentgenographic abnormalities may become apparent after a few months or several years of exposure.[22] Fully developed changes consist of a fine to coarse reticular pattern widely distributed throughout the lungs (Figure 12–9), sometimes with a nodular component.[99] Lung volume may be greatly decreased, and the pleura may become thickened; spontaneous pneumo-

thorax is a frequent complication (Figure 12–9).

Breathlessness is the chief symptom and may be severely disabling. Death may occur from pulmonary insufficiency.[99]

INHALATION DISEASES CAUSED BY NOXIOUS GASES AND SOLUBLE AEROSOLS

Several gases and liquids in a finely dispersed state can produce acute and sometimes chronic damage of the air passages and pulmonary parenchyma. The reaction produced depends upon the chemical composition of the gas or aerosol and the intensity and duration of exposure. Soluble gases such as sulfur dioxide, ammonia, and chlorine tend to cause irritation of the mucous membrane of the eyes and upper respiratory tract, whereas less soluble gases such as phosgene, nitrogen dioxide, ozone, and high concentrations of oxygen penetrate deeply into the lungs and produce alveolocapillary damage. However, the concentration of the gas and the duration of exposure are the chief factors determining clinical presentation, and under appropriate circumstances any one of these toxic gases can produce immediate or delayed pulmonary edema.[100]

In some instances, the chemical injury may affect only the airways, resulting in fulminating bronchitis and bronchiolitis, sometimes complicated by pneumonia and atelectasis and occasionally rapidly fatal.[100] Patients who survive the acute insult may feel relatively well for about 3 weeks and then suffer abrupt clinical deterioration, with cough, shortness of breath, and fever. This delayed development represents the effects of bronchiolitis fibrosa obliterans. The small bronchi and bronchioles are plugged with cellular fibrinous exudate, which subsequently undergoes organization by ingrowth of fibroblasts from the bronchiolar walls, resulting in complete occlusion.

Toxic substances that are ingested or injected may reach the lungs by way of the bloodstream and cause damage to alveolocapillary membranes. Such poisons include the aromatic hydrocarbons, the herbicide paraquat, and a growing number of therapeutic chemicals used chiefly in the treatment of neoplasia.

Although the exact mechanisms by which various gases and fumes cause cell injury are still largely unknown, the results of animal experiments strongly implicate oxidizing agents (oxidants) in the pathogenesis. Subcellular biochemical and structural changes found in lungs exposed to ozone, nitrogen dioxide, and high concentrations of oxygen are similar. The herbicide paraquat and irradiation therapy also cause cellular damage in the lung by virtue of their oxidizing properties.

PULMONARY DISEASE RESULTING FROM OXYGEN THERAPY

Only in the past 20 years or so have physicians become aware of the fact that oxygen therapy for respiratory disease may in itself produce pathologic changes in the lungs that are of clinical and physiologic importance.[101]

Newborn infants with hyaline membrane disease who are kept alive with oxygen therapy and artificial ventilation may evidence pathologic and roentgenologic changes that could be attributed to healing of the acute syndrome, the toxic effects of oxygen, the effects of intermittent positive pressure ventilation, or a combination of these factors.[101] In a study of 32 cyanotic infants in respiratory failure secondary to hyaline membrane disease who received artificial ventilation with 100 per cent oxygen, Northway and his colleagues[101] recognized four stages with more or less distinct pathologic and roentgenographic manifestations. *Stage 1*, seen in the first 2 or 3 days after the onset of symptoms, presented the classic picture of hyaline membrane disease of the newborn. *Stage 2* developed from the fourth to the tenth day after onset and was a period of apparent regeneration. Pathologically both necrosis and repair of the alveolar epithelium were seen. Hyaline membranes persisted and there was coalescence of emphysematous areas. The roentgenographic appearance was one of almost complete opacification of both lungs, usually associated with a well-defined air bronchogram. *Stage 3* was observed in infants between 10 and 20 days after the onset of symptoms. Pathologically, alternating areas of atelectasis and emphysema were observed, creating a "spongy" appearance. Roentgenographically, the nearly complete opacification of lung parenchyma characteristic of the second stage was replaced by multiple small, round radiolucencies resembling bullae, distributed widely throughout both lungs. The roentgenographic appearance simulated a sponge. *Stage 4* developed in infants who survived longer than 1 month and who required continuous oxygen therapy. Pathologically, large emphysematous areas were associated with "tributary" bronchioles that showed marked hypertrophy of their smooth muscle. The chest roentgenogram revealed enlargement of the radiolucent areas seen in stage 3.

In *adults*, it has been suggested that oxygen therapy in high concentrations may be responsible for intra-alveolar hemorrhage, hyaline membrane formation, and alveolar and interstitial fibroblastic proliferation.[102, 103] Because of these observations, emphasis has been placed on the desirability of administering oxygen in lower concentrations, while at the same time monitoring arterial P_{O_2}; preference has been given to the use of compressed air rather than oxygen in pressure-cycle ventilators.

In a study of 70 patients receiving oxygen therapy by artificial ventilation, Nash and associates[102] described two histologic phases, the exudative and the proliferative. The former was characterized by capillary congestion, proteinaceous alveolar material, intra-alveolar hemorrhage, and a fibrinous exudate with well-defined hyaline membranes lining all portions of the acinar air spaces. In the proliferative phase, there was a severe degree of alveolar and interlobular septal fibroblastic proliferation, early fibrosis, and hyperplasia of alveolar lining cells. In both infants and adults, it is difficult to ascribe pathologic changes to oxygen poisoning alone, since many of these patients have organ failure as well, with its attendant severe metabolic disturbances. In addition, many are subjected to positive pressure respiration before death.

PULMONARY DISEASE RESULTING FROM OZONE INHALATION

Unlike most other gases described in this section, ozone has not produced serious acute disease in humans to the best of our knowledge. Nevertheless, there is abundant evidence that even low concentrations of O_3 can produce structural changes in animal lungs and functional changes in both animal and human lungs. Ozone constitutes 90 per cent of the measured oxidant in photochemical smog,[104] and in certain urban areas the concentration of ozone in the atmosphere in particles per million (ppm) is equal to that shown previously to cause structural and physiologic changes. Even higher concentrations of ozone are found within airplanes at altitudes above 30,000 ft, in proximity to high-tension electrical discharges from welding in air or oxygen, and in various industries in which this gas is used as an oxidation agent.[105]

A number of investigators[106, 107] have shown that acute exposure of normal volunteers to low concentrations of ozone (0.3 to 0.9 ppm) results in symptoms of dry cough, chest discomfort, and impaired pulmonary function. Considerable variation is observed among individuals in their symptomatic and functional responses, explainable on the basis of hyper-reactivity of airways in some and by tolerance developed from prolonged exposure to pollution in others.[106] Brief and light exercise while breathing ozone is more consistently associated with impaired function.

PULMONARY DISEASE RESULTING FROM NITROGEN DIOXIDE INHALATION

Like ozone, nitrogen dioxide (NO_2) is a component of photochemical smog, and although its concentration is insufficient to cause serious concern, it possesses an effect identical to that of ozone on pulmonary parenchymal cells and thus represents a potential hazard to humans.

The dangers of exposure to a high concentration of oxides of nitrogen have been known for many years in industry, but not until 1956 were they recognized in relation to recently filled silos.[108] In industry, bronchopulmonary disease occurs from exposure to fuming nitric acid,[109] or, in mining, in association with explosives.[109] There is little doubt, however, that from an epidemiologic viewpoint silo-filler's disease is the most important condition resulting from nitrogen dioxide inhalation.

For 3 to 10 days after a silo has been filled, the fresh silage produces nitric oxide which, on contact with the air, oxidizes to form nitrogen dioxide and its polymer, nitrogen tetroxide. These two gases, being heavier than air, remain just above the silage and are apparent as a brownish-yellow "cloud." Anyone who enters the silo during this period will inhale nitrogen dioxide with resultant lung damage; the severity will be in proportion to the duration and level of exposure. Mild exposure produces only inflammation of the bronchial and bronchiolar mucosa. With very intense exposure, acute pulmonary edema may develop rapidly and may prove fatal.

The course following moderate to severe exposure is triphasic.

1. *The first phase* demonstrates an immediate reaction within the lungs consisting of acute, severe fibrinous bronchiolitis and peribronchiolitis, sometimes with denuding of the epithelium of these airways. The clinical picture is characterized by the abrupt onset of cough, dyspnea, weakness, and a choking feeling that usually persist. Acute pulmonary edema may develop within 4 to 24 hours (Figure 12–10), but usually clears completely if the patient survives.

2. *The second phase* is an *asymptomatic period* lasting from 2 to 5 weeks, although cough, malaise, and shortness of breath may persist during the period of remission. Weakness may become more severe. The chest roentgenogram is normal.

3. *The third phase* becomes manifest 2 to 5 weeks after the initial exposure.[110] During this period the acute bronchiolitis and peribronchiolitis become more organized, with resulting *bronchiolitis fibrosa obliterans*. This stage is characterized roentgenographically by a "miliary nodulation" whose appearance tends to lag somewhat behind the recurrence of symptoms. Multiple discrete nodular opacities of varying size are scattered diffusely throughout the lungs, to a point of confluence in the more severe cases.[108, 111] The nodules may disappear as the clinical course progresses to a stage of chronic pulmonary insufficiency, although they usually persist for a considerable time after the acute symptoms have subsided,[1390] Clinically, the third stage is characterized by fever, chills, progressive shortness of breath, cough, and cyanosis. Moist rales and sibilant rhonchi may be heard on auscultation. A neutrophilic leukocytosis develops in most cases, and the arterial blood P_{CO_2} may be elevated.[108] At this stage, the patient may die of pulmonary insufficiency or may recover more or less completely. Irreversible pulmonary insufficiency may become chronic and give rise to obstructive impairment of pulmonary function.[111]

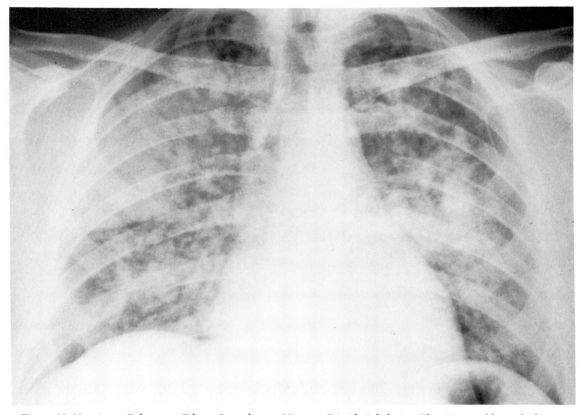

Figure 12–10. **Acute Pulmonary Edema Secondary to Nitrogen Dioxide Inhalation.** This 40-year-old man had spent 6 hours with several other men in an enclosed space on board ship attempting to remove a propeller with cutting torches. Such a procedure is known to be associated with accumulation of nitrogen dioxide. Toward the end of the 6 hours, the patient noted the onset of nausea, vomiting, headache, and productive cough. This posteroanterior roentgenogram reveals extensive involvement of both lungs by a process characteristic of air-space edema. The chest roentgenogram had returned to normal 4 days later so that the process clearly was one of edema. Two months after this roentgenogram, pulmonary function tests were normal with the exception of slight decrease in FRC, and the patient had slight residual shortness of breath on exertion.

PULMONARY DISEASE RESULTING FROM SULFUR DIOXIDE INHALATION

Sulfur dioxide (SO_2) is a highly soluble gas whose major importance in pulmonary disease is as an atmospheric pollutant; continuous exposure to low concentrations in an urban environment may play a role in the pathogenesis of chronic obstructive pulmonary disease. Accidental exposure to high concentrations may occur in pulp and paper factories and refrigeration plants, and in the oil refining and fruit preserving industries.[10] It is probable that high concentrations of SO_2 produce the same triphasic picture as does NO_2.[112] We have seen a pulp mill worker who was accidentally exposed to the fumes rising from a vat of concentrated sulfuric acid, resulting in acute pulmonary edema that resolved within a few days. Three months later he manifested evidence of severe obstructive lung disease caused by extensive

bronchiolitis fibrosa obliterans and generalized bronchiectasis.

PULMONARY DISEASE RESULTING FROM INHALATION OF A VARIETY OF TOXIC SUBSTANCES

The intensely irritant gases *ammonia, chlorine,* and *phosgene,* if inhaled in sufficient concentration, result in pulmonary edema and acute bronchitis and bronchiolitis. Death from pulmonary edema may occur, usually within the first 24 hours. If the patient survives the initial acute episode, recovery tends to be complete[113, 114] although bronchiectasis may develop, especially following ammonia inhalation. *Vaporized mercury* poisoning causes severe tracheobronchitis, bronchiolitis, and pneumonitis and is particularly serious in infants in whom the damage to the airways may prove fatal. When inhaled, the fumes of *zinc chloride* may cause severe damage to the tracheobronchial tree and lung parenchyma, sometimes resulting in death within hours. Patients who survive tend to develop rapidly progressive diffuse interstitial pulmonary fibrosis. Poisoning with the insecticide *chlorinated camphene* can result in extensive bilateral "allergic" bronchopneumonia, sometimes associated with blood eosinophilia. Poisoning with the organophosphate insecticides, *parathion* and *malathion*, occurs most commonly in agricultural workers during or shortly after the spraying of crops. The pathophysiologic consequences result from excessive cholinergic activity, and death may result from central nervous system depression or from diaphragmatic paralysis, the latter being compounded by bronchoconstriction and hypersecretion.

These and other less common causes of pulmonary damage resulting from inhalation of toxic substances are described in some detail in the text *Diagnosis of Diseases of the Chest* (pages 1537 to 1541).

BRONCHOPULMONARY DISEASE ASSOCIATED WITH BURNS

Of 932 burn patients admitted to the Massachusetts General Hospital over a 20-year period, 181 experienced respiratory difficulty and 89 (49 per cent) of these had abnormal chest roentgenograms.[115] The roentgenographic changes consisted of patchy pulmonary opacities thought to be caused by pulmonary edema. In 75 patients, the changes were presumed to be produced by the inhalation of noxious gases, probably products of incomplete combustion. Generally, the incidence of such complications correlates with the severity of the burn and with a history of being in an enclosed space. During the first 24 hours, complications result from upper airway edema caused by direct heat injury or toxic products, usually in patients with head and neck burns. Complications that develop 2 to 5 days after the burn consist of atelectasis, pulmonary edema, and pneumonia. Atelectasis may result from mucous plugging of even large bronchi, presumably as a result of excessive smoke inhalation.[116] Complications arising after 5 days include bronchopneumonia, pulmonary embolism,[117] and ARDS.[118] Peters[119] has stated that when chemical tracheobronchitis occurs in patients with serious cutaneous burns, the mortality is exceedingly high, ranging from 48 to 86 per cent; a patient's condition usually follows a staged progression that is proportional to the extent and severity of the tracheobronchitis.

The toxic products responsible for pulmonary complications are carried in smoke, which consists of a suspension of small particles in hot air and gases and possesses both particulate and gaseous fractions. The particles are made up of carbon, which is coated with combustible products such as organic acids and aldehydes. The gaseous fraction has an extremely variable composition, depending upon the material that is burning, although carbon monoxide and carbon dioxide are the main constitutents and are always present. There are many others, and a list of toxic combustion products of common materials has recently been published.[120] Although most toxic products of inhaled smoke are unidentified, polyvinyl chloride (PVC) has been implicated as a major cause of serious pulmonary parenchymal damage because of its release of hydrogen chloride gas while burning. This substance is a plastic solid widely used as a rubber substitute, as a covering for electric and telephone wire and cable, and in many other manufactured products.[121] When heated to over 225°C, PVC thermally degrades and releases hydrochloric acid. The effect of the acid in the gas phase is largely restricted to irritability, chiefly affecting the upper respiratory tract, whereas loosely bound hydrochloric acid condensed on soot aerosol gains access to the lung parenchyma.[121] In addition to the acute lung damage that results from exposure to burning PVC, there is evidence that this substance may produce an interstitial granulomatosis and fibrosis,[123, 172] and an immunologically-determined multisystem disorder manifested by Raynaud's phenomenon, acro-osteolysis, thrombocytopenia, portal fibrosis, and hepatic and pulmonary dysfunction. Prolonged exposure to low concentrations has been shown to cause angiosarcoma of the liver.

Despite the foregoing, Putman and his colleagues[122] have emphasized that the standard chest roentgenogram is an insensitive means of determining pulmonary injury by smoke inhalation; from a study of 21 patients with acute smoke inhalation, these authors found that determination of blood carboxyhemoglobin and arterial blood gas levels is a more important parameter in the clinical evaluation of these patients than is the chest roentgenogram.

CARBON MONOXIDE POISONING

Carbon monoxide is an odorless gas formed by incomplete combustion of carbon-containing matter. It is produced in high concentration in fires, in which circumstances its inhalation is probably the commonest cause of death. Other sources of this gas include faulty heaters, exhausts from automobiles, inhalation of tobacco smoke, mine explosions, and the burning of charcoal briquets in confined spaces such as trailers, station wagons, and cellars.

The deleterious effects of carbon monoxide in humans appear to be attributable to two factors: (1) tissue hypoxia resulting from the formation of carboxyhemoglobin (COHb), which reduces the oxygen transport capacity of the blood and causes a shift of the oxyhemoglobin dissociation curve to the left, thus curtailing the amount of oxygen available to the tissues; and (2) a direct cytotoxic effect. Characteristically, clinical symptoms develop when carboxyhemoglobin saturation reaches 20 per cent; unconsciousness occurs at about 60 per cent and death at about 80 per cent. If acute carbon monoxide poisoning does not end fatally, follow-up studies have demonstrated neurologic damage characterized by personality deterioration and memory impairment.[124]

Of possibly even greater significance than acute carbon monoxide poisoning is the morbidity associated with long-term exposure to low concentrations of this gas. The blood carboxyhemoglobin level of healthy nonsmoking individuals is roughly 0.5 per cent, a figure that rises to about 3 per cent with increased hemolysis.[125] By contrast, the average COHb of a smoker who smokes one pack a day is 5.9 per cent, a figure that may rise to between 10 and 20 per cent with heavy smoking.[125] It is obvious that such individuals will develop significant hypoxia, particularly if they live at high altitudes. The percentage of inspired carbon monoxide may be increased in heavy traffic, since car exhausts contain between 1 and 7 per cent CO; automobile drivers involved in accidents have higher levels of COHb than controls.

In acute carbon monoxide poisoning, abnormalities may be detected on the chest roentgenogram and consist chiefly of pulmonary edema, usually interstitial in location.

THESAUROSIS

In its broad connotation, this term designates storage in the body of unusual amounts of normal or foreign material. However, since the original descriptions by Bergmann and associates in 1958 and 1962,[126, 127] the term has come to be restricted to pulmonary disease resulting from the inhalation of hair spray and character-

ized by a granulomatous pulmonary infiltration closely resembling sarcoidosis.

An attempt to produce pulmonary disease in dogs by heavy, long-term exposure to commercial hair spray[128] resulted in no significant pulmonary abnormality. However, in a follow-up study of beauticians, Gowdy and Wagstaff[129] found that 21 per cent had an abnormal chest roentgenogram when first seen and that 40 per cent showed abnormalities four years later. On the basis of health department records, these authors felt that beauticians had a 10- to 20-fold increase in the risk of developing roentgenographic abnormalities in their lungs. The patients described by Bergmann and his colleagues[126, 127] manifested roentgenographic and pathologic changes identical to those of sarcoidosis, although they complained of cough and dyspnea. In some of these patients the disease cleared within a few months of removal from exposure, but others had residual diffuse fibrosis. Schraufnagel and his colleagues[130] have recently reported a radiologic/pathologic correlative study of two patients who admitted using an inordinate quantity of hair spray. Pathologically, both patients manifested interstitial granulomas indistinguishable from sarcoidosis. Roentgenographically, the pattern was similar in the two patients, consisting of a fine micronodularity distributed widely throughout both lungs and simulating the pattern produced by alveolar microlithiasis and talcosis of intravenous drug abuse. In a review of 31 cases in the literature, these authors found that eight manifested a micronodular pattern roentgenographically, similar to their own two patients.

Roentgenographic clearing tends to occur fairly rapidly following discontinuance of exposure; a favorable response has also been observed with corticosteroid therapy.[130]

CADMIUM POISONING

Animal studies[131] and epidemiologic investigations in man have proven conclusively that exposure to cadmium fumes can damage the kidneys. Evidence for the development of pulmonary disease in humans is less convincing, but recent reports support the possibility that obstructive disease can develop in long-term workers.[132, 133]

FLUOROCARBON AND HYDROCARBON POISONING

These chemicals are toxic whether inhaled, ingested, or aspirated. The most serious effects on the lungs from the volatile fluorocarbons and hydrocarbons derive from the sniffing of glue, or from the inhalation of freons used as propellants for a variety of sprays.[134] Inhalation of glue or the contents of aerosol cans from plastic bags is usually deliberate and is done by young male teenagers; it may prove fatal. There are three essential components of aerosol sprays—the propellant, the solvent, and the active ingredient—and each of these may be hazardous to health. Agents used by teenagers for "kicks" include various cements, glues, lacquers, paints, fingernail polish remover, lighter and cleaning fluid, gasoline, antifreeze, and virtually all commercial products packaged in aerosol cans.[134] When inhaled in high concentrations, volatile hydrocarbons induce euphoria and hallucinations with subsequent central nervous system depression. The major health hazard lies in their action on the myocardium. Not only may conduction be impaired, but cardiac muscle becomes sensitive to sympathomimetic amines, resulting in arrhythmias. This sensitization may be intensified by hypoxemia, hypercapnia, stress, or physical activity. From the foregoing, it can be seen that the toxicity of the chlorinated volatile hydrocarbons is not primarily pulmonary; however, they diffuse through the alveolocapillary membrane and are carried into the bloodstream to the myocardium, where they cause arrhythmias, and to the kidneys and liver, where they cause cellular damage.

Hydrocarbon pneumonitis results from the aspiration or ingestion of halogenated aromatic hydrocarbons. It has been estimated that 25 per cent of all poisonings in children result from the ingestion of petroleum products. The most common offending agent is kerosene and less frequently gasoline, furniture polish, lighter fluid, cleaning fluid, insecticides, and other household materials. The pathogenesis of the pulmonary disease is controversial. Two mechanisms are possible, both starting from the premise that the child *ingested* the hydrocarbon rather than aspirated it: (1) the offending material is absorbed from the gastrointestinal tract, and, in its passage through the lungs, causes toxic capillary damage that leads to edema; and (2) during the vomiting that almost inevitably follows ingestion, gastric contents are aspirated. A number of experiments have been carried out on animals to discover which of these mechanisms is operative,[138] and it appears very likely that in the majority of cases of hydrocarbon pneumonitis, the insult occurs as a result of aspiration of gastric contents. Since such aspiration is a frequent complication of gastric la-

vage, it has been suggested that any attempts at this procedure to remove hydrocarbon compounds from the stomach should be preceded by placement of a cuffed endotracheal tube.

Roentgenographic changes in the lungs occur in 70 to 90 per cent of children who ingest hydrocarbon compounds. They usually appear within an hour of the ingestion of kerosene,[139] but somewhat later with furniture polish. The severity of the pulmonary abnormality varies and is dependent on the amount ingested. The typical roentgenographic pattern is one of patchy air-space consolidation characteristic of alveolar edema, involving predominantly the basal portions of the lungs, and usually bilaterally symmetrical.[139] Whatever the pathogenesis, there is little doubt that the pathologic changes in the lungs are those of toxic edema. Whether this occurs from the alveolar face as a result of aspiration or is a direct effect of circulating poison on the capillaries seems to be of little moment.

Roentgenographic resolution tends to be slow (up to 2 weeks)[139] and usually lags well behind clinical improvement. Pneumatoceles may develop as a consequence of bronchial or bronchiolar obstruction.

In the absence of witnesses to the incident, the diagnosis may be suspected from the smell of the offending agent on the child's breath. Vomiting follows shortly after ingestion and presumably is associated with aspiration. Symptoms usually are mild, but there is correlation between the amount of kerosene ingested, the severity of clinical symptoms, and the extent of roentgenographic signs.

EPOXIDE POISONING

Epoxides are ubiquitous substances that occur naturally in industry and the environment and *in vivo* as metabolites in certain biochemical pathways.[135] In the recent medical literature,[136, 137] an epoxy resin containing a catalyst known as trimellitic anhydride (TMA) has been implicated in the etiology of immediate and delayed asthma and in a syndrome characterized by pulmonary hemorrhage and edema and anemia. It has been suggested that the pulmonary edema-anemia syndrome may be immunologically mediated.[137]

PARAQUAT POISONING

The ingestion of 200 ml or more of concentrated solution of this herbicide in suicide attempts results in death in 24 hours or less, necropsy revealing extensive cellular necrosis of the liver, heart, and kidneys.[140] Accidental poisoning usually occurs from imbibing a mouthful (15 to 20 ml) of concentrated paraquat solution, commonly from an unlabeled container. In such circumstances, death usually results from respiratory failure 5 to 10 days after ingestion.

Although this substance has been used as a spray from airplanes, there is no evidence that lung disease results from inhalation, presumably because the particle size is too large.[141]

Pathologically, there is evidence of capillary congestion, alveolar edema, and hyaline membrane formation, with accumulation in the alveoli of electron-dense material that resembles lamellar bodies and surfactant.[141] In patients who live longer than 10 days, lung structure becomes entirely disorganized and replaced by many small cysts measuring 0.5 to 2.0 mm in diameter and lined by fibrous tissue.[142] In addition to the lung, the main target organs are the kidney (acute tubular necrosis), the liver (midzone necrosis), the heart (myocarditis), and the adrenals (cortical necrosis).

Roentgenographic changes characteristically appear 3 to 7 days after ingestion and consist initially of fine granular opacities, both discrete and confluent, situated predominantly in the lower lung zones. Roentgenographic changes characteristically progress rapidly to a pattern resembling severe pulmonary edema.[143] Once roentgenographic abnormalities have developed in the chest the chances of survival appear relatively small.

Clinically, the immediate effects of severe poisoning consist of vomiting, abdominal pain, and burning of the mouth and throat; these symptoms are followed shortly by renal and hepatic failure. Respiratory failure develops 5 to 10 days later, sometimes after a period of apparent recovery. Once the lung is involved, death is usual but not invariable.

INHALATION DISEASES UNRELATED TO DUSTS OR FUMES

ASPIRATION OF SOLID FOREIGN BODIES

Aspiration of solid foreign bodies into the tracheobronchial tree occurs almost exclusively in small children under 3 years of age. More than 85 per cent of the aspirated foreign bodies are of vegetable origin, the peanut being by far the most common.[144] Almost equally treacherous is timothy or barley grass. Any child who coughs and wheezes during the summer months should be suspected of having aspirated one of these grasses.

A wide variety of *roentgenographic changes* may be produced in the lungs. When the foreign body is nonreactive, such as a tooth, it may be discovered only incidentally on routine chest roentgenography. In the majority of cases, however, changes in the lungs reflect the presence of partial or complete bronchial obstruction. The lower lobes are involved almost exclusively, and the right more often than the left, in a ratio of 2 to 1. The roentgenographic findings in the 160 patients reported by Brown and his associates[144] were as follows:

Obstructive overinflation	109	(68.1%)
Collapse	22	(13.8%)
"Infiltration"	17	(10.6%)
Radiopaque foreign body	15	(9.4%)
Bronchiectasis with recurrent		
local pneumonitis	3	
Pneumomediastinum	2	
Pneumothorax	1	

The number of patients with "obstructive overinflation" in this study is surprising. Since it can be very difficult to obtain roentgenograms of the chest in infants and young children at a point of maximal inspiration, particularly if there is respiratory distress and consequent tachypnea, we suspect that in the majority of cases the affected lung was *not* overinflated at TLC but that it revealed increased radiolucency as a result of oligemia occasioned by hypoxic vasoconstriction (a reflex reduction in perfusion in response to reduced ventilation). Since collapse was such an uncommon feature of these cases, it must be concluded that collateral air drift from adjacent normal lung parenchyma must have been a potent force in the majority of cases. In a patient in whom a foreign body impacts in a major bronchus, a roentgenogram exposed at inspiration may reveal no abnormality if insufficient time has elapsed for much air to be absorbed. In such circumstances, a roentgenogram exposed at full expiration will show air trapping on the affected side and contralateral shift of the mediastinum. Because of the difficulty in communicating with infants and very young children and the resultant problems in obtaining good quality expiratory roentgenograms, Capitanio and Kirkpatrick[145] have adopted lateral decubitus roentgenography as a satisfactory alternative. They point out that when a child is placed on his or her side. the dependent hemithorax is splinted, restricting movement of the thoracic cage on that side. As a consequence, in normal children inflation of the dependent lung tends to be less than that of the upper lung. However, when air trapping is present in a dependent lung, the affected lobe or segment tends to remain hyperlucent. Fluoroscopic examination will accomplish the same thing, revealing mediastinal "swing" and restricted diaphragmatic excursion on the affected side on deep respiration.

Bronchiectasis is an occasional complication of long retention of a foreign body.

Clinically, although almost all of these patients remember choking on aspiration,[144] it may require much persistence to elicit the history, particularly when the episode occurred a long while before. Foreign bodies composed of vegetable matter, particularly peanuts and other material high in fatty acid, tend to cause an acute inflammatory response within a few hours or at the most a few days, leading to early bronchial obstruction with its usual symptoms and signs. It is noteworthy, however, that an asymptomatic interval may follow aspiration, particularly when no bronchi are obstructed, and such a latent period can extend to several months or even years when bone or inorganic matter has been aspirated. A particularly dramatic presentation of the lodgment of aspirated food in the upper airways is the café coronary, so called because of its resemblance to myocardial infarction.[146]

ASPIRATION PNEUMONIA

The term "aspiration pneumonia" is employed by some to denote the inflammatory response in the lungs to infectious material aspirated from the mouth. This form of pneumonia is frequently caused by anaerobic organisms in patients with poor oral hygiene and commonly is associated with acute lung abscess. This type of aspiration is reviewed in Chapter 6 (*see* page 286). In this section we will deal exclusively with the results of regurgitation from the gastrointestinal tract.

Aspiration of foreign materials from the stomach or esophagus, usually food or its breakdown products, may give rise to various changes in the lung, including atelectasis, pneumonia, and lung abscess. As might be expected, gravity is the major factor affecting the anatomic distribution of pulmonary changes. Thus, the posterior segments of the upper and lower lobes are most commonly affected, particularly in debilitated or bedridden patients.

CHRONIC ASPIRATION PNEUMONIA

In contrast to the acute catastrophic events seen in Mendelson's syndrome (*see* page 505), a more chronic insidious type of aspiration occurs in various conditions, including hypopharyngeal (Zenker's) diverticulum, benign or malignant esophageal stenosis or stricture, achalasia, congenital or acquired tracheoesophageal fistula, and neuromuscular disturbances in swallowing.[147] In all of these, the pulmonary manifestations are the same.

Pathologic changes obviously depend upon the nature of the aspirated material. If gastric juice is included with solid material, an acute chemical pneumonitis usually results with polymorphonuclear infiltration, destruction of epithelial cells, and alveolar edema.[148] If the aspirate is contaminated by anaerobic organisms, a suppurative lung abscess may develop. When aspiration of food is more chronic and repeated, fibrotic and granulomatous reaction occurs in the interstitial tissues of the lung. The granulomas frequently contain foreign body giant cells.

Roentgenographically, the changes usually occur segmentally, involving one or more of the posterior segments of the upper or lower lobes. Some degree of atelectasis is present in almost all cases, and the picture is typical of "bronchopneumonia" (Figure 12–11). Serial roentgenography over a period of months or years shows much variation in the anatomic distribution of segments involved, disease clearing rather slowly in one segment and appearing anew in another.

The patient may be unaware of having aspirated, since such episodes often occur during sleep or following surgical anesthesia,[149] and the disease process may be so insidious that medical help is not sought for some time.

Clinically, productive cough and low-grade fever are present in most cases. Choking on swallowing is an important clue, particularly when tracheoesophageal fistula is present. Definitive diagnosis depends upon identification of the specific abnormality through roentgenologic study of the esophagus with barium.

LIPOID PNEUMONIA

Lipids may accumulate in the lungs from either endogenous or exogenous sources.[150] Accumulation of endogenous lipids constitutes an uncommon group of diseases, including cholesterol pneumonitis (with or without bronchial obstruction), fat embolism, pulmonary alveolar

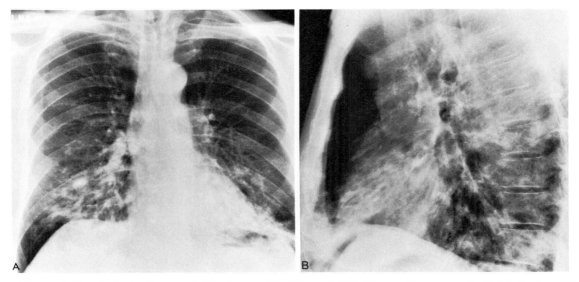

Figure 12–11. Aspiration Pneumonia (Carcinoma of the Pharynx). This 54-year-old man was admitted to the hospital for investigation of an oropharyngeal mass that proved, on biopsy, to be primary carcinoma. Roentgenograms of the chest on admission were normal. During his hospitalization, he developed cough and low-grade fever. Chest roentgenograms in posteroanterior (*A*) and lateral (*B*) projection revealed extensive inhomogeneous, segmental consolidation of both lower lobes, the middle lobe, and the lingula. The possibility that this was caused by aspiration was considered and a barium swallow was performed. Aspiration of barium into the trachea through the larynx was readily demonstrated.

proteinosis, histiocytosis-X, and the lipid storage diseases. These conditions are entirely different in nature from the exogenous forms and are considered elsewhere in this book (*see* page 662). The term "lipoid (lipid) pneumonia" is restricted here to exogenous disease caused by the aspiration of various vegetable, animal, or mineral oils into the lungs.

Mineral oil is undoubtedly the commonest offending agent. A variety of different clinical situations predispose to chronic oil aspiration—for example, the use of mineral oil in infants with feeding difficulties, by old people who are constipated, or by patients with dysphagia caused by neurologic lesions, hypopharyngeal (Zenker's) diverticulum, or achalasia. Oily nose drops are not used as widely as formerly, but cases of lipoid pneumonia are still seen secondary to nasal medication containing liquid paraffin.

Pathologically, the initial reaction to irritative oils, particularly animal fatty acids, is hemorrhagic bronchopneumonia. Secondary bacterial infection may occur, with resulting suppuration and, in some cases, empyema. By contrast, mineral oil, which is a relatively bland substance, occasions no more than a chronic insidious reaction in the lungs. When aspirated, it passes to the peripheral air spaces of the lungs where it is emulsified, the microscopic droplets appearing as free lipid or as intracytoplasmic droplets in macrophages. As the process ma-

tures, alveolar septal thickening becomes pronounced as a result of congestion, infiltration of lymphocytes and plasma cells, increase in reticulin, and fibrosis. Later, the normal lung architecture is replaced by pools of oil surrounded by a giant cell foreign body reaction. Macrophages filled with oil droplets reach the lymphatics, with resultant hyperplasia of lymphoid tissue in the lung and mediastinum. The abnormality is basically a fibrosing process and therefore is usually associated with loss of volume of affected segments.

Roentgenographically, the typical pattern depicts alveolar consolidation. Depending on the quantity of oil aspirated, the resultant air-space shadows may be confluent or discrete—and, in fact, isolated acinar shadows may form a distinctive feature during the early stages. The oil is taken from the alveolar spaces by macrophages that pass into the interstitial space, so that a predominantly interstitial pattern may develop. Although the roentgenographic pattern varies, its most common form shows relatively homogeneous consolidation of one or more segments, in most cases in the lower lobes but sometimes in the midzones, and often with precise segmental limitation (Figure 12–12).[150] The consolidated area may be several centimeters in diameter, with poorly defined or fairly sharply circumscribed margins. Another almost as common manifestation is a peripheral mass with either indistinct or well-circumscribed

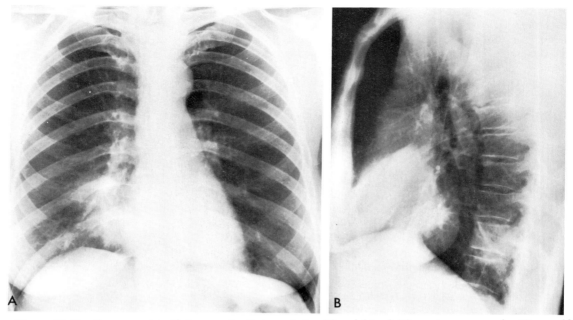

Figure 12–12. Exogenous Lipoid Pneumonia. Posteroanterior (A) and lateral (B) roentgenograms of a 53-year-old asymptomatic woman reveal rather poorly defined shadows of homogeneous density situated in the middle lobe, the anterior segment of the right lower lobe, and the posterior basal segment of the left lower lobe. Thorough clinical and laboratory investigations failed to reveal the cause of these shadows. Ten years later, the patient died following rupture of a congenital berry aneurysm of the anterior cerebral artery. Necropsy revealed inhalation lipid pneumonitis of both lower lobes and the middle lobe. (Courtesy of Dr. George Genereux, University Hospital, Saskatoon, Saskatchewan.)

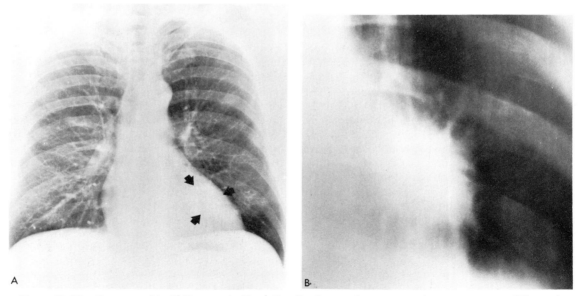

Figure 12–13. Exogenous Lipoid Pneumonia Simulating Carcinoma. A posteroanterior roentgenogram (A) reveals a poorly defined homogeneous opacity in the posterior portion of the left lower lobe (arrows). A tomogram in anteroposterior projection (B) shows a multitude of linear strands extending outward into contiguous lung, creating an appearance usually identified with bronchogenic carcinoma. The resected lobe revealed lipoid pneumonia. The patient was an asymptomatic 42-year-old man who had used oily nose drops for many years.

margins closely simulating peripheral broncho-genic carcinoma (Figure 12–13).[151] This lesion also develops chiefly in the dependent portions of the lung, although sometimes in the middle lobe or lingula. Withdrawal of the medication may be followed by slow but progressive roent-genographic resolution.

Clinically, in most cases the patient is asymp-tomatic and the abnormality is discovered on a screening chest roentgenogram, although some patients complain of chronic cough and pleuritic pain. The diagnosis may be suspected from a history of exposure to oily substances, particu-larly if obstructive esophageal disease is pres-ent. The finding of fat droplets in macrophages in the sputum adds weight to the diagnosis,[152] although fat may be identified in the sputum of normal subjects and its presence is not incon-trovertible evidence of pulmonary disease. Transthoracic percutaneous fine-needle aspira-tion biopsy or bronchoscopic biopsy will gen-erally establish the diagnosis with reasonable certainty; in fact, the latter procedure is pref-erable in some cases to exclude the possibility of an obstructing endobronchial neoplasm.[153, 154]

DRUG-INDUCED PULMONARY DISEASE

Iatrogenic pulmonary disease induced by drugs has received much attention in recent years and is a subject that has been well re-viewed.[155-160] The seriousness of the problem is indicated by the estimation that approximately 5 per cent of all inpatients suffer adverse drug reactions severe enough to cause marked mor-bidity, prolong hospitalization, result in per-manent sequelae, or contribute to a fatal out-come. More than 40 drugs or groups of drugs have been listed as potential agents,[155] and many of these have been dealt with in other sections of this book.

Six major reactions to drug therapy may occur in the lungs, and a host of different drugs may be associated with each. A complete listing can be obtained from the review articles referenced previously, particularly the 1979 review by De-meter and his colleagues.[156] In the following list of the six reactions, only a few examples of the most important drugs are indicated.

Bronchospasm (spasmodic asthma): ASA, in-domethacin, penicillin, tetracycline, erythro-mycin, and several other antibiotics.

Hypersensitivity pneumonitis (with or with-out peripheral eosinophilia): nitrofurantoin (acute phase), sulfonamides, PAS, penicillin.

Noncardiogenic pulmonary edema: heroin/morphine, methadone, propoxyphene, ASA.

Systemic lupus erythematosus: procainamide, hydralazine, penicillin, tetracycline, strepto-mycin, PAS.

Pulmonary vasculitis: penicillin, sulfona-mides, thiouracil.

Interstitial or air-space pneumonitis or both: A wide variety of antineoplastic drugs (*see be-low*), gold, amphotericin B, nitrofurantoin (chronic phase).

In this section we are concerned primarily with therapeutic agents that result in interstitial and alveolar cellular infiltration and fibrosis. The most common offending chemotherapeutic agents are the antineoplastic drugs, a state-of-the-art review of which has recently been pub-lished (Table 12–2).[159] In the following pages, only the most important of these drug reactions will be described in some detail.

BUSULFAN

This chemotherapeutic agent (trade name, Myleran) is used chiefly in the treatment of chronic granulocytic leukemia and was the first of this group to be incriminated as a cause of diffuse interstitial pulmonary fibrosis. The pul-monary disease may develop as early as 1 year after the initiation of therapy but more com-monly requires up to 4 years.[15] Pathologically, there has been observed intra-alveolar fibrosis and large atypical alveolar mononuclear cells. Electron microscopy has shown these bizarre atypical cells to be type II granular pneumo-cytes that have proliferated as a result of chemically-induced alveolitis. The chest roent-genogram shows a diffuse reticular pattern, sometimes with a superimposed acinar pattern indicating combined interstitial and air-space involvement (Figure 12–14); the disease may clear partly or completely following withdrawal of the drug. When such a pattern develops in a patient being treated with this drug, the differential diagnosis must include opportunistic infection in a compromised host (chiefly *Pneu-mocystis carinii* pneumonia). *Pneumocystis* pneumonia may be very difficult to exclude short of lung biopsy, since cessation of immu-nosuppressive therapy may also result in roent-genographic resolution of infection. Symptoms of busulfan-induced pulmonary disease include dyspnea, fever, weakness, weight loss, and a dry hacking cough. There may be sufficient disease to cause respiratory insufficiency. Pul-monary function tests show a restrictive defect with lowered diffusing capacity.[15]

TABLE 12–2. CLINICAL AND PATHOLOGICAL FEATURES OF ANTICANCER DRUG-INDUCED PNEUMONITIS*

Drug	Clinical Appearance	Chest Roentgenogram	Pathological Features	Mechanism
Alkylating Agents				
Busulfan	2% to 10% overall incidence; insidious onset after 4 yr (8 mo-10 yr), rarely after stopping the drug; fever, dyspnea, cough, rales—75%; pigmentation, weight loss, weakness—50%	Alveolar and interstitial pattern	Severe alveolar epithelial atypia; occasional bizarre granular pneumocytes; interstitial infiltrate and fibrosis	Directly toxic radiation predisposes
Cyclophosphamide	Rare reports; subacute onset after 3 wk-3 yr, also after stopping the drug; 2-50 g, more common after 10 g; reversible if drug taken for <3 mo; acute cardiac pulmonary edema; allergic reactions	Interstitial pattern	Similar to busulfan	Direct toxicity; possible hypersensitivity
Chlorambucil	Rare reports; subacute; after 6-22 mo of therapy	Same	Similar to busulfan; fibrosis may predominate	Direct
Melphalan	Few reports; appears after 1-48 mo of therapy; more common in patients older than 70 yr	Same	Alveolar epithelial atypia is more common than fibrosis	Direct
Nitrosoureas				
Carmustine	1.5%-20% incidence; transient; undocumented cases; after 4 mo-3 yr of therapy and after stopping carmustine therapy; prior lung disease and total dose >1,500 mg/sq m increase the risk	Same	Fibrosis may predominate; minimal atypia	Direct
Semustine	1 case; subacute; dyspnea and nonproductive cough	Same	Interstitial fibrosis; epithelial cuboidalization in alveoli	Direct
Antibiotics				
Bleomycin sulfate	3%-5% incidence; dose and schedule related (>450 mg), after mo of therapy or after stopping therapy; fever, cough; rales may precede roentgenographic changes; 10% mortality; rare low-dose toxicity; hypersensitivity pneumonitis variant	Interstitial pattern, often with alveolar superimposition	Interstitial edema and fibrosis; less cellular atypia; widespread alveolar destruction; squamous metaplasia and dysplasia of terminal bronchioles	Direct; hypersensitivity variant
Mitomycin	Less than a dozen cases; 5%-12% incidence after 6 mo of therapy; no fever, no dose relation; resolves after stopping drug therapy and starting steroid therapy	Interstitial pattern; rare pleural effusions	Similar to busulfan	Direct
Antimetabolites				
Methotrexate	More than 40 case reports; occurs from 12 days-5 yr after beginning therapy; possibly dose and schedule related (20 mg/wk); fever, headache; malaise; cough; dyspnea; eosinophilia—50%	Alveolar and interstitial pattern; rarely hilar adenopathy and pleural effusions	Interstitial and alveolar infiltrate of lymphocytes, eosinophils, and plasma cells; occasional poorly formed noncaseating granulomas; fibrosis may predominate	Direct, allergic
Mercaptopurine	Rare; acute onset	Interstitial	Alveolar epithelial proliferation; round cell infiltrate	Possibly direct
Azathioprine	One case; patient had previously received cyclophosphamide	Interstitial		Possibly direct
Cytarabine	Most common if given within 30 days of death; dyspnea during drug administration; abrupt onset of symptoms; gastrointestinal toxicity coexists	Interstitial and alveolar pattern	Interstitial and alveolar; proteinaceous with extravasation of RBCs; no inflammatory cells	Possible direct; hypoalbuminemia
Other Drugs				
Procarbazine hydrochloride	Acute onset within days of first dose, oral or intravenous; fever, chills, eosinophilia, arthralgias, and urticaria	Pleuroparenchymal pattern	Changes complicated by administration of other pulmonary toxins	Allergic
Zinostatin	Single case; dyspnea	Interstitial	Endothelial prominence affecting small vessels; thrombus formation; intimal thickening	Unknown

*Reproduced with minor modifications from Batist, G., and Andrews, J. L.: Pulmonary toxicity of antineoplastic drugs. J.A.M.A., *246*:1449, 1981, with permission of the authors and editor. Copyright 1981, American Medical Association.

In one study of 588 patients allocated at random to a 2-year course of therapy with busulfan, cyclophosphamide, or placebo following surgery for bronchial carcinoma,[162] roentgenographic appearances consistent with busulfan lung were identified in *none* of the 195 patients receiving a mean dose of 464 mg of busulfan over 301 days or of the 192 patients who received cyclophosphamide, but in one of the 201 patients who had received placebo! The reader may derive his or her own conclusions from this provocative study.

BLEOMYCIN

This antineoplastic, antimicrobial agent is associated with an incidence of pulmonary disease ranging from 2.6 per cent to approximately 10 per cent of treated patients, with most series in the 3 to 5 per cent range.[163] The death rate is roughly 50 per cent.[163] Although it has been suggested that the incidence of pulmonary toxicity is reduced by restricting the total dose to less than 500 mg, a number of instances have been reported of the development of proved

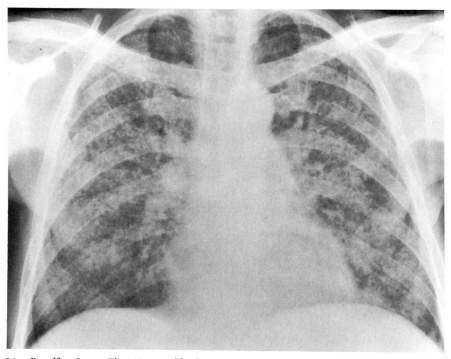

Figure 12–14. Busulfan Lung. This 61-year-old white woman was being treated for chronic myeloid leukemia with busulfan in a dose of 2 mg three times a day. At the time of this roentgenogram, she was complaining of severe exertional dyspnea and showed signs of congestive heart failure. The posteroanterior roentgenogram reveals a widespread coarse reticulonodular pattern throughout both lungs without anatomic predominance. The pattern suggests a predominant interstitial abnormality. The major functional abnormality was a reduction in diffusing capacity to less than half of that predicted. The patient died approximately 1 year later, and at necropsy there was observed generalized fibrous thickening of the alveolar walls with preservation of lung architecture.

interstitial fibrosis in patients who received less than 200 mg.[164] A recent prospective study of 13 patients, followed with pulmonary function testing for a period of six months, concluded that the risk of bleomycin toxicity can be reduced when the drug is given by a continuous infusion.[165]

Pathologically, bleomycin pneumonitis possesses characteristics similar if not identical to those of busulfan lung. Hemorrhage, fibrinous exudate, and occasionally hyaline membranes are present within the alveoli; alveolar epithelial cells contain bizarre hyperchromatic nuclei. There is infiltration of the interstitium by lymphocytes, plasma cells, eosinophils, and fibroblasts. In some areas advanced interstitial fibrosis can be identified.

Roentgenographic abnormalities in the chest consist of a reticular pattern that tends to progress to alveolar consolidation (Figure 12–15).[164] These changes may develop prior to, synchronous with, or following the appearance of clinical symptoms of cough and shortness of breath on exertion, both of which denote pulmonary

toxicity.[163] Pulmonary involvement may progress rapidly to fatal pulmonary insufficiency.[164] Early pulmonary involvement can be detected by a decrease in forced vital capacity and diffusing capacity at a time when the chest roentgenogram is still normal. Prior radiotherapy predisposes to bleomycin toxicity.[163, 164]

CYCLOPHOSPHAMIDE

This medication appears to be a rare cause of pulmonary alveolitis and fibrosis, judging from a recent report that recognized ten well-authenticated cases in the literature.[166]

METHOTREXATE

Pulmonary disease complicating intermittent therapy with this drug has a remarkably high incidence. In the Joint Leukemia Study,[167] pulmonary symptoms developed in 38 (41 per cent) of 93 children receiving maintenance metho-

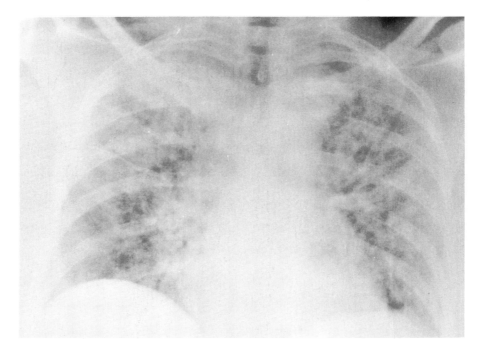

Figure 12–15. Acute Pulmonary Reaction to Bleomycin. Four months prior to the roentgenograms illustrated, histiocytic lymphoma was discovered in the left clavicle of this 55-year-old woman. Shortly thereafter, a 6-week course of chemotherapy was instituted that included a total of 198 units of bleomycin, 10.6 mg of vincristine, and 65 mg daily of prednisone. At the end of the 6-week course, she was begun on maintenance therapy with cyclophosphamide, 100 mg daily. Shortly thereafter, she noted the onset of weakness, dry cough, and a stuffy nose. She had a fever of 103°F, severe leukopenia (total white blood count 700 per cu mm), and was found to be anergic. At this time, a posteroanterior roentgenogram shows extensive disease throughout both lungs, the pattern of which suggests diffuse interstitial and air-space involvement of the parenchyma. An open lung biopsy was performed that day, sections being taken from the lingula and left lower lobe. Histologically, there was evidence of multifocal and diffuse interstitial pneumonitis with marked proliferation of alveolar lining cells. These cells were not only more numerous and larger than normal but contained nuclei whose bizarre appearance suggested drug-induced damage. A few intranuclear inclusion bodies were identified, chiefly in multinucleated cells. Hyaline membrane formation was present in some alveoli. There was no evidence of *Pneumocystis carinii* organisms. The final pathologic diagnosis was "extensive interstitial pneumonitis with rare inclusion body formation." Shortly thereafter, the patient developed acute respiratory failure from which recovery was prolonged.

trexate therapy. In contrast to other chemotherapeutic antineoplastic agents, this drug appears to initiate an acute allergic granulomatous reaction that subsides despite continuation of therapy.[168] In some cases, however, chronic interstitial fibrosis develops.[169] Although pathologic changes have not been extensively documented because of the self-limited nature of the disease, in one patient who was subjected to open lung biopsy, aggregates of mixed inflammatory cells were located both interstitially and in the alveoli, chiefly in the latter.[170] Large mononuclear cells predominated and there were noncaseating granulomas with giant cells. Clusters of lymphocytes and eosinophils were also present. The appearance was felt to be that of an "allergic granulomatous pneumonia." The roentgenographic changes are fairly characteristic and should suggest the diagnosis in the proper clinical setting. Initially, the chest roent-

genogram reveals a diffuse reticular pattern indicating widespread interstitial disease. This progresses rapidly to patchy acinar consolidation which, in time, reverts once again to an interstitial pattern followed by complete resolution.[170] Roentgenologically demonstrable disease may be present for periods ranging from a few days to a year. Paratracheal and hilar lymph nodes sometimes undergo a remarkable increase in size.[171]

The duration of maintenance methotrexate therapy before the development of symptoms ranges from less than 1 month to 5 years; the usual dose is 25 to 50 mg weekly.[168] Symptoms consist of the abrupt onset of fever, cough, dyspnea, and headache. Respiratory distress may be very severe and the patient may be cyanotic. There are usually no abnormal physical findings on examination of the chest. A moderate blood eosinophilia is common.[168]

Blood gas analysis in patients with methotrexate-induced pulmonary disease may show severe hypoxemia. Since acute *Pneumocystis carinii* pneumonia can produce an identical roentgenographic picture and similar clinical manifestations, this must constitute the most important differential possibility.[170] In fact, we know of no way of distinguishing the two conditions short of pathologic examination of tissue obtained by one of the various biopsy techniques.

REFERENCES

1. Stuart, B. O.: Deposition of inhaled aerosols. Arch. Intern. Med., *131*:60, 1973.
2. Davies, C. N.: The handling of particles by the human lungs. Br. Med. Bull., *19*:49, 1963.
3. Gross, P., and Detreville, R. T. P.: The lung as an embattled domain against inanimate pollutants. A precis of mechanisms. Am. Rev. Respir. Dis., *106*:684, 1972.
4. Vallyathan, N. V., Green, F. H. Y., and Craighead, J. E.: Recent advances in the study of mineral pneumoconiosis. Pathol. Annu., *15*(Pt.2):77, 1980.
5. Roub, L. W., Dekker, A., Wagenblast, H. W., and Reece, G. J.: Pulmonary silicatosis: a case diagnosed by needle-aspiration biopsy and energy-dispersive x-ray analysis. Am. J. Clin. Pathol., *72*:871, 1979.
6. Winner, P. C., and Blanchard, J. D.: Assessing the work environment for agents that may cause occupational pulmonary disease. Clin. Chest Med., *2*:317, 1981.
7. Weill, H.: Epidemiologic methods in the investigation of occupational lung disease. Am. Rev. Respir. Dis., *112*:1, 1975.
8. Amandus, H. E., Reger, R. B., Pendergrass, E. P., Dennis, J. M., and Morgan, W. K. C.: The pneumoconioses: Methods of measuring progression. Chest, *63*:736, 1973.
9. UICC-Cincinnati classification of the radiographic appearances of pneumoconioses. A cooperative study by the UICC committee. Chest, *58*:57, 1970.
10. Morgan, W. K. C., and Seaton, A.: Occupational Lung Diseases. Philadelphia, W. B. Saunders Co., 1975, p. 241.
11. Lapp, N. L.: Lung disease secondary to inhalation of nonfibrous minerals. Clin. Chest Med., *2*:219, 1981.
12. Hatch, T. F.: Significance of occupational history in diagnosis of silicosis. Radiology, *50*:746, 1948.
13. Ziskind, M., Jones, R. N., and Weill, H.: Silicosis. Am. Rev. Respir. Dis., *113*:643, 1976.
14. Buechner, H. A., and Ansari, A.: Acute silicoproteinosis. A new pathologic variant of acute silicosis in sandblasters, characterized by histologic features resembling alveolar proteinosis. Dis. Chest, *55*:274, 1969.
15. Bates, D. V., Macklem, P. T., and Christie, R. V.: Respiratory Function in Disease; An Introduction to the Integrated Study of the Lung. 2nd ed., Philadelphia, W. B. Saunders Co., 1971.
16. Felson, B.: Chest Roentgenology, Philadelphia, W. B. Saunders Co., 1973.
17. Greening, R. R., and Heslep, J. H.: The roentgenology of silicosis. Semin. Roentgenol. *2*:265, 1967.
18. Pendergrass, E. P.: Caldwell Lecture, 1957—Silicosis and a few of the other pneumoconioses: Observations of certain aspects of the problem, with emphasis on the role of the radiologist. Am. J. Roentgenol., *80*:1, 1958.
19. Bellini, F., and Ghislandi, E.: "Egg-shell" calcifications at extrahilar sites in a silicotuberculotic patient. Med. Lav., *51*:600, 1960.
20. Dee, P., Suratt, P., and Winn, W.: The radiographic findings in acute silicosis. Radiology, *126*:359, 1978.
21. Renzetti, A. D., Jr., Kobayashi, T., Bigler, A., and Mitchell, M. N.: Regional ventilation and perfusion in silicosis and in the alveolar-capillary block syndrome. Am. J. Med., *49*:5, 1970.
22. Becklake, M. R.: Pneumoconioses. *In* Fenn, W. O., and Rahn, H. (eds.): Handbook of Physiology, Section III, Vol. 2. Baltimore, Waverly Press, 1965, pp. 1601–1614.
23. Brink, G. C., Grzybowksi, S., and Lane, G. B.: Silicotuberculosis. Can. Med. Assoc. J., *82*:959, 1960.
24. Preger, Leslie, et al.: Asbestos-Related Disease. New York, Grune and Stratton, 1978.
25. Craighead, J. E., and Mossman, B. T.: The pathogenesis of asbestos-associated diseases. N. Engl. J. Med., *306*:1446, 1982.
26. Becklake, M. R.: Exposure to asbestos and human disease. N. Engl. J. Med., *306*:1480, 1982.
27. Becklake, M. R.: Asbestos-related diseases of the lung and other organs: Their epidemiology and implications for clinical practice. Am. Rev. Respir. Dis., *114*:187, 1976.
28. Peacock, P. R., Biancifiori, C., and Bucciarelli, E.: Examination of lung smears for asbestos bodies in 109 consecutive lung necropsies in Perugia. Eur. J. Cancer, *5*:155, 1969.
29. Selikoff, I. J., and Hammond, E. C.: Asbestos bodies in the New York City population in two periods of time. *In* Shapiro, H. A. (ed.): International Conference on Pneumoconiosis, Johannesburg, 1969. London, Oxford University Press, 1970, p. 99.
30. Gross, P., deTreville, R. T. P., Cralley, L. J., and Davis, J. M. G.: Pulmonary ferruginous bodies. Development in response to filamentous dusts and a method of isolation and concentration. Arch. Pathol., *85*:539, 1968.
31. Selikoff, I. J., Churg, J., and Hammond, E. C.: The occurrence of asbestosis among insulation workers in the United States. Ann. N.Y. Acad. Sci., *132*:139, 1965.
32. Parkes, W. R.: Asbestos-related disorders. Br. J. Dis. Chest, *67*:261, 1973.
33. Hourihane, D. O'B., Lessof, L., and Richardson, P. C.: Hyaline and calcified pleural plaques as an index of exposure to asbestos. A study of radiological and pathological features of 100 cases with a consideration of epidemiology. Br. Med. J., *1*:1069, 1966.
34. Turner-Warwick, M., and Parkes, W. R.: Circulating rheumatoid and antinuclear factors in asbestos workers. Br. Med. J., *3*:492, 1970.
35. Botham, S. K., and Holt, P. F.: The mechanism of formation of asbestos bodies. J. Pathol. Bacteriol., *96*:443, 1968.
36. Freundlich, I. M., and Greening, R. R.: Asbestosis and associated medical problems. Radiology, *89*:224, 1967.
37. Fletcher, D. E., and Edge, J. R.: The early radiological changes in pulmonary and pleural asbestosis. Clin. Radiol., *21*:355, 1970.

38. Sargent, E. N., Jacobson, G., and Gordonson, J. S.: Pleural plaques: A signpost of asbestos dust inhalation. Semin. Roentgenol., 12:287, 1977.

38a. Sargent, E. N., Gordonson, J., Jacobson, G., Birnbaum, W., and Shaub, M.: Bilateral pleural thickening: A manifestation of asbestos dust exposure. Am. J. Roentgenol., 131:579, 1978.

39. Anton, H. C.: Multiple pleural plaques: Part II. Br. J. Radiol., 41:341, 1968.

40. Solomon, A.: Radiology of asbestosis. Environ. Res., 3:320, 1970.

41. Gaensler, E. A., and Kaplan, A. I.: Asbestos pleural effusion. Ann. Intern. Med., 74:178, 1971.

42. Sluis-Cremer, G. K., and Webster, I.: Acute pleurisy in asbestosis exposed persons. Environ. Res., 5:380, 1972.

43. Epler, G. R., McLoud, T. C., and Gaensler, E. A.: Prevalence and incidence of benign asbestos pleural effusion in a working population. J.A.M.A., 247:617, 1982.

44. Solomon, A., Goldstein, B., Webster, I., and Sluis-Cremer, G. K.: Massive fibrosis in asbestosis. Environ. Res., 4:430, 1971.

45. Mintzer, R. A., Gore, R. M., Vogelzang, R. L., and Holz, S.: Rounded atelectasis and its association with asbestos-induced pleural disease. Radiology, 139:567, 1981.

46. Kleinfeld, M., Messite, J., and Shapiro, J.: Clinical, radiological, and physiological findings in asbestosis. Arch. Intern. Med., 117:813, 1966.

47. McDonald, J. C., Liddell, F. D. K., Gibbs, G. W., Eyssen, G. E., and McDonald, A. D.: Dust exposure and mortality in chrysotile mining, 1910–75. Br. J. Ind. Med., 37:11, 1980.

48. Murphy, R. L. H., Jr., Ferris, B. G., Jr., Burgess, W. A., Worcester, J., and Gaensler, E. A.: Effects of low concentrations of asbestos. Clinical, environmental, radiologic and epidemiologic observations in shipyard pipe coverers and controls. N. Engl. J. Med., 285:1271, 1971.

49. McDonald, J. C.: Asbestos and lung cancer: has the case been proven? Chest, 78:(Suppl.):374, 1980.

50. Enterline, P. E.: Attributability in the face of uncertainty. Chest, 78:(Suppl.):377, 1980.

51. Sluis-Cremer, G. K.: The relationship between asbestosis and bronchial cancer. Chest, 78:(Suppl.):380, 1980.

52. Selikoff, I. J., and Hammond, E. C.: Asbestos and smoking. (Editorial.) J.A.M.A., 242:458, 1979.

53. Berry, G.: Mortality of workers certified by pneumoconiosis medical panels as having asbestosis. Br. J. Ind. Med., 38:130, 1981.

54. Enticknap, J. B., and Smither, W. J.: Peritoneal tumours in asbestosis. Br. J. Ind. Med., 21:20, 1964.

55. Rabinowitz, J. G., Efremidis, S. C., Cohen, B., et al.: A comparative study of mesothelioma and asbestosis using computed tomography and conventional chest radiography. Radiology, 144:453, 1982.

56. Kleinfeld, M., Messite, J., and Tabershaw, I. R.: Talc pneumoconiosis. A.M.A. Arch. Ind. Health, 12:66, 1955.

57. Kleinfeld, M., Messite, J., Kooyman, O., and Zaki, M. H.: Mortality among talc miners and millers in New York State. Arch. Environ. Health, 14:663, 1967.

58. Seaton, A., Lamb, D., Brown, W. R., Sclare, G., and Middleton, W. G.: Pneumoconiosis of shale miners. Thorax, 36:412, 1981.

59. Olscamp, G., Herman, S. J., and Weisbrod, G. L.: Nepheline rock dust pneumoconiosis: a report of two cases. Radiology, 142:29, 1982.

60. Morgan, W. K. C., and Lapp, N. L.: Respiratory disease in coal miners. Am. Rev. Respir. Dis., 113:531, 1976.

61. Green, F. H. Y., and Laqueur, W. A.: Coal workers' pneumoconiosis. Pathol. Annu., 15:333, 1980.

62. Naeye, R. L., Mahon, J. K., and Dellinger, W. S.: Rank of coal and coal workers' pneumoconiosis. Am. Rev. Respir. Dis., 103:350, 1971.

63. Seaton, A., Dodgson, J., Dick, J. A., and Jacobsen, M.: Quartz and pneumoconiosis in coalminers. Lancet, 2:1272, 1981.

64. Gough, J., and Heppleston, A. G.: The pathology of the pneumoconioses. In King, E. J., and Fletcher, C. M. (eds.): Industrial Pulmonary Diseases: A symposium held at the Post-graduate Medical School of London, 18–20 September 1957 and 25–27 March 1958. London, J. & A. Churchill, 1960, pp. 23–26.

65. Bennett, J. G., Dick, J. A., Kaplan, Y. S., et al.: The relationship between coal rank and the prevalence of pneumoconiosis. Br. J. Ind. Med., 36:206, 1979.

66. Soutar, C. A., Turner-Warwick, M., and Parkes, W. R.: Circulating antinuclear antibody and rheumatoid factor in coal pneumoconiosis. Br. Med. J., 3:145, 1974.

67. Lippman, M., Eckert, H. L., Hahon, N., and Morgan, W. K. C.: Circulating antinuclear and rheumatoid factors in coal miners. A prevalence study in Pennsylvania and West Virginia. Ann. Intern. Med., 79:807, 1973.

68. Wagner, J. C., and McCormick, J. N.: Immunological investigations of coal workers' disease. J. R. Coll. Physicians Lond., 2:49, 1967.

69. Pearson, D. J., Mentnech, M. S., Elliott, J. A., et al.: Serologic changes in pneumoconiosis and progressive massive fibrosis of coal workers. Am. Rev. Respir. Dis., 124:696, 1981.

70. Fisher, E. R., Watkins, G., Lam, N. V., et al.: Objective pathological diagnosis of coal workers' pneumoconiosis. J.A.M.A., 245:1829, 1981.

71. Gough, J., James, W. R. L., and Wentworth, J. E.: A comparison of the radiological and pathological changes in coalworkers' pneumoconiosis. J. Fac. Radiol., 1:28, 1949.

72. Gough, J., and Heppleston, A. G.: The pathology of the pneumoconioses. In King, E. J., and Fletcher, C. M. (eds.): Industrial Pulmonary Diseases: A symposium held at the Post-graduate Medical School of London, 18–20 September 1957 and 25–27 March 1958. London, J. & A. Churchill, 1960, pp. 23–26.

73. Lyons, J. P., and Campbell, H.: Relation between progressive massive fibrosis, emphysema, and pulmonary dysfunction in coalworkers' pneumoconiosis. Br. J. Ind. Med., 38:125, 1981.

74. Ryder, R., Lyons, J. P., Campbell, H., and Gough, J.: Emphysema in coal workers' pneumoconiosis. Br. Med. J., 3:481, 1970.

75. Lyons, J. P., Ryder, R., Campbell, H., and Gough, J.: Pulmonary disability in coal workers' pneumoconiosis. Br. Med. J., 1:713, 1972.

76. Shennan, D. H., Washington, J. S., Thomas, D. J., et al.: Factors predisposing to the development of progressive massive fibrosis in coal miners. Br. J. Ind. Med., 38:321, 1981.

77. Morgan, W. K. C.: Respiratory disease in coal miners. J.A.M.A., 231:1347, 1975.

78. Cochrane, A. L., and Moore, F.: A 20-year follow-up

of men aged 55–64 including coal-miners and foundry workers in Staveley, Derbyshire. Br. J. Ind. Med., 37:226, 1980.

79. Morgan, W. K. C., Lapp, N. L., and Seaton, D.: Respiratory disability in coal miners. J.A.M.A., 243:2401, 1980.

80. Ball, J.: The natural history and management of coal workers' pneumoconiosis. In King, E. J., and Fletcher, C. M. (eds.): Industrial Pulmonary Diseases: A symposium held at the Post-graduate Medical School of London, 18–20 September 1957 and 25–27 March 1958. London, J. & A. Churchill, 1960, pp. 241–254.

81. Gilson, J. C., and Hugh-Jones, P.: Lung function in coalworkers' pneumoconiosis. Medical Research Council, Special Report 290, HMSO London, 1955.

82. Morgan, W. K. C., Handelsman, L., Kibelstis, J., Lapp, N. L., and Reger, R.: Ventilatory capacity and lung volumes of U.S. coal miners. Arch. Environ. Health, 28:182, 1974.

83. Musk, A. W., Cotes, J. E., Bevan, C., and Campbell, M. J.: Relationship between type of simple coalworkers' pneumoconiosis and lung function. A nine-year follow-up study of subjects with small rounded opacities. Br. J. Ind. Med., 38:313, 1981.

84. Lyons, J. P., and Campbell, H.: Relation between progressive massive fibrosis, emphysema, and pulmonary dysfunction in coal workers' pneumoconiosis. Br. J. Ind. Med., 38:125, 1981.

85. McLaughlin, A. I., G.: Iron and other radiopaque dusts. In King, E. J., and Fletcher, C. M. (eds.): Industrial Pulmonary Diseases: A symposium held at the Post-graduate Medical School of London, 18–20 September 1957 and 25–27 March 1958. London, J. & A. Churchill, 1960, pp. 146–167.

86. McLaughlin, A. I. G., and Harding, H. E.: The causes of death in iron and steel workers (non-foundry). Br. J. Ind. Med., 18:33, 1961.

87. Sander, O. A.: The nonfibrogenic (benign) pneumoconioses. Semin. Roentgenol., 2:312, 1967.

88. Robertson, A. J.: Pneumoconiosis due to tin oxide. In King, E. J., and Fletcher, C. M. (eds.): Industrial Pulmonary Diseases: A symposium held at the Post-graduate Medical School of London, 18–20 September 1957 and 25–27 March, 1958. London, J. & A. Churchill, 1960, pp. 168–184.

89. Cooper, D. A., Pendergrass, E. P., Vorwald, A. J., Mayock, R. L., and Brieger, H.: Pneumoconiosis among workers in an antimony industry. Am. J. Roentgenol., 103:495, 1968.

90. Heuck, F., and Hoschek, R.: Cer-pneumoconiosis. Am. J. Roentgenol., 104:777, 1968.

91. Hasan, F. M., and Kazemi, H.: Chronic beryllium disease: A continuing epidemiologic hazard. Chest, 65:289, 1974.

92. Deodhar, S. D., Barna, B., and Van Ordstrand, H. S.: A study of the immunologic aspects of chronic berylliosis. Chest, 63:309, 1973.

93. DeNardi, J. M., Van Ordstrand, H. S., and Curtis, G. H.: Berylliosis. Summary and survey of all clinical types in ten year period. Cleve. Clin. Q., 19:171, 1952.

94. American College of Chest Physicians Report of the Section on Nature and Prevalence Committee on Occupational Diseases of the Chest: Beryllium disease. Dis. Chest, 48:550, 1965.

95. Dudley, H. R.: The pathologic changes of chronic beryllium disease. A.M.A. Arch. Ind. Health, 19:184, 1959.

96. Gary, J. E., and Schatzki, R.: Radiological abnormal-

ities in chronic pulmonary disease due to beryllium. A.M.A. Arch. Ind. Health, 19:117, 1959.

97. Gaensler, E. A., Verstraeten, J. M., Weil, W. B., et al.: Respiratory pathophysiology in chronic beryllium disease. Review of thirty cases with some observations after long-term steroid therapy. A.M.A. Arch. Ind. Health, 19:132, 1959.

98. Norris, G. F., and Peard, M. C.: Berylliosis: Report of two cases, with special reference to the patch test. Br. Med. J., 1:378, 1963.

99. Edling, N. P. G.: Aluminium pneumoconiosis. A roentgendiagnostic study of five cases. Acta Radiol., 56:170, 1961.

100. Conner, E., Dubois, A., and Comroe, J., Jr.: Acute chemical injury of the airway and lungs. Anesthesiology, 23:538, 1962.

101. Northway, W. H., Jr., Rosan, R. C., and Porter, D. Y.: Pulmonary disease following respirator therapy of hyaline-membrane disease. Bronchopulmonary dysplasia. N. Engl. J. Med., 276:357, 1967.

102. Nash, G., Blennerhassett, J. B., and Pontoppidan, H.: Pulmonary lesions associated with oxygen therapy and artificial ventilation. N. Engl. J. Med., 276:368, 1967.

103. Balentine, J. D.: Pathologic effects of exposure to high oxygen tensions. A review. N. Engl. J. Med., 275:1038, 1966.

104. Cross, C. E., De Lucia, A. J., Reddy, A. K., Hussain, M. Z., Chow, C.-K., and Mustafa, M. G.: Ozone interactions with lung tissue. Biochemical approaches. Am. J. Med., 60:929, 1976.

105. Editorial: Ozone in smog. Lancet, 2:1077, 1975.

106. Hackney, J. D., Linn, W. S., Mohler, J. G., Pedersen, E. E., Breisacher, P., and Russo, A.: Experimental studies on human health effects of air pollutants. II. Four-hour exposure to ozone alone and in combination with other pollutant gases. Arch. Environ. Health, 30:379, 1975.

107. Bates, D. V., Bell, G. M., Burnham, C. D., et al.: Short-term effects of ozone on the lung. J. Appl. Physiol., 32:176, 1972.

108. Lowry, T., and Schuman, L. M.: "Silo-filler's disease"—a syndrome caused by nitrogen dioxide. J.A.M.A., 162:153, 1956.

109. Becklake, M. R., Goldman, H. I., Bosman, A. R., and Freed, C. C.: The long-term effects of exposure to nitrous fumes. Am. Rev. Tuberc., 76:398, 1957.

110. Ramirez-R. J., and Dowell, A. R.: Silo-filler's disease: Nitrogen dioxide-induced lung injury. Long-term follow-up and review of the literature. Ann. Intern. Med., 74:569, 1971.

111. Cornelius, E. A., and Betlach, E. H.: Silo-filler's disease. Radiology, 74:232, 1960.

112. Woodford, D. M., Coutu, R. E., and Gaensler, E. A.: Obstructive lung disease from acute sulfur dioxide exposure. Respiration, 38:238, 1979.

113. Ploysongsang, Y., Beach, B. C., and DiLisio, R. E.: Pulmonary function changes after acute inhalation of chlorine gas. South. Med. J., 75:23, 1982.

114. Montague, T. J., and Macneil, A. R.: Mass ammonia inhalation. Chest, 77:496, 1980.

115. Phillips, A. W., Tanner, J. W., and Cope, O.: Burn therapy. IV. Respiratory tract damage (an account of the clinical, x-ray and postmortem findings) and the meaning of restlessness. Ann. Surg., 158:799, 1963.

116. Pietak, S. P., and Delahaye, D. J.: Airway obstruction following smoke inhalation. Can. Med. Assoc. J., 115:329, 1976.

117. Achauer, B. M., Allyn, P. A., Furnas, D. W., and

Bartlett, R. H.: Pulmonary complications of burns: The major threat to the burn patient. Ann. Surg., 177:311, 1973.

118. Kangarloo, H., Beachley, M. C., and Ghahremani, G. G.: The radiographic spectrum of pulmonary complications in burn victims. Am. J. Roentgenol., 128:441, 1977.

119. Peters, W. J.: Inhalation injury caused by the products of combustion. C.M.A. Journal, 125:249, 1981.

120. Done, A. K.: The toxic emergency: Where there's smoke, there may be more than fire. Emerg. Med., 13:111, 1981.

121. Dyer, R. F., and Esch, V. H.: Polyvinyl chloride toxicity in fires. Hydrogen chloride toxicity in fire fighters. J.A.M.A., 235:393, 1976.

122. Putman, C. E., Loke, J., Matthay, R. A., and Ravin, C. E.: Radiographic manifestations of acute smoke inhalation. Am. J. Roentgenol., 129:865, 1977.

123. Lilis, R.: Vinyl chloride and polyvinyl chloride exposure and occupational lung disease. Chest, 78:826, 1980.

124. Smith, J. S., and Brandon, S.: Morbidity from acute carbon monoxide poisoning at three-year follow-up Br. Med. J., 1:318, 1973.

125. Astrup, P.: Some physiological and pathological effects of moderate carbon monoxide exposure. Br. Med. J., 4:447, 1972.

126. Bergmann, M., Flance, I. J., and Blumenthal, H. T.: Thesaurosis following inhalation of hair spray: A clinical and experimental study. N. Engl. J. Med., 258:471, 1958.

127. Bergmann, M., Flance, I. J., Cruz, P. T., et al.: Thesaurosis due to inhalation of hair spray. Report of twelve new cases, including three autopsies. N. Engl. J. Med., 266:750, 1962.

128. Giovacchini, R. P., Becker, G. H., Brunner, M. J., and Dunlap, F. E.: Pulmonary disease and hairspray polymers. Effects of long-term exposure of dogs. J.A.M.A., 193:298, 1965.

129. Gowdy, J. M., and Wagstaff, M. J.: Pulmonary infiltration due to aerosol thesaurosis. A survey of hairdressers. Arch. Environ. Health, 25:101, 1972.

130. Schraufnagel, D. E., Paré, J. A. P., and Wang, N.-S.: Micronodular pulmonary pattern: Association with inhaled aerosol. Am. J. Roentgenol., 137:57, 1981.

131. Palmer, K. C., Snider, G. L., and Hayes, J. A.: Cellular proliferation induced in the lung by cadmium aerosol. Am. Rev. Respir. Dis., 112:173, 1975.

132. DeSilva, P. E., and Donnan, M. B.: Chronic cadmium poisoning in a pigment manufacturing plant. Br. J. Ind. Med., 38:76, 1981.

133. Lauwerys, R. R., Roels, H. A., Buchet, J.-P., Bernard, A., and Stanescu, D.: Investigations on the lung and kidney function in workers exposed to cadmium. Environ. Health Perspect., 28:137, 1979.

134. Wyse, D. G.: Deliberate inhalation of volatile hydrocarbons: A review. Can. Med. Assoc. J., 108:71, 1973.

135. Manson, M. M.: Epoxides—is there a human health problem? Br. J. Ind. Med., 37:317, 1980.

136. Herbert, F. A., and Orford, R.: Pulmonary hemorrhage and edema due to inhalation of resins containing tri-mellitic anhydride. Chest, 76:546, 1979.

137. Patterson, R., Addington, W., Banner, A. S., et al.: Antihapten antibodies in workers exposed to trimellitic anhydride fumes: A potential immunopathogenetic mechanism for the trimellitic anhydride

pulmonary disease-anemia syndrome. Am. Rev. Respir. Dis., 120:1259, 1979.

138. Wolfe, B. M., Brodeur, A. E., and Shields, J. B.: The role of gastrointestinal absorption of kerosene in producing pneumonitis in dogs. J. Pediatr., 76:867, 1970.

139. Brünner, S., Rovsing, H., and Wulf, H.: Roentgenographic changes in the lungs of children with kerosene poisoning. Am. Rev. Respir. Dis., 89:250, 1964.

140. Cooke, N. J., Flenley, D. C., and Matthew, H.: Paraquat poisoning. Q. J. Med., 42:683, 1973.

141. Kimbrough, R. D.: Toxic effects of the herbicide paraquat. Chest, 65(Suppl.):65S, 1974.

142. Thurlbeck, W. M., and Thurlbeck, S. M.: Pulmonary effects of paraquat poisoning. Chest, 69(Suppl):276, 1976.

143. Davidson, J. K., and MacPherson, P.: Pulmonary changes in paraquat poisoning. Clin. Radiol., 23:18, 1972.

144. Brown, B. St. J., Ma, H., Dunbar, J. S., and MacEwan, D. W.: Foreign bodies in the tracheobronchial tree in childhood. J. Can. Assoc. Radiol., 14:158, 1963.

145. Capitanio, M. A., and Kirkpatrick, J. A.: The lateral decubitus film. An aid in determining air-trapping in children. Radiology, 103:460, 1972.

146. Berkmen, Y. M.: Aspiration and inhalation pneumonias. Semin. Roentgenol., 15:73, 1980.

147. Hughes, R. L., Freilich, R. A., Bytell, D. E., Craig, R. M., and Moran, J. M.: Aspiration and occult esophageal disorders: Clinical conference in pulmonary disease from Northwestern University Medical School; Chicago, Chest, 80:489, 1981.

148. Wynne, J. W., Ramphal, R., and Hood, C. I.: Tracheal mucosal damage after aspiration: A scanning electron microscope study. Am. Rev. Respir. Dis., 124:728, 1981.

149. Broe, P. J., Toung, T. J. K., and Cameron, J. L.: Aspiration pneumonia. Surg. Clin. North Am., 60:1551, 1980.

150. Genereux, G. P.: Lipids in the lungs: Radiologic-pathologic correlation. J. Can. Assoc. Radiol., 21:2, 1970.

151. Kennedy, J. D., Costello, P., Balikian, J. P., and Herman, P. G.: Exogenous lipoid pneumonia. A.J.R., 136:1145, 1981.

152. Sundberg, R. H., Kirschner, K. E., and Brown, M. J.: Evaluation of lipoid pneumonia. Dis. Chest, 36:594, 1959.

153. Lipinski, J. K., Weisbrod, G. L., and Sanders, D. E.: Exogenous lipoid pneumonitis. J. Canad. Assoc. Radiol., 31:92, 1980.

154. Lipinski, J. K., Weisbrod, G. L., and Sanders, D. E.: Exogenous lipoid pneumonitis: Pulmonary patterns. Am. J. Roentgenol., 136:931, 1981.

155. Rosenow, E. C., III: The spectrum of drug-induced pulmonary disease. Ann. Intern. Med., 77:977, 1972.

156. Demeter, S. L., Ahmad, M., and Tomashefski, J. F.: Drug-induced pulmonary disease. Part I. Patterns of response. Part II. Categories of drugs. Part III. Agents used to treat neoplasms or alter the immune system including a brief review of radiation therapy. Clev. Clin. Q., 46:89, 1979.

157. Seltzer, S. E., and Herman P. G.: Drug-induced pulmonary reactions associated with abnormal chest radiograph. J.C.E. Radiol., 1:25, 1979.

158. Sostman, H. D., Putman, C. E., and Gamsu, G.:

Diagnosis of chemotherapy lung. Am. J. Roentgenol., *136*:33, 1981.

159. Batist, G., and Andrews, J. L., Jr.: Pulmonary toxicity of antineoplastic drugs. J.A.M.A., *246*:1449, 1981.

160. Morrison, D. A., and Goldman, A. L.: Radiographic patterns of drug-induced lung disease. Radiology, *131*:299, 1979.

161. Heard, B. E., and Cooke, R. A.: Busulphan lung. Thorax, *23*:187, 1968.

162. Stott, H., Stephens, R., Fox, W., Simon, G., and Roy, D. C.: An investigation of the chest radiographs in a controlled trial of busulphan, cyclophosphamide, and a placebo after resection for carcinoma of the lung. Thorax, *31*:265, 1976.

163. Samuels, M. L., Johnson, D. E., Holoye, P. Y., and Lanzotti, V. J.: Large-dose bleomycin therapy and pulmonary toxicity. A possible role of prior radiotherapy. J.A.M.A., *235*:1117, 1976.

164. Iacovino, J. R., Leitner, J., Abbas, A. K., Lokich, J. J., and Snider, G. L.: Fatal pulmonary reaction from low doses of bleomycin. An idiosyncratic tissue response, J.A.M.A., *235*:1253, 1976.

165. Cooper, K. R., and Hong, W. K.: Prospective study of the pulmonary toxicity of continuously infused bleomycin. Cancer Treat. Rep., *65*:419, 1981.

166. Collis, C. H.: Lung damage from cytotoxic drugs. Cancer Chemother. Pharmacol., *4*:17, 1980.

167. Cooperative study: Acute lymphocytic leukemia in children. Maintenance therapy with methotrexate administered intermittently. Acute Leukemia Group B. J.A.M.A., *207*:923, 1969.

168. Whitcomb, M. E., Schwarz, M. I., and Tormey, D. C.: Methotrexate pneumonitis: Case report and review of the literature. Thorax, *27*:636, 1972.

169. Henderson, J. and Paré, J. A. P.: Unpublished data, 1976.

170. Everts, C. S., Westcott, J. L., and Bragg, D. G.: Methotrexate therapy and pulmonary disease. Radiology, *107*:539, 1973.

171. Sostman, H. D., Matthay, R. A., Putman, C. E., and Smith, G. J. W.: Methotrexate-induced pneumonitis. Medicine, *55*:371, 1976.

172. Cordasco, E. M., Demeter, S. L., Kerkay, J., et al.: Pulmonary manifestations of vinyl and polyvinyl chloride (interstitial lung disease): newer aspects. Chest, *78*:828, 1980.

173. Whitwell, F., Newhouse, M. L., and Bennett, D. R.: A study of the histological cell types of lung cancer in workers suffering from asbestosis in the United Kingdon. Br. J. Ind. Med., *31*:298, 1974.

13

Diseases of the Thorax Caused by External Physical Agents

Trauma to the thorax may result in a wide variety of effects on the thoracic wall, diaphragm, mediastinum, and bronchopulmonary system. The results may be direct (for example, fractures of the ribs, spine, or shoulder girdles, traumatic diaphragmatic hernia, esophageal rupture, and pulmonary contusion or laceration) or indirect (such as air embolism resulting from the escape of air into pulmonary veins subsequent to parenchymal laceration).

This chapter deals with all effects of trauma on the thorax, both direct and indirect. Since the manifestations in the lungs, pleura, mediastinum, diaphragm, and chest wall are quite different, each of these is considered separately, although as might be anticipated a great deal of overlap occurs. Also, the effects of penetrating and nonpenetrating trauma may be quite different and thus require separate consideration. In the section on penetrating trauma, the postoperative chest is dealt with in some detail. "Trauma" is used here in its broad sense to indicate all affections of the thorax resulting from *external physical agents;* thus, irradiation injury is included in this category.

EFFECTS ON THE LUNGS OF NONPENETRATING TRAUMA

PULMONARY PARENCHYMAL CONTUSION

Pulmonary contusion consists of the exudation of edema fluid and blood into the parenchyma of the lung in both its air-space and interstitial components,[1, 2] and is the most common pulmonary complication of blunt chest trauma. In nonpenetrating injuries it occurs more frequently than rib fracture[1, 2] and, indeed, rib fractures are frequently absent.

Roentgenographically, the pattern varies from irregular, patchy areas of air-space consolidation (Figure 13–1) to diffuse and extensive homogeneous consolidation. As might be expected, there is no conformity to lobes or segments.[1] Although the major change is usually in the lung directly deep to the traumatized areas, it may develop also, or even predominantly, on the opposite side, as a result of a contrecoup effect. Changes are apparent roentgenographically soon after trauma (almost invariably within 6 hours). Resolution typically occurs rapidly, improvement being noted within 24 to 48 hours[2] and clearing usually being complete within 3 or 4 days (Figure 13–1).[1–3]

Clinically, the findings are seldom striking; in fact, symptoms may be entirely absent or may be masked by the many other injuries the patient may have.[4] Hemoptysis is said to occur in 50 per cent of cases, and there may be mild fever; shortness of breath may develop following severe contusion.

PULMONARY PARENCHYMAL LACERATION, TRAUMATIC LUNG CYST, AND HEMATOMA

Closed chest trauma can result in the development of one or more cystic spaces within the lung that may remain air-filled or may fill partly or completely with blood. The trauma usually is blunt and often severe, as in automobile accidents. Children and young adults seem to be particularly prone, probably because of the greater flexibility of their thoracic walls. In a recent review of the literature,[5] of 40 cases of traumatic lung cysts, 88 per cent occurred in patients under the age of 30 years.

Three mechanisms have been suggested to explain the development of traumatic lung

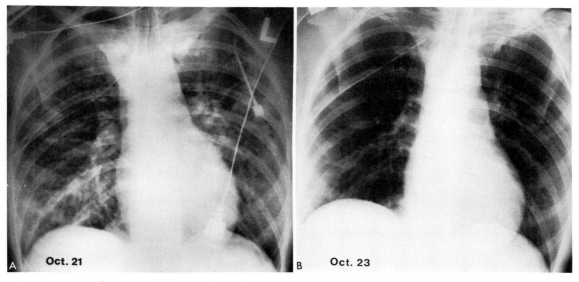

Figure 13–1. Pulmonary Contusion with Rapid Resolution. Shortly after his arrival in the emergency room following an automobile accident, this 22-year-old man showed roentgenographic evidence of poorly defined patchy air-space consolidation throughout both lungs *(A)*. The appearance is one of pulmonary edema of any cause, although the history and normal cardiac size obviously favor traumatic contusion. Complete clearing had occurred 48 hours later *(B)*.

cysts. (1) The physical force ruptures alveolar tissue, and the inherently elastic lung parenchyma recoils from the ruptured area, leaving a spherical cystic lesion. (2) Sudden compression of an area of lung closes off a segment of the peripheral bronchial tree and creates within it a bursting, explosive-like pressure that is expended in the rupture of successive alveolar walls within the lobules supplied by the occluded bronchus. (3) The propagation of a concussion wave creates shearing stresses that tear the substance of the lung.[1]

These lesions may be apparent roentgenographically immediately after trauma but more commonly are not seen until a few hours or even several days later, usually because their presence is masked by surrounding pulmonary contusion.[6]

Roentgenographically, they may appear as single or multiple lesions, unilocular or multilocular, ranging from oval to spherical and from 2 cm up to as large as 14 cm in diameter. Usually these cystic spaces are located subpleurally in peripheral areas of the lung. Their appearance depends in large measure on whether hemorrhage has occurred into them. Approximately half the lesions present as thin-walled air-filled cavities with or without fluid levels, and the remainder present as homogenous, well-circumscribed masses of water density—pulmonary hematomas (Figure 13–2). Bleeding into a cyst results from rupture of

capillaries. They may be single or multiple (Figure 13–3). Pneumothorax may occur occasionally.

A characteristic of these lesions is their tendency to persist for a long time, frequently up to 4 months. However, they generally decrease progressively in size.

There are no symptoms directly attributable to these lesions *per se,* unless they become infected, which is rare.[5] Pulmonary hematomas indistinguishable from those caused by closed chest trauma sometimes develop following segmental or wedge resection of the lung.

FRACTURES OF THE TRACHEA AND BRONCHI

Fractures of the tracheobronchial tree usually result from blunt trauma to the anterior chest in vehicular accidents; the incidence is highest in males under 40 years of age. In adults particularly, the trauma is severe enough to result in fractures of the first three ribs; this was observed in an astonishing 91 per cent of patients in one series.[7] In children, rib fractures are seldom seen, presumably owing to the resiliency of the rib cage. Fractures of the intrathoracic trachea are horizontal and usually occur just above the carina.[2, 3] Fractures of the bronchi (*synonyms:* rupture, transection) constitute 80 per cent of tracheobronchial injuries.[3] They are usually horizontal and complete and

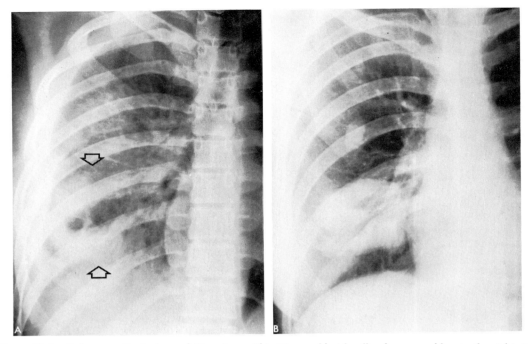

Figure 13–2. Pulmonary Contusion and Hematoma. This 15-year-old girl suffered a severe blow to the right side of her chest in a car accident. Three hours after the accident, an anteroposterior roentgenogram (A) demonstrates extensive consolidation of the parenchyma of the right lung due to pulmonary contusion (the left lung was clear). In addition to the diffuse opacity, an indistinctly defined shadow of greater density is present in the right base *(arrows)*, containing a central radiolucency; there is a large hemothorax. Three weeks later (B), the general opacity caused by contusion has completely cleared, as has the hemothorax. However, there remains a large, sharply circumscribed, lobulated shadow containing an air-fluid level that represents the laceration and hematoma vaguely visible in (A). A much smaller hematoma can be identified in the lung directly above the major lesion. Complete clearing did not occur until 6 months later. (Courtesy of Dr. J. G. Monks, Rosetown Union Hospital, Rosetown, Saskatchewan.)

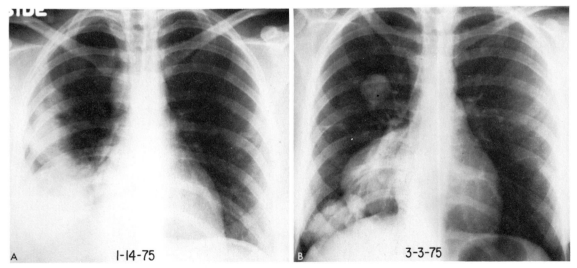

Figure 13–3. Multiple Unilateral Pulmonary Hematomas. This 17-year-old white girl was involved in a two-car collision in which she sustained fractures of her right scapula and humerus. The day after admission, an anteroposterior roentgenogram (A) revealed extensive parenchymal consolidation in the lower two-thirds of the right lung in nonsegmental distribution; the left lung was clear. There was some widening of the superior mediastinum, undoubtedly from venous hemorrhage. Two months later, a roentgenogram in posteroanterior projection (B) revealed multiple, sharply circumscribed homogeneous nodules in the right lung ranging from 1 to 6 cm in diameter (12 discrete nodules can be identified). No cavitation was present and the left lung remained clear. Seven months after the injury, all signs of disease had disappeared. (Courtesy of Dr. John D. Armstrong, Jr., University of Utah College of Medicine and Valley West Hospital, Salt Lake City, Utah.)

involve the main-stem bronchi 1 to 2 cm distal to the carina.[2, 3] This complication of trauma is very uncommon but is one of the most serious intrathoracic visceral injuries resulting from closed chest trauma. Unfortunately its rarity probably contributes to the infrequency with which it is recognized early. The right main bronchus is affected more frequently than the left, and the pulmonary vessels are rarely damaged.[8]

Roentgenologically, the most common finding is pneumothorax, although this is not present in 30 per cent of cases,[9] probably because fracture commonly affects the bronchi within the mediastinum and the mediastinal parietal pleura remains intact. Pneumothorax may be very large and characteristically does not respond to chest tube drainage because of the free communication between the fractured airway and pleural space.[10] Escape of air into the mediastinum may lead to mediastinal and deep cervical emphysema; the combination of a large pneumothorax and mediastinal emphysema in the absence of pleural effusion serves as a useful diagnostic criterion. Displacement of fracture ends may lead to bronchial obstruction and atelectasis of an entire lung (Figure 13–4),[2] but it is important to recognize that atelectasis may be a late development, and the discovery of such a change some time after an accident should strongly suggest the diagnosis. Fractures of one or more of the first three ribs should provide additional confirmatory evidence.

Symptoms and signs include cyanosis, pain, hemoptysis, shock, and cough. Air usually is identifiable in the subcutaneous tissues, initially involving the neck and upper thorax and later becoming generalized. When pneumothorax has developed, a large air leak may prevent expansion of the lung, even with intercostal tube suction. Such a situation should strongly suggest the diagnosis.

In approximately 10 per cent of patients, tracheobronchial fracture is unassociated with roentgenographically demonstrable abnormality or with much in the way of symptoms or signs.[3] It is probable that in such cases the bronchial sheath is preserved, thus preventing passage of air into the mediastinum or pleura. Thus, the consequence of the trauma may not become evident until the patient presents with atelectasis of a lobe or lung as a result of bronchial stenosis. Bronchoscopy is superior to bronchography in the early stages of the injury,[11] although the latter procedure may be of value in the assessment of bronchial deformity in later, more chronic stages (Figure 13–4). In either

stage, tomography may be of help in revealing large defects in the trachea or major bronchi.

The overall mortality of tracheobronchial injury resulting from blunt trauma is approximately 30 per cent, more than half of these patients dying within 1 hour of injury.[12] Early diagnosis is extremely important, since primary surgical repair results in anatomic and functional restoration.[13]

LUNG TORSION

This rare complication of trauma occurs almost invariably in children, presumably because of the easy compressibility of their thoracic cage. The trauma usually is severe, such as when a child is run over by a vehicle, and torsion occurs most often when the major force is applied to the compressible lower thorax. The lung is twisted through 180 degrees, so that its base comes to lie at the apex of the hemithorax and its apex at the base. The diagnosis should be obvious from the roentgenographic appearance of the chest. The pattern of pulmonary vascular markings is altered in a predictable manner, the main lower lobe artery sweeping upward toward the apex and the lower lung vessels being comparatively diminutive. If the torsion is not relieved, vascular supply is compromised and the lung becomes roentgenographically opaque as a result of exudation of edema fluid and blood into the air spaces.[2, 14]

ATELECTASIS

Post-traumatic collapse of a lobe—or very occasionally of a whole lung—is not common, but when present constitutes a cause of significant venoarterial shunting at a time when a patient's clinical status may be in balance. The cause of the atelectasis is not always clear, although it is probable that most cases are owing to bronchial obstruction from blood clots or mucous plugs. In such circumstances, bronchoscopy will readily reveal the cause and permit prompt relief of the obstruction.

ADULT RESPIRATORY DISTRESS SYNDROME

The ominous consequences of prolonged shock in the immediate post-traumatic period are those of the adult respiratory distress syndrome of any etiology and have been thoroughly described in Chapter 10 (*see* page 512).

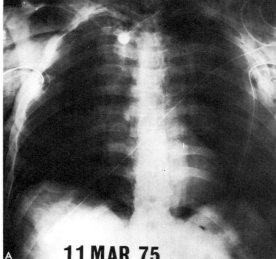

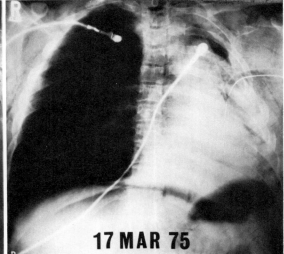

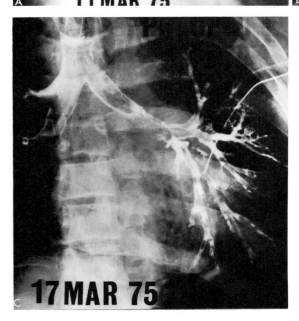

Figure 13–4. **Fracture of the Left Main Bronchus.** On admission to the hospital following a severe crushing injury to his chest, this 33-year-old man showed roentgenographic evidence *(A)* of severe subcutaneous and mediastinal emphysema and fractures of multiple left ribs, including the first, second, and third (not visible on the illustration). Bilateral pneumothorax had been treated in the emergency room by intubation. At this time, both lungs were well expanded. Six days later *(B)*, there had occurred almost total collapse of the left lung. Bronchoscopy revealed an obstruction in the midportion of the left main bronchus. The obstructing material resembled a blood clot, although in some areas the bronchoscopist thought he was looking at the edge of a cartilaginous ring. Bronchography performed shortly thereafter *(C)* revealed severe deformity and narrowing of the distal end of the left main-stem bronchus just before its bifurcation *(arrows)*. At thoracotomy, the left main bronchus was found to be completely disrupted just proximal to its bifurcation and this was repaired by end-to-end anastomosis. Both bronchoscopy and bronchography three months later revealed a stricture of the left main bronchus at the site of anastomosis, reducing its lumen by approximately half. (Courtesy of Dr. Harold Stolberg, Hamilton Civic Hospitals, Hamilton, Ontario.)

EFFECTS ON THE PLEURA OF NONPENETRATING TRAUMA

Hemothorax and pneumothorax are common manifestations of nonpenetrating trauma, and each may develop from a variety of causes.

HEMOTHORAX

Blood may enter the pleural space from injury to the chest wall, diaphragm, lung, or mediastinum. Although hemorrhage may result from laceration of the parietal or visceral pleura by fractured ribs, hemothorax or pneumothorax (or both) may occur in closed chest trauma without evidence of fracture. When blood enters the pleural space it coagulates rapidly, but, presumably as a result of physical agitation produced by movement of the heart and lungs, the clot may be defibrinated and leave fluid indistinguishable roentgenologically from effusion from any other cause.[2, 15] As in empyema, loculation tends to occur early in hemothorax, increasing still further the difficulty of obtaining needle drainage. The importance of the site of hemorrhage in relation to the quantity of hemothorax has been emphasized:[2] when bleeding is from a vessel in the chest wall, diaphragm, or mediastinum, the hemothorax tends to increase despite the quantity of blood present. When the blood comes from the pulmonary vasculature the expanding hemothorax compresses the lung, with resultant pulmonary tamponade that may produce hemostasis.

PNEUMOTHORAX

Pneumothorax complicating trauma may occur without roentgenographic evidence of rib fracture. When fracture is present the likely mechanism is laceration of the visceral pleura by rib fragments, and in such circumstances hemothorax may be expected as a concomitant finding. When no fractures are visible the usual mechanism is pulmonary *interstitial* emphysema secondary to pulmonary trauma and parenchymal laceration. This explanation also provides adequate reason for the occurrence of pneumomediastinum and subcutaneous emphysema without rib fracture.

When a pneumothorax is small and the visceral pleural line is poorly visualized, roentgenography at full expiration may reveal the partially collapsed lung to better advantage. When a patient's condition does not warrant roentgenography in the erect position, examination in the lateral decubitus position permits identification of very small quantities of gas in the pleural space;[16] in the supine position, small collections of gas are usually situated at the base of the hemithorax just above the diaphragm.

EFFECTS ON THE MEDIASTINUM OF NONPENETRATING TRAUMA

The abnormalities with which we are primarily concerned in nonpenetrating trauma to the mediastinum include pneumomediastinum, hemorrhage, rupture of the aorta and major vessels, perforation of the esophagus, and rupture of the thoracic duct. Traumatic abnormalities of the heart and pericardium are not within the scope of this book.

PNEUMOMEDIASTINUM

Traumatic pneumomediastinum may develop after closed chest trauma, and in such circumstances probably is produced by the same mechanism as spontaneous pneumomediastinum—the rupture of alveoli into the perivascular sheath as a result of an abrupt increase in pressure. Pneumomediastinum may also follow traumatic rupture of the esophagus (most commonly during diagnostic instrumentation) or fracture of the tracheobronchial tree; in the former case, the mediastinal emphysema may be associated with acute mediastinitis.

The roentgenographic signs are identical to those of pneumomediastinum from any cause (*see* Chapter 16).

MEDIASTINAL HEMORRHAGE

The majority of cases of mediastinal hemorrhage result from trauma, usually of a severe nature, such as that associated with an automobile accident. Less common causes include rupture of an aortic aneurysm,[17] faulty insertion of central venous lines, and extension of blood from the retropharyngeal soft tissues secondary to trauma or to spontaneous hemorrhage associated with coagulation disorders. Undoubtedly the majority of cases of mediastinal hemorrhage go unrecognized, the amount of bleeding being insufficient to produce symptoms and signs.

Roentgenologically, hemorrhage typically results in uniform, symmetrical widening of the mediastinum in any of its compartments. Local accumulation of blood in the form of a hematoma is manifested by a homogeneous mass that may project to one or both sides of the mediastinum and may be situated in any compartment.[17]

RUPTURE OF THE THORACIC AORTA AND ITS BRANCHES

Rupture of the aorta is a well-recognized sequela of closed chest injury, approximately 70 per cent of incidences following severe automobile accidents.[18] Because of the variable mobility of different portions of the aorta, sudden deceleration produces shearing stresses, the more mobile anterior portion of the aortic arch being "whipped" on the more fixed posterior arch and paraspinal aorta.[19] Approximately 95 per cent of all aortic ruptures occur in the region of the aortic isthmus at the site of the ligamentum arteriosum;[19] the remaining 5 per cent are immediately above the aortic valve. Immediate death is the usual result of aortic rupture, only 10 to 20 per cent of all patients with this injury living longer than 1 hour[19] and less than 5 per cent living long enough for a chronic traumatic aneurysm to develop. Surprisingly, complete transection of the aorta may be associated with survival.[20]

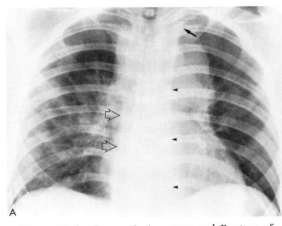

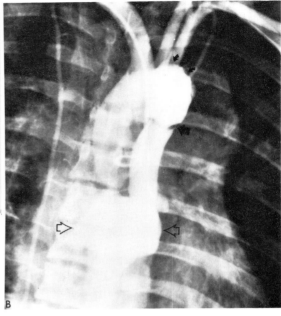

Figure 13–5. Traumatic Aneurysm and Rupture of the Thoracic Aorta. This 16-year-old boy crashed into a telephone pole in an automobile traveling at 85 mph. Shortly after his arrival in the emergency room, a chest roentgenogram in anteroposterior projection *(A)* revealed marked widening of the upper mediastinum and loss of visualization of the aortic knob. A wide paravertebral opacity *(arrowheads)* extends up to the apex, creating an early extrapleural apical cap *(arrow)*. Note also the widening of the right paravertebral stripe *(open arrows)*. The suspicion of aortic rupture was confirmed by aortography *(B)*. The site of primary aortic laceration is indicated by a *thick arrow,* the irregular bulge immediately above *(small arrows)* representing dissection proximally. Several centimeters distally is a large, well-circumscribed collection of contrast medium *(open arrows)*, which represents an extra-aortic hematoma from a second rupture. The patient exsanguinated following section of the mediastinal pleura at thoracotomy.

Pathologically, the tear usually begins in the intima and proceeds outward. The most minimal lesion is a transverse intimal tear, the more severe lesions involving the media and even all layers of the aortic wall.

Plain roentgenograms of the chest almost invariably reveal widening of the superior mediastinum due to hemorrhage (Figure 13–5), although such hemorrhage may eventually prove to be of venous origin owing either to direct trauma or to iatrogenic causes such as malpositioning of a central venous line.[21] The contour of the aortic knob is generally invisible, an important sign that should alert the roentgenologist to the possibility of aortic rupture. However, it must be emphasized that in some cases the shadow of the aortic knuckle is preserved and this must not be construed as evidence excluding the diagnosis.[22] As the hematoma enlarges, the left main bronchus may be deviated anteriorly, inferiorly, and to the right, and the trachea may be displaced to the right. These signs are said to be present in about 75 per cent of patients.[18] Recent studies[23, 24] have emphasized the importance of identifying displacement of the nasogastric tube to the right; in fact, Gerlock and associates[24] found that when both the trachea and nasogastric tube were shifted to the right, the patient had a 96 per cent probability of having an acute rupture of the thoracic aorta. Displacement of the right paraspinous interface has also been found to be a highly reliable sign of aortic rupture (Figure 13–5): in a retrospective review of the roentgenographic findings in 14 patients with proven acute traumatic rupture of the aorta, Peters and Gamsu[25] found displacement of the right paraspinous interface in eight; the sign was not seen roentgenographically in any patient who did not have evidence of rupture on thoracic aortography. Another sign of potential value in diagnosis is the left apical extrapleural cap (Figure 13–5). A potential space exists between the isthmus of the aorta and the parietal pleura of the left lung. Provided that the parietal pleura is intact, extravasated blood may track cephalad along the course of the left subclavian artery between the parietal pleura and the extrapleural soft tissues, resulting in a homogeneous opacity over the apex of the left hemithorax—the extrapleural apical cap.[26] This may be one of the earliest roentgenologic manifestations of aortic rupture. In a recent prospective and retrospective study of 45 patients with traumatic rupture of the aorta in which the value of the left apical cap was assessed, Simeone and his colleagues[27] found that in seven cases a left apical cap was the only clearly visible abnormality; in 11 patients a cap was present together with a poorly defined aortic knob, while in 13 cases there was the additional finding of mediastinal widening. In 14 cases, all of the classic signs of aortic rupture were present except for an apical cap. In this same series, of 32 aortograms performed, 12 were solely because of an apical cap; two were positive for aortic rupture and ten negative, suggesting that the left apical cap *by itself* constitutes an unreliable sign of acute aortic rupture. Hemothorax complicating traumatic rupture of the aorta is common and is almost invariably left-sided.[15] Another sign that has been suggested recently as a possible indicator of aortic tear is widening of the right paratracheal stripe to a diameter greater than 5 mm.[20] Fracture of the first and second ribs, formerly considered a potential indicator of aortic/brachiocephalic trauma, is now considered an unreliable sign on the strength of several well-documented studies.[29–31]

Early recognition of aortic rupture is imperative in view of the poor survival rates of undiagnosed patients with this type of injury. Approximately 20 per cent of patients with aortic rupture survive the initial trauma, although the majority of survivors have a thin-walled aneurysm, which, if untreated, will rupture within 2 weeks in approximately 60 per cent and within 10 weeks in 90 per cent.[20] For any patient who has suffered severe chest trauma and in whom any of the above signs is present (including simple widening of the upper mediastinum), aortography (preferably by the transaxillary approach) is imperative to establish the diagnosis and to reveal the anatomic extent of the rupture.

Occasionally, mediastinal hemorrhage following severe chest trauma can result from damage to one of the great vessels arising from the aortic arch.[32]

PERFORATION OF THE ESOPHAGUS

Rupture of the esophagus from closed chest trauma is rare and results in changes localized to the mediastinum and the pleura.[15] Of considerably greater frequency is the rupture that occurs as a complication of esophagoscopy or gastroscopy,[33] overzealous dilatation of a stricture or achalasia, or disruption of the suture line following esophageal resection and anastomosis. The usual result of esophageal rupture is acute mediastinitis manifested roentgeno-

graphically by mediastinal widening, usually more evident superiorly and typically possessing a smooth, sharply defined margin. Air may be visible within the mediastinal compartments, and this constitutes one of the earliest and most important signs of esophageal perforation. If the mediastinal pleura is ruptured, there is early development of hydrothorax or hydropneumothorax. If pleural integrity is maintained, mediastinal changes develop rapidly and pleural effusion develops late.[34] In any of these circumstances, identification of ingested material (such as milk) in pleural fluid is diagnostic. In the majority of cases the site of rupture must be identified precisely—and sometimes with considerable difficulty—by roentgenographic evidence of extravasation of ingested contrast material. The type of contrast medium to be employed in such a study is still somewhat controversial, although we concur with other observers[35] that because it provides better contrast, barium is the agent of choice in this difficult diagnostic situation.

Chills and high fever are common, and effects of obstruction of the superior vena cava may be apparent. Physical examination usually reveals subcutaneous emphysema in the soft tissues of the neck or Hamman's sign on auscultation over the apex of the heart. When the diagnosis is not suspected initially and treatment is not instituted promptly, the inflammation may progress to abscess formation, with subsequent perforation of the abscess into a bronchus or the pleural cavity. Prognosis correlates closely with early diagnosis and immediate treatment.

RUPTURE OF THE THORACIC DUCT

Rupture of the thoracic duct, resulting in chylothorax, may develop from surgical trauma, nonpenetrating injuries, or penetrating wounds from a bullet or knife.[2, 15] The anatomic course of the thoracic duct establishes on which side the chylothorax develops. As it enters the thorax the duct lies slightly to the right of the midline, so that rupture in its lower third—the unusual site in crushing injuries—leads to right-sided chylothorax. The duct crosses the midline to the left in the midthorax, so that its disruption above this point as a result of crushing injury or, more commonly, surgical trauma, tends to produce left-sided chylothorax. Chylothorax resulting from nonpenetrating thoracic trauma may be bilateral.

Several days may elapse between the time of chest trauma and of roentgenographically demonstrable pleural fluid,[2, 15] a time lag that should strongly suggest this entity. The reason is that initially the extravasated chyle is confined to the mediastinal space and ruptures into the pleural space only when the accumulation has acquired sufficient pressure.

The rupture of large quantities of chyle from the mediastinum into the pleural space may give rise to the abrupt onset of respiratory difficulty. Thoracentesis yielding milky fluid of high fat content confirms the diagnosis, and the precise site of rupture may be established by lymphangiography.

EFFECTS ON THE DIAPHRAGM OF NONPENETRATING TRAUMA

The only abnormality of the diaphragm occurring as a result of trauma is rupture or tear. This may be caused by direct penetrating injury or blunt nonpenetrating trauma to the abdomen or thorax, the number of cases attributable to each type of trauma being roughly equal.[36] The most common causal trauma is an automobile accident or falling from a height. In some cases herniation occurs at the time of the accident, but its presence is masked by injuries to other organs. In other cases, major herniation of abdominal contents may occur into the thorax without associated signs or symptoms, being detected months or years later on a screening chest roentgenogram. It has been estimated that nine out of ten traumatic diaphragmatic hernias are overlooked at the time of injury.

Although traumatic hernias account for only a small percentage of all diaphragmatic hernias (approximately 5 per cent[37]), 90 per cent of strangulated hernias are of traumatic origin.[3] In 90 to 98 per cent of cases, the left hemidiaphragm is affected.[36] The right hemidiaphragm is protected by the liver, which dissipates the force of indirect trauma and prevents laceration. The central and posterior portions of the left hemidiaphragm are most commonly involved. The hernial contents depend on the size and position of the rupture. They may include omentum, stomach, small and large intestine, spleen, kidney, and even pancreas. As might be anticipated, there is no peritoneal sac. Roentgenographically, the left hemidiaphragm cannot be traced and abnormal shadows are visible in the left hemithorax (Figure 13–6). These depend on the nature of hernial contents and are commonly inhomogeneous, owing to the presence of gas-containing bowel, usually with fluid levels. In contrast to Bochdalek hernias, a portion of the stomach is commonly present (Figure 13–6). The roentgenographic appearance may simulate eventration or diaphragmatic paralysis, and differentiation may be possible only by barium examination of the

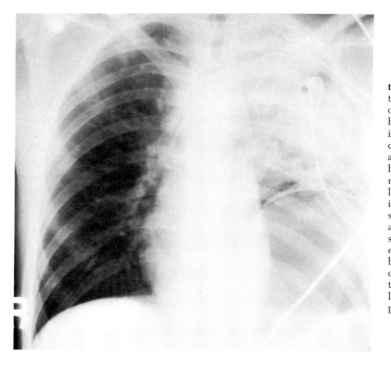

Figure 13–6. Acute Traumatic Rupture of the Left Hemidiaphragm. An anteroposterior roentgenogram of the chest of this 20-year-old man, taken shortly after his arrival in the emergency room following severe trauma to the left side of the chest in a motor accident, reveals a large air-containing viscus occupying the lower half of the left hemithorax. The upper margin of the air-containing space simulates an elevated left hemidiaphragm but in fact represents the wall of a herniated stomach. The left lung shows massive airlessness, whose etiology is confused somewhat by the fact that the tip of the endotracheal tube lies in the right main bronchus. (Is the airlessness due to severe contusion or atelectasis or both?) A left thoracotomy was performed and a large laceration of the left hemidiaphragm repaired.

gastrointestinal tract. Of major differential importance is the fact that with hernia, afferent and efferent loops of bowel are constricted as they traverse the orifice in the diaphragm whereas in eventration or paralysis the loops typically are widely separated.

In the less than 10 per cent of cases in which rupture occurs in the right hemidiaphragm, a portion of the liver may herniate through the rent and create a mushroom-like mass within the right hemithorax, the herniated liver being constricted by the tear.

Traumatic diaphragmatic hernia usually is suspected on roentgenographic examination following injury, although it is surprising how often an unsuspected diaphragmatic tear is found at thoracotomy or laparotomy performed for some other purpose.[36] Toombs and his colleagues[38] have emphasized the importance of computed tomography in the study of patients following acute chest trauma: in their series of 20 patients, many abnormalities were discovered on CT that were not apparent on conventional roentgenograms, including one case of acute rupture of the diaphragm.

The majority of hernias give rise to symptoms, although they may not be noted for months or even years after the traumatic episode. Immediate symptoms consist of severe substernal pain, vomiting, shock, and dyspnea resulting from lung compression. The most frequent associated injuries are rupture of the spleen, perforation of a hollow abdominal viscus, and fractured ribs. Intestinal obstruction as a result of strangulation occurs most commonly in cases of long-standing hernia.

EFFECTS ON THE CHEST WALL OF NONPENETRATING TRAUMA

FRACTURES OF THE RIBS

Fractures of the rib cage as a result of blunt trauma most commonly involve the fourth to tenth ribs. The severity of the trauma required to fracture the first three ribs may result in serious intrathoracic damage, including torsion of the lung and tracheobonchial fracture. On the other hand, *isolated* first-rib fractures, owing to the nature of the trauma, are unlikely to be associated with tracheobronchial or aortic rupture but are frequently accompanied by maxillofacial or neurologic injuries.[29]

The possibility of hemothorax, pneumothorax, or hemopneumothorax complicating severe rib fracture renders it desirable—if not necessary—to perform chest roentgenography several hours after trauma. The fracture of multiple ribs may result in a "flail" chest, which may lead rapidly to severe respiratory failure.

Cough fractures of the ribs occur more often in women than in men and almost invariably involve the sixth to ninth ribs, most often the seventh and usually in the posterior axillary line.

FRACTURES OF THE SPINE

Fractures of thoracic vertebral bodies may result in extraosseous hemorrhage and the development of unilateral or bilateral paraspinal masses. Although the fracture is usually evident roentgenographically, the major evidence of its presence may be deformity of the contiguous paraspinal soft tissues.

POST-TRAUMATIC HERNIA OF THE LUNG

Protrusion of a portion of lung through an abnormal aperture of the thoracic cage may be congenital or traumatic in origin and may be cervical, thoracic, or diaphragmatic in position. The protrusion is covered by both parietal and visceral pleura. Congenital hernias occur most frequently in the supraclavicular fossa, less often at the costochondral junction. Traumatic hernias may follow chest trauma or surgery, and in a small percentage of cases the weakened area is the result of inflammatory or neoplastic damage to the thoracic cage. The most common location of post-traumatic herniation is the parasternal region just medial to the costochondral junction, where the intercostal musculature is thinnest. The patient usually complains of a bulge appearing during coughing and straining, and in most cases the diagnosis is evidenced by the clinical finding of a soft crepitant mass that develops under these conditions and disappears during expiration or rest. Chest roentgenograms reveal pulmonary parenchymal tissue herniating through an obvious defect in the rib cage, or through a supraclavicular fossa. Optimal visualization requires the Valsalva maneuver and tangential roentgenographic projection in most cases.

PULMONARY EFFECTS OF NONTHORACIC TRAUMA

A number of pleuropulmonary abnormalities occur as a consequence of trauma whose pathogenesis is unrelated to direct injury to the thorax (although chest injury may have occurred as well). Some of these effects are specific to trauma, including traumatic fat embolism, traumatic air embolism, and neurogenic pulmonary edema (following severe trauma to the head), while others are nonspecific, such as pulmonary thromboembolism and adult respiratory distress syndrome (shock lung).

Except for pulmonary thromboembolism, each of the aforementioned abnormalities is associated with pulmonary edema. If there is suspicion that the chest was also injured, the only condition that need be considered in differential diagnosis is severe pulmonary contusion. Sometimes this differentiation can be difficult, although contusion tends to be less diffuse and to clear more rapidly. Each of these conditions has been discussed elsewhere in the book.

EFFECTS ON THE THORAX OF PENETRATING TRAUMA

PENETRATING WOUNDS OF THE THORAX

The usual roentgenographic appearance of the path of a bullet through lung parenchyma is a rather poorly defined homogeneous shadow which, as might be expected, is more or less circular when viewed in the direction in which the bullet passed and longitudinal when viewed in perpendicular projection. The indistinct definition is caused by hemorrhage and edema into the parenchyma surrounding the bullet track. The hemorrhage usually clears in a few days, leaving a "longitudinal" hematoma that may not resolve for several weeks or months. Resolution usually is complete and without residua. In a small percentage of cases a central radiolucency may be apparent along the bullet's course.

Penetrating wounds of the thorax from a knife or bullet may induce traumatic pneumothorax, although the searing effect of a bullet as it passes through the pleura may cauterize the tissues sufficiently to prevent escape of air into the pleural space.

THE POSTOPERATIVE CHEST

ROENTGENOGRAPHIC MANIFESTATIONS

The number of requests for roentgenographic examination of the chest with mobile apparatus at a patient's bedside has increased enormously in recent years, partly because of a remarkable growth of intensive care units and partly because of the introduction of complex cardiovascular surgical procedures that require close surveillance postoperatively. The roentgenographic abnormalities with which we are primarily concerned in the immediate postoperative period are those following thoracotomy, a subject that has recently been excellently reviewed by Goodman.[34]

Although changes observed in the soft tissues of the chest wall, the thoracic cage, the pleura, the mediastinum, the diaphragm, and the lungs are in many ways interdependent and therefore should be considered together in interpretation, it serves a useful purpose to deal with them separately.

Soft Tissues of the Chest Wall. Surgical emphysema, manifested by linear streaks of gas density along the lateral chest wall and frequently in the neck, is almost invariably apparent for 2 or 3 days postoperatively. It need only cause concern when it is present in exceptionally large quantities, in which circumstance the gas may be coming from the mediastinum as a result of pulmonary interstitial and mediastinal emphysema

Thoracic Cage. The absence of a rib, usually the fifth or sixth, is frequently but not invariably a finding following thoracotomy. Nowadays the ribs often are spread rather than resected in both pulmonary and cardiac procedures, so that an intact rib cage is quite compatible with prior thoracotomy; ribs that have been spread may be fractured. Sternotomy is evidenced only by the presence of wire sutures.

Median sternotomy has become the principal surgical approach to the heart and great vessels, and one of the feared postoperative complications is sternal dehiscence. Attention has been drawn to a roentgenologic sign that has been thought by some to indicate the presence of sternal dehiscence, the "midsternal stripe."[40] This stripe consists of a thin lucent line of variable length oriented vertically in the midline of the sternum. On the strength of one thorough study,[41] however, it is clear that the midsternal stripe possesses little or no significance in establishing the presence of sternal dehiscence.

Pleura. The most common roentgenographic abnormality in the postoperative period is pleural effusion. During the 2 or 3 days after thoracotomy little or no fluid is evident, since the pleural space is effectively drained. Following removal of the drainage tube, however, a small amount of fluid often appears, only to disappear quite quickly during convalescence. Minimal residual pleural thickening may remain, particularly over the lung base.

The accumulation of fluid in larger than expected amounts may result from a variety of causes, including poor positioning of the drainage tube, hemorrhage from an intercostal vessel, or infection (empyema). In the presence of pleural adhesions, fluid may loculate in areas that are not in communication with the drainage tube, a finding that is particularly common following pleural decortication. In such circumstances, absorption of the fluid may be prolonged, sometimes for several weeks. Such local intrapleural collections are not of major importance unless the accumulation is very large or infected.

Pneumothorax postoperatively may be due to a variety of causes. Lack of communication with the drainage tube is probably the most common cause, particularly if the gas is loculated. Other causes include leakage into the pleural space from a blown bronchial stump (bronchopleural fistula) or from a bare area of lung following wedge or segmental resection of lung.

The incidence of bronchopleural fistula as a complication of pulmonary resection is approximately 2 per cent[42] and the mortality rate ranges from 16 to 22 per cent.[42, 43] It occurs as a result of necrosis of the bronchial stump and is most common after right pneumonectomy. Characteristically, it is heralded by the sudden onset of dyspnea and expectoration of bloody fluid during the first 10 days postoperatively. The chest roentgenogram reveals an unexpected disappearance of fluid as a reflection of emptying of the pleural space by way of the tracheobronchial tree. With the introduction of a modern stapling machine to effect closure of the bronchus, fistulas are becoming much less frequent.

Mediastinum. The two major abnormalities of the mediastinum that occur in the postoperative period are enlargement and displacement. Enlargement results from the accumulation of either gas or fluid. Persistence of pneumomediastinum in the absence of any other potential cause should raise the suspicion of interstitial pulmonary emphysema associated with some form of pulmonary disease.[44]

Position of the mediastinum is one of the most important indicators of pulmonary abnormality during the postoperative period. Displacement may occur toward or away from the side of the thoracotomy. Ipsilateral displacement is an expected finding following pneumonectomy, although position depends to some extent on whether a chest tube has been inserted into the empty pleural space for suction.[39] Following removal of part of a lung, e.g., one lobe, mediastinal displacement is temporary, the normal midline position being regained as the remainder of the lung undergoes compensatory overinflation. Excessive displacement toward the operated side may be a sign of atelectasis in the ipsilateral lung. In the case of pneumonectomy, ipsilateral mediastinal displacement is progressive and permanent (*see* further on). Mediastinal displacement *away* from the operated side may occur as a result of atelectasis in the contralateral lung or an accumulation of excessive fluid or gas in the ipsilateral pleural space.

The status of the chest roentgenogram following pneumonectomy has been clarified by Hanson and his colleagues on the basis of an unpublished review of 110 cases. Within 24 hours of pneumonectomy, the ipsilateral pleural space is air-containing, the mediastinum is shifted slightly to the ipsilateral side, and the hemidiaphragm is slightly elevated (in virtually all these cases a chest tube had been inserted for pleural drainage) (Figure 13–7). The postpneumonectomy space then begins to fill with serosanguineous fluid and fibrin in a progressive and normally predictable manner at a rate of approximately two rib spaces a day. The majority of the 110 cases studied by Hanson and his colleagues showed 80 to 90 per cent obliteration of the space at the end of 2 weeks and complete obliteration by 2 to 4 months. Obliteration of the space occurs not only as a result of fluid accumulation but by progressive ipsilateral displacement of the mediastinum and elevation of the hemidiaphragm. Mediastinal displacement is an almost invariable finding and constitutes the most reliable indicator of a normal postoperative course. It generally requires 6 to 8 months to reach its maximum. Failure of the mediastinum to shift in the postoperative period almost always indicates an abnormality in the postpneumonectomy space—bronchoplural fistula, empyema (Figure 13–8), hemorrhage, or occasionally chylothorax.

In Hanson and his associates' series, the character of the fluid level was found to have little or no diagnostic or prognostic significance, the contour of the air-fluid interface being less important than the appearance of bubbles or a drop in the level of fluid by more than 2 cm. The most sensitive indicator of *late* complications was found to be a return to the midline of a previously shifted mediastinum, particularly the tracheal air column. This indicated the

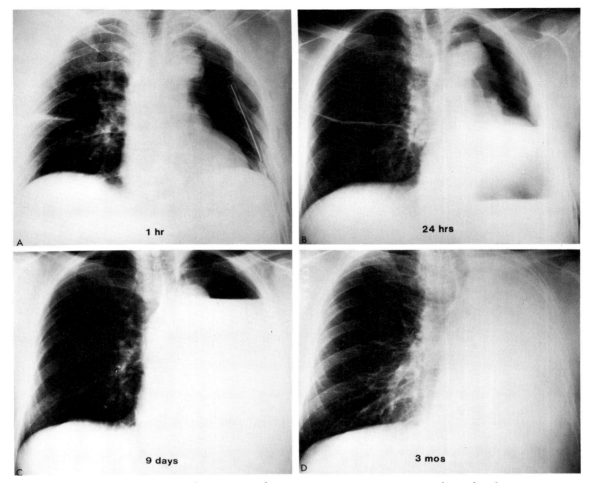

Figure 13–7. Postpneumonectomy Course, Normal. An anteroposterior roentgenogram obtained in the supine position at the bedside 1 hour following left pneumonectomy (A) reveals a slight reduction in the volume of the left hemithorax. The space is air-filled and the mediastinum is in the midline. At 24 hours, a roentgenogram in the erect position (B) shows moderate elevation of the left hemidiaphragm (as indicated by the gastric air bubble), a moderate shift of the mediastinum to the left, and a prominent air-fluid level in the plane of the third interspace anteriorly. By 9 days (C), fluid had filled approximately two-thirds of the cavity of the left hemithorax, but the mediastinum was still displaced to the left (note the curvature of the tracheal air column). By 3 months (D), the left hemithorax had become completely airless. Note the persistent shift of the mediastinum to the left and the prominent curve of the air column of the trachea.

presence within the postpneumonectomy space of an expanding process such as recurrent neoplasm, bronchopleural fistula, or empyema.

Diaphragm. Following pneumonectomy or lobectomy, the ipsilateral hemidiaphragm is almost invariably elevated during the first few postoperative days. Following pneumonectomy, this elevation persists along with ipsilateral mediastinal shift, despite accumulation of fluid in the pleural space. Following lobectomy, diaphragmatic elevation and mediastinal displacement disappear over a period of several days or weeks as the remainder of the ipsilateral lung undergoes compensatory overinflation.

Elevation of the hemidiaphragm may result from a number of pathologic states within the lungs, including atelectasis, acute bronchopneumonia, and pulmonary thromboembolism. Differentiation of these conditions may be difficult from roentgenographic signs alone, although the time interval following surgery may be of some assistance (*see* further on).

Depression of one hemidiaphragm is a very uncommon postoperative abnormality and is invariably caused by a massive pneumothorax or hydrothorax.

Lungs. The chest roentgenogram following thoracotomy may reveal changes to be anticipated from the nature of the surgical procedure. For example, following lobectomy, rearrangement of fissures often results in displacement, which must not be misinterpreted as evidence

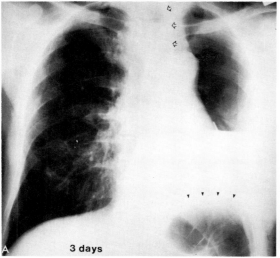

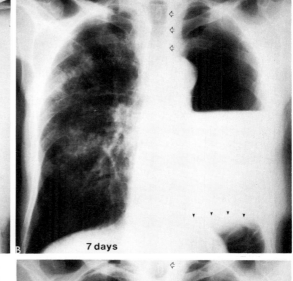

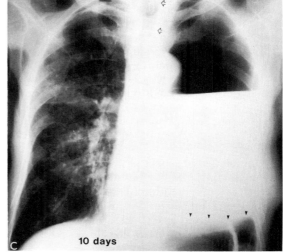

Figure 13–8. Postpneumonectomy Course Complicated by Empyema. Three days following left pneumonectomy *(A)*, the amount of fluid that has accumulated, the position of the left hemidiaphragm *(arrowheads)*, and the shift of the tracheal air column to the left *(open arrows)* are all consistent with a normal postoperative course (compare with Figure 13–7). At 7 days *(B)*, however, the left hemidiaphragm *(arrowheads)* has undergone some depression and the tracheal air column *(open arrows)* has returned to the midline. Such a change should suggest empyema, bronchopleural fistula, pleural hemorrhage, or conceivably chylothorax. By 10 days *(C)*, the left hemidiaphragm *(arrowheads)* had become concave superiorly and the mediastinum and tracheal air column *(open arrows)* had shifted further to the right. Proved left-sided empyema.

of atelectasis. Similarly, the vascular markings become more widely spaced and lung density is reduced as a result of compensatory overinflation, signs that must not be confused with those resulting from atelectasis or from reduced perfusion due to pulmonary embolism.

Undoubtedly the most common pulmonary complication of surgical procedures is atelectasis, whether the surgery is thoracic or abdominal. Atelectasis may vary widely in extent and may affect multiple small lobular units whose airlessness causes insufficient density to be appreciated roentgenologically. In such circumstances, atelectasis may be evidenced only by the demonstration on pulmonary function testing of decreased lung volume, increased venous admixture, or decreased pulmonary compliance. The mechanisms of development of postoperative atelectasis also vary considerably. The

most common cause is mucous plugging from retained secretions. Gamsu and his colleagues[45] have recently documented a disruption of mucociliary clearance and pooling of mucus associated with atelectasis following major surgery. A loss of surfactant is considered to be responsible for atelectasis occurring postoperatively in patients undergoing cardiopulmonary bypass for open heart surgical procedures.[46] For as yet unexplained reasons, this adhesive atelectasis shows a most unusual predilection for the left lower lobe.

Any local pulmonary opacity identified in the postoperative period must be regarded as one of the big four—atelectasis, pneumonia (either bacterial or aspiration in type), infarction, or edema. The manifestations of these complications are no different from those that develop in a nonsurgical setting.

CLINICAL MANIFESTATIONS

Factors that determine morbidity and mortality after thoracotomy and resectional surgery are numerous and include: (1) the general health of the patient, (2) preoperative evaluation, including assessment of lung function, (3) management by the anesthesiologist, (4) the extent of the surgery, (5) the technical ability of the surgeon, and (6) postoperative care.

The general health of the patient undoubtedly plays a role in the successful outcome of the operation. Not infrequently the requirement for surgery is urgent if not emergent, permitting incomplete if any correction of existing disorders. If a reasonable interval exists between the decision for surgery and the operation itself, there is little doubt that the prognosis can be improved with proper preparation,[47] at least in patients with either chronic bronchitis or obesity. Since it has been shown that the majority of patients with bronchogenic carcinoma (the most common indication for pulmonary resectional surgery) have coincident chronic bronchitis, it is imperative that these patients be encouraged to discontinue cigarette smoking some days prior to surgery; scheduling surgery late in the morning to permit time for cough to clear accumulated mucus is an additional precautionary technique.

A fundamental aspect of preoperative preparation is a clinical and physiologic assessment of the patient's breathing reserve, both to determine the likelihood of survival after resectional surgery and to avoid creating a respiratory cripple.[48] An experienced physician or surgeon may feel confident in making such a judgment on the basis of history and by observing the patient as he or she walks through corridors and up stairs. However, most physicians feel more comfortable with an objective determination of pulmonary function (*see* further on).

The anesthiologist and the anesthetic employed can exert a significant influence over the incidence of postoperative complications. In a review of disturbances in gas exchange during anesthesia, Rehder and associates[49] found that functional residual capacity (FRC) decreases and that chest wall mechanics are altered; both oxygenation and CO_2 elimination are impaired, and both venous admixture and alveolar dead space are increased. Serious hypoxia can result if artificial ventilation is discontinued while the respiratory center is still depressed by anesthetics or narcotics.

It is probable that the extent of surgical resection exerts considerable influence on outcome. For example, mortality is higher following pneumonectomy than lobectomy, but this may simply be a reflection of the area of gas exchange available to a patient whose remaining lung tissue is probably affected by COPD. The surgical approach is also important. For example, it has been demonstrated that when the pleura is opened, airway resistance increases abruptly, whereas if entry is by way of the mediastinum by splitting the sternum, airway conductance is not disturbed.[50]

Pulmonary dysfunction is an invariable accompaniment of thoracic and upper abdominal surgery. A decrease occurs in all lung volumes and in compliance. Perfusion of nonventilated alveoli is reflected in hypoxemia. These changes become maximal 48 to 72 hours after surgery and usually clear completely within 7 days without clinical evidence of their presence.[51] They probably result from persistent shallow breathing initiated by pain, narcotic drugs, and general anesthesia. Pain inhibits coughing and prevents effective expectoration, in addition to reducing lung volume. The major preventive measure to overcome physiologic dysfunction is encouragement of the patient by the physician, nurse, or therapist to cough and to inspire deeply in order to renew surfactant and to clear the airways.

Assessment of Operative Risk

Although it might appear logical to assume that a careful evaluation of pulmonary function would prove useful in the selection of patients for resectional surgery, there are no convincing data to support such a contention. Patients with abnormal pulmonary function studies are more likely to get into trouble after surgery, particularly if preoperative and postoperative care is neglected.[52] Pulmonary function test values that indicate a high risk of developing postoperative cardiopulmonary complications include: (1) vital capacity less than 1.0 liter; (2) FEV_1 less than 0.5 liter (3) maximal midexpiratory flow less than 0.6 liter per second; (4) maximum voluntary ventilation (MVV, MBC) less than 50 per cent of predicted; (5) PaO_2 less than 55 mm Hg; and (6) elevated preoperative PCO_2.[53]

THORACIC COMPLICATIONS OF NONTHORACIC SURGERY

The major thoracic complications of abdominal surgery are atelectasis, pneumonia, thromboembolism, subphrenic abscess, cardiogenic pulmonary edema, and ARDS.[54] Atelectasis is undoubtedly the commonest of these and in the majority of patients is related to retention of secretions and mucous plugging of airways. Retention is undoubtedly abetted by diminished diaphragmatic excursion caused by splinting as a result of pain or occasionally caused by a large pneumoperitoneum following laparotomy. Similar effects may follow peritoneal dialysis.

In a review of the risks of abdominal and thoracic surgery in patients with chronic obstructive pulmonary disease, Gaensler and Weisel[55] point out that the prevalence of postoperative pulmonary complications is greater after abdominal than after thoracic surgery. Whether the same prevalence would exist in subjects without COPD is not known, but the overall incidence of complications following any form of surgery is clearly greater in patients with disturbed pulmonary function.

In one series of 132 male patients over the age of 47, all of whom were cigarette smokers and lived in an industrial environment, some degree of respiratory complication developed in 85.6 per cent during the 10 days after upper abdominal surgery as judged clinically.[56] On the second day 52.5 per cent demonstrated some roentgenographic abnormality, almost half of these being of major severity. A clinical assessment of 785 patients who underwent major surgical procedures under general anesthesia revealed a considerably lower incidence of chest complications (5 per cent).[57] However, when surgery was carried out on the upper abdomen, the complication rate rose to 10 per cent, and when surgery was performed on the gastrojejunal or biliary tracts, the incidence of complications more than doubled (21 per cent).

The roentgenographic and clinical features of acute pneumonia and pulmonary embolism are no different from those observed in other clinical settings. Subphrenic abscess, although uncommon, is almost always a complication of abdominal surgery.

COMPLICATIONS OF INTUBATION AND MONITORING APPARATUS

The intubation and monitoring apparatus to be discussed include chest tubes for drainage of the pleural space, nasogastric tubes, venous catheters for measurement of central venous pressure (CVP) or for hyperalimentation, arterial catheters for measurement of pulmonary arterial and wedge pressures (Swan-Ganz), and the intra-aortic assist balloon.[58] Complications associated with endotracheal and tracheostomy tubes have already been discussed in relation to large airway obstruction (*see* page 526).

CHEST DRAINAGE TUBES

Complications of chest drainage tubes are uncommon and usually are readily apparent clinically. It should be appreciated that a drainage tube inserted anterolaterally and directed posteriorly will drain the posterior pleural space but, with the patient lying in a supine position, will not drain a pneumothorax situated anteriorly. Similarly, a drainage tube in any position will not drain a loculated accumulation of fluid or gas in an area not in communication with the tube's holes. Occasionally a tube will be situated entirely within the chest wall or even within the abdominal cavity, in which case its malposition should be readily apparent roentgenographically.

NASOGASTRIC TUBES

Since the majority of nasogastric tubes are opaque, any malposition should be readily apparent roentgenographically. The two most common misplacements are coiling within the esophagus and incomplete insertion, in both of which the function of the nasogastric tube is clearly not being served. A complication of far greater clinical importance is the faulty insertion of the nasogastric tube into the tracheobronchial tree rather than into the esophagus, particularly if the tube is meant for hyperalimentation; the injection of large amounts of fluid into the lungs rather than the stomach can have disastrous consequences.

MONITORING APPARATUS

Hemodynamic monitoring is an important aspect of contemporary intensive care of the critically ill patient. In an excellent review of catheter insertion techniques, complications, and troubleshooting in hemodynamic monitoring, Baigrie and Morgan[59] state that potential problems fall into two general categories, those related to technical pitfalls and those related to patient complications.

Percutaneous Central Venous Catheters

The increasing use of catheters to monitor central venous pressure and to provide a route

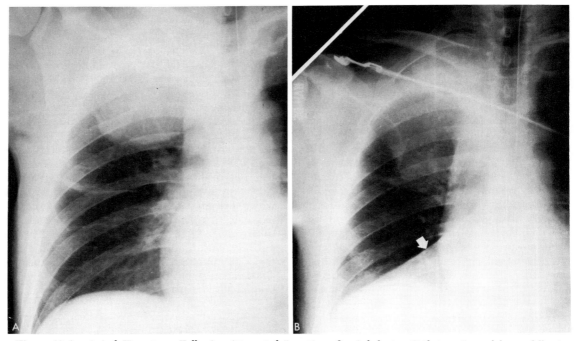

Figure 13–9. Apical Hematoma Following Attempted Insertion of a Subclavian Catheter. Several hours following attempted insertion of a right subclavian catheter, an anteroposterior roentgenogram *(A)* reveals a large homogeneous mass occupying the upper third of the right hemithorax (a previous roentgenogram was normal). One week later *(B)*, the opacity was slightly larger and less well defined. Coincidentally, there had developed complete airlessness of the right lower lobe caused by atelectasis, presumably from an obstructing mucous plug *(arrow* points to downwardly displaced major fissure).

for hyperalimentation has brought to light a number of complications with which the physician should be thoroughly familiar. Some of these pertain to the catheterization procedure itself, either early or late, and relate to abnormalities within or around the vein catheterized. Others—perhaps the majority—arise from incorrect positioning of the tip of the catheter. Complications of central venous catheterization have recently been the subject of an excellent review.[60] The major complications of aberrant positioning are as follows:

1. *Inaccurate venous pressure measurements:* Pressure recorded in the jugular vein is not equivalent to central venous pressure. However, since it is often within the normal range and may show only slightly diminished dynamics, it is unlikely that the malposition of the catheter will be recognized clinically.

2. *Thrombophlebitis:* A catheter that is allowed to remain in the internal jugular vein will frequently traumatize the vessel because of its torqued tip, resulting in thrombophlebitis and occasionally perforation.

3. *Perforation of a vein:* A vein may be perforated either at the time of insertion or some time later owing to gradual erosion of a relatively thin-walled intrathoracic vessel by the catheter tip. Depending on the vein involved and the reason for catheter insertion (monitoring of pressure or hyperalimentation), the result may be mediastinal hemorrhage, hemothorax, pneumothorax, massive hydrothorax, or extrapleural hematoma (Figure 13–9).

4. *Perforation of the myocardium:* Of the 300 patients studied by Langston,[61] the tip of the central venous catheter was in the right atrium or right ventricle in 40 (13 per cent). This is obviously an extremely hazardous position for any catheter, particularly one with a firm or sharp tip, since perforation of the right atrium or ventricle may result in fatal pericardial tamponade (from either blood or infused fluid). Also, such a catheter may readily cause arrhythmias, as is well recognized by physicians who regularly perform cardiac catheterization in the laboratory.

5. *Catheter coiling, knotting, and breaking:* Coiled catheters traumatize the vein and are much more likely to perforate, break, and embolize; they also show a much greater tendency to twist into knots, and although such knots sometimes can be manipulated free. this is not always possible.

It is obvious that all these complications of aberrant central venous catheters may be prevented by roentgenographic monitoring of their position immediately after insertion.

Indwelling Balloon-Tipped Pulmonary Arterial Catheters (Swan-Ganz)

Flow-directed balloon-tipped catheters for monitoring circulatory hemodynamics in critically ill patients have been used with increasing frequency since their first description in 1970.[62] Complications of these catheters include atrial and ventricular dysrhythmias, rupture of the balloon, knotting of the catheter, perforation of the pulmonary artery, and thromboembolism and infarction.[63, 64] The last-named complication is undoubtedly the most frequent, some form of pulmonary ischemic lesion being observed in nine (7.2 per cent) of 125 patients in one series.[63] Thromboembolism may result from one or more of four mechanisms: (1) irritation of the endothelium of a major pulmonary artery by the catheter balloon results in thrombus formation on the roughened endothelium and subsequent embolization; (2) prolonged inflation of the balloon for recording of wedge pressure results in peripheral ischemia and infarction; (3) formation of thrombus around the distal end of the catheter with subsequent embolization; and (4) tightening of a large intracardiac loop of the catheter by hemodynamic action may propel the tip of the catheter to a point where it occludes a small peripheral artery with resultant infarction (Figure 13–10). The last mechanism can be avoided if the technique described by Swan and associates is strictly adhered to—the balloon is inflated as soon as a large caliber vein is encountered and the catheter is permitted to float into the pulmonary artery.

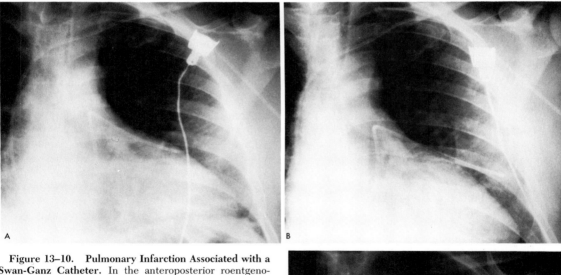

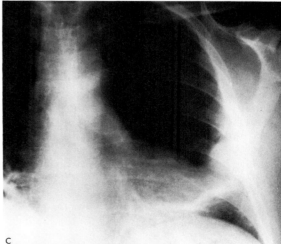

Figure 13–10. Pulmonary Infarction Associated with a Swan-Ganz Catheter. In the anteroposterior roentgenogram illustrated in (A), a Swan-Ganz catheter is in position in the left lower lobe, its tip in a position consistent with subsegmental artery. Twenty-four hours later (B), the intrapulmonary extent of the catheter had increased considerably, such that its tip now lies less than 2 cm from the visceral pleural surface. Several days later (C), a wedge-shaped opacity had appeared in the left axillary lung zone highly suggestive of a pulmonary infarct; its position corresponds precisely to what was undoubtedly an impacted Swan-Ganz catheter tip.

In a recent review of the risk factors of pulmonary artery flow-guided catheters in the perioperative period, Katz and his colleagues[65] concluded that such monitoring in critically ill patients is a relatively safe procedure. Of 392 patients assessed, the incidence of all complications was very low except for bacteremia, found in 21 patients (5 per cent), and pulmonary thromboembolism, observed in 16 patients (4 per cent). None of the complications was directly responsible for death.

Intra-aortic Counterpulsation Balloon

This catheter has been gaining increased popularity for use in conditions characterized by low output cardiac decompensation and cardiogenic shock. It provides augmentation of diastolic coronary artery perfusion as well as reduced impedance to ventricular injection.[66, 67] Reported complications resulting from the use of this device include:[58, 67] damage to the aorta including dissection, laceration of the wall, and subadventitial hematoma formation; red blood cell destruction; embolic phenomena; vascular insufficiency of the catheterized limb; and balloon rupture with secondary gas embolism. The most common complication observed by the radiologist is improper positioning.[58] The ideal position of the tip is just distal to the origin of the left subclavian artery. A more proximal position can occlude the left subclavian artery and one more distal may result in decreased effectiveness of diastolic counterpulsation.

RADIATION INJURIES OF THE LUNG

It seems reasonably safe to assume that within the therapeutic range of doses usually administered, the pulmonary parenchyma reacts to ionizing radiation in up to 100 per cent of patients. The incidence of pulmonary effects of radiation therapy varies considerably from series to series, largely as a result of semantic confusion. The term "radiation pneumonitis" is used by some to denote a roentgenographic abnormality and by others to describe a clinical syndrome. We take the position that the lung may be affected in the absence of a roentgenographically demonstrable abnormality,[69] suggesting that pulmonary function testing may be a more sensitive means of determining the extent of damage. Damage to the lungs may follow radiation therapy directly to the lungs or to any part of the thorax, including the medias-

tinum and chest wall. In only a relatively small number of patients—possibly no more than 5 to 15 per cent—does such therapy result in respiratory symptoms.[68]

There are many variables that affect the reaction, including the volume of lung tissue irradiated, the radiation dose administered, the time over which it is given, and the quality of the radiation.

Volume of Lung Irradiated. This is considered by some to be perhaps the most important factor leading to lung damage.[70, 71] It has been estimated that a 3000 rads total dose delivered in fractions to 25 per cent of total lung volume probably would not produce symptoms, whereas an identical dose delivered in the same manner to the entire volume of both lungs would probably prove fatal.[70]

Effect of Dosage. It is probable that if the lungs are normal before the administration of ionizing radiation, the effects (as measured by symptoms and signs, roentgenologic changes, and physiologic tests) will be proportionate to the amount of radiation delivered.[69] Radiation pneumonitis seldom occurs with a dose of less than 2000 rads,[72] although there are exceptions. Doses in excess of 6000 rads given over a period of 5 to 6 weeks almost invariably lead to severe radiation pneumonitis.

Time-Dose Factor. The radiation effect on the lung is related less to the total dose than to the rate of which it is delivered, since fractionation permits repair of sublethal damage between fractions.[68] This biologic effect of relative equivalent therapy takes into account the total dose absorbed, the number of fractions, and the time elapsed between first and last treatments.[73]

Other Factors. Other variables that influence biologic pulmonary damage include retreatment, associated chemotherapy, and corticosteroid withdrawal;[68, 74] each of these factors apparently increases susceptibility. There is little evidence to support the clinical impression that patients with chronic bronchitis are more likely to develop radiation pneumonitis than those without bronchial abnormality.

In addition to the effects of roentgen therapy, radiation injury to the lungs may also follow inhalation of beta-emitting radionuclides.[75]

PATHOGENESIS

Radiation may damage genetic material (such as DNA itself) and nongenetic macromolecules (such as proteins and polysaccharides). The effect on genetic material becomes manifest when tissue cells are called upon to reproduce and thus will be most evident in cells with a rapid turnover rate and least obvious in highly differentiated cells. In the lungs, the cells most sensitive to radiation-induced chromosomal defects are capillary endothelial, bronchial, and alveolar type II cells. As a result of radiation damage regeneration of these cells is impeded, with subsequent distortion of architecture by deposition of collagen and eventual fibrosis.

All lung tissues, including type I alveolar epithelial cells, may show the effects of radiation on nongenetic material, with resultant increased permeability of membranes, fragmentation of connective tissue, and the immediate functional disturbances these changes induce. Fibrotic replacement may subsequently result in irreversible functional derangement.[68]

It has been suggested[76] that the involvement of lung tissue outside the radiation field might indicate a delayed hypersensitivity immune reaction in response to an antigen resulting from intensive irradiation. The extraordinary latent period for the reaction, the histologic pattern, the involvement of unirradiated lung, and the beneficial response to corticosteroid therapy seem to support this hypothesis.

PATHOLOGIC CHANGES

In humans the earliest reports of pathologic changes have derived from patients who died 4 to 12 weeks after completion of radiation therapy, at a time when secondary changes from superimposed infection or heart failure are difficult to separate from the effects of radiation. Two stages of radiation damage are recognizable—the early or acute reaction (radiation pneumonitis) and the late or fibrotic stage. The *acute reaction* is characterized pathologically by desquamation of alveolar and bronchiolar cells and by exudation into alveolar spaces of plasma, which forms protein-rich hyaline membranes.[77, 78] The vascular lesions are evidenced by engorgement and thrombosis of capillaries and arterioles, and the alveolar septa are thickened by deposits of immature connective tissue and by lymphocytic infiltration.[79, 80] The *late* or *fibrotic stage* is characterized by an almost complete replacement of normal parenchyma by dense fibrous tissue.[80] A combination of several stages of pathologic change within the same tissue sample or a combination of atypical septal cell proliferation, vascular changes, and widespread hyaline membranes has been sug-

gested as a pathologic criterion for the diagnosis of late stage radiation damage.

ROENTGENOGRAPHIC MANIFESTATIONS

Pulmonary disease is seldom if ever manifested either symptomatically or roentgenographically while the patient is receiving radiation therapy. In fact, changes are seldom apparent roentgenographically until at least 1 month after cessation of treatment and in many cases until as long as 4 to 6 months.[81]

Acute radiation pneumonitis is manifested roentgenographically by consolidation of lung parenchyma, usually associated with considerable loss of volume. Depending on the severity of the reaction and therefore on the dose delivered, the resultant opacity may be patchy or confluent. The volume of lung affected usually but not always corresponds to the area irradiated, and thus there is no tendency to segmental or lobar distribution. In fact the margins of affected lung usually bear a close relationship to the position of the radiation ports.[82] Loss of volume may be severe, caused either by extensive bronchiolar plugging or more likely by a loss of surfactant (adhesive atelectasis), but despite this the major and segmental bronchi are more or less unaffected and an air bronchogram is almost invariably present (Figure 13–11).[72, 81]

The late or chronic stage of radiation damage is characterized by fibrosis (Figure 13–11). The affected lung shows severe loss of volume, with obliteration of all normal architectural markings, and the peripheral parenchyma may be airless and opaque as a result of replacement by fibrous tissue. It has been stated that radiation fibrosis generally is well established and stable 9 to 12 months after the completion of radiation therapy.

Roentgenographically demonstrable pleural effusion is very uncommon,[72, 83] even though effusions are often present at necropsy; fairly extensive thickening of the pleura may be seen both roentgenologically and pathologically.[72] The development of pericardial effusion following radiation therapy to the mediastinum is not uncommon; of note is the fact that it may not occur until years after the radiotherapeutic incident.[84, 85]

CLINICAL MANIFESTATIONS

Many patients with roentgenographic evidence of radiation damage remain asympto-

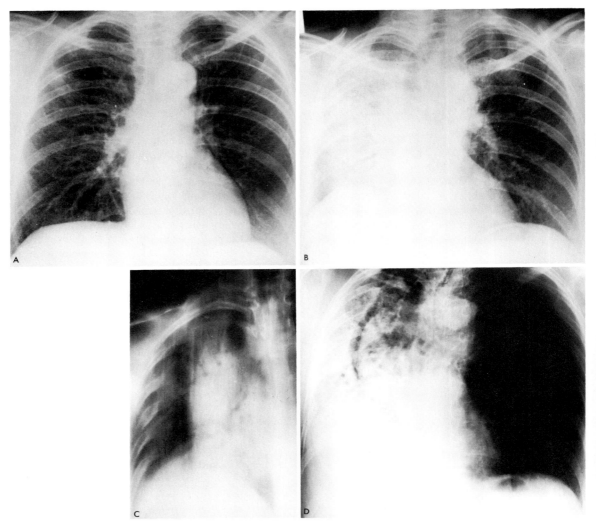

Figure 13–11. Acute Radiation Pneumonitis and Subsequent Fibrosis. This 52-year-old woman presented with a large ulcerated mass in the right breast that proved on biopsy to be carcinoma. Preoperative cobalt teletherapy was administered to the breast and mediastinum in a dosage of approximately 3,000 rads. The breast was then removed and over a period of 6 weeks postoperative cobalt therapy administered to the right lung in a dosage of 5,100 rads and to the mediastinum of 3,500 rads. A posteroanterior roentgenogram *(A)* at the end of the postoperative radiation therapy revealed no significant abnormalities. Three weeks later, however, a remarkable change had occurred in the appearance of the chest *(B)*, the right lung having undergone severe loss of volume as evidenced by elevation of the hemidiaphragm and shift of the mediastinum. The underlying density is rather granular in nature and an air bronchogram is identified within it, seen to better advantage in the anteroposterior tomogram of the right hemithorax illustrated in *C*. A posteroanterior roentgenogram approximately 1 month later *(D)* revealed severe loss of volume of the right lung. The pattern observed earlier had changed to a very coarse inhomogeneous pattern in which extensive bronchiectasis was readily apparent.

matic.[72] Radiation pneumonitis rarely produces symptoms during the 1-month period after termination of therapy, and when they do develop it is commonly between 2 and 3 months and occasionally as late as 6 months after the completion of therapy. Symptoms generally have an insidious onset and consist of nonproductive cough, weakness, fever, and shortness of breath on exertion. Cough may be very troublesome

and occur in spasms. The patient may have a sensation of inability to inspire to TLC and when encouraged to do so will invariably cough. Chest pain develops occasionally but hemoptysis is rare.[72, 81] Weakness and fever may be major complaints, the latter usually being low grade but sometimes high and spiking.[68] Dyspnea is usually mild and noted only on exertion but may occasion extreme respiratory distress.

Death may be caused by respiratory insufficiency.

Acute radiation pneumonitis may persist for up to 1 month and can either resolve completely or progress to pulmonary fibrosis. In a minority of patients, fibrosis develops insidiously without an acute phase being recognized. With the onset of fibrosis, symptoms of the acute pneumonitis gradually abate.

The institution of radiation therapy of an endobronchial neoplasm can induce edema and acute obstruction of the airway lumen. In our experience and that of others,[90] this effect can have diastrous consequences if the tumor is in the trachea. This complication can be prevented by preliminary treatment with prednisolone or mustine hydrochloride. The development of new primary neoplasms following radiotherapy and chemotherapy is well recognized.[86, 87] Since such lesions may occur coincidentally with the malignancy under treatment or in an area outside the treatment field, they do not necessarily represent complications of therapy.

Repeated small doses of radiation received either as treatment of disease or as a result of occupational exposure appear to result in an increased incidence of visceral malignancy including bronchogenic carcinoma.[88, 89]

PULMONARY FUNCTION STUDIES

It is important to appreciate that in many patients receiving radiation therapy pulmonary function improves initially, presumably due to the therapeutic effect on malignant tissue within the thorax.[80] The major impairment in function is restrictive in nature; vital capacity and flow rates are decreased, the former to a proportionately greater degree. Diffusing capacity is decreased when a large volume of lung is involved; it may return to normal as the acute process subsides but more commonly remains decreased as fibrosis ensues.[69, 80]

REFERENCES

1. Williams, J. R., and Bonte, F. J.: Pulmonary damage in nonpenetrating chest injuries. Radiol. Clin. North Am., *1*:439, 1963.
2. Reynolds, J., and Davis, J. T.: Injuries of the chest wall, pleura, pericardium, lungs, bronchi and esophagus. Radiol. Clin. North Am., *4*:383, 1966.
3. Wiot, J. F.: The radiologic manifestations of blunt chest trauma. J.A.M.A., *231*:500, 1975.
4. Hussey, H. H.: Editorial: Pulmonary contusion. J.A.M.A., *230*:264, 1974.
5. Ganske, J. G., Dennis, D. L., and Vanderveer, J. B.,

6. Williams, J. R., and Stembridge, V. A.: Pulmonary contusion secondary to nonpenetrating chest trauma. Am. J. Roentgenol., *91*:284, 1964.
7. Burke, J. F.: Early diagnosis of traumatic rupture of the bronchus. J.A.M.A., *181*:682, 1962.
8. Collins, J. P., Ketharanathan, V., and McConchie, I.: Rupture of major bronchi resulting from closed chest injuries. Thorax, *28*:371, 1973.
9. Eijgelaar, A., and Homan van der Heide, J. N.: A reliable early symptom of bronchial or tracheal rupture. Thorax, *25*:120, 1970.
10. Harvey-Smith, W., Bush, W., and Northrop, C.: Traumatic bronchial rupture. Am. J. Roentgenol., *134*:1189, 1980.
11. Tyson, M. D., Watson, T. R., Jr., and Sibley, J. R.: Traumatic bronchial rupture with plastic repair. N. Engl. J. Med., *258*:160, 1958.
12. Chesterman, J. T., and Satsangi, P. N.: Rupture of the trachea and bronchi by closed injury. Thorax, *21*:21, 1966.
13. Weisel, W., Watson, R. R., and O'Connor, T. M.: Longterm follow-up study of patients with bronchial anastomosis or tracheal replacement. Chest, *61*:141, 1972.
14. Daughtry, D. C.: Traumatic torsion of the lung. N. Engl. J. Med., *256*:385, 1957.
15. Williams, J. R., and Bonte, F. J.: The Roentgenological Aspect of Non-Penetrating Chest Injuries. Springfield, Ill., Charles C Thomas, 1961.
16. Paredes, S., and Hipona, F. A.: The radiologic evaluation of patients with chest trauma. Med. Clin. North Am., *59*:37, 1975.
17. Raphael, M. J.: Mediastinal haematoma. A description of some radiological appearances. Br. J. Radiol., *36*:921, 1963.
18. Fishbone, G., Robbins, D. I., Osborn, D. J., and Grnja, V.: Trauma to the thoracic aorta and great vessels. Radiol. Clin. North Am., *11*:543, 1973.
19. Sanborn, J. C., Heitzman, E. R., and Markarian, B.: Traumatic rupture of the thoracic aorta. Roentgenpathological correlations. Radiology, *95*:293, 1970.
20. Parmley, L. F., Mattingly, T. W., Manion, W. C., and Jahnke, E. J., Jr.: Nonpenetrating traumatic injury of the aorta. Circulation, *17*:1086, 1958.
21. Hewes, R. C., Smith, D. C., and Lavine, M. H.: Iatrogenic hydromediastinum simulating aortic laceration. Am. J. Roentgenol., *133*:817, 1979.
22. Sherbon, K. J.: Traumatic rupture of the thoracic aorta—The radiologist's responsibility. Australas. Radiol., *164*:164, 1975.
23. Tisnado, J., Tsai, F. Y., Als, A., and Roach, J. F.: A new radiographic sign of acute traumatic rupture of the thoracic aorta: Displacement of the nasogastric tube to the right. Radiology, *125*:603, 1977.
24. Gerlock, A. J., Jr., Muhletaler, C. A., Coulam, C. M., and Hayes, P. T.: Traumatic aortic aneurysm: Validity of esophageal tube displacement sign. Am. J. Roentgenol., *135*:713, 1980.
25. Peters, D. R., and Gamsu, G.: Displacement of the right paraspinous interface: A radiographic sign of acute traumatic rupture of the thoracic aorta. Radiology, *134*:599, 1980.
26. Simeone, J. F., Minagi, H., and Putman, C. E.: Traumatic disruption of the thoracic aorta: Significance of the left apical extrapleural cap. Radiology, *117*:265, 1975.
27. Simeone, J. F., Deren, M. M., and Cagle, F.: The value of the left apical cap in the diagnosis of aortic

(top of right column) Jr.: Traumatic lung cyst: Case report and literature review. J. Trauma, *21*:493, 1981.

rupture. A prospective and retrospective study. Radiology, *139*:35, 1981.

28. Woodring, J. H., Pulmano, C. M., and Stevens, R. K.: The right paratracheal stripe in blunt chest trauma. Radiology, *143*:605, 1982.

29. Yee, E. S., Thomas, A. N., and Goodman, P. C.: Isolated first rib fracture: Clinical significance after blunt chest trauma. Ann. Thorac. Surg., *32*:278, 1981.

30. Fisher, R. G., Ward, R. E., Ben-Menachem, Y., Mattox, K. L., and Flynn, T. C.: Arteriography and the fractured first rib: Too much for too little? A. J. R., *138*:1059, 1982.

31. Woodring, J. H., Fried, A. M., Hatfield, D. R., Stevens, R. K., and Todd, E. P.: Fractures of first and second ribs: Predictive value for arterial and bronchial injury. A. J. R., *138*:211, 1982.

32. Eller, J. L., and Ziter, F. M. H., Jr.: Avulsion of the innominate artery from the aortic arch. An evaluation of roentgenographic findings. Radiology, *94*:75, 1970.

33. Leading article: Traumatic perforation of oesophagus. Br. Med J., *1*:524, 1972.

34. Parkin, G. J. S.: The radiology of perforated oesophagus. Clin. Radiol., *24*:324, 1973.

35. Vessal, K., Montali, R. J., Larson, S. M., Chaffee, V., and James, A. E., Jr.: Evaluation of barium and Gastrografin as contrast media for the diagnosis of eosphageal ruptures or perforations. Am. J. Roentgenol., *123*:307, 1975.

36. Ebert, P. A., Gaertner, R. A., and Zuidema, G. D.: Traumatic diaphragmatic hernia. Surg. Gynecol. Obstet., *125*:59, 1967.

37. Marchand, P.: Traumatic hiatus hernia. Br. Med. J., *1*:754, 1962.

38. Toombs, B. D., Sandler, C. M., and Lester, R. G.: Computed tomography of chest trauma. Radiology, *140*:733, 1981.

39. Goodman, L. R.: Postoperative chest radiograph: II. Alterations after major intrathoracic surgery. Am. J. Roentgenol., *134*:803, 1980.

40. Escovitz, E. S., Okluski, T. A., and Lapayowker, M. S.: The midsternal stripe: A sign of dehiscence following median sternotomy. Radiology, *121*:521, 1976.

41. Berkow, A. E., and Demos, T. C.: The midsternal stripe and its relationship to postoperative sternal dehiscence. Radiology, *121*:525, 1976.

42. Williams, N. S., and Lewis, C. T.: Bronchopleural fistula: a review of 86 cases. Br. J. Surg., *63*:520, 1976.

43. Malave, G., Foster, E. D., Wilson, J. A., and Munro, D. D.: Bronchopleural fistula—present-day study of an old problem. A review of 52 cases. Ann. Thorac. Surg., *11*:1, 1971.

44. Westcott, J. L., and Cole, S. R.: Interstitial pulmonary emphysema in children and adults: Roentgenographic features. Radiology, *111*:367, 1974.

45. Gamsu, G., Singer, M. M., Vincent, H. H., Berry, S., and Nadel, J. A.: Postoperative impairment of mucous transport in the lung. Am. Rev. Respir. Dis., *114*:673, 1976.

46. Templeton, A. W., Almond, C. H., Seaber, A., Simmons, C., and MacKenzie, J.: Postoperative pulmonary patterns following cardiopulmonary bypass. Am. J. Roentgenol., *96*:1007, 1966.

47. Van De Water, J. M.: Preoperative and postoperative techniques in the prevention of pulmonary complications. Surg. Clin. North Am., *60*:1339, 1980.

48. Hechtman, H. B., Krausz, M. M., Utsunomiya, T., and Valeri, C. R.: Preoperative assessment of the high risk surgical patient. Surg. Clin. North Am., *60*:1349, 1980.

49. Rehder, K., Sessler, A. D., and Marsh, H. M.: General anesthesia and the lung. Am. Rev. Respir. Dis., *112*:541, 1975.

50. Ghia, J., and Andersen, N. B.: Pulmonary function and cardiopulmonary bypass. J.A.M.A., *212*:593, 1970.

51. Bartlett, R. H., Gazzaniga, A. B., and Geraghty, T. R.: Respiratory maneuvers to prevent postoperative pulmonary complications. J.A.M.A., *224*:1017, 1973.

52. Stein, M., and Cassara, E. L.: Preoperative pulmonary evaluation and therapy in surgery patients. J.A.M.A., *211*:787, 1970.

53. Hodgkin, J. E., Dines, D. E., and Didier, E. P.: Preoperative evaluation of the patient with pulmonary disease. Mayo Clin. Proc., *48*:114, 1973.

54. Goodman, L. R.: Postoperative chest radiograph: I. Alterations after abdominal surgery. Am. J. Roentgenol., *134*:533, 1980.

55. Gaensler, E. A., and Weisel, R. D.: The risks in abdominal and thoracic surgery in COPD. Postgrad. Med., *54*:183, 1973.

56. Collins, C. D., Darke, C. S., and Knowelden, J.: Chest complications after upper abdominal surgery: Their anticipation and prevention. Br. Med. J., *1*:401, 1968.

57. Wightman, J. A. K.: A prospective survey of the incidence of postoperative pulmonary complications. Br. J. Surg., *55*:85, 1968.

58. Ravin, C. E., Putman, C. E., and McLous, T. C.: Hazards of the intensive care unit. Am. J. Roentgenol., *126*:423, 1976.

59. Baigrie, R. S., and Morgan, C. D.: Hemodynamic monitoring: catheter insertion techniques, complications and trouble-shooting. C.M.A. Journal, *121*:885, 1979.

60. Mitchell, S. E., and Clark, R. A.: Complications of central venous catheterization. Am. J. Roentgenol., *133*:467, 1979.

61. Langston, C. S.: The aberrant central venous catheter and its complications. Radiology, *100*:55, 1971.

62. Swan, H. J. C., Ganz, W., Forrester, J., Marcus, H., Diamond, G., and Chonette, D.: Catheterization of the heart in man with use of a flow-directed balloon-tipped catheter. N. Engl. J. Med., *283*:447, 1970.

63. Foote, G. A., Schabel, S. I., and Hodges, M.: Pulmonary complications of the flow-directed balloon-tipped catheter. N. Engl. J. Med., *290*:927, 1974.

64. McLoud, T. C., and Putman, C. E.: Radiology of the Swan-Ganz catheter and associated pulmonary complications. Radiology, *116*:19, 1975.

65. Katz, J. D., Cronau, L. H., Barash, P. G., and Mandel, S. D.: Pulmonary artery flow guided catheters in the perioperative period. Indications and complications. J.A.M.A., *237*:2832, 1977.

66. Brown, B. G., Goldfarb, D., Topaz, S. R., and Gott, V. L.: Diastolic augmentation by intra-aortic balloon. Circulatory hemodynamics and treatment of severe, acute left ventricular failure in dogs. J. Thorac. Cardiovasc. Surg., *53*:789, 1967.

67. Hyson, E. A., Ravin, C. E., Kelley, M. J., and Curtis, A. M.: Intraaortic counterpulsation balloon: radiographic considerations. Am. J. Roentgenol., *128*:915, 1977.

68. Gross, N. J.: Pulmonary effects of radiation therapy. Ann. Intern. Med., *86*:81, 1977.

69. Cooper, G., Jr., Guerrant, J. L., Harden, A. G., and Teates, D.: Some consequences of pulmonary irradiation. Am. J. Roentgenol., *85*:865, 1961.

70. Rubin, P., and Casarett, G. W.: Clinical Radiation Pathology, Vol. I. Philadelphia, W. B. Saunders Co., 1968.

71. Bloomer, W. D., and Hellman, S.: Normal tissue responses to radiation therapy. N. Engl. J. Med., 293:80, 1975.

72. Lougheed, M. N., and Maguire, G. H.: Irradiation pneumonitis in the treatment of carcinoma of the breast. J. Can. Assoc. Radiol., 11:1, 1960.

73. Wara, W. M., Phillips, T. L., Margolis, L. W., and Smith, V.: Radiation pneumonitis: A new approach to the derivation of time-dose factors. Cancer, 32:547, 1973.

74. Parris, T. M., Knight, J. G., Hess, C. E., and Constable, W. C.: Severe radiation pneumonitis precipitated by withdrawal of corticosteroids: A diagnostic and therapeutic dilemma. Am. J. Roentgenol., 132:284, 1979.

75. Leading article: Case of acute radiation injury. Br. Med. J., 2:574, 1974.

76. Roswit, B., and White, D. C.: Severe radiation injuries of the lung. Am. J. Roentgenol., 129:127, 1977.

77. Jennings, F. L., and Arden, A.: Development of radiation pneumonitis. Time and dose factors. Arch. Pathol., 74:351, 1962.

78. Bennett, D. E., Million, R. R., and Ackerman, L. V.: Bilateral radiation pneumonitis, a complication of the radiotherapy of bronchogenic carcinoma. (Report and analysis of seven cases with autopsy.) Cancer, 23:1001, 1969.

79. Teates, C. D.: The effects of unilateral thoracic irradiation on pulmonary blood flow. Am. J. Roentgenol., 102:875, 1968.

80. Deeley, T. J.: The effects of radiation on the lungs in the treatment of carcinoma of the bronchus. Clin. Radiol., 11:33, 1960.

81. Smith, J. C.: Radiation pneumonitis. A review. Am. Rev. Respir. Dis., 87:647, 1963.

82. Polansky, S. M., Ravin, C. E., and Prosnitz, L. R.: Pulmonary changes after primary irradiation for early breast carcinoma. Am. J. Roentgenol., 134:101, 1980.

83. Whitcomb, M. E., and Schwarz, M. E.: Pleural effusion complicating intensive mediastinal radiation therapy. Am. Rev. Respir. Dis., 103:100, 1971.

84. Gomm, S. A., and Stretton, T. B.: Chronic pericardial effusion after mediastinal radiotherapy. Thorax, 36:149, 1981.

85. Applefeld, M. M., Cole, J. F., Pollock, S. H., et al.: The late appearance of chronic pericardial disease in patients treated by radiotherapy for Hodgkin's disease. Ann. Intern. Med., 94:338, 1981.

86. Sadove, A. M., Block, M., Rossof, A. H., et al.: Radiation carcinogenesis in man: New primary neoplasms in fields of prior therapeutic radiation. Cancer, 48:1139, 1981.

87. Nelson, D. F., Cooper, S., Weston, M. G., and Rubin, P.: Second malignant neoplasms in patients treated for Hodgkin's disease with radiotherapy or radiotherapy and chemotherapy. Cancer, 48:2386, 1981.

88. Doll, R.: Radiation hazards: 25 years of collaborative research. Br. J. Radiol., 54:179, 1981.

89. Smith, P. G., and Doll, R.: Mortality from cancer and all causes among British radiologists. Br. J. Radiol., 4:187, 1981.

90. Cameron, S. J., Grant, I. W. B., Lutz, W., and Pearson, J. G.: The early effect of irradiation on ventilatory function in bronchial carcinoma. Clin. Radiol., 20:12, 1969.

14

DISEASES OF THE CHEST
OF UNKNOWN ORIGIN

SARCOIDOSIS

Sarcoidosis (*synonyms:* Boeck's sarcoid, Bes-nier-Boeck-Schaumann's disease) is a disease of unknown etiology, difficult to define in precise terms. It is characterized pathologically by the noncaseating granuloma, whose presence in many organs, including the lung, liver, spleen, lymph nodes, skin, and bone, creates a complex clinical and roentgenologic picture usually indicative of the diagnosis. It is to be emphasized, however, that the demonstration of noncaseating granulomas does not in itself constitute absolute evidence of the disease, since such lesions are by no means specific. For example, it is not uncommon to find local noncaseating granulomas—or "sarcoid lesions"—in the skin or in various organs, in association with such diseases as carcinoma, Hodgkin's disease, and ulcerative colitis, or secondary to trauma. It is this lack of specificity that makes definition so difficult and creates the necessity for careful distinction between the pathologic findings of a noncaseating granuloma and the clinical-roentgenologic-pathologic disseminated disease known as sarcoidosis.[1]

INCIDENCE AND EPIDEMIOLOGY

In the majority of cases, the presence of sarcoidosis is first identified on a screening chest roentgenogram of asymptomatic individuals. Approximately 50 per cent of patients with sarcoidosis are symptomless when the disease is first recognized; only 25 per cent present with respiratory symptoms, usually dyspnea.[2] The disease appears to be more common in

temperate than in tropical climates.[2] Sarcoidosis is extremely rare in Southeast Asia. A mass community roentgenographic survey of 3.6 million persons in Taiwan did not uncover a single case,[3] although four confirmed cases have recently been described in Hong Kong Chinese persons.[4] The disease appears to be more prevalent in rural areas, a distribution that has been particularly noted in the southeastern United States. Sarcoidosis is rarely seen in African or South American Negroes or mulattoes, whereas the black population of the United States is unusually susceptible. This is particularly true in black women, in whom the estimated incidence is 10 to 17 times that in Caucasians.[1, 5] A disproportionately high incidence has also been observed among Puerto Ricans living in the United States.[6]

The sex incidence varies in different series, showing no predominance in some and a definite female predominance in others.[1, 2] Although the disease may occur at any age, it is recognized most commonly in patients between the ages of 20 and 40.[2, 5] Reports in the American medical literature[7] suggest that sarcoidosis in children, although infrequent, is more commonly associated with symptoms; for example, in an analysis of the clinical and radiologic characteristics of pulmonary sarcoidosis in 26 children ranging in age from 2.5 to 17 years (mean, 13 years), Merten and his colleagues[8] found that 25 (96 per cent) were symptomatic at the time of diagnosis. This discrepancy in clinical manifestations between children and adults has also been reported by others.[9] In very young children under the age of four years, the incidence of symptoms referable to the joints, skin, and eyes is unusually high, with most of the reported cases being Caucasian.[9, 10]

ETIOLOGY AND PATHOGENESIS

The lungs and hilar lymph nodes are the structures most commonly involved (in 80 to 90 per cent of cases in large series),[1, 5] strongly suggesting that the etiologic agent enters the body via the lungs, probably by inhalation, and from there dissemination occurs to other organs and tissues. Despite this possible evidence, the etiology remains obscure. Several theories have been proposed and these have been discussed in considerable detail by Scadding in his comprehensive review of the subject.[2] At the time of this writing, the two most likely hypotheses are: (1) an infectious etiology, in which a variety of organisms have been implicated, including *Mycobacterium tuberculosis*,[2] atypical mycobacteria,[11] and other transmissible agents;[12–14] and (2) an immunologic reaction to an unidentified antigen or antigens.[15] Rather than discussing these theoretical possibilities further, we feel that it would be of greater value to present in some detail certain aspects of the pathogenesis of the disease concerning which a considerable body of new information has surfaced in recent years. Much of what follows has been gleaned from an edited transcript of an NIH Conference on the subject moderated by Crystal and published in 1981.[16]

Morphologically, the hallmark of pulmonary sarcoidosis is the granuloma, and in fact the diagnosis cannot be made without demonstrable granuloma formation. However, it has become increasingly apparent that preceding the formation of granulomas there occurs an active alveolitis (interstitial pneumonitis) characterized by an accumulation of inflammatory and immune-effector cells in the interstitium. The cell population of the alveolitis is almost entirely mononuclear, consisting of monocytes, macrophages, and lymphocytes in approximately equal numbers.[17] The stimulus for the accumulation of these cells is unknown, although there is considerable evidence to indicate the mechanism by which monocytes are attracted to the interstitium (*see* further on). Although the effector role of monocytes and macrophages is unknown, there is solid evidence that sarcoidosis is distinguished by the presence of large numbers of activated T-lymphocytes, which probably play a major role in pathogenesis.[17]

Much of the information regarding the cell population and activity of the alveolitis of sarcoidosis has accumulated through the technique of bronchopulmonary lavage in addition to histologic examination of tissue. For example, it is known that the cell populations of patients with sarcoidosis differ markedly from those of normal subjects.[18] In normal lungs, the cell population consists of 90 per cent alveolar macrophages, less than 10 per cent lymphocytes, and less than 1 per cent polymorphonuclear leukocytes. By contrast, in the 45 patients with biopsy-proven pulmonary sarcoidosis who were studied by Crystal and his colleagues,[16] there was a marked increase in the proportion of lymphocytes, averaging 33 ($\pm$ 6) per cent; in those patients with clinical evidence of active disease, the proportion of lymphocytes was even higher (55 [$\pm$ 8] per cent). In total numbers, the alveolitis was characterized by an increase in the number of both lymphocytes and mononuclear phagocytes (monocytes and macrophages).

In normal lungs, the percentage of lung lymphocytes that are T-lymphocytes ranges from 65 to 80 per cent, whereas in sarcoid lungs this amounts to 90 ($\pm$ 4) per cent,[18] the majority being of the "helper" variety.[19] Associated with this excess of T-lymphocytes in the lung is a peripheral blood T-lymphocytopenia; by contrast, in normal subjects the proportion of T-lymphocytes in lung and blood is the same. Further, in sarcoidosis the proportion of lung lymphocytes that are B-lymphocytes is significantly reduced while the proportion in the blood is increased. Sarcoid lung has 20 to 25 times more T-lymphocytes than B-lymphocytes.[18] It is of some interest that recent studies by J. D. Fulmer (personal communication) have shown an excess of T-lymphocytes in the lungs of patients with acute idiopathic pulmonary fibrosis and acute histiocytosis-X; by contrast, in the chronic phase of these diseases, T-lymphocytosis disappears and is replaced by polymorphonuclear leukocytosis.

In contrast to the evidence for an overactive cell–mediated immune response at sites of disease activity, cutaneous anergy and decreased phytohemagglutinin-induced lymphoblastic transformation are found in most patients with active sarcoidosis.[20] This apparent paradox may be explained by the lymphocytopenia in the peripheral blood, consisting mostly of suppressor cells that are the activated fighting helper cells being held at the sites of disease activity.[21] In the peripheral blood, B-lymphocyte overactivity is reflected in increased levels of immunoglobulins and kappa and lambda chains, often accompanied by circulating immune complexes.

The mechanism by which monocytes accumulate in excess numbers in the lungs is a function of T-lymphocytes. It has been shown that these cells elaborate a specific substance, monocyte chemotactic factor, that attracts blood monocytes.[22, 23] The T-lymphocytes of sarcoid lung secrete 25 times as much monocyte chemotactic factor as the T-lymphocytes of peripheral blood, thus establishing a gradient between lung and blood that results in a virtually continuous supply of monocytes in lung tissue. In addition, neutrophils are rarely found in sarcoid lung, presumably because T-lymphocytes secrete a leukocyte inhibitory factor.[22]

The excess numbers of activated macrophages that accumulate in the lungs of patients with sarcoidosis are known to produce increased quantities of lysozyme and angiotensin-converting enzyme. Although blood levels of these enzymes are also increased, evidence is not at all convincing that these blood levels reflect the intensity of the alveolitis.

As already pointed out, the granulomas that are requisite to the diagnosis of sarcoidosis appear to evolve subsequent to the phase of active alveolitis.[17] As shown by Rosen and associates,[25] developing granulomas are composed of a loose collection of inflammatory and immune-effector cells of which monocytes, macrophages, and lymphocytes predominate over epithelioid cells. As the granuloma matures, there occurs an increase in the number of epithelioid cells (derived from the mononuclear phagocyte system) and a corresponding decrease in the number of mononuclear phagocytes and lymphocytes. Thus, alveolitis and granulomas are present in inverse proportions—the greater the amount of alveolitis the fewer the granulomas, and vice versa.[17] Multinucleated giant cells, commonly of the Langhans' type, are frequently found among the epithelioid cells within the granulomas and are presumed to develop from epithelioid cells themselves.[17] In more mature granulomas, fibroblasts may be present in considerable numbers at the periphery of the lesions and presumably are responsible for the fibrosis that constitutes the end stage of the granulomas in some patients. In the study by Rosen and his colleagues,[25] fibrosis was much more frequent (82 per cent) in biopsy specimens in which interstitial pneumonitis was absent than when it predominated (32 per cent) or was prominent (60 per cent).

Specific histocompatibility antigens (HLA) have not been associated with increased susceptibility to sarcoidosis, but two different studies[26, 27] have shown an excess of HLA B8 in patients whose disease spontaneously resolved (notably those presenting with erythema nodosum and arthralgia) but not in those showing residual damage.

In summary, sarcoidosis consists initially of an alveolitis characterized by diffuse infiltration of lung parenchyma by mononuclear cells including monocytes, macrophages, and lymphocytes. Bronchopulmonary lavage accurately characterizes this cell population and acts as a useful monitor of the activity of the alveolitis. It is probable that the major effector cell is a "helper" T-lymphocyte that elaborates monocyte chemotactic factor which attracts blood monocytes. Progression of the disease is characterized by gradual resolution of the alveolitis and its replacement by multinucleated giant cell granulomas. Granulomas may undergo complete resolution leaving no residua, as in the majority of cases, or may undergo progressive fibrosis terminating in the end-stage lung; the eventual outcome is at least partly dependent on HLA.

PATHOLOGIC CHARACTERISTICS

In order of frequency, organs involved in disseminated sarcoidosis are the lungs, liver, spleen, heart, and bone marrow,[1] the lungs being by far the most commonly affected and their incidence of involvement being approximated or equaled only by the lymph nodes. Affection of the skin and eye is not uncommon.

In the lungs, as discussed above, it is now recognized that noncaseating granuloma formation—the histologic hallmark of sarcoidosis—is preceded by a stage of nongranulomatous interstitial pneumonitis or alveolitis.[16, 25] Rosen and his colleagues carried out a histologic study of biopsy tissue from 128 patients with clinical findings consistent with sarcoidosis with the view of determining the incidence of interstitial pneumonitis in relation to granuloma formation. They classified interstitial pneumonitis as "predominating" if it was present in a greater amount than granulomas, as "prominent" if it was present in a lesser amount than granulomas but nevertheless quite conspicuous, and as "absent" if it was present in a very minimal amount or not at all. The biopsy specimens revealed interstitial pneumonitis predominating in 31 (24 per cent) of the 128 patients, prominent in 48 (38 per cent), and absent in 49 (38 per cent). Their findings appear to indicate that interstitial pneumonitis represents an early lesion and possibly the initial lesion in pulmonary sarcoidosis.

Noncaseating granulomas typically develop in relation to the lymphatic channels in the peribronchiolar and subpleural interstitial tissues and along the interlobular septa. Multiple deposits are scattered throughout the interstitium of the lung, including the alveolar walls, but seldom if ever within the parenchymal air spaces. Individual deposits are microscopic in size and although commonly discrete, they may conglomerate to form masses 3 to 4 cm in diameter. The lung parenchyma between nodules usually is normal, although conglomeration may markedly distort the lung architecture. Lesions in the parenchymal interstitial tissue may produce much more distortion of atria and alveoli without actually destroying them. Blood vessels may be affected, although the endothelium commonly remains intact and, therefore, thrombosis rarely occurs. Granulomas may also be seen in the walls of larger bronchi.

Microscopically, the granuloma consists of groups of large epithelioid cells with little or no surrounding cuff of inflammatory cells that is so characteristic of granulomas of infectious origin. Caseous necrosis does not occur, but the center of the nodule may contain a small amount of eosinophilic necrotic material. Multinucleated giant cells are common, particularly in fibrotic lesions. Their nuclei are usually at the periphery and their cytoplasm frequently contains inclusion bodies. Three types of inclusion bodies have been described—the asteroid, the lamellated or conchoidal body (Schaumann body), and, occasionally, anisotropic particles. None of these inclusion bodies is specific for sarcoidosis, since they are seen in other forms of granulomatous and foreign body reaction. Lymphocytes, occasionally plasma cells, and rarely neutrophils and eosinophils may be present within the nodule itself or around its periphery.

It is reasonably certain that these granulomatous lesions can heal without significant residua. However, fibrosis may occur, apparently starting in the periphery of the nodule and proceeding toward the center, the granuloma becoming gradually transformed into a relatively acellular mass of hyaline material. Extensive pulmonary fibrosis ensues in a small percentage of cases. The end result is widespread interstitial fibrosis, bronchiolectasis, and distortion of lung architecture.[28] Such fibrosis may be associated with irregular areas of pulmonary emphysema.

ROENTGENOGRAPHIC MANIFESTATIONS

The roentgenologic changes in thoracic sarcoidosis may usefully be classified for descriptive purposes into four groups or stages:

Stage 0. No demonstrable abnormality.

Stage 1. Hilar and mediastinal lymph node enlargement without pulmonary abnormality.

Stage 2. Hilar and mediastinal lymph node enlargement plus diffuse pulmonary disease.

Stage 3. Diffuse pulmonary disease unassociated with node enlargement.

This classification does not provide for that stage of the disease characterized by diffuse fibrosis and the end-stage lung, and it might be reasonable to consider this pattern as stage 4. The majority of patients (as many as 88 per cent in one series[29]) have lymph node enlargement with or without parenchymal involvement.

LYMPH NODE ENLARGEMENT WITHOUT PULMONARY ABNORMALITY

Bilateral hilar lymph node enlargement occurs in 75 to 90 per cent of patients with sarcoidosis, in approximately equal numbers with and without diffuse parenchymal disease.[30] Of 150 patients with proved sarcoidosis studied by Kirks and his colleagues,[31] lymph node enlargement was present as the sole abnormality in 65 (43.3 per cent) and in association with pulmonary disease in 61 (40.7 per cent). Although symptoms are present in about 50 per cent of patients with hilar lymph node enlargement, in most cases they are referable to involvement elsewhere.[30] Node enlargement usually is localized to the bronchopulmonary, tracheobronchial, and paratracheal groups and is almost always symmetric bilaterally (Figure 14–1). In our experience, paratracheal lymph node enlargement is far more often bilateral than right-sided only. The right paratracheal zone is much more clearly visualized on posteroanterior roentgenograms than the left because the latter is obscured by the superimposed aorta and brachiocephalic vessels. Enlargement of posterior mediastinal nodes is very uncommon in our experience, although the incidence in reported series varies greatly (only one of 62 patients in one series[32] but in six [20 per cent] of 30 cases in another series[33]). Unilateral hilar lymph node enlargement is uncommon, being reported in 3 to 5 per cent of proved cases.[34] Occasionally, enlarged hilar and carinal nodes can compress the major bronchi.

The contour of the outer borders of enlarged hila usually is lobulated, particularly on the right side. Calcification of hilar lymph nodes has been reported in roughly 5 per cent of patients[34] and in some cases is said to resemble the eggshell calcification of silicosis.[34] Paratracheal node enlargement seldom if ever occurs without concomitant enlargement of hilar nodes. This bilaterally symmetric hilar and paratracheal lymph node enlargement contrasts sharply with the node enlargement that char-

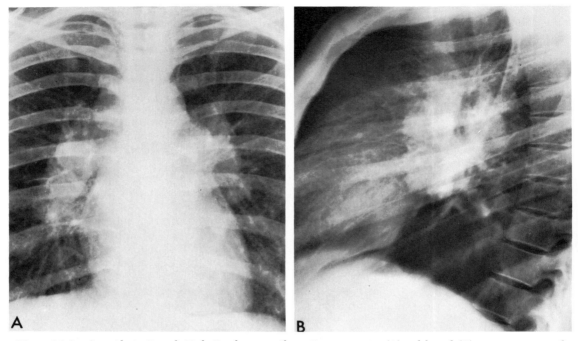

Figure 14–1. Sarcoidosis: Lymph Node Involvement Alone. Posteroanterior *(A)* and lateral *(B)* roentgenograms of a 32-year-old asymptomatic woman demonstrate marked enlargement of both hila, the lobulated contour being typical of lymph node enlargement. The azygos node is enlarged, as are nodes in the aortopulmonary window. The lungs are clear.

acterizes lymphomas. In lymphomas, enlargement tends to occur predominantly in the anterior and paratracheal groups; when it involves the hilar nodes, it is predominantly unilateral and asymmetric. Also, retrosternal node enlargement is common in lymphoma and fairly uncommon in sarcoidosis, being observed in only ten (16 per cent) of the 62 patients studied by Bein and associates.[32] However, the possibility of sarcoidosis should not be dismissed when such node enlargement is present, particularly when it is associated with enlargement of hilar nodes. An additional contrasting feature of sarcoidosis and lymphoma is that in the former the onset of diffuse lung disease is commonly associated with a diminution in lymph node size or at least with cessation of their growth, a finding not observed in lymphoma.

It is important to appreciate the fact that the designation "hilar and mediastinal lymph node enlargement without pulmonary disease" applies to *roentgenographic* evidence alone and not to pathologic or pulmonary function evidence. In a recent report of 21 consecutive patients with this stage of the disease who underwent open lung biopsy, Rosen and his colleagues[35] found typical sarcoid granulomas in all. Similarly, pulmonary function impairment

is a common finding in the absence of roentgenographically apparent lung abnormality.

Seventy to 80 per cent of patients with hilar lymph node enlargement, with or without visible pulmonary involvement, will eventually show complete roentgenographic resolution without residua.

DIFFUSE PULMONARY DISEASE WITH OR WITHOUT LYMPH NODE ENLARGEMENT

Approximately 16[31] to 25 per cent[30] of patients with pulmonary sarcoidosis present with pulmonary disease without hilar lymph node enlargement. In the majority of cases the pulmonary abnormality is diffuse and evenly distributed throughout the lungs. Three basic patterns of disease can be recognized: the reticulonodular pattern, the "acinar" pattern, and large nodules.

The Reticulonodular Pattern

This roentgenographic pattern may range from purely nodular to purely reticular but usually is a combination of both (Fig. 14–2).[30, 31] The reticulation may be in the form of a very fine or a very coarse network. A so-called miliary pattern is uncommon.

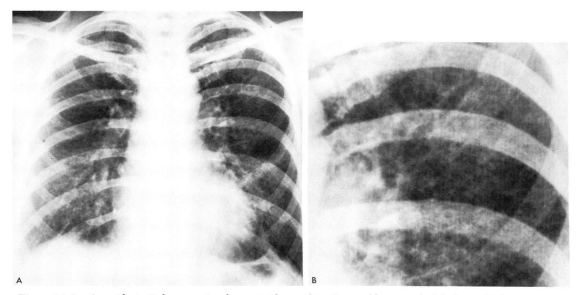

Figure 14–2. Sarcoidosis: Pulmonary Involvement Alone. This 47-year-old woman had had a radical mastectomy 6 years previously for carcinoma of the breast. For the past 2 years she had noted increasing dyspnea on exertion, which lately was interfering with housework. Because of the history, the diagnosis of lymphangitic carcinoma was suspected clinically. A posteroanterior roentgenogram *(A)* and a magnified view of the upper portion of the left lung *(B)* revealed a diffuse reticular pattern throughout both lungs, unassociated with mediastinal or hilar lymph node enlargement. The diagnosis of sarcoidosis was established from a scalene node biopsy.

The "Acinar" Pattern

This consists chiefly of indistinctly defined opacities measuring up to 6 or 7 mm in diameter, thus possessing features of acinar shadows. They may be discrete or coalescent and in the latter circumstance may be associated with an air bronchogram.[31] This pattern is frequently associated with a reticulonodular pattern elsewhere in the lungs. Sometimes confluence of

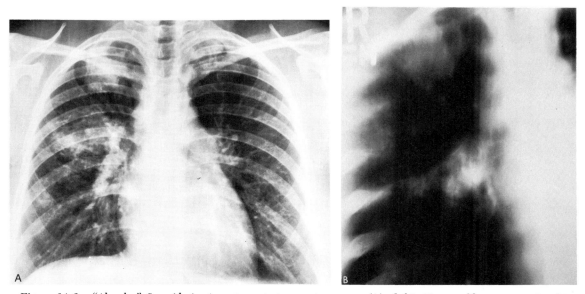

Figure 14–3. "Alveolar" Sarcoidosis. A posteroanterior roentgenogram *(A)* of this 26-year old asymptomatic white woman reveals two poorly defined homogeneous opacities in the right lung, one in the apex and the other in the parahilar zone. Paratracheal (and possibly hilar) lymph nodes are enlarged bilaterally, but there is no evidence of diffuse lung disease. A tomogram in anteroposterior projection *(B)* shows the masses to be homogeneous in density, except for a calcified lymph node in the parahilar opacity. Transbronchial biopsy of the lower lesion revealed noncaseating granulomas consistent with sarcoidosis.

acinar shadows can produce large areas of consolidation (Figure 14–3) or scattered, hazy consolidations with irregular borders. The presence of bullae and fibrosis in upper lung zones sometimes creates an appearance suggesting cavitary tuberculosis. It is probable that this appearance represents the persistence of fibrotic contraction following clearing of diffuse disease. Approximately one-third of the 150 patients studied by Kirks and his associates[31] eventually showed complete roentgenographic resolution of their pulmonary disease, the remainder showing either persistence of the acinar pattern for the duration of follow-up or progression to pulmonary fibrosis. The acinar pattern is observed more frequently in black than in white patients.

Large Nodules

An occasional case of sarcoidosis proved by biopsy or by a positive Kveim reaction shows large, dense, round lesions simulating metastatic neoplasm.[20] This pattern, consisting of sharply marginated nodular opacities with an average diameter greater than 1 cm, was observed in only three of the 150 patients studied by Kirks and associates;[31] all were black.

When diffuse pulmonary disease and lymph node enlargement coexist, their roentgenographic appearance is no different from that of separate involvement. However, in such circumstances, the two manifestations differ greatly in their temporal relationship in different patients. Diffuse pulmonary disease usually appears when hilar node enlargement is present, although the latter may be regressing. Node enlargement may disappear and be replaced by diffuse pulmonary involvement, either concurrently or as remotely as several years later; or it may remain, and diffuse pulmonary involvement may be superimposed upon it. So far as we are aware, there has been no report to indicate that hilar lymph node enlargement may develop *subsequent to* pulmonary parenchymal disease.

The relationship between the roentgenographic stage of the disease and the predominance of alveolitis or interstitial pneumonitis in relation to granuloma formation has received scant attention to date. However, in their retrospective study of 128 biopsy specimens from patients with sarcoidosis, Rosen and his colleagues[25] found that interstitial pneumonitis present in greater amount than granulomas occurred with significantly greater frequency in roentgenographic stage 1 (9/22 specimens; 41

per cent) than in stage 2 (10/54; 19 per cent) or stage 3 (5/29; 17 per cent). No other significant relationships were observed.

Other Roentgenographic Abnormalities

Cavitation is very uncommon, being observed in only eight (0.6 per cent) of the approximately 1180 cases reviewed by Mayock and associates.[5] The pathogenesis of cavitation in pulmonary sarcoidosis has not been clearly established but may relate to the expulsion of hyaline material or ischemic necrotic tissue from the center of large conglomerate sarcoid granulomas.[36] It is important to eliminate all other causes of cavitation before accepting sarcoidosis as the underlying condition. *Atelectasis* is a rare manifestation of pulmonary sarcoidosis. It may be associated with obstructive pneumonitis and is caused by endobronchial lesions that may be suspected if the overall roentgenologic or clinical picture suggests general sarcoidosis. *Pleural effusion* is uncommon but probably not to the extent that was once thought. The effusion is an exudate containing a predominance of lymphocytes.[37] Pleural biopsy often reveals noncaseating granulomas, and it has been postulated that the pathogenesis of pleural effusion is probably related to extensive involvement of both the visceral and parietal pleura by granulomatous disease. *Spontaneous pneumothorax* has been reported, presumably resulting from rupture of a bleb or bulla developing as a consequence of pulmonary fibrosis.[38]

Osseous involvement is said to occur in approximately 10 to 15 per cent of cases as judged roentgenologically. Characteristically, the small bones of the hands are predominantly involved, the pattern being chiefly lytic and consisting of cystic lesions and a lacelike trabecular pattern. However, it appears that the osseous manifestations of sarcoidosis are protean. They may be osteolytic, osteoblastic, or a combination of the two, and they may appear in a wide variety of skeletal elements. The only feature common to almost all cases is a strong predilection for blacks.

PULMONARY FIBROSIS

When pulmonary changes have been present for more than two years, resolution is the exception rather than the rule. Although there is disagreement as to what percentage of patients with pulmonary sarcoidosis develop irreversible pulmonary changes, an incidence of 20 per cent probably is reasonably accurate.[29, 38] Scarring usually is rather coarse, in the form of irregular linear strands extending outward from the hila toward the periphery and usually possessing considerable upper zonal predominance (Figure 14–4). It is commonly more uneven in its distribution than the reticulonodular pattern characteristic of the active stage and usually is associated with well-defined structural changes in the lungs, including bleb or bulla formation, bronchiectasis, and general emphysema. When fibrosis and emphysema are severe, changes in the heart and pulmonary vasculature are typical of pulmonary hypertension and cor pulmonale. In contrast to the predominance of lymphocytes in the bronchial lavage of patients with active sarcoidosis, those with advanced disease and fibrosis may manifest an excess of neutrophils.[40]

CLINICAL MANIFESTATIONS

It is impossible to state precisely in what percentage of these patients symptoms develop, but we would estimate the incidence at approximately 50 per cent of cases. Patients with roentgenographic evidence of hilar lymph node enlargement alone are almost always asymptomatic in our experience, although some authors would not concur.[20] Symptoms are often associated with multisystem involvement; they develop insidiously in the majority of cases and frequently are constitutional in type, consisting of weight loss, fatigue, weakness, and malaise. Fever occurs in about 17 per cent of cases on average.[5]

Symptoms of *pulmonary involvement* develop in 20 to 50 per cent of cases and include dry cough and shortness of breath.[20] Hemoptysis is rare. Auscultatory signs usually are absent in the early stages of the disease, although a few scattered rales may be heard in some cases. With the development of pulmonary fibrosis, crepitations may become more widespread and the breath sounds may become bronchial. Direct involvement of the *heart* is characterized by paroxysmal arrhythmias.[41] The incidence of myocardial involvement in necropsied cases is approximately 20 per cent,[1, 41] but this involvement may be unassocated with symptoms and is diagnosed clinically in less than 5 per cent of cases. The most common arrhythmia other than premature ventricular beats is ventricular tachycardia. Complete heart block is the most common conduction disturbance. The presence of arrhythmias in young individuals should suggest the diagnosis of myocardial sarcoidosis.

Enlargement of *peripheral lymph nodes* is said to be clinically evident in 73 per cent of cases,[5] but it is probable that involvement of peripheral nodes, whether clinically palpable

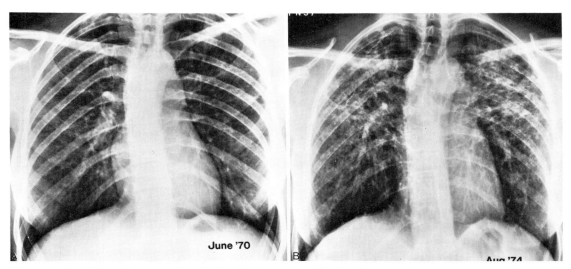

Figure 14–4. Diffuse Pulmonary Sarcoidosis with Progressive Fibrosis. The initial chest roentgenogram *(A)* of this 37-year-old woman reveals a rather coarse reticular pattern throughout both lungs with definite upper zonal predominance. There is no evidence of hilar or mediastinal lymph node enlargement. Open lung biopsy showed noncaseating granuloma consistent with a diagnosis of sarcoidosis. Three years later, the reticulation had become more marked and there had occurred an upward displacement and flaring of lower zone vessels, indicating the fibrotic nature of the upper zone disease. This was still more evident 1 year later *(B)*. Note that despite the fibrotic nature of the disease, there had occurred no overall reduction in lung volume, chiefly because of overinflation of lower zone parenchyma

or not, occurs at some time in every case of sarcoidosis. Lymph node biopsies from regions such as the scalene area, even when nodes are not palpable, are positive in 80 per cent of cases.[42] Palpable lymph nodes are found more often in series that include a large number of black patients. They are found most frequently in the cervical area but may also be felt in the axillae, epitrochlear regions, and the groin.[2]

The incidence of *ocular involvement* is approximately 20 per cent.[5] The characteristic lesion is uveitis, although involvement of the conjunctiva, sclera, retina, and lens may occur, resulting in cataracts and glaucoma.

Cutaneous involvement probably occurs in no more than one-third of cases.[5] Skin lesions are particularly common in blacks and consist of slightly raised nodules, often purplish in hue (lupus pernio), usually about the face, neck, shoulders, digits, and sometimes the mucous membranes of the nose. Large plaques resembling psoriasis may develop over the trunk or extremities. Lupus pernio and skin plaques usually are associated with a chronic persistent course. In the series reported by Sharma,[43] roentgenologic resolution of pulmonary disease occurred in only 22 per cent of the patients with skin plaques and in none of those with lupus pernio. A particular interesting form of cutaneous involvement in sarcoidosis is erythema nodosum, which consists of transitory, raised, slightly painful erythematous lesions, usually on the skin of the lower extremities. An acute onset of sarcoidosis characterized by fever, arthralgia, hilar lymph node enlargement, and erythema nodosum is a fairly common mode of presentation in Europe and often is referred to as Löfgren's syndrome.[44]

The incidence of *hepatic and splenic involvement* depends on whether the figures are obtained from clinical or postmortem studies. Whereas necropsy reveals sarcoid granulomas at these sites in approximately 70 per cent of cases,[1] and liver and spleen are palpable clinically in only about 25 per cent of cases. Although involvement of the liver seldom is of a degree sufficient to impair function, enlargement of the spleen may be so severe as to necessitate splenectomy because of hypersplenism or because of its effects as a space-occupying mass.[1]

Bone and joint involvement may occur with or without skin lesions.[5] Kaplan[45] has described three forms of joint involvement: (1) migratory polyarthritis associated with erythema nodosum, fever, and hilar lymph node enlargement; (2) single or recurrent episodes of polyarticular or monarticular arthritis; and (3)

persistent arthritis. The most frequent form is that which occurs acutely and is associated with fever and often with erythema nodosum. This is an arthralgia rather than an arthritis and tends to involve the larger joints, particularly the ankles, wrists, elbows, and knees. Symptoms range in duration from a few days to several weeks, and the patient typically is free of disability. Arthritis is uncommon and usually is seen in patients with multiple system involvement. Bone involvement in sarcoidosis frequently is associated with cutaneous manifestations, particularly the form known as lupus pernio;[2] bone pain is rare. A case has been reported recently in which migratory polyarthralgia was associated with painful clubbing of fingers and toes, bilateral and symmetrical.[46]

The combination of parotid gland involvement, uveitis, and pyrexia is called uveoparotid fever. Although uveitis is common and the volume of saliva and enzyme secretion from parotid and submaxillary glands often is decreased, enlargement of the *exocrine glands* is rare. Involvement of the lacrimal glands may result in keratoconjunctivitis sicca and duct obstruction. Granulomatous infiltration of the *kidneys* rarely leads to impairment of function; renal insufficiency usually develops as a result of hypercalcemia, nephrocalcinosis, and nephrolithiasis but has also been reported in association with interstitial sarcoid nephritis.[47, 48]

Central nervous system involvement occurs in 5 per cent of patients.[49] The most characteristic intracranial localization is in the hypothalamus, with resultant impaired hormonal secretion from the anterior or posterior lobes or both.[49] Involvement of the facial nerves causes unilateral or bilateral facial palsy, a manifestation that sometimes is associated with uveoparotid fever. Direct involvement of the *endocrine glands* is relatively uncommon. Cases have been described in which hypercalcemia resulted from primary hyperparathyroidism rather than from the more common increased absorption of calcium owing to enhanced sensitivity to vitamin D. Symptomatic involvement of the *gastrointestinal tract* is very rare.[2] Infiltration of *skeletal muscle* may give rise to weakness.

PULMONARY FUNCTION TESTS

Pulmonary function impairment in sarcoidosis is common, even in the absence of roentgenographically apparent lung abnormality.[50] The pattern is predominantly one of restriction, at least in the earlier stages of the disease: vital capacity and functional residual capacity are reduced, the alveolar-arterial oxygen gradient is increased, diffusing capacity is decreased, and there are ventilation-perfusion abnormalities.[51] Slight or considerable reduction in compliance is seen, even in asympatomatic patients with no roentgenographic evidence of pulmonary disease. One of the most common findings is a low diffusing capacity, which may remain reduced when other function tests have improved and after symptoms have disappeared and the chest roentgenogram has returned to normal.[52] In a large percentage of such cases, lung biopsy reveals interstitial granulomatous or fibrotic disease. From studies of the fine structural morphometry of such lungs, the disturbances in blood–air gas transfer have been attributed to ventilation-perfusion inequality rather than to a diffusion defect.[53] In addition to these disturbances in function, some patients, particularly those with a roentgenographic pattern suggesting fibrosis, manifest clear evidence of an obstructive component.[54] The FEV_1-FVC ratio may be decreased and many patients show frequency dependence of dynamic compliance[55] and elevated ratios of closing volume to vital capacity.[54] In one study, 10 to 20 patients with sarcoidosis showed increased responsiveness to methacholine bronchial provocation compared to normal controls.[56]

Sequential roentgenographic studies of 64 patients with proved sarcoidosis showed that, when individuals are used as their own controls, overall profusion of opacities correlates highly with physiologic changes over time.[57]

LABORATORY INVESTIGATION

Approximately 2 per cent of unselected patients with clinically diagnosed and biopsy confirmed sarcoidosis have *hypercalcemia*. This comparatively low incidence does not indicate the true situation, however, since the majority of patients with untreated sarcoidosis whose calcium levels are normal can be shown by special studies to have abnormal calcium metabolism.[58] The disturbance appears to bear little relationship to osseous involvement, resulting chiefly from an increase in absorption of calcium from the gastrointestinal tract because of increased sensitivity to vitamin D. However, both influences may be operative to a greater or lesser extent. The hypercalcemia usually can be corrected by corticosteroid therapy, which serves to differentiate it from the hypercalcemia

of hyperparathyroidism. Although the majority of patients show only slight elevation in the serum calcium level, in a small number the levels pose a threat to life. The most significant effect is on the kidneys, in which nephrocalcinosis and nephrolithiasis may develop and may impair renal function.

Fifty per cent or more of patients have elevated levels of *serum globulins* during the active phase of the disease,[5] including abnormalities in gamma globulin, alpha$_2$ globulin, alpha$_2$ and gamma globulin, and beta globulin alone or in combination with alpha$_2$ or gamma globulin fractions.

A variety of other biochemical changes have been reported in sarcoidosis, usually in the form of elevated serum concentrations as a reflection of disease activity. Serum alkaline phosphatase has been found to be increased in 30 to 45 per cent of patients.[5] Many groups of investigators[59–62] have reported significant elevation of serum angiotensin I–converting enzyme (ACE) in patients with active sarcoidosis, particularly those with pulmonary involvement; however, as pointed out previously, evidence that increased blood levels of this enzyme (or of lysozyme) reflect intensity of the alveolitis is not at all convincing.[16] Increased levels of serum ACE are not specific for sarcoidosis,[63] having been observed in other granulomatous diseases. However, in one study of a variety of noninfectious granulomas, Katz and his colleagues[64] found normal ACE values in all patients except those with sarcoidosis. Serum levels of alpha$_1$-antitrypsin have also been found to be raised in patients with untreated active sarcoidosis but not in those with inactive disease or in healthy age- and sex-matched controls.[65]

Mayock and associates[5] found hemoglobin values below 11 g per 100 ml in 22 per cent of their patients. Leukopenia is common, white cell counts below 5000 per cu mm being observed in approximately 30 per cent of cases. Eosinophilia greater than 5 per cent occurs in about one-third of cases.

DIAGNOSIS AND DIFFERENTIAL DIAGNOSIS

Patients with sarcoidosis may present with a wide variety of symptoms and signs involving many organs and tissues.[1] Most commonly, ocular disturbances, enlarged peripheral lymph nodes, skin eruptions, and respiratory symptoms are the reasons for the patient's consulting a physician. Presenting complaints may be constitutional in nature and include weakness and loss of weight and appetite. However, the majority of patients are asymptomatic when first seen and the disease is discovered on a screening chest roentgenogram. A mode of presentation less common in North America than in Europe and the British Isles is the syndrome of erythema nodosum with hilar lymph node enlargement, often associated with fever and arthralgia. This syndrome has been accepted as synonymous with sarcoidosis whether or not pathologic proof is forthcoming, and with this we are in complete agreement. There is a strong female sex predominance in this association. Erythema nodosum may occur also in association with tuberculous, fungal, and streptococcal infections and as a reaction to drugs.

Although the clinical picture in sarcoidosis usually is nonspecific, the diagnosis can be made with confidence in most cases when tissue biopsy reveals noncaseating granuloma, especially if the Kveim test is positive. It should be remembered, however, that certain other granulomatous diseases, particularly tuberculosis, coccidioidomycosis, histoplasmosis, cryptococcosis, and brucellosis, may present a pathologic and clinical picture similar to that of sarcoidosis.

It is of course vital to recognize that the histologic identification of noncaseating granulomas on biopsy specimens may establish the diagnosis of sarcoidosis but generally provides little information regarding the intensity of the alveolitis. Similarly, neither chest roentgenograms nor pulmonary function studies can estimate with any degree of accuracy the activity of alveolitis.[66] For this assessment, it is now generally agreed that bronchoalveolar lavage and gallium scanning are required procedures. As previously discussed, analysis of lavage data not only characterizes the type of cells present but also estimates the overall intensity of the alveolitis.[16a] Further, it has been shown that when the proportion of T-lymphocytes remains low over a period of time, there is little change in lung function, whereas when the proportion of lung T-lymphocytes remains high, lung function can be expected to deteriorate.[16a] With regard to ^{67}Ga uptake patterns, Line[67] has stated that in patients with sarcoidosis there is a significant association of gallium uptake and the proportion of lung effector cells that are lymphocytes; and that the association of gallium uptake with the proportion of effector cells that are T-lymphocytes is even stronger. Thus, it may be concluded that although gallium scanning is not diagnostically specific, it can nevertheless be employed to characterize the severity and anatomic location of alveolitis and can be used repetitively to provide a longitudinal assessment of the degree of inflammation in lung parenchyma.[67]

BIOPSY TECHNIQUES

Frequently the diagnosis can be established pathologically from a biopsy of a characteristic skin lesion or a palpable supraclavicular lymph node. In the absence of such lesions and when mediastinal and hilar lymph node enlargement is apparent roentgenographically (with or without pulmonary involvement), lymph nodes can usually be obtained either from the scalene group (positive in 75 to 80 per cent of cases)[42] or from the mediastinum by mediastinoscopy (positive in 95 to 100 per cent of cases).[69, 70] There is little doubt that transbronchial biopsy of peripheral bronchi can be performed with minimal risk and may show a highly significant yield.[71, 72] Koerner and associates[71] obtained positive peripheral transbronchial biopsies in 21 of 23 patients without significant complications, a success rate almost identical to the experience at the medical center of the University of Alabama in Birmingham, where positive biopsies were obtained in 22 of 25 patients over a one-year period (unpublished data). Peripheral transbronchial biopsy yields tissue approximately 1 mm in diameter, and, as previously emphasized, such a specimen is inadequate to exclude the presence of tuberculosis.[73] Open-lung biopsy undoubtedly produces the most satisfactory tissue specimens but is probably associated with a higher morbidity and mortality than the other procedures referred to.

THE KVEIM TEST

This test consists of the intradermal injection of 0.1 to 0.2 ml of crude saline suspension of sarcoid tissue, usually obtained from the spleen of patients with active sarcoidosis. A positive reaction is the development of a sarcoid granuloma in the injection area. The test site should be marked and that area biopsied 4 to 6 weeks after the injection.[74] The incidence of positive reactions in pathologically proved cases varies from series to series, although most investigators find the incidence of positive reaction in patients with active disease to range from 70 to 84 per cent. Positive reactivity is considerably higher in patients with bilateral hilar lymph node enlargement than in those with diffuse pulmonary disease alone. Certain specific diseases, including Crohn's disease, ulcerative colitis, celiac disease, and tuberculous lymphadenitis, are reported to show a significant incidence of false positive reactions.[76]

It is obvious that Kveim sensitivity does not replace lymph node or skin biopsy as a means of confirming a clinically suspected diagnosis of sarcoidosis. However, it serves as a complementary technique in substantiating the diagnosis, particularly in patients with atypical clinical presentations and biopsy evidence of noncaseating granulomas.

CLINICAL COURSE AND PROGNOSIS

As has been stated, the etiologic agent of sarcoidosis almost certainly enters the body through the lungs, from where it may disseminate to virtually any organ or tissue. Judging from the asymptomatic condition of some patients who have general lymph node enlargement and organ involvement, it can be assumed that dissemination is much more widespread than is usually suggested by the clinical findings. It is our opinion that the majority of patients with this disease probably are asymptomatic and remain so throughout the course of their illness.

Considerable variability exists in the prognostic assessment of patients with sarcoidosis. Although this results partly from a poorly understood variation in geographic and ethnic background in the occurrence of the disease, there is little doubt that the source of the subjects studied and the length of clinical observation following diagnosis are much more important aspects determining the final outcome. The black population in the United States appears to be more susceptible to the disease, and it has been suggested that their prognosis is poor.[77] However, studies originating in Philadelphia[78] and Washington[79] do not support this contention. The incidence of severe disability appears to be increased in patients with persistent skin lesions,[77] in those with an intermittent course with frequent relapses, and in young children.[7] An onset of the disease with erythema nodosum and bilateral hilar lymph node enlargement, with or without low-grade fever, almost invariably indicates a favorable prognosis.[30, 80] When bilateral hilar lymph node enlargement is associated with diffuse pulmonary disease (stage 2), less than half of affected patients show complete resolution; when interstitial disease is present alone (stage 3), less than a quarter of patients show complete resolution.[80] The overall mortality rate ranges from 5 to 10 per cent, and in patients followed up for many years, the percentage is probably closer to 10.[77, 78, 80] Death is usually caused by cardiac decompensation as a result of cor pulmonale secondary to pulmonary fibrosis. Superimposed tuberculosis is common and, in the days before chemotherapy was used, was frequently fatal. Since tuberculin reactivity undergoes little change when active sarcoidosis becomes inactive, the development of tuberculin sensitivity in patients with sarcoidosis means superimposed tuberculosis.

Approximately 65 per cent of patients recover completely or have only minimal residual disease.[1, 77] Some degree of permanent disability remains in 20 to 25 per cent of patients, the majority from pulmonary fibrosis, some from eye or skin involvement, and a few from renal insufficiency or irreversible damage to the central nervous system.

Indications for treatment include progressive pulmonary impairment, progressive loss of visual acuity, myocardial sarcoidosis associated with electrocardiographic evidence of conduction defects, central nervous system involvement, cutaneous lesions other than erythema nodosum, and persistent hypercalcemia or hypercalciuria with renal insufficiency.[81] Corticosteroid therapy appears to be beneficial for those manifestations of the disease generally considered immunologic in type, such as hypercalcemia and uveitis.[82] It is less obviously of benefit in the presence of pulmonary involvement, although it may result in transitory roentgenologic and, occasionally, functional improvement. The syndrome of erythema nodosum, with or without arthralgia, can usually be controlled with noncorticosteroid anti-inflammatory agents.[82]

DIFFUSE FIBROSING ALVEOLITIS, CHRONIC INTERSTITIAL PNEUMONIA, IDIOPATHIC PULMONARY FIBROSIS, AND THE END-STAGE LUNG

This rather complex heading indicates the state of semantic variability, if not confusion, currently surrounding the whole subject of diffuse interstitial inflammation and fibrosis. As originally defined by Scadding[83, 84] and with the suggested addition of the adjective "diffuse" by Gough, the generic name "fibrosing alveolitis" was intended to refer to a broad general category of disease of the pulmonary parenchyma characterized by an inflammatory process beyond the terminal bronchiole, having as its essential features (1) cellular thickening of the alveolar walls with a strong tendency to fibrosis and (2) the presence of large mononuclear cells, presumably of alveolar origin, within the alveolar spaces.[85] According to Scadding and Hinson,[85] the two essential features are present in varying proportions in different patients and probably at different stages in the same patient. Features such as other forms of cellular exudate, fibrinous exudate, and hyaline membrane formation may be observed in the more acute cases. In chronic cases there may be varying degrees of fibrotic destruction of lung architecture leading to anatomic changes such as excess of smooth muscle, hyperplasia of bronchiolar epithelium to line residual air spaces, and honeycombing. Despite these possible additional features, however, the term "diffuse fibrosing alveolitis" was intended to refer to a general category of disease with only two essential characteristics—thickening of the alveolar walls and the presence of mononuclear cells within the alveoli.

By contrast, Liebow and Carrington[86] have encompassed what appears to be a larger group of interstitial "diseases" under the heading of the diffuse interstitial pneumonias. This designation implies that the most significant or persistent component of a tissue response in the lung is situated in the interalveolar septa and more proximal supporting tissues. There is widespread but almost never uniform thickening of the walls of the distal air spaces, whose size may be either decreased or increased. These authors recognize five relatively distinct entities, distinguishable according to histologic, and to some extent roentgenologic and clinical, criteria.[86] (1) classic or "usual" interstitial pneumonia (UIP); (2) bronchiolar interstitial pneumonia (BIP), a diffuse lesion similar to UIP but with superimposed, probably nonbacterial, bronchiolitis obliterans; (3) desquamative interstitial pneumonia (DIP), in which there is striking proliferation of macrophages and desquamation of granular pneumocytes into the distal air spaces of the lungs, associated with a minor but probably important interstitial infiltrate of plasma cells, eosinophils, and lymphocytes; (4) lymphoid interstitial pneumonia (LIP), in which there is an infiltration of parenchymal interstitium and air spaces with lymphoid cells in a pattern difficult to distinguish from lymphoma; and (5) giant cell interstitial pneumonia (GIP), consisting of an interstitial infiltration of somewhat variegated small and large mononuclear cells associated with large numbers of irregular, phagocytic giant cells. Although each of these diseases appears to be histologically distinct, all may converge following long-standing and persistent activity toward an appearance that lacks specificity by both roentgenologic and pathologic criteria—diffuse interstitial pulmonary fibrosis, honeycombing, and the end-stage lung.

An excessive deposition of fibrous tissue in the interstitium of the lungs occurs in a wide variety of diseases. Many may be recognized as distinct entities because of specific pathologic changes in the lungs in addition to the fibrosis, because of associated nonpulmonary abnormalities, or because of a combination of these two. These diseases include:

1. The granulomatoses, including tuberculosis, the mycoses, sarcoidosis, and the extrinsic allergic alveolitides.

2. The collagen-vascular diseases, particularly scleroderma, rheumatoid disease, polymyositis, and Sjögren's syndrome.

3. The pneumoconioses, including the many diseases associated with exposure to inorganic dusts, particularly silica and asbestos.

4. Conditions associated with long-standing postcapillary hypertension and recurrent pulmonary edema with subsequent organization of the edema fluid in the interstitium and the alveolar spaces.

5. Irradiation damage to the lungs.

6. Neoplastic invasion of the interstitium of the lung, particularly lymphangitic.

7. Drug-induced fibrosis, including that caused by busulfan, bleomycin, and methotrexate.

8. Various diseases of undertermined origin in which some degree of interstitial fibrosis commonly occurs at the late or end stage of the disease, including alveolar microlithiasis, idiopathic pulmonary hemosiderosis and Goodpasture's syndrome, von Recklinghausen's neurofibromatosis, histiocytosis-X, alveolar proteinosis, and adult respiratory distress syndrome.

These diseases are discussed individually in the sections appropriate to their etiology. The discussion here is limited to the diffuse interstitial pneumonias and interstitial fibrosis in which the major clinical, roentgenologic, and pathologic changes are confined to the lungs and are not manifested elsewhere in the body. Acute diffuse interstitial pneumonia or fibrosis is a condition originally described by Hamman and Rich,[87] consisting of a syndrome that has traditionally borne their names. If the progress of the signs and symptoms of interstitial pneumonia is rapid, leading to death in less than a year, it is appropriate to use the term "Hamman-Rich syndrome." However, the majority of cases of diffuse interstitial fibrosis reported subsequent to the original descriptions manifested a much more chronic course. It is a contradiction to speak of "chronic" Hamman-Rich disease and, with the exception of the occasional case in which an acute course of the disease can be accurately documented, it is recommended that the eponym be dropped in favor of one of the more descriptive terms "idiopathic pulmonary fibrosis," "diffuse interstitial pneumonia," or "diffuse fibrosing alveolitis."

Diffuse fibrosing alveolitis shows no sex predominance and a broad age incidence. On average, however, the disease probably affects men slightly more often than women, and most patients are between the ages of 40 and 70 years.[88]

ETIOLOGY

Although diffuse interstitial fibrosis is commonly termed idiopathic, there is considerable evidence that the pathologic changes result from a nonspecific reaction to a variety of stimuli. It is thought by many to be a hypersensitivity or autoimmune disease because of the finding of hyperglobulinemia, autoantibodies, a positive Coombs test, or blood eosinophilia.[89] In addition, the cellular infiltration with lymphocytes, plasma cells, and mononuclear cells suggest a disorder of the immune mechanism.[89] The existence of collagen diseases in other family members further supports such a concept. However, in one series of six patients with cryptogenic fibrosing alveolitis,[90] none showed evidence of immunologic damage on immunofluorescent staining of biopsied pulmonary lesions.

A familial form of diffuse interstitial fibrosis has been reported in which transmission is by a simple mendelian autosomal dominant characteristic.[91] Designated "familial fibrocystic pulmonary dysplasia," this condition possesses pathologic characteristics identical to those of the nonfamilial form of diffuse interstitial fibrosis. Another familial disease in which pathologic changes are observed that are indistinguishable from those of cryptogenic interstitial pneumonia

is von Recklinghausen's neurofibromatosis.[92] Certain drugs and poisons, notably busulfan, bleomycin, methotrexate, and paraquat, have been implicated as precipitating factors.

From their study of 369 patients with all types of interstitial pneumonia seen during the 20-year period from 1950 to 1970, Gaensler and his colleagues[93] found the cause of the disease to be unknown in 45 per cent (more than one-third of these patients were classified as having UIP and somewhat less than one-third as having DIP). Among the remaining 55 per cent, by far the most common causes of interstitial pneumonia were the collagen-vascular diseases and the pneumoconioses, each accounting for about 20 per cent of the entire group.

CHRONIC INTERSTITIAL PNEUMONIA

In the following pages, we will discuss the pathologic, roentgenologic, and clinical aspects of each of the five varieties of diffuse interstitial pneumonia as defined by Liebow and Carrington,[86] ending with what appears to be the final common pathway—diffuse interstitial pulmonary fibrosis and the end-stage or honeycomb lung.

"USUAL" INTERSTITIAL PNEUMONIA (UIP)

Undoubtedly the most common of the diffuse interstitial pneumonias, UIP is believed to begin with diffuse damage to alveolar walls, reflected *morphologically* by edema and proteinaceous exudate in the interstitium and hyaline membrane formation in the alveoli. Shortly thereafter, there is cellular infiltration of monocytes and lymphocytes, sometimes associated with plasma cells, eosinophils, and neutrophils, in both interstitium and air spaces. At this stage the general architecture of the lungs is preserved. Necrosis of alveolar lining cells may be extensive but is soon followed by regeneration of alveolar epithelium, which relines the damaged alveoli and grows over coagulated masses of alveolar exudate, thus incorporating such masses into the alveolar wall.[93] Shortly after the appearance of regenerating epithelial cells, fibroblasts can be identified in both the interstitium and the alveoli. If the insult continues unabated, proliferation of fibroblasts and deposition of collagen fibers generally increase in prominence, usually accompanied by smooth muscle proliferation. The eventual result is progressive disorganization of pulmonary architecture, severe interstitial fibrosis, and the honey-comb or end-stage lung (*see* further on). In a study in which the cellular yield on bronchopulmonary lavage was compared in a number of pulmonary diseases and correlated with histologic study of biopsy material,[94] a striking lymphocytosis was found in patients with diffuse idiopathic interstitial lung disease and not in control subjects or patients with a variety of other diseases. Other investigators[95] have found an excess of lymphocytes in bronchoalveolar lavage only in those patients with interstitial fibrosis who are responding to treatment. Most patients with fibrosing alveolitis show a predominance of polymorphonuclear neutrophils in bronchial washings, in contrast to the abundance of lymphocytes found in patients with sarcoidosis and hypersensitivity pneumonitis.[88, 95, 96] The accumulation of neutrophils in the lungs has been attributed to the release of chemotactic factor by alveolar macrophages that have been activated by immune complexes deposited in lung tissue.[97]

Roentgenologically, it is clear that the manifestations of the earliest stages of the disease (as described morphologically) have not been adequately documented. It is probable that the earliest discernible changes roentgenologically are those attributable to interstitial pulmonary fibrosis. As might be expected, the roentgenographic pattern varies with the stage of the disease. The earliest manifestation consists of fine reticulation, predominantly in the lung bases. As fibrosis progresses, the reticular or reticulonodular pattern becomes more coarse until the end-stage appearance of honeycombing is manifested. We have been repeatedly impressed by the progressive loss of lung volume apparent in serial roentgenographic studies over 2 to 3 years and consider that diffuse reticular disease with increasing elevation of the diaphragm—signs that occur much less frequently in other forms of diffuse interstitial fibrosis—strongly suggests the diagnosis of either UIP or scleroderma. Apart from this progressive loss of volume, there is nothing specific about the roentgenographic pattern in UIP.

Clinically, symptoms include progressive dyspnea, nonproductive cough, weight loss, and fatigue.[89, 93] Sputum is typically sparse but may be blood-streaked. Symptoms develop insidiously without much in the way of constitutional disturbances, particularly in older patients.[98] Clubbing of the fingers is very common, being observed in 35 (83 per cent) of 42 patients in one study.[89] Clubbing may antedate symptoms and other signs of pulmonary disease. Cyanosis

and pulmonary hypertension may be present in the early stages of the disease but usually denote the end stages. They lead to cor pulmonale, cardiac decompensation, and occasionally secondary polycythemia. Physical examination of the chest usually reveals no abnormalities in the early stages of the disease. Later, however, diffuse crepitations of a very superficial quality frequently are heard, predominantly over the lung bases. DeRemee and coworkers[99] call these crepitations "Velcro" rales because of their resemblance to the sound produced by tearing apart mated strips of Velcro adhesive, a substance commonly found on blood pressure cuffs. The combination of these fine rales, clubbing of the fingers, and dyspnea (but no orthopnea) is virtually diagnostic of UIP. The blood of these patients contains increased levels of immunoglobulins and various non–organ-specific antibodies such as antinuclear protein (ANF) and antiglobulin (rheumatoid factor). Scadding[98] has estimated that about one-third of patients with fibrosing alveolitis have antinuclear protein and one-third rheumatoid factor, usually in low titers; only a few have both.

BRONCHIOLITIS OBLITERANS AND DIFFUSE INTERSTITIAL PNEUMONIA (BIP)

Pathologically, the major difference between BIP and UIP is the presence of obliterating bronchiolitis in the former. Changes in the alveoli are identical to those of UIP, with the addition of large numbers of fat-filled large mononuclear cells within the interstitium and alveoli representing endogenous lipoid (cholesterol) pneumonia. Since the latter change is a frequent manifestation of airway obstruction of any etiology, the reason for recognizing BIP as a distinct entity is the presence of the extensive background of interstitial pneumonia.[86] BIP is thus characterized by three morphologic abnormalities—interstitial pneumonia and fibrosis, obliterating bronchiolitis, and endogenous lipoid pneumonia. The etiology of the bronchiolar lesion is not clear, although the morphologic similarity of the bronchiolar and alveolar changes would suggest that the two lesions are caused by the same agent.

Roentgenologically, Liebow and Carrington[86] describe "streaked, flamelike lesions which tend to predominate in the upper lobes." We have seen one case of biopsy-confirmed BIP in which homogeneous consolidation of the axillary portion of both upper zones was the major roentgenographic abnormality.

Clinically, the course of the disease is said to be rapid and relentless, terminating in severe respiratory insufficiency.[86]

DESQUAMATIVE INTERSTITIAL PNEUMONIA (DIP)

This disease of unknown etiology is the second commonest form of chronic diffuse interstitial pneumonia and, in contrast to UIP in which the inflammation is predominantly interstitial, is characterized by a heavy accumulation of mononuclear cells, mostly macrophages, in the distal air spaces of the lungs.[100] It is mostly a disease of adults, although by 1970 five cases had been described in children.[101] Some investigators believe that DIP is not a distinct entity but is simply an early stage of UIP.[85, 88] Scadding and Hinson[85] described a pathologic spectrum in 16 patients with diffuse fibrosing alveolitis in which changes ranged from relatively pure desquamation of alveolar lining cells with minimal alveolar wall thickening (thus resembling Liebow's DIP) to predominant thickening of alveolar walls associated with only sparse desquamation of alveolar cells. These authors were able to find little support for the sharp contrast between DIP and UIP suggested by Liebow and his associates.[100] They suggested that a more appropriate designation for the two patterns of disease would be a desquamative type and a mural type of fibrosing alveolitis. In a study of 29 patients with idiopathic pulmonary fibrosis,

Crystal and his coworkers[88] concluded that DIP most likely represents an early stage of idiopathic pulmonary fibrosis, whereas UIP represents a later stage (Figure 14–5). Necropsy examination of the lungs of patients for whom a diagnosis of DIP was established earlier by biopsy has revealed diffuse pulmonary fibrosis unassociated with the desquamative features noted earlier on biopsy.[102] However, the prognosis is better for those patients showing a desquamative pattern. Although the process is often irreversible, it tends to pursue a more benign course than most other chronic diffuse interstitial pneumonias.[85, 93, 103] Over a follow-up period of 10 years, Davis and his associates[103] found an uncorrected mortality rate of 87 per cent for 31 patients with UIP and of only 16 per cent for 20 patients with DIP. In some patients the disease is reversible and leaves no residue, sometimes abating spontaneously but more often in response to corticosteroid therapy.[100, 103]

The etiology of DIP is unknown, and it is possible that it represents a reaction to a variety of initiating factors. In some instances the onset consists of an acute respiratory infection,[104] suggesting a mycoplasmal or viral etiology. Autoantibodies are identified and symptoms and signs suggesting immunologic disease occur even more commonly in DIP than in UIP.

Pathologically, as a result of loss of type I alveolar epithelial cells and proliferation of type II cells, the alveoli are lined by large cuboidal cells. The alveolar spaces are filled with large

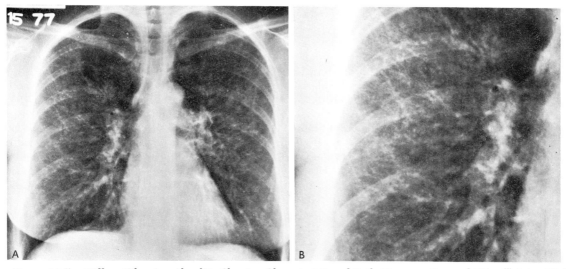

Figure 14–5. **Diffuse Fibrosing Alveolitis Showing Characteristics of Both Desquamative and "Usual" Interstitial Pneumonitis.** A posteroanterior roentgenogram *(A)* and a magnified view of the right midzone *(B)* reveal a rather coarse reticular pattern throughout both lungs, without anatomic predilection. There is no evidence of hilar lymph node enlargement, pleural effusion, or cardiomegaly. This 37-year-old white woman complained of increasing dyspnea on exertion over the past several months. An open lung biopsy was performed.

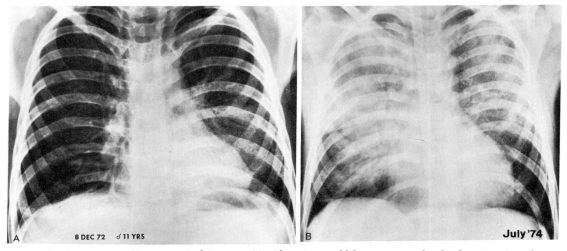

Figure 14–6. Desquamative Interstitial Pneumonitis. This 11-year-old boy was seen for the first time in February, 1972; he complained of increasing shortness of breath on exertion. A posteroanterior roentgenogram (A) revealed an exceedingly fine reticular pattern, more marked on the left and in the lower zones. The pattern of disease in the right lower zone suggested the presence of several bullae. There was no definite evidence of lymph node enlargement. Open lung biopsy was performed, and the histologic diagnosis was desquamative interstitial pneumonitis. The disease was relentlessly progressive, both clinically and roentgenologically. By July, 1974, the patient was in respiratory failure and a roentgenogram (B) showed marked extension of the disease, which now was affecting chiefly the mid- and upper lung zones. Although in some areas a reticular pattern can still be identified, much of the opacity is now homogeneous and is associated with an air bronchogram, suggesting extensive involvement of air spaces. The patient died shortly thereafter.

mononuclear cells that have been shown by electron microscopy to be mostly macrophages.[88, 102, 105] In Gaensler and associates' series,[104] some of the desquamated cells within or lining the alveoli were giant cells. Slight thickening of the parenchymal interstitial tissue occurs, with infiltration of the interalveolar septa by eosinophils and sometimes plasma cells, and with well-marked collections of lymphocytes in all but the earliest stages.[104, 105, 106]

Although DIP generally pursues a more benign course than the other interstitial pneumonias, it can also take the final common pathway of smooth muscle proliferation, hyperplasia of epithelium, severe interstitial fibrosis, honeycombing, and the end-stage lung.[86, 93, 102]

Roentgenologically, the changes have been described as a "ground-glass" opacification of the lungs, bilaterally symmetric, and most severe in the basal zones (Figure 14–6).[100] However, in their follow-up study of 37 cases, Feigin and Friedman[107] found only six to possess the "classic" appearance of hazy, ground-glass opacities in lower lung zones; the most common roentgenographic appearance in their series was rather nonspecific, consisting of irregular opacities most numerous in the lung bases. Gaensler and his colleagues reported increased thickness and loss of definition of basal vascular markings.[104] Triangular opacities extending into both lung bases from the hila and consisting of combined reticulonodular and acinar patterns (indicating combined interstitial and air space disease) have been reported to be suggestive of the diagnosis.[108] Progressive loss of lung volume appears to be a major finding in many cases.[93] In Gaensler and associates' series,[104] spontaneous pneumothorax developed in three of the 12 cases, bilateral pleural effusion in two, and cor pulmonale in three. As with many other diffuse interstitial diseases of the lung, roentgenograms may be perfectly normal despite symptoms of moderate severity. In the large series reviewed by Davis and associates,[103] chest roentgenograms described as "normal by any standards" were seen in 15 per cent of patients with DIP and 7 per cent of those with UIP. Roentgenographic changes are almost invariably diffuse.

Clinically, symptoms consist of dyspnea, weight loss, and nonproductive cough.[109] Arthralgia and myalgia may be present.[109] Physical findings in the chest may be absent or may be limited to basal rales. Finger clubbing is present in about half the cases.

LYMPHOID INTERSTITIAL PNEUMONIA (LIP)

This condition is characterized by a widespread, focally massive, lymphoid infiltration of the lung that is often exceedingly difficult to distinguish from pulmonary lymphoma.[86]

Pathologically, LIP is uniquely interstitial, the alveolar septa and peribronchiolar and perivenous interstitium showing extensive infiltration, the latter often massively. The cellular infiltrate tends to be a mixture of the dominant small lymphocytes, with plasma cells and occasional large mononuclear cells.[86] Heavy mononuclear infiltration may be associated with bronchiolar obstruction, the distal parenchyma showing evidence of endogenous lipoid "pneumonia."

According to Liebow and Carrington,[86] features that would suggest LIP rather than lymphoma include a relative paucity of mitoses, absence of involvement of structures such as the perichondrium or cartilage, the relative absence of infiltration of the pleura, and the absence of involvement of local lymph nodes or extrapulmonary tissues. However, lymph node enlargement, with or without hepatosplenomegaly, has been noted in five of 18 reported cases.[110]

Roentgenologically, the findings are not in any way specific judging from descriptions in the literature. Liebow and Carrington[86] describe linear and branching opacities in the periphery of the lungs early in the course of the disease, consistent with septal (Kerley) lines and corresponding to septal and peribronchial lymphocytic infiltration. As the disease progresses, consolidation tends to be more central and more homogeneous, reflecting heavy interstitial infiltration that impinges upon and even obliterates alveoli. Eventually, there is the stage of honeycombing and the end-stage lung.

Clinically, three of the 13 patients described by Carrington and Liebow[111] were less than 14 years of age. Sex distribution was equal. Dyspnea was the major complaint of all patients and was almost always associated with cough. Cyanosis and clubbing were noted in roughly half the patients. Some patients with a diffuse lymphocytic type of interstitial disease have an associated monoclonal gammopathy, usually IgM but occasionally IgG in type.[112, 113] In fact, Genereux has informed us in a personal communication that he has seen a case of LIP in which immunofluorescent staining revealed IgG in alveolar walls.

GIANT CELL INTERSTITIAL PNEUMONIA (GIP)

This rare but apparently histologically distinctive form of interstitial pneumonia is characterized by the presence within alveoli of innumerable bizarre giant cells 40 to 60 μ in diameter containing up to 25 small dark nuclei.[86, 114] In addition, there are a few irregular large mononuclear cells. The interstitial tissues are thickened by fibrosis and by a predominantly lymphocytic and plasmacytoid infiltrate.[114] The giant cells tend to be very large, to a point of nearly filling an alveolus, and are so remarkably phagocytic as to suggest the description "cannibalistic."[86]

Roentgenologically, changes in the three patients studied by Liebow and Carrington[86] consisted of "streaked and mottled nodular densities that extend from the hilum to the very periphery of the lung, without perihilar concentration." The chest roentgenograms of the three patients reported by Reddy and associates[114] showed bilateral nodular opacities of varying density, more prominent in midlung zones.

Clinically, complaints include cough, dyspnea, fever, fatigue, and weight loss. Pulmonary rales and finger clubbing have been reported.[114] In contrast to the situation in children, adults do not appear to have defective immunologic systems.[114]

PULMONARY FUNCTION IN DIFFUSE INTERSTITIAL PNEUMONIA

Earlier studies of pulmonary function in patients with all varieties of diffuse interstitial pneumonia revealed a predominantly restrictive insufficiency, with reduction in VC and FRC and relatively normal values for maximal breathing capacity and FEV. In more recent reports,[115, 116] airway conductance and FEV_1-FVC, measured directly, have been shown to be normal. In some patients, a considerable increase in elastic recoil results in supernormal bronchial air flow, particularly as reflected in the maximal midexpiratory flow. Patients tend to hyperventilate, largely as a result of an increase in the physiologic dead space, and alveolar ventilation appears to be increased. Compliance is reduced, the maximal negative intrathoracic pressure (elastic recoil) being either normal or increased. The work of breathing is increased. Diffusing capacity is characteristically reduced, often to less than 50 per cent of predicted values.[115, 117] Arterial blood gas analysis reveals hypoxemia and a normal or low PCO_2. In the earlier stages of the disease, hypoxemia may not be detected in resting subjects. In the later stages, PCO_2 levels may rise above normal, an ominous finding. Hypoxemia is caused chiefly by $\dot{V}/\dot{Q}$ inequality. Approximately 20 per cent of the hypoxemia observed on exercise can be explained on a diffusion basis.[118] Measurement of the A-a O_2 gradient on exercise is considered particularly useful in following up patients receiving therapy.[119] Pulmonary function tests carried out before and after corticosteroid therapy indicate a beneficial effect during the early stages of the disease[103] and negligible response when the stage of honeycombing has been reached.

The prognosis in patients with diffuse interstitial pneumonia varies considerably and is directly related to the degree of fibrosis.[103] Approximately 20 per cent of patients with idiopathic pulmonary fibrosis die from a cardiac disorder, but most succumb to primary respiratory failure, often precipitated by infection.[120] However, it is not unusual for patients to survive for at least 5 years—and some as long as 15 years—after diagnosis.

Bronchoalveolar lavage may provide useful information in determining prognosis and a response to therapy in patients with fibrosing alveolitis. For example, Rudd and his associates[95] found a direct relationship between the number of lymphocytes obtained on lavage and the response to therapy: patients who did not respond and who showed a poor prognosis on follow-up had an excess of neutrophils and eosinophils on bronchoalveolar lavage. Other investigators[121] have described an association between the intensity of neutrophil alveolitis and prognosis, patients in whom more than 10 per cent of lavage cells are polymorphonuclear neutrophils showing an accelerated deterioration in function.

DIFFUSE PULMONARY FIBROSIS AND THE END-STAGE LUNG

The lung can respond to injury in only a limited manner. With persistent injury from a wide variety of different causes, pathologic changes that may be easily distinguished in the early stages of disease converge toward a common pathway that terminates in the end-stage lung. This terminal state totally lacks specificity by roentgenologic, pathologic, and usually pathophysiologic criteria.[122]

Little is known about the factors that lead to severe pulmonary interstitial fibrosis and destruction of pulmonary parenchymal structure. It is not even certain that the fibrogenic response to injury is a healing process. The pathologic characteristics of the many diffuse interstitial pneumonias have already been described, specifically with reference to their early or active stages. As the process advances, the sequence of events is fairly uniform and predictable: alveolar obliteration occurs, with the formation of epithelium-lined cystic spaces into which dilated bronchioles lead.[122] The general picture thus appears to be one of obliteration of the distal pulmonary structures and dilatation of those more proximal. Squamous metaplasia of the epithelium sometimes develops. In addition to the extensive proliferation of fibrous tissue at this end stage, muscular hyperplasia may be present in the alveolar walls, the pleura, and the walls of the bronchi, blood vessels, and lymphatics. Grossly, the lungs are characteristically small and firm but may be enlarged when emphysematous changes prevail. The pleura is moderately thickened and possesses a hobnail appearance not unlike that in Laennec's cirrhosis of the liver. The cut surface shows an irregular cystic pattern resembling a honeycomb. The multiple thick-walled cysts seldom measure more than 5 mm in diameter.

Roentgenologically, the end-stage lung is characterized by a coarse reticular or reticulonodular pattern throughout the lungs and thick-walled cystic spaces 3 to 10 mm in diameter creating a honeycomb pattern (Figure 14–7). There is little doubt that these cysts represent the thick-walled, epithelium-lined cystic spaces so characteristic of this disease morphologically. We are strongly of the opinion that the designation honeycomb lung should not be applied to any pattern in which the cystic spaces measure less than 5 or 6 mm in diameter. If this restriction is applied, the differential diagnostic possibilities can be reduced to relatively few diseases (scleroderma, histiocytosis-X, pulmonary myomatosis, rheumatoid lung, and rarely, sarcoidosis and berylliosis). We submit that this is the only way to bring some order to the confusion that surrounds diffuse interstitial lung disease.

As with any disease characterized by diffuse fibrosis, the passage of time may permit appreciation of progressive loss of lung volume.

Osseous metaplasia may occur as an occasional late manifestation of severe interstitial fibrosis (Figure 14–7).[122] Another infrequent but important "complication" is neoplasia. It has been suggested that the neoplastic proliferation results from atypical regenerative changes in either bronchiolar or alveolar epithelium, a situation that commonly exists in the honeycomb lung. Adenocarcinoma appears to be the most frequent cell type, although alveolar cell carcinoma, epidermoid carcinoma, and anaplastic carcinoma have also been reported.[122] Bronchogenic carcinoma is seen often enough in

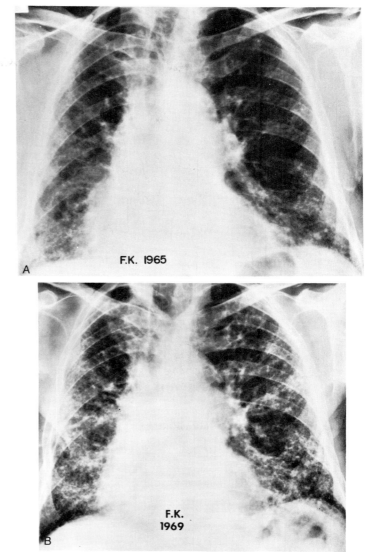

Figure 14–7. Calcification (Ossification) in Fibrosing Alveolitis. In 1961, this 74-year-old man had no symptoms referable to his chest, and a chest roentgenogram was normal. Four years later (A), a coarse reticular pattern had developed throughout both lungs, with some basal predominance. Four years later (B) the reticular pattern had become more marked and its calcific nature more evident. At necropsy, there was widespread disorganization of lung architecture and diffuse interstitial and alveolar fibrosis characteristic of the end-stage lung. Trabeculae of bone were present within the dense fibrous tissue. (Courtesy of Dr. George Genereux, Saskatoon, Saskatchewan.)

cases of diffuse interstitial pulmonary fibrosis to represent more than a coincidence.[123, 124]

NEUROFIBROMATOSIS AND DIFFUSE PULMONARY DISEASE

Von Recklinghausen's neurofibromatosis is an organic neurocutaneous syndrome consisting of multiple neurofibromas and cutaneous café au lait spots. Despite the fact that neurofibromatosis is a congenital abnormality, the pulmonary disease typically does not become evident until the patient reaches adulthood. The incidence of pulmonary involvement is approximately 10 per cent.[125]

The pulmonary manifestations consist of diffuse interstitial pulmonary fibrosis and bullae, either alone or in combination (Figure 14–8). The interstitial fibrosis characteristically involves both lungs symmetrically with some basal predominance, whereas the bullae usually are asymmetric and tend to upper lobe predominance. In some cases bullae are unassociated with roentgenographic evidence of interstitial fibrosis, although it should be noted that interstitial fibrosis has been seen in all patients with bullae whose lungs have been examined histologically.[125, 126]

Of obvious assistance in roentgenologic diagnosis is the presence of numerous cutaneous nodules projected over the lungs or seen in profile on the chest wall (Figure 14–8). In

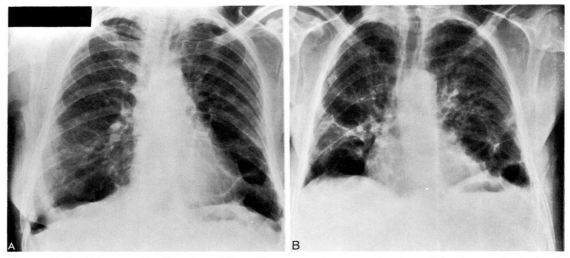

Figure 14–8. Pulmonary Manifestations of Neurofibromatosis. Posteroanterior views of the chest on inspiration (A) and expiration (B) reveal numerous bullae in the lower portion of both lungs, most evident on the expiratory film because of air trapping. A background of diffuse reticulation is present, suggesting interstitial pulmonary fibrosis. Along the lateral chest wall in (A) are numerous nodular opacities representing cutaneous neurofibromas.

addition, extrapulmonary stigmata may be observed, including scoliosis, ribbon deformity of the ribs, and mediastinal masses.

Clinically, respiratory symptoms tend to be mild.[125] The most frequent complaint is dyspnea on exertion. Pulmonary function tests usually reveal evidence of obstruction, although a restrictive pattern may be dominant. Diffusing capacity is often decreased.[125]

The etiology and pathogenesis of interstitial fibrosis in patients with neurofibromatosis are unknown, although a genetic factor seems highly probable.

ANKYLOSING SPONDYLITIS AND UPPER LOBE PULMONARY FIBROSIS

An uncommon manifestation of ankylosing spondylitis is pulmonary fibrosis, which uniquely affects the upper lobes only. All affected patients in one study[127] had total spinal ankylosis and half manifested peripheral joint involvement. Ankylosing spondylitis affects males predominantly and results in fixation of the thoracic cage in an inspiratory position. Patients with ankylosing spondylitis have always been considered susceptible to pulmonary tuberculosis.

The few available pathologic descriptions have indicated the presence of a rather nonspecific interstitial and alveolar fibrosis, with infil-

tration by chronic inflammatory cells, primarily lymphocytes.[128] The more severe the fibrosis, the greater the tendency for the development of bronchial dilatation, bullae, and cavities.[129] Roentgenologically, the early changes are said to consist of "spotty irregular opacities."[127] Eventually, there are coalescence of opacities, considerable shrinkage, and a final appearance that simulates chronic fibrotic pulmonary tuberculosis. The disease is almost invariably bilateral. The reported incidence of cavitation varies considerably. In many cases cavitation is associated with *Aspergillus* mycetoma formation, in which circumstances exsanguination may occur.[129]

By the time these patients develop upper lobe fibrosis, they have severe spondylitis associated with marked rigidity. In all reported cases, an intensive search for an etiologic agent, particularly *Mycobacterium tuberculosis*, has proved negative. The reported isolation of *Mycobacterium fortuitum* in two cases[130] and of *Mycobacterium scrofulaceum* in one case[131] probably reflects superimposed infection.

LYMPHANGIOMYOMATOSIS AND TUBEROUS SCLEROSIS

These two conditions are considered together because of the great similarities in their pathologic, roentgenologic, and clinical manifestations in the lungs.[132] The common denominator of the two conditions is progressive, widespread proliferation of smooth muscle in the pleura, alveolar septa, walls of bronchi and bronchioles, pulmonary vessels, and lymphatics, together with similar changes in lymph nodes, especially those in the posterior mediastinum or retroperitoneal space or both. These morphologic abnormalities result in a characteristic roentgenographic triad of gradually progressive diffuse interstitial lung disease, recurrent chylous pleural effusion (and sometimes chylous ascites), and recurrent pneumothorax.

Tuberous sclerosis is an inherited disorder of mesodermal development. Inheritance is considered to occur through a dominant gene with variable or incomplete expression. The condition is manifested by a characteristic, rather bizarre group of findings including mental defects, epilepsy, retinal phacoma, angiomyolipomas of the kidneys, rhabdomyomas of the heart, intracranial calcifications, sclerotic lesions of bones, and various skin lesions, notably adenoma sebaceum and subungual fibromas. Extrapulmonary manifestations usually appear in infancy or early childhood, and 75 per cent of patients so affected die before their twentieth year.[166]

Pulmonary lymphangiomyomatosis (synonyms: pulmonary myomatosis, intrathoracic angiomyomatous hyperplasia, pulmonary leiomyosarcoma, lymphangiomatous malformation, and lymphangiopericytoma) is only part of a general syndrome characterized by excessive accumulation of muscle in relation to extrapulmonary lymphatics.[134] Pulmonary involvement occurs exclusively in females at an age ranging from 17 to 47 years.[134] A familial incidence has not been reported.

The *pathologic changes* in the lungs are characterized by multiple cysts usually measuring a few millimeters in diameter but occasionally larger. The walls of the cysts are formed largely by masses of smooth muscle cells and partly by bronchiolar epithelium. A hamartomatous proliferation of smooth muscle is also found in the pleura and alveolar septa and around blood vessels and lymphatics. Focal emphysema develops at least partly as a result of the marked narrowing of small airways by burgeoning masses of muscle in their walls.[134] Vessels may be totally occluded by smooth muscle, providing an explanation for pulmonary hemorrhage and hemosiderosis in the interstitial tissues.[134] Intra- and extrapulmonary lymphatics often are dilated, and there are lymphocytes and proliferated smooth muscle cells within their walls. The thoracic duct may be largely obliterated,

resulting in chylothorax, chyloperitoneum, and occasionally chylopericardium. Lymph nodes in the mediastinum and retroperitoneal space may contain much smooth muscle, resulting in impairment of lymph flow and the development of chylous effusions.[134] Fibrous tissue may be increased in the lungs of some patients, but the pathologic picture as a whole is quite different from that of diffuse idiopathic interstitial fibrosis.[134] Although muscular hyperplasia can be a feature of many cases of idiopathic pulmonary fibrosis, it is seldom as extensive as in lymphangiomyomatosis and does not manifest the intimate relationship to lymphatic spaces. In addition, mesodermal tumors composed of smooth muscle and other elements (termed variously angiomyolipomas, lymphangiomyomas, and hemangiomyomas) are occasionally present in patients with pulmonary lymphangiomyomatosis.

The *roentgenographic pattern* in the lungs is identical in lymphangiomyomatosis and tuberous sclerosis and is indistinguishable from that of idiopathic pulmonary fibrosis, with the exception of the effects on lung volume. Characteristically, in diffuse interstitial fibrosis, there is progressive loss of lung volume whereas in lymphangiomyomatosis and tuberous sclerosis volume tends to be increased (Figure 14–9).[134] The basic pattern is coarse reticulonodular in type and tends to be generalized (Figure 14–9), although in two patients we studied it was more prominent in the lung bases. The late roentgenographic pattern is one of honeycombing. Pleural effusions may be unilateral or bilateral and typically are large and recurrent. All are chylous on direct examination. Effusions may be present in the absence of lung involvement. Spontaneous pneumothorax is common. The identification of numerous sclerotic lesions (or sometimes cystic rarefactions) throughout the bony skeleton, together with the other typical changes, should establish the diagnosis beyond reasonable doubt. Further confirmation may be had by the roentgenologic demonstration of renal enlargement secondary to angiomyolipomas, or of intracranial calcifications.

Clinically, in both lymphangiomyomatosis and tuberous sclerosis, the presenting complaint is increasing shortness of breath, frequently associated with pneumothorax and sometimes with repeated hemoptysis. Chylous effusions tend to be common in lymphangiomyomatosis and rare in tuberous sclerosis.[134, 135] Although chyloperitoneum and chylopericardium are present sometimes, the most common site of chylous effusion is the pleural space. The central nervous system stigmata of tuberous

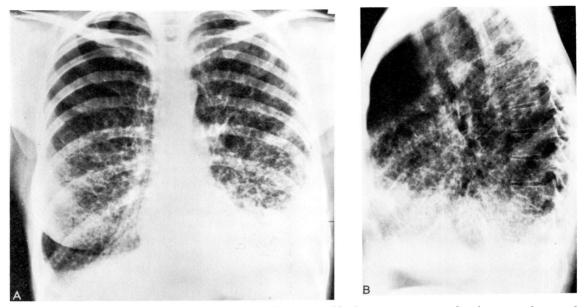

Figure 14–9. Pulmonary Lymphangiomyomatosis. This 24-year-old white woman presented with a 2-year history of increasing cough and dyspnea, the latter having become very severe just prior to admission. Roentgenograms in posteroanterior (A) and lateral (B) projection reveal a coarse reticulation throughout both lungs, with considerable basal and midzone predominance. In the lower lung zones particularly, there are multiple thick-walled cystic spaces ranging from 5 to 10 mm in diameter. This is the basic pattern of "honeycomb lung." There are bilateral pleural effusions, larger on the left. The heart is not enlarged. The patient died shortly after this examination. At necropsy, the pulmonary architecture was grossly disorganized and consisted of a multitude of cystic air-containing spaces ranging in diameter from 0.4 to 1.0 cm. All lobes were affected more or less uniformly. Histologically, much of the parenchyma was replaced by smooth muscle cells arranged in broad, interweaving bands. The cystic spaces were incompletely lined by type I and type II pneumocytes and by low columnar epithelium. Chylous pleural effusions were present bilaterally. The thoracic duct, retroperitoneal lymphatic channels, and cisterna chyli were the site of lymphagiectasia and smooth muscle proliferation. Multiple angiomyolipomas were present in the kidneys. (Courtesy of Dr. Melvin Figley, University of Washington Hospital, Seattle.)

sclerosis include mental retardation, epilepsy, and cerebral calcifications, and are present in less than half the cases.[133] Pulmonary tuberous sclerosis is more likely to be associated with involvement of other organs, including the kidneys, eyes, bones, heart, thyroid, and ovaries.[133]

Abnormalities of pulmonary function are similar in the two disorders. The pattern typically is one of obstruction, with reduction in VC and increase in FRC and RV. FEV_1-FVC usually is well below the predicted normal. Hypoxemia is common and may be severe, although P_{CO_2} almost invariably is decreased.[133, 134]

PULMONARY DISEASE CHARACTERIZED BY EXCESS ACCUMULATION OF LIPIDS

Lipids may accumulate in the lungs from either endogenous or exogenous sources. The latter chiefly results in lipoid pneumonia, a condition caused by the aspiration of various vegetable, animal, or mineral oils into the lungs. Lipoid pneumonia was discussed in Chapter 12 (see page 604). In this section, we will deal with a group of diseases characterized by the accumulation within the lungs of excess lipids of endogenous origin, including cholesterol pneumonitis, pulmonary alveolar proteinosis, and the lipid storage diseases (histiocytosis-X and Gaucher's disease).

CHOLESTEROL PNEUMONITIS

Two forms of cholesterol pneumonitis can be recognized, depending on the presence or absence of airway obstruction.[136]

CHOLESTEROL PNEUMONITIS ASSOCIATED WITH BRONCHIAL OBSTRUCTION

In the presence of inflammation, any form of chronic bronchial obstruction may be associated with secondary cholesterol degeneration. Probably the most common example is the obstructive pneumonitis that results from bronchogenic carcinoma. However, this form of endogenous lipoid pneumonia can also be an integral pathologic feature of diffuse disease such as bronchiolitis obliterans and diffuse interstitial pneumonia (BIP). Pathologically, the condition is manifested by the presence of fat-filled large mononuclear cells in the interstitium and alveoli. Since the accumulation of cholesterol is incidental to the obstructing process, its presence is not roentgenographically identifiable.

CHOLESTEROL PNEUMONITIS UNASSOCIATED WITH BRONCHIAL OBSTRUCTION

Genereux[136] recognized two forms of cholesterol pneumonitis in the absence of bronchial obstruction—primary and secondary. The secondary form develops frequently in association with pre-existing pulmonary diseases such as peripheral neoplasms, lung abscesses, infarcts, and bronchiectasis, the cholesterol accumulating in lung parenchyma at the periphery of such processes. The primary form of nonobstructive cholesterol pneumonitis is a rather poorly defined entity characterized by segmental or lobar consolidation and atelectasis, a patent airway system, and extensive cholesterol deposits. Although its etiology is unknown, the condition bears sufficient resemblance to so-called inflammatory pseudotumor (unresolved pneumonia or carnified lung) to raise the question whether the accumulation of lipid is not merely a reaction to a nonspecific parenchymal insult.

PULMONARY ALVEOLAR PROTEINOSIS

This rare but fascinating disease has been recognized only relatively recently, having been reported for the first time by Rosen and his colleagues[137] in 1958. It is a disease of unknown etiology characterized by the deposition within the air spaces of the lung of a somewhat granular material high in protein and lipid content. The alveolar walls and interstitial tissue characteristically are normal or almost so. This disease occurs predominantly in patients between the ages of 20 and 50, although a recent report of three cases in children[138] cites ten references to the disease in infants and children; males are most often affected in the ratio of 2 to 1. Six well-documented sibships with alveolar proteinosis have been described, one including four siblings.[139] This appears to constitute strong evidence for a genetic basis for the disease, the

possible inheritance being autosomal recessive, at least in some cases.

The *morphologic changes* are confined to the lungs. Postmortem, the lungs are heavy and firm and the normal architecture is preserved. Microscopically, the walls of the bronchioles and alveoli are normal or at most slightly thickened by lymphocytic infiltration.[140] The alveoli are filled with a granular, flocculent, proteinaceous material that is rich in lipids and stains a deep pink by the periodic acid–Schiff method. PAS-positive granules, probably consisting of mucopolysacharides, may be seen in swollen alveolar epithelial cells. Rosen and his colleagues[137] postulated that the material in the alveoli was derived from or excreted by these lining septal cells. Acicular crystals and laminated bodies, which stain with varying intensity and which are believed to be cellular fragments, are seen in the material that fills the alveoli.

Analysis of the insoluble material obtained by pulmonary lavage of patients with alveolar proteinosis has shown that lipids constitute 55 per cent of the dry weight.[141] McClenhan and his associates[142] concluded that the alveolar material represents an accumulation of modified normal surfactant and serum rather than abnormal lipids or protein or disproportionate quantities of normal lipids. They postulated that type II alveolar epithelial cells produced an excess of intra-alveolar coagulum, which was poorly cleared by defective macrophages.

Alveolar proteinosis has been described in infants[143] usually in association with lymphopenia, immunoglobulin deficiencies, or thymic alymphoplasia. There also appears to be an increased incidence in patients with hematologic malignancy or lymphoma.[144] The patient whose roentgenograms are illustrated in Figure 14–10 died of chronic myelogenous leukemia 18 years after the diagnosis of alveolar proteinosis was first made.

Since the majority of patients recover from alveolar proteinosis and their chest roentgenograms return to normal, it is thought that the intra-alveolar material is partly expectorated and partly phagocytized and removed by the lymphatics.[145]

With rare exceptions the *roentgenographic pattern* is bilateral and symmetrical[146] and is identical in both distribution and character to that of pulmonary edema (Figure 14–10). Since the process is one of air-space consolidation, the basic lesion is the acinar shadow. Confluence of acinar shadows is the rule, with the production of irregular, rather poorly defined, patchy shadows scattered widely throughout the lungs. In many cases the shadows are distrib-

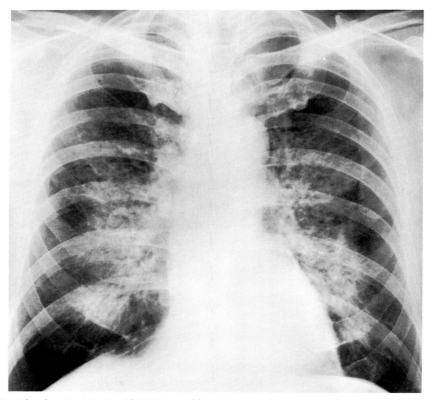

Figure 14–10. Alveolar Proteinosis. This 63-year-old man noted the onset of dyspnea and dry cough 5 months previously. A posteroanterior roentgenogram reveals involvement of the central and midzones of both lungs by patchy air-space consolidation which in many areas is confluent. The disease possesses a "butterfly" pattern of distribution, the peripheral zones of the lungs being spared. An air bronchogram is visible. Cardiac size is normal. Pulmonary function tests revealed normal values except for diffusing capacity, which was reduced by about 50 per cent. Lung biopsy showed the alveolar spaces to be filled with granular, eosinophilic material. The alveolar walls were normal. The patient was placed on corticosteroid therapy, and his chest roentgenogram returned to normal in 5 months. (Courtesy of Dr. Adolf Glay, St. Mary's Hospital, Montreal.)

uted in a "butterfly" or "bat's wing" pattern (Figure 14–10). Occasionally, for unknown reasons, the roentgenographic pattern may simulate diffuse interstitial lung disease despite pathologic confirmation of its predominantly alveolar location.[147] In children, as might be expected, acinar nodules are considerably smaller than in adults, and this should be taken into consideration in pattern recognition.[138]

Resolution usually is complete roentgenographically but may occur asymmetrically and in a spotty fashion and may even be associated with the development of new foci of air-space consolidation in areas not previously affected.[145] Neither hilar nor mediastinal lymph node enlargement, nor pleural effusion, occurs at any stage of the disease.

Clinically, approximately one-third of cases are asymptomatic. The remainder manifest a variety of symptoms, the most frequent being shortness of breath on exertion, usually pro-

gressive in severity and unassociated with orthopnea. Cough is often present and usually is dry but may be associated with "chunky" gelatinous or even purulent expectoration. Hemoptysis rarely occurs. Fatigue, weight loss, and pleuritic pain may be present,[137, 145] and a low-grade fever is said to develop at the onset of the illness in 50 per cent of patients.[137] Physical signs usually are conspicuous by their absence, although clubbing of the fingers and toes is not uncommon.

Although it is difficult to be precise about prognosis, several reviews of the literature suggest that the disease is fatal in about one-third of cases, death resulting from either respiratory failure or superimposed infection. Opportunistic organisms that appear to show an affinity for the constituents of the alveolar material include *Nocardia,* aspergilli, and cryptococci.

Irrigation of the tracheobronchial tree has been employed with success as a means of removing proteinaceous material and on occasion has been life-saving;[137, 145, 148, 149] in fact, pulmonary lavage has been employed successfully in a patient with a severely low PaO_2 by using partial cardiopulmonary bypass.[150] Normal saline alone is as effective a solution as one containing heparin and acetylcysteine.

Pulmonary function studies may be completely normal or there may be a reduction in diffusing capacity, vital capacity, and lung compliance.

HISTIOCYTOSIS-X

In 1953, Lichtenstein[151] grouped together under this heading three diseases that he considered to possess similar morphologic characteristics—Letterer-Siwe disease, Hand-Schüller-Christian disease, and eosinophilic granuloma. The designation "X" by Lichtenstein indicated the lack of knowledge of the etiology of this disease at that time, and so far as we are aware, little, if any, progress has been made in this area. In a recent report of 17 patients with histiocytosis-X,[152] 12 were found to be immunologically abnormal, as evidenced by the presence of circulating lymphocytes spontaneously cytotoxic to cultured human fibroblasts or of antibody to autologous erythrocytes; the patients also had a notable lack of histamine H_2 surface receptors on their T-lymphocytes, suggesting a suppressor-cell deficiency. These markers of cell-mediated immunodeficiency were reversed following intramuscular injections of an extract of thymus gland. Histiocytosis-X is characterized morphologically by granulomatous infiltration of alveolar septa and bronchial walls by a distinctive cell, the histiocyte. The histiocyte is a large pale cell containing a faintly eosinophilic cytoplasm and a rounded nucleus with a distinct nucler membrane. These cells often present a foamy appearance and may contain sudanophilic material. Eosinophils and giant cells are scattered among the histiocytes. The histologic appearance suggests inflammation rather than neoplasia. The later stages of the disease are characterized by the deposition of reticulum and collagen and are dominated by fibrosis.

Histiocytosis-X tends to be a multisystem disease and may involve many organs and tissues, including lymph nodes, lung, skin, central nervous system, liver, spleen, stomach, intestine, kidney, and bone. The distinction between the three varieties depends partly on age of onset and partly on the organ systems involved

but chiefly on the clinical presentation and course of the disease. *Letterer-Siwe disease* occurs in infants and children and is characterized by widespread dissemination and a fulminating fatal course. *Hand-Schüller-Christian disease* usually becomes manifest during childhood or adolescence and progresses much more slowly, so that most affected persons live into adult life; occasionally, it presents in adulthood.[153] One or all of the classic triad of signs (exophthalmus, diabetes insipidus, and osteolytic lesions of the skull) may be present. *Eosinophilic granuloma* is a disease of adults; it may disseminate widely throughout the body but is more commonly localized to the lungs or the bones or both. It is not always possible to fit histiocytosis-X into one of these categories. In fact, in any one patient interconversion may occur from one form to another. The variety with which we are primarily concerned is eosinophilic granuloma.

Eosinophilic granuloma occurs most frequently in Caucasians and only rarely has been described in blacks. There appears to be a distinct predominance in young adult males, an incidence that may relate to the fact that the majority of the diagnoses are based on lung biopsy, a procedure more likely to be carried out on young people and perhaps particularly those in the armed forces.

Although our knowledge of *morphologic characteristics*, particularly in the early stages, is based on small bits of tissue obtained at biopsy, it may be reasonably assumed that the pathologic changes are similar throughout the lungs. During the early or active stage of the disease the lungs show widespread granularity or nodularity, individual foci measuring up to a few millimeters in diameter. These foci consist of aggregates of a wide variety of cells. The predominant cells have large vesicular nuclei, prominent nucleoli, and abundant pale eosinophilic cytoplasm that occasionally is vacuolated. Giant cells, eosinophils, lymphocytes, and polymorphonuclear cells may be intermingled with the histiocytes. The granulomatous lesions are rather vascular and usually are predominantly in the peribronchial and perivascular interstitial tissues and in the septa beneath the pleura.[154] General involvement of the alveolar walls occurs in the later stages of the disease. Histochemically, the foamy histiocytes contain chiefly cholesterol.

As the disease progresses, fibrosis replaces the granulomatous process, with resultant gross disorganization of lung architecture and the development of the characteristic multiple small

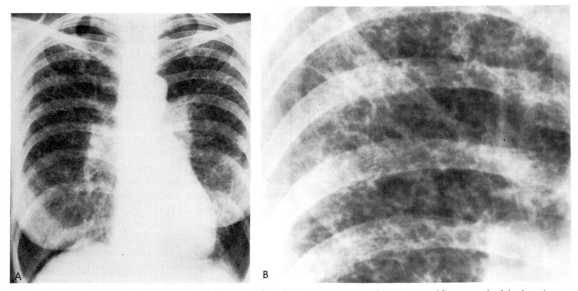

Figure 14–11. Histiocytosis-X (Eosinophilic Granuloma). For many years this 57-year-old woman had had a chronic cough productive of small amounts of whitish-green sputum. During the last three to four years she had experienced increasing shortness of breath on exertion, to a point that she could climb only one flight of stairs before stopping. A posteroanterior roentgenogram *(A)* and a magnified view of the upper portion of the right lung *(B)* reveal a rather coarse reticular pattern that is more prominent in the upper than in the lower lung zones. A honeycomb pattern is suggested in the upper zones. Lung volume appears slightly increased; there are no other findings of note. Histologic sections from an open biopsy revealed gross distortion of lung architecture, normal parenchyma being replaced by broad cellular bands consisting of fibroblasts, histiocytes, and foamy macrophages. In places these bands were associated with a heavy eosinophilic infiltration. There were many giant cells. The prominent histiocytic and eosinophilic infiltrate, associated with fibrosis, cyst formation, and vasculitis, was felt to be consistent with the diagnosis of eosinophilic granuloma.

cysts that tend to give the lung a honeycomb appearance. In the later stages, the histologic appearance is entirely nonspecific. Although a few histiocytes may still be visible in the walls of the cystic spaces, eosinophilic infiltration is often minimal or absent and there may be nothing to suggest the origin of the disease as eosinophilic granuloma, particularly in biopsy specimens.[155]

The *roentgenographic pattern* in the lungs varies with the stage of the disease. Involvement is characteristically diffuse and bilaterally symmetric. Unlike many other diffuse diseases of the lungs, eosinophilic granuloma does not affect the bases predominantly and, in fact, tends to be more extensive in the upper zones.[156] The granulomatous or active stage of the disease is manifested by a nodular pattern, individual lesions ranging from 1 to 10 mm in diameter and presumably representing the individual granulomatous foci observed histologically.

In later stages, the pattern may become reticulonodular (Figure 14–11). The end stage is characterized by a very coarse reticular pattern which in the upper lung zones particularly,

often assumes a cystic appearance characteristic of the honeycomb pattern (Figure 14–11). These cysts usually measure about 1 cm in diameter. We feel that this honeycomb pattern is highly suggestive of eosinophilic granuloma, particularly when it is located mostly in the upper lung zones. In our experience, the progressive loss of lung volume that is so characteristic of diffuse fibrosing alveolitis is seldom seen in eosinophilic granuloma. Even during the active stage of the disease, hilar and mediastinal lymph node enlargement occurs rarely in adults[154, 156] but may be present in children.[157] The same may be said of pleural effusion.[158] However, spontaneous pneumothorax is frequent[156] and may be the first indicator of pulmonary disease, occasionally in the absence of demonstrable abnormality in the lungs.[157] Concomitant involvement of bones and lungs is not uncommon. The diffuse micronodular pattern considered to represent prefibrotic granulomatous infiltration may regress or even completely resolve.

Clinically, at least a third of patients with pulmonary eosinophilic granuloma are asymptomatic when the diagnosis is made, the disease being discovered on screening roentgenography. Symptoms vary widely. Nonspecific constitutional symptoms, including fatigue, weight loss, and fever, may be observed in up to 30 per cent of patients. Approximately two-thirds have a cough, which usually is nonproductive. Dyspnea is present in only about 40 per cent of cases. Hemoptysis is extremely rare. Chest pain caused either by spontaneous pneumothorax or by an osteolytic rib lesion occurs in about 25 per cent. The association of diabetes insipidus and diffuse lung disease, although occurring in only 10 to 25 per cent of cases, should immediately suggest the diagnosis.[156] Physical findings are of little help in diagnosis. The identification of Langerhans' cells in broncho-alveolar lavage has been suggested as a useful technique in diagnosis.[159]

Pulmonary function studies usually reveal a restrictive type of insufficiency with decreased vital capacity, normal residual volume,[28] and normal flow rates. Patients tend to hyperventilate, and the combination of low diffusing capacity and increased physiologic dead space indicates the presence of ventilation-perfusion inequality. It is usual for relatively good pulmonary function to be maintained in cases of eosinophilic granuloma, even when roentgenography reveals extensive abnormality, a state of affairs that seldom obtains in diffuse idiopathic fibrosis.[28]

Although the course of the pulmonary disease varies considerably, often it is rather benign, changing little over the years and manifesting little or no evidence of its presence symptomatically despite persisting abnormality roentgenographically. It is usually stated that in adults the course is insidious and associated with a good prognosis. However, in a follow-up of 12 proved cases, Lewis[156] reported that five had died of the disease and that severe incapacitation from respiratory insufficiency had developed in another two. Our own experience with a few cases tends to support this rather poor prognosis in contrast to the figures reported by others.

GAUCHER'S DISEASE

This disease represents an inborn error of metabolism resulting from a deficiency of β-glucosidase, the enzyme that catalyzes glucosylceramide.[160] This produces an accumulation of this substance in reticuloendothelial cells, whose appearance becomes altered to form Gaucher's cells. These cells, which contain cy-

toplasmic bodies that usually stain strongly for acid phosphatase, accumulate in organs of the reticuloendothelial system, particularly the liver, spleen and lymph nodes, and in the bones and lungs. The majority of patients are female and over 95 per cent are Jews.

In a review of the literature, Wolson[160] found ten case reports of patients with Gaucher's disease in whom pulmonary involvement of one form or another was demonstrated. The roentgenographic manifestations are said to consist of a diffuse reticulonodular or miliary pattern affecting both lungs diffusely.[160] Necropsy examination reveals complete consolidation of lung parenchyma by enormous numbers of Gaucher's cells.

The closely related lipid storage disorder, Niemann-Pick disease, is a syndrome resulting from an inborn error of phospholipid metabolism. Roentgenographic manifestations in the chest are said to consist of a widespread nodular pattern throughout both lungs.[161]

PULMONARY ALVEOLAR MICROLITHIASIS

This rare, curious disease of unknown etiology is characterized by the presence within the alveoli of myriad tiny calculi ("calcispherytes"). The definitive work on the subject was published by Sosman and his colleagues in 1957[162] on the basis of 26 cases collected from many centers throughout the world. The disease has been identified in premature stillborn twins,[163] indicating that the condition may originate *in utero*. It is probable that in the majority of cases the disease begins in early life. There is no obvious sex predominance.[162]

Although the etiology of the disease remains obscure, a familial occurrence has been noted in more than half the reported cases.[162, 163] This familial incidence has been almost completely restricted to siblings, and in only two instances has the disease been diagnosed in both a parent and a child.[164] Although the familial incidence would implicate an inborn error of metabolism, environmental factors have also been postulated. Theories based on a metabolic disturbance have been proposed but are difficult to substantiate in view of the consistently normal serum calcium and phosphorus levels in reported series.[165]

Morphologically, microliths range from 0.01 to 3.0 mm in diameter. They are almost invariably intra-alveolar, although there is evidence suggesting that they may be formed in the

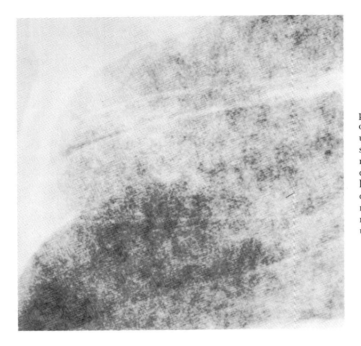

Figure 14–12. Alveolar Microlithiasis. A posteroanterior roentgenogram of this 40-year-old asymptomatic man revealed a remarkably uniform opacification of both lungs. On close scrutiny this can be seen to be produced by a multitude of tiny, discrete opacities of calcific density (the figure is a detail view of the right lower zone from a two to one primary magnification image). Multiple function tests were normal except for a reduction in RV of 800 ml, representing the displacement of pulmonary volume by the calcispherytes.

alveolar walls and subsequently be extruded into the alveolar air spaces. Chemical analysis reveals chiefly calcium and phosphorus and no silicon or iron. The composition appears to be very similar to that of bone, the major constituent being apatite, a tricalcium phosphate in one or more of its many forms. In fact, alveolar microlithiasis has been shown to manifest intense uptake of bone imaging tracer (^{99m}Tc diphosphonate).[166]

In the early stages of the disease the alveolar walls appear perfectly normal. In later stages, interstitial fibrosis associated with giant cell formation thickens the alveolar walls. Blebs and bullae often form, particularly in the apices.[162] Pulmonary hypertension and cor pulmonale may develop, in association with right ventricular dilatation and hypertrophy.

Roentgenographically, there is no other pulmonary disease whose pattern is so characteristic and diagnostic as alveolar microlithiasis. Although there is considerable variation from patient to patient depending on the severity of affliction, the fundamental pattern is one of a very fine sandlike micronodulation diffusely involving both lungs (Figure 14–12). Regardless of the effect of superimposition or summation of shadows, individual deposits are usually identifiable, particularly with magnification roentgenography. They are extremely sharply defined and measure less than 1 mm in diameter. The overall density is greater over the lower than upper zones, probably because of in-

creased thickness of lung rather than selectively greater involvement. The opacities may be so numerous as to appear confluent, and a normally exposed chest roentgenogram shows the lungs as almost uniformly white, often with total obliteration of the mediastinal and diaphragmatic contours. The contrast between the extreme density of the lung parenchyma on one side of the pleura and the ribs on the other may create the illusion of a "black" pleural line.

In their classic paper, Sosman and his colleagues[161] suggested that in many patients the microliths continue to form and perhaps increase in size as the disease progresses. However, there is no doubt that the disease may become "arrested" and the deposition of concentrations cease. We have had the opportunity of studying two brothers in whom the extensive changes apparent roentgenographically were stationary for 30 years.

Clinically, the majority of patients are asymptomatic when their disease is first discovered. The diagnosis is usually made on the basis of the typical pattern on a screening chest roentgenogram. Symptoms may be absent even when the chest roentgenogram reveals the lungs to be almost solid and white, with little visible air-containing parenchyma. In no other condition is the lack of association between roentgenologic and clinical findings so striking as in pulmonary alveolar microlithiasis.

The first symptom to develop in advanced cases is dyspnea on exertion; cough and expectoration are uncommon.[162] As the disease progresses, respiratory insufficiency may develop, with cyanosis, clubbing of the fingers, and clinical signs of right ventricular hypertrophy and failure. The physical signs usually are unrevealing except in the late stages, when breath sounds may be decreased, particularly at the bases.

Pulmonary function studies vary considerably from case to case, depending upon both the extent of replacement of alveolar air by concretions and the presence or absence of interstitial fibrosis. During the several years in which we have followed our two cases, the only significant finding has been a reduction in residual volume caused by the physical presence of calculi in the pulmonary air spaces. Other investigators[167] have observed a decrease in maximal breathing capacity, an increase in residual volume, and a decrease in diffusing capacity.

REFERENCES

1. Longcope, W. T., and Freiman, D. G.: A study of sarcoidosis. Based on a combined investigation of 160 cases including 30 autopsies from the The Johns Hopkins Hospital and Massachusetts General Hospital. Medicine, 31:1, 1952.
2. Scadding, J. G.: Sarcoidosis. London, Eyre and Spottiswoode, 1967.
3. Hsing, C. T., Han, F. C., Liu, H. C., and Chu, B. Y.: Sarcoidosis among Chinese. Am. Rev. Respir. Dis., 89:917, 1964.
4. Panna Lal Nandi, Man Cheuk Au, and Guan Bee Ong: Sarcoidosis among Chinese. Chest, 80:74, 1981.
5. Maycock, R. L., Bertrand, P., Morrison, C. E., and Scott, J. H.: Manifestations of sarcoidosis. Analysis of 145 patients, with a review of nine series selected from the literature. Am. J. Med., 35:67, 1963.
6. Keller, A. Z.: Anatomic sites, age attributes, and rates of sarcoidosis in U.S. veterans. Am. Rev. Respir. Dis., 107:615, 1973.
7. Kendig, E. L., and Brummer, D. L.: The prognosis of sarcoidosis in children, Chest, 70:351, 1976.
8. Merten, D. F., Kirks, D. R., and Grossman, H.: Pulmonary sarcoidosis in childhood. Am. J. Roentgenol., 135:673, 1980.
9. Kendig, E. L., Jr.: Sarcoidosis. Am. J. Dis. Child., 136:11, 1982.
10. Hetherington, S.: Sarcoidosis in young children. Am. J. Dis. Child., 136:13, 1982.
11. Mankiewicz, E.: The relationship of sarcoidosis to anonymous bacteria. (Proc. Third Internat. Conf. on Sarcoidosis.) Acta Med. Scand., 425(Suppl.):68, 1964.
12. Mitchell, D. N., Rees, R. J. W., and Goswami, K. K. A.: Transmissible agents from human sarcoid and Crohn's disease tissues. Lancet, 2:761, 1976.
13. Mitchell, D. N., and Rees, R. J. W.: The nature and physical characteristics of a transmissible agent from human sarcoid tissue. Ann. N.Y. Acad. Sci., 278:233, 1976.
14. Mitchell, D. N., and Rees, R. J. W.: Further observations on the nature and physical characteristics of transmissible agents from human sarcoid and Crohn's disease tissues. In Williams, W. J., and Davies, B. H. (eds.): Eighth International Conference on Sarcoidosis and Other Granulomatous Disease. Cardiff, U.K., Alpha Omega Publishing Ltd., 1978, p. 121.
15. James, D. G.: Modern concepts of sarcoidosis. Chest, 64:675, 1973.
16. Crystal, R. G., Roberts, W. C., Hunninghake, G. W., Gadek, J. E., Fulmer, J. D., and Line, B. R.: Pulmonary sarcoidosis: A disease characterized and perpetuated by activated lung T-lymphocytes. Ann. Intern. Med., 94:73, 1981.
16a. Crystal, R. G.: Skin testing, blood studies, and bronchoalveolar lavage to assess activity. Ann. Intern. Med., 94:73, 1981.
17. Roberts, W. C.: Morphologic aspects of pulmonary sarcoidosis: In Crystal, R. G., moderator: Pulmonary sarcoidosis: A disease characterized and perpetuated by activated lung T-lymphocytes. Ann. Intern. Med., 94:73, 1981.
18. Hunninghake, G. W.: Characterization of the alveolitis of sarcoidosis. In Crystal, R. G., moderator: Pulmonary sarcoidosis: A disease characterized and perpetuated by activated lung T-lymphocytes. Ann. Intern. Med., 94:73, 1981.
19. Hunninghake, G. W., and Crystal, R. G.: Pulmonary sarcoidosis. A disorder mediated by excess helper T-lymphocyte activity at sites of disease activity. N. Engl. J. Med., 305:429, 1981.
20. Kataria, Y. P., Shaw, R. A., and Campbell, P. B.: Sarcoidosis: an overview II. Clin. Notes Respir. Dis., 20:3, 1982.
21. James, D. G., and Williams, W. J.: Immunology of sarcoidosis. Am. J. Med., 72:5, 1982.
22. Gadek, J. E.: Maintenance of the alveolitis of sarcoidosis. In Crystal, R. G., moderator: Pulmonary sarcoidosis: A disease characterized and perpetuated by activated lung T-lymphocytes. Ann. Intern. Med., 94:73, 1981.
23. Hunninghake, G. W., Gadek, J. E., Young, R. C., Jr., et al.: Maintenance of granuloma formation in pulmonary sarcoidosis by T-lymphocytes within the lung. N. Engl. J. Med., 302:594, 1980.
24. Crystal, R. G.: Skin testing, blood studies, and bronchoalveolar lavage to assess activity. In Crystal, R. G., moderator: Pulmonary sarcoidosis: A disease characterized and perpetuated by activated lung T-lymphocytes. Ann. Intern. Med., 94:73, 1981.
25. Rosen, Y., Athanassiades, T. J., Moon, S., and Lyons, H. A.: Nongranulomatous interstitial pneumonitis in sarcoidosis. Relationship to development of epithelioid granulomas. Chest, 74:122, 1978.
26. Smith, M. J., Turton, C. W. G., Mitchell, D. N., et al.: Association of HLA B8 with spontaneous resolution in sarcoidosis. Thorax, 36:296, 1981.
27. Neville, E.: HLA antigens and disease. Mt. Sinai J. Med., 44:772, 1977.
28. Bates, D. V., Macklem, P. T., and Christie, R. V.: Respiratory Function in Disease; An Introduction to the Integrated Study of the Lung, 2nd ed. Philadelphia, W. B. Saunders Co., 1971.
29. Smellie, H., and Hoyle, C.: The natural history of pulmonary sarcoidosis. Q. J. Med., 29:539, 1960.
30. Ellis, K., and Renthal, G.: Pulmonary sarcoidosis: Roentgenographic observations on course of disease. Am. J. Roentgenol., 88:1070, 1962.
31. Kirks, D. R., McCormick, V. D., and Greenspan, R.

H.: Pulmonary sarcoidosis. Roentgenologic analysis of 150 patients. Am. J. Roentgenol., *117*:777, 1973.

32. Bein, M. E., Putman, C. E., McLoud, T. C., and Mink, J. H.: A reevaluation of intrathoracic lymphadenopathy in sarcoidosis. Am. J. Roentgenol., *131*:409, 1978.

33. Schabel, S. I., Foote, G. A., and McKee, K. A.: Posterior lymphadenopathy in sarcoidosis. Radiology, *129*:591, 1978.

34. Rabinowitz, J. G., Ulreich, S., and Soriano, C.: The usual unusual manifestations of sarcoidosis and the "hilar haze"—a new diagnostic aid. Am. J. Roentgenol., *120*:821, 1974.

35. Rosen, Y., Amorosa, J. K., Moon, S., Cohen, J., and Lyons, H. A.: Occurrence of lung granulomas in patients with stage I sarcoidosis. Am. J. Roentgenol., *129*:1083, 1977.

36. Gorske, K. J., and Fleming, R. J.: Mycetoma formation in cavitary pulmonary sarcoidosis. Radiology, *95*:279, 1970.

37. Beekman, J. F., Zimmet, S. M., Chun, B. K., Miranda, A. A., and Katz, S.: Spectrum of pleural involvement in sarcoidosis. Arch. Intern. Med., *136*:323, 1976.

38. McCort, J. J., and Paré, J. A. P.: Pulmonary fibrosis and cor pulmonale in sarcoidosis. Radiology, *62*:496, 1954.

39. Murray, R. O., and Jacobson, H. G.: The Radiology of Skeletal Disorders; Exercises in Diagnosis. Baltimore, Williams & Wilkins, 1971.

40. Roth, C., Huchon, G. J., Arnoux, A., et al.: Bronchoalveolar cells in advanced pulmonary sarcoidosis. Am. Rev. Respir. Dis., *124*:9, 1981.

41. Editorial: Myocardial sarcoidosis. Lancet, *2*:1351, 1972.

42. Editorial: "Diagnosis" of sarcoidosis. N. Engl. J. Med., *267*:103, 1962.

43. Sharma, O. P.: Cutaneous sarcoidosis: Clinical features and management. Chest, *61*:320, 1972.

44. Löfgren, S., and Lundbäck, H.: The bilateral hilar lymphoma syndrome. I. A study of the relation to age and sex in 212 cases. II. A study of the relation to tuberculosis and sarcoidosis in 212 cases. Acta Med. Scand., *142*:259, 1952.

45. Kaplan, H.: Sarcoid arthritis: A review. Arch. Intern. Med., *112*:924, 1963.

46. West, S. G., Gilbreath, R. E., and Lawless, O. J.: Painful clubbing and sarcoidosis. J.A.M.A., *246*:1338, 1981.

47. King, B. P., Esparza, A. R., Kahn, S. I., and Garella, S.: Sarcoid granulomatous nephritis occurring as isolated renal failure. Arch. Intern. Med., *136*:241, 1976.

48. Bear, R. A., Handelsman, S., Lang, A., et al.: Clinical and pathological features of six cases of sarcoidosis presenting with renal failure. Can. Med. Assoc. J., *121*:1367, 1979.

49. Delaney, P.: Neurologic manifestations in sarcoidosis. Review of the literature, with a report of 23 cases. Ann. Intern. Med., *87*:336, 1977.

50. Young, R. L., and Krumholz, R. A., with the technical assistance of Harkleroad, L. E.: A physiologic roentgenographic disparity in sarcoidosis. Dis. Chest, *50*:81, 1966.

51. Kent, D. C., and Spence, W.: Physiologic abnormalities in pulmonary sarcoidosis. Dis. Chest, *46*:680, 1964.

52. Leading article: Pulmonary function in sarcoidosis. Br. Med. J., *1*:710, 1967.

53. Divertie, M. B., Cassan, S. M., O'Brien, P. C., and Brown, A. L., Jr.: Fine structural morphometry of diffuse lung diseases with abnormal blood-air gas transfer. Mayo Clin. Proc., *51*:42, 1976.

54. Miller, A., Teirstein, A. S., Jackler, I., Chuang, M., and Siltzbach, L. E.: Airway function in chronic pulmonary sarcoidosis with fibrosis. Am. Rev. Respir. Dis., *109*:179, 1974.

55. Renzi, G. D., Renzi, P. M., Lopez-Majano, V., and Dutton, R. E.: Airway function in sarcoidosis: effect of short-term steroid therapy. Respiration, *42*:98, 1981.

56. Bechtel, J. T., Starr, T., III, Dantzker, D. R., and Bower, J. S.: Airway hyperreactivity in patients with sarcoidosis. Am. Rev. Respir. Dis., *1241*:759, 1981.

57. McLoud, T. C., Epler, G. R., Gaensler, E. A., Burke, G. W., and Carrington, C. B.: A radiographic classification for sarcoidosis: physiologic correlation. Invest. Radiol., *17*:129, 1982.

58. Reiner, M., Sigurdsson, G., Nunziata, V., Malik, M. A., Poole, G. W., and Joplin, G. F.: Abnormal calcium metabolism in normocalcaemic sarcoidosis. Br. Med. J., *2*:1473, 1976.

59. Lieberman, J.: Elevation of serum angiotensin-converting-enzyme (ACE) level in sarcoidosis. Am. J. Med., *59*:365, 1975.

60. Fanburg, B. L., Schoenberger, M. D., Bachus, B., and Snider, G. L.: Elevated serum angiotensin I converting enzyme in sarcoidosis. Am. Rev. Respir. Dis., *114*:525, 1976.

61. Rohrbach, M. S., and DeRemee, R. A.: Pulmonary sarcoidosis and serum angiotensin-converting enzyme. Mayo Clin. Proc., *57*:64, 1982.

62. Gupta, R. G., Oparil, S., and Szidon, J. P.: Clinical significance of serum angiotensin-converting enzyme levels in sarcoidosis. J. Lab. Clin. Med., *93*:940, 1979.

63. Studdy, P., Bird, R., and James, D. G.: Serum angiotensin-converting enzyme (sace) in sarcoidosis and other granulomatous disorders. Lancet, *2*:1331, 1978.

64. Katz, P., Fauci, A. S., Yeager, H., Jr., and Reen, B. M.: Serum angiotensin-converting enzyme and lysozyme in granulomatous diseases of unknown cause. Ann. Intern. Med., *94*:359, 1981.

65. Young, R. C., Jr., Headings, V. E., Bose, S., Harden K. A., Crockett, E. D., Jr., and Hackney, R. L. Jr.: Alpha₁ antitrypsin levels in sarcoidosis: Relationship to disease activity. Chest, *64*:39, 1973.

66. Fulmer, J. D.: Roentgenograms and physiologic studies to assess activity. *In* Crystal, R. G., moderator: Pulmonary sarcoidosis: A disease characterized and perpetuated by activated lung T-lymphocytes. Ann. Intern. Med., *94*:73, 1981.

67. Line, B. R.: Gallium scanning to assess activity. *In* Crystal, R. G., moderator: Pulmonary sarcoidosis: A disease characterized and perpetuated by activated lung T-lymphocytes. Ann. Intern. Med., *94*:73, 1981.

68. Kent, D. C.: Recurrent unilateral hilar adenopathy in sarcoidosis. Am. Rev. Respir. Dis., *91*:252, 1965.

69. Mikhail, J. R., Mitchell, D. N., Drury, R. A. B., and Sutherland, I.: A comparison of the value of mediastinal lymph node biopsy and the Kveim test in sarcoidosis. Am. Rev. Respir. Dis., *104*:544, 1971.

70. Munkgaard, S., and Neukirch, F.: Comparison of biopsy procedures in intrathoracic sarcoidosis. Acta Med. Scand., *205*:179, 1979.

71. Koerner, S. K., Sakowitz, A. J., Appelman, R. I., Becker, N. H., and Schoenbaum, S. W.: Transbronchial lung biopsy for the diagnosis of sarcoidosis. N. Engl. J. Med., *293*:268, 1975.

72. Poe, R. H., Israel, R. H., Utell, M. J., and Hall, W. J.: Probability of a positive transbronchial lung biopsy result in sarcoidosis. Arch. Intern. Med., *139*:761, 1979.

73. Leading article: Diagnosis of pulmonary sarcoidosis. Br. Med. J., *4*:540, 1975.

74. Leading article: The Kveim test. Br. Med. J., *2*:604, 1971.

75. American Thoracic Society: Brummer, D. L., Chairman, Chaves, A. D., Cugell, D. W., Marks, C. E., Pierce, A. K., Ross, J. C., Utz, J. P., Young, R. C., Jr., and Ziskind, M. M.: The Kveim test. A statement by the committee on therapy. Am. Rev. Respir. Dis., *103*:435, 1971.

76. Editorial: The Kveim controversy. Lancet, *2*:750, 1971.

77. Sones, M., and Israel, H. L.: Course and prognosis of sarcoidosis. Am. J. Med., *29*:84, 1960.

78. Israel, H. L.: Prognosis of sarcoidosis. Ann. Intern. Med., *73*:1038, 1970.

79. Young, R. C., Jr., Titus-Dillon, P. Y., Schneider, M. L., Shelton, T. G., Hackney, R. L., Jr., and Harden, K. A.: Sarcoidosis in Washington, D.C., Clinical observations in 105 black patients. Arch. Intern. Med., *125*:102, 1970.

80. Siltzbach, L. E., James, D. G., Neville, E., Turiaf, J., Battesti, J. P., Sharma, O. P., Hosoda, Y., Mikami, R., and Odaka, M.: Course and prognosis of sarcoidosis around the world. Am. J. Med., *57*:847, 1974.

81. American Thoracic Society: Brummer, D. L., Chairman, Chaves, A. D., Cugell, D. W., Marks, C. E., Pierce, A. K., Ross, J. C., Utz, J. P., Young, R. C., Jr., and Ziskind, M. M.: Treatment of sarcoidosis. A statement by the committee on therapy. Am. Rev. Respir. Dis., *103*:433, 1971.

82. Mitchell, D. N., and Scadding, J. G.: Sarcoidosis. Am. Rev. Respir. Dis., *110*:774, 1974.

83. Scadding, J. G.: Fibrosing alveolitis. Br. Med. J., *2*:686, 1964.

84. Scadding, J. G.: Fibrosing alveolitis. Br. Med. J., *2*:941, 1964.

85. Scadding, J. G., and Hinson, K. F. W.: Diffuse fibrosing alveolitis (diffuse interstitial fibrosis of the lungs). Thorax, *22*:291, 1967.

86. Liebow, A. A., and Carrington, C. B.: The interstitial pneumonias. In Simon, M., Potchen, E. J., and Le May, M. (eds.): Frontiers of Pulmonary Radiology. New York, Grune & Stratton, 1969, p. 102.

87. Hamman, L., and Rich, A. R.: Fulminating diffuse interstitial fibrosis of the lungs. Trans. Am. Clin. Climatol. Assoc., *51*:154, 1935.

88. Crystal, R. G., Fulmer, J. D., Roberts, W. C., Moss, M. L., Line, B. R., and Reynolds, H. Y.: Idiopathic pulmonary fibrosis. Ann. Intern. Med., *85*:769, 1976.

89. Stack, B. H. R., Grant, I. W. B., Irvine, W. J., and Moffat, M. A. J.: Idiopathic diffuse interstitial lung disease: A review of 42 cases. Am. Rev. Respir. Dis., *92*:939, 1965.

90. Dill, J., Ghose, T., Landrigan, P., MacKeen, A. D., and MacNeil, A. R.: Cryptogenic fibrosing alveolitis. Chest, *67*:411, 1975.

91. Solliday, N. H., Williams, J. A., Gaensler, E. A., Coutu, R. E., and Carrington, C. B.: Familial chronic interstitial pneumonia. Am. Rev. Respir. Dis., *108*:193, 1973.

92. Patchefsky, A. S., Atkinson, W. G., Hoch, W. S., Gordon, G., and Lipshitz, H. I.: Interstitial pulmonary fibrosis and von Recklinghausen's disease: An ultrastructural and immunofluorescent study. Chest, *64*:459, 1973.

93. Gaensler, E. A., Carrington, C. B., and Coutu, R. E.: Chronic interstitial pneumonias. Clin. Notes Respir. Dis., *10*:3, 1972.

94. Carrington, C. B., Gaensler, E. A., Coutu, R. E., FitzGerald, M. X., and Gupta, R. G.: Usual and desquamative interstitial pneumonia. Chest, *69*:261, 1976.

95. Rudd, R. M., Haslam, P. L., and Turner-Warwick, M.: Cryptogenic fibrosing alveolitis: Relationships of pulmonary physiology and bronchoalveolar lavage to response to treatment and prognosis. Am. Rev. Respir. Dis., *124*:1, 1981.

96. Weinberger, S. E., Kelman, J. A., Elson, N. A., et al.: Bronchoalveolar lavage in interstitial lung disease. Ann. Intern. Med., *89*:459, 1978.

97. Hunninghake, G. W., Gadek, J. E., and Lawley, T. J.: Mechanisms of neutrophil accumulation in the lungs of patients with idiopathic pulmonary fibrosis. J. Clin. Invest., *68*:259, 1981.

98. Scadding, J. G.: Diffuse pulmonary alveolar fibrosis. Thorax, *29*:271, 1974.

99. DeRemee, R. A., Harrison, E. G., Jr., and Andersen, H. A.: The concept of classic interstitial pneumonitis-fibrosis (CIP-F) as a clinicopathologic syndrome. Chest, *61*:213, 1972.

100. Liewbow, A. A., Steer, A., and Billingsley, J. G.: Desquamative interstitial pneumonia. Am. J. Med., *39*:369, 1965.

101. Rosenow, E. C., III, O'Connell, E. J., and Harrison, E. G., Jr.: Desquamative interstitial pneumonia in children. Report of two cases. Am. J. Dis. Child., *120*:344, 1970.

102. Patchefsky, A. S., Israel, H. L., Hoch, W. S., and Gordon, G.: Desquamative interstitial pneumonia: relationship to interstitial fibrosis. Thorax, *28*:680, 1973.

103. Davis, G. S., Brody, A. R., Landis, J. N., Graham, W. G. B., Craighead, J. E., and Green, G. M.: Quantitiation of inflammatory activity in interstitial pneumonitis by bronchofiberoscopic pulmonary lavage. Chest, *69*:265, 1976.

104. Gaensler, E. A., Goff, A. M., and Prowse, C. M.: Desquamative interstitial pneumonia. N. Engl. J. Med., *274*:113, 1966.

105. Valdivia, E., Hensley, G., Wu, J., Leroy, E. P., and Jaeschke, W.: Morphology and pathogenesis of desquamative interstitial pneumonitis. Thorax, *32*:7, 1977.

106. Liebow, A. A.: New concepts and entities in pulmonary disease. *In* Liebow, A. A., and Smith, D. E. (eds.): The Lung. Baltimore, Williams and Wilkins, 1968, pp. 333–365.

107. Feigin, D. S., and Friedman, P. J.: Chest radiography in desquamative interstitial pneumonitis: A review of 37 patients. Am. J. Roentgenol., *134*:91, 1980.

108. Lemire, P., Bettez, P., Gelinas, M., and Raymond, G.: Patterns of desquamative interstitial pneumonia (D. I. P.) and diffuse interstitial pulmonary fibrosis (D. I. P. F.). Am. J. Roentgenol., *115*:479, 1972.

109. Patchefsky, A. S., Banner, M., and Freundlich, I. M.: Desquamative interstitial pneumonia. Significance of intranuclear viral-like inclusion bodies. Ann. Intern. Med., *74*:322, 1971.

110. Binette, J. P., and Montes, M.: Lymphoid interstitial pneumonia. Can. Med. Assoc. J., *114*:810, 1976.

111. Carrington, C. B., and Liebow, A. A.: Lymphocytic interstitial pneumonia. Am. J. Pathol., *48*:36A, 1966.

112. Halprin, G. M., Ramirez-R., Jr., and Pratt, P. C.: Lymphoid interstitial pneumonia. Chest, *62*:418, 1972.

113. Liebow, A. A., and Carrington, C. B.: Duffuse pulmonary lymphoreticular infiltrations associated with dysproteinemia. Med. Clin. North Am., *57*:809, 1973.

114. Reddy, P. A., Gorelick, D. F., and Christianson, C. S.: Giant cell interstitial pneumonia (GIP). Chest, *58*:319, 1970.

115. Ostrow, D., and Cherniack, R. M.: Resistance to airflow in patients with diffuse interstitial lung disease. Am. Rev. Respir. Dis., *108*:205, 1973.

116. Schofield, N. McC., Davies, R. J., Cameron, I. R., and Green, M.: Small airways in fibrosing alveolitis. Am. Rev. Respir. Dis., *113*:729, 1976.

117. Boushy, S. F., and North, L. B.: Pulmonary function in infiltrative lung disease. Chest, *64*:448, 1973.

118. Wagner, P. D., Dantzker, D. R., Dueck, R., dePolo, J. L., Wasserman, K., and West, J. B.: Distribution of ventilation-perfusion ratios in patients with interstitial lung disease. Chest, *69*:256, 1976.

119. Fulmer, J. D., Roberts, W. C., and Crystal, R. G.: Diffuse fibrotic lung disease: A correlative study. Chest, *69*:263, 1976.

120. Stack, B. H. R., Choo-Kang, Y. F. J., and Heard, B. E.: The prognosis of cryptogenic fibrosing alveolitis. Thorax, *27*:535, 1972.

121. Strumpf, I. J., Feld, M. K., Cornelius, M. J., et al.: Safety of fiberoptic bronchoalveolar lavage in evaluation of interstitial lung disease. Chest, *80*:268, 1981.

122. Genereux, G. P.: The end-stage lung. Radiology, *116*:279, 1975.

123. Beaumont, F., Jansen, H. M., Elema, J. D., et al.: Simultaneous occurrence of pulmonary interstitial fibrosis and alveolar cell carcinoma in one family. Thorax, *36*:252, 1981.

124. Turner-Warwick, M., Lebowitz, M., Burrows, B., and Johnson, A.: Cryptogenic fibrosing alveolitis and lung cancer. Thorax, *35*:496, 1980.

125. Webb, W. R., and Goodman, P. C.: Fibrosing alveolitis in patients with neurofibromatosis. Radiology, *122*:289, 1977.

126. Klatte, E. C., Franken, E. A., and Smith, J. A.: The radiographic spectrum in neurofibromatosis. Semin. Roentgenol., *11*:17, 1976.

127. Chakera, T. M. H., Howarth, F. H., Kendall, M. J., Lawrence, D. S., and Whitfield, A. G. W.: The chest radiograph in ankylosing spondylitis. Clin. Radiol., *26*:455, 1975.

128. Wolson, A. H., and Rohwedder, J. J.: Upper lobe fibrosis in ankylosing spondylitis. Am. J. Roentgenol., *124*:466, 1975.

129. Weiss, W., Boucot, K. R., Cooper, D. A., Carnahan, W. J., and Seidman, H.: The risk of lung cancer according to cell type and cigarette dosage. Abstract American Thoracic Society. Am. Rev. Respir. Dis., *103*:881, 1971.

130. Gacad, G., and Massaro, D.: Pulmonary fibrosis and group IV mycobacteria infection of the lungs in ankylosing spondylitis. Am. Rev. Respir. Dis., *109*:274, 1974.

131. Libshitz, H. I., and Atkinson, G. W.: Pulmonary cystic disease in ankylosing spondylitis: Two cases with unusual superinfection. J. Can. Assoc. Radiol., *29*:266, 1978.

132. Silverstein, E. F., Ellis, K., Wolff, M., and Jaretzki, A., III: Pulmonary lymphangiomyomatosis. Am. J. Roentgenol., *120*:832, 1974.

133. Harris, J. O., Waltuck, B. L., and Swenson, E. W.: The pathophysiology of the lungs in tuberous sclerosis. A case report and literature review. Am. Rev. Respir. Dis., *100*:379, 1969.

134. Corrin, B., Liebow, A. A., and Friedman, P. J.: Pulmonary lymphangiomyomatosis. Am. J. Pathol., *79*:348, 1975.

135. Stovin, P. G. I., Lum, L. C., Flower, C. D. R., Darke, C. S., and Beeley, M.: The lungs in lymphangiomyomatosis and in tuberous sclerosis. Thorax, *30*:497, 1975.

136. Genereux, G. P.: Lipids in the lungs: Radiologic-pathologic correlation. J. Can. Assoc. Radiol., *21*:2, 1970.

137. Rosen, S. H., Castleman, B., and Liebow, A. A.: Pulmonary alveolar proteinosis. N. Engl. J. Med., *258*:1123, 1958.

138. McCook, T. A., Kirks, D. R., Merten, D. F., et al.: Pulmonary alveolar proteinosis in children. Am. J. Roentgenol., *137*:1023, 1981.

139. Teja, K., Cooper, P. H., Squires, J. E., and Schnatterly, P. T.: Pulmonary alveolar proteinosis in four siblings. N. Engl. J. Med., *305*:1390, 1981.

140. Divertie, M. B. Brown, A. L., Jr., and Harrison, E. G., Jr.: Pulmonary alveolar proteinosis. Two cases studied by electron microscopy. Am. J. Med., *40*:351, 1966.

141. Sahu, S., DiAugustine, R. P., and Lynn, W. S.: Lipids found in pulmonary lavage of patients with alveolar proteinosis and in rabbit lung lamellar organelles. Am. Rev. Respir. Dis., *114*:177, 1976.

142. McClenahan, J. B., and Mussenden, R.: Pulmonary alveolar proteinosis. Arch. Intern. Med., *133*:284, 1974.

143. Colón, A. R., Jr., Lawrence, R. D., Mills, S. D., and O'Connell, E. J.: Childhood pulmonary alveolar proteinosis (PAP). Am. J. Dis. Child., *121*:481, 1971.

144. Green, D., Dighe, P., Ali, N. O., and Katele, G. V.: Pulmonary alveolar proteinosis complicating chronic myelogenous leukemia. Cancer, *46*:1763, 1980.

145. Ramirez, J.: Pulmonary alveolar proteinosis. A roentgenologic analysis. Am. J. Roentgenol., *92*:571, 1964.

146. Mendenhall, E., Jr., Solu, S., and Easom, H. F.: Pulmonary alveolar proteinosis. Am. Rev. Respir. Dis., *84*:876, 1961.

147. Miller, P. A., Ravin, C. E., Smith, G. J. W., and Osborne, D. R. S.: Pulmonary alveolar proteinosis with interstitial involvement. Am. J. Roentgenol., *137*:1069, 1981.

148. Jenkins, D. W., Teichner, R. L., Griggs, G. W., and Byrd, R. B.: Alveolar proteinosis. Lavage in the presence of bronchopleural fistula. J.A.M.A., *234*:74, 1975.

149. Ramirez, J.: Alveolar proteinosis: Importance of pulmonary lavage. Am. Rev. Respir. Dis., *103*:666, 1971.

150. Freedman, A. P., Pelias, A., Johnston, R. F., et al.: Alveolar proteinosis lung lavage using partial cardiopulmonary bypass. Thorax, *36*:543, 1981.

151. Lichtenstein, L.: Histiocytosis X: Integration of eosinophilic granuloma of bone, "Letterer-Siwe disease," and "Schüller-Christian disease" as related

manifestations of a single nosologic entity. Arch. Pathol., *56*:84, 1953.

152. Osband, M. E., Lipton, J. M., Lavin, P., et al.: Histiocytosis-X—Demonstration of abnormal immunity, T-cell histamine H2–receptor deficiency, and successful treatment with thymic extract. N. Engl. J. Med., *304*:146, 1981.

153. Kaufman, A., Bukberg, P. R., Werlin, S., and Young, I. S.: Multifocal eosinophilic granuloma ("Hand-Schuller-Christian disease"). Report illustrating H-S-C chronicity and diagnostic challenge. Am. J. Med., *60*:541, 1976.

154. Knudson, R. J., Badger, T. L., and Gaensler, E. A.: Eosinophilic granuloma of the lung. Med. Thorac. *23*:248, 1966.

155. Enriquez, P., Dahlin, D. C., Hayles, A. B., and Henderson, E. D.: Histiocytosis X: A clinical study. Mayo Clin. Proc., *42*:88, 1967.

156. Lewis, J. G.: Eosinophilic granuloma and its variants with special reference to lung involvement. A report of 12 patients. Q. J. Med., *33*:337, 1964.

157. Carlson, R. A., Hattery, R. R., O'Connell, E. J., and Fontana, R. S.: Pulmonary involvement by histiocytosis X in the pediatric age group. Mayo Clin. Proc., *51*:542, 1976.

158. Tittel, P. W., and Winkler, C. F.: Chronic recurrent pleural effusion in adult histiocytosis-X. Br. J. Radiol., *54*:68, 1981.

159. Verea-Hernando, H., Fontan-Bueso, J., Martin-Egana, M. T., and Arnal-Monreal, F.: Langerhans

cells in bronchoalveolar lavage in the late stages of pulmonary histiocytosis X. Chest, *81*:130, 1982.

160. Wolson, A. H.: Pulmonary findings in Gaucher's disease. Am. J. Roentgenol., *123*:712, 1975.

161. Lachman, R., Crocker, A., Schulman, J., and Strand, R.: Radiological findings in Niemann-Pick disease. Radiology, *108*:659, 1973.

162. Sosman, M. C., Dodd, G. D., Jones, W. D., and Pillmore, G. U.: The familial occurrence of pulmonary alveolar microlithiasis. Am. J. Roentgenol., *77*:947, 1957.

163. Caffrey, P. R., and Altman, R. S.: Pulmonary alveolar microlithiasis occurring in premature twins. J. Pediatr., *66*:758, 1965.

164. Drinković, I., Strohal, K., and Sabljica, B.: Mikrolithiasis alveolaris pulmonum. (Pulmonary alveolar microlithiasis.) Fortschr. Roentgenstr., *97*:180, 1962.

165. O'Neill, R. P., Cohn, J. E., and Pellegrino, E. D.: Pulmonary alveolar microlithiasis—a family study. Ann. Intern. Med., *67*:957, 1967.

166. Brown, M. L., Swee, R. G., Olson, R. J., and Bender, C. E.: Pulmonary uptake of ^{99m}Tc diphosphonate in alveolar microlithiasis. Am. J. Roentgenol., *131*:703, 1978.

167. Oka, S., Shiraishi, K., Ogata, K., Goto, Y., Yasuda, T., and Yanagihara, H.: Pulmonary alveolar microlithiasis. Report of three cases. Am. Rev. Respir. Dis., *93*:612, 1966.

15

Diseases of the Pleura

Although to our knowledge the precise incidence of pleural abnormality in association with chest disease is unknown, it is seen in a sufficient proportion of roentgenograms of hospital patients that its importance cannot be overestimated. Pleural effusion—the most important if not the most frequent abnormality observed—may occur alone without other changes in the thorax or may accompany abnormalities of the lungs, mediastinum, or chest wall. In the former circumstance, diagnosis may prove exceedingly difficult, even with bacteriologic, biochemical, and pathologic investigative techniques. When effusion occurs as part of a complex of roentgenographic changes, however, it may provide an important diagnostic clue. Often its cause is immediately apparent—for example, when it accompanies enlargement of the heart and is the result of cardiac decompensation, or when it occurs as a hemothorax in association with multiple rib fractures following trauma to the chest wall. Just as often, however, an effusion constitutes one facet of a complex of roentgen signs that tries the diagnostic skills of the physician.

PLEURAL EFFUSION

Since the etiologic diagnosis of pleural effusion depends largely upon whether or not there is other disease in the lungs, mediastinum, diaphragm, or chest wall, the approach to differential diagnosis must be along different lines when effusion is the sole abnormality and when one or more of these structures is affected. Justification for this approach can be found in a report by Rabin and Blackman[1] of 78 cases of bilateral pleural effusion of widely varying etiology. Only 29 showed additional roentgenographic shadows that directed attention to a specific etiology. In the remaining 49 cases, almost two-thirds of the series, no other abnormalities were apparent that might aid in diagnosis of the disease causing the effusion. It is important to note that underlying pulmonary or mediastinal disease is not always detectable on the first available roentgenograms. Large effusions may mask parenchymal shadows or mediastinal masses, and these may become evident only when fluid has been removed or when CT or special roentgenography in the supine or lateral decubitus position renders the underlying lung or mediastinal contour visible.

CLINICAL MANIFESTATIONS

Pleural pain is a frequent manifestation of "dry" pleurisy but usually disappears when effusion develops. A dry cough often persists and may be productive if there is an associated pneumonia. Dyspnea is common; if it is severe and associated with decreased respiratory reserve, it may require immediate thoracentesis for relief. Physical examination reveals dullness or flatness on percussion and a decrease or absence of breath sounds. When dullness or percussion is shifting, this sign by itself is diagnostic. Breath sounds may be bronchial at the interface between dependent fluid and aerated lung.

Depending upon the presence and nature of underlying pulmonary disease, the results of pulmonary function studies in cases of pleural effusion are so variable that little information of value has been published. In the absence of underlying pulmonary disease, the effects of pleural effusion on pulmonary function reflect the combination of a space-occupying process and a reduction in lung volume as a consequence of relaxation atelectasis. The space-occupying process reduces all subdivisions of lung volume, including TLC, FRC, and VC, although ventilatory ability may be little impaired when the other lung is normal and there is no pleural pain inhibiting chest movement.

PLEURAL EFFUSION CAUSED BY INFECTION

Pleural infections usually produce an exudative effusion—*i.e.*, with a protein content greater than 3 g per 100 ml. The inflammatory reaction results in increased capillary permeability, causing protein loss from capillaries. According to Black,[2] reabsorption of fluid and protein by the lymphatics may be impaired when fibrin deposition and inflammatory thickening of the pleural membrane occur. By far the commonest etiologic agents of infectious pleural effusion are the bacteria. Although the fungi, viruses, and parasites are much less common causes, the identification of pleural effusion with each of these etiologic agents is of considerable diagnostic significance.

BACTERIA

MYCOBACTERIUM TUBERCULOSIS

In many areas of the world, tuberculosis remains the most common cause of pleural effusion in the absence of demonstrable pulmonary disease. In some areas of the United States, tuberculous pleural effusion is becoming a rarity. For example, of 108 patients with pleural effusion studied at the Mayo Clinic,[3] only one had effusion of tuberculous etiology. Tuberculous pleural effusion occurs most commonly in young adults as an uncomplicated serous effusion. Although it may complicate established pulmonary tuberculosis—when its presence invariably indicates activity of the pulmonary disease—it also presents as uncomplicated "pleurisy with effusion." Pleural effusion as a manifestation of primary tuberculosis occurs more commonly in adults than in children.

The onset of tuberculous pleurisy with effusion may be insidious, heralded only by mild pleuritic pain, perhaps with low-grade fever, a slight unproductive cough, weight loss, and easy fatigability. More often the onset is acute, with chest pain, fever, and prostration, suggesting acute pneumonia.[4]

The long-term prognosis in cases of tuberculous pleurity with effusion is influenced to a considerable extent by the method of treatment. Simple bed rest often results in complete absorption of the pleural fluid and apparently complete restoration of the patient's health to normal, but the incidence of subsequent active pulmonary tuberculosis is high. By contrast, although short-term results are similar and occur no more rapidly with chemotherapy, the incidence of subsequent pulmonary tuberculosis is much less with this treatment.[5]

Aspiration typically yields clear, straw-colored fluid, containing more than 3 g protein per 100 ml. The effusion is seldom bloody or even pink, although erythrocytes may be visible microscopically. Lymphocytes predominate, amounting to more than 70 per cent of total white cells, although polymorphonuclear forms may be more numerous during the early stages. It is fairly safe to consider effusions containing more than 50 per cent polymorphonuclears as being of nontuberculous etiology. A low pleural fluid glucose content (less than 25 mg per 100 ml) suggests a tuberculous etiology but also may be present in association with bacterial pneumonias, rheumatoid disease, and bronchogenic carcinoma.

A *presumptive* diagnosis of tuberculous pleural effusion may be made with a combination of a positive tuberculin test and a predominantly lymphocytic response in the pleural fluid. In roughly 60 to 80 per cent of patients with proved tuberculosis, pleural biopsy specimens reveal granulomas.[6] Although this finding is virtually diagnostic, definitive diagnosis requires the identification of acid-fast organisms in the tissue specimen or a positive culture of pleural fluid or tissue. The incidence of positive culture from pleural fluid is surprisingly low, being found in only 20 to 25 per cent of proved cases, whereas cultures of biopsy specimens are positive in from 55 to 80 per cent of patients.[7]

BACTERIA OTHER THAN MYCOBACTERIUM TUBERCULOSIS

It is probable that pleural effusion is a common accompaniment of acute pneumonia, although its presence is frequently unrecognized because of its small amount. The recorded incidence of parapneumonic effusion probably would increase sharply if roentgenograms were obtained in the lateral decubitus position in all cases. Parapneumonic effusions usually are "benign" serous exudates that resolve spontaneously. When the underlying pneumonia is of bacterial (nontuberculous) origin, a predominance of polymorphonuclear leukocytes will be present and in a few patients the fluid will become grossly cloudy and then frankly purulent (empyema). When empyema develops or when a serous effusion becomes loculated, drainage is required.[8] According to Light, there are four main indications for tube drainage: (1) the presence of gross pus; (2) organisms visible on Gram staining; (3) a glucose level in the pleural fluid of less than 50 mg per 100 ml; or (4) a pleural fluid pH level of less than 7.20. In about one-third of empyemas, tube drainage alone proves inadequate and open drainage with rib resection is required.[9]

As in the bacterial pneumonias, the types of organisms responsible for empyema vary with the host's state of health. In the western world, as a result of the control of tuberculosis and the availability of antibiotics effective against pyogenic infections, most empyemas are now caused by *Staphylococcus aureus*, enteric gram-negative bacilli, and anaerobic bacteria. Acid-fast bacteria, *Streptococcus pneumoniae*, and *Str. pyogenes* are uncommonly isolated on culture.[10] In patients who acquire infections in the community, the most frequent organisms are anaerobes and staphylococci, whereas in hospitalized patients, gram-negative bacilli predominate. Not uncommonly, pus aspirated from the pleural cavity in patients with empyema is sterile, a finding that may reflect the administration of antimicrobial drugs before admission. Perhaps more often, negative results are caused by a failure to culture pleural fluid anaerobically. When such culture is performed, at least one-third of cases will show positive growth.[9, 10] Of 83 cases of empyema studied in three different hospitals with a special interest in anaerobic infection, pleural fluid culture isolated anaerobic bacteria exclusively in 29 cases (35 per cent), anaerobes mixed with aerobic or facultative bacteria in 34 cases (41 per cent), and aerobic or facultative bacteria exclusively in the remaining 20 cases (24 per cent).[10]

Although most patients with empyema are febrile and manifest blood neutrophilia, the compromised host and patients receiving corticosteroid therapy may be afebrile and have a normal white count.

KLEBSIELLA, ENTEROBACTER, AND SERRATIA

GENERA. Most instances of *Klebsiella-Enterobacter-Serratia* infections occur in elderly hospital patients who have been compromised by major medical or surgical illnesses. By contrast, most cases of pneumonia caused by *Klebsiella* types I, III, IV, and V develop in alcoholic or otherwise debilitated patients and are rarely hospital-acquired. Pleural effusion in the form of empyema frequently complicates acute pneumonia caused by these organisms. The character of the effusion varies from mildly to frankly purulent.

STAPHYLOCOCCUS AUREUS. In infants and young children, pleural effusion in the form of empyema develops in almost every case of acute staphylococcal pneumonia, being observed in over 90 per cent of cases. In young patients, the change in roentgenologic findings characteristically is extremely rapid, from minimal to very extensive involvement within a few hours. Pleural effusion or empyema occurs in approximately 50 per cent of adult patients and is a useful sign in differentiating staphylococcal from other forms of pneumonia.[11] Pneumatoceles appear as distinctive, generally thin-walled cystic spaces, ranging from 1 cm in diameter to the volume of a hemithorax. Their pathogenesis is thought to involve check-valve obstruction of a small bronchus or of a peribronchial abscess.

STREPTOCOCCUS PYOGENES. Streptococcal pneumonia is uncommon but when present is associated with a high incidence of pleural effusion. For example, Welch and associates[12] observed effusion in 19 of 20 patients with acute β-hemolytic streptococcal pneumonia in a military population. The pleural fluid varies from serous effusion to frank pus. In children particularly, acute streptococcal pneumonia is commonly preceded by acute viral disease, especially the exanthems.

STREPTOCOCCUS PNEUMONIAE. In contrast to its frequency in acute *Streptococcus pyogenes* pneumonia, roentgenographically demonstrable pleural effusion is uncommon in cases of acute pneumonia caused by *Streptococcus pneumoniae*, at least on posteroanterior and lateral roentgenograms exposed in the erect position. Fourteen (11 per cent) of 123 patients considered to have pneumococcal pneumonia on the basis of smears and roentgenologic appearance were found to have effusion or empyema.[13] However, since no large series of cases of acute pneumococcal pneumonia appears to have been studied by lateral decubitus roentgenography, the true incidence of associated effusion is unknown.

FRANCISELLA TULARENSIS. This organism is responsible for tularemia, a disease that is most common in rodents and small mammals. Insects act as both reservoirs and vectors. Of the four main clinical forms of the disease, ulceroglandular, oculoglandular, typhoidal, and pulmonary, the last two most frequently include pulmonary and pleural involvement, ranging from 50 to 75 per cent.[14] The combination of parenchymal consolidation (sometimes distinctive), enlarged hilar lymph nodes, and pleural effusion should permit a reasonably firm *presumptive* diagnosis. Rising serum agglutinin titers against *Francisella tularensis* or isolation of the organism from sputum or pleural fluid is necessary for *positive* diagnosis.

OTHER BACTERIA. Several other bacteria of varying species that are uncommon or rare causes of pleuropulmonary disease in humans have a high incidence of associated pleural effusion. The effusions are commonly purulent and are frequently associated with acute pneumonia, sometimes with abscess formation. Acute pneumonias in which effusion or empyema is particularly common include those caused by *Bacillus anthracis*, *Malleomyces mallei*, *Escherichia coli*, *Salmonella* species, and *Haemophilus influenzae*. Pleural effusion is not a prominent manifestation of legionnaires' disease.[15]

FUNGI

ACTINOMYCES ISRAELII AND NOCARDIA SPECIES. These are clearly the two most important "fungi" in the etiology of pleural effusion. They may be considered together, since their roentgenologic characteristics are identical. Pulmonary involvement is an invariable accompaniment, usually in the form of acute air-space pneumonia. Abscess formation is common. The infection extends into the pleura, producing empyema, and subsequently may transgress the parietal pleura to involve the chest wall, with rib destruction and subcutaneous abscess formation (empyema necessitatis).

Pleural effusion caused by other fungi is very uncommon.

VIRUSES AND MYCOPLASMA

Although roentgenographic demonstration of pleural effusion in viral and *Mycoplasma* pneumonia was formerly considered rare, Fine and his coworkers[16] achieved this in 12 (20 per cent) of 59 patients with serologically proved *Mycoplasma*, viral, or cold agglutinin–positive pneumonia. In four cases, however, this required roentgenography of patients in the lateral decubitis position. The overall incidence of effusion in their series was roughly the same in *Mycoplasma* pneumonia, influenzal pneumonia, and in pneumonia associated with elevated cold agglutinin titers.

PARASITES

ENTAMEBA HISTOLYTICA. Pleuropulmonary involvement in amebiasis is almost invariably secondary to liver abscess, with transmission of the infection into the thorax by way of the portal vein or diaphragmatic lymphatics or occasionally by direct extension through the diaphragm into the pleural space and eventually into the lung. Pleuropulmonary disease is said to occur in 15 to 20 per cent of patients with liver involvement.[17] The pleural effusion is usually serofibrinous. The pulmonary lesion may cavitate, providing communication between the bronchial tree and the liver abscess—a bronchohepatic fistula—in which case fluid of typical "chocolate sauce" appearance may be seen on thoracentesis or in the sputum. This fluid contains blood, cytolyzed liver tissue, and small solid particles of liver parenchyma. The rapid response to specific antiamebic therapy makes early diagnosis vital.

PNEUMOCYSTIS CARINII. Roentgenographic evidence of pleural effusion in *Pneumocystis* infestation is said to be rare.[18] However, Forrest[19] reported pleural effusion in two of 14 cases of proved *Pneumocystis* pneumonia, and one of our patients with combined *Pneumocystis* and cytomegalovirus pneumonia had small bilateral pleural effusions.

ECHINOCOCCUS GRANULOSUS (HYDATID DISEASE). Pleural effusion is uncommon in hydatid disease.[20] It occurs when a pulmonary hydatid cyst ruptures into the pleural space rather than into its usual site, the bronchial tree. In most cases, since air also is present, the roentgenographic appearance is of a hydropneumothorax. Scolices and daughter cysts floating on the surface of the fluid produce irregularities of the fluid surface, creating the "water lily" sign or "sign of the camalote." It is relatively easy to recover hooklets from the pleural fluid or sputum in cases in which a cyst has ruptured.

PLEURAL EFFUSION CAUSED BY IMMUNOLOGIC DISEASE

Only three of the collagen diseases are important causes of pleural effusion: systemic lupus erythematosus (SLE), Wegener's granulomatosis, and rheumatoid disease. Pleural effusion in cases of polyarteritis nodosa, scleroderma, or dermatomyositis probably results from other causes (*e.g.*, heart failure) and not from the primary disease.

SYSTEMIC LUPUS ERYTHEMATOSUS

Effusions are bilateral in about half the cases and, when unilateral, are predominantly left-sided.[21] They are usually small but may be massive. Winslow and his colleagues[21] stress the importance of pleuritis as an early manifestation of SLE. Of 57 cases reported by these authors, pleural effusion occurred in 42; in three of these, pleuritis appeared as an isolated first sign, and in 16 others it was associated with only minor antecedent symptoms. In 23 of the 42 cases the effusion was bilateral, either simultaneously or alternately, and in 13 of the 19 cases of unilateral effusion it was on the left side. Levin[22] has emphasized the importance of distinguishing pleural effusion due to direct involvement of the pleura by SLE from that associated with lupus nephrosis. The former characteristically is accompanied by pain and splinting, whereas the serous effusions of nephrosis are painless. When the effusion is attributable to direct pleural involvement, it is probable that inflammation and fibrinoid necrosis of vessel walls of the pleura produce increased capillary permeability, resulting in pleural effusion with a relatively high protein concentration. By contrast, when the effusion results from the nephrotic syndrome secondary to SLE, it will be a transudate. The fluid usually possesses no significant biochemical findings.

The most common associated roentgenologic finding is enlargement of the cardiovascular silhouette, which is said to occur in 35 to 50 per cent of all cases.[23] Pulmonary involvement is entirely nonspecific in nature. Its reported incidence varies widely. Except as a terminal event, when pneumonia may be extensive, the pulmonary changes consist of nonspecific basal "pneumonitis" or atelectasis, usually in the lung bases. Although there is nothing specific about the roentgenographic pattern of systemic lupus, the combination of bilateral pleural effusion with nonspecific enlargement of the cardio-vascular silhouette should at least suggest the diagnosis. Confirmation depends upon the demonstration of antinuclear or anti-DNA antibodies.

WEGENER'S GRANULOMATOSIS

Pleural effusion is said to occur fairly frequently in this disease (in six of 11 cases in one series),[24] although it is greatly overshadowed by the pulmonary manifestations. The typical roentgenographic pattern in the lungs is that of rounded opacities, usually sharply circumscribed, ranging from a few millimeters to 9 cm in diameter. They are usually bilateral and widely distributed, with no predilection for any lung zone.

RHEUMATOID DISEASE

Pleural abnormality probably is the most frequent manifestation of rheumatoid disease in the thorax.[25] Of 516 patients with rheumatoid arthritis in one series,[26] 108 (21 per cent) gave a history of pleurisy and 17 (3.3 per cent) had pleural effusions for which no other cause could be found.

The most noteworthy aspect of pleural effusion in rheumatoid disease is its predominance in men. For example, 24 of 25 patients studied by Carr and Mayne[27] were males, a sex incidence similar to that of all reported series and especially remarkable since the incidence of rheumatoid arthritis in females is about twice that in males. Although effusions usually appear some time after the clinical onset of rheumatoid arthritis, they may antedate both signs and symptoms of joint disease. They are usually unilateral, slightly more often on the right side. The only unique characteristic of the pleural effusion roentgenographically is its tendency to remain relatively unchanged for many months or even years.[27]

The fluid is typically an exudate, usually turbid and greenish-yellow,[27] with a predominantly lymphocytic cellular reaction. In some cases polymorphonuclear leukocytes are found in abundance. Characteristically, the glucose content is very low (20 to 25 mg or less per 100 ml), despite normal blood glucose levels, and does not rise following intravenous infusion of glucose.[27] It has been estimated that pleural fluid glucose levels below 30 mg per 100 ml are found in 70 to 80 per cent of patients with rheumatoid disease.[28] Although elevated levels of rheumatoid factor in pleural fluid have been found in a significant number of cases without apparent associated rheumatoid disease, some authors consider that the finding of rheumatoid arthritis cells in pleural fluid is evidence of a rheumatoid etiology.[29]

It has been shown that the detection of immune complex levels in pleural fluid by various techniques can be useful in confirming whether or not the etiology of a disease is of collagen-vascular type, and that it may even help in distinguishing lupus erythematosus and rheumatoid disease as the initiating cause.[30]

Empyema is surprisingly common in rheumatoid pleuropulmonary disease[31] and probably follows a discharge into the pleural cavity of necrotic material from rheumatoid nodules.

The incidence of coexistent pulmonary disease and pleural effusion in rheumatoid disease is not known, but it seems that they tend to occur independently. For example, there was no evidence of pulmonary disease in 19 of Carr and Mayne's 25 patients with rheumatoid effusion.[27]

Symptoms relating to the effusion vary and often are absent. Of 25 patients described by Carr and Mayne,[27] 13 were asymptomatic, six had typical pleural pain, and two experienced a dull ache in the thorax. Shortness of breath was the presenting complaint in six patients, and in only two did chills and fever suggestive of acute infection herald the onset.

PLEURAL EFFUSION CAUSED BY ASBESTOS

It is probable that the benign pleural effusion that is related to chronic asbestos exposure is frequently undiagnosed. Two recent studies[32, 33] have shown that the latent period from exposure to the development of pleural effusion is shorter than for other asbestos-related disorders. Prevalence among workers is dose-related. Effusions usually are small and hemorrhagic and persist for several months; one out of three recur. One-quarter to two-thirds of patients are asymptomatic (*see* page 587 for further information).

PLEURAL EFFUSION CAUSED BY NEOPLASMS

The importance of cancer as an etiologic agent in pleural effusion is reflected in Rabin and Blackman's report of 78 cases of bilateral effu-

sion associated with a heart of normal size.[1] Thirty-five (44.9 per cent) were due to cancer, 19 being metastatic, 13 lymphoma, and three primary carcinoma of the lung. Of these 35 patients, 13 (almost 40 per cent) showed no roentgenographic abnormality of the thorax other than pleural effusion.

BRONCHOGENIC CARCINOMA

Pleural involvement in primary bronchogenic carcinoma is not uncommon, effusion having been observed in 8 per cent of patients in one large series[34] and in 15 per cent of another.[35] As a cause of pleural effusion, these neoplasms are nearly always associated with roentgenographically demonstrable pulmonary abnormality. Bronchogenic carcinoma causing combined pulmonary disease and pleural effusion may manifest itself as local increase in density in two ways: (1) as a peripheral mass, commonly but not always contiguous to the visceral pleura, and (2) as obstructive pneumonitis ("drowned lung"). There may or may not be roentgenographic evidence of enlargement of hilar or mediastinal lymph nodes.

The recovery of malignant cells from pleural fluid of patients with proved bronchogenic carcinoma is generally regarded as evidence of inoperability. If cells are not found—a common event, judging from the series reported by Rosenblatt and Lisa[36] in which 22 per cent of patients with pleural effusion and bronchogenic carcinoma had no evidence of metastatic pleural involvement—the significance of the effusion is controversial. A reasonable explanation exists for fluid formation without direct neoplastic involvement—for example, as a result of venous obstruction secondary to compression by tumor, or, perhaps more likely, from the inflammatory component of obstructive pneumonitis. However, Brinckman's analysis of patients with pleural effusion complicating otherwise operable bronchogenic carcinoma[37] suggests that effusion is an ominous finding even when cells are not recovered. Thoracotomy revealed extrapulmonary spread of the disease in 17 of 21 such patients. Although Brinkman's results seem to render thoracotomy questionable in such patients, effusion should not be regarded as categorical evidence of inoperability if all other findings favor operation, especially if there is roentgenographic evidence of obstructive pneumonitis or venous obstruction.

It has been suggested that two specific procedures are underused in the diagnosis of malignant pleural effusion: one is the use of thoracoscopy to identify suitable areas for direct pleural biopsy,[38–40] and the other is chromosome analysis of cells present in pleural fluid.[41]

BRONCHIOLAR CARCINOMA

Pleural effusion is not uncommon with this neoplasm, being observed in 8 to 10 per cent of cases,[42] always in association with pulmonary involvement. The parenchymal disease may vary from a small nodule in the same or opposite lung to massive consolidation. Pleural effusion associated with widespread pulmonary disease may cause difficulty in roentgenologic differential diagnosis, particularly between metastatic carcinoma and lymphoma. Enlargement of hilar and mediastinal lymph nodes favors the diagnosis of lymphoma but does not exclude metastatic carcinoma or bronchiolar carcinoma. *Positive* diagnosis depends on the recovery of typical cells from the pleural fluid or sputum or on lung or lymph node biopsy.

LYMPHOMA AND LEUKEMIA

The incidence of pleural effusion in patients with Hodgkin's disease ranges from 16[43] to 28 per cent,[44] and in those with non–Hodgkin's lymphoma from 16[43] to 20 per cent.[45] Opinion differs concerning the precise mechanisms by which pleural fluid accumulates in cases of lymphoma, the main point of controversy being the obstructive influence of mediastinal lymph nodes. Judging from the results of a number of studies,[43–47] it must be concluded that the cause of pleural effusion is highly variable, possibly being lymphatic obstruction, venous obstruction, secondary pulmonary infection, direct involvement of the pleura by neoplasm, or a combination of these. Obviously, chylothorax must be excluded from this statement, since this condition results largely from obstruction of the thoracic duct. Such effusions contain high concentrations of neutral fat and fatty acid.

In leukemia, pleural effusion is usually unilateral and as a roentgenographic abnormality is second only to mediastinal lymph node enlargement in frequency. Although effusion may be found in up to 25 per cent of patients, probably it is due to actual leukemic infiltration in no more than 5 per cent. It is more likely caused by obstructed lymphatics, cardiac failure, or infection, since it is most common in chronic forms of the disease. However, in acute leukemia, particularly in children, general pleural thickening or local pleural thickening simulating plaques may be caused by leukemic infiltration.[48]

METASTATIC CARCINOMA

Rabin and Blackman's report of 78 cases of bilateral pleural effusion[1] included 19 caused by metastatic neoplasm, in seven cases without other demonstrable abnormality in the lungs or mediastinum. Primary origin of the neoplasms varied; the majority were from the breast, others being from the pancreas, stomach, ovary, kidney, and bladder.

In one series of 122 patients with breast carcinoma and pleural effusion,[49] the median survival was 6 months after the onset of effusion. Ipsilateral effusion occurred in 83 per cent of the patients.

Of 52 cases of metastatic carcinoma to the pleura reported by Meyer,[50] effusion was present in only 31, the remainder being nodular deposits only. This author feels, with apparent justification, that effusions develop as a result of neoplastic infiltration of the mediastinal lymph nodes, with resultant lymphatic obstruction. If Meyer's conclusion is valid, it would lend some support to Stewart's thesis[51] that a pleural exudate of high protein content is removed from the pleural space by the lymphatics by bulk flow. Provided that the lymphatic channels are not obstructed and the rate of fluid formation is not too great, it might be logically assumed that, in this way, the pleural space could be kept dry (or ideally moist) and that if lymphatic drainage were obstructed, pleural fluid would accumulate. Meyer[50] provided further support for a close link between lymphatic obstruction and pleural effusion with metastatic carcinoma when he observed that effusions do not develop with metastatic *sarcoma*. In this condition lymphatic metastases seldom occur. It should be emphasized that mediastinal nodes may be involved by metastatic neoplasm and thereby create lymphatic obstruction and resultant pleural effusion, without clear-cut roentgenographic evidence of their enlargement. This fact is of importance in differential diagnosis when repeated examination of fluid from such an effusion detects no malignant cells. In these cases, positive diagnosis must await discovery of the site of the primary neoplasm.

The pleural effusions of metastatic cancer are characteristically exudates, of relatively high protein content and with a specific gravity of

1.018 or greater. Blood content varies from none to heavy (of Meyer's 31 cases, only nine were grossly hemorrhagic). Glucose content usually is higher than 80 mg per 100 ml, a finding that may be of value in differentiating these effusions from those of tuberculous etiology.

PRIMARY NEOPLASMS OF THE PLEURA

There are two types of pleural mesothelioma—local benign and diffuse malignant. The former is associated with pleural effusion uncommonly (two of 17 cases reported by Hutchinson and Friedenberg[52]) and the latter almost invariably. The pleural fluid is usually bloody and may contain detectable quantities of hyaluronic acid. This acid may be demonstrated in the tissue of both benign and malignant mesotheliomas by both histochemical[53] and biochemical[54] methods. Roentgenographically, the local variety appears as a soft tissue mass of varied size, lying peripherally and contiguous to the pleura, usually at an obtuse angle to the chest wall. The diffuse malignant type commonly presents as thickening of the pleura throughout much of the hemithorax, but the early development of massive effusion often obscures the underlying pleural abnormality. In the diffuse variety, despite massive opacification the hemithorax may show little change in volume. Or volume may even be reduced, a peculiarity that has been attributed to a combination of compression and obstructive atelectasis secondary to invasion of the medial aspect of the lung, with resulting bronchial compression and occlusion. This combination of changes is seen also in obstructing bronchogenic carcinoma with massive collapse and pleural effusion, and differential diagnosis usually is between these two entities.

PRIMARY NEOPLASMS OF THE CHEST WALL

Pleural effusion in multiple myeloma is uncommon but may be associated with roentgenographic changes distinctive enough to permit strongly *presumptive* diagnosis. Destructive lesions in one or more ribs may be associated with soft tissue masses, which commonly protrude into the thorax and indent the pleura and lung. The ribs may be expanded, a finding that is almost pathognomonic of myeloma.

Malignant bone tumors arising in the ribs or

(occasionally) thoracic spine may extend into the thoracic cavity and lead to pleural effusion. Primary mesenchymal neoplasms originating in the tissues of the intercostal spaces may have the same effect. The combination of an expanding lesion of the chest wall and pleural effusion is highly *suggestive* of the diagnosis, although roentgenologic differentiation from myeloma other than multiple may be impossible.

PLEURAL EFFUSION CAUSED BY THROMBOEMBOLIC DISEASE

As a roentgenographic manifestation of thromboembolic disease, pleural effusion is as common as, if not more common than, parenchymal consolidation.[55] In our experience it nearly always indicates infarction. The parenchymal shadow may be diminutive or hidden by the fluid,[56, 57] confusing the diagnostic possibilities to such an extent that an embolic episode will be suggested only if there is a high index of suspicion. The amount of pleural fluid is frequently small but may be abundant. It is more often unilateral.[58] Pleural fluid usually develops and absorbs synchronously with the infarction but sometimes appears later and clears sooner.[59] The pleural fluid almost invariably is serosanguineous and possesses a protein concentration higher than 3 g per 100 ml.

The pulmonary changes are varied. In a study of 72 patients following pulmonary embolism Stein and his associates[55] observed roentgenographic abnormalities in the chest in 60: pleural effusion in 33, homogeneous opacities resembling pneumonia in 27, elevation of the hemidiaphragm (usually with some parenchymal abnormality) in 21, and line shadows in 19.

PLEURAL EFFUSION CAUSED BY CARDIAC DECOMPENSATION

Probably one of the most common forms of pleural effusion is that associated with increase in hydrostatic pressure in the venous circulation, either pulmonary or systemic or both. It occurs most commonly with cardiac decompensation but may be seen also with constrictive pericarditis[60, 61] or obstruction of the superior vena cava or azygos vein. The mechanisms whereby the effusions develop are complex and are related not only to increased hydrostatic pressure but also to influences such as altered capillary permeability (secondary to anoxia) and reduced lymphatic drainage. Considerable confusion and difference of opinion have existed as to whether the development of hydrothorax in human cardiac decompensation is attributable predominantly to failure of the right side of the heart (systemic venous hypertension), the left side of the heart (pulmonary venous hypertension), or a combination of the two. We have felt for some time that right-sided or left-sided cardiac failure in relatively "pure" form seldom leads to hydrothorax and that decompensation of both sides of the heart is required. In 1970, Mellins and his colleagues[62] reported a study on dogs, in which they found that a significantly larger amount of pleural fluid accumulated after systemic venous hypertension than after pulmonary venous hypertension, and the largest amount of fluid accumulated with combined systemic and venous hypertension. Although one cannot categorically apply these results to humans, they at least lend considerable support to the contention that the clinical situation most favorable for the development of pleural effusion is decompensation of both sides of the heart.

For some unknown reason, hydrothorax is much more prone to develop in the right pleural space than in the left, but it may be bilateral. Associated roentgenologic evidence of cardiac enlargement with or without pulmonary venous hypertension usually makes the diagnosis obvious. The fluid is usually clear and light yellow and is a transudate, with low protein content and a specific gravity of 1.015 or less.

A roentgenologic finding peculiar to hydrothorax associated with congestive heart failure is the so-called phantom tumor, in which fluid tends to localize (not loculate) in an interlobar pleural fissure. These "disappearing tumors" occur most frequently in the right horizontal fissure. The mechanism of this localization is not clear, but it seems likely that it has nothing to do with pleural adhesions.

PLEURAL EFFUSION CAUSED BY TRAUMA

Hemothorax is a common manifestation of nonpenetrating trauma and may develop from a variety of causes. Blood may enter the pleural space from injury to the chest wall, diaphragm, lung, or mediastinum. Although hemorrhage may result from laceration of the parietal or visceral pleura by fractured ribs, hemothorax may occur (with or without associated pneumothorax) in closed chest trauma without evidence of fracture. When blood enters the pleural space it coagulates rapidly, but, presumably as a result of physical agitation produced by movement of the heart and lungs, the clot may be defibrinated and leave fluid indistinguishable roentgenologically from effusion of any other cause.[63] When a solid clot does remain it may prove a hindrance to adequate thoracentesis, a procedure that should be carried out thoroughly to prevent later troublesome fibrothorax. As in empyema, loculation tends to occur early in hemothorax, increasing still further the difficulty of obtaining needle drainage. Reynolds and Davis[63] emphasized the importance of the site of hemorrhage in relation to the quantity of hemothorax. When bleeding is from a vessel in the chest wall, diaphragm, or mediastinum, the hemothorax tends to increase despite the quantity of blood present. When the blood comes from the pulmonary vasculature the expanding hemothorax compresses the lung, with resultant pulmonary tamponade that may produce hemostasis.

Other causes of pleural fluid accumulation following trauma, each considered elsewhere in this book, include rupture of the aorta, esophageal perforation, rupture of the thoracic duct, thoracotomy, and malpositioning of central venous and Swan-Ganz[64] catheters. An association has recently been reported between recurrent left-sided pleural effusions and silent splenic hematomas following trauma.[65]

PLEURAL EFFUSION CAUSED BY DISEASE ARISING OUTSIDE THE THORAX

There are many diseases in which pleural effusion develops without direct extension of the offending organism or cell into the thorax. They are intra-abdominal or retroperitoneal in location and involve the transfer of fluid from below the diaphragm through diaphragmatic lymphatics into the pleural space.

In 1929 Lemon and Higgins[66] described lymphatic channels that carry particulate matter from the peritoneum to the thorax and found that those of the right hemidiaphragm are larger and carry more fluid than those of the left. More recently, it has been shown that, in the presence of ascites, carbon particles or radioiodinated serum albumin instilled into the peritoneal space passes into the pleural space[67] and that flow is always from the peritoneum to the pleura and never in the reverse direction.[67, 68]

It is probable that in some patients fluid transfer from the peritoneal to the pleural space occurs by way of diaphragmatic lymphatics and in others by way of diaphragmatic defects. The question inevitably arises as to why all cases of ascites are not associated with pleural effusion, and, to the best of our knowledge, the answer has not been found.

PANCREATITIS

Although not a true "infection," acute, chronic, or relapsing pancreatitis is sometimes associated with pleural effusion, often without roentgenographic evidence of other intrathoracic abnormality. Effusions are predominantly left-sided.[69] Of considerable diagnostic importance is the amylase content of the effusions, which is high and usually greater than in the serum.[69] The importance of this observation in any patient with severe epigastric pain is obvious.

PLEURAL EFFUSION FOLLOWING ABDOMINAL SURGERY

The development of small pleural effusions is common after abdominal surgery. Light and George[70] carried out a study of 200 patients 48 to 72 hours following surgery in whom roentgenograms were obtained in the right and left lateral decubitus positions. Pleural effusion was identified in 97 patients (49 per cent), being less than 4 mm in thickness in 50 patients, 4 to 10 mm in 26, and greater than 10 mm in 21. The incidence was higher following surgery on the upper abdomen, in patients with postoperative atelectasis on the side on which the surgery was performed, and in patients with free abdominal fluid.

SUBPHRENIC ABSCESS

Small pleural effusions are often found in cases of acute subphrenic infection, being observed in 37 (79 per cent) of 47 cases reported by Miller and Talman.[71] Associated findings include elevation and restriction of movement of the ipsilateral hemidiaphragm (95 per cent in the above series) and basal "plate" atelectasis or pneumonitis (79 per cent). This combination of findings should strongly suggest the diagno-sis, especially in the postoperative period after laparotomy or following rupture of a hollow abdominal viscus.

MEIGS-SALMON SYNDROME

In 1934 Salmon[72] described the association of pleural effusion with benign pelvic tumors, a report that antedated by 3 years that by Meigs and Cass[73] of seven cases of ovarian fibromas associated with ascites and hydrothorax. The syndrome is now known to be associated with a wide variety of primary pelvic neoplasms, including fibroma, thecoma, granulosa cell tumors, Brenner tumors, cystadenoma, adenocarcinoma, and even extraovarian pelvic tumors such as fibromyoma of the uterus. According to Meigs,[68] the first four of these neoplasms are those with which the syndrome is most commonly associated. In 1945 Dockerty[74] reviewed the literature and found that almost 40 per cent of ovarian neoplasms measuring more than 6 cm in diameter were associated with ascites and that hydrothorax occurred in 2 to 3 per cent of these.

The effusions vary widely in amount and may be massive; they occur more frequently on the right but may be left-sided or bilateral. Although usually a transudate, the fluid occasionally contains blood. The importance of Meigs' syndrome lies in the fact that neither pleural effusion nor ascites is necessarily an ominous sign in cases of pelvic neoplasm, even when the growth is malignant. Removal of the pelvic tumor is usually followed by disappearance of the hydrothorax and the ascites.

NEPHROTIC SYNDROME AND OTHER CAUSES OF DIMINISHED PLASMA OSMOTIC PRESSURE

Pleural effusion is common in the nephrotic syndrome. The main influence leading to pleural transudation is diminution in the plasma osmotic pressure, thereby upsetting the fine balance that normally keeps the pleural space "dry." The fluid is a transudate. The nephrotic syndrome is one of the few abnormalities with a high incidence of atypical location of pleural effusion, commonly in the subpulmonic space. Of 19 cases of pleural effusion in the nephrotic syndrome and acute glomerulonephritis studied by Cavina and Vichi,[75] the effusion was subpulmonic in ten. The reasons underlying this high incidence are obscure. Clearly, the fact that the effusion is a transudate is not significant in this regard, since a wide variety of fluids (including blood) sometimes behave similarly.

CIRRHOSIS OF THE LIVER

Of 200 consecutive cases of cirrhosis of the liver associated with ascites, Johnston and Loo[67] found 12 (6 per cent) to have hydrothorax. The effusion was right-sided in eight patients, bilateral in two, and left-sided in two. According to Black,[2] there are at least three possible mechanisms for the development of pleural effusion in patients with cirrhosis—hypoproteinemia, azygos hypertension, and transfer of peritoneal fluid to the pleural cavity. It is probable that the chief mechanism is the transfer of ascitic fluid through the diaphragm by way of either the lymphatics or diaphragmatic defects.

ACUTE GLOMERULONEPHRITIS

The incidence of pleural effusions in association with acute glomerulonephritis in children is fairly high, having been observed in 42 of 76 children studied by Kirkpatrick and Fleisher.[76] It is postulated that these effusions relate to alterations in extracellular fluid volume, but the evidence that they are not infectious in origin is not clearly documented.

UREMIC PLEURITIS

Both the pericardium and pleura may become inflamed in patients with uremia. The pleuritis is not necessarily fibrinous; in some patients, the fluid is an exudate containing high levels of protein and LDH, suggesting that there must be some disruption of the pleural membrane.[77] Affected patients sometimes complain of pain, and friction rubs frequently are heard on auscultation.

MYXEDEMA

Abnormal accumulations of pleural fluid are known to occur in patients with myxedema even in the absence of cardiovascular, renal, or other causes of fluid retention. Most often the effusion occurs in the pericardium, but it may also develop in the pleural space. It has no distinctive roentgenographic characteristics.

CHYLOTHORAX

Chylothorax designates an increase in pleural fluid that is high in lipid content. The fluid is characteristically "milky" in appearance, although not all milky effusions are truly chylous in nature.[78, 79] *Chylous* effusion is caused by the escape of chyle into the pleural space from obstruction of the thoracic duct. *Chyliform (or pseudochylous) effusion* results from fatty degeneration of malignant cells in pleural fluid. Chylous effusion is high in neutral fat and fatty acid but low in cholesterol whereas chyliform effusion is low in neutral fat and high in cholesterol and lecithin.[78] This distinction is of obvious diagnostic and therapeutic importance. At one time it was thought that the histologic identification of fat globules in milky pleural fluid stained by Sudan dyes confirmed the diagnosis of chylothorax, but this is now known to be erroneous. The simultaneous analysis of fasting samples of serum and pleural fluid by lipoprotein electrophoresis readily distinguishes chylous from pseudochylous effusion.[80]

The commonest cause of chylothorax is trauma. It may result from open or closed chest trauma but more commonly is iatrogenic and follows thoracotomy. Since the thoracic duct crosses to the left of the spine between the fifth and seventh thoracic vertebrae, it is particularly vulnerable to traumatic injury during surgery on the left hemithorax near the hilum. Postoperative chylothorax is particularly common in children undergoing surgery for congenital heart disease.[81] Obstruction of the thoracic duct by lymphoma or bronchogenic carcinoma tends to cause right-sided chylothorax when the lower portion of the duct is invaded and left-sided chylothorax when the upper half is affected. Sometimes chylothorax occurs spontaneously;[82] of 92 cases of chylothorax reviewed by Schmidt,[82] fully one-third were idiopathic. Bilateral chylothorax usually is caused by neoplasm, trauma, or lymphangiomyomatosis. Lymphangiography is said to play an important role in the investigation of patients with chylothorax.[83]

PNEUMOTHORAX

The roentgenographic signs of pneumothorax were discussed in Chapter 4 (*see* page 232). The present section deals chiefly with the incidence, mechanisms of production, and etiology of spontaneous pneumothorax.

Spontaneous pneumothorax occurs most commonly in men in the third and fourth decades of life.[84] In one study of 176 episodes in 153 patients,[85] there was a male to female ratio of eight to one. There was no unilateral predominance and only five episodes were bilateral. Although the male predominance is unexplained, West[86] has attributed the increased incidence in patients with a tall thin stature to the mechanical stresses that he believes increase at the apex of the lung with increasing lung height, an observation that has been supported by statistics obtained from a Mayo Clinic study.[87] Spontaneous pneumothorax is sometimes associated with demonstrable blebs or bullae at the lung apices. The frequency of recurrence of spontaneous pneumothorax on the same side is surprisingly high, amounting to roughly 30 per cent.[88] In approximately 10 per cent of cases, spontaneous pneumothorax will develop subsequently on the contralateral side.[88]

Pleural effusion coincident with pneumothorax seems to occur less frequently than might be anticipated. For example, Lindskog and Halasz[84] found fluid in only 19 (26 per cent) of their 72 patients before diagnostic or therapeutic manipulation. Of the 15 effusions aspirated, 11 were serous and four were bloody.

Symptoms and Signs

Chest pain and dyspnea, either alone or in combination, are the classic symptoms of spontaneous pneumothorax. Dyspnea, which may be severe, may disappear within 24 hours regardless of whether the collapsed lung undergoes partial re-expansion. The major physical sign suggesting pneumothorax is a marked decrease or absence of breath sounds despite normal or increased resonance on percussion. Even with a small pneumothorax (approximately 20 per cent) in patients with otherwise normal lungs, the relative difference in breath sounds between the two hemithoraces will suggest the diagnosis. However, in patients with emphysema whose breath sounds are already greatly reduced and in whom percussion is normal or increased, the presence of pneumothorax may be very difficult to recognize by physical signs.

The effect of pneumothorax on pulmonary function depends largely on its size. It is noteworthy that reduction in lung volumes and flow rates may be influenced at least partly by pleural pain. In a study of 12 patients with spontaneous pneumothorax, Norris and associates[89] found nine to have a P_{O_2} below 80 mm Hg. The physiologic dead space was normal but there was an increased A-a gradient for oxygen. The authors concluded that there was an increased anatomic shunt.

Pathogenesis of Spontaneous Pneumothorax

Spontaneous pneumothorax almost always is the result of rupture of an air-containing space within or immediately deep to the visceral pleura. This is commonly a pleural bleb, a small cystic space seldom exceeding 1 to 2 cm in diameter and most frequently situated over the lung apex. The pathogenesis of bleb formation usually is attributed to the dissection of air from a ruptured alveolus through interstitial tissue into the thin fibrous layer of visceral pleura, where it accumulates in the form of a cyst. The immediate cause of rupture of a pleural bleb is unknown. It is clearly not related to exceptional effort, since the majority of patients are at rest when spontaneous pneumothorax occurs. For many years pulmonary tuberculosis was regarded as the underlying cause of most spontaneous pneumothoraces, but long ago this incorrect theory was discarded. On average, it seems that in about 50 per cent of cases there is no roentgenographic evidence of disease[90] although tomography may reveal small blebs that are invisible on plain roentgenograms.

Although spontaneous pneumothorax occurs most frequently in otherwise healthy young adults as a result of rupture of visceral pleural blebs, it can also be associated with innumerable pulmonary diseases. In adults the following list gives some idea of the broad spectrum of diseases associated with spontaneous pneumothorax but is by no means complete (no attempt is made to indicate incidence): spasmodic asthma, staphylococcal septicemia, pulmonary infarction, sarcoidosis, idiopathic pulmonary hemosiderosis, pulmonary alveolar proteinosis, Marfan's syndrome, familial fibrocystic pulmonary dysplasia, chronic interstitial pulmonary fibrosis, histiocytosis-X, coccidioidomycosis, echinococcal disease, primary carcinoma of the lung, pulmonary metastases (including those from carcinoma of the pancreas and adrenal, Wilms' tumor, and particularly osteogenic and other types of sarcoma), diffuse emphysema, Shaver's disease (bauxite pneumoconiosis), Wegener's granulomatosis, and acute bacterial pneumonia. An unusual condition is recurrent spontaneous pneumothorax associated with menses (catamenial pneumothorax).[91] Despite the highly convincing evidence that endometriosis is responsible for these pneumothoraces, the precise mechanism for their development is by no means clear. This entity was first described in 1958, and since then, 59 cases have been reported in the English literature.[92] Four additional cases recently reported[92] support the significant role that diaphragmatic defects and endometriosis play in the pathogenesis of this unusual condition; at thoracotomy, numerous small perforations of the right hemidiaphragm were found in three patients, two of whom had associated endometriosis of that diaphragm. However, the finding of endometrial tissue in the diaphragm or parietal pleura cannot logically account for this phenomenon, and involvement of lung and visceral pleura occurs in only a minority of cases. The pneumothorax is almost invariably right-sided. A recent report of catamenial pneumothorax in two sisters is of some interest.[93]

A nonspecific morphologic reaction to pleural injury from pneumothorax consists of histiocytic, eosinophilic, and giant cell infiltration of the pleura;[94] the reaction has been said to closely resemble histiocytosis-X.

When spontaneous pneumothorax is associated with primary carcinoma of the lung, it is important to recognize the roentgenographic signs of bronchial obstruction in addition to those of the collapse produced by pneumothorax. A previously normal lung that has undergone total collapse as a result of pneumothorax should show an air bronchogram. In the presence of an endobronchial obstructing lesion, no air bronchogram will be visible and the collapsed lung will be of homogeneous density. Similarly, when a bronchus is obstructed, the volume of the involved hemithorax decreases as the pneumothorax is absorbed, with ipsilateral mediastinal shift and hemidiaphragmatic elevation. Occasionally, a mucous plug may obstruct a bronchus during expansion of the lung and, as a result, the affected segments will fail to inflate with the remainder of the lung. The importance of appreciating this complication is obvious.

TRAUMATIC PNEUMOTHORAX

Pneumothorax complicating trauma may occur without roentgenographic evidence of rib fracture. When fracture is present the likely mechanism is laceration of the visceral pleura by rib fragments, and in such circumstances hemothorax may be expected as a concomitant finding. When no fractures are visible the probable mechanism is pulmonary interstitial emphysema secondary to pulmonary contusion or parenchymal laceration. This explanation also provides adequate reason for the occurrence of pneumomediastinum and subcutaneous emphysema without rib fracture.

Traumatic pneumothorax is frequently iatrogenic—for example, as a result of the passage of air into the mediastinum by way of cervical fascial planes following tracheostomy, or following attempted insertion of a central venous catheter into the subclavian vein. Patients being assisted by artificial ventilation are particularly at risk for the development of pneumothorax, more so when volume cycled machines and positive end-expiratory pressure (PEEP) are used, or when marginal alveoli are inflamed as a result of infection, infarction, or aspiration of gastric contents. Alveolar rupture is more likely to occur when very high peak inspiratory pressures are employed to ventilate patients with severely obstructed airways or noncompliant lungs.

PLEURAL THICKENING

All diseases other than pleural effusion that cause widening or "thickening" of the pleural line are considered here. Lesions include such widely diverse entities as pleural plaques, fibrin bodies, benign and malignant neoplasms, and pleural calcification.

LOCAL PLEURAL THICKENING

The most common cause of local thickening of the pleura is a remote serous effusion that heals by fibrosis. Since pleural effusions of infectious etiology are invariably basal, it is not surprising that this is the anatomic location of most cases of residual pleural thickening of this type. The usual roentgenographic abnormality is partial obliteration or blunting of the posterior and lateral costophrenic sulci. Thickening of the pleural line may extend for a variable distance up the lateral and posterior thoracic walls, diminishing gradually toward the apex and seldom amounting to more than 1 to 2 mm in width. Such minor changes are of significance only in that they indicate previous active pleuritis.

Of the same character but in a different location is the curved shadow of unit density frequently visualized in the apex of one or both lungs, in the concavity formed by the first and second ribs. Euphemistically called the "apical cap," it is sometimes ascribed to tuberculosis, despite convincing evidence to the contrary. Renner and his colleagues[95] studied the visceral pleura and subpleural parenchyma of 113 left lungs obtained at necropsy. Premortem roentgenograms of 104 were available for correlation. In no case was there histologic evidence of tuberculosis. The commonest pathologic finding (in 20.3 per cent of cases) was nonspecific fibrous scarring of apical lung parenchyma that merged with the visceral pleura. The frequency of scarring observed pathologically increased significantly with age, suggesting to the authors that such local pleural thickening and subpleural scarring might be related to healing of pulmonary disease in the presence of chronic ischemia. Care should be taken to recognize the possibility that apical pleural thickening may be an early manifestation of much more serious disease—apical pulmonary cancer, or Pancoast tumor. Suspicion should be enhanced when the apical abnormality is predominantly unilateral.

The local pleural thickening that characterizes the pleural plaques of asbestos-related disease is discussed later (*see* page 688).

LOCAL PLEURAL MASSES

Masses arising from the pleura or situated within the pleural space are of widely varying etiology and all are uncommon. *Pleural hyaloserositis* is a local, identical manifestation in the pleura of the cartilagelike whitish thickenings that occur on the liver and spleen. Because of its sugar icing appearance, it is termed "Zuckerguss."[96] These deposits tend to arise from the parietal pleura and histologically are composed of hyaline sclerotic tissue; they may become calcified. *Fibrin bodies* are tumorlike concentrations of fibrin that sometimes develop in a serofibrinous pleural effusion. These bodies are round, oval, or of irregular shape and are seldom more than 3 to 4 cm in diameter. They usually become evident following absorption of a pleural effusion.

Benign pleural neoplasms are very uncommon. Subpleural *lipomas* composed of normal adult fat have been reported to arise from connective tissues deep to the parietal pleura. By far the most important benign neoplasm of the pleura is *local mesothelioma*. In contrast to the high degree of malignancy of the diffuse variety, local lesions are almost always benign. They may arise from either the parietal or visceral pleura but more commonly from the latter.[97] Symptoms attributable to the tumor itself are often insignificant, although large lesions may give rise to dyspnea or chest pain. Initially, symptoms may be extrathoracic, chiefly in the form of finger clubbing and hypertrophic osteoarthropathy.[97] In fact, the association of hypertrophic osteoarthropathy and a large local intrathoracic mass should strongly suggest the possibility of benign pleural mesothelioma. This association is much greater than with bronchogenic carcinoma. Pathologically, these lesions occur in two forms: (1) predominantly fibrous, usually well encapsulated, nodular, and yellowish-white, often highly vascular, and attached by a relatively narrow pedicle; (2) a benign epithelial form, usually bearing papillary projections with fibrovascular stalks covered with mesothelial cells similar in appearance to epithelial cells.[97]

Roentgenologically, these lesions are sharply circumscribed somewhat lobular masses of homogeneous density, from 2 to 15 cm in diameter. They tend to form an obtuse angle with the chest wall, a finding important to establishment of the extrapulmonary origin of a thoracic mass. There is a tendency for these lesions to change position with respiration or needling,[98] regardless of their site of origin.

GENERAL PLEURAL THICKENING

Three distinct entities must be considered under this heading—fibrothorax, the pleural disease associated with asbestosis, and diffuse mesothelioma.

FIBROTHORAX

Healing of a massive hemothorax or pyothorax may be associated with deposition of a thick layer of dense fibrous tissue, almost always on the visceral pleura. The thickness of the pleural "peel" may be 2 cm or more around a whole lung, resulting in marked decrease in volume of the hemithorax and creating a severe impediment to ventilation. Calcification occurs frequently on the *inner* aspect of the peel and provides an indicator by which the thickness of the peel may be measured.

Aberrations in pulmonary function associated

with fibrothorax and the remarkable improvement to be anticipated from decortication have been discussed in detail by Bates and his colleagues.[99] The physiologic pattern is one of restriction, with decrease in lung volumes and diffusing capacity. In contrast to restrictive interstitial lung disease, however, the maximal static pulmonary recoil pressure is not elevated.

The degree to which unilateral fibrothorax impairs ventilation of the underlying lung can be gauged, at least roughly, by assessing pulmonary vascularity. If the pulmonary vessels of the affected lung are smaller than those of the opposite side, it can be assumed that the reduction in perfusion has occurred in response to reduced ventilation and resulting hypoxic vasoconstriction. If the vascularity of the two lungs is roughly symmetric, it is reasonable to assume that vasoconstriction has not occurred and that ventilation is therefore preserved. We have frequently been impressed by the fact that the degree of pleural thickening does not bear a close relationship to reduced ventilation and perfusion. In other words, a thick pleural peel does not necessarily imply reduced ventilation any more than a thin peel.

PLEURAL DISEASE ASSOCIATED WITH ASBESTOSIS

There are three types of roentgenographic changes in the pleura in asbestos-exposed individuals: plaque formation, diffuse pleural thickening, and pleural effusion. Each of these may occur alone or in combination with the others. These pleural manifestations dominate the picture roentgenographically in the majority of series.[100] Of 56 cases described by Freundlich and Greening,[100] 48 per cent showed pleural thickening alone, 41 per cent showed combined pleural and parenchymal manifestations, and only 11 per cent showed parenchymal changes alone.

Pleural plaques usually are bilateral and tend to follow the rib contours.[101] They are fibrotic processes that begin in the deepest part of the parietal pleura and morphologically are ivory white in color. They may be smooth or nodular in contour and may measure up to 1 cm in thickness, although they usually are thinner (*see* Figure 12–6, page 586). They occur most commonly on the aponeurotic portion of the diaphragm, on the posterolateral chest wall between the seventh and tenth ribs, and on the lateral chest wall between the sixth and ninth ribs.[102]

Origin from the parietal pleura is in contrast to the visceral pleural involvement that characterizes previous hemothorax or empyema. The earliest appearance of a pleural plaque is as a thin line of unit density visible under a rib in the axillary region, usually the seventh or eighth rib, on one or both sides. The plaques may be very difficult to visualize, particularly when viewed *en face*, and tangential roentgenograms may be necessary (*see* Figure 12–7, page 587). In fact, the frequency with which plaques occur along the posterolateral or anterolateral portion of the thorax suggested to Fletcher and Edge[102] that oblique projections of the thorax should be standard in the roentgenographic investigation of patients suspected of having asbestosis. The greatest problem in the diagnosis of early plaque formation lies in distinguishing them from normal companion shadows of the chest wall—muscle and fat shadows that may be identified in as many as 75 per cent of normal posteroanterior roentgenograms along the convexity of the thorax inferiorly. In fact, sometimes it is impossible to differentiate pleural plaques from companion shadows with conviction. Despite these difficulties, it is clear that noncalcified plaques occur often enough to be regarded as virtually diagnostic of asbestos-related disease.

Although uncalcified pleural plaque formation is the commonest roentgenographic manifestation of asbestos-related disease, the most striking and characteristic abnormality is calcification of pleural plaques. The frequency of pleural calcification is variable. Anton[103] found calcified and noncalcified plaques in roughly equal numbers in his 40 patients, whereas Freundlich and Greening[100] observed calcification in only 21 per cent of their 56 patients. Calcified plaques vary from small linear or circular shadows usually situated over the diaphragmatic domes (Figure 15–1) to complete encirclement of the lower portion of the lungs. No portion of the pleura is immune to calcification, although the commonest site is the diaphragm.[104]

Diffuse pleural thickening may occur alone or in combination with pleural plaques. It is almost invariably bilateral but varies considerably in extent, sometimes covering both lungs diffusely but more frequently affecting only a quarter or half the vertical height of each lung. In contrast to pleural plaques, it is fairly uniform in thickness and thus can be recognized only over the convexity of the lungs.

The third pleural manifestation of asbestos-related disease not often appreciated, is *pleural*

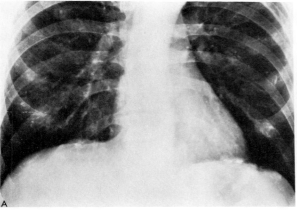

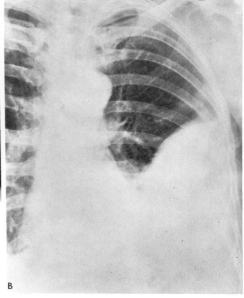

Figure 15–1. Malignant Mesothelioma Associated with Asbestos-related Pleural Plaques. This 60-year-old man had worked in the asbestos mines of Quebec for many years and showed roentgenographic evidence of calcification of the diaphragmatic pleura bilaterally *(A)*. There was no convincing evidence of pulmonary disease roentgenologically. Approximately 6 months after the roentgenogram illustrated in *(A)* the patient presented with pain in the left side of his chest. A posteroanterior roentgenogram *(B)* revealed a large left-sided pleural effusion associated with an irregular, poorly defined mass in the lateral portion of the left hemithorax. Proved malignant mesothelioma.

effusion. In recent years, two series of cases of acute pleurisy in asbestos-exposed individuals have been reported, one of nine patients[105] and the other of 12.[106] In the latter series, the effusion was present in 21 per cent of all patients with asbestosis seen in the author's laboratory. Such effusions are frequently recurrent, usually bilateral, and often associated with chest pain.[106] In all cases, the fluid was a sterile, serous, or blood-tinged exudate. Pathologic examination of the pleura in many of these cases revealed nonspecific pleuritis and thickening, sometimes associated with rare asbestos bodies and fibers. In the majority of cases, the pleural effusion was associated with asbestos involvement of the lung parenchyma. As pointed out by Gaensler and Kaplan[106] the diagnosis of asbestos pleural effusion must be made with caution and only following exclusion of other diagnostic possibilities. The major differential diagnoses must include tuberculosis and mesothelioma. Of the 12 patients in the Gaensler and Kaplan series, the presence of mesothelioma was recognized in one patient 9 years after the first documented effusion. Of four cases in another series,[107] two eventually developed mesothelioma. Differentiation from a tuberculous pleural effusion can only be made with confidence if culture of the effusion is persistently negative for *M. tuberculosis* or if the effusion improves spontaneously without therapy.

DIFFUSE PLEURAL MESOTHELIOMA

In recent years there have been many reports concerning this disease and its relationship to asbestosis,[100, 101, 108–110] pointing to an association between an industrial hazard and pleuropulmonary cancer that must surely represent one of the closest known relationships of its kind. The incidence of neoplasia in asbestos-exposed individuals appears to relate to the type of asbestos involved. This is particularly true for mesothelioma, in which the most commonly implicated dust is crocidolite. It is generally agreed that the risk of developing mesothelioma is somewhat less in exposure to amosite and considerably less for chrysotile than for crocidolite.[111] Despite thorough search, mesothelioma has not been found to be associated with anthophyllite asbestos production in Finland.[112]

Although mesothelial neoplasms are not invariably associated with asbestos exposure, careful history-taking will reveal such exposure in approximately 80 per cent of patients.[113] The presence of parenchymal fibrosis or pleural plaques (or both) may suggest the diagnosis but even these clues sometimes are absent.

Pathologically, the characteristic appearance of pleural mesothelioma is of a thick, gray-white mass encasing the lung and extrinsically compressing the bronchi. The neoplasm tends to invade locally but seldom metastasizes to distant

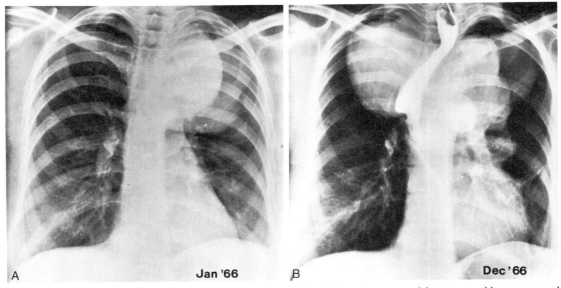

Figure 15–2. Malignant Mesothelioma. The initial posteroanterior (A) roentgenogram of this 45-year-old woman reveals a large homogeneous mass arising from the mediastinal aspect of the left upper hemithorax. The obtuse angle at which the mass relates to the mediastinum suggests an origin from either the pleura or the mediastinum. Since one of the differential diagnostic possibilities was aortic aneurysm, an aortogram was performed but was normal except for displacement of the aorta and its major branches by the mass. A large malignant mesothelioma was resected at thoracotomy. Almost 1 year later (B) the left-sided mass had recurred and had extended through the posterior mediastinum into the right hemithorax.

sites. Histologically, the neoplasm may be predominantly epithelial or mesenchymal in type or may show characteristics of both. Epithelial cells are cuboidal and form tubulopapillary structures, whereas mesenchymal stromal cells resemble those of spindle-cell sarcomas. Difficulty may be encountered in differentiating primary pleural mesothelioma from pleural metastasis by light microscopy. However, electron microscopy may prove helpful in determining the origin of the neoplasm.

Surprisingly, asbestos bodies can be identified within these neoplasms in only about 25 per cent of cases.[114] This is in contrast to bronchogenic carcinoma associated with asbestosis, in which situation asbestos bodies often are found in the neoplasm.[115]

Roentgenographically, the commonest presentation of pleural mesothelioma is of irregular, nodular opacities around the periphery of the lung, either over the convexity or along the mediastinum or diaphragm (Figure 15–2). Such opacities may or may not be associated with pleural effusion. When effusion is present, it frequently obscures the underlying neoplasm (Figure 15–1). In contrast to other forms of pleural effusion, that associated with mesothelioma is frequently not accompanied by significant shift of the mediastinum to the contralat-

eral side, a peculiarity that has two possible explanations: (1) the formation of a large pleural "peel" acts in a restrictive capacity, preventing inflation of the lung on full inspiration and thus reducing volume; and (2) local invasion of the medial aspect of the lung by the neoplasm can occlude bronchi and result in atelectasis. This pattern of massive pleural effusion unassociated with mediastinal shift can also occur with primary bronchogenic carcinoma accompanied by obstructive atelectasis and metastatic pleural effusion, and it is obviously important to differentiate these two causes. In a recently reported computed tomographic study of five patients with proven pleural mesothelioma,[116] it was shown that in all cases conventional chest roentgenography underestimated the extent of disease; in each case CT revealed an extensive, pleural-based mass surrounding the lung, spreading into the fissures, and extending into the mediastinum and sometimes the contralateral chest, abdomen, and chest wall. It is clear that CT is superior to other investigative techniques in the assessment of the extent of these neoplasms.

Clinically, patients with pleural mesothelioma may present with vague chest or shoulder ache or with true pleuritic pain. As the disease progresses, shortness of breath, weight loss, and a dry hacking cough may become evident. Physical examination often reveals clubbing, retraction of the thorax, and dullness on percussion. Pleural fluid may be either straw-colored or serosanguineous, in roughly equal numbers.

The prognosis is extremely poor, survival seldom exceeding 2 years from the time of diagnosis. The majority of patients die within the first year of the onset of symptoms.[113]

The incidence of peritoneal mesotheliomas also is greater in patients with asbestosis.[117] Enticknap and Smither[117] described 11 patients with peritoneal neoplasms, all of whom had worked in the same asbestos factory. A number of studies have shown an increased incidence of gastrointestinal[110] and laryngeal[118] carcinoma in asbestos workers.

REFERENCES

1. Rabin, C. B., and Blackman, N. S.: Bilateral pleural effusion. Its significance in association with a heart of normal size. J. Mt. Sinai Hosp., *24*:45, 1957.
2. Black, L. F.: The pleural space and pleural fluid. Mayo Clin. Proc., *47*:493, 1972.
3. Storey, D. D., Dines, D. E., and Coles, D. T.: Pleural effusion. A diagnostic dilemma. J.A.M.A., *236*:2183, 1976.
4. Levine, H., Szanto, P. B., and Cugell, D. W.: Tuberculous pleurisy. An acute illness. Arch. Intern. Med., *122*:329, 1968.
5. Pines, A.: The results of chemotherapy in the treatment of tuberculous pleural effusions. Br. Med. J., *2*:863, 1957.
6. Scerbo, J., Keltz, H., and Stone, D. J.: A prospective study of closed pleural biopsies. J.A.M.A., *218*:377, 1971.
7. Klockars, M., Pettersson, T., Riska, H., and Hellström, P.-E.: Pleural fluid lysozyme in tuberculous and non-tuberculous pleurisy. Br. Med. J., *1*:1381, 1976.
8. Light, R. W.: Management of parapneumonic effusions. Chest, *70*:325, 1976.
9. Varkey, B., Rose, H. D., Kutty, C. P., and Politis, J.: Empyema thoracis during a ten-year period: Analysis of 72 cases and comparison to a previous study (1952 to 1967). Arch. Intern. Med., *141*:1771, 1981.
10. Bartlett, J. G., Gorbach, S. L., Thadepalli, H., and Finegold, S. M.: Bacteriology of empyema. Lancet, *1*:338, 1974.
11. Wiita, R. M., Cartwright, R. R., and Davis, J. G.: Staphylococcal pneumonia in adults. A review of 102 cases. Am. J. Roentgenol., *86*:1083, 1961.
12. Welch, C. C., Tombridge, T. L., Baker, W. J., and Kinney, R. J.: Beta-hemolytic streptococcal pneumonia: Report of an outbreak in a military population. Am. J. Med. Sci., *242*:157, 1961.
13. Brewin, A., Arango, L., Hadley, W. K., and Murray, J. F.: High-dose penicillin therapy and pneumococcal pneumonia. J.A.M.A., *230*:409, 1974.
14. Dennis, J. M., and Boudreau, R. P.: Pleuropulmonary tularemia: Its roentgen manifestations. Radiology, *68*:25, 1957.
15. Swartz, M. N.: Clinical aspects of legionnaires' disease. Ann. Intern. Med., *90*:492, 1979.
16. Fine, N. L., Smith, L. R., and Sheedy, P. F.: Frequency of pleural effusions in Mycoplasma and viral pneumonias. N. Engl. J. Med., *283*:790, 1970.
17. Webster, B. H.: Pleuropulmonary amebiasis. A review with an analysis of ten cases. Am. Rev. Respir. Dis., *81*:683, 1960.
18. Capitanio, M. A., and Kirkpatrick, J. A., Jr.: *Pneumocystis carinii* pneumonia. Am. J. Roentgenol., *97*:174, 1966.
19. Forrest, J. V.: Radiographic findings in *Peneumocystis carinii* pneumonia. Radiology, *103*:539, 1972.
20. Rakower, J., and Milwidsky, H.: Hydatid pleural disease. Am. Rev. Respir. Dis., *90*:623, 1964.
21. Winslow, W. A., Ploss, L. N., and Loitman, B.: Pleuritis in systemic lupus erythematosus: Its importance as an early manifestation in diagnosis. Ann. Intern. Med., *49*:70, 1958.
22. Levin, D. C.: Proper interpretation of pulmonary roentgen changes in systemic lupus erythematosus. Am. J. Roentgenol., *111*:510, 1971.
23. Bulgrin, J. G., Dubois, E. L., and Jacobson, G.: Chest roentgenographic changes in systemic lupus erythematosus. Radiology, *74*:42, 1960.
24. Gonzalez, L., and Van Ordstrand, H. S.: Wegener's granulomatosis: Review of 11 cases. Radiology, *107*:295, 1973.
25. Sievers, K., Aho, K., Hurri, L., and Perttala, Y.: Studies of rheumatoid pulmonary disease. A comparison of roentgenological findings among patients with high rheumatoid factor titers and with completely negative reactions. Acta Tuberc. Scand., *45*:21, 1964.
26. Walker, W. C., and Wright, V.: Rheumatoid pleuritis. Ann. Rheum. Dis., *26*:467, 1967.
27. Carr, D. T., and Mayne, J. G.: Pleurisy with effusion in rheumatoid arthritis, with reference to the low concentration of glucose in pleural fluid. Am. Rev. Respir. Dis., *85*:345, 1962.
28. Lillington, G. A., Carr, D. T., and Mayne, J. G.: Rheumatoid pleurisy with effusion. Arch. Intern. Med., *128*:764, 1971.
29. Mays, E. E.: Rheumatoid pleuritis: Observations in eight cases and suggestions for making the diagnosis in patients without the "typical findings." Dis. Chest, *53*:202, 1968.
30. Halla, J. T., Schrohenloher, R. E., and Volanakis, J. E.: Immune complexes and other laboratory features of pleural effusions: A comparison of rheumatoid arthritis, systemic lupus erythematosus, and other diseases. Ann. Intern. Med., *92*:748, 1980.
31. Sybers, R. G., Sybers, J. L., Dickie, H. A., and Paul, L. W.: Roentgenographic aspects of hemorrhagic pulmonary-renal disease (Goodpasture's syndrome). Am. J. Roentgenol., *94*:674, 1965.
32. Robinson, B. W. S., and Musk, A. W.: Benign asbestos pleural effusion: diagnosis and course. Thorax, *36*:896, 1981.
33. Epler, G. R., McLoud, T. C., and Gaensler, E. A.: Prevalence and incidence of benign asbestos pleural effusion in a working population. J.A.M.A., *247*:617, 1982.
34. Emerson, G. L., Emerson, M. S., and Sherwood, C. E.: The natural history of carcinoma of the lung. J. Thorac. Cardiovasc. Surg., *37*:291, 1959.
35. Cohen, S., and Hossain, S. A.: Primary carcinoma of the lung. A review of 417 histologically proved cases. Dis. Chest, *49*:67, 1966.

36. Rosenblatt, M. B., and Lisa, J. R.: Cancer of the Lung. Pathology, Diagnosis and Treatment. New York, Oxford University Press, 1956.

37. Brinkman, G. L.: The significance of pleural effusion complicating otherwise operable bronchogenic carcinoma. Dis. Chest, 36:152, 1959.

38. Boutin, C., Viallat, J. R., Cargnino, P., and Farisse, P.: Thoracoscopy in malignant pleural effusions. Am. Rev. Respir. Dis., 124:588, 1981.

39. Williams, T., and Thomas, P.: The diagnosis of pleural effusions by fiberoptic bronchoscopy and pleuroscopy. Chest, 80:566, 1981.

40. Loddenkemper, R.: Thoracoscopy: results in noncancerous and idiopathic pleural effusions. Poumon-Coeur, 37:261, 1981.

41. Falor, W. H., Ward, R. M., and Brezler, M. R.: Diagnosis of pleural effusions by chromosome analysis. Chest, 81:193, 1982.

42. Ludington, L. G., Verska, J. J., Howard, T., Kypridakis, G., and Brewer, L. A., III: Bronchiolar carcinoma (alveolar cell), another great imitator; a review of 41 cases. Chest, 61:622, 1972.

43. Vieta, J. O., and Craver, L. F.: Intrathoracic manifestations of the lymphomatoid diseases. Radiology, 37:138, 1941.

44. Fisher, A. M. H., and Kendall, B., and Van Leuven, B. D.: Hodgkin's disease. A radiological survey. Clin. Radiol, 13:115, 1962.

45. Molander, D. W., and Pack, G. T.: Treatment of lymphosarcoma. In Pack, G. T., and Ariel, I. M. (eds.): Treatment of Cancer and Allied Diseases, 2nd ed., vol. 9. Lymphomas and Related Diseases. New York, Harper & Row, 1964, pp. 131–167.

46. Stolberg, H. O., Patt, N. L., MacEwen, K. F., et al.: Hodgkin's disease of the lung. Roentgenologic-pathologic correlation. Am. J. Roentgenol., 92:96, 1964.

47. Martin, J. J.: The Nisbet Symposium: Hodgkin's disease. Radiological aspects of the disease. Australas. Radiol., 11:206, 1967.

48. Siegel, M. J., Shackelford, G. D., and McAlister, W. H.: Pleural thickening: An unusual feature of childhood leukemia. Radiology, 138:367, 1981.

49. Raju, R. N., and Kardinal, C. G.: Pleural effusion in breast carcinoma: Analysis of 122 cases. Cancer, 48:2524, 1981.

50. Meyer, P. C.: Metastatic carcinoma of the pleura. Thorax, 21:437, 1966.

51. Stewart, P. B.: The rate of formation and lymphatic removal of fluid in pleural effusions. J. Clin. Invest., 42:258, 1963.

52. Hutchinson, William B., and Friedenberg, M. J.: Intrathoracic mesothelioma. Radiology, 80:937, 1963.

53. Arai, H., Endo, M., Sasai, Y., Yokosawa, A., Sato, H., Motomiya, M., and Konno, K.: Histochemical demonstration of hyaluronic acid in a case of pleural mesothelioma. Am. Rev. Respir. Dis., 111:699, 1975.

54. Motomiya, M., Endo, M., Arai, H., Yokosawa, A., Sato, H., and Konno, K.: Biochemical characterization of hyaluronic acid from a case of benign, localized, pleural mesothelioma. Am. Rev. Respir. Dis., 111:775, 1975.

55. Stein, G. N., Chen, J. T., Goldstein, F., et al.: The importance of chest roentgenography in the diagnosis of pulmonary embolism. Am. J. Roentgenol., 81:255, 1959.

56. Fleischner, F. G.: Pulmonary embolism. Can. Med. Assoc. J., 78:653, 1958.

57. Torrance, D. J., Jr.: Roentgenographic signs of pulmonary artery occlusion. Am. J. Med. Sci., 237:651, 1959.

58. Fleischner, F. G.: Pulmonary embolism. Clin. Radiol., 13:169, 1962.

59. Figley, M. M., Gerdes, A. J., and Ricketts, H. J.: Radiographic aspects of pulmonary embolism. Semin. Roentgenol., 2:389, 1967.

60. Cornell, S. H., and Rossi, N. P.: Roentgenographic findings in constrictive pericarditis. Analysis of 21 cases. Am. J. Roentgenol., 102:301, 1968.

61. Good, J. T., Jr., Moore, J. B., Fowler, A. A., and Sahn, S. A.: Superior vena cava syndrome as a cause of pleural effusion. Am. Rev. Respir. Dis., 125:246, 1982.

62. Mellins, R. B., Levine, O. R., and Fishman, A. P.: Effect of systemic and pulmonary venous hypertension on pleural and pericardial fluid accumulation. J. Appl. Physiol., 29:564, 1970.

63. Reynolds, J., and Davis, J. T.: Injuries of the chest wall, pleura, pericardium, lungs, bronchi and esophagus. Radiol. Clin. North Am., 4:383, 1966.

64. Hart, U., Ward, D. R., Gillilian, R., and Brawley, R. K.: Fatal pulmonary hemorrhage complicating Swan-Ganz catheterization. Surgery, 91:24, 1982.

65. Koehler, P. R., and Jones, R.: Association of left-sided pleural effusions and splenic hematomas. Am. J. Roentgenol., 135:851, 1980.

66. Lemon, W. S., and Higgins, G. M.: Lymphatic absorption of particulate matter through the normal and paralyzed diaphragm. An experimental study. Am. J. Med. Sci., 178:536, 1929.

67. Johnston, R. F., and Loo, R. V.: Hepatic hydrothorax. Studies to determine the source of the fluid and report of thirteen cases. Ann. Intern. Med., 61:385, 1964.

68. Meigs, J. V.: Pelvic tumors other than fibromas of the ovary with ascites and hydrothorax. Obstet. Gynecol., 3:471, 1954.

69. Hammarsten, J. F., Honska, W. L., Jr., and Limes, B. J.: Pleural fluid amylase in pancreatitis and other diseases. Am. Rev. Tuberc., 79:606, 1959.

70. Light, R. W., and George, R. B.: Incidence and significance of pleural effusion after abdominal surgery. Chest, 69:621, 1976.

71. Miller, W. T., and Talman, E. A.: Subphrenic abscess. Am. J. Roentgenol., 101:961, 1967.

72. Salmon, U. J.: Benign pelvic tumors associated with ascites and pleural effusion. J. Mt. Sinai Hosp., 1:169, 1934.

73. Meigs, J. V., and Cass, J. W.: Fibroma of the ovary with ascites and hydrothorax. With a report of seven cases. Am. J. Obstet. Gynecol., 33:249, 1937.

74. Dockerty, M. B.: Ovarian neoplasms. A collective review of the recent literature. Int. Abstr. Surg., 81:179, 1945.

75. Cavina, C., and Vichi, G.: Radiological aspects of pleural effusions in medical neuropathy in children. Ann. Radiol. Diag., 31:163, 1958.

76. Kirkpatrick, J. A., Jr., and Fleisher, D. S.: The roentgen appearance of the chest in acute glomerulonephritis in children. J. Pediatr., 64:492, 1964.

77. Gilbert, L., Ribot, S., Frankel, H., Jacobs, M., and Mankowitz, B. J.: Fibrinous uremic pleuritis: A surgical entity. Chest, 67:53, 1975.

78. Latner, A. L.: Cantarow and Trumper—Clinical Biochemistry, 7th ed. Philadelphia, W. B. Saunders Co., 1975.

79. Hesseling, P. B., and Hoffman, H.: Chylothorax: A review of the literature and report of 3 cases. S. Afr. Med. J., *60*:675, 1981.

80. Seriff, N. S., Cohen, M. L., Samuel, P., and Schulster, P. L.: Chylothorax: Diagnosis by lipoprotein electrophoresis of serum and pleural fluid. Thorax, *32*:98, 1977.

81. Higgins, C. B., and Reinke, R. T.: Postoperative chylothorax in children with congenital heart disease. Clinical and roentgenographic features. Radiology, *119*:409, 1976.

82. Schmidt, A.: Chylothorax. Review of 5 years' cases in the literature and report of a case. Acta Chir. Scand., *118*:5, 1959.

83. Freundlich, I. M.: The role of lymphangiography in chylothorax. A report of six nontraumatic cases. Am. J. Roentgenol., *125*:617, 1975.

84. Lindskog, G. E., and Halasz, N. A.: Spontaneous pneumothorax. A consideration of pathogenesis and management with review of seventy-two hospitalized cases. A.M.A. Arch. Surg., *75*:693, 1957.

85. Inouye, W. Y., Berggren, R. B., and Johnson, J.: Spontaneous pneumothorax: treatment and mortality. Dis. Chest, *51*:67, 1967.

86. West, K.: Distribution of mechanical stress in the lung, a possible factor in localization of pulmonary disease. Lancet, *1*:839, 1971.

87. Melton, L. J., Hepper, N. G. G., and Offord, K. P.: Influence of height on the risk of spontaneous pneumothorax. Mayo Clin. Proc., *56*:678, 1981.

88. Hickok, D. F., and Ballenger, F. P.: The management of spontaneous pneumothorax due to emphysematous blebs. Surg. Gynecol. Obstet., *120*:499, 1965.

89. Norris, R. M., Jones, J. G., and Bishop, J. M.: Respiratory gas exchange in patients with spontaneous pneumothorax. Thorax, *23*:427, 1968.

90. Ruckley, C. V., and McCormack, R. J. M.: The management of spontaneous pneumothorax. Thorax, *21*:139, 1966.

91. Shearin, R. P. N., Hepper, N. G. G., and Payne, W. S.: Recurrent spontaneous pneumothorax concurrent with menses. Mayo Clin. Proc., *49*:98, 1974.

92. Slasky, B. S., Siewers, R. D., Lecky, J. W., and Zajko, A.: Catamenial pneumothorax: The roles of diaphragmatic defects and endometriosis. A.J.R., *138*:639, 1982.

93. Hinson, J. M., Jr., Brigham, K. L., Daniell, J.: Catamenial pneumothorax in sisters. Chest, *80*:634, 1981.

94. Askin, F. B., McCann, B. G., Kuhn, C.: Reactive eosinophilic pleuritis: A lesion to be distinguished from pulmonary eosinophilic granuloma. Arch. Pathol. Lab. Med., *101*:187, 1977.

95. Renner, R. R., Markarian, B., Pernice, N. J., and Heitzman, E. R.: The apical cap. Radiology, *110*:569, 1974.

96. Galatius-Jensen, F., and Halkier, E.: Radiological aspects of pleural hyalo-serositis. Br. J. Radiol., *38*:944, 1965.

97. Blount, H. ·C., Jr.: Localized mesothelioma of the pleura. A review with six new cases. Radiology, *67*:822, 1956.

98. Hayward, R. H.: Migrating lung tumor. Chest, *66*:77, 1974.

99. Bates, D. V., Macklem, P. T., and Christie, R. V.: Respiratory Function in Disease: An Introduction to the Integrated Study of the Lung, 2nd ed. Philadelphia, W. B. Saunders Co., 1971.

100. Freundlich, I. M., and Greening, R. R.: Asbestosis and associated medical problems. Radiology, *89*:224, 1967.

101. Hourihane, D. O., Lessof, L., and Richardson, P. C.: Hyaline and calcified pleural plaques as an index of exposure to asbestos. A study of radiological and pathological features of 100 cases with a consideration of epidemiology. Br. Med. J., *1*:1069, 1966.

102. Fletcher, D. E., and Edge, J. R.: The early radiological changes in pulmonary and pleural asbestosis. Clin. Radiol., *21*:355, 1970.

103. Anton, H. C.: Multiple pleural plaques, part II. Br. J. Radiol., *41*:341, 1968.

104. Solomon, A.: Radiology of asbestosis. Environ. Res., *3*:320, 1970.

105. Sluis-Cremer, G. K., and Webster, I.: Acute pleurisy in asbestosis exposed persons. Envir. Res., *5*:380, 1972.

106. Gaensler E. A., and Kaplan, A. I.: Asbestos pleural effusion. Ann. Intern. Med., *74*:178, 1971.

107. Eisenstadt, H. B.: Benign asbestos pleurisy. J.A.M.A., *192*:419, 1965.

108. Enterline, P., DeCoufle, P., and Henderson, V.: Respiratory cancer in relation to occupational exposures among retired asbestos workers. Br. J. Ind. Med., *30*:162, 1973.

109. Whitwell, F., Newhouse, M. L., and Bennett, D. R.: A study of the histological cell types of lung cancer in workers suffering from asbestosis in the United Kingdom. Br. J. Ind. Med., *31*:298, 1976.

110. Becklake, M. R.: Asbestos-related diseases of the lung and other organs: Their epidemiology and implications for clinical practice. Am. Rev. Respir. Dis., *114*:187, 1976.

111. Editorial: Asbestosis and malignant disease. N. Engl. J. Med., *272*:590, 1965.

112. Meurman, L. O., Kiviluoto, R., and Hakama, M.: Mortality and morbidity among the working population of anthophyllite asbestos miners in Finland. Br. J. Ind. Med., *31*:105, 1974.

113. Borow, M., Conston, A., Livornese, L., and Schalet, N.: Mesothelioma following exposure to asbestos. A review of 72 cases. Chest, *64*:641, 1973.

114. Hourihane, D. O.: A biopsy series of mesotheliomata, and attempts to identify asbestos within some of the tumors. Ann. N.Y. Acad. Sci., *132*:647, 1965.

115. Demy, N. G., and Adhler, H.: Asbestosis and malignancy. Am. J. Roentgenol., *100*:597, 1967.

116. Alexander, E., Clark, R. A., Colley, D. P., and Mitchell, S. E.: CT of malignant pleural mesothelioma. Am. J. Roentgenol., *137*:287, 1981.

117. Enticknap, J. B., and Smither, W. J.: Peritoneal tumors in asbestosis. Br. J. Ind. Med., *21*:20, 1964.

118. Libshitz, H. I., Wershba, M. S., Atkinson, G. W., and Southard, M. E.: Asbestosis and carcinoma of the larynx. A possible association. J.A.M.A., *228*:1571, 1974.

16

Diseases of the Mediastinum

Although mediastinal diseases constitute only a small fraction of diseases that affect the thorax, their differential diagnosis is difficult because of their common roentgenographic manifestation—widening of the mediastinal silhouette. The majority of mediastinal diseases have an insidious onset and may be present for a long while without occasioning symptoms or signs. In a small percentage of cases, symptoms may be abrupt in onset and alarming in acuity. An example is the acute mediastinitis that follows esophageal rupture. Between these two extremes of clinical presentation are those patients who complain of a mild sensation of pressure in the retrosternal area or who seek medical aid because of symptoms resulting from compression of the air-, blood-, or food-conducting systems within this narrow space.

The diagnosis of mediastinal disease may be very easy or extremely difficult. Of all differential diagnostic considerations, the anatomic location of lesions within the three mediastinal compartments is possibly of the greatest importance, and the reader is urged to refresh his memory about these anatomic subdivisions and normal mediastinal landmarks by referring to the appropriate section in Chapter 1. Similarly, methods and techniques for the investigation of mediastinal abnormalities are described in detail in Chapter 2. Briefly, although investigative algorithms will vary somewhat from institution to institution, it can be stated with some conviction that once mediastinal widening is identified on conventional roentgenograms of the chest and the cause is not immediately apparent, the most productive procedure to conduct next is computed tomography. This conclusion was supported by a recent study by Baron and his colleagues,[1] in which CT was employed in the study of 71 patients for assessment of a widened mediastinum: CT correctly identified normal variants, soft-tissue masses, or vascular abnormalities as the cause of the mediastinal

widening in 92 per cent of the patients. In 58 per cent of the cases, a specific and correct diagnosis was made that obviated further and more invasive diagnostic evaluation. The recommendation made by these authors is one with which we are in complete agreement: invasive diagnostic procedures should be reserved for the minority of cases in which CT is indeterminate or in which additional information is required prior to surgery. Conclusions similar to those of Baron and his colleagues were reached by a Mallinckrodt group from a CT study of 23 pediatric patients with mediastinal abnormalities:[2] CT provided additional diagnostic information in 82 per cent of the patients, and in 65 per cent, the CT findings contributed to a change in clinical management.

For those readers interested in delving more deeply into diseases of the mediastinum, particularly with regard to radiologic correlations with anatomy and pathology, the monograph by Heitzman is highly recommended.[3]

MEDIASTINITIS

Infections of the mediastinum may be acute or chronic, the former sometimes progressing to abscess formation and often being fulminating and lethal. Chronic mediastinitis usually is granulomatous, the result of tuberculous or mycotic infection. In addition, there is a group of mediastinopathies of unknown cause characterized by the accumulation of dense fibrous tissue, sometimes associated with similar deposits elsewhere in the body, notably the retroperitoneal space.

ACUTE MEDIASTINITIS

Acute infections of the mediastinum are rare and in the majority of patients result from

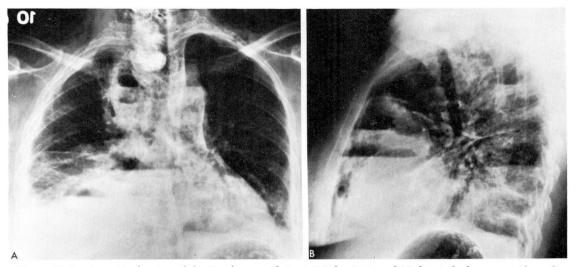

Figure 16–1. **Acute Perforation of the Esophagus with Acute Mediastinitis and Mediastinal Abscesses.** Three days before the roentgenograms illustrated, this 41-year-old woman swallowed a fork and shortly thereafter developed severe retrosternal pain and fever. Posteroanterior (A) and lateral (B) roentgenograms in the erect position reveal an irregularly widened upper mediastinum and multiple air fluid levels within the mediastinum anteriorly and posteriorly. There are bilateral pleural effusions and probable bilateral lower lobe pneumonia. Several days later, barium administered by mouth opacified the whole of the esophagus but showed a large sinus tract extending into the mediastinum posteriorly. Recovery was prolonged but complete.

esophageal perforation. The esophagus may perforate from a variety of causes, including erosion from a primary carcinoma or an impacted foreign body, as a complication of esophagoscopy (particularly when accompanied by biopsy), or spontaneously (usually after vomiting).[4] A less common cause of acute mediastinitis is direct extension of infection from adjacent soft tissues (the retropharyngeal space, lungs, pleura, lymph nodes, or pericardium).

The main roentgenographic manifestation of acute mediastinitis is widening of the mediastinum, usually more evident superiorly, and typically having a smooth, sharply defined margin. When the mediastinitis has resulted from esophageal rupture, gas may be visible within the mediastinal compartment as well as in the soft tissues of the neck.[5] There may be an associated pneumothorax or hydropneumothorax, more commonly on the left. Multiple abscesses may develop (Figure 16–1). The diagnosis is rapidly confirmed roentgenologically by the demonstration of extravasation of ingested contrast material into the periesophageal space or pleura.[5]

The diagnosis should be suspected clinically in any patient in whom severe retrosternal pain develops abruptly and radiates to the neck and whose history points to one of the pathogeneses described. Chills and high fever are common, and the effects of obstruction of the superior vena cava may be apparent. Physical examination of a patient whose esophagus has perforated commonly reveals subcutaneous emphysema in the soft tissues of the neck or a "Hamman sign" on auscultation over the apex of the heart. When the diagnosis is not suspected initially and treatment is not instituted promptly, the inflammation may progress to abscess formation, with subsequent perforation of the abscess into the esophagus, a bronchus, or the pleural cavity.

The prognosis in cases of acute mediastinitis resulting from esophageal rupture is poor; in one series of 39 cases, 15 patients died.[4]

CHRONIC MEDIASTINITIS

Since the specific etiology of chronic mediastinitis usually is unknown, it serves little useful purpose to subdivide cases into two groups depending on whether mediastinal involvement is predominantly granulomatous or fibrotic, especially since the roentgenologic and clinical manifestations are similar or identical.

Although in the majority of instances the etiology of the *granulomatous inflammation* is not established, it is probable that histoplasmosis and tuberculosis are the most common causes.[6] In a review of the literature, Goodwin and associates[7] found 38 cases of mediastinal granulomatosis that were attributed to etiologically proved healing granulomatous disease of lymph nodes, 26 caused by histoplasmosis and 12 by mycobacterial infection. Almost invariably the inflammatory process develops in the upper half of the mediastinum, usually anterior to the trachea and near the hila. The more extensive lesions extend from the innominate veins superiorly to the root of a lung.[6] The amount of cellular infiltration and caseation varies widely; the inflammation is usually associated with considerable fibrosis.

Roentgenographically, the most common manifestation is general widening of the upper half of the mediastinum, with a somewhat lobulated paratracheal mass projecting more to the right than to the left. Calcification occurs in some cases. In a minority of patients, parenchymal disease or bronchopulmonary lymph node enlargement indicates the pulmonary origin of the mediastinal disease. In some cases the mediastinal silhouette is normal, and the roentgenographic manifestations result from bronchial or vascular obstruction (Figure 16–2).[8]

Most patients are asymptomatic. Of the 103 cases reviewed by Schowengerdt and associates,[6] only 27 manifested symptoms or signs relating to involvement of mediastinal structures. Obstruction of the superior vena cava was present in 14 patients and of the esophagus in nine; in two there was compression of the tracheobronchial tree, in one a bronchoesophageal fistula, and in one compression and obliteration of pulmonary veins. These various manifestations of obstruction may occur alone or in combination.[7] Benign superior vena caval syndrome is much less common than the malignant variety. Pulmonary arterial hypertension usually results from obstruction of large central pulmonary veins, with consequent pulmonary venous hypertension and eventual arteriolar vasoconstriction. However, it can also be caused by direct encroachment on central pulmonary arteries.[9]

Definitive diagnosis requires examination of lymph nodes biopsied from the scalene area or of tissue from the mediastinum. In addition to routine morphologic examination, such tissue should be cultured for acid-fast and mycotic organisms.

Sclerosing mediastinitis (idiopathic mediastinal fibrosis) probably has several etiologies, and although the responsible organism rarely is isolated, the majority of cases most likely represent the end-stages of chronic granulomatous infection. In a review of 77 cases,[6] the etiology was positively established in only three (histoplasmosis in two and tuberculosis in one).

One of the distinctive characteristics of some cases of sclerosing mediastinitis is its association

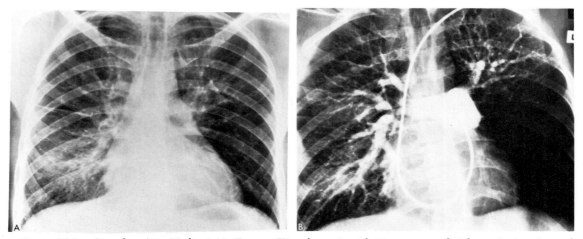

Figure 16–2. Granulomatous Mediastinitis Due to Histoplasmosis with Encasement of Pulmonary Arteries and Veins. A posteroanterior roentgenogram *(A)* reveals interstitial edema throughout the right lung and left upper zone. Septal lines are present in the right costophrenic angle. A striking disparity in density of the lower half of the two lungs is observed, the left being relatively radiolucent and, in fact, markedly oligemic. A pulmonary arteriogram *(B)* shows almost complete occlusion of the left interlobar artery with virtually no perfusion of the left lower lobe and lingula. Although there appears to be good opacification of the arteries of the right lung, the truncus anterior and interlobar arteries show concentric narrowing medial to the hilum. The venous phase of the angiogram is not available, but it is almost certain that the pulmonary veins are affected in the same manner, resulting in venous hypertension and the interstitial edema apparent on the plain roentgenogram. (Courtesy of Dr. M. J. Palayew, Jewish General Hospital, Montreal.)

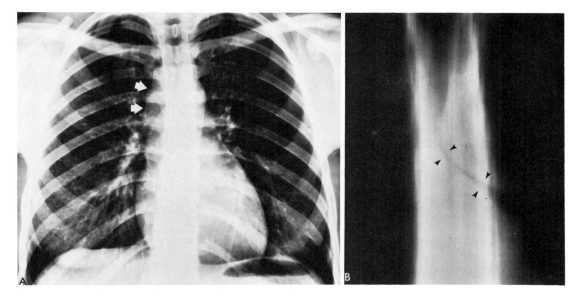

Figure 16–3.   Sclerosing Mediastinitis with Involvement of Major Airways.   Five months prior to the roentgenograms illustrated, this 19-year-old girl had noted the onset of shortness of breath on exertion, nonproductive cough, and recurrent wheezing episodes precipitated by physical exertion or exposure to cold air. Pulmonary function studies revealed a significant impairment of flow rates. The clinical diagnosis was bronchial asthma. A roentgenogram of her chest in posteroanterior projection (A) reveals normal appearance of her lungs. A smooth, well-defined homogeneous mass is seen in the right tracheobronchial angle, obscuring the shadow of the azygos vein (*arrow*). In addition, there is a suggestion of narrowing of the air column of the main bronchi. A tomogram of the carinal region in anteroposterior projection (B) reveals a severe degree of stenosis of the whole length of the left main bronchus (*arrowheads*). The lower 2 cm of the trachea and right main bronchus are similarly but less severely affected. Biopsies of mediastinal tissue and lymph node obtained at mediastinoscopy revealed findings consistent with fibrosing mediastinitis. At right thoracotomy, a diffuse mass with ill-defined edges was found extending from the posterior wall of the superior vena cava over the trachea, into the mediastinum behind the trachea, and downward around the right upper lobe bronchus and into the mediastinum. Only partial resection of the mass was possible because of technical problems. The region of the left main bronchus could not be explored. Histologically, the tissue was composed of collagenous fibrosis with slight focal lymphocytic infiltration. The etiology was not established and the final diagnosis was idiopathic sclerosing mediastinitis. Information regarding the patient's subsequent course is not available. (Courtesy of Dr. Murray Mazer, St. Boniface General Hospital, St. Boniface, Manitoba.)

with a similar fibrotic process elsewhere—retroperitoneal fibrosis, pseudotumor of the orbit, Riedel's struma, and ligneous perityphlitis of the cecum.[10] The number of reported cases with combinations of these idiopathic sclerosing lesions is sufficient to indicate that this association is more than coincidental. Mediastinal and retroperitoneal fibrosis have also been reported during treatment with methysergide, a drug used for the alleviation of headache.[11] The disease almost invariably regresses when the drug is withdrawn.

The anatomic region of the mediastinum involved in sclerosing mediastinitis is the same as in granulomatous disease, comprising the paratracheal zone, the carina, and the hilum of one or both lungs. Morphologically, the process presents as a mass or plaque of woody, white fibrous tissue resembling a pancake in the anterior portion of the upper mediastinum, usually more on the right side. The mass usually

obstructs the superior vena cava or innominate veins and may constrict the aorta, the pulmonary arteries or veins, the esophagus, or portions of the tracheobronchial tree (Figure 16–3).[12] When mediastinal and retroperitoneal fibrosis coexist, the two are remote anatomically.

The roentgenographic manifestations of sclerosing mediastinitis are identical to those of the granulomatous variety. Symptoms and signs are present more often in cases of the sclerotic form of chronic mediastinitis than when the reaction is predominantly granulomatous. Of the 77 cases reviewed by Schowengerdt and coworkers[6] and judged to be examples of fibrous mediastinitis, in 64 (83 per cent) adjacent mediastinal structures were affected. The superior vena cava was obstructed in 49 patients, making this by far the most common obstructive manifestation.

Precise diagnosis requires histologic examination of tissue removed at mediastinoscopy or thoracotomy. Differentiation from neoplasm may be impossible by inspection alone, and histologic examination is mandatory.

PNEUMOMEDIASTINUM

Pneumomediastinum connotes the presence of gas in the mediastinal space. It is rare in adults (except in intensive care units) and undoubtedly is most common in newborn infants. Etiology and pathogenesis are varied and may be considered under three headings—spontaneous, traumatic, and following rupture of the esophagus or tracheobronchial tree.

The *spontaneous* occurrence is the most common mechanism of pneumomediastinum, both in neonates and in adults. In adults it occurs predominantly in males during the second and third decades of life. In both age groups, the mechanism probably is the same: rupture of marginally situated alveoli whose bases relate to blood vessels. Many patients who develop mediastinal emphysema have no clear-cut evidence of underlying lung disease. In some, a precipitating event cannot be identified, the diagnosis being made following the discovery of subcutaneous emphysema in the soft tissues of the neck or from a chest roentgenogram obtained because of retrosternal discomfort.[13] In most patients, however, the development of pneumomediastinum can be related to an incident that resulted in a sudden rise in intra-alveolar pressure, often with concomitant airway narrowing. Physiologic mechanisms that exert stress on alveolar walls and cause rupture include deep respiratory and Valsalva maneuvers, coughing, and vomiting. In the majority of instances, rupture probably occurs as a result of check-valve bronchiolar obstruction secondary to bronchiolitis. For example, pulmonary interstitial emphysema and pneumomediastinum are frequent complications of hyaline membrane disease in neonates and of measles and giant-cell pneumonia in children.[14] Other conditions that have been reported to be associated with pneumomediastinum include asthma, diabetic ketoacidosis (with accompanying vomiting and hyperventilation), parturition, and athletic competition.[13, 15]

Whatever the cause of the rupture, air passes into the interstitial tissues of the lung and tracks through the interstitial space to the hilum and mediastinum.[16] Air may also extend peripherally toward the visceral pleura and rupture into the pleural space. Pneumothorax frequently oc- curs with pneumomediastinum, particularly in the neonatal period, being identified in 25 of 40 cases in one series.[17] Pneumothorax may also result from rupture of the mediastinal pleura when sufficient gas accumulates in this compartment. Sometimes air within the interstitial tissues of the lung ("interstitial emphysema") can be detected roentgenographically. Since gas in the interstitial tissues of otherwise normal lung should not be apparent because of lack of contrast, to visualize it requires the presence of disease in contiguous parenchyma, a feature of particular note in neonates with the respiratory distress syndrome.[18]

When sufficient gas accumulates in mediastinal compartments, pressure may build up and impede blood flow, particularly in low pressure veins. Respiratory embarrassment also may result from the presence of large amounts of gas in the pulmonary interstitial space, resulting in "stiff" lungs. Either or both of these mechanisms may lead to the syndrome of "mediastinal air block."[16] Such a build-up of pressure occurs only when gas is prevented from passing into the neck, a situation particularly prone to occur in the neonatal period. More frequently—and almost invariably in adults—air escapes from the mediastinum by way of the fascial planes of the great vessels into the neck and anterior chest wall, producing subcutaneous emphysema. Occasionally, pneumomediastinum (usually severe) is associated with roentgenographic evidence of extraperitoneal gas, commonly in a subphrenic location; although formerly it was thought that this gas reached the extraperitoneal space via vascular sheaths posteriorly, Kleinman and his colleagues[19] have shown that the route is anterior rather than posterior and that dissection occurs along internal mammary vessels enclosed between the sternocostal origins of the diaphragm.

Traumatic pneumomediastinum may develop after closed chest trauma and in such circumstances probably has the same mechanism of production as in spontaneous pneumomediastinum—the rupture of alveoli into the perivascular sheath as a result of an abrupt increase in pressure. Pneumomediastinum may also follow traumatic rupture of the esophagus or fracture of the tracheobronchial tree.

Rupture of the esophagus occurs most frequently during episodes of severe vomiting[20] but may occur spontaneously during labor, severe asthmatic attacks, or strenuous exercise. (Each one of these three events can cause pneumomediastinum without esophageal rupture.) When rupture is associated with vomiting

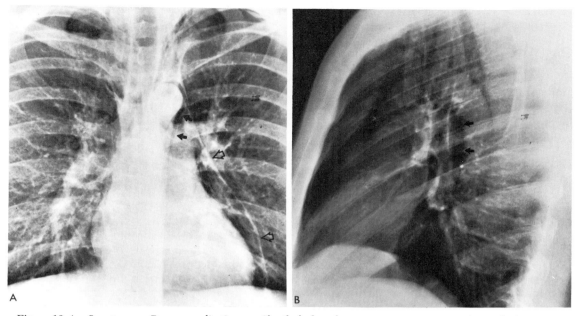

Figure 16–4. Spontaneous Pneumomediastinum. Shortly before these roentgenograms were obtained, this 20-year-old man had noted an abrupt onset of fairly severe retrosternal pain. Views of the chest in posteroanterior (*A*) and lateral (*B*) projections reveal a long linear opacity roughly paralleling the left heart border in posteroanterior projection (*open arrows*), representing the laterally displaced mediastinal pleura. In addition, considerable gas is present around the aortic arch and proximal descending thoracic aorta (*solid arrows* in both projections). In lateral projection, note the gas outlining the anterior surface of the heart and the brachiocephalic vessels.

(Boerhaave's syndrome),[20] the usual site is in the lower 8 cm of the esophagus, an area relatively unsupported by connective tissue. The classic tear is vertical and involves the left posterolateral wall.[20]

Roentgenographic signs of pneumomediastinum are usually easy to detect, especially in infants. In posteroanterior projection, the mediastinal pleura is displaced laterally, creating a longitudinal line shadow parallel to the heart border and separated from the heart by gas. This shadow is usually more evident on the left side (Figure 16–4). A longitudinal gas shadow may be identified adjacent to the thoracic aorta also. In lateral projection, a layer of extrapulmonary gas almost always can be identified in the retrosternal region, and, in infants, this may be the only convincing sign of pneumomediastinum. In infants with a large accumulation of gas, the thymus may be well outlined and may be displaced upward. When gas becomes interposed between the heart and diaphragm in cases of pneumomediastinum, it permits visualization of the central portion of the diaphragm in continuity with the lateral portions, creating "the continuous diaphragm sign."[21]

The *symptoms and signs* resulting from pneumomediastinum depend largely upon the amount of air in the mediastinal space and the presence or absence of associated infection. In infants, mediastinal emphysema is usually benign and only rarely is associated with respiratory failure or cardiovascular collapse. In the adult, the diagnosis may be suggested by a history of abrupt onset of retrosternal pain radiating to the shoulders and down both arms, usually preceded by some occurrence, such as a spasm of coughing, sneezing, or vomiting, which resulted in excessive increase in intrathoracic pressure. The pain usually is aggravated by respiration and sometimes by swallowing. Dyspnea may be severe. Physical examination usually reveals the presence of air in the subcutaneous tissues of the neck or over the thoracic wall. Hamman's sign may be detected on auscultation over the apex of the heart. This sign, consisting of a crunching or clicking noise synchronous with the heart beat, has been estimated to occur in approximately 50 per cent of cases and is heard best when the patient is in the left lateral decubitus position.[22]

Patients in whom air does not freely escape from the mediastinum into the neck, notably neonates, may have engorged neck veins, a rapid, thready pulse, and significant systemic hypotension.

MEDIASTINAL HEMORRHAGE

The majority of cases of mediastinal hemorrhage result from trauma, usually of a severe nature such as that associated with an automobile accident and resultant chest cage compression. Less common causes include rupture of an aortic aneurysm and extension of blood from the retropharyngeal soft tissues secondary to trauma or spontaneous hemorrhage associated with coagulation disorders. Undoubtedly the majority of cases of mediastinal hemorrhage go unrecognized, the amount of bleeding being insufficient to produce symptoms and signs.

Roentgenologically, hemorrhage typically results in uniform, symmetric widening of the mediastinum in any of its compartments. Local accumulation of blood in the form of a hematoma is manifested by a homogeneous mass that may project to one or both sides of the mediastinum and may be situated in any compartment.[23]

MEDIASTINAL MASSES

The diseases of the mediastinum that have been described to this point show little or no predilection for a specific anatomic zone within the mediastinum. By contrast, a wide variety of lesions that present as "masses" show a strong predilection for one of the three mediastinal compartments. Thus it is logical to classify mediastinal masses on the basis of anatomic location. It is stressed that any classification based on anatomic location implies that a specific lesion has a *predilection* for a specific compartment. It should be clear that overlap is bound to occur and all that is implied is that lesions occur *predominantly* in one or another compartment.

Almost half of all patients with mediastinal masses are asymptomatic, the abnormality being discovered on a screening chest roentgenogram.[24, 25] A review of 1064 cases of "primary mediastinal tumors" seen over a 40-year period at the Mayo Clinic[24] showed that the great majority of patients were adults, only 8 per cent being under 15 years of age at the time of diagnosis. There was no sex predominance. In all cases, the diagnosis was established at thoracotomy and the incidence of the various tumors was as follows: neurogenic tumors, thymomas, and benign cysts—60 per cent; malignant lymphoma, teratoma, granuloma, or intrathoracic goiter—30 per cent; and some type of benign or malignant mesenchymal tumor—10 per cent.

The following section represents little more than a brief outline of a very broad topic. The interested reader is directed to the accumulated experience of the Mayo[24] and Cleveland[25] Clinics.

MEDIASTINAL MASSES SITUATED PREDOMINANTLY IN THE ANTERIOR COMPARTMENT

The anterior mediastinal compartment is bounded anteriorly by the sternum and posteriorly by the pericardium, aorta, and brachiocephalic vessels. It contains the thymus gland, anterior mediastinal lymph nodes, and mesenchymal tissue. It is the most common site of mesenchymal neoplasms, of intrathoracic thyroid and parathyroid hyperplasias and neoplasms, and, of course, of thymomas.

THYMOMA

The majority of tumors that are constructed of the cell types existing in the normal thymus are solid lymphoepithelial neoplasms, although some are cystic. Occasionally, they contain an abundance of fat and are known as thymolipomas. Solid thymomas are the most frequently occurring anterior mediastinal neoplasms, and approximately one-third are malignant;[26] they seldom attain the size of teratomas.[27] They may occur at any age but are rare in children.

Pathologically, thymomas arise from both epithelial and thymocytic elements of the thymic parenchyma. They are usually divided into four types, based on the predominant cell—lymphocytic, epithelial, lymphoepithelial (mixed), and spindle cell (epithelial variant).[24, 25] The various cell types occur with approximately equal frequency.[24] Hassall's corpuscles are infrequent or absent in the lymphocytic and epithelial types, whereas the spindle cell variety is composed of a mixture of mature Hassall's corpuscles and epithelial cells resembling fibroblasts. It is virtually impossible in individual cases to establish whether these lesions are benign or malignant by histologic examination alone. More reliable criteria in determining prognosis are the gross characteristics of local invasion or complete encapsulation.

Thymolipomas are benign neoplasms of the fatty tissue within the thymus and are said to constitute 2 to 9 per cent of thymic tumors. Grossly, the tumor is yellowish, soft, and pliable, and often is lobate. Histologically, the tumor consists of adult adipose tissue inter-

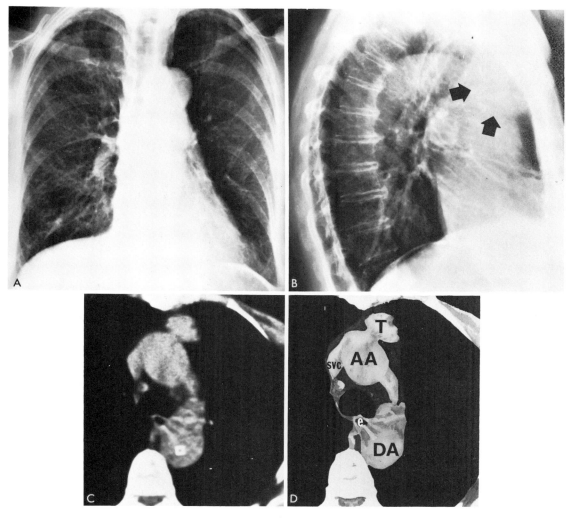

Figure 16–5. Anterior Mediastinal Thymoma in a 73-Year-Old Woman with Myasthenia Gravis. Posteroanterior *(A)* and lateral *(B)* roentgenograms reveal a poorly defined mass in the anterior mediastinum, seen to poor effect on the PA view but obvious in lateral projection *(arrows)*. A CT scan immediately below the transverse arch of the aorta *(C)* and a diagrammatic representation of the scan *(D)* demonstrate the mass to relate to the anterolateral aspect of the ascending aorta; the mass is only partly demarcated from the aorta. A contrast scan revealed increased attenuation within the mass but to a value considerably less than that observed in the aorta, indicating that the mass was a solid, vascularized tumor. T = Thymoma; AA = ascending aorta; DA = descending aorta; svc = superior vena cava; e = esophagus.

spersed with areas of normal, hyperplastic, or atrophic thymic tissue.[28] Characteristically, thymolipomas can grow to huge proportions, 68 per cent of reported cases being heavier than 500 g, 23 per cent over 2000 g, and one reported tumor weighing over 12,000 g.[28] The majority of patients are asymptomatic.

Roentgenologically, most thymomas are visualized near the junction of the heart and great vessels (Figure 16–5). They are round or oval, and their margins are smooth or lobulated.[29] They may protrude to one or both sides of the mediastinum and tend to displace the heart and great vessels posteriorly. They may be solid or

cystic (Figure 16–6), the distinction being readily discernible on nonenhanced and contrast-enhanced CT scans. In some cases calcification is apparent at the periphery of the lesion or throughout its substance. Thymolipomas often grow very large in size and, as a result of their soft, pliable consistency, tend to slump toward the diaphragm. They adapt themselves to the diaphragmatic contour, thus becoming largely inferior in position and leaving the superior mediastinal space clear.[28]

Roentgenographic techniques that aid in the identification and assessment of thymic tumors include conventional roentgenography in pos-

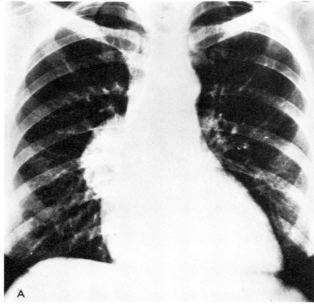

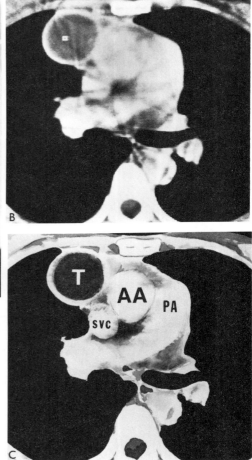

Figure 16–6. Cystic Thymoma. A posteroanterior roentgenogram *(A)* on this 50-year-old asymptomatic woman reveals a large homogeneous mass protruding to the right side of the mediastinum. It was situated in the anterior mediastinum as revealed on lateral projection (not illustrated) and was not calcified. A CT scan at the level of the main pulmonary artery *(B)* and a diagrammatic representation of the scan *(C)* reveal a large mass relating anteriorly to the angle formed by the ascending aorta and superior vena cava. This scan was obtained following injection of contrast material and reveals increased attenuation of the periphery of the mass but no change in the density of its center, whose attenuation approximated water. T = Thymoma; AA = ascending aorta; PA = main pulmonary artery; svc = superior vena cava.

teroanterior, oblique and lateral projection, lateral tomography, and computed tomography. In a Mayo Clinic study of 69 cases of thymoma,[26] although CT did not reveal any lesions that were not suspected from other roentgenographic studies, it clarified significant anatomic relations and, perhaps more importantly, demonstrated adherence and invasion as signs of malignancy. In patients with myasthenia gravis, it is probable that CT will yield considerable diagnostic information in influencing patient management.[30-32] Two recent articles dealing with computed tomography of the normal and abnormal thymus are highly recommended to those readers desiring more information on this important subject.[35, 36]

There is a close relationship between thymic neoplasms and myasthenia gravis. Approximately 15 per cent of patients with myasthenia gravis have thymic tumors and approximately 25 to 50 per cent of patients with thymic tumors have myasthenia gravis [24, 25, 33, 34] In the absence

of myasthenia gravis, most patients with thymomas are asymptomatic.[24]

Although malignant thymomas can spread by implantation and by direct extension, distant metastases are very uncommon. The recurrence rate following surgical removal is high.[33] In patients with myasthenia gravis removal of a thymoma seldom results in complete abatement of symptoms, although approximately 50 per cent of patients show some degree of remission.[25, 33]

GERMINAL CELL NEOPLASMS

This group of tumors includes benign dermoid cysts, benign and malignant teratomas, endodermal sinus tumors, seminomas, choriocarcinomas, and embryonal carcinomas. They are considered to arise from primitive germ cell rests whose journey along the urogenital ridge to the primitive gonad was interrupted in the mediastinum.[37] In the majority of cases, they become manifest only in adolescence or early adulthood, although they are presumably present from birth. Of the 106 germinal cell neoplasms reported from the Mayo Clinic in 1971,[24] 86 were benign. One hundred of the 106 tumors were located in the anterior mediastinum. Teratomas are much more common than other varieties of germinal cell tumors, with an incidence about equal to that of thymomas.

DERMOID CYST AND TERATOMA

These tumors may be solid or cystic and approximately 30 per cent are malignant.[38] The term "dermoid cyst" should be reserved for those cases in which the tumor consists only of epidermis and its appendages. Teratomas contain ectodermal, mesodermal, and endodermal derivatives, the malignant varieties being largely endodermal in origin. The majority of cystic lesions are benign, and most of the solid lesions are malignant. Teratomas and dermoid cysts occur early in life, perhaps more frequently in young adults than in children. There is no sex predilection.[38] Compared with other sites of origin, the mediastinum is a very uncommon location for teratomas; the majority of lesions arise in the ovarian or sacrococcygeal region.

Roentgenologically, the majority of dermoid cysts and teratomas are visualized in the anterior mediastinum close to the origin of the major vessels from the heart. Benign lesions are round or oval and are smooth in contour. By contrast, the malignant lesions tend to be lobulated. They may become large—on average, considerably larger than thymomas (other than thymolipomas). Calcification may be present around the periphery of the lesion, particularly in dermoid cysts, but since such calcification may also occur in thymomas, this finding is of no differential diagnostic value. The diagnosis of dermoid cyst may be made with certainty in the very occasional case in which bone or a tooth is demonstrated within the lesion. Computed tomography is said to be superior to other imaging methods in the investigation of benign cystic teratomas;[39] specific CT characteristics include a fatty mass with a denser dependent element, and globular calcification, bone, or teeth situated within a solid protuberance into the cystic cavity.

It is important to recognize that rapid increase in size of these tumors does not necessarily indicate malignancy. Hemorrhage into a dermoid cyst or cystic teratoma may increase its size rapidly and give rise to severe retrosternal pain or discomfort. When a cyst ruptures into the trachea or a bronchus, its contents are expectorated. If the expectorated material contains hair (trichoptysis), the diagnosis of dermoid cyst can be made with certainty.

Dermoid cysts and teratomas of the mediastinum seldom occasion symptoms, usually being discovered on a screening chest roentgenogram. Tumors that grow large may give rise to shortness of breath, cough, and a sensation of pressure or pain in the retrosternal area.

SEMINOMA

This rare neoplasm is thought to originate from aberrant germ cells in the anterior mediastinum. It occurs almost exclusively in young men, the average age being 27 years.[40] The cell structure and histologic pattern are identical to those of testicular seminoma and ovarian dysgerminoma. The neoplasm may be well encapsulated or may invade local tissues and give rise to distant metastases.[41]

Roentgenologically, this mediastinal mass cannot be distinguished from malignant teratoma. It tends to have a lobulated margin and may protrude from one or both sides of the mediastinum.[40, 41]

The clinical picture is not distinctive; patients may be asymptomatic or may have symptoms and show signs of local pressure.

PRIMARY CHORIOCARCINOMA

This variety of germinal cell neoplasm has a mediastinal origin even more rarely than seminoma. Of 17 choriocarcinomas seen at the Mayo Clinic over a period of 10 years, only one originated in the mediastinum.[37] By 1975 a total of 23 primary mediastinal choriocarcinomas had been reported, almost all in men.[42] The peak age incidence is between 20 and 30 years. An extragonadal origin should not be accepted unless examination of serial sections of the testicles has excluded the possibility that the mediastinal lesion is metastatic.[43]

Pathologically, the tumor typically is a rounded, lobulated mass, occasionally with a thin capsule. Histologically, syncytial trophoblasts predominate;[44] necrosis is common. Richardson and his colleagues[45] have noted a tendency to misinterpret extragonadal germ cell cancers as adenocarcinoma or as undifferentiated large-cell carcinoma; they point out that this error can be obviated by identifying elevated levels of the beta subunit of human chorionic gonadotropin or of alpha-fetoprotein, or by immunoperoxidase staining of the tissue for these markers.

The roentgenographic appearance is not distinctive, depicting an anterior mediastinal mass with a somewhat lobulated contour expanding the mediastinum unilaterally or bilaterally.

Growth tends to be extremely rapid. This neoplasm usually occasions symptoms of dyspnea, hemoptysis, hoarseness, stridor, dysphagia, and Horner's syndrome.[37] Gynecomastia is reported to occur in about two-thirds of cases,[44] invariably associated with elevated gonadotropin levels and a positive urinary Aschheim-Zondek test[37] The prognosis is extremely poor, death occurring in most cases within four to six weeks of the time of diagnosis.

THYROID MASSES

Although extension of goiter into the thorax is seen in only 1 to 3 per cent of cases of thyroidectomy,[46] thyroid masses nevertheless constitute a significant percentage of anterior mediastinal masses. These lesions usually are nodular colloid goiters, and thyrotoxicosis may be present in some cases; carcinoma is uncommon.[25]

Seventy-five to 80 per cent of these masses arise from a lower pole or the isthmus of the thyroid and extend into the anterior mediastinum in front of the trachea. The remainder arise from the posterior aspect of either thyroid lobe and extend into the posterior mediastinum behind the trachea, innominate vein, and innominate or subclavian arteries.[47] In the posterior mediastinum they are situated almost exclusively on the right. The mass typically is well encapsulated, often showing degeneration, cystic changes, and calcification. A recent report[48] sites five characteristic CT features of substernal thyroid: (1) anatomic continuity with the cervical thyroid, (2) focal calcifications, (3) a relatively high CT number, (4) a rise in CT number after bolus administration of contrast medium, and (5) prolonged enhancement after contrast administration. The authors suggest that while not all of the features may be present, a combination should permit accurate diagnosis in most cases.

Roentgenographically, the appearance is that of a sharply defined, smooth or lobulated mass of homogeneous density.[23] Anterior mediastinal goiters displace the trachea posteriorly and laterally, whereas those in the posterior mediastinum displace the trachea anteriorly and the esophagus posteriorly and laterally. Calcification within the mass is fairly common. Radioactive isotopic studies are diagnostic when positive, but these lesions are seldom functioning.[47]

The majority of patients with intrathoracic goiters are asymptomatic,[24, 25] the abnormality being discovered on a screening chest roentgenogram. When present symptoms relate to tracheal compression and include respiratory distress (which may be worsened by certain movements of the neck), inspiratory and expiratory stridor, and hoarseness. Physical examination usually reveals evidence of a goiter ascending into the neck when the patient swallows.

PARATHYROID MASSES

The presence of parathyroid glands within the mediastinum is best explained on the basis of their migration along with the thymus gland during embryonic life. Normally they are so small as to be invisible roentgenographically, and it is only when they enlarge as a result of neoplasia or hyperplasia that they may be demonstrable.

Parathyroid masses may become sufficiently large to widen the mediastinal silhouette, usually unilaterally.[29] They rarely calcify. If neither standard roentgenography nor CT reveals a mass, and the barium-filled esophagus is not displaced in cases of known hyperparathyroidism in which surgical exploration of the neck has revealed no evidence of a hyperfunctioning gland, arteriography may be required to reveal a mediastinal lesion.[49] While angiography appears to be more sensitive than CT in localizing mediastinal glands, it has been stated that CT is very useful in identifying glands in patients with previous failed explorations.[50]

MESENCHYMAL NEOPLASMS

Mesenchymal neoplasms of the mediastinum are rare and include lipoma, fibroma, hemangioma, and lymphangioma.

Lipoma, like other mesenchymal tumors of the mediastinum, may occur in any of the three mediastinal compartments but are seen most commonly anteriorly. Certain roentgenographic features may aid in their diagnosis. Since the density of fat is lower than that of other soft tissues, the roentgenographic density of lipomas often—but not always—is less than that of other mediastinal masses. Should doubt exist on evidence provided by standard roentgenograms, CT will almost invariably reveal the tumors' fatty nature (see Figure 16–7, page 706).[51-53] Because of their pliability, these tumors almost never give rise to symptoms.[38]

An unusual abnormality is the mediastinal accumulation of fat that occurs in association with Cushing's syndrome[54] and with long-term corticosteroid therapy.[54, 55] Corticosteroids mobilize and redistribute reserve fatty tissue, resulting in the excessive deposition of fat in the upper mediastinum and in both pleuropericardial angles. Mediastinal widening tends to be smooth and symmetric and extends from the thoracic inlet to the hila bilaterally. It is important that the abnormality be correctly identified in order to avoid subjecting patients to unwarranted investigation or useless surgery.

Benign fibrous tissue tumors (*fibroma*) are found most commonly in the anterior mediastinum, whereas the malignant counterpart (*fibrosarcoma*) is more commonly situated posteriorly.[29] There are no distinctive roentgenographic features. Pleural effusion may occur with either the benign or malignant variety.

Both benign and malignant neoplasms of blood vessels—*hemangioma, endothelioma, hemangiosarcoma*, and *hemangiopericytoma*—are rare. Hemangiomas tend to occur in the anterior mediastinum and may be multiple. Phleboliths may be identified within them, a virtually diagnostic sign.[29] Adjacent ribs may become hypertrophied or eroded.

Lymphangiomas may occur in two forms: a cavernous or cystic variety that often extends into the neck and occurs in infants (*hygroma*), and a variety that occurs later in life in the lower anterior mediastinum and does not communicate with the neck. Histologically, these lesions are thin-walled, cystic, multilocular tumors lined by endothelial cells and containing clear, yellow fluid.[24] Because of their soft, yielding consistency, they seldom produce symptoms, even when the tumors are large. Chylothorax develops in some cases.

MEDIASTINAL MASSES SITUATED PREDOMINANTLY IN THE MIDDLE COMPARTMENT

The middle mediastinal compartment contains the heart, pericardium, all the major vessels leaving and entering this organ, plus the trachea and main bronchi, paratracheal and tracheobronchial lymph nodes, the phrenic nerves, and the upper portions of the vagus nerves.

LYMPH NODE ENLARGEMENT

Lymph node enlargement is undoubtedly the most common cause of mediastinal enlargement, and, with the exception of lymph node hyperplasia, its various etiologies have been described elsewhere in the book. These include lymphoma (*see* page 430), leukemia (*see* page 440), metastases (*see* page 444), sarcoidosis (*see* page 643), granulomatous mediastinitis (*see* page 695), and, rarely, infectious mononucleosis (*see* page 337). With the exception of Hodgkin's disease, in which involvement of anterior mediastinal and retrosternal nodes is common, the anatomic distribution of lymph node enlargement in all these diseases is predominantly midmediastinal.

LYMPH NODE HYPERPLASIA

This unusual condition, originally described by Castleman[56] in 1954 and since then by other investigators,[40, 57] is of unknown etiology. The enlarged lymph nodes have a distinctive histologic appearance. Hochholzer and associates[40] recently reported finding 47 cases of this lesion in the literature and an additional 35 in the files of the U.S. Armed Forces Institute of Pathology. The patients' ages ranged from 8 to 58 years, and there was no sex predominance.

Lymph node hyperplasia usually presents as a solitary mass in the mediastinum, the hilar regions, or the peripheral lymph node areas. The microscopic appearance is one of lymphoid follicles scattered widely throughout the mass instead of only in the peripheral cortical zones as in normal lymph nodes. Penetration of the enlarged nodes by capillaries is a feature of the disease.

The roentgenographic appearance is one of a solitary mass, with a smooth or lobulated contour, in any of the three mediastinal compartments but most commonly in the middle and posterior ones.[24] Calcification has not been reported. The major differential diagnosis is neurogenic tumor, from which lymph node hyperplasia may be indistinguishable, even angiographically.[58] Although these masses may grow extremely large—up to 16 cm in diameter[40]—they seldom cause symptoms.

PRIMARY TRACHEAL NEOPLASMS

Although bronchogenic carcinoma is usually manifested in the mediastinum in the form of metastases to lymph nodes from a primary lesion in the lung, rarely the carcinoma arises in the trachea or main bronchi just distal to the bifurcation and thus is situated within the middle mediastinum. If the neoplasm extends outward into the paratracheal space, it may widen the mediastinum to one or the other side. An irregular shaggy mass is usually evident within the tracheal air column on standard roentgenograms or on tomograms.

Symptoms include cough, hemoptysis, and sometimes severe dyspnea and wheezing; stridor may be apparent.

BRONCHOGENIC CYST

Congenital bronchial cysts of the mediastinum were described in detail in Chapter 5 (*see* page 239) and are reviewed only briefly here. These cysts usually are discovered in childhood or early adult life. Although it is generally accepted that the majority are situated in the vicinity of the carina in relation to one of the major airways (*see* Figure 16–14, page 715), many arise in the midportion of the posterior mediastinum. Almost all have only a single cavity. They contain milky white or dirty brown mucoid material and rarely communicate with the tracheobronchial tree. Although these cysts may grow very large without occasioning symptoms, even small ones may cause tracheobronchial obstruction in infants and children.[23] They may undergo an abrupt increase in size as a result of hemorrhage or infection, or rarely they may undergo spontaneous disappearance.

MASSES SITUATED IN THE ANTERIOR CARDIOPHRENIC ANGLE

Masses in the vicinity of the cardiophrenic angle on either side, although anteriorly situated, relate to the heart and therefore are truly in the middle mediastinum. Accumulations of fat that normally occupy these angles may attain a considerable size. Pleuropericardial fat pads are always bilateral but may be asymmetric, that on the right usually being the larger. When the nature of such a mass is in question, the diagnosis can be made with ease by CT scanning (Figure 16–7).

The differential diagnosis of masses occupying the anterior cardiophrenic angle is extensive. It includes lesions arising within the lung parenchyma, in the visceral or parietal pleural membranes or pleural space, within the space between the pericardium and the mediastinal pleura (usually but not invariably fat), within the pericardium or contiguous myocardium (*e.g.*, cardiac aneurysm), within the diaphragm, from beneath the diaphragm (hernia), and finally tumors such as teratomas or thymomas that much more frequently occupy anatomic sites elsewhere in the mediastinum. Lesions arising in any of these anatomic regions conceivably can produce roentgenographic shadows of a similar nature. Only three will be consid-

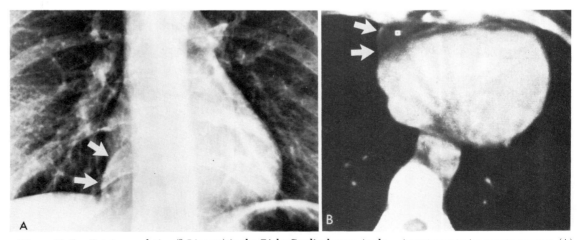

Figure 16–7. Fat Accumulation (? Lipoma) in the Right Cardiophrenic Angle. A posteroanterior roentgenogram (*A*) of a 53-year-old asymptomatic woman reveals a smooth, sharply demarcated opacity in the right cardiophrenic angle (*arrows*). Its roentgenographic density is no different from that of contiguous mediastinum. A CT scan at the level of the mass (*B*) shows the mass to be of very low attenuation (*arrows*), indicating its fatty nature

ered here—pleuropericardial cyst, hernia through the foramen of Morgagni, and enlargement of diaphragmatic lymph nodes.

PLEUROPERICARDIAL (MESOTHELIAL) CYSTS

Mesothelial cysts (pericardial or pleuropericardial cysts and diverticula) probably are congenital and result from aberrations in the formation of the coelomic cavities. Of the 72 cysts reviewed by the Mayo Clinic group,[24] 54 were in the cardiophrenic angles and 53 were on the right side. Microscopically, the cyst walls are composed of fibrous connective tissue and are lined by a single layer of mesothelial cells. They seldom communicate with the pericardial cavity, and they contain clear or serous fluid.

Roentgenographically, the great majority of pericardial cysts are smooth in contour and round or oval. Lateral projection may reveal a tear-drop configuration due to insertion of the cyst in the interlobar fissure between the middle and lower lobes. In the majority of cases they range in diameter from 3 to 8 cm. The cystic nature of these masses can be confirmed by CT, thus obviating needless thoracotomy.[59]

Symptoms are almost invariably absent. although a very large cyst may give rise to a sensation of retrosternal pressure or to dyspnea.[46]

HERNIA THROUGH THE FORAMEN OF MORGAGNI

The foramina of Morgagni are small triangular deficiencies in the diaphragm, a few centimeters from the midline on each side, between muscle fibers originating from the xiphisternum and the seventh rib (*see* Figure 1–57, page 85). When larger than normal they may permit herniation of abdominal contents into the thorax. Herniation is almost invariably right-sided, since the left foramen is protected by the pericardium. Hernial contents include omentum, liver, or small or large bowel. When the hernial sac is filled with liver, the roentgenographic shadow is homogeneous and usually indistinguishable from a large pleuropericardial fat pad. When the hernial sac contains omentum, the density of the mass may indicate its fatty nature. In such circumstances the transverse colon occupies a high position within the abdomen, peaking anteriorly and superiorly in the vicinity of the hernia. Thus barium examination of the colon is virtually diagnostic (Figure 16–8). When the hernial sac contains small or large bowel, the presence of gas-containing loops usually permits ready diagnosis that may, if necessary, be confirmed by barium examination.

Patients usually are asymptomatic but occasionally complain of retrosternal pain or gastrointestinal or respiratory symptoms.[60] Strangulation of hernial contents occurs rarely.

ENLARGEMENT OF DIAPHRAGMATIC LYMPH NODES

The diaphragmatic group of parietal lymph nodes is normally not visualized on chest roentgenograms because of the small size of the nodes and their investment with fat and loose pleural reflections. However, when enlarged, these lymph nodes displace the pleura laterally and produce a smooth, round or lobulated mass projecting out of the cardiophrenic angle. In patients with Hodgkin's disease particularly, enlargement of these nodes causes opacities that simulate pleuropericardial fat pads. Such node enlargement may occur as the initial presentation of patients with Hodgkin's disease,[61] although Castellino and Blank[61] have noted such enlargement more often during relapse of the disease. Thus it is important to compare the cardiophrenic angles on serial chest roentgenograms, considering this area a potential site of recurrent disease. Similarly, a reduction in the size of nodes can constitute convincing evidence of the effectiveness of therapy.

DILATATION OF THE MAIN PULMONARY ARTERY

Dilatation of the main pulmonary artery may be of sufficient degree to suggest a mediastinal neoplasm.[62] Although the great majority of cases are associated with either pulmonary arterial hypertension or left-to-right shunt, some are poststenotic and related to pulmonary valve stenosis.[62] A few are idiopathic. Idiopathic dilatation invariably does not give rise to symptoms and is unassociated with evidence of hemodynamic abnormality roentgenologically or during cardiac catheterization.[62]

Roentgenographic manifestations depend upon the cause of the dilatation. Physical examination of patients with a severe degree of dilatation may reveal a widely split second heart sound, varying little with respiration.

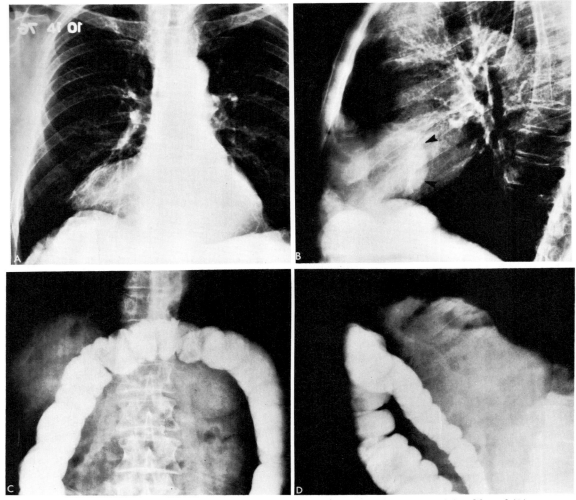

Figure 16–8. Hernia of Omentum Through the Foramen of Morgagni. Posteroanterior *(A)* and lateral *(B)* roentgenograms of this 73-year-old asymptomatic man reveal a large, fairly sharply circumscribed mass in the right cardiophrenic angle *(arrows* in *B)*. In posteroanterior projection the mass appears homogeneous in density, but in lateral projection it is somewhat inhomogeneous. Its central portion is slightly more radiolucent, suggesting tissue of fat density. Anteroposterior *(C)* and lateral *(D)* projections of the abdomen following barium enema reveal moderate elevation of the transverse colon, whose superior aspect lies contiguous to the diaphragm anteriorly. This deformity of the colon is characteristic of herniation of omentum through the foramen of Morgagni.

DILATATION OF THE MAJOR MEDIASTINAL VEINS

DILATATION OF THE SUPERIOR VENA CAVA (SVC)

The great majority of cases of SVC dilatation are the result of raised central venous pressure, commonly from cardiac decompensation, cardiac tamponade due to pericardial effusion, or constrictive pericarditis. The roentgenographic appearance is distinctive—a smooth, well-defined widening of the right side of the mediastinum. The azygos vein is almost always dilated as well, and this is a more dependable sign of

systemic hypertension because the diameter of the vein in the right tracheobronchial angle can be precisely measured. (The azygos is dilated when its diameter is greater than 10 mm when the patient is erect or 14 to 15 mm when the patient is recumbent.)

DILATATION OF THE AZYGOS AND HEMIAZYGOS VEINS

There are many causes of enlargement of the azygos and hemiazygos veins: intrahepatic and extrahepatic portal vein obstruction, anomalous pulmonary venous drainage, acquired occlusion of the inferior or superior vena cava, azygos continuation (infrahepatic interruption) of the inferior vena cava, persistence of the left superior vena cava, hepatic vein obstruction (Budd-Chiari syndrome or veno-occlusive disease of the liver), and elevated central venous pressure of any etiology.[63] The last is by far the most common cause and results from cardiac decompensation, tricuspid valvular lesions, acute pericardial tamponade, or constrictive pericarditis. Congenital infrahepatic interruption (azygos continuation) of the inferior vena cava is often associated with congenital cardiac malformation, with errors in abdominal situs, or with asplenia or polysplenia.[64] Whereas formerly angiography (via the inferior vena cava) was the method of choice in establishing the diagnosis of azygos and hemiazygos continuation (Figure 16–9), it has been shown recently that ultrasonographic examination can be pathognomonic, thus obviating an interventional procedure.[65]

Roentgenographically, dilatation of the azygos vein is evidenced by a round or oval shadow in the right tracheobronchial angle exceeding

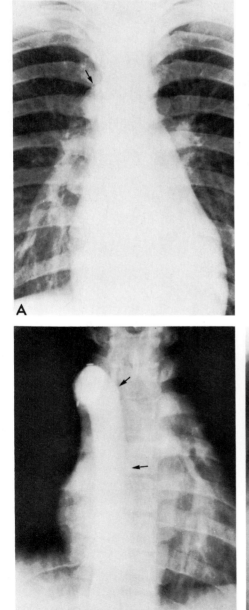

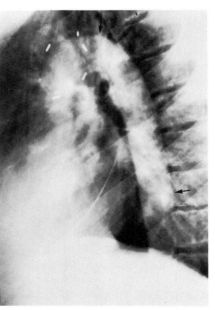

Figure 16–9. Azygos Continuation (Infradiaphragmatic Interruption) of the Inferior Vena Cava. A posteroanterior roentgenogram *(A)* of a 19-year-old asymptomatic man reveals a smooth homogeneous mass situated in the right tracheobronchial angle *(arrow)*. On the basis of this roentgenogram, this mass could be an enlarged azygos vein or an enlarged azygos lymph node. The right femoral vein was catheterized by the Seldinger technique. Anteroposterior *(B)* and lateral *(C)* roentgenograms following injection of contrast medium demonstrate a broad vessel in the right posterior mediastinum *(arrows in both projections)*. At the level of the right tracheobronchial angle, the vessel turns anteriorly to empty into the superior vena cava.

A

B

C

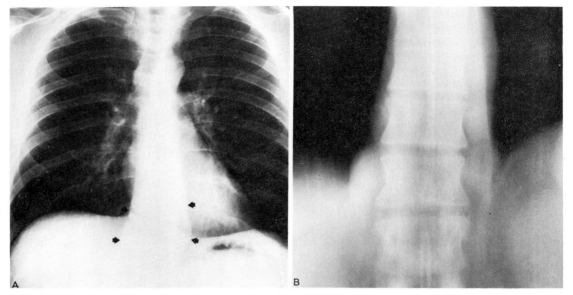

Figure 16–10. **Proximal Interruption (Azygos and Hemiazygos Continuation) of the Inferior Vena Cava.** A screening chest roentgenogram *(A)* of this 31-year-old asymptomatic man revealed an increased width of the paraspinal soft tissues in the lower thoracic region bilaterally *(arrows)*. The shadow of the azygos vein in the right tracheobronchial angle measured 10 mm, the upper limits of normal. An anteroposterior tomogram of the lower thoracic spine in the supine position *(B)* shows the bilateral opacities to be greater in width than on the erect study and to be somewhat lobulated in contour. In the recumbent position, the diameter of the azygos vein had increased to 24 mm, a marked degree of dilatation. Following insertion of a catheter into the inferior vena cava, contrast medium was injected. Excellent opacification of the inferior vena cava was observed up to the level of the renal veins, but flow proximal to that point was by way of markedly dilated azygos and hemiazygos veins. Within the thorax, the hemiazygos vein passed across the midline to join the azygos at the level of T8. The markedly dilated azygos then continued cephalad to terminate in the superior vena cava at its familiar location in the right tracheobronchial angle.

10 mm on roentgenograms obtained in the erect position or 14 mm on tomograms obtained in the supine position. In a correlative study of 54 adult patients ranging in age from 23 to 77, Preger and his colleagues[66] related the width of the azygos vein to central venous pressure. They found that when the diameter of the azygos vein was greater than 15 mm as measured on an anteroposterior chest roentgenogram obtained in the supine position, the central venous pressure was greater than 10 cm of water.

A dilated azygos vein can be differentiated from an enlarged azygos lymph node fairly easily by comparing the diameter of the shadow on roentgenograms exposed in the erect and supine positions. Dilatation of the posterior portions of the azygos or hemiazygos veins may result in widening and irregularity of the paraspinal line, on the right and left side, respectively (Figure 16–10).[67] Extreme tortuosity of a dilated azygos arch has been known to simulate a pulmonary mass on a lateral roentgenogram.[68]

The symptoms and signs of azygos and hemiazygos vein dilatation depend entirely on the cause. Most patients with congenital absence (infradiaphragmatic interruption) of the inferior vena cava are asymptomatic, but some have symptoms or signs attributable to the associated congenital heart disease.

DILATATION OF THE AORTA OR ITS BRANCHES

ANEURYSMS OF THE THORACIC AORTA

Aortic aneurysms may be classified as arteriosclerotic, syphilitic, traumatic, dissecting (secondary to cystic medial necrosis), poststenotic (coarctation of the aorta), and "mycotic."

Aneurysms of the *ascending arch* may be saccular or fusiform, the former usually extending anteriorly and to the right (Figure 16–11). When large enough, such an aneurysm may erode the sternum and give rise to a prominent thumping pulsation over the anterior chest wall—thus the designation, "aneurysm of signs." An aneurysm of the *transverse arch* tends to compress contiguous structures, resulting in a brassy cough, hemoptysis, hoarseness, and cyanosis of the face and upper extremities and thus is sometimes referred to as the "aneurysm of symptoms." It produces a mass in the midmediastinum that characteristically obliterates the aortic window. Aneurysms of the *descending arch* and of the *descending thoracic aorta* may become large without occasioning symptoms but may erode the vertebral column. Aneurysms of the descending aorta are most often arteriosclerotic in origin. During aortography only a small portion of the aneurysm may be outlined with contrast medium because of partial obliteration of the aneurysmal cavity by a thrombus.

Calcification of the walls of thoracic aneurysms is relatively common (Figure 16–11). At one time, the presence of calcification in the supravalvular portion of the ascending arch was highly suggestive of syphilis, but nowadays, such calcification is much more frequently associated with advanced atherosclerosis and with aortic valve disease.

Traumatic aneurysms of the thoracic aorta typically involve the posterior portion of the descending arch just beyond the origin of the left subclavian artery. They tend to project to the left (*see* complete description in Chapter 13).

Dissecting aneurysms may occur at any site in the thoracic aorta but originate most often in the ascending arch. Their highest incidence is in patients with Marfan's syndrome (cystic medial necrosis of the aorta), aortic coarctation, hypertension, or during pregnancy. Arteriosclerosis may be present because of the age of most of these patients but is more likely a coincidental finding than a significant contributing factor in the dissection. Hemorrhage into the tissues surrounding the dissection may be revealed by widening or obliteration of the paraspinal shadow at any point along the descending aorta. In a number of studies reported recently,[69–73] dynamic CT scanning has been shown to be the procedure of choice in the initial investigation of these patients (Figure 16–12). Findings include localized increase in aortic caliber, displaced intimal calcifications, intimal flaps, differential time density between the two lumens, and false channels. Despite the accuracy of CT, however, aortography will still be required in some cases prior to surgery.

Dissecting aneurysms usually cause severe retrosternal pain that radiates through to the back, and sometimes syncope. Physical examination may reveal evidence of acute peripheral arterial occlusion, aortic insufficiency, or bruits over the affected portion of aorta.

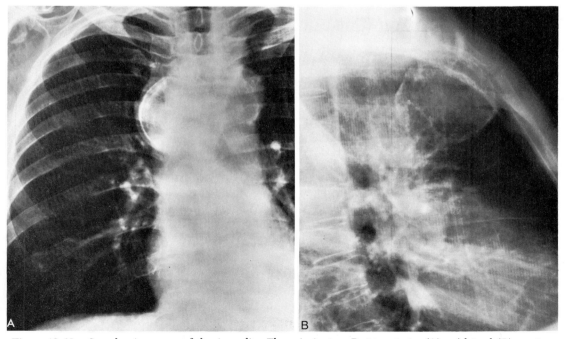

Figure 16–11. Saccular Aneurysm of the Ascending Thoracic Aorta. Posteroanterior (*A*) and lateral (*B*) roentgenograms of this 52-year-old asymptomatic man reveal a well-circumscribed mass situated in the anterior mediastinum and projecting entirely to the right. Its wall is densely calcified. The etiology of the aneurysm was not established.

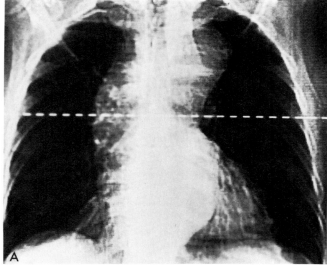

Figure 16–12. **Dissecting Aneurysm of the Ascending Aorta.** A scout view of the thorax obtained at the time of computed tomography (A) reveals a markedly elongated dilated thoracic aorta. Following injection of contrast medium, a CT scan obtained at the level of the dashed line (B) and a diagrammatic representation of the scan (C) reveal dense opacification of the true lumen of the aorta (AA in C), anterolateral to which is a large half-moon–shaped false channel (D in C), representing the dissection. AA = Ascending aorta; D = dissection; PA = pulmonary artery; svc = superior vena cava.

BUCKLING AND ANEURYSM OF THE INNOMINATE ARTERY

Both of these conditions present as a smooth well-defined mass in the right superior paramediastinal area, extending upward from the aortic arch. Buckling is a relatively common condition that occurs in patients with hypertension or arteriosclerosis or both. The innominate artery is about 5 cm long and is firmly fixed proximally at its origin from the aorta and distally by the subclavian and carotid arteries. When the thoracic aorta elongates and dilates as a result of atherosclerosis, the arch moves cephalad, carrying with it the origin of the innominate artery. Because of its fixation superiorly, the innominate artery buckles to the right.[74] When the artery buckles posteriorly and laterally, it occasionally impresses deeply into the lung, becoming almost completely surrounded by lung parenchyma and thus simulating a mass.[75] The diagnosis may be suggested roentgenographically by the association of elongation and tortuosity of the thoracic aorta, although CT or aortography may be required

sometimes to establish the vascular nature of the opacity. Occasionally, a similar appearance may be present in the left superior paramediastinal area as a result of buckling of the left common carotid artery.[76]

MEDIASTINAL MASSES SITUATED PREDOMINANTLY IN THE POSTERIOR COMPARTMENT

The posterior mediastinal compartment lies between the pericardium and the anterior aspect of the vertebral column. It contains the descending thoracic aorta, the esophagus, the thoracic duct, the lower portion of the vagus nerves, and the posterior group of mediastinal lymph nodes. Since by definition the posterior limit of the mediastinum is formed by the anterior surface of the vertebral column, the paravertebral zones and posterior gutters are anatomically excluded. However, since these areas contain structures of importance in the etiology of posterior mediastinal masses—including the sympathetic nerve chains and peripheral nerves—these zones customarily are included with the posterior mediastinum.

Approximately 30 per cent of posterior mediastinal tumors are malignant neoplasms.[46]

NEUROGENIC NEOPLASMS

Neoplasms of neural origin can originate from the nerve sheath, the nerve cell, or from all nerve elements (axon, sheath, cells, and connective tissue).[24] Nerve sheath tumors are the most common of these and are almost invariably benign. Neoplasms arising from nerve elements other than the sheath are more frequently malignant.[24] Neoplasms of neural origin are commonly divided into three groups:

1. Those arising from peripheral nerves, *i.e.*, neurofibromas and neurilemomas. Neurofibromas arise from endoneural tissue, and neurilemomas (schwannomas) from the sheath of Schwann. Mediastinal neurofibromas may be associated with neurofibromas elsewhere in the body (von Recklinghausen's neurofibromatosis).

2. Those arising from sympathetic ganglia, *i.e.*, ganglioneuromas, neuroblastomas, and sympathicoblastomas. The first of these is benign, and the last two are increasingly malignant, undifferentiated varieties of ganglion cell neoplasms, the last being composed of embryonal sympathicoblasts.

3. Those arising from paraganglionic cells, *i.e.*, pheochromocytomas and paragangliomas

(chemodectomas). These neoplasms may be benign or malignant. Chemodectomas are believed to originate from the aortic bodies that are innervated by the sensory branches of the vagus nerve. A number of aortic bodies are situated between the pulmonary artery and the aorta.[77]

With the exception of chemodectoma, neurogenic neoplasms are almost invariably located in the posterior mediastinum, anywhere from the thoracic inlet to the diaphragm. Neurofibromas and neurilemomas constitute by far the great majority of neurogenic neoplasms in adults, and ganglioneuromas and neuroblastomas are the most common in children.

Roentgenographically, the appearance of all neurogenic neoplasms is very similar—sharply circumscribed round or oval shadows of homogeneous density in the paravertebral zones on one or the other side (Figure 16–13). The presence of calcification can aid in the differentiation of neurogenic tumors from other posterior mediastinal tumors, at least in children, being relatively common in primary and rare in secondary neoplasms.[78] Although the presence of calcium is helpful in distinguishing a neoplasm from a cyst, it is not a reliable indicator of either the benignity or malignancy of a neoplasm.[79] The ribs or vertebrae are eroded in some cases, just as often by benign as by malignant neoplasms. A neurofibroma that originates in a nerve root within the spinal canal may be shaped like a dumbbell or an hourglass, part being inside and part outside the spinal canal. In such circumstances the intervertebral

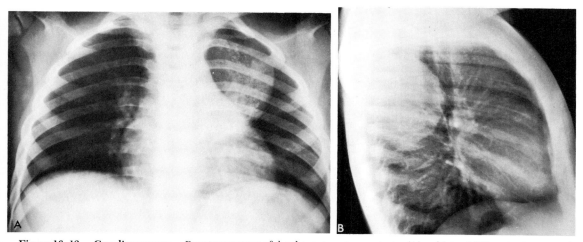

Figure 16–13.   Ganglioneuroma.   Roentgenograms of the thorax in anteroposterior *(A)* and lateral *(B)* projections reveal a smooth, sharply circumscribed mass situated in the left paravertebral gutter superiorly. The mass contains numerous speckled deposits of calcium throughout its substance. The spine was normal. Histologically, the mass proved to be a well-differentiated, juvenile ganglioneuroma. The patient was an asymptomatic 5-year-old boy. (Courtesy of Bernadette Nogrady, Montreal Children's Hospital.)

foramen may be expanded. Pleural effusion occurs in some cases and, like bone erosion, does not necessarily signify malignancy.[23]

In the majority of patients, neurogenic neoplasms do not give rise to symptoms and are identified on screening chest roentgenograms.[46] Compression of intercostal nerves or tracheobronchial airways can give rise to pain or dyspnea in a minority of patients.

MENINGOCELE (MENINGOMYELOCELE)

This rare anomaly of the spinal canal consists of herniation of the leptomeninges through an intervertebral foramen. The lesions are usually single and may be situated anywhere between the thoracic inlet and the diaphragm. A meningocele contains cerebrospinal fluid only; a meningomyelocele contains nerve elements also.

These lesions show no features that distinguish them from solid neurogenic neoplasms. An associated kyphoscoliosis is frequent,[80] the meningocele usually being situated at the apex of the curvature on its convex side. Enlargement of the intervertebral foramen is a very common finding. Association with generalized neurofibromatosis is common but is of little differential value since posterior mediastinal neurofibroma and neurofibrosarcoma may also be part of von Recklinghausen's disease.

Myelography usually shows the contrast medium passing into the meningocele.[23] The extent and nature of the lesion and the presence of associated bony erosion can be well established by CT, with or without metrizamide myelography.[81]

NEURENTERIC CYST

This rare derivative of the foregut, known also as archenteric cyst and the "split notochord syndrome,"[82] results from incomplete separation of endoderm from the notochordal plate during early embryonic life.[83] Histologically, the cyst wall contains both gastrointestinal and neural elements. The epithelium most commonly resembles small intestine, stomach, or esophagus. The cyst is connected by a stalk to the meninges and commonly to a portion of the gastrointestinal tract. If attachment is to the esophagus within the thorax, communication is rare. However, if attachment is to the gastrointestinal tract within the abdomen, in most cases there is communication so that the cyst may contain

gas and may opacify with barium during examination of the upper gastrointestinal tract.

The roentgenographic appearance is of a sharply defined, round or oval lobulated mass of homogeneous density, frequently associated with congenital defects of the thoracic spine.[23, 84] Neurenteric cysts typically produce symptoms, including pain, and therefore become manifest early in life.

GASTROENTERIC CYST

Like bronchogenic and neurenteric cysts, gastroenteric cysts develop from the foregut and sometimes are grouped with bronchogenic cysts under the term "bronchoesophageal cysts."[84] Also known as intramural esophageal cysts or esophageal duplication,[82] they represent a failure of complete vacuolation of the originally solid esophagus to produce a hollow tube. They are lined by esophageal, gastric, or small intestinal mucosa in contrast to bronchial cysts, which are lined by bronchial mucosa (Figure 16–14). The majority are detected in infancy or childhood and are said to be more common in males.[38] Peptic ulceration may occur in the gastrointestinal mucosa and may cause pain.[38]

These rare lesions occur in the paraspinal region of the posterior mediastinum. They are usually round or oval and are homogeneous in density. Communication with the gastrointestinal tract may allow the passage of gas into the cyst and probably results from perforation of the cyst into the esophageal lumen in association with peptic ulceration.[23] In the majority of cases, these lesions produce no symptoms.

PRIMARY LESIONS OF THE ESOPHAGUS

Esophageal lesions that may present roentgenographically as mediastinal masses or as causes of mediastinal widening include neoplasms, diverticula, esophageal hiatus hernia, and megaesophagus.

Neoplasms of the Esophagus. Primary carcinoma of the esophagus rarely becomes large enough to be visible but may obliterate the aortic window or cause deformity of the superior or inferior pleuroesophageal stripes as viewed in posteroanterior projection. Thickening of the posterior tracheal stripe has been emphasized as a reliable sign of mediastinal disease,[85] specifically as a sign of squamous-cell carcinoma of the esophagus.[87] CT may be of considerable

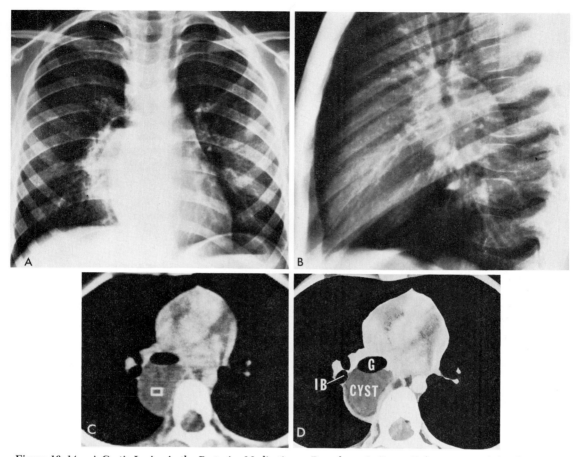

Figure 16–14.   A Cystic Lesion in the Posterior Mediastinum: Bronchogenic Cyst.   Posteroanterior *(A)* and lateral *(B)* roentgenograms of the chest of this eight-year-old white girl reveal a large, fairly well demarcated mass projecting to the right of the mediastinum and containing a prominent fluid level. A CT scan was performed to clarify the anatomic extent of the lesion although its cystic nature was well recognized. Following injection of contrast medium, a CT scan obtained approximately 4 cm below the carina *(C)* and a diagrammatic representation of the scan *(D)* revealed the mass to relate to the medial aspect of the right intermediate bronchus and to completely obliterate the azygoesophageal recess. The periphery of the mass opacifies although its central portion is of low attenuation, indicating its fluid nature. Histologically, the mass was a typical bronchogenic cyst. IB = Intermediate bronchus; G = gas in cyst. (Standard roentgenograms courtesy of Dr. Guy Hicks, Birmingham Children's Hospital.)

value in identifying the extent of mediastinal spread in patients with carcinoma of the esophagus.[86] A benign neoplasm of the esophagus (which is rare) may grow large and present as a rounded mass projecting to one or both sides of the posterior mediastinum (Figure 16–15).[88]

Esophageal Diverticula.   Diverticula occur in the pharyngeal region (Zenker's), in the midthoracic region as a result of cicatricial contraction from healing histoplasmosis or tuberculosis (traction diverticulum), and in the lower esophagus as a result of outpouching of the mucosa through defects in the muscular wall at the point of entry of blood vessels (pulsion diverticulum). Unlike the other two varieties, traction diverticula seldom if ever are visible on plain roentgenograms. Zenker's diverticu-

lum originates between the transverse and oblique fibers of the inferior pharyngeal constrictor muscle and thus is a pharyngeal rather than an esophageal diverticulum. It may become large enough to be identified in the superior mediastinum on plain roentgenograms, frequently containing an air-fluid level. Symptoms include dysphagia, chronic cough due to aspiration, and in some cases recurrent aspiration pneumonia.

Diverticula arising from the lower third of the esophagus are almost always congenital in origin and present as round, cystlike structures to the right of the midline just above the diaphragm. An air-fluid level is present in most cases. Barium studies are diagnostic.

Megaesophagus.   Of the many causes of dil-

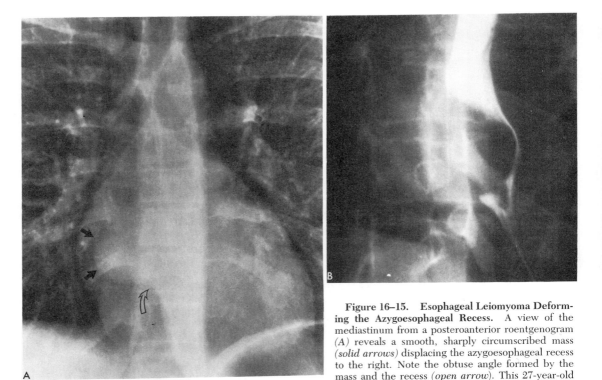

Figure 16–15. Esophageal Leiomyoma Deforming the Azygoesophageal Recess. A view of the mediastinum from a posteroanterior roentgenogram (A) reveals a smooth, sharply circumscribed mass (*solid arrows*) displacing the azygoesophageal recess to the right. Note the obtuse angle formed by the mass and the recess (*open arrow*). This 27-year-old woman complained of mild retrosternal discomfort on swallowing solid food. Barium opacification of the esophagus (B) reveals a sharply circumscribed deformity of the barium column in a configuration typical of an extramucosal intramural lesion. Proved leiomyoma.

atation of the esophagus—inflammatory stenosis, scleroderma, carcinoma, and achalasia—the last-named causes the most severe generalized dilatation. The dilated esophagus is apparent as a shadow projecting entirely to the right side of the mediastinum. Since it is behind the heart, it does not cause a silhouette sign with that structure. The trachea may be bulged anteriorly. An air-containing esophagus may be identified on standard roentgenograms of some patients with scleroderma.

Esophageal Hiatus Hernia. Standard roentgenograms of the chest often reveal the herniated portion of stomach directly behind the heart and slightly to the right of the midline. A fluid level is present in many cases. When the diagnosis is in doubt on the basis of evidence provided by plain roentgenograms, barium opacification confirms the presence or absence of the hernia.

DISEASES OF THE THORACIC SPINE

Neoplasms. A wide variety of primary neoplasms of bone and cartilage may involve the thoracic spine and posterior rib cage, including osteochondroma, aneurysmal bone cyst, chon-

drosarcoma, osteogenic sarcoma, Ewing's tumor, myeloma, and, perhaps most commonly, metastatic neoplasm. In a few cases, the major roentgenographic finding is an extraosseous soft tissue mass, and identification of the primary bone lesion requires careful roentgenographic study. The lymphomas, particularly Hodgkin's disease, may be manifested roentgenologically as a fusiform paraspinal soft tissue mass produced by enlargement of the posterior parietal group of lymph nodes; in such cases, contiguous vertebrae may be eroded by extranodal invasion.

Infectious Spondylitis. Tuberculous and nontuberculous spondylitis are often associated with a paraspinal mass caused by inflammation and abscess formation in contiguous soft tissues. Commonly, there is a bilateral fusiform mass in the paravertebral zone, with its maximal diameter at the point of major bone destruction.

Fracture with Hematoma Formation. Fractures of thoracic vertebral bodies may result in extraosseous hemorrhage and the development of unilateral or bilateral paraspinal masses. Although the fracture is usually visible roentgenographically, the major evidence of its presence may be deformity of the contiguous paraspinal soft tissues.

EXTRAMEDULLARY HEMATOPOIESIS

Although rare, this mediastinal abnormality should be borne in mind in any case of a paravertebral mass in a patient with severe anemia, with or without splenomegaly and hepatomegaly.[40, 89] Extramedullary hematopoiesis occurs as a compensatory phenomenon in various diseases in which there is inadequate production or excessive destruction of blood cells. The origin of extramedullary hematopoiesis in the paravertebral regions is obscure but it has been postulated that it represents an extension from marrow cavities or perhaps from lymph nodes or embryonic rests.[89]

The characteristic roentgenographic finding is of multiple masses, smooth or lobulated in contour and of homogeneous density, situated in the paravertebral regions, either unilaterally or bilaterally,[29] usually below the seventh thoracic vertebra. A presumptive diagnosis usually can be made when this roentgenographic finding is present in patients with severe anemia and splenomegaly.

The presence of extramedullary hematopoiesis within the thorax usually occasions no symptoms.

REFERENCES

1. Baron, R. L., Levitt, R. G., Sagel, S. S., and Stanley, R. J.: Computed tomography in the evaluation of mediastinal widening. Radiology, *138*:107, 1981.
2. Siegel, M. J., Sagel, S. S., and Reed, K.: The value of computed tomography in the diagnosis and management of pediatric mediastinal abnormalities. Radiology, *142*:149, 1982.
3. Heitzman, E. R.: The Mediastinum: Radiologic Correlations with Anatomy and Pathology. St. Louis, C. V. Mosby Co., 1977.
4. Craddock, D. R., Logan, A., and Mayell, M.: Traumatic rupture of the oesophagus and stomach. Thorax, *23*:657, 1968.
5. Christoforidis, A., and Nelson, S. W.: Spontaneous rupture of esophagus with emphasis on the roentgenologic diagnosis. Am. J. Roentgenol., *78*:574, 1957.
6. Schowengerdt, C. G., Suyemoto, R., and Main, F. B.: Granulomatous and fibrous mediastinitis. A review and analysis of 180 cases. J. Thorac. Cardiovasc. Surg., *57*:365, 1969.
7. Goodwin, R. A., Nickell, J. A., and Des Prez, R. M.: Mediastinal fibrosis complicating healed primary histoplasmosis and tuberculosis. Medicine, *51*:227, 1972.
8. Wieder, S., White, T. J., III, Salazar, J., et al.: Pulmonary artery occlusion due to histoplasmosis. A.J.R., *138*:243, 1982.
9. Arnett, E. N., Bacos, J. M., Macher, A. M., et al.: Fibrosing mediastinitis causing pulmonary arterial hypertension without pulmonary venous hypertension. Clinical and necropsy observations. Am. J. Med., *63*:634, 1977.
10. Comings, D. E., Skubi, K.-B., Eyes, J. V., and Motulsky, A. G.: Familial multifocal fibrosclerosis. Findings suggesting that retroperitoneal fibrosis, mediastinal fibrosis, sclerosing cholangitis, Riedel's thyroiditis, and pseudotumor of the orbit may be different manifestations of a single disease. Ann. Intern. Med., *66*:884, 1967.
11. Graham, J. R., Suby, H. I., LeCompte, P. R., and Sadowsky, N. L.: Fibrotic disorders associated with methysergide therapy for headache. N. Engl. J. Med., *274*:359, 1966.
12. Nelson, W. P., Lundberg, G. D., and Dickerson, R. B.: Pulmonary artery obstruction and cor pulmonale due to chronic fibrous mediastinitis. Am. J. Med., *38*:279, 1965.
13. Munsell, W. P.: Pneumomediastinum: A report of 28 cases and review of the literature. J.A.M.A., *202*:689, 1967.
14. Gilmartin, D.: Mediastinal emphysema in Melbourne children. With particular reference to measles and giant-cell pneumonia. Australas. Radiol., *15*:27, 1971.
15. Morgan, E. J., and Henderson, D. A.: Pneumomediastinum as a complication of athletic competition. Thorax, *36*:155, 1981.
16. Macklin, M. T., and Macklin, C. C.: Malignant interstitial emphysema of the lungs and mediastinum as an important occult complication in many respiratory diseases and other conditions: An interpretation of the clinical literature in the light of laboratory experiment. Medicine, *23*:281, 1944.
17. Rudhe, U., and Ozonoff, M. B.: Pneumomediastinum and pneumothorax in the newborn. Acta Radiol. (Diagn.), *4*:193, 1966.
18. Macpherson, R. I., Chernick, V., and Reed, M.: The complications of respirator therapy in the newborn. J. Can. Assoc. Radiol., *23*:91, 1972.
19. Kleinman, P. K., Brill, P. W., and Whalen, J. P.: Anterior pathway for transdiaphragmatic extension of pneumomediastinum. Am. J. Roentgenol., *131*:271, 1978.
20. Rogers, L. F., Puig, A. W., Dooley, B. N., and Cuello, L.: Diagnostic considerations in mediastinal emphysema: A pathophysiologic-roentgenologic approach to Boerhaave's syndrome and spontaneous pneumomediastinum. Am. J. Roentgenol., *115*:495, 1972.
21. Levin, B.: The continuous diaphragm sign. A newly-recognized sign of pneumomediastinum. Clin. Radiol., *24*:337, 1973.
22. Gray, J. M., and Hanson, G. C.: Mediastinal emphysema: Aetiology, diagnosis, and treatment. Thorax, *21*:325, 1966.
23. Leigh, T. F.: Mass lesions of the mediastinum. Radiol. Clin. North Am., *1*:377, 1963.
24. Wychulis, A. R., Payne, W. S., Clagett, O. T., and Woolner, L. B.: Surgical treatment of mediastinal tumors. A 40-year experience. J. Thorac. Cardiovasc. Surg., *62*:379, 1971.
25. Benjamin, S. P., McCormack, L. J., Effler, D. B., and Groves, L. K.: Primary tumors of the mediastinum. Chest, *62*:297, 1972.
26. Brown, L. R., Muhm, J. R., and Gray, J. E.: Radiographic detection of thymoma. Am. J. Roentgenol., *134*:1181, 1980.
27. Herlitzka, A. J., and Gale, J. W.: Tumors and cysts of the mediastinum. Survey of one hundred and seventy-four mediastinal tumors treated surgically during the past eighteen years at the University of Wisconsin hospitals. A.M.A. Arch. Surg., *76*:697, 1958.
28. Teplick, J. G., Nedwich, A., and Haskin, M. E.:

Roentgenographic features of thymolipoma. Am. J. Roentgenol., *117*:873, 1973.

29. Leigh, T. F., and Weens, H. S.: Roentgen aspects of mediastinal lesions. Semin. Roentgenol., *4*:59, 1969.

30. Mink, J. H., Bein, M. E., Sukov, R., et al.: Computed tomography of the anterior mediastinum in patients with myasthenia gravis and suspected thymoma. Am. J. Roentgenol., *130*:239, 1978.

31. Moore, A. V., Korobkin, M., Powers, B., et al.: Thymoma detection by mediastinal CT: Patients with myasthenia gravis. A.J.R., *138*:217, 1982.

32. Fon, G. T., Bein, M. E., Mancusco, A. A., et al.: Computed tomography of the anterior mediastinum in myasthenia gravis. Radiology, *142*:135, 1982.

33. Bertelsen, S., Malmstrøm, J., Heerfordt, J., and Pedersen, H.: Tumours of the thymic region. Symptomatology, diagnosis, treatment, and prognosis. Thorax, *30*:19, 1975.

34. Rosenthal, T., Hertz, M., Samra, Y., and Shahin, N.: Thymoma: Clinical and additional radiologic signs. Chest, *65*:428, 1974.

35. Baron, R. L., Lee, J. K. T., Sagel, S. S., and Peterson, R. R.: Computed tomography of the normal thymus. Radiology, *142*:121, 1982.

36. Baron, R. L., Lee, J. K. T., Sagel, S. S., and Levitt, R. G.: Computed tomography of the abnormal thymus. Radiology, *142*:127, 1982.

37. Wenger, M. E., Dines, D. E., Ahmann, D. L., and Good, C. A.: Primary mediastinal choriocarcinoma. Mayo Clin. Proc., *43*:570, 1968.

38. Lyons, H. A., Calvy, G. L., and Sammons, B. P.: The diagnosis and classification of mediastinal masses. I. A Study of 782 cases. Ann. Intern. Med., *51*:897, 1959.

39. Friedman, A. C., Pyatt, R. S., Hartman, D. S., et al.: CT of benign cystic teratomas. A.J.R., *138*:659, 1982.

40. Hochholzer, L., Theros, E. G., and Rosen, S. H.: Some unusual lesions of the mediastinum: Roentgenologic and pathologic features. Semin. Roentgenol., *4*:74, 1969.

41. Steinmetz, W. H., and Hays, R. A.: Primary seminoma of the mediastinum. Report of a case with an unusual site of metastasis and review of the literature. Am. J. Roentgenol., *86*:669, 1961.

42. Cohen, B. A., and Needle, M. A.: Primary mediastinal choriocarcinoma in a man. Chest, *67*:106, 1975.

43. Fine, G., Smith, R. W., Jr., and Pachter, M. R.: Primary extragenital choriocarcinoma in the male subject. Case report and review of the literature. Am. J. Med., *32*:776, 1962.

44. Leading article: Primary mediastinal choriocarcinoma. Br. Med. J., *2*:135, 1969.

45. Richardson, R. L., Schoumacher, R. A., Mehmet, F. F., et al.: The unrecognized extragonadal germ cell cancer syndrome. Ann. Intern. Med., *94*:181, 1981.

46. Daniel, R. A., Jr., Diveley, W. L., Edwards, W. H., and Chamberlain, N.: Mediastinal tumors. Ann. Surg., *151*:783, 1960.

47. Rietz, K.-A., and Werner, B.: Intrathoracic goiter. Acta Chir. Scand., *119*:379, 1960.

48. Glazer, G. M., Axel, L., and Moss, A. A.: CT diagnosis of mediastinal thyroid. A.J.R., *138*:495, 1982.

49. Hardy, J. D., Snaveley, J. R., and Langford, H. G.: Low intrathoracic parathyroid adenoma. Large functioning tumor representing fifth parathyroid, opposite eighth dorsal vertebra with independent arterial supply and opacified at operation with arteriogram. Ann. Surg., *159*:310, 1965.

50. Krudy, A. G., Doppman, J. L., Brennan, M. F., et al.: The detection of mediastinal parathyroid glands by comuted tomography, selective arteriography, and venous sampling. An analysis of 17 cases. Radiology, *140*:739, 1981.

51. Homer, M. J., Wechsler, R. J., and Carter, B. L.: Mediastinal lipomatosis. CT confirmation of a normal variant. Radiology, *128*:657, 1978.

52. Chalaoui, J., Sylvestre, J., Dussault, R. G., et al.: Thoracic fatty lesions: Some usual and unusual appearances. Can. Med. Assoc. J., *32*:197, 1981.

53. Mendez, G., Jr., Isikoff, M. B., Isikoff, S. K., and Sinner, W. N.: Fatty tumors of the thorax demonstrated by CT. A.J.R., *133*:207, 1979.

54. Price, J. E., Jr., and Rigler, L. G.: Widening of the mediastinum resulting from fat accumulation. Radiology, *96*:497, 1970.

55. van de Putte, L. B. A., Wagenaar, J. P. M., and San, K. H.: Paracardiac lipomatosis in exogenous Cushing's syndrome. Thorax, *28*:653, 1973.

56. Castleman, B. (ed.): Case Records of the Massachusetts General Hospital, Case 40011. N. Engl. J. Med., *250*:26, 1954.

57. Tung, K. S. K., and McCormack, L. J.: Angiomatous lymphoid hamartoma. Report of five cases with a review of the literature. Cancer, *20*:525, 1967.

58. Hammond, D. I.: Giant lymph node hyperplasia of the posterior mediastinum. J. Can. Assoc. Radiol., *30*:256, 1979.

59. Pugatch, R. D., Braver, J. H., Robbins, A. H., and Faling, L. J.: CT diagnosis of pericardial cysts. Am. J. Roentgenol., *131*:515, 1978.

60. Paris, F., Tarazona, V., Casillas, M., et al.: Hernia of Morgagni. Thorax, *28*:631, 1973.

61. Castellino, R. A., and Blank, N.: Adenopathy of the cardiophrenic angle (diaphragmatic) lymph nodes. Am. J. Roentgenol, *114*:509, 1972.

62. Buckingham, W. B., Sutton, G. C., and Meszaros, W. T.: Abnormalities of the pulmonary artery resembling intrathoracic neoplasms. Dis. Chest, *40*:698, 1961.

63. Bernal-Ramirez, M., Hatch, H. B., Jr., and Bower, P. J.: Interruption of the inferior vena cava with azygos continuation. Chest, *65*:469, 1974.

64. Berdon, W. E., and Baker, D. H.: Plain film findings in azygos continuation of the inferior vena cava. Am. J. Roentgenol., *104*:452, 1968.

65. Garris, J. B., Kangarloo, H., and Sample, W. F.: Ultrasonic diagnosis of infrahepatic interruption of the inferior vena cava with azygos (hemiazygos) continuation. Radiology, *134*:179, 1980.

66. Preger, L., Hooper, T. I., Steinbach, H. L., and Hoffman, J. I. E.: Width of azygos vein related to central venous pressures. Radiology, *93*:521, 1969.

67. Floyd, G. D., and Nelson, W. P.: Developmental interruption of the inferior vena cava with azygos and hemiazygos substitution. Unusual radiographic features. Radiology, *119*:55, 1976.

68. Rockoff, S. D., and Druy, E. M.: Tortuous azygos arch simulating a pulmonary lesion. A.J.R., *138*:577, 1982.

69. Godwin, J. D., Herfkens, R. L., Skiöldbrand, C. G., et al.: Evaluation of dissections and aneurysms of the thoracic aorta by conventional and dynamic CT scanning. Radiology, *136*:125, 1980.

70. Gross, S. C., Barr, I., Eyler, W. R., et al.: Computed tomography in dissection of the thoracic aorta. Radiology, *136*:135, 1980.

71. Egan, T. J., Neiman, H. L., Herman, R. J., et al.: Computed tomography in the diagnosis of aortic aneurysm dissection or traumatic injury. Radiology, *136*:141, 1980.

72. Lardé, D., Belloir, C., Vasile, N., et al.: Computed tomography of aortic dissection. Radiology, *136*:147, 1980.

73. Heiberg, E., Wolverson, M., Sundaram, M., et al.: CT findings in thoracic aortic dissection. Am. J. Roentgenol., *136*:13, 1981.

74. Schneider, H. J., and Felson, B.: Buckling of the innominate artery simulating aneurysm and tumor. Am. J. Roentgenol., *85*:1106, 1961.

75. Christensen, E. E., Landay, M. J., Dietz, G. W., and Brinley, G.: Buckling of the innominate artery simulating a right apical lung mass. Am. J. Roentgenol., *131*:119, 1978.

76. Sandler, C. M., Toombs, B. D., and Lester, R. G.: Buckling of the left common carotid artery simulating mediastinal neoplasm. Am. J. Roentgenol., *133*:312, 1979.

77. Surakiatchanukul, S., Goodsitt, E., and Storer, J.: Chemodectoma of the aortic body. Chest, *60*:464, 1971.

78. Bar-Ziv, J., and Nogrady, M. B.: Mediastinal neuroblastoma and ganglioneuroma. The differentiation between primary and secondary involvement on the chest roentgenogram. Am. J. Roentgenol., *125*:380, 1975.

79. Reed, J. C., Hallet, K. K., and Feigin, D. S.: Neural tumors of the thorax: Subject review from the AFIP. Radiology, *126*:9, 1978.

80. Miles, J., Pennybacker, J., and Sheldon, P.: Intrathoracic meningocele. Its development and association with neurofibromatosis. J. Neurol. Neurosurg. Psychiatr., *32*:99, 1969.

81. Healy, J. F., Wells, M. V., Carlstrom, T., and Rosenkrantz, H.: Lateral thoracic meningocele demonstrated by computerized tomography. Comput. Tomogr., *4*:159, 1980.

82. Kirwan, W. O., Walbaum, P. R., and McCormack, R. J. M.: Cystic intrathoracic derivatives of the foregut and their complications. Thorax, *28*:424, 1973.

83. Madewell, J. E., Sobonya, R. E., and Reed, J. C.: Neurenteric cyst. RPC from the AFIP. Radiology, *109*:707, 1973.

84. Ochsner, J. L., and Ochsner, S. F.: Congenital cysts of the mediastinum: 20-year experience with 42 cases. Ann. Surg., *163*:909, 1966.

85. Bachman, A. L., and Teixidor, H. S.: The posterior tracheal band: A reflector of local superior mediastinal abnormality. Part 1. Br. J. Radiol., *48*:352, 1975.

86. Daffner, R. H., Halber, M. D., Postlethwait, R. W., et al.: CT of the esophagus. II. Carcinoma. Am. J. Roentgenol., *133*:1051, 1979.

87. Putman, C. E., Curtis, A. M., Westfried, M. and McLoud, T. M.: Thickening of the posterior tracheal stripe: A sign of squamous cell carcinoma of the esophagus. Radiology, *121*:533, 1976.

88. Cohen, A. M., and Cunat, J. S.: Giant esophageal leiomyoma as a mediastinal mass. J. Can. Assoc. Radiol., *32*:129, 1981.

89. Da Costa, J. L., Loh, Y. S., and Hanam, E.: Extramedullary hemopoiesis with multiple tumor-stimulating mediastinal masses in hemoglobin E–thalassemia disease. Chest, *65*:210, 1974.

17

Diseases of the Diaphragm and Chest Wall

The thoracic cage, including the chest wall and diaphragm, serves the dual purpose of enclosing and protecting the contents of the thorax and of producing the movements that effect the pleural pressure changes necessary to respiration. A multitude of diseases and anomalies affect the chest wall and diaphragm, and whether primary or secondary they may affect either or both major functions of the thoracic cage.

THE DIAPHRAGM

The normal anatomy, physiology, and roentgenology of the diaphragm are discussed in detail in Chapter 1, and it is suggested that the reader refresh his memory of these subjects before proceeding. In addition, certain aspects of the physiology of the diaphragm are described in Chapter 18, with reference to paralysis of both hemidiaphragms and alveolar hypoventilation.

ABNORMALITIES OF DIAPHRAGMATIC POSITION OR MOTION

PARALYSIS OF THE DIAPHRAGM

Paralysis of the diaphragm results from interruption of nerve impulses through the phrenic nerve, most commonly caused by invasion from neoplasm, usually of bronchogenic origin. Various benign conditions may be responsible,[1] but the second largest number of cases are those that in the absence of discoverable etiology must be labeled "idiopathic."[1] In such cases the paralysis occurs almost invariably on the right side and usually in males.

In a review of the roentgenologic manifestations of unilateral diaphragmatic paralysis, Alexander[2] described four cardinal signs: elevation of a hemidiaphragm above the normal range; diminished, absent, or paradoxical motion during respiration; paradoxical motion under conditions of augmented load such as sniffing; and finally, mediastinal swing during respiration. Roentgenographically, the elevated hemidiaphragm presents an accentuated dome configuration in both posteroanterior and lateral projections (Figure 17–1). Since its peripheral points of attachment are fixed, the costophrenic and costovertebral sulci tend to be narrowed and sharpened.

Patients with a paralyzed hemidiaphragm may be asymptomatic but frequently complain of dyspnea on effort. Vital capacity and total lung capacity are reduced by 25 to 50 per cent.

EVENTRATION

Eventration is a congenital anomaly consisting of failure of muscular development of part or all of one or both hemidiaphragms.[3] In some cases it may be difficult or impossible to differentiate eventration from diaphragmatic paralysis and, in fact, there is a tendency to use the terms synonymously.

Pathologically, an eventrated diaphragm consists of a thin membranous sheet attached peripherally to normal muscle at points of origin from the rib cage. It occurs almost exclusively on the left side, a point that may be of value in the differentiation from diaphragmatic paralysis. The latter has an approximately equal incidence on both sides, except when "idiopathic," in which circumstance it occurs almost invariably on the right side.[1] Somewhat more common than total eventration is partial eventration, usually of the anteromedial portion of the right

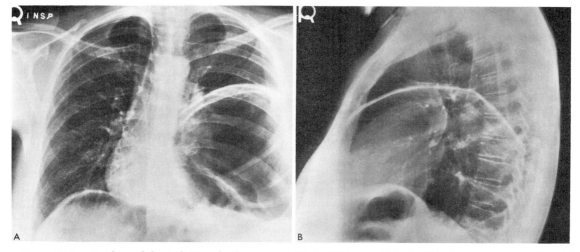

Figure 17–1. Paralysis of the Left Hemidiaphragm Associated with Severe Colonic Dilatation Secondary to Sigmoid Volvulus. Posteroanterior *(A)* and lateral *(B)* roentgenograms reveal a remarkable degree of elevation of the left hemidiaphragm. Severely dilated loops of colon are situated beneath this hemidiaphragm and to a lesser extent beneath the right one. The mediastinum is displaced considerably into the right hemithorax.

hemidiaphragm.[3] The *roentgenologic signs* of eventration are identical to those described for diaphragmatic paralysis.

Clinically, eventration of the diaphragm characteristically does not give rise to symptoms and is discovered on a screening chest roentgenogram. The major exception occurs in neonates, in whom hemidiaphragmatic elevation and mediastinal shift may be severe enough to result in ventilatory, cardiovascular, and gastrointestinal embarrassment. In such circumstances, surgical correction may be life-saving.[3]

DIAPHRAGMATIC HERNIAS

Herniation of abdominal or retroperitoneal organs or tissues into the thorax may occur through congenital or acquired weak areas in the diaphragm or through rents resulting from traumatic rupture. By far the most common diaphragmatic hernia is that which occurs through the esophageal hiatus.

HERNIA THROUGH THE ESOPHAGEAL HIATUS

It is clearly outside the scope of this work to discuss hiatus hernia in detail. Although it is the most common form of diaphragmatic hernia in the adult, its effects relate almost entirely to the gastrointestinal tract and only seldom is its presence manifested by changes in the chest roentgenogram. In infants, esophageal hiatus hernias are less common than hernias through the foramen of Bochdalek but are more common than those through the foramen of Morgagni.[4]

The diagnosis of hiatus hernia requires thorough barium study of the esophagogastric junction. Plain roentgenograms of the chest may show a mass in the posteroinferior mediastinum, usually containing a fluid level (Figure 17–2). Incarceration of such hernial contents is frequent. The development of acute upper gastrointestinal tract symptoms in a patient with a herniated stomach that has undergone volvulus should immediately raise the suspicion of acute strangulation, caused by torsion greater than 180 degrees with resultant impairment of gastric blood supply. This complication is life-threatening and necessitates immediate surgical intervention.

HERNIA THROUGH THE FORAMEN OF BOCHDALEK

In infants, herniation through the pleuroperitoneal hiatus is not only the most common form of diaphragmatic hernia but also is by far the most serious. When large, it is associated with a high death rate unless surgically corrected. Between 80 and 90 per cent of Bochdalek hernias occur on the left side,[4] partly because of the fact that defects in the right hemidiaphragm are protected by the liver.

Closure of the posterolateral portion of the diaphragm by fusion of the pleuroperitoneal

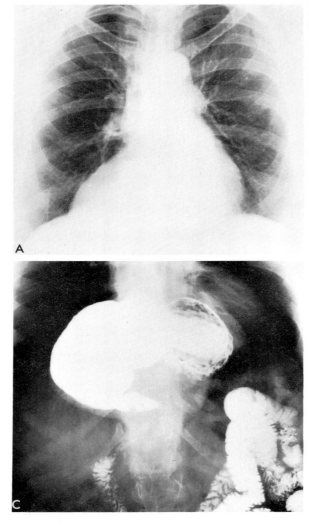

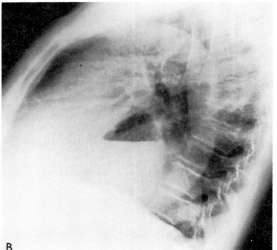

Figure 17–2. Hiatus Hernia. Posteroanterior *(A)* and lateral *(B)* roentgenograms reveal a large soft tissue mass in the posterior mediastinum, projecting to the right as a smooth, well-defined shadow in the plane of the cardiophrenic angle. A prominent air-fluid level is present within it. Note the downward displacement of the right hemidiaphragm. Roentgenography following ingestion of barium *(C)* shows herniation of the whole stomach through the esophageal hiatus into the posterior mediastinum; in the process the stomach has undergone complete organoaxial volvulus. The shadow projected in the plane of the right cardiophrenic angle on the posteroanterior roentgenogram is caused by the rotated greater curvature of the stomach. The patient is a 65-year-old woman who had no definite symptoms referable to the hernia.

membrane with the septum transversum normally occurs by the eighth week of fetal life. Since the intestines return from the yolk stalk to the abdominal cavity during the tenth week, herniation through the pleuroperitoneal hiatus may occur if the intestines return prematurely before the eighth week or if there is delayed or incomplete closure of the pleuroperitoneal membrane.[5]

The size of the defect ranges widely. When large, as with complete or almost complete absence of a hemidiaphragm, the entire abdominal contents, including the stomach, may be in the left hemithorax, thereby interfering with normal lung development and resulting in hypoplasia. Following repair of a unilateral defect, the ipsilateral lung may reinflate and develop normally or may have suffered permanent destruction, particularly of the lower lobe.[6]

The roentgenographic manifestations depend almost entirely on hernial contents and thus on the size of the defect. In infants in whom the defect is large, the roentgenographic appearance is characteristic (Figure 17–3). The ipsilateral hemidiaphragm is partly or completely obscured; multiple radiolucencies representing gas-containing loops of intestine—some containing fluid levels—are seen within the hemithorax; the heart and mediastinum are shifted into the opposite hemithorax and the ipsilateral lung is compressed and airless; and there is partial or complete absence of intestinal gas within the abdomen.[4] In some patients the presentation may be delayed: in a recent report of seven infants ranging in age from 2 to 20 months with left-sided congenital diaphragmatic hernia,[7] the roentgenographic findings were classic in only one patient; in two patients acute pneumonia was simulated; in three, gastric volvulus; and in one, pneumothorax. When the defect is small—in which circumstances it is usually discovered roentgenographically in asymptomatic adults—the hernial contents are usually retroperitoneal fat, a portion of the spleen or kidney, or omentum.

Large Bochdalek hernias are a rare cause of acute respiratory distress in neonates, usually resulting in death unless surgical correction is performed promptly. If infants survive without surgical correction, there is the added danger of strangulation of herniated bowel.[4] It is vital to note that the roentgenographic presentation of congenital right diaphragmatic hernia may be delayed for several days after birth.

HERNIA THROUGH THE FORAMEN OF MORGAGNI

Morgagni (retrosternal or parasternal) hernia is a rare form of congenital diaphragmatic hernia, constituting less than 10 per cent in most series.[4] The foramina of Morgagni are small clefts bounded by diaphragmatic muscle fibers originating from the sternum medially and from the seventh costal cartilages laterally. They are triangular, the base being formed by the anterior thoracic wall and the apex being directed posteriorly. The clefts contain the mammary vessels and normally are filled with loose areolar connective tissue and fat. Since the foramen relates to the heart on the left side, the majority of herniations occur on the right.

Although these defects are developmental in origin, it is probable that herniation requires the additional mechanism of obesity, at least in adults. In contrast to Bochdalek hernias, a peritoneal sac is present in most cases. Usually the content of the hernial sac is omentum.

Roentgenographically, the typical appearance is that of a smooth, well-defined opacity in the right cardiophrenic angle. In the majority of patients the shadow is of homogeneous density in which circumstance the herniated viscus is usually liver; the diagnosis in these cases can be confirmed noninvasively by radionuclide scanning.[8] Occasionally, the opacity is inhomogeneous as a result of either an air-containing loop of bowel or the predominantly fatty nature of the hernial contents. In the latter situation the hernia is likely to contain omentum, and a barium enema study will reveal the transverse colon to be situated high in the abdomen with a peak situated anteriorly and superiorly (*see* Figure 16–8, page 708), a finding that is virtually diagnostic.

The majority of hernias through the foramen of Morgagni do not give rise to symptoms.

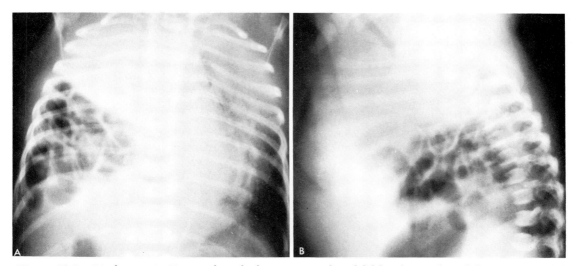

Figure 17–3. Diaphragmatic Hernia Through the Foramen of Bochdalek. This newborn baby was referred for roentgenography of the chest when it was noted in the nursery that he was cyanotic and showed chest retraction, subcostal indrawing, and grunting respiration. These roentgenograms in anteroposterior (A) and lateral (B) projections demonstrate numerous loops of air-filled bowel in the posteroinferior portion of the right hemithorax. The right lung above the hernia contents is airless, and the mediastinum is displaced considerably to the left. Only the lower portion of the left lung appears to be air-containing. At thoracotomy, the right hemithorax was found to contain the liver, stomach, small intestine, kidneys, and adrenal gland; the right lung was severely hypoplastic. The hernial contents were returned to the abdomen and a large right pleuroperitoneal foramen was closed. The infant died 2 days later.

When the sac contains portions of the gastrointestinal tract, strangulation and obstruction may occur.

SUBPHRENIC ABSCESS

Although formerly subphrenic abscess occurred predominantly in young patients after incidents such as perforation of the appendix and developed chiefly in the posterior subphrenic space of the right hemidiaphragm, recent reports suggest that subphrenic infection now occurs as frequently after abdominal surgery, that its incidence on either side is approximately equal,[9] and that it involves the anterior and posterior subphrenic spaces equally as often. Meyers[10] has shown that the main pathway by which infection spreads to and from the upper and lower peritoneal compartments is the right paracolic gutter. Superiorly, the right paracolic gutter is continuous with the subhepatic space and its posterosuperior extension, Morrison's pouch, and from there with the right subphrenic space.[10] Thus, an abscess in the right subhepatic space often spreads to the right subphrenic space. Subphrenic abscesses on the left side occur chiefly in the anterior subphrenic space; the left anterior compartment is bounded on the right by the falciform ligament so that an abscess here may extend across the midline into the right upper quadrant.[11] Such a collection can simulate an abscess in the lesser sac; however, left anterior subphrenic abscesses are immediately subdiaphragmatic, whereas lesser sac abscesses that extend to the right of the midline are not usually contiguous with the diaphragm.[11]

Roentgenologic signs of subphrenic abscess include abnormalities within the lung, the pleural space, the subphrenic space, and the diaphragm itself. In an analysis of the signs in 48 cases of subphrenic abscess, Miller and Talman[12] reported the following findings:

Elevation of the ipsilateral hemidiaphragm	44/47	(95%)
Restriction of diaphragmatic motion	33/36	(92%)
Fixation of the hemidiaphragm	19/36	(53%)
Pleural effusion	37/47	(79%)
Basal pulmonary opacity (pneumonitis or atelectasis or both)	33/47	(70%)

Gas was identified in the abscess cavity in 30 per cent and displacement of intra-abdominal viscera in 35 per cent of these 48 patients. In a more recent retrospective study of the roentgenographic findings in 82 patients with proven subphrenic abscess,[13] conventional roentgenograms revealed extraluminal gas or a soft-tissue mass in 58 patients (71 per cent), the diagnosis being suggested in the majority. Procedures of value in confirming the diagnosis included barium examination of the gastrointestinal tract (particularly in abscesses situated on the left), computed tomography, gallium scanning, and ultrasonic examination.

A subphrenic abscess should be suspected in any patient with chronic fever, vague upper abdominal pain, loss of weight, and sometimes chills and anemia.[9] It should be borne in mind that considerable time may elapse between the causal episode and the development of symptoms.

THE CHEST WALL

ABNORMALITIES OF THE RIBS

CONGENITAL ANOMALIES

Congenital anomalies of the ribs, including fusion of two or more ribs and various types of bifid ribs, are relatively common and are of little or no significance. Of potentially greater importance is the anomalous accessory rib, usually arising from the seventh cervical vertebrae. In many cases cervical ribs give rise to no symptoms, but when they compress subclavian vessels or the brachial plexus the symptoms may be disabling. The diagnosis of cervical rib syndrome is certain when there is roentgenographic evidence of a cervical rib associated with the typical symptoms and signs of pain and weakness of the arm, swelling of the hand, and variation in the intensity of the pulses in the two arms when the affected extremity is in certain positions. This syndrome may be mimicked by the effects of other lesions that compress structures at the cervicothoracic inlet, including the scalenus anticus, costoclavicular, hyperabduction, subcoracoid, pectoralis minor, and the first thoracic rib syndromes.[14]

NOTCHING AND EROSION

Pathologic notching of ribs may occur on the inferior or superior aspect, much more often the former. By far the most common cause is coarctation of the aorta, which typically produces notching several centimeters lateral to the costovertebral junction on the inferior as-

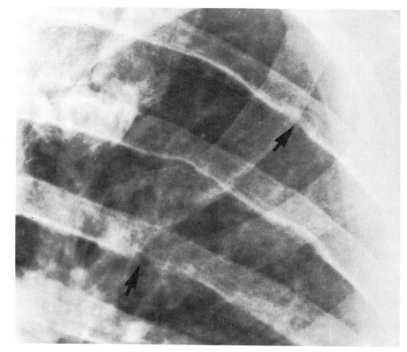

Figure 17–4. Rib Notching: Coarctation of the Aorta. A magnified view of the left upper ribs demonstrates numerous defects of the inferior surfaces of ribs four to eight bilaterally *(arrows)*. Proven coarctation of the aorta in a 58-year-old man.

pect of ribs three to nine (Figure 17–4). These notches are caused by erosion from pulsating, dilated intercostal arteries taking part in collateral arterial flow. These arteries may become extremely tortuous and may even extend to and erode the superior aspects of contiguous ribs. Rib notching secondary to coarctation of the aorta seldom is seen in patients before the age of 6 or 7 years and usually is not well developed until the early teens. Rib notching may occur in other conditions also, particularly the tetralogy of Fallot, unilateral on the left side in most cases.

It is difficult to improve upon the classification of causes of rib notching formulated by Boone and his colleagues:[15]

I. Arterial
    A. Aortic obstruction
        1. Coarctation of the aortic arch
        2. Thrombosis of the abdominal aorta
    B. Subclavian artery obstruction
        1. Blalock-Taussig operation
        2. "Pulseless disease"
    C. Widened arterial pulse pressure (?)
    D. Decreased pulmonary blood supply
        1. Tetralogy of Fallot
        2. Pulmonary atresia (pseudotruncus)
        3. Ebstein's malformation
        4. Pulmonary valve stenosis
        5. Unilateral absence of the pulmonary artery
        6. Pulmonary emphysema

II. Venous
    A. Superior vena cava obstruction
III. Arteriovenous
    A. Pulmonary arteriovenous fistula
    B. Intercostal arteriovenous fistula
IV. Neurogenic
    A. Intercostal neurinoma
V. Osseous
    A. Hyperparathyroidism
VI. Idiopathic
VII. Normal

Notching or erosion of the *superior* aspects of the ribs is considerably less common than that of the inferior aspects, but we suspect that it may be present more often than is generally recognized because of its more subtle roentgenologic appearance. This subject has been reviewed by Sargent and his colleagues,[16] who classified superior marginal rib defects into three main etiologic groups, related to an imbalance of osteoblastic-osteoclastic activity:

I. Disturbance of osteoblastic activity (decreased or deficient bone formation)
    A. Paralytic poliomyelitis (bulbar or spinal)
    B. Collagen diseases (rheumatoid arthritis, scleroderma, lupus erythematosus, Sjögren's disease)
    C. Localized pressure (rib retractors, chest tubes, multiple hereditary exostoses, neurofibromatosis, thoracic neu-

roblastoma, and coarctation of the
aorta with superior *and* inferior rib
erosion)
    D. Osteogenesis imperfecta
    E. Marfan's syndrome
    F. Radiation damage
II. Disturbance of osteoclastic activity (increased bone resorption)
    A. Hyperparathyroidism
    B. Hypervitaminosis D (?)
III. Idiopathic (no demonstrable associated etiology)

INFLAMMATORY DISEASES

Primary osteomyelitis of the ribs is rare and may be difficult to appreciate roentgenologically until bone destruction is advanced. More commonly, osteomyelitis is secondary to infectious processes in the lung (usually of tuberculous or fungal etiology) or to empyema (empyema necessitatis). Tuberculous involvement of the rib cage is characterized by destructive lesions associated with a periosteal reaction and a soft tissue mass. Tuberculous osteitis is said to be the most common inflammatory lesion of a rib and occasionally is the first manifestation of the disease.[17]

Costochondral osteochondritis (Tietze's syndrome) is characterized by painful, nonsuppurative swelling of one or more costochondral or costosternal joints.[18] The etiology of this rare, benign, self-limited process is unknown. Involved cartilage is said to be histologically normal. The second ribs are most commonly involved. The affected ribs may show evidence of periosteal reaction and increased size and density anteriorly. Subperiosteal new bone formation tends to occur along the superior aspects of the affected ribs.

The clinical picture is that of painful nonsuppurative swelling of one or more upper rib cartilages, without apparent cause and in some cases alternating between remission and exacerbation.

ABNORMALITIES OF THE STERNUM

PECTUS EXCAVATUM

This common deformity of the sternum, also known as "funnel chest," consists of depression of the sternum such that the ribs on each side protrude anteriorly more than the sternum itself. It is generally believed that pectus excavatum results from a genetically determined abnormality of the sternum and related portions of the diaphragm. Although some authors regard this anomaly as a potential cause of cardiac or respiratory symptoms, the majority of patients are symptom-free except for the anxiety occasioned by the physical deformity.[19] Occasionally, multiple congenital defects may be associated with pectus excavatum.

The roentgenographic manifestations are easily recognized (Figure 17–5). In posteroanterior projection, the heart is seen to be displaced to the left and rotated in a way suggestive of a "mitral configuration." The parasternal soft tissues of the anterior chest wall, which are seen in profile instead of *en face*, are apparent as increased density over the inferomedial portion of the right hemithorax and should not be mistaken for disease of the right middle lobe, even though the right heart border is obscured by a silhouetting effect (Figure 17–5). The degree of sternal depression is easily seen on lateral roentgenograms.

In a study of 54 children with pectus excavatum, Guller and Hable[19] identified a heart murmur in 44 per cent, the most frequent murmur simulating pulmonic stenosis and probably resulting from kinking of the pulmonary artery. Increased splitting of the second heart sound was frequently observed, and in association with the pulmonic murmur suggested atrial septal defect. The electrocardiogram usually showed increased left-sided potentials, presumably as a result of leftward displacement of the heart. Although auscultatory, electrocardiographic, and roentgenographic abnormalities suggestive of significant heart disease were frequent in this series, the authors considered that all 54 children had normal hearts. Most surgeons are of the opinion that surgical correction is seldom indicated and then only to prevent psychologic upset resulting from cosmetic deformity.[20]

PECTUS CARINATUM

The reverse of pectus excavatum is pectus carinatum or "pigeon breast," a congenital or acquired deformity in which the sternum protrudes anteriorly more than normal. The most common cause of acquired pectus carinatum is congenital atrial or ventricular septal defect,[21] the combination being observed in approximately 50 per cent of patients. Another acquired cause of pectus carinatum is prolonged and severe asthma dating from early childhood.

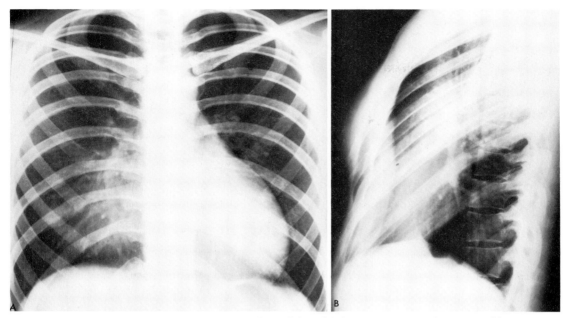

Figure 17–5. Pectus Excavatum. Posteroanterior *(A)* and lateral *(B)* roentgenograms of a 20-year-old asymptomatic woman reveal severe funnel chest deformity. The mediastinum is displaced to the left; in posteroanterior projection the inferomedial portion of the right lung shows a poorly defined increase in density caused by superimposition over the right lung of the soft tissues within the sternal depression. The right heart border is obscured.

The great majority of patients with congenital pectus carinatum are asymptomatic.

ABNORMALITIES OF THE THORACIC SPINE

ABNORMALITIES OF CURVATURE (KYPHOSCOLIOSIS)

Abnormalities of curvature of the thoracic spine may be predominantly lateral (scoliosis), predominantly posterior (kyphosis), or a combination of the two (kyphoscoliosis). Abnormalities of curvature, particularly scoliosis, are common, but deformity of a sufficient degree to lead to symptoms and signs referable to the heart and lungs is rare. Respiratory or cardiovascular embarrassment seldom occurs in cases of simple scoliosis or kyphosis and when present usually indicates a severe degree of kyphoscoliosis. Etiologically, abnormalities of curvature may be divided into three major groups:

1. *Congenital,* including anomalies of the thoracic spine such as hemivertebrae and various hereditary disorders.

2. *Paralytic.*

3. *Idiopathic,* which includes the majority of patients with severe kyphoscoliosis. Cases in this group are unassociated with congenital de-

fects or other diseases to which the abnormal curvature may be ascribed (Figure 17–6). This variety shows a female sex predominance of 4 to 1.

The major complications of severe kyphoscoliosis are pulmonary arterial hypertension and cor pulmonale. Pathologic studies of the lungs of patients so affected reveal small lungs with reduction in both functioning parenchyma and the pulmonary vascular bed.[22] Severe muscular hypertrophy of the pulmonary arteries is common and is presumably caused by hypoxemia.

Apart from the spinal curvature itself, the roentgenographic changes in severe kyphoscoliotic cardiopulmonary disease are extremely difficult to assess. In the great majority of cases the scoliotic curvature is convex to the right. Assessment of cardiac enlargement and of the state of the pulmonary vasculature may be exceedingly difficult because of the severe deformity of the thoracic cage.

Most children with kyphoscoliosis are asymptomatic,[23] and the presence of cardiac abnormalities should suggest primary heart disease independent of the kyphoscoliosis. There is a tendency for disability to relate to an increasing angle of scoliosis and to age.[24] Symptoms and signs of respiratory and cardiac failure usually do not appear until the fourth or fifth decade.

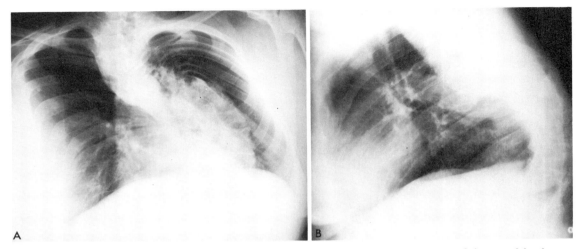

Figure 17–6. Kyphoscoliosis. Posteroanterior *(A)* and lateral *(B)* roentgenograms reveal severe deformity of the thoracic skeleton, the spine possessing a marked scoliosis to the left in the midthoracic region and a severe kyphos in the mid and lower regions. Deformity of the rib cage is as might be anticipated from the thoracic curvature. The 48-year-old woman had no significant complaints referable to the respiratory tract; her thoracic deformity was the result of a remote poliomyelitis. Pulmonary function tests revealed remarkably normal values, there being only a slight reduction in VC and FRC.

Once failure has become manifest the clinical course is usually rapidly downhill, characterized by repeated episodes of cardiac failure, often precipitated by pulmonary infection. However, even adults with severe kyphoscoliosis may remain asymptomatic. In a study of 500 patients, Godfrey[25] found that cardiorespiratory failure did not occur if the vital capacity remained greater than 40 per cent of predicted.

Tests of pulmonary function characteristically reveal a decrease in VC and TLC and normal or increased values of RV.[23, 26] In patients with cor pulmonale, TLC may be reduced to as low as 2 liters.[27] Flow is reduced only in proportion to the reduction in VC, and direct measurement of airway resistance reveals normal values.[27] Arterial blood gases are almost invariably abnormal in adults and occasionally in adolescents.[23] In the more advanced cases it is common to find both hypoxemia and hypercapnia, a combined form of respiratory failure that can be attributed either to alveolar hypoventilation secondary to shallow respiration or to $\dot{V}/\dot{Q}$ imbalance.[26] Studies with radioactive xenon have indicated defects in both ventilation and perfusion.[28] Lung compliance is reduced in most patients.

ANKYLOSING SPONDYLITIS

Involvement of the thoracic spine by ankylosing spondylitis results in fixation of the chest cage in an inspiratory position and leads to overinflation and restriction of pulmonary function. The typical patient with ankylosing spondylitis who is seen by the physician is a young male with a history of onset of symptoms early in the third decade of life. Although peripheral joint involvement develops eventually in about 18 to 25 per cent of cases, there is little question that ankylosing spondylitis is an entity distinct from rheumatoid arthritis;[34] however, although both diseases probably have an autoimmune pathogenesis in common.

Pathologically, ankylosing spondylitis consists of synovitis, chondritis, and juxta-articular osteitis of the sacroiliac, apophyseal, and costovertebral articulations. Progression of the disease is marked by erosion of subchondral bone, destruction of cartilage, and eventual bony ankylosis. Calcification and ossification deep to the paraspinal ligaments are late changes. Aortic valvulitis develops in approximately 4 per cent of patients,[34, 35] an incidence that increases to 10 per cent in patients who have had the disease for 30 years.[35]

In addition to the characteristic changes in the thoracic skeleton, the chest roentgenogram reveals general pulmonary overinflation. In approximately 1 to 2 per cent of patients pleuropulmonary manifestations develop, most commonly in the form of upper lobe fibrotic and bullous disease (*see* page 660).[36] These fibrobullous lesions sometimes contain mycetomas and occasionally are the result of atypical mycobacterial infection.

The clinical picture is characterized by intermittent or continuous low back pain, sometimes associated with constitutional symptoms such as fatigue, weight loss, anorexia, and low-grade fever. As the disease progresses upward and involves the thoracic spine, the patient may complain of chest pain that is sometimes accentuated during respiration. As the spine fuses, the kyphotic curvature gradually increases and chest expansion progressively diminishes. Few patients complain of dyspnea.

The pattern of pulmonary function is one of restriction and overinflation, the result of fixation of the thorax in an expanded position. VC is reduced, often to 70 per cent or less of predicted values; RV and FRC are usually but not always increased.[29] Mixing efficiency and flow resistance are normal. Maximal static inspiratory transpulmonary pressure is diminished, as in emphysema. Ventilation-perfusion relationships are usually normal.[29]

NEOPLASMS OF THE CHEST WALL

Primary neoplasms of the soft tissues of the chest wall are exceedingly rare, the most common benign lesion being lipoma and the most common malignant neoplasm being fibrosarcoma.[30–32] The point of origin of a *lipoma* in the chest wall establishes its mode of presentation. When it originates adjacent to the parietal pleura, it causes a soft tissue mass that indents the lung and possesses a contour characteristic of its extrapulmonary origin. When it arises outside the rib cage it presents as a palpable soft tissue mass that may be visualized roentgenographically if viewed in profile or, if of sufficient size, even *en face*. The density of lipomas is intermediate between that of air and soft tissue. Therefore, when a lipoma relates to lung parenchyma it may not be readily distinguishable roentgenographically from other soft tissue masses, whereas when it relates to the soft tissues of the chest wall, the contrast with contiguous soft tissues usually permits its identification as of fat origin.

A soft tissue neoplasm of the chest wall may be identified roentgenographically in asymptomatic subjects or may become evident clinically as a soft tissue mass outside the chest wall. If the tumor occasions pain it is likely to be malignant. Evaluation of the extent of such neoplasms can be facilitated by computed tomography.[33]

Neoplasms of the thoracic skeleton are uncommon. Ochsner and his colleagues[31] reported 134 such cases, representing only 5 per cent of all neoplasms of bones and joints studied from 1953 to 1956. Of the 134 cases, 84 (63 per cent) were primary (48 benign and 36 malignant) and the remainder metastatic. The majority of the latter were from primaries in the lung and breast. In the younger age group, the most common benign primary neoplasms were eosinophilic granuloma and aneurysmal bone cyst and the most common malignant neoplasm was Ewing's sarcoma.

Of the 134 cases reported by Ochsner and his coworkers,[31] the following characteristics were noted: (1) *rib* lesions were most commonly metastatic, chiefly from the lung and breast; (2) most of those arising in the *sternum* were malignant, most commonly chondrosarcoma; (3) involvement of the *clavicles* was most often by metastatic neoplasm, benign neoplasms being the next most common; (4) in the *scapulae*, primary neoplasms were more numerous than metastatic ones and the majority were benign; and (5) involvement of the *thoracic vertebrae* was almost invariably metastatic in origin.

Primary neoplasms of the thoracic skeleton may be conveniently divided into those that are cartilaginous or osteogenic in origin and those that are hematopoietic or reticuloendothelial. Of the *cartilaginous and osteogenic* neoplasms, osteochondroma is the most common benign type. The most common malignant neoplasm is chondrosarcoma, while osteogenic sarcoma and synovioma are less common.[31] Among the *hematopoietic and reticuloendothelial* neoplasms, the most common benign variety is fibrous dysplasia (Figure 17–7), although eosinophilic granuloma, hemangioma, and aneurysmal bone cyst also occur.[31] Involvement of the rib cage by Paget's disease presents a typical roentgenographic appearance similar to that in any other bone. Myeloma is the most frequent malignant neoplasm, followed by Hodgkin's disease, Ewing's sarcoma, and reticulum cell sarcoma.[31] In older patients, particularly males, the association of a destructive lesion of one or more ribs with a soft tissue mass that protrudes into the thorax and indents the lung is highly suggestive of myeloma. However, a similar appearance can be created by primary lung carcinoma invading the chest wall and by other primary chest wall neoplasms. Advanced myelomatosis of the rib cage may be associated with expansion of bone (Figure 17–8). The majority of benign neoplasms of the thoracic skeleton occasion no symptoms and usually are detected in asymptomatic subjects on a screening chest roentgenogram. However, a pathologic fracture may cause a patient to seek medical advice. Malig-

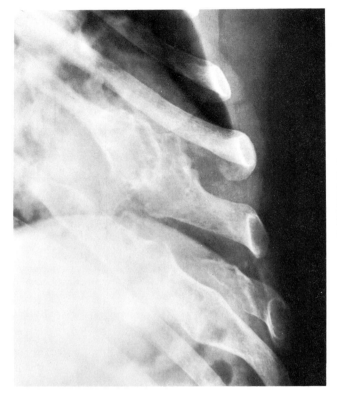

Figure 17–7. Polyostotic Fibrous Dysplasia of the Left Rib Cage. An oblique view of the left rib cage reveals considerable expansion and distortion of ribs along the lower axillary lung zone (one rib has been removed). The left innominate bone and left tibia were affected in a similar manner. Bone involvement is thus unilateral, representing the osseous manifestation of Albright's syndrome.

Figure 17–8. Multiple Myeloma of the Rib Cage. A posteroanterior roentgenogram reveals extensive destruction of virtually all ribs bilaterally. Note that several of the ribs have been expanded, a common feature in multiple myeloma of ribs.

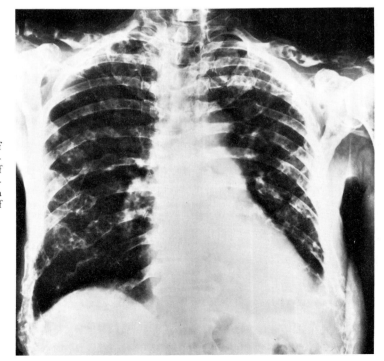

nant neoplasms may cause pain and may be palpable. Roentgenologic assessment may be of value in suggesting the diagnosis, but definitive diagnosis requires close correlation between the histologic and roentgenologic appearances of the neoplasm.

REFERENCES

1. Riley, E. A.: Idiopathic diaphragmatic paralysis. A report of eight cases. Am. J. Med., 32:404, 1962.
2. Alexander, C.: Diaphragm movements and the diagnosis of diaphragmatic paralysis. Clin. Radiol., 17:79, 1966.
3. Chin, E. F., and Lynn, R. B.: Surgery of eventration of the diaphragm. J. Thorac. Surg., 32:6, 1956.
4. Reed, J. O., and Lang, E. F.: Diaphragmatic hernia in infancy. Am. J. Roentgenol., 82:437, 1959.
5. Whittaker, L. D., Jr., Lynn, H. B., Dawson, B., and Chaves, E.: Hernias of the foramen of Bochdalek in children. Mayo Clin. Proc., 43:580, 1968.
6. Morris, J., J., Black, F. O., and Stephenson, H. E., Jr.: The fate of the unexpanded lung in congenital diaphragmatic hernia. Report of a case. Dis. Chest, 48:649, 1965.
7. Siegel, M. J., Shackelford, G. D., and McAlister, W. H.: Left-sided congenital diaphragmatic hernia: Delayed presentation. Am. J. Roentgenol., 137:43, 1981.
8. Robinson, A. E., Gooneratne, N. S., Blackburn, W. R., and Brogdon, B. G.: Bilateral anteromedial defect of the diaphragm in children. Am. J. Roentgenol., 135:301, 1980.
9. Rosenberg, M.: Chronic subphrenic abscess. Lancet, 2:379, 1968.
10. Meyers, M. A.: The spread and localization of acute intraperitoneal effusions. Radiology, 95:547, 1970.
11. Halvorsen, R. A., Jones, M. A., Rice, R. P., and Thompson, W. M.: Anterior left subphrenic abscess: Characteristic plain film and CT appearance. A.J.R., 139:283, 1982.
12. Miller, W. T., and Talman, E. A.: Subphrenic abscess. Am. J. Roentgenol., 101:961, 1967.
13. Connell, T. R., Stephens, D. H., Carlson, H. C., and Brown, M. L.: Upper abdominal abscess: A continuing and deadly problem. Am. J. Roentgenol., 134:759, 1980.
14. Siegel, R. S., and Steichen, F. M.: Cervicothoracic outlet syndrome. Vascular compression caused by congenital abnormality of thoracic ribs: A case report. J. Bone Joint Surg., 49A:1187, 1967.
15. Boone, M. L., Swenson, B. E., and Felson, B.: Rib notching: its many causes. Am. J. Roentgenol., 91:1075, 1964.
16. Sargent, E. N., Turner, A. F., and Jacobson, G.: Superior marginal rib defects. An etiologic classification. Am. J. Roentgenol., 106:491, 1969.
17. Wolstein, D., Rabinowitz, J. G., and Twersky, J.: Tuberculosis of the rib. J. Can. Assoc. Radiol., 25:307, 1974.
18. Skorneck, A. B.: Roentgen aspects of Tietze's syndrome. Painful hypertrophy of costal cartilage and bone—osteochondritis? Am. J. Roentgenol., 83:748, 1960.
19. Guller, B., and Hable, K.: Cardiac findings in pectus excavatum in children: Review and differential diagnosis. Chest, 66:165, 1974.
20. Clark, J. B., and Grenville-Mathers, R.: Pectus excavatum. Br. J. Dis. Chest, 56:202, 1962.
21. Davies, H.: Chest deformities in congenital heart disease. Br. J. Dis. Chest, 53:151, 1959.
22. Naeye, R. L.: Kyphoscoliosis and cor pulmonale. A study of the pulmonary vascular bed. Am. J. Pathol., 38:561, 1961.
23. Weber, B., Smith, J. P., Briscoe, W. A., et al.: Pulmonary function in asymptomatic adolescents with idiopathic scoliosis. Am. Rev. Respir. Dis., 111:389, 1975.
24. Bjure, J., Grimby, G., Kasalicky, J., et al.: Respiratory impairment and airway closure in patients with untreated idiopathic scoliosis. Thorax, 25:451, 1970.
25. Godfrey, S.: Respiratory and cardiovascular consequences of scoliosis. Respiration, 27(Suppl.):67, 1970.
26. Kafer, E. R.: Respiratory function in paralytic scoliosis. Am. Rev. Respir. Dis., 110:450, 1974.
27. Bates, D. V., Macklem, P. T., and Christie, R. V.: Respiratory Function in Disease; an Introduction to the Integrated Study of the Lung, 2nd ed. Philadelphia, W. B. Saunders Co., 1971.
28. Bake, B., Bjure, J., Kasalichy, J., and Nachemson, A.: Regional pulmonary ventilation and perfusion distribution in patients with untreated idiopathic scoliosis. Thorax, 27:703, 1972.
29. Travis, D. M., Cook, C. D., Julian, D. G., et al.: The lungs in rheumatoid spondylitis. Gas exchange and lung mechanics in a form of restrictive pulmonary disease. Am. J. Med., 29:623, 1960.
30. Ochsner, A., Sr., and Ochsner, A., Jr.: Tumors of the thoracic wall. In Spain, D. M. (ed.): Diagnosis and Treatment of Tumors of the Chest. New York, Grune & Stratton, 1960, pp. 209–239.
31. Ochsner, A. Jr., Lucas, G. L., and McFarland, G. B., Jr.: Tumors of the thoracic skeleton. Review of 134 cases. J. Thorac. Cardiovasc. Surg., 52:311, 1966.
32. Omell, G. H., Anderson, L. S., and Bramson, R. T.: Chest Wall Tumors. Radiol. Clin. North Am., 11:197, 1973.
33. Gouliamos, A. D., Carter, B. L., and Emami, B.: Computed tomography of the chest wall. Radiology, 134:433, 1980.
34. Boland, E. W.: Ankylosing spondylitis. In Hollander, J. L. (ed.): Arthritis and Allied Conditions, 17th ed. Philadelphia, Lea & Febiger, 1966, pp. 633–655.
35. Graham, D. C., and Smythe, H. A.: The carditis and aortitis of ankylosing spondylitis. Bull. Rheum. Dis., 9:171, 1958.
36. Jessamine, A. G.: Upper lung lobe fibrosis in ankylosing spondylitis. Can. Med. Assoc. J., 98:25, 1968.

18

Respiratory Disease
Associated With a Normal
Chest Roentgenogram

DISEASES OF THE
LUNG PARENCHYMA

In Chapter 1 the limitations of roentgeno-graphic visibility in alveolar and interstitial pulmonary disease are discussed. Even in ideal circumstances, with technically perfect roentgenograms interpreted carefully by experienced observers, lesions may be so minute as to be imperceptible or may be hidden behind or juxtaposed to bony or vascular shadows. A solitary uncalcified lesion less than 6 mm in diameter is rarely appreciated and then usually only in retrospect, when the lesion has grown and is detected on subsequent roentgenograms. Pathologically proved nodules as large as 2 cm in diameter may be overlooked, particularly if they are situated over the convexity of the lung or in the paramediastinal areas where the rib cage, large vessels, and mediastinal contents tend to obscure their image. By contrast, multiple micronodular opacities measuring no more than 1 or 2 mm in diameter are usually appreciated, possibly because of the effect of super-imposition. Reference is made throughout this book to those diseases that at some stage of their development or regression fail to cast detectable roentgenographic shadows. No attempt is made in this chapter to review all these conditions, but attention is directed to those in which a normal chest roentgenogram is more than an occasional finding.

LOCAL DISEASES

In contrast to bacterial pneumonia, in which roentgenographic evidence of disease usually is present with the onset of symptoms, when the acute local disease is confined to the interstitium of the lungs (as in nonbacterial pneumonia) symptoms may precede roentgenographic signs by at least 48 hours.[1]

Chronic pulmonary disease may be present and active for months and even years before it becomes roentgenographically visible. It has been estimated that a local tuberculous infection is not roentgenographically detectable until 2 or 3 months after initial infection, and bronchogenic carcinoma undoubtedly is present for years before it becomes visible. In both of these diseases, the establishment of a positive diagnosis by sputum analysis in the presence of a normal chest roentgenogram has been repeatedly documented.

GENERAL DISEASES

Diffuse granulomatous and fibrotic diseases of the lungs may be present with a normal chest roentgenogram. In miliary tuberculosis fever, general malaise, and headaches may develop some weeks before roentgenologic abnormality, and in some instances the minute pulmonary lesions are not detected before death. In diseases such as *sarcoidosis, eosinophilic granuloma,* and *scleroderma* a diffuse reticular or reticulonodular pattern may be visible during the granulomatous and edematous phase, only to disappear during the fibrotic stage. However, particularly in *scleroderma*, no lesions may be roentgenographically visible even when symptoms and disturbances of pulmonary function indicate involvement of the lung interstitium. Cases of *sarcoidosis* have been reported in which chest roentgenograms were normal despite abnormal findings in biopsy specimens or pulmonary function abnormalities consisting of reduction in compliance, vital capacity, and diffusing capacity. Patients with *diffuse interstitial fibrosis* (fibrosing alveolitis) and *farmer's lung* have been shown to have pathologic evidence of interstitial fibrosis in the absence of roentgenographic abnormality. Normal pulmonary function tests and chest roentgenograms have also been reported in cases of diffuse interstitial *leukemic infiltration* of the lungs. In patients who die of leukemia, parenchymal infiltration is commonly observed pathologically (in approximately 25 per cent of cases)[2] but seldom roentgenographically. It has been estimated that infiltration with leukemic cells is sufficiently extensive to produce symptoms and disturb pulmonary function in less than 3 per cent of cases.[2]

Pulmonary vascular disease may be of significant degree without roentgenographic manifestations—for example, the extensive obstruction of the vasculature in *thromboembolic disease,* the prehypertensive stage of *arteritis* as a manifestation of scleroderma or rheumatoid arthritis, and the severe proliferation of the intima of pulmonary arterial vessels of all sizes, as has been reported in *polymyositis.*

DISEASES OF THE PLEURA

The chest roentgenogram may be normal in cases of acute pleuritis. However, dry pleurisy often is associated with diaphragmatic elevation and reduction in diaphragmatic excursion. Effusions as large as 300 ml may not be visible on standard posteroanterior and lateral chest roentgenograms exposed in the erect position. However, films exposed in the lateral decubitus position can reveal effusions of 100 ml or less, and special roentgenographic techniques may show as little as 10 to 15 ml, an amount that may be visible even in healthy subjects.

DISEASES OF THE AIRWAYS

Many patients with disease of the conducting airways have normal chest roentgenograms. In *chronic bronchitis* this is more the rule than the exception. Many patients with *asthma* have overinflated lungs, particularly during acute attacks, but chest roentgenograms may appear entirely normal during remission. In fact, the presence of overinflation during attacks may be difficult to appreciate without comparison with films obtained during remission. Approximately 7 per cent of patients with *bronchiectasis* fail to show evidence of this disease on standard chest roentgenograms. Patients with *emphysema,* particularly in the advanced stages of the disease, show distinctly abnormal roentgenograms. However, pathologic-roentgenologic correlative studies have shown that patients with mild to moderate emphysema may have completely normal films.[3, 4]

Patients with various types of *endobronchial masses* that only partly obstruct an airway may have normal chest roentgenograms, at least when films are exposed at full inspiration. (More commonly, the volume of lung parenchyma distal to the partial obstruction is *smaller* than normal, whether or not its density is increased.) Obviously, in such circumstances a roentgenogram exposed following full expiration, preferably forced, will reveal air trapping in lung parenchyma distal to the partial obstruction. When the obstruction is in the trachea or a major bronchus, dyspnea and generalized wheezing may suggest the diagnosis of asthma.

ALVEOLAR HYPOVENTILATION

The term "hypoventilation" is used to designate inadequate alveolar ventilation, either local or general, as reflected in reduced PaO_2 values while the patient breathes room air, with or without a rise in $PaCO_2$. It is obvious that in those instances in which ventilation-perfusion inequality leads to *regional* "hypoventilation" and hypoxemia, an absence of hypercapnia indicates that the overall ventilation is adequate and that, in fact, alveolar ventilation to certain areas is relatively increased to compensate for the carbon dioxide retention resulting from reduced ventilation to other areas.

Pulmonary diseases that lead to alveolar hypoventilation with hypoxemia and normal or lowered $PaCO_2$ have been discussed elsewhere in various sections of this book. Respiratory failure associated with hypercapnia occurs in two broad groups of disorders, those of *pulmonary* origin (Table 18–1) and those of *nonpulmonary* origin (Table 18–2). In this chapter we will deal with disorders of ventilatory control and the neuromuscular diseases—those abnormalities of the central nervous and neuromuscular systems that characteristically reduce overall ventilation and result in both hypoxemia and hypercapnia. Recent electromyographic studies of the pharyngeal and diaphragmatic

TABLE 18–1. Airway/Pulmonary Causes of Respiratory Failure with Hypercapnia

Upper Airway Obstruction

ACUTE

Infection (pharyngitis, tonsillitis, epiglottitis, laryngotracheitis)

Edema (irritant gases, angioneurotic edema)

Retropharyngeal hemorrhage (trauma, postoperative, hemophilia, acute leukemia)

Foreign bodies

CHRONIC

Postintubation stenoses (fibrosis, granulation tissue, tracheomalacia)

Tumors (squamous-cell carcinoma, cylindroma)

Vocal cord paralysis

Hypertrophied tonsils and adenoids

Pharynx (sleep deprivation syndrome of obesity)

Micrognathia

Lower Airway Obstruction

ACUTE

Infection (acute bronchiolitis)

Edema (pulmonary venous hypertension, capillary leakage)

Bronchospasm (asthma and anaphylactoid reactions)

CHRONIC

Emphysema

Chronic bronchitis

Extensive bronchiectasis

Cystic fibrosis

Familial dysautonomia

---

muscles during sleep have shown simultaneous reduction in electrical activity,[5, 6] indicating that central neural drive plays a major role in occlusive apneic episodes caused by upper airway disease; this is true whether the disease be purely functional or partly the result of local pathology. This form of ventilatory failure is seen most commonly in obese patients and results in sleep deprivation and the hypersomnia–sleep apnea syndrome.[7] Disorders of the mechanism that drives the chest "bellows" are considered under two headings: those that result from defective ventilatory control and those caused by an inadequate respiratory pump (Table 18–2). It will become apparent in the discussion that follows that such a division is purely arbitrary, since considerable overlap occurs between these functions.

The chest roentgenogram is within normal limits in the majority of cases of hypoventilation resulting from central nervous system or neuromuscular disease. In those instances in which hypoventilation is caused by diaphragmatic paralysis the diaphragm is elevated, but very commonly this finding is ignored on the supposition that the chest roentgenogram was exposed at a position of incomplete inspiration.

TABLE 18–2. Nonairway/Pulmonary Causes of Respiratory Failure with Hypercapnia

Disorders of Ventilatory Control

A. CEREBRAL DYSFUNCTION

1. Infection (encephalitis), trauma, vascular
2. Status epilepticus, tetanus, Parkinson's disease
3. Narcotic and sedative overdose (e.g., barbiturates, glutethimide, phenothiazines and benzodiazepines, tricyclic antidepressants)

B. RESPIRATORY CENTER DYSFUNCTION

1. Impaired brain stem controller:

Idiopathic hypoventilation of the obese

Idiopathic hypoventilation of the non-obese

Myxedema

Metabolic alkalosis (compensatory)

Sudden infant death syndrome?

2. Ablation of afferent and efferent spinal pathways:

Bilateral high cervical cordotomy

Cervical spinal cord trauma

Transverse myelitis

Multiple sclerosis

Parkinson's disease

C. PERIPHERAL RECEPTOR DYSFUNCTION

1. Carotid body destruction (bilateral carotid endarterectomy and carotid body resection for asthma)
2. Bilateral damage to afferent nerves (Arnold-Chiari syndrome with syringomyelia)
3. Familial dysautonomia (?)
4. Diabetic neuropathy (?)
5. Tetanus(?)

Disorders of the Respiratory Pump

A. NEUROMUSCULAR DISEASE

1. Anterior horn cells:

Poliomyelitis

Amyotrophic lateral sclerosis

2. Peripheral nerves:

Landry-Guillain-Barré syndrome

Acute intermittent porphyria

Paralytic shellfish poisoning

Myxedema (?)

3. Respiratory muscles:

Respiratory muscle fatigue

Myotonic muscular dystrophies

Nonmyotonic muscular dystrophies

Acid maltase deficiency

Connective tissue (autoimmune) diseases (polymyositis and systemic lupus erythematosus)

Hypokalemia (in treatment of diabetes with insulin, renal tubular acidosis)

Hypophosphatemia

Idiopathic rhabdomyolysis (myoglobinuria)

4. Myoneural junction:

Myasthenia gravis

Myasthenialike syndromes (medications—particularly antibiotics—and associated neoplasm)

Clostridium botulinum poisoning

Fish poisoning (ciguatera)

B. CHEST CAGE DISORDERS

1. Flail chest
2. Kyphoscoliosis
3. Thoracoplasty

Patients who hypoventilate, and particularly those with a raised diaphragm, are subject to atelectasis and pneumonia, and in fact such complications may be responsible for bringing the primary disease to the attention of the physician. In severe prolonged hypoventilation states, cor pulmonale may develop. This may be reflected in the chest roentgenogram by diminution of the peripheral vasculature and enlargement of the hilar and cardiac shadows.

DISTURBANCES OF VENTILATORY CONTROL

REGULATION OF RESPIRATION

Some basic knowledge of normal ventilatory control is required in order to comprehend the various disorders of this system. This subject has recently been reviewed by Berger and his associates[8-10] and by Derenne and his co-workers,[11] and the interested reader is referred to these treatises for more detailed information. The respiratory controller consists of two anatomically and functionally separate systems, operating as controls for voluntary and automatic breathing. *Voluntary ventilation* can be altered from a control situated within the cerebral cortex (Figure 18–1). *Automatic breathing* originates from a highly complex accumulation of interconnected nerve cell groups situated in the brain stem. The dorsal respiratory group (DRG) of neurons appears to play an important role in the regulation of respiration, since it is the primary projection site of numerous afferent fibers.

Numerous sensors, both chemical and neurogenic, play major roles in the regulation of respiration. These include the peripheral chemoreceptors located in the carotid and aortic bodies, central chemoreceptors that are believed to lie near the ventrolateral surface of the medulla, receptors situated in the upper airways and lungs, and perhaps reflexes arising from intercostal muscle spindles and the diaphragmatic tendon.[11]

The carotid and aortic body chemoreceptors respond to decreased PaO_2 and increased $PaCO_2$. Afferent fibers from the carotid body travel in the ninth cranial nerve and those from the aortic body in the tenth cranial nerve, both groups ending in the DRG of the medulla (Figure 18–1).

There is abundant evidence for a central chemosensitive organ in the medulla that responds to acidification of brain extracellular

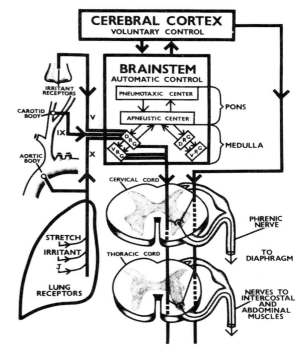

Figure 18–1. Schematic Representation of the Respiratory Controller. The respiratory controller is made up of voluntary (cerebral cortical) and automatic (brainstem) centers. The efferent fibers from each run in distinct spinal cord pathways, as depicted on the right side of the drawing. A variety of interconnections exist between the cortical control and the different components of the brainstem control. The sensors or receptors are shown on the left side of the diagram, the afferent input ending in the dorsal respiratory group (DRG) of neurons in the medulla. Not depicted are afferent fibers ascending in the phrenic nerve from the diaphragm and in the spinal cord from nerve endings in intercostal muscles. *See* text for further description.

fluid by carbon dioxide, although its neurohistology and neurophysiology are poorly understood.

A multitude of receptors that affect respiration exist in the upper airways and lungs. Three types of receptors have been recognized in the lungs—stretch, irritant, and type J (Figure 18–1). The pulmonary *stretch receptors* are thought to lie within the smooth muscle of the airways, and are activated by distention of the lung, producing the classic Hering-Breuer inspiratory inhibitory reflex. *Irritant receptors* are believed to be interspersed among airway epithelial cells and, when stimulated by endogenous or exogenous chemical irritants, induce hyperpnea. *Type J (juxtapulmonary-capillary) receptors* are located in the walls of the pulmonary capillaries and are activated by an increase in the volume of pulmonary interstitial fluid and perhaps by an increase in pulmonary capillary pressure such as is thought to occur during exercise. Fibers from all three classes of lung receptors travel in the tenth cranial nerve to the ipsilateral DRG located within the medulla.[8]

In addition to the more obvious feedback networks that regulate respiration, breathing also may be modified by stimuli that arise from a variety of cerebral cortical centers and from proprioceptive receptors throughout the body. There is good evidence that the latter type of sensors may be the primary initiators of the hyperventilation that occurs with exercise.

Projecting axons from the automatic (involuntary) controller in the brain stem descend in the ventrolateral spinal white matter. Fibers that are involved in voluntary respiration originate in the cortex and travel separately in the dorsolateral columns of the spinal cord. Impulses from cortical and brain stem centers are integrated at the level of the spinal respiratory motoneurons in the anterior horns, the site of transmission of local spinal reflexes (Figure 18–1). Impaired automatic control with maintenance of normal voluntary breathing occurs following bilateral cordotomy performed for the relief of pain. This procedure interrupts the spinothalamic tracts and results in ablation of respiratory axons, including those that both ascend and descend in the ventrolateral spinal cord. It causes the syndrome of "Ondine's curse," in which the patient breathes relatively normally during the day but experiences long periods of apnea at night (*see* further on).

In recent years a variety of methods have been devised to determine the output of the respiratory controller. Major interest has centered around the response to hypercapnia by performing diaphragmatic electromyography and by measuring mouth occlusion pressures shortly after the onset of an inspiratory effort. Recent studies show a good linear correlation in ventilatory response to these methods of assessment.

DISORDERS OF THE CENTRAL NERVOUS SYSTEM

Many disorders that affect the central nervous system are associated with respiratory depression, acting directly or indirectly on the respiratory center with resultant hypoventilation. These include the ingestion of various drugs, organic brain disease, myxedema, and metabolic alkalosis, as well as an idiopathic type that may or may not be associated with obesity.

Although narcotic and analgesic agents in prescribed amounts are perhaps the drugs most responsible for hypoventilation and respiratory failure in patients with underlying chronic lung disease, only rarely do they cause hypoventilation in individuals with normal lungs. In the latter circumstance, drug-induced hypoventilation usually occurs in adults in suicide attempts and in children following accidental ingestion.

Traumatic, infectious, or vascular brain damage may produce either an increase or a decrease in minute ventilation, the latter commonly following an initial stage of overventilation. In patients with organic brain disease, it is probable that increased intracranial pressure caused at least partly by edema may play a role in hypoventilation, since artificial ventilation enables some of these patients to survive an acute episode of respiratory failure. Subsequently, they return to a state of spontaneous ventilation with normal blood gas levels.

Coma is not uncommon in myxedema, occurring usually in elderly obese females.[12] Another form of respiratory depression that results in hypoventilation is that caused by metabolic alkalosis. These changes appear to represent a compensatory mechanism that permits a rise in CO_2 content and PCO_2 and thereby enables the acid-base balance to return to normal.

IDIOPATHIC HYPOVENTILATION IN THE OBESE (PICKWICKIAN SYNDROME)

The syndrome of cyanosis, polycythemia, and obesity was originally described by Kerr and Lagen[13] in 1936. It was given the name "pickwickian syndrome" by Burwell and his colleagues in 1956 because of the similar appearance and behavior of their patient to the fat boy in the novel *Pickwick Papers* by Charles Dickens.[14]

Various mechanisms have been postulated to explain the underventilation that occurs in obese patients who manifest both hypoxemia and hypercapnia. It is probable that more than one factor is operative in most cases. In most, a major cause is believed to be upper airway obstruction that significantly reduces alveolar ventilation when the patient is in the supine position. A lowered expiratory reserve volume[15, 16] may play a part by promoting an extremely low $\dot{V}/\dot{Q}$ ratio at the bases. The work of breathing may be greatly increased by the fat deposits enveloping the chest[17] and even infiltrating the muscle of the chest wall. Chronic bronchitis, even of mild degree, when added to these functional disturbances (decrease in expiratory reserve volume and increase in the work of breathing) could aid in the production of hypoventilation and respiratory failure. In most—if not all—cases it is likely that there is some disturbance of the respiratory center itself, which then becomes less sensitive to carbon dioxide. It has even been suggested that narcolepsy and the pickwickian syndrome are *primarily* the result of disturbance of the respiratory center. There seems little doubt that obesity itself plays at least a part, since reduction in weight invariably results in considerable improvement and in some cases complete cure.[16]

IDIOPATHIC HYPOVENTILATION IN THE NONOBESE

Alveolar hypoventilation occurs in some patients who are not obese, apparently as a result of a defect in the brain stem controller. Approximately 50 per cent of the patients have a history of prior central nervous system disease, usually encephalitis, Parkinson's disease, syringomyelia, or neurosyphilis.[18] This entity constitutes Ondine's curse,[19] in which gas exchange is normal or almost so when the patient is awake and under voluntary ventilatory control but in which respiratory failure and even death may ensue during sleep.[18] Idiopathic alveolar hypoventilation in nonobese patients represents a diagnosis of exclusion, since prior central nervous system disease, upper airway obstruction, or neuromuscular disorder must first be ruled out before the diagnosis is acceptable.

DISORDERS OF THE PERIPHERAL CHEMORECEPTORS AND CERVICAL SPINAL CORD

In humans, peripheral chemoreceptors situated chiefly in the carotid bodies account for virtually all the hypoxic drive. Bilateral carotid endarterectomy or removal of both carotid bodies, a "therapeutic procedure" that has been advocated (without proven benefit) for bronchial asthma, may abolish compensatory hyperventilation when such patients become hypoxemic.

Lesions of the spinal cord can interfere with both afferent and efferent spinal pathways. Either trauma or transverse myelitis in the cervical cord may result in quadriplegia. Transection of the cord below the level of the fifth cervical vertebra causes intercostal muscle paralysis but does not interfere with diaphragmatic function. Cervical cordotomy may interfere with respiratory function and result in sleep-induced apnea and even sudden death. This surgical procedure is used to relieve intractable pain and results in section of efferent pathways to the phrenic nerve nuclei; there is evidence that respiratory control mechanisms are also disturbed, probably as a result of ablation of reticular formation spinal tracts.[20]

DISTURBANCES OF THE RESPIRATORY PUMP

For descriptive purposes, it is useful although somewhat arbitrary to visualize ventilatory control (including peripheral receptors, afferent axons to central controller, and efferent spinal cord pathways) as terminating in the anterior horn cells, where impulses that serve voluntary and automatic control integrate with spinal reflexes (*see* Figure 18–1). The respiratory pump thus includes not only the rib cage and muscles of respiration but also its electrical connections. Disturbances of the respiratory pump can result from disease of the anterior horn cells, the phrenic and intercostal nerves, the myoneural junctions, or the respiratory muscles themselves.

The respiratory muscles are divided into three distinct groups with different mechanisms of action—the diaphragm, the intercostal and accessory muscles, and the abdominal muscles.[11, 21] Although these are involved in both inspiration and expiration, only impairment of the inspiratory muscles results in pathophysiology. Expiration is largely passive, and expiratory flow limitation results from alteration in the mechanical properties of the lungs rather than from muscle failure. The diaphragm is the principal muscle of inspiration. It probably acts alone during quiet breathing, the intercostal and accessory muscles being recruited only when the demand for ventilation increases. The abdominal muscles play an important role in augmenting ventilation when exertion increases O_2 requirements. Contraction during expiration displaces the abdominal contents inward and upward, lengthening the diaphragmatic muscle and decreasing its radius, thus improving the efficiency of the diaphragm as a pressure generator.

When it contracts, the diaphragm not only pushes down on the abdominal viscera and displaces the abdominal wall outward but it also lifts and expands the rib cage. The degree of thoracic expansion depends upon abdominal pressure. If the abdominal muscles are contracted, descent of the diaphragm is restricted and rib cage movement accentuated. At the end of a quiet expiration, the diaphragm is relaxed and pleural and abdominal pressures are equal. On inspiration, intrapleural pressure becomes more negative and abdominal pressure more positive, i.e., transdiaphragmatic pressure dif-

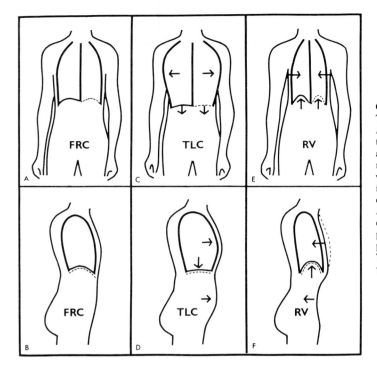

Figure 18–2. Schematic Depiction of Chest Cage and Diaphragmatic Movements Throughout the Respiratory Cycle: Normal. Anteroposterior (A) and lateral (B) views show the position of the chest wall and diaphragm at resting lung volume (FRC). At full inspiration (C and D), the diaphragm contracts with resultant expansion of the chest cage, increase in intra-abdominal pressure, and a consequent protrusion of the abdominal wall. At full expiration (E and F), abdominal muscle contraction causes a rise in intra-abdominal pressure and elevation of the relaxed diaphragm. FRC = functional residual capacity; TLC = total lung capacity; RV = residual volume.

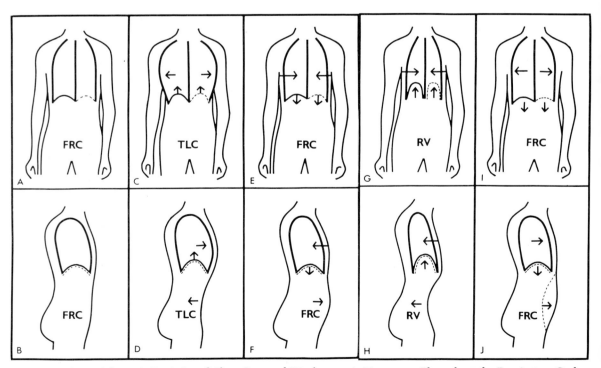

Figure 18–3. Schematic Depiction of Chest Cage and Diaphragmatic Movements Throughout the Respiratory Cycle: Bilateral Diaphragmatic Paralysis. On inspiration to TLC from FRC (A to D), the increased negative intrapleural pressure "sucks" the diaphragm up and draws the abdominal wall in. On expiration to FRC (E and F), the diaphragm descends and the abdomen protrudes. With a deeper expiration to RV accompanied by active contraction of the abdominal muscles (G and H), the diaphragm rises. Subsequently, during the first part of inspiration to FRC (I and J), abdominal muscle recoil is associated with descent of the flaccid diaphragm, creating the false impression of active contraction.

ference increases (ΔPdi). Normally this pressure difference exceeds 25 cm H_2O at a position of maximum inspiration. When the abdominal muscles are relaxed, this increase in pressure causes protrusion of the abdominal wall (Figure 18–2).

When the diaphragm is paralyzed as a result of either neuropathic or myopathic disorders, it is totally flaccid. With each inspiratory effort of the external intercostal and accessory muscles of respiration, the rib cage expands, lowering intrapleural pressure and "sucking" the diaphragm into the thorax, a most inefficient form of breathing (Figure 18–3A–D). This upward movement of the diaphragm results in an equal reduction of abdominal and pleural pressure, so that transdiaphragmatic pressure difference remains at zero. The fall in abdominal pressure in turn induces indrawing of the abdominal wall (Figure 18–3D).

Diaphragmatic dysfunction does not have to be total to provoke symptoms and signs. Disability from a weakened muscle may be accentuated or precipitated by an increased load on the respiratory system, such as that occasioned by exercise or concomitant COPD. With the exception of sudden and complete diaphragmatic paralysis such as occurs following upper cervical spinal cord transection, diaphragmatic muscle fatigue is probably the final common pathway to all conditions leading to respiratory failure with hypercapnia.

Bilateral phrenic paralysis can be caused by a variety of primary muscular and neurogenic disorders (*see* further on) and almost invariably produces symptoms and signs. If paralysis is confined to one hemidiaphragm, symptoms and signs may be absent. Unilateral paralysis usually is detected on a screening chest roentgenogram, the affected hemidiaphragm being markedly elevated and showing fluoroscopic evidence of parodoxical motion on "sniffing" (Figure 18–4A–D). If a patient with these findings manifests symptoms, it is probable that both hemidiaphragms are involved in an asymmetric manner, permitting relatively greater elevation of one side.

Involvement of the diaphragm is often a late manifestation of a generalized neuromuscular disease. Symptoms consist of shortness of breath on exertion, disturbed sleep, morning headache, and daytime fatigue and somnolence. Some patients are unable to lie flat.[22] Bilateral paralysis is associated with paradoxical movement of the abdominal wall during inspiration. Patients should be examined in the supine position and should not be made aware that their pattern of breathing is being observed. During inspiration (Figure 18–3A–D) the chest cage expands and the abdominal wall moves inward; during expiration (Figure 18–3E and F) the abdomen distends and the chest wall contracts.

A number of objective methods are available

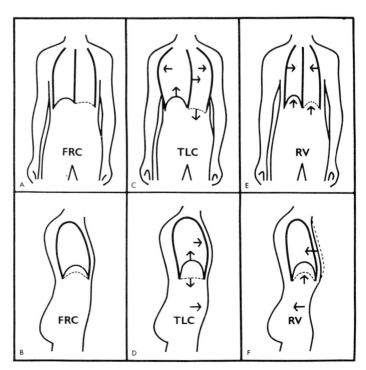

Figure 18–4. Schematic Depiction of Chest Cage and Diaphragmatic Movements Throughout the Respiratory Cycle: Right Hemidiaphragmatic Paralysis. At FRC (A and B), the right hemidiaphragm is elevated. On full inspiration to TLC (C and D), the left hemidiaphragm actively contracts and descends, whereas the flaccid right hemidiaphragm passively elevates in response to the more negative intrapleural pressure. On full expiration to RV (E and F), a rise in intra-abdominal pressure evokes an even greater elevation of the paralyzed right hemidiaphragm.

for the detection of diaphragmatic paralysis. These tests are useful not only in the assessment of the degree of weakness quantitatively but in establishing the cause of disability when physical findings are equivocal. Procedures used to determine the efficiency of the respiratory pump include pulmonary function tests, fluoroscopic evaluation of diaphragmatic motion, measurement of the movements of the chest and abdominal walls by magnetometry, the assessment of muscle activity by surface and esophageal electromyography, and the measurement of transdiaphragmatic pressures by balloons in the stomach and esophagus.

Fluoroscopic examination may be of some value in assessing unilateral diaphragmatic paralysis by revealing paradoxical motion on deep breathing and, more particularly, on sniffing (Figure 18–4). However, as pointed out in Chapter 17, such changes should be interpreted with some degree of caution. In contrast to the situation that pertains when only one hemidiaphragm is affected, when the *entire* diaphragm is paralyzed and there is no functioning diaphragmatic muscle, fluoroscopic examination of the patient in the erect position may reveal some downward displacement of the diaphragm on inspiration, a phenomenon that occurs in some patients who employ the passive recoil of the abdominal wall to assist inspiration. Active contraction of the abdominal muscles during a complete expiration is associated with upward displacement of the diaphragm (Figure 18–3G and H). At the onset of inspiration the abdominal muscles relax, decreasing abdominal pressure. This permits the diaphragm to descend passively during inspiration, thus producing the false impression of active muscle contraction (Figure 18–3I and J).[23] This maneuver appears early in the inspiratory phase, from below FRC to the resting expiratory level (FRC), at which point the increasing negative intrapleural pressure causes the flaccid diaphragm to move upward and the abdominal wall inward (Figure 18–3C and D).

Magnetometry measures the anteroposterior dimensions of the rib cage and abdomen simultaneously and separately during the respiratory cycle and is a useful method of recording diaphragmatic paralysis.[24]

Phrenic nerve conduction can be measured by recording the diaphragmatic muscle action potential with either esophageal electrodes or surface electrodes over the lateral chest wall. A positive response in the presence of suspected diaphragmatic paralysis indicates that the disorder is myopathic rather than neuropathic.

Routine pulmonary function tests may suggest the possibility of respiratory neuromuscular disease. When the lung parenchyma is normal and patient cooperation complete, a decrease in TLC or increase in RV (thus a decrease in VC) may indicate respiratory muscle weakness. Flow rates may also reflect neurogenic or myopathic disorders. Most laboratories include flow-time or flow-volume curves as screening procedures. Since early flow is effort-dependent and late flow effort-independent (reflecting flow in small airways), a relative dysfunction in the first part of the forced vital capacity suggests a neuromuscular defect.[25] It is important to remember that upper airway obstruction may also produce a similar pattern of predominantly reduced FEV_1 (*see page 523*).

Maximum inspiratory and expiratory pressures are useful indices of respiratory muscle strength. Although this is a simple test, its performance requires patient cooperation.

Initially patients with neuromuscular respiratory disease hyperventilate, but this is inevitably succeeded by hypoventilation as the disease progresses. However, even severe hypoxemia and hypercapnia can be corrected in these patients by voluntary hyperventilation. In patients with severe weakness or complete paralysis of the diaphragm, assumption of the supine position causes further deterioration in gas exchange. The explanation for this lies in the change in gravitational forces. The weight of the abdominal organs displaces the flaccid diaphragm upward into the thoracic cavity and thus further reduces the effectiveness of the remaining inspiratory muscles.[23] In addition, a further drop in PaO_2 and a rise in $PaCO_2$ often occur during sleep, when control of breathing is solely automatic.[23] The presence of hypoxemia and hypercapnia, in spite of a remaining potential for the respiratory pump to restore gas exchange to normal, can only be interpreted as a disturbance of respiratory control. There appears to be a resetting of central or peripheral sensors (or both) and perhaps a deficiency of tendon receptor response in diaphragmatic muscle.

Perhaps the most effective means of identifying weakness or paralysis of the diaphragm is the measurement of transdiaphragmatic pressure (Pdi). This is accomplished by recording pressures in balloons placed in both the esophagus and stomach. Gastric and esophageal pressure devices and EMG have recently been incorporated into a single catheter.[26] In normal subjects the change of Pdi (ΔPdi) that develops during the course of a maximum inspiration exceeds 25 cm H_2O. In the presence of complete diaphragmatic paralysis Pdi undergoes no change in full inspiration. If the diaphragm is weaker than normal, recorded values will be considerably below normal.

In patients with neuromuscular disease the determination of respiratory drive by CO_2 response curves and mouth occlusion pressures may reveal a deficiency. However, this is not a direct measurement of respiratory muscle function. When values are abnormal, it can be assumed that either the respiratory controller is defective or there is a disturbance of receptor input.

In addition to specific disease entities that result in weakness and eventual paralysis, the diaphragm, like any skeletal muscle, may tire, a state that is potentially reversible. Diaphragmatic fatigue occurs most commonly in advanced COPD[27] and is manifested by asynchronous breathing, an important criterion of prognosis and a finding that some investigators view as an indication for artificial ventilation.[27]

DISORDERS OF THE ANTERIOR HORN CELLS AND PERIPHERAL NERVES

Anterior horn cell involvement in disease may result in acute or chronic respiratory failure (*see* Table 18–2). The hereditary hepatic porphyrias are inborn errors of porphyrin metabolism inherited as mendelian autosomal dominants, which may be associated with ascending paralysis and respiratory failure. Remissions may be followed by further exacerbations but not necessarily affecting the respiratory musculature.

Acute polyneuritis (Landry-Guillain-Barré syndrome) can be associated with acute or subacute hypoventilation. Of all the neuromuscular diseases, Guillain-Barré syndrome is probably the commonest cause of respiratory failure. Although in some respects this disease is a diagnosis of exclusion, there is an accepted clinical presentation that includes symmetric ascending paralysis and a lack of cellular response in the cerebrospinal fluid. It shows a striking predilection for patients under the age of 26 years of either sex.

Paralytic shellfish poisoning is caused by the ingestion of bivalve mollusks (oysters, clams, and mussels) that are contaminated with the neurotoxins of the dinoflagellates *Gonyaulax catanella* and *Tamarensis saxitoxin*. The neurotoxin produced by these parasites blocks the propagation of nerve and muscle action potentials.

MYONEURAL AND RESPIRATORY MUSCLE DISORDERS

The diseases that lead to blockage at the myoneural junction, with consequent acute or chronic hypoventilation, are myasthenia gravis, the myasthenialike syndrome associated with neoplasms and various medications, and infection caused by *Clostridium botulinum*. The defect in myasthenia gravis has now been established as postsynaptic rather than presynaptic, *i.e.*, in the muscle rather than the nerve.[28] Although most experimental evidence suggests that antiacetylcholine receptor antibodies are responsible for the pathophysiologic response at the myoneural junction,[29] in some cases of myasthenia there is the additional (or perhaps exclusive) factor of a T cell–dependent cellular immunity to receptor that may be responsible for destruction of the postsynaptic apparatus.[30]

Myasthenialike syndromes occur in association with neoplasia, the administration of various antibiotics, and antiseizure therapy. Respiratory paralysis caused by antibiotics may develop within 1 to 24 hours after the administration of these drugs, usually in patients with renal disease or myasthenia gravis. In most cases the respiratory failure is of short duration, spontaneous ventilation being resumed within 24 hours.[31] Penicillamine, a drug used in the treatment of rheumatoid arthritis and Wilson's disease, may be associated with the development of myasthenia gravis.

Organophosphate poisoning caused by the insecticides Parathion and Malathion results from inhibition of acetylcholinesterase at nerve endings. Acetylcholine accumulates at cholinergic synapses resulting in an initial stimulation and a later inhibition of synaptic transmission, with consequent fatigue and paralysis of the diaphragm.

Although types A and B botulism, caused by *Clostridium botulinum*, have traditionally been regarded as the organisms responsible for acute respiratory failure, this complication is also seen in type E botulism following ingestion of contaminated canned fish.[32-35] The endotoxin from this organism blocks the release of acetylcholine in the cholinergic system. A recent report from the Centers for Disease Control, Atlanta, has emphasized the necessity for early intubation in these patients.[36]

Fish causing ciguatera (barracuda, red snapper, amberjack, and grouper) produce ciguatoxin, which has been shown to inhibit human red cell cholinesterase *in vitro*. Respiratory paralysis occurs occasionally, presumably from the same mechanism that has been reported in organophosphate poisoning.

We have seen examples of myasthenia-like syndromes associated with carcinoma, but in no instance has the respiratory musculature been involved, nor are we aware of any published reports of respiratory failure occurring in such circumstances.

Respiratory muscle disorders that give rise to hypoventilation and a particularly insidious type of chronic respiratory failure are myotonic and progressive muscular dystrophy.[37, 38] This complication develops in approximately 10 per cent of patients with myotonic muscular dystrophy. A myopathy that is being increasingly recognized as a cause of respiratory failure is that resulting from acid maltase deficiency,[39] a type II glycogen storage disease.

Although polymyositis and dermatomyositis are more commonly associated with problems of aspiration consequent upon pharyngeal muscle paralysis, in some cases involvement of the diaphragm leads to acute or chronic hypoventilation. Muscular weakness has been postulated as the mechanism that leads to "shrinking" of the lungs in patients with systemic lupus erythematosus.[40] In this disease serial chest roentgenograms may reveal progressive loss of lung volume unassociated with other abnormalities of the lung parenchyma.

Acute flaccid paralysis requiring artificial ventilation has been reported to occur in association with hypophosphatemia, with hypokalemia and with renal tubular acidosis. In these circumstances artificial ventilation is required while electrolyte disturbance is being corrected.

CLINICAL MANIFESTATIONS

The diseases that result in disturbances of ventilatory control and those that limit respiratory muscle function may be associated with similar symptoms and signs. Essential to the establishment of the correct diagnosis is a careful neurologic examination. Various measurements of respiratory drive and respiratory muscle function have been devised that are useful in defining the pathophysiology, and these have already been described. This section summarizes the clinical findings that are common to the two groups of disorders (see Table 18–2) and the clinical features that may suggest certain specific causes.

Patients complain of anxiety, lethargy, headache, dyspnea, and sometimes a feeling of suffocation. In cases in which ventilation is severely restricted, confusion may be apparent and coma and death· can supervene rapidly.

Cyanosis may or may not be present, depending upon the degree of hypoventilation. Appreciation of the degree of alveolar ventilation clinically is unreliable except when apnea has occurred, by which time the patient will be severely cyanotic.

Epileptic seizures may be responsible for severe tissue hypoxia and transitory lactic acidosis. This diagnosis is easily made clinically. Tetanus is now largely a disease found in developing countries; however, in areas such as New York City, where drug addiction is a major problem, tetanus has undergone a resurgence. In this complicated setting, intubation or tracheostomy is invariably required for ventilatory support.[41] Puncture wounds and lacerations acquired on the farm or in the garden are common sites of infection. The development of tetanic spasm may require the use of paralyzing drugs. Patients with mild tetanus experience trismus (inability to open the mouth) and hypertonicity of the chest wall and abdominal muscles; those with moderate and severe disease have tetanic spasms in addition. Even those with mild disease manifest hypoxemia and hyperventilation associated with metabolic acidosis and a restrictive pattern of pulmonary function.

A traumatic, infectious, or vascular etiology of brain damage associated with respiratory failure is usually clearly indicated by a history of trauma, fever, rigidity of neck muscles, or local neurologic signs. The mechanism of the hyperventilation that occurs in some cases is nonchemical and probably is related to central neurologic damage; the prognosis is poor.[42] It is of interest that patients with cerebrovascular accidents who hyperventilate tend to have a *lower* Po_2 than those with a normal respiratory pattern, despite a normal chest roentgenogram.[43] Similar findings have been noted in unconscious patients following head injury,[44] suggesting that seriously ill patients must have interstitial pulmonary edema, either neurogenic in origin or resulting from aspiration of gastric juices.

Drug intoxication should be strongly suspected in any patient admitted to the hospital in a semicomatose or comatose state. Methods for identifying the drug and for estimating its blood levels can prove useful in the management of the poisoned patient. Examination of the pupils may aid in diagnosis; they are usually responsive to light in barbiturate poisoning and fixed and dilated in glutethimide poisoning. Patients who die from sedative drug overdose commonly manifest extensive air-space consolidation of their lungs, either from bacterial pneumonia or from edema secondary to gastric juice aspiration. Dialysis and forced diuresis are not required in the management of the great majority of these patients; in fact, complications are less frequent when supportive care alone is used.

Poliomyelitis should be suspected as the cause of acute respiratory failure when symptoms of bulbar palsy are present in an unvaccinated individual. Patients with porphyria also may have bulbar symptoms and may give a history of previous attacks of abdominal pain. The diagnosis is supported when other members of the family are known to be afflicted, and confirmation can be obtained by the discovery of porphyrin precursors in the urine.

Polyneuritis (Landry-Guillain-Barré syndrome) usually begins with peripheral muscular weakness, a finding that should alert the physician to the necessity for frequent measurements of vital capacity and arterial blood gases in order to detect the onset of respiratory failure (which may develop abruptly). Although the prognosis usually is good, ventilatory support may have to be provided for prolonged periods.

Prior to the onset of hypoventilation, patients with myasthenia and myasthenialike syndromes usually manifest paresthesia, diplopia, dysphagia, ptosis, general weakness, respiratory fatigability, and dyspnea. In some cases these disorders of the myoneural junction are brought to the attention of the physician after a surgical procedure in which the additive effect of sedation and muscle relaxants results in a long period of inadequate ventilation postoperatively. Botulism also produces a myoneural form of muscular paralysis. In the early stages of the disease the diagnosis can be suspected when a history is obtained of recent ingestion of suspicious-tasting food removed from a distended plastic container or can.

Ciguatera (poisoning by fish) and shellfish poisoning are manifested by vomiting, diarrhea, dry mouth, a metallic taste, myalgia, arthralgia, blurred vision, photophobia, transient blindness, and paresthesias around the mouth and lips.

Polymyositis usually involves the proximal muscles and frequently is associated with skin changes similar to those seen in scleroderma. The measurement of serum enzymes—including transaminase (SGOT and SGPT), aldolase, and creatine phosphokinase—and electromyographic studies are of help in diagnosis.

Hypokalemia should be suspected as a cause of muscle paralysis in situations where potassium loss might be excessive.

Diseases leading to chronic hypoventilation of neuromuscular origin include myxedema, the idiopathic forms of respiratory center depression seen in both obese and nonobese individuals, and destruction of the anterior horn cells in poliomyelitis and amyotrophic lateral sclerosis. In addition, the muscular dystrophies, and occasionally polymyositis and myasthenia gravis, may be responsible for prolonged underventilation. Cases of underventilation due to these neuromuscular diseases may go unrecognized for a long time, particularly if the hypoxemia is not severe enough to cause cyanosis. These patients may complain of dyspnea and fatigability on exertion, or of recurrent headache, particularly in the morning upon waking, perhaps due to raised intracranial pressure resulting from increased circulating carbon dioxide during sleep. Somnolence may be very disabling. It occurs more commonly in obese hypoventilators, although it may be present in any patient with respiratory failure. It is not uncommon for the diagnosis of chronic hypoventilation, particularly of the idiopathic type, to be made because of the finding of polycythemia or cor pulmonale. In the obese patient with upper airway obstruction, somnolence during the day may be attributed to sleep deprivation at night, and it seems likely that the worsening of blood gas exchange that occurs in the supine position, even in patients who are not obese, satisfactorily explains the tendency to fall asleep during the day. In the idiopathic hypoventilation syndrome, with or without obesity, blood gas values may be restored to normal limits after the patient has taken two or three deep breaths. In the hypoventilation syndrome, respiratory arrest or pulmonary embolism are the commonest causes of death.

Chronic respiratory failure caused by disorders of the anterior horn cells or by muscular dystrophies usually is readily recognized because of a prolonged history of muscle wasting and weakness.

Patients with chronic hypoventilation may show electrocardiographic evidence of right ventricular hypertrophy and in some instances cardiac failure due to cor pulmonale. In nerve cell and muscle disorders, pulmonary function tests reveal restriction, reflected predominantly in reduction in vital capacity.

VENOARTERIAL SHUNTS

EXTRAPULMONARY VENOARTERIAL SHUNTS

Oxygen transport to the tissues may be inadequate despite normal structure and function of lung parenchyma. In these circumstances, the hypoxemia is caused by shunting of venous blood into arterial channels, and blood gas analysis reveals reduced PO_2 with normal or reduced PCO_2. The most common cause of shunting is congenital heart disease. In this section we are concerned primarily with extrapulmonary venoarterial shunts in which the standard chest roentgenogram is normal.

A form of venoarterial shunting, which in some cases at least is extrapulmonary in type, is that found in patients with advanced cirrhosis of the liver. These patients usually have normal chest roentgenograms, and evidence of shunting lies in the results of arterial blood gas analysis, which reveals mild to moderate hypoxemia and compensated respiratory alkalosis. There is reason to believe that more than one mechanism is responsible for the hypoxemia associated with liver cirrhosis. In some instances venous blood in the portal system may reach the left side of the heart through anastomotic channels with pulmonary veins.[45, 46] In others, severe arterial dilatation has been identified in the lungs of patients who have died of cirrhosis.[47] In addition, spider nevi can be detected on the pleura.[47] Studies carried out in our laboratories in patients with advanced cirrhosis and severe hypoxemia have shown that the majority do not have significant absolute shunts but rather ventilation/perfusion defects.[48] In experimental portal cirrhosis in dogs[49] and in studies of lymph flow in the thoracic duct in humans with hepatic cirrhosis[50, 51] there has been demonstrated a marked outpouring of fluid from liver sinusoids; this has resulted in lymph flow overloads for the thoracic duct system, permitting back-up of fluid in the pulmonary lymphatics and resultant $\dot{V}/\dot{Q}$ disturbance.

In some cases of hepatic cirrhosis, small nodular and linear opacities can be identified roentgenographically in the lung bases.[47]

The hypoxemia observed in patients with hepatic cirrhosis is more severe in the sitting than in the recumbent position (orthodeoxia), a phenomenon that can be explained by either increased pressure in the thoracic duct in the erect position or increased basilar blood flow in those patients with shunts. Most patients with advanced cirrhosis of the liver present with symptoms and signs attributable to the liver damage, the hypoxemia and hypocapnia rarely being severe enough to produce symptoms or signs. Secondary polycythemia may occur occasionally and, in the absence of blood gas analysis, may be confused with erythrocytosis associated with hepatomas.

PULMONARY VENOARTERIAL SHUNTS

In addition to those patients with cirrhosis of the liver who have normal chest roentgenograms and whose hypoxemia is caused by arteriovenous shunts or excessive pulmonary lymph, there are some patients in whom, during the postoperative period, blood is shunted from pulmonary artery to pulmonary vein and yet whose chest roentgenograms reveal nothing of note. In such cases, impairment of ventilation-perfusion ratios may be demonstrated.

METHEMOGLOBINEMIA AND CARBON MONOXIDE POISONING

Oxygen transport to the tissues may be reduced as a result of methemoglobinemia or carbon monoxide poisoning. Methemoglobinemia may result from exposure to drugs or chemicals that act by increasing the rate of hemoglobin oxidation or by overstimulating the intraerythrocyte mechanisms that protect hemoglobin against oxidation.[52] It may also result from impairment of the patient's capacity to reduce hemoglobin, either on an enzymatic or chemical basis. Acquired methemoglobinemia has been reported to follow the ingestion of well water containing high concentrations of nitrate.[53]

Two types of hereditary methemoglobinemia have been described, one caused by enzymatic lack and the other associated with an abnormal type of hemoglobin (hemoglobin M). Methemoglobinemia causes no alteration in the chest roentgenogram. Patients usually present with symptoms and signs caused by tissue anoxia, including headache, nausea, dizziness, pounding pulse, or listlessness. The congenital variety of the disease is associated with mental retardation.[52]

Carbon monoxide poisoning may lead to either an acute respiratory emergency or, when lower concentrations of the gas have been inhaled, a more chronic presentation characterized by abnormal behavior. Carboxyhemoglobin levels of 10 to 15 per cent have been found in heavy cigarette and cigar smokers. These concentrations are also considered to be responsible for a reversible form of secondary polycythemia. The acute variety usually results from excessive inhalation of exhaust fumes from automobiles. In such cases the patient may be comatose when found, with cherry-red skin and mucous membranes.

ALVEOLAR HYPERVENTILATION

Normally, alveolar ventilation is proportional to the metabolic requirements of the tissues. In response to fever or exertion of any type, an increased demand for oxygen at the tissue level results in increased alveolar ventilation. Similarly, thyrotoxicosis and moving from sea level to a high altitude evoke physiologic responses in an attempt to maintain adequate oxygen supply to tissues. Hyperventilation may be described as ventilation in excess of the capacity required to maintain P_{CO_2} between 35 and 45 mm Hg.

ETIOLOGY AND PATHOGENESIS

Hyperventilation with reduction in the P_{CO_2} to 35 mm Hg or less may result from both pulmonary and extrapulmonary causes. In the majority of instances, excessive ventilation is of psychogenic origin.

Organic Pulmonary Disease

Hyperventilation and hypocapnia may occur in patients with bronchial asthma, pneumonia, pulmonary embolism, and diffuse granulomatous or fibrotic interstitial disease. In cases of organic pulmonary disease, hypocapnia is usually associated with hypoxemia. An exception to this rule occurs in some patients with diffuse fibrosis of the lungs when the P_{O_2} may be normal at rest and fall only with exercise.

Extrapulmonary Disorders

Excessive ventilation leading to hypocapnia may occur as a result of various nonpulmonary disorders. These include organic disorders of the central nervous system, disease states resulting in metabolic acidosis, drug ingestion (particularly salicylates), ammonium chloride therapy, mechanical ventilation during anesthesia or in patients unable to breathe spontaneously, and psychological disturbances.

The central nervous system disorders that may lead to hyperventilation include cerebrovascular accidents, brain trauma, meningitis, and encephalitis. In many cases of organic brain disease, hypoxemia and hypercapnia develop as increasing intracranial pressure depresses the respiratory center. In such patients, blood gas analysis during the initial stage may indicate respiratory alkalosis caused by hyperventilation; later, respiratory acidosis may develop as the H^+ ion concentration rises as a result of hypoventilation and carbon dioxide retention.

Hyperventilation in primary metabolic acidosis results from stimulation of the respiratory center and carotid bodies by an increase in H^+ ion concentration. The major cause for this type of hyperventilation is the ketosis associated with uncontrolled diabetes and renal failure.

The ingestion of salicylates in large enough quantities to provoke hyperventilation usually occurs accidentally in children but sometimes constitutes a suicidal attempt in young adults or an abuse of prescribed medication in the elderly.[54] The acid-base disorder most often consists of a mixed respiratory alkalosis and an anion gap-type metabolic acidosis. In a minority of cases uncomplicated respiratory alkalosis and metabolic acidosis are also seen.[54] Although in young people salicylate intoxication is generally considered to be a benign disease with a low mortality rate, such is not the case in the elderly.[54]

Hyperventilation with compensated or uncompensated hypocapnia may also be iatrogenic in origin. This is a common occurrence during controlled ventilation in anesthetized patients and occurs in a small percentage of persons maintained on artificial respiration, particularly if they have normal lungs.

Cheyne-Stokes respiration is a nonpulmonary form of hyperventilation recognizable clinically by the contrast between periods of hyperventilation and of apnea. Tidal volume progressively increases during the hyperpneic phase and subsequently decreases without change in respiratory rate. This form of periodic breathing occurs in patients with left ventricular failure or impaired cerebrovascular circulation. The subject of feedback control systems with particular reference to ventilatory control and Cheyne-Stokes breathing has been discussed at some length by Cherniack and Longobardo,[56] and the interested reader is referred to this review for more detail.

By far the most common cause of hyperventilation is of psychological origin. Psychogenic hyperventilation varies in degree and clinical presentation. It occurs in a wide variety of persons, from those who complain of dyspnea occurring at rest and who require frequent deep respiratory efforts to the hysterical patient who overbreathes to the extent of inducing coma or tetany.

With the exception of hyperventilation caused by pulmonary disease, the various forms of alveolar hyperventilation are unassociated with roentgenographically apparent alteration in the lungs. In fact, even organic pulmonary disease, particularly in association with pulmonary embolism, may not be evident roentgenographically.

CLINICAL MANIFESTATIONS

Patients with diffuse interstitial pulmonary disease may complain of dyspnea on exertion, but the overventilation at rest that is detectable by arterial blood gas analysis rarely produces symptoms. Hyperpnea occasioned by pulmonary embolic episodes is often recognized as a transitory dyspneic sensation. Many of the patients who are overventilating as a result of central nervous system lesions or metabolic acidosis are semicomatose or comatose, and then the excessive respirations are often an inconsequential feature of a much more complex problem. The symptoms and signs manifested by individuals who hyperventilate for a psychological reason readily lead to a diagnosis. Dyspnea is usually noted at rest and when associated with exertion is characteristically seen to follow rather than to occur during effort. The majority of patients with psychogenic hyperventilation describe their shortness of breath as an inability to "get enough air down into their lungs," although some complain of a smothering feeling at night just before falling asleep or immediately on waking. Chest pain is common and has been attributed to either an overdistended stomach or to overuse of intercostal muscles. Most patients with psychogenic dyspnea complain of giddiness, numbness, tingling of the extremities, headaches, premature heartbeats producing palpitations, and gastrointestinal symptoms including dryness of the mouth, belching, abdominal bloating, and gas pains, often with difficulty in swallowing.[55] The hyperventilation syndrome may be precipitated by anxiety over organic disease.

Spirometry often confirms the diagnosis of psychogenic hyperventilation strongly suspected on clinical grounds. The characteristic pattern is highly irregular breathing punctuated by deep periodic inspirations. In the majority of instances arterial blood gas analysis shows reduction in the PCO_2, usually with proportional reduction in bicarbonate levels. Electrocardiograms may reveal depression of the ST segment and reduction or inversion of the T wave in any or all leads.[55] When hyperventilation is severe the electroencephalogram may record slowed activity.

Occasionally one encounters primary respiratory alkalosis due to extrapulmonary organic disease in patients in whom lactic acidosis develops, presumably as a "compensatory" mechanism to the alkalotic state.

REFERENCES

1. Rigler, L. G.: Roentgen examination of the chest. Its limitations in the diagnosis of disease. J.A.M.A., 142:773, 1950.
2. Resnick, M. E., Berkowitz, R. D., and Rodman, T.: Diffuse interstitial leukemic infiltration of the lungs producing the alveolar-capillary block syndrome. Report of a case, with studies of pulmonary function. Am. J. Med., 31:149, 1961.
3. Thurlbeck, W. M., Henderson, J. A., Fraser, R. G., and Bates, D. V.: Chronic obstructive lung disease. A comparison between clinical, roentgenologic, functional and morphologic criteria in chronic bronchitis, emphysema, asthma and bronchiectasis. Medicine, 49:81, 1970.
4. Thurlbeck, W. M., and Simon, G.: Radiographic appearance of the chest in emphysema. Am. J. Roentgenol., 130:429, 1978.
5. Önal, E., Lopata, M., and O'Connor, T. D.: Diaphragmatic and genioglossal electromyogram responses to isocapnic hypoxia in humans. Am. Rev. Resp. Dis., 124:215, 1981.
6. Önal, E., Lopata, M., and O'Connor, T.: Pathogenesis of apneas in hypersomnia-sleep apnea syndrome. Am. Rev. Resp. Dis., 125:167, 1982.
7. Phillipson, E. A.: Control of breathing during sleep. Am. Rev. Resp. Dis., 118:909, 1978.
8. Berger, A. J., Mitchell, R. A., and Severinghaus, J. W.: Regulation of respiration (first of three parts). N. Engl. J. Med. 297:92, 1977.
9. Berger, A. J., Mitchell, R. A., and Severinghaus, J. W.: Regulation of respiration (second of three parts). N. Engl. J. Med., 297:138, 1977.
10. Berger, A. J., Mitchell, R. A., and Severinghaus, J. W.: Regulation of respiration (third of three parts). N. Engl. J. Med., 297:194, 1977.
11. Derenne, J-Ph., Macklem, P. T., and Roussos, Ch. L.: The respiratory muscles: Mechanics, control and pathophysiology. I. Am. Rev. Resp. Dis., 118:119, 373, 581, 1978.
12. Forester, C. F.: Coma in myxedema. Report of a case and review of the world literature. Arch. Intern. Med., 111:734, 1963.
13. Kerr, W. J., and Lagen, J. B.: The postural syndrome related to obesity leading to postural emphysema and cardiorespiratory failure. Ann. Intern. Med., 10:569, 1936.
14. Burwell, C. S., Robin, E. D., Whaley, R. D., and Bickelmann, A. G.: Extreme obesity associated with alveolar hypoventilation—a Pickwickian syndrome. Am. J. Med., 21:811, 1956.
15. Holley, H. S., Milic-Emili, J., Becklake, M. R., and Bates, D. V.: Regional distribution of pulmonary ventilation and perfusion in obesity. J. Clin. Invest., 46:475, 1967.
16. Bedell, G. N., Wilson, W. R., and Seebohm, P. M.: Pulmonary function in obese persons. J. Clin. Invest., 37:1049, 1958.
17. Kaufman, B. J., Ferguson, M. H., and Cherniack, R.

M.: Hypoventilation in obesity. J. Clin. Invest., 38:500, 1959.

18. Mellins, R. B., Balfour, H. H., Jr., Turino, G. M., and Winters, R. W.: Failure of automatic control of ventilation (Ondine's curse). Report of an infant born with this syndrome and review of the literature. Medicine, 49:487, 1970.

19. Severinghaus, J. W., and Mitchell, R. A.: Ondine's curse—failure of respiratory center automaticity while awake. Clin. Res., 10:122, 1962.

20. Kuperman, A. S., Krieger, A. J., and Rosomoff, H. L.: Respiratory function after cervical cordotomy. Chest, 59:128, 1971.

21. Luce, J. M., and Culver, B. H.: Respiratory muscle function in health and disease. Chest, 81:82, 1982.

22. Blythe, J. A., Griffin, J. P., and Gonyea, E. F.: Bilateral diaphragmatic paralysis in association with neurogenic disease. Arch. Intern. Med., 137:1455, 1977.

23. Newsom Davis, J., Goldman, M., Loh, L., and Casson, M.: Diaphragm function and alveolar hypoventilation. Q. J. Med., 45:87, 1976.

24. Konno, K., and Mead, J.: Measurement of the separate volume changes of rib cage and abdomen during breathing. J. Appl. Physiol., 22:407, 1967.

25. Goldstein, R. L., Hyde, R. W., Lapham, L. W., Gazioglu, K., and de Papp, Z. G.: Peripheral neuropathy presenting with respiratory insufficiency as the primary complaint. Problem of recognizing alveolar hypoventilation due to neuromuscular disorders. Am. J. Med., 56:443, 1974.

26. Önal, E., Lopata, M., Ginzburg, A. S., and O'Connor, T. D.: Diaphragmatic EMG and transdiaphragmatic pressure measurements with a single catheter. Am. Rev. Resp. Dis., 124:563, 1981.

27. Sharp, J. T.: Diaphragmatic function and respiratory failure. Chest, 71:566, 1977.

28. Mulder, D. W.: Myasthenia gravis. Mayo Clin. Proc., 52:334, 1977.

29. Engel, A. G., Lambert, E. H., and Howard, F. M., Jr.: Immune complexes (IgG and C3) at the motor end-plate in myasthenia gravis: Ultrastructural and light microscopic localization and electrophysiologic correlations. Mayo Clin. Proc., 52:267, 1977.

30. Richman, D. P., Patrick, J., and Arnason, B. G.: Cellular immunity in myasthenia gravis. Response to purified acetylcholine receptor and autologous thymocytes. N. Engl. J. Med., 294:694, 1976.

31. Lindesmith, L. A., Baines, R. D., Jr., Bigelow, D. B., and Petty, T. L.: Reversible respiratory paralysis associated with polymyxin therapy. Ann. Intern. Med., 68:318, 1968.

32. Koenig, M. G., Spickard, A., Cardella, M. A., and Rogers, D. E.: Clinical and laboratory observations on type E botulism in man. Medicine, 43:517, 1964.

33. Whittaker, R. L., Gilbertson, R. B., and Garrett, A. S., Jr.: Botulism, type E. Report of eight simultaneous cases. Ann. Intern. Med., 61:448, 1964.

34. Armstrong, R. W., Stenn, F., Dowell, V. R., Jr., Ammerman, G., and Sommers, H. M.: Type E botulism from home-canned gefilte fish. J.A.M.A., 210:303, 1969.

35. Canada Diseases Weekly Report. Botulism in Canada— Summary for 1981. Vol. 8–7:33, 1982.

36. Hughes, J. M., Blumenthal, J. R., Merson, M. H., Lombard, G. L., Dowell, V. R., Jr., and Gangarosa, E. J.: Clinical features of types A and B foodborne botulism. Ann. Intern. Med., 95:442, 1981.

37. Kilburn, K. H., Eagan, J. T., Sieker, H. O., and Heyman, A.: Cardiopulmonary insufficiency in myotonic and progressive muscular dystrophy. N. Engl. J. Med., 261:1089, 1959.

38. Inkley, S. R., Oldenburg, F. C., and Vignos, P. J., Jr.: Pulmonary function in Duchenne muscular dystrophy related to stage of disease. Am. J. Med., 56:297, 1974.

39. Engel, A. G., Gomez, M. R., Seybold, M. E., and Lambert, E. H.: The spectrum and diagnosis of acid maltase deficiency. Neurology, 23:95, 1973.

40. Gibson, G. J., Edmonds, J. P., and Hughes, G. R. V.: Diaphragm function and lung involvement in systemic lupus erythematosus. Am. J. Med., 63:926, 1977.

41. Heurich, A. E., Brust, J. C. M., and Richter, R. W.: Management of urban tetanus. Med. Clin. North Am., 57:1373, 1973.

42. Lane, D. J., Rout, M. W., and Williamson, D. H.: Mechanism of hyperventilation in acute cerebrovascular accidents. Br. Med. J., 3:9, 1971.

43. Rout, M. W., Lane, D. J., and Wollner, L.: Prognosis in acute cerebrovascular accidents in relation to respiratory pattern and blood gas tensions. Br. Med. J., 3:7, 1971.

44. Moss, I. R., Wald, A., and Ransohoff, J.: Respiratory functions and chemical regulation of ventilation in head injury. Am. Rev. Resp. Dis., 109:205, 1974.

45. Wolfe, J. D., Taskins, D. P., Holly, F. E., Brachman, M. B., and Genovesi, M. G.: Hypoxemia of cirrhosis. Detection of abnormal small pulmonary vascular channels by a quantitative radionuclide method. Am. J. Med., 63:746, 1977.

46. Ellman, B. A., Curry, T. S., III, Glotzbach, R. E., and Simpson, P. R.: Systemic embolization as a complication of transhepatic venography. Radiology, 141:67, 1981.

47. Berthelot, P., Walker, J. G., Sherlock, S., and Reid, L.: Arterial changes in the lungs in cirrhosis of the liver—lung spider nevi. N. Engl. J. Med., 274:291, 1966.

48. Ruff, F., Hughes, J. M. B., Stanley, N., McCarthy, D., Greene, R., Aronoff, A., Clayton, L., and Milic-Emili, J.: Regional lung function in patients with hepatic cirrhosis. J. Clin. Invest., 50:2403, 1971.

49. Levy, M.: Sodium retention and ascites formation in dogs with experimental portal cirrhosis. Am. J. Physiol., 233:F572, 1977.

50. Dumont, A. E., and Witte, M. H.: Contrasting patterns of thoracic duct lymph formation in hepatic cirrhosis. Surg. Gynecol. Obstet., 122:524, 1966.

51. Dumont, A. E., and Mulholland, J. H.: Flow rate and composition of thoracic-duct lymph in patients with cirrhosis. N. Engl. J. Med., 263:471, 1960.

52. Jaffé, E. R.: Hereditary methemoglobinemias associated with abnormalities in the metabolism of erythrocytes. Am. J. Med., 41:786, 1966.

53. Comly, H. H.: Cyanosis in infants caused by nitrates in well water. J.A.M.A., 129:112, 1945.

54. Anderson, R. J., Potts, D. E., Gabow, P. A., Rumack, B. H., and Schrier, R. W.: Unrecognized adult salicylate intoxication. Ann. Intern. Med., 85:745, 1976.

55. Rice, R. L.: Symptom patterns of the hyperventilation syndrome. Am. J. Med., 8:691, 1950.

56. Cherniack, N. S., and Longobardo, G. S.: Cheyne-Stokes Breathing: An instability in physiologic control. N. Engl. J. Med., 288:952. 1973.

19

Tables of Differential Diagnosis and Decision Trees

GENERAL COMMENTS

This book is based on two premises: (1) that one of the early steps in the diagnosis of diseases of the chest should be an assessment of the pattern of changes revealed on a chest roentgenogram; and (2) that correlation of these findings with the clinical history and with abnormalities revealed by physical examination, laboratory investigation, pulmonary function testing, and special investigations will yield a positive diagnosis in the majority of cases. If this proposition is accepted, clearly it is necessary to evaluate the chest roentgenogram on a basis of pattern recognition in which individual patterns can be related to pathogenesis and thence to etiology.

From the 17 *Tables of Differential Diagnosis* included in the second edition of *Diagnosis of Diseases of the Chest*, we have selected nine that we believe are referred to most frequently in working out a differential diagnosis of diseases of that pattern. Within the tables the classification of disease is on an etiologic basis, categories being arranged in the same order as the chapters in the book—developmental, infectious, immunologic, neoplastic, and so forth. Each table includes *all* common diseases and the *majority* of uncommon diseases which produce that particular pattern.

The *Decision Trees* approach differential diagnosis in a somewhat different way. While the correct recognition of a roentgenographic pattern goes partway toward solving a diagnostic problem, with only few exceptions is it possible to make a definitive diagnosis without knowledge of the clinical state of the patient and without the benefit of roentgenologic/clinical correlation. Since the *Tables of Differential Diagnosis* include only minimal reference to

clinical status, we have created a series of algorithms that introduce into the diagnostic equation the clinical presentation of the patient. An algorithm can be broadly defined as a step-by-step procedure for solving a problem, and in the present context is analogous to a "decision tree." The decision trees which follow each table are designed in such a way that the trunk of the tree represents the specific roentgenographic pattern of disease. The first divisions or "branches" of the tree consist of a variety of clinical presentations that categorize the important diseases producing that roentgenographic pattern. Continuing up the branch leads to the diagnosis that most likely fits that particular combination of roentgenographic pattern and clinical presentation. One further step up the tree brings one to the methods that are recommended for establishing that particular diagnosis.

In each decision tree, there is a maximum of eight branches; thus, no more than eight diagnostic possibilities are considered for any one pattern. We have recognized the danger of attempting to keep the differential considerations under sufficient control that the final product would not appear too "pat" and oversimplified. We have attempted to select those conditions which, on the basis of *probability*, are most likely to cause each specific pattern. Nevertheless, we wish to emphasize that *for any specific roentgenographic pattern differential diagnosis cannot be restricted only to the conditions listed in the decision trees* (the tables can be referred to for a listing of all diagnostic possibilities).

The Tables of Differential Diagnosis *are designed to be used in the following manner. First, refer to the descriptions of the characteristics of each specific pattern that precede the* tables and to the roentgenograms that manifest that pattern. When a specific roentgenographic pattern is recognized, the appropriate table is consulted and reviewed. The headings in each table are intended to provide a brief review of the characteristics of each disease that might aid in differentiating it from others that cause the same pattern. Thus, the most likely diagnostic possibilities are selected. Page references on the right-hand side of each table indicate the section in the text in which the disease is discussed in detail.

The Decision Trees can be referred to either in conjunction with the tables or independently. Obviously, they can be used only when sufficient clinical information is available. To facilitate appreciation of the likeliest possibilities in each of the decision trees, the diseases that are the most frequent cause of each pattern are shaded and printed in boldface type.

TABLE 19–1

CYSTIC AND CAVITARY DISEASE

This table includes all forms cf pulmonary disease characterized by circumscribed air-containing spaces with distinct walls. This broad definition includes such entities as blebs, bullae, and cystic bronchiectasis. Fluid levels may be present or absent. Cavities may be single or multiple.

	ETIOLOGY	ANATOMIC DISTRIBUTION	CHARACTER OF WALL
DEVELOPMENTAL	Intralobar bronchopulmonary sequestration	Two-thirds of cases left lower lobe, one-third right lower lobe. Almost in-variably contiguous to diaphragm.	May be thin- or thick-walled.
	Bronchogenic cyst	Medial third of lower lobes.	Thin-walled.
	Congenital cystic adenomatoid mal-formation	No definite predilection.	Multiple air-containing cysts scattered irregularly through a mass of unit density.
INFECTIOUS	**Bacteria** *Staphylococcus aureus*	No lobar predilection.	Tends to be thick with ragged inner lining.
	Klebsiella-Enterobacter-Serratia genera	Upper lobes predominate.	Tends to be thick with ragged inner lining.
	Mycobacterium species	Apical and posterior re-gions of upper lobes and apical region of lower lobes.	Tends to be of moderate thickness. Inner lining generally smooth.
	Pseudomonas aeruginosa *Escherichia coli*	Predominantly lower lobes.	Highly variable.
	Bacillus proteus	Predominantly upper lobes.	Tends to be thick, with ragged inner lining.

TABLE 19–1—CYSTIC AND CAVITARY DISEASE / 751

ADDITIONAL FINDINGS	COMMENTS
Air-fluid levels may be present. The cyst volume may change on serial roentgenographic examinations. Cyst may be masked by pneumonia in surrounding parenchyma.	Cyst may be solitary but more commonly multilocular or multiple. (*See* page 238.)
An air-fluid level may be present. When pneumonitis leads to communication between cyst and the bronchial tree, the cavity may be masked by the surrounding pneumonia.	Seventy-five per cent of bronchogenic cysts eventually become air-containing as a result of communication with contiguous lung. (*See* page 239.)
An expanding process, causing enlargement of affected lung and hemithorax.	Volume of lung affected varies considerably. (*See* page 242.)
Pleural effusion (empyema) with or without bronchopleural fistula (pyopneumothorax) almost invariable in children and may occur in adults.	In adults, cavities result from tissue necrosis; in children, air-containing spaces commonly due to pneumatocele formation. Staphylococcal pyemia may lead to multiple small abscesses widely distributed throughout both lungs. (*See* page 269.)
Pleural effusion (empyema) may be present. Cavity rarely contains large masses of necrotic lung—acute lung gangrene.	Abscess formation in acute pneumonia. Cavities are usually single but tend to be multilocular. Multiple cavities may be present if pneumonia is multilobar. (*See* page 276.)
Cavities may be multiple.	Cavitation tends to be a more prominent feature of atypical mycobacterial disease than of mycobacterium tuberculosis. (*See* page 295.)
Empyema frequent.	Often the result of bacteremia from an extrathoracic focus (GU tract). Tends to occur in debilitated states (alcoholism or diabetes). (*See* page 274.)
May be associated with loss of volume of affected lobe. Pleural effusion uncommon.	(*See* page 279.)

Table continued on following page

TABLE 19-1. *(Continued)*

	ETIOLOGY	ANATOMIC DISTRIBUTION	CHARACTER OF WALL
	Salmonella species	——	——
	Streptococcus pneumoniae	Upper lobe predilection.	Thick, with ragged inner lining.
	Pseudomonas pseudomallei	Upper lobes predominate.	Moderately thick.
	Malleomyces mallei	No lobar predilection.	Highly variable.
	Anaerobic organisms	Posterior portion of both lungs.	Tends to be thick with ragged inner lining.
	Fungi *Actinomyces israelii* *Nocardia* species }	Lower lobe predilection, bilateral.	Generally thick-walled.
INFECTIOUS *(Cont.)*	*Histoplasma capsulatum*	Predominantly upper lobes.	Variable.
	Coccidioides immitis	Predominantly upper lobes.	Tends to be very thin-walled.
	Blastomyces dermatitidis	No predilection.	Variable, but generally thick-walled.
	Cryptococcus neoformans	Predominantly lower lobes.	Variable, but generally thick-walled.
	Sporotrichum schenckii *Geotrichum* species }	Upper lobe predilection.	Characteristically thin-walled.
	Zygomycetes group	Not distinctive.	——
	Aspergillus species *Candida albicans* }	——	——

TABLE 19–1—CYSTIC AND CAVITARY DISEASE / **753**

TABLE 19–1. *(Continued)*

ADDITIONAL FINDINGS	COMMENTS
Frequently associated with empyema.	*(See* page 279.)
The cavity may contain large irregular masses of necrotic lung—acute lung gangrene.	A rare complication of fulminating pneumococcal pneumonia. *(See* page 267.)
Effusions rare.	*(See* page 276.)
Empyema.	*(See* page 276.)
Cavities frequently multiple. Empyema common.	Tend to be associated with debilitation, alcoholism, and poor oral hygiene. *(See* page 286.)
Pleural effusion (empyema) is common as is extension into the chest wall with or without rib destruction.	Roentgenographic patterns of these two organisms are indistinguishable. *(See* pages 315 and 316.)
Cavities may be multiple.	No clear-cut distinguishing roentgenographic features from postprimary tuberculosis. *(See* page 302.)
These thin-walled cavities tend to occur in the asymptomatic form of the disease following "fleeting" pneumonitis.	Not to be confused with cavitating nodules which tend to be somewhat thicker walled and frequently multiple *(see* Table 19–4). *(See* page 307.)
Cavitation occurs in about 15 per cent of cases. Pleural effusion and hilar lymph-node enlargement very uncommon.	*(See* page 310.)
Cavitation occurs in about 15 per cent of cases. Pleural effusion and hilar lymph-node enlargement very uncommon.	*(See* page 312.)
———	*(See* page 321.)
———	*(See* page 319.)
———	Primary disease of the lungs sometimes cavitates; however, more often these organisms are opportunistic invaders in the form of fungus balls (mycetoma) in chronic debilitating disease with cavitating pneumonic lesions of other etiology. *(See* pages 317 and 314.)

Table continued on following page

TABLE 19–1. *(Continued)*

	ETIOLOGY	ANATOMIC DISTRIBUTION	CHARACTER OF WALL
INFECTIOUS *(Cont.)*	**Parasites** *Entamoeba histolytica* (amebiasis)	Almost restricted to right lower lobe.	Generally thick-walled with irregular ragged inner lining.
	Paragonimus westermani	No predilection.	Characteristically thin-walled, with local elevation or hump on inner lining.
	Echinococcus granulosus (hydatid cyst)	Lower lobe predilection.	Air may dissect between ectocyst and endocyst, creating a halo; or contents of cyst may be expelled into bronchial tree, leaving a thin-walled cystic space.
IMMUNOLOGIC	Wegener's granulomatosis	Widely distributed and bilateral, with no predilection for upper or lower lung zones.	Usually thick, with irregular inner lining. In time, cavities may become thin-walled cystic spaces.
	Rheumatoid necrobiotic nodule	Peripheral subpleural parenchyma, commonly in lower lobes.	Thick with smooth inner lining. With remission of the arthritis, cavities may become thin-walled and gradually disappear.
NEOPLASTIC	Bronchogenic carcinoma	Clear-cut predilection for upper lobes, both lungs being affected equally.	Tends to be thick, with an irregular, nodular inner lining (mural nodules). Thin-walled cavities simulating bronchogenic cysts occur occasionally.
	Hematogeneous metastases	Cavitation occurs more frequently in upper than in lower lobe lesions.	May be thin- or thick-walled.
	Hodgkin's disease	Lower lobe predilection.	Thin- or thick-walled.

TABLE 19-1—CYSTIC AND CAVITARY DISEASE / **755**

TABLE 19-1. *(Continued)*

ADDITIONAL FINDINGS	COMMENTS
Right pleural effusion almost invariable.	Organisms enter thorax via right hemidiaphragm from liver abscess. (*See* page 339.)
In addition to cavities, there may be isolated nodular shadows containing vacuoles. Pleural effusion rarely.	Organisms enter thorax via diaphragm from peritoneal space. (*See* page 348.)
Irregularities of fluid layer caused by collapsed membranes (water-lily sign or sign of the camalote). Hydropneumothorax occasionally.	(*See* page 345.)
Cavities commonly multiple but all masses do not necessarily cavitate.	Cavitation occurs eventually in from one-third to one-half of patients. With treatment, cavitary lesions may disappear or heal with scar formation. (*See* page 382.)
Pleural effusion or spontaneous pneumothorax.	Well circumscribed masses are more frequently multiple than solitary and range in size from 3 mm to 7 cm. Cavitary nodules wax and wane in concert with frequently associated subcutaneous nodules. (*See* page 370.)
Chunks of necrotic cancer occasionally may become detached and lie free within the cavity, simulating fungus ball.	Cavitation occurs in 2 to 10 per cent of bronchogenic carcinomas, most commonly in lesions peripherally located. The majority are squamous-cell in type (adenocarcinomas and large cell undifferentiated carcinomas cavitate occasionally, small cell carcinomas rarely if ever). (*See* page 413.)
Cavitation may involve only a few of multiple nodules throughout the lungs, such nodules characteristically showing considerable variation in size.	Cavitation in metastatic neoplasms less common (4 per cent) than in primary neoplasms (9 per cent). Occurs more frequently in squamous-cell neoplasms but also in adenocarcinoma (particularly from the large bowel) and sarcoma. (*See* page 445.)
Cavities are frequently multiple. Commonly associated with mediastinal and hilar lymph-node enlargement.	Cavitation occurs characteristically in peripheral parenchymal consolidation. (*See* page 430.)

Table continued on following page

TABLE 19–1. *(Continued)*

	ETIOLOGY	ANATOMIC DISTRIBUTION	CHARACTER OF WALL
THROMBOEMBOLIC	Septic embolism	Lower lobe predilection predominantly posterior and lateral segments.	Usually thin-walled but may be thick, with shaggy inner lining.
INHALATIONAL	Silicosis—complicated (large opacities)	Strong predilection for upper lobes.	Tends to be thick with irregular inner lining.
	Coal-worker's pneumoconiosis—complicated (large opacities)	Strong predilection for upper lobes.	Tends to be thick with irregular inner lining.
AIRWAYS DISEASE	Blebs or bullae	Predilection for upper lobes, particularly extreme apex.	Thin-walled.
	Cystic bronchiectasis	Predilection for lower lobes.	Thin-walled.
TRAUMATIC	Pulmonary parenchymal laceration (traumatic lung cyst)	Characteristically in the peripheral subpleural parenchyma immediately underlying the point of maximum injury.	Typically thin-walled.
IDIOPATHIC	Sarcoidosis	No predilection.	No typical characteristics.

TABLE 19–1 — CYSTIC AND CAVITARY DISEASE / **757**

TABLE 19–1. *(Continued)*

ADDITIONAL FINDINGS	COMMENTS
Prominent feeding artery, associated pleural effusion, raised diaphragm, or multiple lesions may suggest the diagnosis. A mass of necrotic lung may separate and lie within the cavity, simulating intracavitary fungus ball.	A rare manifestation which may be misdiagnosed unless clinical picture and associated roentgenographic findings suggest the possibility. (*See* page 468.)
Background of nodular or reticulonodular disease is inevitable although serial examinations may reveal diminution in the number of nodules due to incorporation into the massive consolidation. Hilar lymph-node enlargement is the rule, with or without eggshell calcification.	Cavitation in conglomerate lesions may be the result of either superimposed tuberculosis or ischemic necrosis. (*See* page 578.)
Background of simple coal-worker's pneumoconiosis throughout the remainder of the lungs.	Cavitation in conglomerate shadows is due to either superimposed tuberculosis or ischemic necrosis. (*See* page 590.)
With infection, fluid levels may develop. In some cases, roentgenologic evidence of diffuse emphysema will be present.	The thinness of the wall is the main differentiating feature from true cavitation. (*See* page 553.)
Usually considerable loss of volume of affected segment or segments.	"Cavities" represent severely dilated segmental bronchi. Usually multiple and commonly with air-fluid levels. (*See* page 558.)
The presence of laceration may be masked by surrounding pulmonary contusion. In some cases of bullet or knife wounds of the lung, a central radiolucency may be observed along the course of the bullet track, simulating a cavity when viewed in the same direction as the wound.	Approximately half these lesions present as thin-walled air-filled cavities (with or without air-fluid levels) and the remainder as pulmonary hematomas. They may be single or multiple, unilocular or multilocular; they are oval or spherical in shape and range from 2 to 14 cm in diameter. (*See* page 616.)
Cavities may contain mycetomas.	True cavitation in sarcoidosis is very uncommon. Important to exclude all other causes of cavitation before accepting the diagnosis. (*See* page 646.)

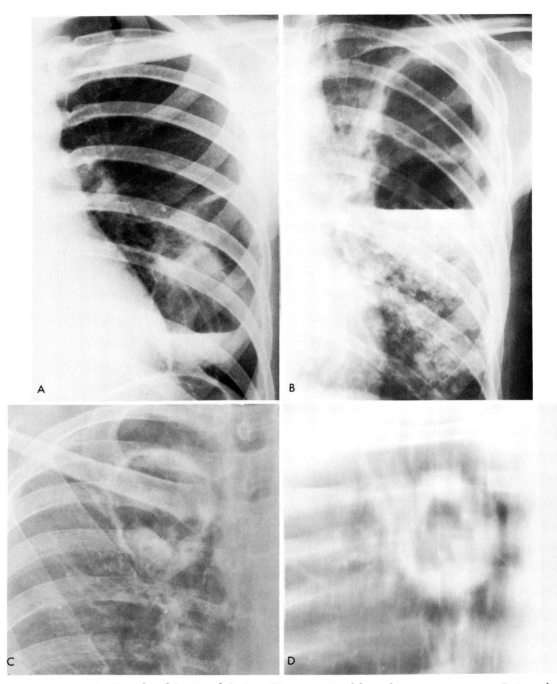

Figure 19–1. Four Examples of Cystic and Cavitary Disease. *A,* Intralobar pulmonary sequestration. *B,* Acute lung abscess *(Staphylococcus aureus).* *C,* Chronic tuberculous cavity containing a mycetoma. *D,* Cavitating bronchogenic carcinoma (tomogram).

DECISION TREE 19–1A

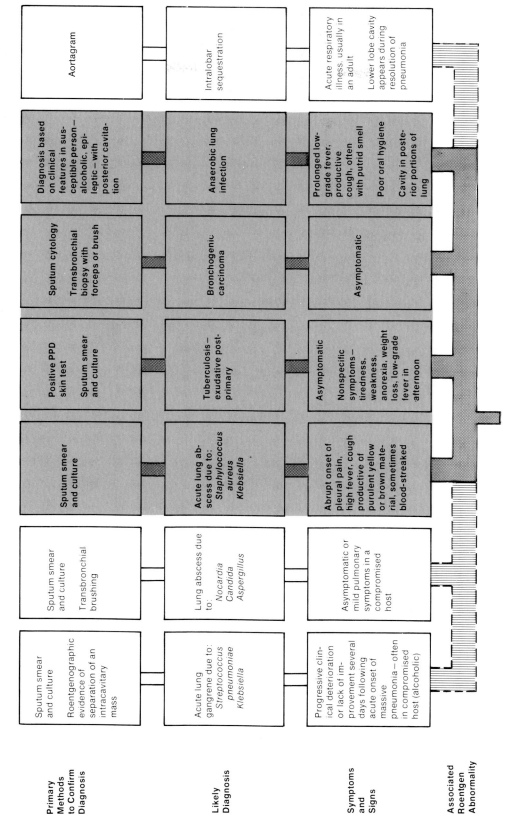

Primary Methods to Confirm Diagnosis	Sputum smear and culture Roentgenographic evidence of separation of an intracavitary mass	Sputum smear and culture Transbronchial brushing	Sputum smear and culture	Positive PPD skin test Sputum smear and culture	Sputum cytology Transbronchial biopsy with forceps or brush	Diagnosis based on clinical features in susceptible person — alcoholic, epileptic — with posterior cavitation		Aortagram
Likely Diagnosis	Acute lung gangrene due to: *Streptococcus pneumoniae* *Klebsiella*	Lung abscess due to: *Nocardia* *Candida* *Aspergillus*	Acute lung abscess due to: *Staphylococcus aureus* *Klebsiella*	Tuberculosis—exudative post-primary	Bronchogenic carcinoma	Anaerobic lung infection		Intralobar sequestration
Symptoms and Signs	Progressive clinical deterioration or lack of improvement several days following acute onset of massive pneumonia—often in compromised host (alcoholic)	Asymptomatic or mild pulmonary symptoms in a compromised host	Abrupt onset of pleural pain, high fever, cough productive of purulent yellow or brown material, sometimes blood-streaked	Asymptomatic Nonspecific symptoms—tiredness, weakness, anorexia, weight loss, low-grade fever in afternoon	Asymptomatic	Prolonged low-grade fever, productive cough, often with putrid smell Poor oral hygiene Cavity in posterior portions of lung		Acute respiratory illness, usually in an adult Lower lobe cavity appears during resolution of pneumonia
Associated Roentgen Abnormality								
Basic Pattern								

Cystic and Cavitary Disease (Usually Solitary)

■ = Common Disease

□ = Uncommon Disease

DECISION TREE 19-1B

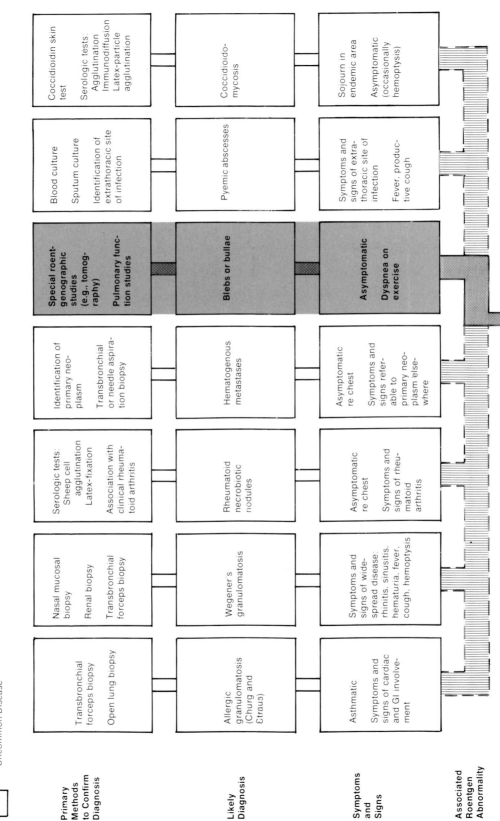

Cystic and Cavitary Disease (Usually Multiple)

| | Common Disease |
| | Uncommon Disease |

Primary Methods to Confirm Diagnosis

| Transbronchial forceps biopsy / Open lung biopsy | Nasal mucosal biopsy / Renal biopsy / Transbronchial forceps biopsy | Serologic tests: Sheep cell agglutination / Latex-fixation / Association with clinical rheumatoid arthritis | Identification of primary neoplasm / Transbronchial or needle aspiration biopsy | Special roentgenographic studies (e.g., tomography) / Pulmonary function studies | Blood culture / Sputum culture / Identification of extrathoracic site of infection | Coccidioidin skin test / Serologic tests: Agglutination / Immunodiffusion / Latex-particle agglutination |

Likely Diagnosis

| Allergic granulomatosis (Churg and Straus) | Wegener's granulomatosis | Rheumatoid necrobiotic nodules | Hematogenous metastases | Blebs or bullae | Pyemic abscesses | Coccidioidomycosis |

Symptoms and Signs

| Asthmatic / Symptoms and signs of cardiac and GI involvement | Symptoms and signs of widespread disease: rhinitis, sinusitis, hematuria, fever, cough, hemoptysis | Asymptomatic re chest / Symptoms and signs of rheumatoid arthritis | Asymptomatic re chest / Symptoms and signs referable to primary neoplasm elsewhere | Asymptomatic / Dyspnea on exercise | Symptoms and signs of extrathoracic site of infection / Fever, productive cough | Sojourn in endemic area / Asymptomatic (occasionally hemoptysis) |

Associated Roentgen Abnormality

Basic Pattern

TABLE 19–2
SOLITARY PULMONARY NODULES
LESS THAN 6 CM IN DIAMETER

For the purposes of this table, the criteria for inclusion in this category are as follows:

1. The presence of a solitary roentgenographic shadow not exceeding 6 cm in its largest diameter.

2. The lesion is fairly discrete but not necessarily sharply circumscribed.

3. It may have any contour (smooth, lobulated, or umbilicated) or shape.

4. It may be calcified or cavitated.

5. Satellite lesions may be present.

6. The lesion is surrounded by air-containing lung; *or* if it is adjacent to the visceral pleural surface over the convexity of the thorax, at least two-thirds of its circumference is contiguous with air-containing lung.

7. Symptoms may be present.

TABLE 19–2. *(Continued)*

	ETIOLOGY	INCIDENCE	LOCATION
	Bronchogenic cyst	Peak incidence third decade; predilection for males and Yemenite Jews.	Lower lobe predilection, most commonly medial third.
	Bronchopulmonary sequestration (intralobar and extralobar)	Rare in this size range.	Almost invariably lower lobe, related to diaphragm.
	Pulmonary arteriovenous fistula	0.6 per cent of Bateson's series. In two-thirds of cases, lesions are single.	More common in lower lobes
DEVELOPMENTAL	Varicosity of a pulmonary vein	Very rare (47 cases reported by 1976).	Medial third of lung (lingular vein on left or medial basal pulmonary vein on right).
	Congenital bronchial atresia	Very rare.	Strong predilection for the apicoposterior bronchus of the left upper lobe.
INFECTIOUS	**Bacteria** *Mycobacterium tuberculosis* (tuberculoma)	Common.	Predilection for upper lobes, the right more often than the left.

TABLE 19-2. *(Continued)*

SIZE AND SHAPE	CALCIFICATION	CAVITATION	COMMENTS
Usually several centimeters; round or oval, smooth, well defined.	Rarely in wall; calcium has been reported in cyst contents.	Yes, when communication occurs with bronchial tree.	Two-thirds of bronchial cysts are pulmonary, one-third mediastinal. Cysts are homogeneous until communication established with contiguous lung, usually because of infection (occurs eventually in 75 per cent of cases). (*See* page 239.)
Commonly measure over 6 cm in diameter (*see* Table 19–3).	No	Common.	(*See* page 238.)
Up to 6 cm; round or oval, slightly lobulated, sharply defined.	Occasionally, probably due to phleboliths.	No	Diagnosis by identification of feeding artery and draining vein. Angiography of *both lungs* imperative if surgery is contemplated in order to identify multiple fistulas not visible on plain roentgenograms. Forty to 65 per cent of cases have hereditary hemorrhagic telangiectasia. (*See* page 247.)
Several centimeters; round or oval, lobulated, well defined.	No	No	Change in size with Valsalva and Mueller procedures. Differential diagnosis from arteriovenous fistula by late filling and slow drainage on pulmonary angiography. (*See* page 249.)
Oval; approximately 2×5 cm; smooth, sharply defined.	No	No	The mass consists of inspissated mucus which accumulates within the bronchus immediately distal to the point of obliteration; the lung parenchyma distal to the occlusion is overinflated due to collateral air drift. (*See* page 242.)
0.5 to 4 cm; round or oval; 25 per cent are lobulated.	Frequent.	Uncommon.	"Satellite" lesions in 80 per cent; the draining bronchus may show irregular thickening of its wall or occasionally bronchostenosis. (*See* page 296.)

Table continued on following page

TABLE 19–2. *(Continued)*

	ETIOLOGY	INCIDENCE	LOCATION
	Fungi *Histoplasma capsulatum* (histoplasmoma)	Common.	More frequently in the lower than in the upper lobes.
	Coccidioides immitis	Uncommon.	Upper lobe predilection.
	Aspergillus fumigatus (mucoid impaction)	Very uncommon; largely restricted to patients with bronchospasm.	Upper lobe predilection.
INFECTIOUS *(Cont.)*	*Cryptococcus neoformans*	Uncommon.	Lower lobe predominance, usually in the periphery.
	Parasites *Echinococcus* (hydatid cyst)	Common in endemic areas.	Lower lobe predilection, right more often than left.
	Dirofilaria immitis	Rare.	No known predilection.

TABLE 19–2. *(Continued)*

SIZE AND SHAPE	CALCIFICATION	CAVITATION	COMMENTS
Seldom more than 3 cm in diameter; round or oval; typically sharply circumscribed.	Common, often central in location, thus producing the "target" appearance.	Rare.	"Satellite" lesions fairly common. Histoplasmomas may be multiple, ranging considerably in size. Associated hilar lymph-node calcification is common. (*See* page 303.)
0.5 to 3.0 cm; round or oval; typically sharply circumscribed.	In some cases.	Common; may be thin- or thick-walled.	(*See* page 308.)
2 to 6 cm (rarely up to 8 cm in diameter); tends to be finger-like but may be Y-shaped or V-shaped in conformity with bronchial subdivision.	No	True cavitation occurs rarely as a result of lung necrosis, although air-fluid levels may be visible within the markedly dilated bronchus.	The mass is caused by mucoid impaction within a proximal segmental bronchus. It tends to be transient in nature, although it may persist unchanged for weeks or even months, or may increase in size while under observation. When the lesion clears, it leaves as a residuum cylindrical or saccular dilatation of the affected bronchi. The impacted bronchus may or may not cause atelectasis of the involved segment; atelectasis frequently is prevented by collateral air drift. (*See* page 318.)
Ranges from 2 to 10 cm (*see* Table 19–3). Sharply circumscribed and homogeneous.	No	Very uncommon.	Commonly pleural based. (*See* page 312.)
Range from 1 to 10 cm (*see* Table 19–3). Almost always well circumscribed. Tendency to bizarre irregular shape.	Very rare.	Common.	(*See* page 345.)
Well circumscribed.	No	Sometimes.	Involvement of larger pulmonary arteries may result in a shadow simulating pulmonary infarction. (*See* page 344.)

Table continued on following page

TABLE 19–2. *(Continued)*

	ETIOLOGY	INCIDENCE	LOCATION
	Rheumatoid necrobiotic nodule	Rare.	In the peripheral subpleural zone, usually lower lobes.
IMMUNOLOGIC			
	Wegener's granulomatosis	Rare.	No predilection.
NEOPLASTIC	Bronchial adenoma	Incidence compared to bronchogenic carcinoma 1:50. Twenty to 25 per cent of all bronchial adenomas present as solitary nodules.	Predilection for right upper and middle lobes and lingula.
	Hamartoma	Constitute approximately 5 per cent of solitary peripheral nodules.	No lobar predilection.
	Leiomyoma Fibroma Lipoma Hemangioma Hemangio-endothelioma Hemangio-pericytoma Chemodectoma Granular-cell myoblastoma Neurogenic neoplasms Chondroma Endometriosis Teratoma Inflammatory pseudotumor	Very rare.	No definite predilection.

TABLE 19–2. *(Continued)*

SIZE AND SHAPE	CALCIFICATION	CAVITATION	COMMENTS
3 mm to 7 cm; well circumscribed, smooth.	No	Common. Cavities possess thick walls and smooth inner lining.	More commonly multiple than solitary. Pleural effusion may be present. Eosinophilia in some patients. Nodules wax and wane in concert with the frequently associated subcutaneous nodules and in proportion to the activity of the rheumatoid arthritis. (*See* page 370.)
A few millimeters to 9 cm. Tend to be well circumscribed.	No	In one-third to one-half of cases.	Much less common manifestation than multiple nodules, although solitary nodules were observed in 4 of 20 cases in one series. (*See* page 382.)
Average 4 cm (range 1 to 10 cm), round or oval, sharply circumscribed, slightly lobulated.	Rare.	Rare.	The remaining 75 per cent of bronchial adenomas relate to a bronchial lumen and lead to segmental atelectasis or obstructive pneumonitis. (*See* page 400.)
The majority are less than 4 cm in diameter; well circumscribed; more often lobulated than smooth in a ratio of 2:1.	Incidence varies widely in reported series, but certainly occurs in a minority of cases. "Popcorn" configuration virtually diagnostic.	No	Ten per cent arise endobronchially and then may cause bronchial obstruction, atelectasis, or obstructive pneumonitis. Serial examination may reveal slow growth. (*See* page 402.)
Up to 6 cm; usually well defined.	Rarely.	No	Rarely these neoplasms may arise within a bronchial wall and thus be manifested roentgenographically by bronchial obstruction and peripheral atelectasis or obstructive pneumonitis. (*See* pages 403–405.)

Table continued on following page

TABLE 19–2. *(Continued)*

	ETIOLOGY	INCIDENCE	LOCATION
NEOPLASTIC *(Cont.)*	Bronchogenic carcinoma	Varies widely; in patients referred for resection, approximately 40 per cent of solitary nodules will be malignant.	Predominantly upper lobes.
	Hematogenous metastasis	3 to 5 per cent of asymptomatic nodules.	Predominantly lower lobes.
	Bronchiolo-alveolar carcinoma	The most common method of presentation of local bronchiolo-alveolar carcinoma.	No predilection.
	Non-Hodgkin's lymphoma	Rare.	No predilection.
	Multiple myeloma (plasmacytoma)	Rare.	No predilection.
	Bronchopulmonary amyloidosis	Extremely rare.	No predilection.
INHALATIONAL	Lipoid pneumonia	Rare.	Usually dependent portion of upper and lower lobes, but sometimes right middle lobe or lingula.
TRAUMATIC	Pulmonary hematoma	Uncommon.	Usually in a peripheral subpleural location.

TABLE 19–2. *(Continued)*

SIZE AND SHAPE	CALCIFICATION	CAVITATION	COMMENTS
Commonly over 2 cm. Margins tend to be ill-defined, lobulated, or umbilicated.	Very rare.	2 to 10 per cent.	Satellite lesions very uncommon. (*See* pages 409 and 419.)
3 mm to 6 cm; smooth or slightly lobulated. Tend to be well circumscribed.	Rarely and only in osteogenic sarcoma or chondrosarcoma.	Occasionally.	In 25 per cent of cases, metastatic lesions to the lungs are solitary. (*See* page 445.)
Range, 1 to 6 cm; round, smooth, or lobulated; may be sharply circumscribed or ill-defined.	No	Rarely.	An air bronchogram or air bronchiologram is a common roentgenographic feature, except in the smaller lesions. Tends to be very slow growing. (*See* page 423.)
3 mm to 6 cm; round, ovoid, triangular or polyhedral; tends to have fuzzy outline.	No	In histiocytic lymphoma, "cyst-like" lesions may occur which resemble cavitation.	May be a manifestation of either primary or secondary disease. (*See* page 436.)
Up to 6 cm; lobulated.	No	No	No distinguishing features from peripheral bronchogenic carcinoma. (*See* page 441.)
Up to 5 cm in diameter.	Occasionally in the periphery.	Occasionally.	This is a plasma cell dyscrasia. (*See* page 443.)
5 mm to 6 cm; sharply circumscribed, smooth or lobulated; sometimes associated with streaky linear opacities radiating outwards from periphery.	No	No	(*See* page 604.)
Size highly variable —commonly 2 cm to 6 cm but may be very large (*see* Table 19–3); oval or round, sharply circumscribed, smooth.	No	A hematoma occurs as a result of hemorrhage into a pulmonary parenchymal laceration or traumatic lung cyst—thus, an air-fluid level may be present as a result of communication with the bronchial tree.	Generally undergo slow but progressive decrease in size, although they may persist for long periods of time, sometimes up to four months. May be multiple. Not uncommonly result from segmental or wedge resection of lung parenchyma. The presence of a hematoma may be masked by surrounding pulmonary contusion. (*See* page 616.)

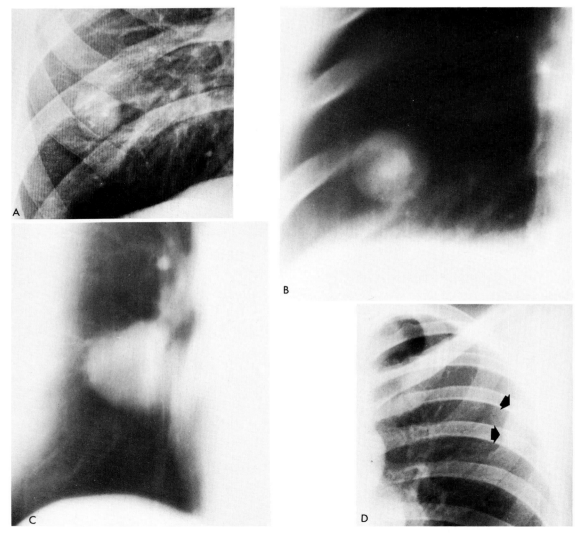

Figure 19–2.   Four Examples of Solitary Nodules Less than 6 cm in Diameter. *A*, Hamartoma (*note* central scattered calcifications). *B*, Histoplasmoma (*note* central target calcification on this AP tomogram). *C*, Primary squamous cell carcinoma of the right lower lobe (tomogram). *D*, Post-traumatic pulmonary hematoma (*arrows*).

DECISION TREE 19–2

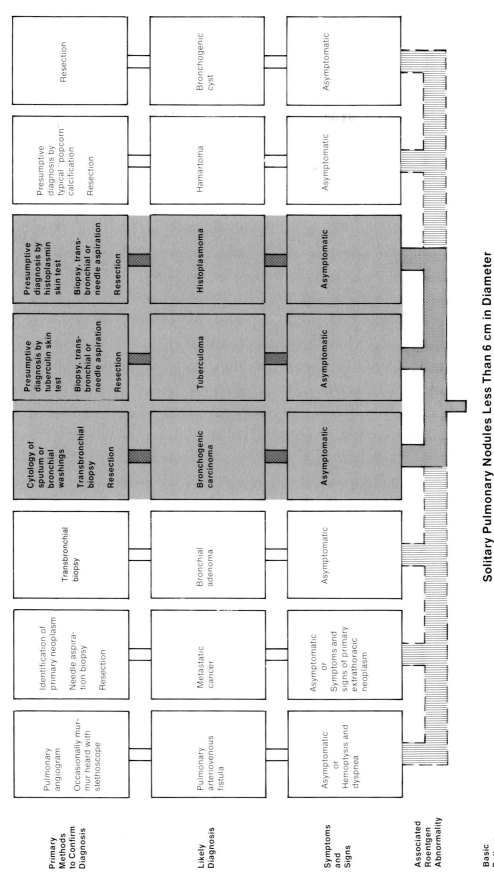

 = Common Disease

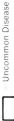 = Uncommon Disease

Primary Methods to Confirm Diagnosis	Pulmonary angiogram Occasionally murmur heard with stethoscope	Identification of primary neoplasm Needle aspiration biopsy Resection	Transbronchial biopsy	Cytology of sputum or bronchial washings Transbronchial biopsy Resection	Presumptive diagnosis by tuberculin skin test Biopsy, transbronchial or needle aspiration Resection	Presumptive diagnosis by histoplasmin skin test Biopsy, transbronchial or needle aspiration Resection	Presumptive diagnosis by typical "popcorn" calcification Resection	Resection
Likely Diagnosis	Pulmonary arteriovenous fistula	Metastatic cancer	Bronchial adenoma	Bronchogenic carcinoma	Tuberculoma	Histoplasmoma	Hamartoma	Bronchogenic cyst
Symptoms and Signs	Asymptomatic or Hemoptysis and dyspnea	Asymptomatic or Symptoms and signs of primary extrathoracic neoplasm	Asymptomatic	Asymptomatic	Asymptomatic	Asymptomatic	Asymptomatic	Asymptomatic
Associated Roentgen Abnormality								
Basic Pattern								

Solitary Pulmonary Nodules Less Than 6 cm in Diameter

TABLE 19-3

SOLITARY PULMONARY MASSES
6 CM OR MORE IN DIAMETER

The general characteristics of lesions included in this table are the
same as for solitary nodules less than 6 cm in diameter. The separation
of a group of entities into this category on the basis of size alone is

	ETIOLOGY	LOCATION
DEVELOPMENTAL	Intralobar broncho-pulmonary sequestration	Two-thirds of cases left lower lobe; one-third of cases right lower lobe; rare elsewhere. Almost invariably contiguous to diaphragm in posterior bronchopulmonary segment.
	Extralobar broncho-pulmonary sequestration	Related to left hemidiaphragm in 90 per cent of cases, lying immediately above, below, or within it.
INFECTIOUS	Acute lung abscess	Predilection for posterior portions of upper or lower lobes.
	Cryptococcus neoformans (cryptococcosis)	Lower lobe predominance, usually in the periphery.
	Blastomyces dermatitidis	No stated predominance.
	Nocardia asteroides	Lower lobe predominance.
	Actinomyces israelii	Lower lobe predominance.
	Echinococcus (hydatid cyst)	Predilection for lower lobes, right more often than left.

TABLE 19-3—SOLITARY PULMONARY MASSES 6 CM OR MORE IN DIAMETER / **773**

perhaps arbitrary but appeared to be necessary in view of the restriction on size imposed by most authorities for inclusion of solitary nodules as so-called coin lesions.

SHAPE	CALCIFICATION	CAVITATION	COMMENTS
Round, oval, or triangular in shape and typically well circumscribed.	No	Frequent.	Enclosed within visceral pleura of affected lung. Although cystic in nature, mass remains homogeneous until communication established with contiguous lung as a result of infection. Supplied by systemic artery and drains via pulmonary veins. (*See* page 238.)
Well-defined homogeneous mass.	No	Seldom.	Frequently associated with other anomalies and sometimes with diaphragmatic eventration. Enclosed within its own visceral pleural layer—therefore seldom infected or air-containing (*cf.* intralobar). Supplied by systemic artery (usually from abdominal aorta) and drains via systemic rather than pulmonary veins (IVC or azygos system). (*See* page 239.)
Tends to be round; somewhat ill-defined when acute but sharply circumscribed when chronic.	No	Almost inevitable.	Usually of staphylococcal etiology. The mass may remain unchanged for many weeks without perforation into bronchial tree. (*See* page 271.)
Tends to be well circumscribed, homogeneous in density and solitary.	No	Reported in 16 per cent of cases.	Commonly pleural based. (*See* page 312.)
Margins tend to be ill-defined.	No	Uncommon.	Frequency of this manifestation varies widely in reported series. May simulate bronchogenic carcinoma. (*See* page 310.)
Indistinguishable from actinomycosis.	No	Frequent.	The initial roentgenographic presentation in 4 of 12 cases in one series, with cavitation in all. (*See* page 316.)
Somewhat ill-defined. Simulates bronchogenic carcinoma.	No	Frequent.	The initial roentgenographic presentation in 6 of 15 cases in one series. (*See* page 315.)
Sharply circumscribed; tends to possess bizarre, irregular shape.	Extremely rare.	Common.	Communication with bronchial tree may produce the "meniscus" sign or sign of the camalote. (*See* page 345.)

Table continued on following page

TABLE 19–3.   *(Continued)*

	ETIOLOGY	LOCATION
IMMUNOLOGIC	Wegener's granulomatosis	No predilection.
	All benign neoplasms listed in Table 19–2	No definite predilection.
	Bronchogenic carcinoma	Predominantly upper lobes.
	Hematogenous metastasis	Predominantly lower lobes.
NEOPLASTIC	Bronchiolo-alveolar carcinoma	No predilection.
	Hodgkin's disease	No predilection.
	Non-Hodgkin's lymphoma	No clear-cut lobar predilection; tends to be more centrally than peripherally located.
	Multiple myeloma (plasmacytoma)	Over the convexity of thorax contiguous to chest wall.
INHALATIONAL	Lipoid pneumonia	Dependent portions of upper and lower lobes (occasionally right middle lobe or lingula).
TRAUMATIC	Pulmonary hematoma	Usually deep to point of maximum trauma.

TABLE 19-3—SOLITARY PULMONARY MASSES 6 CM OR MORE IN DIAMETER / 775

TABLE 19-3. *(Continued)*

SHAPE	CALCIFICATION	CAVITATION	COMMENTS
Well circum-scribed.	No	In one-third to one-half of cases.	Solitary nodules much less common than multiple. The lesion was solitary in 4 of 20 cases in one series. Range from a few millimeters to 9 cm in diameter. (*See* page 382.)
Well circum-scribed, smooth.	Rarely.	No	Any of these neoplasms may reach a large size, particularly chemodectoma, neurogenic tumors, and leiomyoma. (*See* page 400.)
Margins tend to be ill-defined, lobulated, or umbilicated.	No	Fairly common.	Most common method of presentation of large cell carcinoma, somewhat less common in adenocarcinoma and squa-mous-cell carcinoma and very uncom-mon in small cell carcinoma. (*See* page 409.)
Tend to be sharply circum-scribed, somewhat lobulated.	Rare—re-stricted to metastatic osteogenic sarcoma or chondro-sarcoma.	Predominantly in upper lobe lesions but is uncommon.	(*See* page 445.)
Tends to be ill-defined.	No	No	Tend to be very slow growing; may occupy most of the volume of a lobe, but there is no tendency to cross interlobar fissures. Air bronchogram frequent. (*See* page 423.)
Shaggy and ill-defined.	No	Sometimes.	Size ranges widely and may vary with time. An air bronchogram should be visible. (*See* page 430.)
Smooth and fairly sharply circum-scribed.	No	Rare.	May be a manifestation of either primary or secondary lymphocytic lymphoma. Often without associated hilar or medi-astinal lymph-node enlargement. Tends to grow slowly. Rarely obstructs the bronchial tree so that an air bronchogram is almost invariable. (*See* page 436.)
Sharply circum-scribed, possessing an obtuse angle with the chest wall.	No	No	Due to protrusion into the thorax of a primary lesion originating in a rib—thus almost invariably associated with a de-structive lesion of one or more ribs. May reach a very large size. (*See* page 441.)
Well circumscribed, smooth or lobulated. Sometimes with very shaggy outer margin.	No	No	Usually homogeneous in density. Closely simulates peripheral bronchogenic carcinoma. (*See* page 604.)
Sharply circum-scribed, round or oval.	No	No	Hematomas are usually less than 6 cm in diameter but occasionally are very large. Resolution may take several months. (*See* page 616.)

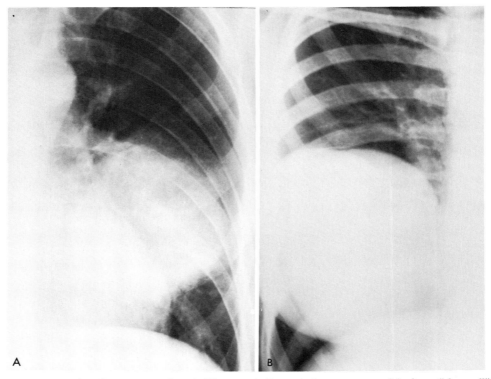

Figure 19–3. **Examples of Masses over 6 cm in Diamter.** *A*, Primary adenocarcinoma of the lung, "clear-cell" in type. *B*, Echinococcus (hydatid) cyst.

DECISION TREE 19-3

■ = Common Disease

□ = Uncommon Disease

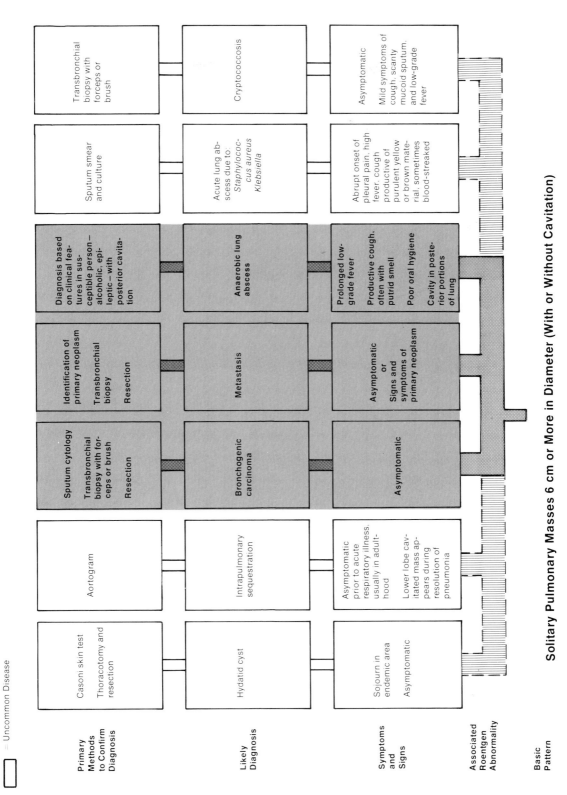

Primary Methods to Confirm Diagnosis	Casoni skin test Thoracotomy and resection	Aortogram	Sputum cytology Transbronchial biopsy with forceps or brush Resection	Identification of primary neoplasm Transbronchial biopsy Resection	Diagnosis based on clinical features in susceptible person—alcoholic, epileptic—with posterior cavitation	Sputum smear and culture	Transbronchial biopsy with forceps or brush
Likely Diagnosis	Hydatid cyst	Intrapulmonary sequestration	Bronchogenic carcinoma	Metastasis	Anaerobic lung abscess	Acute lung abscess due to: *Staphylococcus aureus* *Klebsiella*	Cryptococcosis
Symptoms and Signs	Sojourn in endemic area Asymptomatic	Asymptomatic prior to acute respiratory illness, usually in adulthood Lower lobe cavitated mass appears during resolution of pneumonia	Asymptomatic	Asymptomatic or Signs and symptoms of primary neoplasm	Prolonged low-grade fever Productive cough, often with putrid smell Poor oral hygiene Cavity in posterior portions of lung	Abrupt onset of pleural pain, high fever, cough productive of purulent yellow or brown material, sometimes blood-streaked	Asymptomatic Mild symptoms of cough, scanty mucoid sputum, and low-grade fever
Associated Roentgen Abnormality							
Basic Pattern							

Solitary Pulmonary Masses 6 cm or More in Diameter (With or Without Cavitation)

TABLE 19–4

MULTIPLE PULMONARY NODULES, WITH OR WITHOUT CAVITATION

The individual lesions generally possess the same characteristics as those described in Table 19–3.

Cavitation or calcification may be present or absent in some.or all of the lesions.

	ETIOLOGY	LOCATION	SIZE AND SHAPE
DEVELOPMENTAL	Pulmonary arteriovenous fistula	Lower lobe predilection.	One to several centimeters; round or oval, lobulated, well circumscribed.
INFECTIOUS	Pyemic abscesses	Generalized but more numerous in lower lobes.	Range from 0.5 to 4 cm; usually round and well circumscribed.
	Pseudomonas pseudomallei	No predilection.	4 to 11 mm; irregular and poorly defined.
	Coccidioides immitis	Upper lobe predilection.	0.5 to 3.0 cm; round or oval, well circumscribed.
	Histoplasma capsulatum	No predilection.	0.5 to 3.0 cm. Round and sharply circumscribed.
	Paragonimus westermani	Lower lobe predilection, usually in the periphery.	3 to 4 cm; well circumscribed.
IMMUNOLOGIC	Wegener's granulomatosis	Widely distributed, bilateral, no predilection for upper or lower lung zones.	5 mm to 9 cm; round, sharply circumscribed.
	Rheumatoid necrobiotic nodules	Peripheral subpleural parenchyma, more commonly lower lobes.	3 mm to 7 cm; round, well circumscribed, smooth.

CALCIFICATION	CAVITATION	GENERAL COMMENTS
No	No	Multiple in one-third of all cases. Diagnosis by identification of feeding artery and draining vein; lesions may change in size between Valsalva and Mueller procedures; angiography necessary to identify all fistulas. Forty to 65 per cent of cases associated with hereditary hemorrhagic telangiectasia. (*See* page 247.)
No	Common, usually thick-walled.	Commonly caused by *Staphylococcus aureus*. (*See* page 271.)
No	Common.	Nodules tend to enlarge, coalesce and cavitate as the disease progresses. (*See* page 276.)
Sometimes.	Common; may be thin- or thick-walled.	In approximately 2 per cent of affected patients, multiple cavities may be associated with pneumothorax and empyema. In contrast to tuberculosis, cavitary disease may occur in anterior segment of an upper lobe. (*See* page 307.)
Sometimes.	No	May remain unchanged over many years or may undergo slow growth. Seldom exceed 4 or 5 in number. (*See* page 302.)
Occasionally.	Common.	Multiple ring opacities or thin-walled cysts are characteristic. (*See* page 348.)
No	In one-third to one-half of patients; characteristically thick-walled, with irregular, shaggy inner lining.	May be associated with focal areas of pneumonitis. Typically occurs in patients who manifest no allergic background. Note related but somewhat different condition "allergic granulomatosis." (*See* page 382.)
No	Common, usually with thick walls and smooth inner lining.	Nodules tend to wax and wane in concert with subcutaneous nodules and in proportion to the activity of the rheumatoid arthritis. With remission of arthritis, cavities may become thin-walled and gradually disappear. In Caplan's syndrome, nodules tend to develop rapidly and appear in crops; both cavitation and calcification may occur in this variety of rheumatoid nodule. (*See* page 370.)

Table continued on following page

TABLE 19–4. *(Continued)*

	ETIOLOGY	LOCATION	SIZE AND SHAPE
NEOPLASTIC	Papilloma	No predilection.	Up to several centimeters; round, sharply circumscribed.
	Hematogenous metastases	Predilection for lower lobes.	3 mm to 6 cm or more; typically round and sharply circumscribed.
	Non-Hodgkin's lymphoma	More numerous in lower lung zones.	3 mm to 7 cm; round, ovoid, triangular, or polyhedral, usually with fuzzy outlines.
	Multiple myeloma (plasmacytoma)	No known predilection.	Lobulated.
	Broncho-pulmonary amyloidosis	Widely distributed.	Highly variable.
TRAUMATIC	Multiple pulmonary hematomas	Unilateral or bilateral, generally in lung deep to maximum trauma.	Highly variable. Commonly 2 to 6 cm but may be very large. Sharply circumscribed.
IDIOPATHIC	Sarcoidosis	Widely distributed.	Average diameter greater than 1 cm.

TABLE 19–4. *(Continued)*

CALCIFICATION	CAVITATION	GENERAL COMMENTS
No	Frequent.	Obstruction of airways leads to peripheral atelectasis and obstructive pneumonitis. Diagnosis is suggested by a combination of multiple solid or cavitary lesions throughout the lungs associated with laryngeal or tracheal papillomas. (*See* page 403.)
Rare, but if present, virtually diagnostic of osteogenic sarcoma or chondrosarcoma.	In approximately 4 per cent of cases, more frequently in upper lobes.	Wide range in size of multiple nodules is highly suggestive of the diagnosis. Seldom associated with mediastinal or bronchopulmonary lymph-node enlargement. (*See* page 445.)
No	"Cystlike" lesions may occur in histiocytic lymphoma, simulating cavitation.	A manifestation of *secondary* lymphocytic lymphoma. Mediastinal and bronchopulmonary lymph-node enlargement is associated in some cases. (*See* page 436.)
No	No	(*See* page 441.)
Lesions may be calcified or ossified.	Sometimes.	This is the parenchymal form of the disease. Now regarded as one of the plasma cell dyscrasias. (*See* page 443.)
No	No	Generally undergo slow but progressive decrease in size and may persist for weeks or even months. Initially, hematomas may be masked by surrounding pulmonary contusion. (*See* page 616.)
No	No	A rare pattern in sarcoidosis (in only 3 of 150 patients in one series). Simulates metastases. (*See* page 646.)

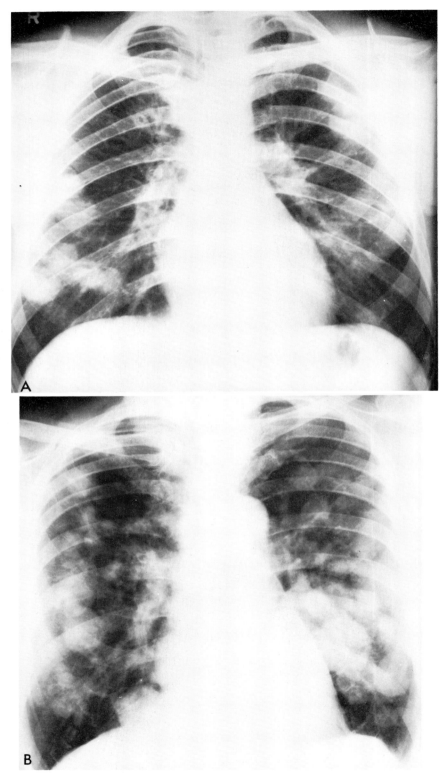

Figure 19–4. **Examples of Multiple Pulmonary Nodules.** *A*, Pyemic abscesses secondary to acute osteomyelitis of the femur caused by *Staphylococcus aureus;* the masses show no evidence of cavitation, although such occurred eventually in the majority of lesions. *B*, Hematogenous metastases from primary fibrosarcoma of the ilium.

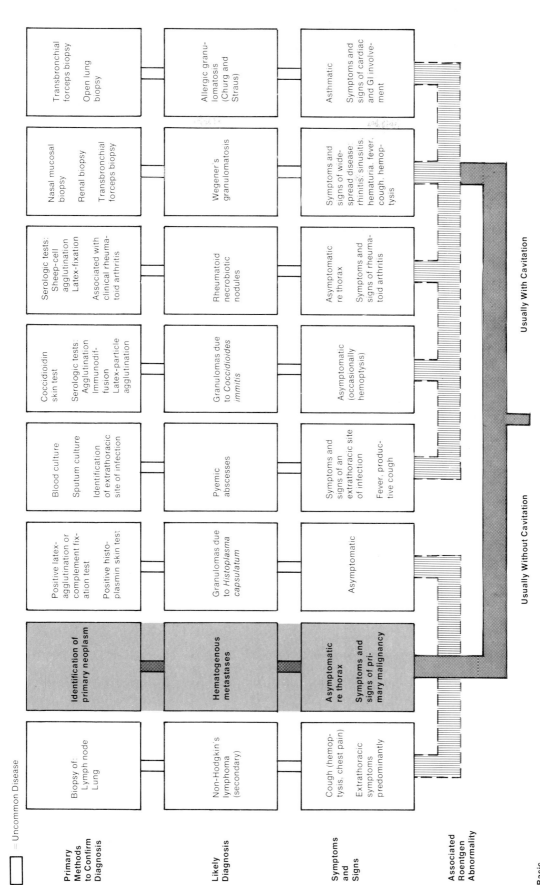

DECISION TREE 19-4

= Common Disease

= Uncommon Disease

Primary Methods to Confirm Diagnosis	Biopsy of: Lymph node Lung	Positive latex-agglutination or complement fixation test Positive histoplasmin skin test	Blood culture Sputum culture Identification of extrathoracic site of infection	Coccidioidin skin test Serologic tests: Agglutination Immunodiffusion Latex-particle agglutination	Serologic tests: Sheep-cell agglutination Latex-fixation Associated with clinical rheumatoid arthritis	Nasal mucosal biopsy Renal biopsy Transbronchial forceps biopsy	Transbronchial forceps biopsy Open lung biopsy
Likely Diagnosis	Non-Hodgkin's lymphoma (secondary)	Granulomas due to *Histoplasma capsulatum*	Pyemic abscesses	Granulomas due to *Coccidioides immitis*	Rheumatoid necrobiotic nodules	Wegener's granulomatosis	Allergic granulomatosis (Churg and Straus)
Symptoms and Signs	Cough (hemoptysis, chest pain) Extrathoracic symptoms predominantly	Asymptomatic	Symptoms and signs of an extrathoracic site of infection Fever, productive cough	Asymptomatic (occasionally hemoptysis)	Asymptomatic re thorax Symptoms and signs of rheumatoid arthritis	Symptoms and signs of widespread disease rhinitis, sinusitis, hematuria, fever, cough, hemoptysis	Asthmatic Symptoms and signs of cardiac and GI involvement

Identification of primary neoplasm

Hematogenous metastases

Asymptomatic re thorax Symptoms and signs of primary malignancy

Associated Roentgen Abnormality

Usually Without Cavitation

Usually With Cavitation

Basic Pattern

Multiple Pulmonary Nodules

783

TABLE 19–5

DIFFUSE PULMONARY DISEASE WITH A
PREDOMINANTLY ACINAR PATTERN

"Diffuse" implies involvement of all lobes of both lungs. Although the disease necessarily is widespread, it need not affect all lung regions uniformly. For example, the lower lung zones may be involved to a greater or lesser degree than the upper, or the central and midportions

	ETIOLOGY	ANATOMIC DISTRIBUTION
	Histoplasma capsulatum	Generalized.
INFECTIOUS	Varicella-zoster virus (chickenpox pneumonia)	Widespread; acinar lesions may be confluent in central areas of lungs.
	Influenza virus	Uniform.
	Pneumocystis carinii	Generalized.
	Ascaris lumbricoides or *Ascaris suum*	Generalized.
IMMUNOLOGIC	Goodpasture's syndrome and idiopathic pulmonary hemorrhage	Widespread but more prominent in perihilar areas and in midlung and lower lung zones.
	Necrotizing alveolitis	Generalized.
NEOPLASTIC	Bronchiolo-alveolar carcinoma	Diffuse.
	Hematogenous metastases	Widespread.
THROMBOEMBOLIC	Traumatic fat embolism	Diffuse, although predominantly peripheral.
	Amniotic fluid embolism	Generalized.
CARDIOVASCULAR	Pulmonary edema	Usually bilateral and symmetric. Cortex of lung may be relatively spared (the "butterfly" pattern).

of the lungs may be more severely affected than the peripheral ("bat's-wing" distribution).

The term "acinar pattern" implies airspace consolidation, which may be confluent and thereby render individual acinar shadows unidentifiable.

Other abnormalities such as pleural effusion and cardiac enlargement may be present.

ADDITIONAL FINDINGS	COMMENTS
Hilar lymph-node enlargement frequent.	Acute widely disseminated histoplasmosis; symptoms may be disproportionately mild. Over a period of years, healing may result in multiple small calcific foci. (*See* page 302.)
Hilar lymph-node enlargement in some cases.	Over a period of many years, healing may result in multiple small calcific foci throughout the lungs. (*See* page 334.)
"Mitral configuration" of the heart may be present.	This pattern in acute influenza virus pneumonia occurs particularly in patients who have mitral stenosis or are pregnant. (*See* page 328.)
No lymph node enlargement or pleural effusion.	Represents an extension of the infection from the interstitium where it originates to alveolar air spaces. (*See* page 341.)
None.	Represents severe edema occasioned by allergic response to the passage of larvae through the pulmonary circulation. (*See* page 343.)
Confluence of opacities may occur—in which circumstances an air bronchogram will be seen. Lymph-node enlargement may be recognized occasionally.	An acinar pattern is seen in relatively pure form in the early stages of these diseases but with passage of the alveolar hemorrhage into the interstitial space, the pattern becomes reticular. (*See* page 360.)
Pleural effusion in 8 to 10 per cent. Mediastinal lymph-node enlargement uncommon.	Diffuse disease occurs more often in a mixed pattern. (*See* page 423.)
———	A rare manifestation of hematogenous metastases. (*See* page 445.)
Fracture of extremities, pelvis, or axial skeleton usually present. Heart size normal.	Lesions appear within one to two days after trauma and resolve within one to four weeks. Absence of cardiac enlargement and of signs of postcapillary hypertension aid in differentiation from pulmonary edema of cardiac origin. (*See* page 469.)
If vascular occlusion is severe enough, the heart may be enlarged as a result of cor pulmonale.	Air-space pulmonary edema indistinguishable from that of any other cause. (*See* page 471.)
Associated findings depend largely on the etiology of the edema—for example, signs of interstitial pulmonary edema (septal lines, and so forth) in edema of cardiac origin.	(*See* page 497.)

Table continued on following page

TABLE 19–5. *(Continued)*

	ETIOLOGY	ANATOMIC DISTRIBUTION
	Acute aspiration pulmonary edema (near-drowning)	Diffuse.
	Hydrocarbon pneumonitis	Predominantly basal, bilaterally.
INHALATIONAL	Noxious gases Silo-filler's disease (NO_2 toxicity)—acute phase Sulfur dioxide Phosgene Acute cadmium poisoning Secondary to burns	Diffuse.
	Acute berylliosis (fulminating variety)	Diffuse.
	Acute berylliosis (insidious variety)	Diffuse.
	Acute silicoproteinosis	Diffuse.
IDIOPATHIC	Adult respiratory distress syndrome	Usually diffuse.
	Pulmonary edema associated with narcotic abuse	Diffuse.
	Alveolar proteinosis	Bilateral and symmetric, commonly in a "butterfly" distribution. Resolution tends to occur asymmetrically.
	Sarcoidosis	Diffuse.

TABLE 19–5. *(Continued)*

ADDITIONAL FINDINGS	COMMENTS
To be noted are the normal cardiac size and the absence of signs of pulmonary venous hypertension.	Roentgenographic pattern is one of diffuse patchy air-space consolidation typical of pulmonary edema. May occur with aspiration of fresh or sea water (in near-drowning), ethyl alcohol, kerosene, and, by far the most common, acid gastric juice (Mendelson's syndrome). (*See* pages 504 to 508.)
A pneumatocele may develop in an occasional patient as a consequence of bronchial or bronchiolar obstruction.	The roentgenographic pattern is characteristic of patchy air-space consolidation due to edema. The hila tend to be indistinct and hazy due to edema. (*See* page 601.)
None.	The widespread acinar pattern is due to acute pulmonary edema which develops within several hours of exposure and which usually clears completely if the patient survives. (*See* pages 598 to 600.)
None.	Morphologic changes consist of severe proteinaceous edema of the lungs. Roentgenologic changes characteristically develop rapidly following an overwhelming exposure. (*See* page 595.)
None.	Roentgenographic changes consist of diffuse bilateral "haziness" with subsequent development of irregular patchy densities scattered widely throughout the lungs; develop one to four weeks after the onset of symptoms. Roentgenographic clearing may take two to three months. (*See* page 595.)
Hilar lymph-node enlargement.	Roentgenographic pattern is similar or identical to that of alveolar proteinosis. An acute, rapidly progressive course is characteristic. Most commonly seen in sandblasters. (*See* page 581.)
None.	Characterized by massive bilateral pulmonary edema, usually associated with normal microvascular pressure. (*See* page 512.)
None.	Most commonly the result of heroin or methadone overdosage. (*See* page 511.)
None.	Differentiated from subacute pulmonary edema on the basis of absence of cardiac enlargement and of signs of pulmonary venous hypertension; Kerley B lines have been reported, however. (*See* page 663.)
Hilar and mediastinal lymph-node enlargement in many cases.	An uncommon pattern in this disease. May be the predominant pattern (in 20 per cent of patients) or associated with a reticulonodular pattern elsewhere in the lungs. (*See* page 645.)

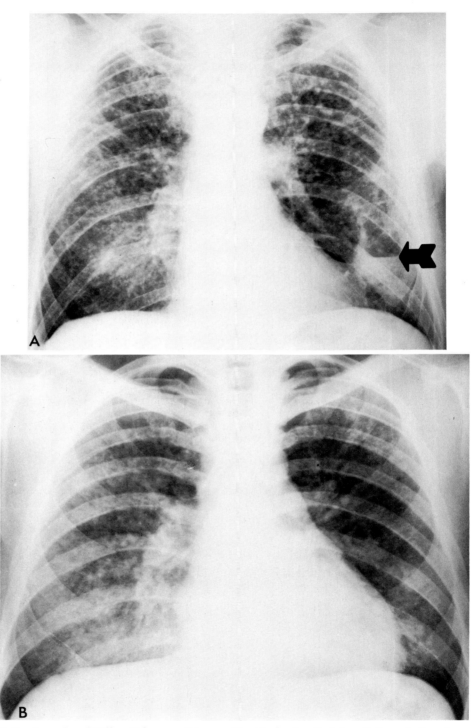

Figure 19–5. Examples of Diffuse Pulmonary Disease with a Predominantly Acinar Pattern. *A*, Bronchogenic spread of *Mycobacterium tuberculosis*; the multiple acinar shadows are caused by widespread endobronchial dissemination of infective material from the left lower lobe abscess (arrow). *B*, Idiopathic pulmonary hemorrhage, acute phase.

DECISION TREE 19-5A

■ = Common Disease

☐ = Uncommon Disease

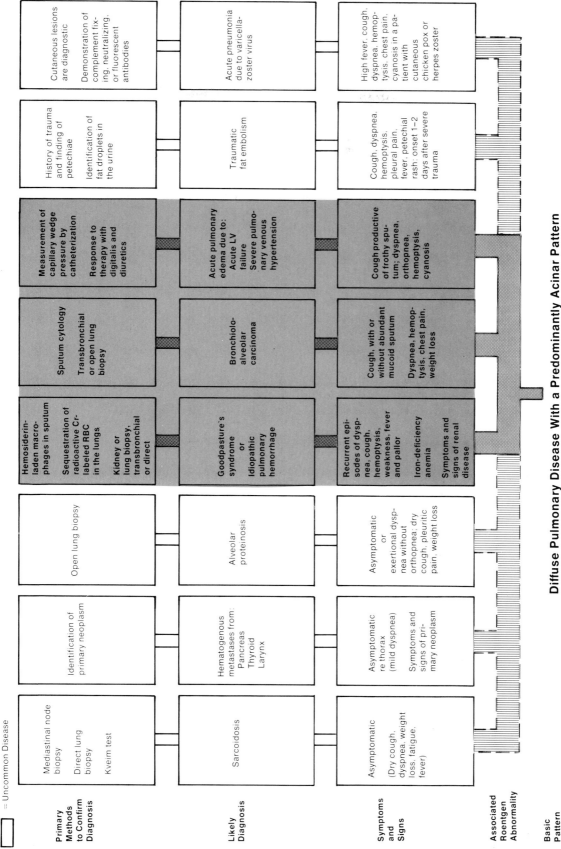

Primary Methods to Confirm Diagnosis	Mediastinal node biopsy Direct lung biopsy Kveim test	Identification of primary neoplasm	Open lung biopsy	**Hemosiderin-laden macrophages in sputum** **Sequestration of radioactive Cr-labeled RBC in the lungs** **Kidney or lung biopsy, transbronchial or direct**	**Sputum cytology** **Transbronchial or open lung biopsy**	**Measurement of capillary wedge pressure by catheterization** **Response to therapy with digitalis and diuretics**	History of trauma and finding of petechiae Identification of fat droplets in the urine	Cutaneous lesions are diagnostic Demonstration of complement fixing, neutralizing, or fluorescent antibodies
Likely Diagnosis	Sarcoidosis	Hematogenous metastases from: Pancreas Thyroid Larynx	Alveolar proteinosis	**Goodpasture's syndrome or Idiopathic pulmonary hemorrhage**	**Bronchiolo-alveolar carcinoma**	**Acute pulmonary edema due to:** **Acute LV failure** **Severe pulmonary venous hypertension**	Traumatic fat embolism	Acute pneumonia due to varicella-zoster virus
Symptoms and Signs	Asymptomatic (Dry cough, dyspnea, weight loss, fatigue, fever)	Asymptomatic re thorax (mild dyspnea) Symptoms and signs of primary neoplasm	Asymptomatic or exertional dyspnea without orthopnea; dry cough, pleuritic pain, weight loss	**Recurrent episodes of dyspnea, cough, hemoptysis, weakness, fever and pallor** **Iron-deficiency anemia** **Symptoms and signs of renal disease**	**Cough, with or without abundant mucoid sputum** **Dyspnea, hemoptysis, chest pain, weight loss**	**Cough productive of frothy sputum; dyspnea, orthopnea, hemoptysis, cyanosis**	Cough, dyspnea, hemoptysis, pleural pain, fever, petechial rash: onset 1-2 days after severe trauma	High fever, cough, dyspnea, hemoptysis, chest pain, cyanosis in a patient with cutaneous chicken pox or herpes zoster
Associated Roentgen Abnormality								
Basic Pattern								

Diffuse Pulmonary Disease With a Predominantly Acinar Pattern

789

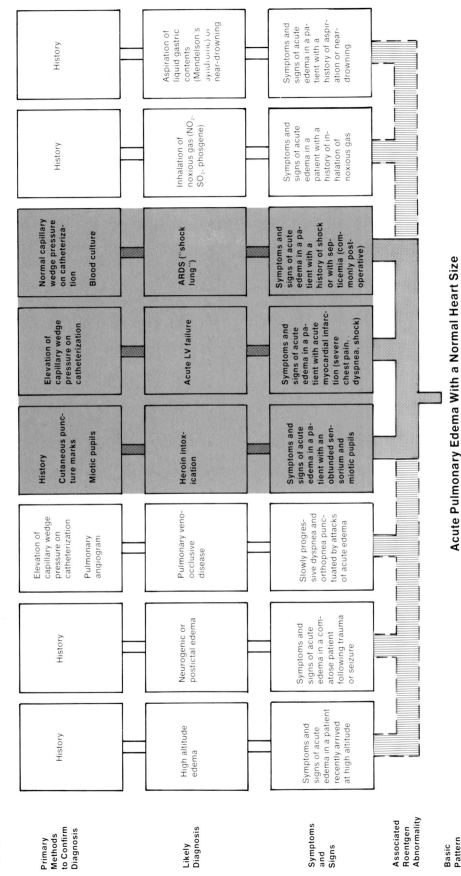

DECISION TREE 19-5B

Acute Pulmonary Edema With a Normal Heart Size

| Primary Methods to Confirm Diagnosis | History | History | History | Elevation of capillary wedge pressure on catheterization / Pulmonary angiogram | History / Cutaneous puncture marks / Miotic pupils | Elevation of capillary wedge pressure on catheterization | Normal capillary wedge pressure on catheterization / Blood culture | History | History |

| Likely Diagnosis | High altitude edema | Neurogenic or postictal edema | Pulmonary venoocclusive disease | Heroin intoxication | Acute LV failure | ARDS ("shock lung") | Inhalation of noxious gas (NO₂, SO₂, phosgene) | Aspiration of liquid gastric contents (Mendelson's syndrome) or near-drowning |

| Symptoms and Signs | Symptoms and signs of acute edema in a patient recently arrived at high altitude | Symptoms and signs of acute edema in a comatose patient following trauma or seizure | Slowly progressive dyspnea and orthopnea punctuated by attacks of acute edema | Symptoms and signs of acute edema in a patient with an obtunded sensorium and miotic pupils | Symptoms and signs of acute edema in a patient with acute myocardial infarction (severe chest pain, dyspnea, shock) | Symptoms and signs of acute edema in a patient with a history of shock or with septicemia (commonly postoperative) | Symptoms and signs of acute edema in a patient with a history of inhalation of noxious gas | Symptoms and signs of acute edema in a patient with a history of aspiration or near-drowning |

Associated Roentgen Abnormality

Basic Pattern

= Common Disease

= Uncommon Disease

790

TABLE 19–6

DIFFUSE PULMONARY DISEASE WITH A PREDOMINANTLY NODULAR, RETICULAR, OR RETICULONODULAR PATTERN

The large number of diseases capable of producing an "interstitial" pattern within the lungs has made this table the longest in the group. As with diseases characterized by an acinar pattern, "diffuse" involvement connotes affection of all lobes of both lungs, although the pattern may be more marked in some areas. Other abnormalities may be present, such as pleural effusion, hilar and mediastinal lymph node enlargement, and cardiac enlargement. The individual patterns may be described as follows.

NODULAR. The purely nodular interstitial diseases of the lungs perhaps are best epitomized by hematogenous infections such as miliary tuberculosis. Since the infecting organism arrives via the circulation and is trapped in the capillary sieve, it must be purely interstitial in location, at least early in its course. The pattern consists of discrete punctate opacities which range from tiny nodules 1 mm in diameter (barely visible roentgenographically) to 5 mm.

RETICULAR. This pattern consists of a network of linear opacities which may be conceived as a series of "rings" surrounding spaces of air density. It is useful to describe a reticular pattern according to the size of the "mesh": the terms fine, medium, and coarse are widely used and appear generally acceptable.

RETICULONODULAR. This pattern may be produced by a mixture of nodular deposits and diffuse linear thickening throughout the interstitial space. In addition, although a linear network throughout the interstitial tissue may appear roentgenographically as a purely reticular pattern, the orientation of some of the linear densities parallel to the x-ray beam may suggest a nodular component.

THE HONEYCOMB PATTERN. In this book, the term "honeycomb pattern" is restricted to a very coarse reticulation in which the air spaces in the "mesh" measure not less than 5 mm in diameter and are surrounded by a thick wall.

TABLE 19–6. *(Continued)*

	ETIOLOGY	ANATOMIC DISTRIBUTION	VOLUME OF THORAX
	Bacteria		
	Mycobacterium tuberculosis	Generalized, uniform.	Unaffected.
	Staphylococcus aureus	Generalized, uniform.	Unaffected.
	Salmonella species	Generalized, uniform.	Unaffected.
	Mycoplasma pneumoniae	Generalized, uniform.	Unaffected.
	Fungi		
	Coccidioides immitis	Generalized, uniform.	Unaffected.
	Cryptococcus neoformans	Generalized, uniform.	Unaffected.
	Blastomyces brasiliensis	Generalized, uniform.	Unaffected.
INFECTIOUS	*Blastomyces dermatitidis*	Generalized, uniform.	Unaffected.
	Histoplasma capsulatum	Generalized, uniform.	Unaffected.
	Viruses		
	Rubeola	Generalized, uniform.	Unaffected.
	Cytomegalovirus	Generalized, uniform.	Unaffected.
	Parasites		
	Schistosoma species (schistosomiasis)	Generalized, uniform.	Unaffected.
	Filaria species (filariasis)	Generalized, uniform.	Unaffected.

TABLE 19–6. *(Continued)*

ADDITIONAL FINDINGS	COMMENTS
None.	Characteristic miliary pattern resulting from hematogenous dissemination. (*See* page 295.)
When of sufficient size, lesions may excavate to produce microabscesses.	Miliary pattern (hematogenous dissemination). (*See* page 269.)
There may be disseminated destructive lesions of bone.	Miliary pattern (hematogenous dissemination). (*See* page 279.)
Kerley B lines in some cases.	The presenting pattern in 28 of 100 cases in one series. Symptoms tend to be mild in contrast to the more common acute segmental disease. (*See* page 325.)
Generalized hematogenous spread may lead to destructive lesions of bone.	Miliary pattern (hematogenous dissemination). (*See* page 307.)
None.	Miliary pattern (hematogenous dissemination). (*See* page 312.)
None.	Hematogenous dissemination with production of miliary pattern is the only pulmonary manifestation of the disease. Seen only in South America. (*See* page 312.)
Thoracic or remote bone involvement.	Miliary pattern (hematogenous dissemination). (*See* page 310.)
Hilar node enlargement in the majority of cases.	The "epidemic" form of the disease, typically developing in groups of people heavily exposed to organisms in caves or in locales of contaminated soil. Acute nodules measuring 3 to 4 mm may heal to form multiple discrete calcifications many years later. (*See* page 302.)
Lymph-node enlargement is common.	Reticulonodular. Primary measles infection of lungs may be associated with secondary bacterial pneumonia. (*See* page 331.)
None.	Early stage manifestation, followed shortly by patchy acinar consolidation. (*See* page 335.)
The central pulmonary arteries may be dilated secondary to vascular obstruction.	Hematogenous dissemination with production of a reticulonodular pattern. (*See* page 348.)
Hilar lymph-node enlargement in some cases.	Tropical pulmonary eosinophilia. Hematogenous dissemination with production of very fine reticulonodular pattern of low density. (*See* page 344.)

Table continued on following page

TABLE 19–6. *(Continued)*

	ETIOLOGY	ANATOMIC DISTRIBUTION	VOLUME OF THORAX
INFECTIOUS *(Cont.)*	*Pneumocystis carinii*	Generalized, uniform.	Unaffected.
	Toxoplasma gondii	Generalized, uniform.	Unaffected.
IMMUNOLOGIC	Idiopathic pulmonary hemosiderosis Goodpasture's syndrome	Usually widespread but may be more prominent in the perihilar areas and the mid and lower lung zones.	May be a slight decrease in late stages of the disease.
	Scleroderma (diffuse systemic sclerosis)	Generalized but more prominent in lung bases.	Serial roentgenographic studies may reveal progressive loss of lung volume.
	Rheumatoid disease	Generalized but more prominent in lung bases.	Serial roentgenographic studies may reveal progressive loss of lung volume.
	Diseases of alveolar hypersensitivity (extrinsic allergic alveolitis) Farmer's lung, etc.	Generalized.	Unaffected.
	Dermatomyositis and polymyositis	Generalized but more prominent in lung bases.	Serial studies may reveal progressive loss of lung volume, particularly if polymyositis involves the muscles of respiration.
	Sjögren's syndrome	Generalized but more prominent in lung bases.	Unaffected.
	Waldenström's macroglobulinemia	Generalized.	Unaffected.

TABLE 19-6. *(Continued)*

ADDITIONAL FINDINGS	COMMENTS
No lymph-node enlargement or pleural effusion.	Early stage manifestation. (*See* page 341.)
Hilar lymph-node enlargement common.	Represents the pattern seen in the early stages of diffuse disease. (*See* page 340.)
None.	Early in the disease, the pattern represents a transition stage from acute hemorrhage into the air spaces to complete resolution, but in the later stages, interstitial fibrosis is permanent. (*See* page 360.)
Associated findings include esophageal dysperistalsis, terminal pulp calcinosis, absorption of distal phalanges, and widening of the periodontal membrane. Pleural effusion uncommon.	The roentgenographic pattern in the early stages consists of a fine reticulation which tends to coarsen and become reticulonodular as the disease progresses. Small cysts measuring up to 1 cm in diameter may be identified in the lung periphery, particularly in the bases. (*See* page 372.)
Incidence of coexisting pleural effusion and pulmonary disease not clear, but the two are probably independent. Roentgenographic evidence of rheumatoid arthritis in most patients.	In the early stages, the roentgenographic pattern is punctate or nodular in character; in the later or fibrotic stage, the pattern consists of medium to coarse reticulation. (*See* page 369.)
Vary somewhat depending on specific disease entity, chiefly regarding hilar and mediastinal lymph-node enlargement.	Considerable similarity exists in the roentgenographic pattern observed in all these diseases, ranging from a diffuse nodular pattern through coarse reticulation characteristic of diffuse interstitial fibrosis. While the pattern is generally "interstitial" in type, involvement of air spaces in the form of acinar opacities may be observed in most if not all during the acute stage of the disease. Irreversible changes of fibrosis tend to occur with continuous or repeated exposure. (*See* pages 388 to 394.)
Additional findings may be those associated with scleroderma or rheumatoid arthritis. When polymyositis involves the muscles of respiration, small volume lungs may be apparent.	In patients with diffuse lung involvement, the roentgenographic pattern is reticular or reticulonodular and may be indistinguishable from the changes of scleroderma or rheumatoid disease. These diseases sometimes occur in conjunction with primary malignancy elsewhere. (*See* page 375.)
This syndrome consists of a triad of keratoconjunctivitis sicca, xerostomia, and recurrent swelling of the parotid gland. Occasionally appears in association with any of the collagen diseases.	One-third of patients show a diffuse reticulonodular pattern similar to that of other collagen diseases characterized by vascular involvement. Joint changes resemble rheumatoid or psoriatic arthritis. Remarkable female sex predominance. (*See* page 376.)
May be associated with localized homogeneous consolidation.	Diffuse reticulonodular pattern is produced by infiltration of interstitium by lymphoid and plasmacytoid cells. (*See* page 442.)

Table continued on following page

TABLE 19–6. *(Continued)*

	ETIOLOGY	ANATOMIC DISTRIBUTION	VOLUME OF THORAX
IMMUNOLOGIC *(Cont.)*	Nitrofurantoin-induced pulmonary disease	Generalized but more prominent in lung bases.	Unaffected.
	Systemic lupus erythematosus	Generalized.	Serial studies may reveal progressive loss of lung volume.
	Necrotizing "sarcoidal" angiitis and granulomatosis	Generalized.	Unaffected.
	Bronchiolo-alveolar carcinoma	Diffuse.	Unaffected.
	Lymphangitic carcinomatosis	Commonly generalized but more prominent in the lower lung zones.	Serial roentgenographic studies may reveal progressive reduction in volume.
	Hodgkin's disease	Generalized.	Unaffected.
NEOPLASTIC	Non-Hodgkin's lymphoma	Diffuse.	Unaffected.
	Leukemia	Diffuse.	Unaffected.
	Waldenström's macroglobulinemia	Diffuse.	Unaffected.
	Bronchopulmonary amyloidosis	Diffuse.	Unaffected.

TABLE 19–6. *(Continued)*

ADDITIONAL FINDINGS	COMMENTS
Pleural effusion in some cases.	Pattern consists of a diffuse fine reticulation. Almost invariably associated with peripheral blood eosinophilia. A similar roentgenographic pattern associated with eosinophilia may occur in the absence of known exciting cause. (*See* page 381.)
Pleural effusions common. Enlargement of cardiovascular silhouette usually due to pericardial effusion.	Etiology of reticular pattern varied. (*See* page 364.)
Hilar and mediastinal lymph node enlargement in some cases.	Predominantly nodular pattern. Nodules may be well-defined or ill-defined. Pattern indistinguishable from sarcoidosis roentgenologically but associated with angiitis pathologically. (*See* page 386.)
Pleural effusion in 8 to 10 per cent, always in association with pulmonary involvement.	The roentgenographic pattern is basically nodular, representing subacinar consolidation. An associated linear or reticular pattern can be caused by lymphangitic spread. Metastatic carcinoma of the pancreas may produce a pattern indistinguishable roentgenologically or morphologically. (*See* page 423.)
Hilar or mediastinal lymph-node enlargement is frequent but is not necessary to the diagnosis. Kerley B lines frequent.	Although the basic change is linear or reticular, there may be a coarse nodular component as well, caused by hematogenous dissemination. (*See* page 445.)
Mediastinal and hilar lymph-node enlargement almost invariably associated.	Differentiation from sarcoidosis or lymphangitic carcinoma may be difficult or impossible on purely roentgenologic grounds. (*See* page 430.)
Pleural effusion in about one-third of cases. Mediastinal and hilar lymph-node enlargement may be inconspicuous or absent.	In some cases of histiocytic lymphoma, this diffuse pattern may be due to Sjögren's syndrome. The roentgenographic pattern may simulate lymphangitic carcinoma. (*See* page 436.)
Mediastinal and hilar lymph-node enlargement may be present but not necessarily. Pleural effusion in some cases.	This is the usual pattern of pulmonary parenchymal involvement, but tends to occur only in the terminal stages of the disease or during blastic crises. (*See* page 440.)
Pleural effusion in about 50 per cent of cases.	This rare lymphoproliferative disorder is one of the plasma cell dyscrasias. (*See* page 442.)
Hilar and mediastinal lymph-node enlargement may be massive, and nodes may be densely calcified.	This is the diffuse alveolar septal form of the disease. (*See* page 443.)

Table continued on following page

TABLE 19–6. *(Continued)*

	ETIOLOGY	ANATOMIC DISTRIBUTION	VOLUME OF THORAX
	Embolism from oily contrast media	Diffuse, uniform.	Unaffected.
THROMBOEMBOLIC	Talc granulomatosis of drug addicts	Usually generalized.	May be reduced in the presence of severe fibrosis.
	Metallic mercury embolism	Predominantly lower lung zones.	Unaffected.
	Schistosomiasis	Generalized.	Unaffected.
	Interstitial pulmonary edema	Diffuse but predominantly lower lung zones.	May be reduced.
CARDIOVASCULAR	Pulmonary fibrosis secondary to chronic postcapillary hypertension	Predominantly mid and lower lung zones.	Unaffected.
	Hemosiderosis secondary to chronic postcapillary hypertension	Predominantly mid and lower lung zones.	Unaffected.
	Transient tachypnea of the newborn	Generalized.	Normal or reduced.
INHALATIONAL	Inorganic dust pneumoconiosis Silicosis (simple)	Generalized but often predominantly mid and upper lung zones.	Little affected.

TABLE 19-6. *(Continued)*

ADDITIONAL FINDINGS	COMMENTS
None.	The typical pattern is finely reticular; complete clearing usually occurs within 48 to 72 hours, although an abnormal pattern may persist for up to 11 days. This complication usually occurs following lymphangiography with ultrafluid Lipiodol. (*See* page 477.)
Pulmonary arterial hypertension and cor pulmonale in advanced cases.	Creates a pure micronodular pattern similar to alveolar microlithiasis. (*See* page 475.)
A local collection of mercury may be present in the heart, usually near the apex of the right ventricle.	Roentgenographic appearance distinctive because of the very high density of the intravascular mercury. May be in the form of spherules or of short tubular opacities. (*See* page 477.)
May be associated with signs of pulmonary arterial hypertension and cor pulmonale.	Presumably results from the passage of ova through vessel walls and the foreign body reaction to them. (*See* page 473.)
Varies with the etiology of the edema, but usually those associated with pulmonary venous hypertension.	Roentgenographic pattern consists of loss of normal sharp definition of pulmonary vascular markings, and thickening of the interlobular septa (Kerley B lines). (*See* page 498.)
Typical cardiac configuration of chronic mitral valve disease. Almost invariably associated with signs of severe pulmonary venous and arterial hypertension. Ossific nodules may be present.	Roentgenographic pattern consists of a rather coarse but poorly defined reticulation. Probably related to recurrent episodes of air-space and interstitial edema and hemorrhage.
Typical cardiac configuration of chronic mitral valve disease. Almost invariably associated with signs of severe pulmonary venous and arterial hypertension. Ossific nodules may be present.	Pattern consists of tiny punctate opacities of low density. The incidence morphologically (25 per cent of cases of mitral stenosis) is much higher than roentgenographically. Usually associated with high levels of pulmonary arterial pressure.
None.	A manifestation of interstitial "edema" resulting from failure of clearance of excess fluid from the lungs at delivery.
Hilar lymph-node enlargement in some cases, uncommonly associated with "eggshell calcification" (5 per cent). Pleural thickening in late stages. Kerley A and B lines are common and may be present without visible nodules.	The roentgenographic pattern ranges from well circumscribed nodular opacities of uniform density ranging from 1 to 10 mm in diameter to a reticular or reticulonodular appearance. (*See* page 580.)

Table continued on following page

TABLE 19–6. (Continued)

	ETIOLOGY	ANATOMIC DISTRIBUTION	VOLUME OF THORAX
	Coal-worker's pneumoconiosis (simple)	Generalized.	Unaffected.
	Asbestosis	In the early stages, predominantly lower lung zones; later generalized.	Normal or slightly reduced.
	Talcosis	Identical to asbestosis.	As with asbestosis.
	Kaolin (china-clay) pneumoconiosis	Generalized.	Unaffected.
INHALATIONAL *(Cont.)*	Chronic berylliosis	Diffuse.	In advanced cases there may be marked loss of lung volume.
	Aluminum pneumoconiosis (aluminosis, bauxitosis, Shaver's disease)	Diffuse.	Considerable loss of lung volume may occur.

	Pneumoconiosis due to radiopaque dusts
	  Siderosis
	  Stannosis (tin oxide)
	  Baritosis (barium sulfate)
	  Antimony
	  Rare earth
	  (cerium, etc.)
		Generalized.	Unaffected.

	Thesaurosis due to hair spray inhalation	Diffuse.	Unaffected.

TABLE 19–6. *(Continued)*

ADDITIONAL FINDINGS	COMMENTS
Enlargement of hilar lymph nodes is present in some cases but is seldom a predominant feature.	The roentgenographic pattern is typically nodular but may be predominantly reticular in the early stages. Nodules range from 1 to 10 mm in size and tend to be somewhat less well defined than in silicosis. (*See* page 590.)
The pleural manifestations dominate the picture roentgenographically and consist of plaque formation or general thickening, with or without calcification.	The roentgenographic pattern may be divided into three stages: a fine reticulation occupying predominantly the lower lung zones and creating a ground-glass appearance of the lungs—the early changes; a stage in which the interstitial reticulation becomes more marked, producing the "shaggy heart" sign; and a late stage in which reticulation is generalized throughout the lungs. Note high incidence of associated neoplasia. (*See* page 583.)
The hallmark of the roentgenologic diagnosis of talcosis is pleural plaque formation—often diaphragmatic in position and massive. Large opacities may develop identical to those seen in silicosis and coalworker's pneumoconiosis.	Pulmonary involvement similar to asbestosis. (*See* page 590.)
Progressive massive fibrosis may occur as a late manifestation, as in silicosis and coalworker's pneumoconiosis.	The roentgenographic pattern ranges from no more than a generalized increase in lung markings to a diffuse nodular or "miliary" mottling. (*See* page 590.)
Focal areas of emphysema may be identified in advanced cases, usually in the upper lobes. Spontaneous pneumothorax occurs in over 10 per cent of patients.	The roentgenographic pattern varies with degree of exposure: if minor, there is a diffuse granular "haziness"; with moderate exposure, the pattern is nodular, the nodules being ill-defined and of moderate size (calcification of nodules has been observed); in advanced cases, the pattern may be chiefly reticular. (*See* page 595.)
Pleural thickening occasionally. Emphysematous bullae develop commonly and are associated with a high incidence of pneumothorax.	The roentgenographic pattern consists of a fine to coarse reticular pattern, sometimes with a nodular component. (*See* page 596.)
Lymph-node enlargement is not a feature.	In siderosis, the roentgenographic pattern is reticulonodular in type, the deposits being of rather low density compared to the silicotic nodule. In the siderosis of silver polishers, a fine stippled pattern is created. If the free silica content of dust is high (siderosilicosis), the pattern is indistinguishable from silicosis. The roentgenographic pattern of the other dusts is basically nodular, the nodules being of very high density. None of these dusts is fibrogenic. (*See* page 593.)
None.	Pattern consists of a fine micronodulation which tends to clear with discontinuance of exposure to hair spray. (*See* page 601.)

Table continued on following page

TABLE 19–6. *(Continued)*

	ETIOLOGY	ANATOMIC DISTRIBUTION	VOLUME OF THORAX
INHALATIONAL (*Cont.*)	Silo-filler's disease (nitrogen dioxide) — third phase	Diffuse.	Unaffected.
AIRWAYS DISEASE	Cystic fibrosis	Generalized, uniform.	Considerable over-inflation.
	"Small airways disease"	Generalized.	Unaffected or slight over-inflation.
	Familial dysautonomia (Riley-Day syndrome)	Generalized.	Increased.
IDIOPATHIC	Sarcoidosis	Usually generalized but in stages of development or resolution may show some lack of uniformity.	Usually unaffected although fibrosis may be associated with emphysema and overinflation.
	"Usual" interstitial pneumonia (UIP) (diffuse fibrosing alveolitis; interstitial pulmonary fibrosis)	There is a predilection for the lower lung zones in the early stages, but becoming more generalized and uniform as the disease progresses.	Sequential studies will show progressive loss of lung volume.
	Histiocytosis-X (eosinophilic granuloma)	Diffuse but with a tendency for predominance of lesions in the upper lung zones.	Usually normal.

TABLE 19–6. *(Continued)*

ADDITIONAL FINDINGS	COMMENTS
None.	This phase is characterized roentgenographically by miliary nodulation whose appearance tends to lag behind the recurrence of symptoms. The multiple discrete nodular shadows of varying size tend to become confluent in the more severe cases. The nodulation may disappear in time although it commonly persists for a considerable period after acute symptoms have subsided. (*See* page 598.)
May be associated with segmental areas of consolidation or atelectasis due to bronchopneumonia or bronchiectasis.	The pattern is one of accentuation of the linear markings throughout the lungs giving a coarse reticular appearance. (*See* page 562.)
Signs of pulmonary arterial hypertension and cor pulmonale in chronic advanced disease.	The roentgenographic pattern is reticulonodular and simulates sarcoidosis (but without hilar lymph-node enlargement). Diagnosis should be suggested when the pulmonary function pattern is obstructive rather than restrictive. (*See* page 561.)
Local areas of segmental consolidation and atelectasis may be present, particularly in the right upper lobe and less frequently the right middle and left lower lobes.	The roentgenographic pattern is identical to that of cystic fibrosis. (*See* page 566.)
Hilar and mediastinal lymph-node enlargement often constitutes the earliest roentgenologic finding, with diffuse lung involvement developing subsequently (with or without disappearance of the node enlargement). In approximately 25 per cent of cases, the pulmonary changes exist alone.	The pattern is usually reticulonodular in type, although ranging from purely nodular to purely reticular. In the approximately 20 per cent of cases which progress to fibrosis the pattern is coarsely reticular, somewhat uneven in distribution and associated with bulla formation and generalized overinflation. (*See* page 644.)
None.	In the early stages the pattern is one of fine reticulation predominantly in the lung bases; the later stage is characterized by a generalized coarse reticular or reticulonodular pattern with "honeycombing" in some cases. (*See* page 653.)
Spontaneous pneumothorax in some cases.	The roentgenographic pattern varies with the stage of the disease, beginning with nodular and progressing to reticulonodular and finally to a typical honeycomb pattern. Probably the most common cause of a honeycomb pattern. (*See* page 665.)

Table continued on following page

TABLE 19–6. *(Continued)*

	ETIOLOGY	ANATOMIC DISTRIBUTION	VOLUME OF THORAX
	Drug-induced pulmonary disease Busulfan Bleomycin Methotrexate	Diffuse.	Unaffected.
	Desquamative interstitial pneumonitis (DIP)	Generalized but showing a distinct predominance in the lower lung zones.	Progressive loss of lung volume in the later stages of the disease.
	Pulmonary lymphangio-myomatosis and tuberous sclerosis	Usually generalized but predominantly basal.	Increased.
	Neurofibromatosis	Generalized.	May be increased.
IDIOPATHIC (*Cont.*)	Lymphoid interstitial pneumonia (LIP)	Generalized.	Unaffected.
	Alveolar microlithiasis	Widespread, although the lower zones show greater opacification due to larger volume of parenchyma.	Unaffected.
	Oxygen toxicity	Generalized, uniform.	Increased.
	Gaucher's disease	Generalized.	Unaffected.

TABLE 19–6. *(Continued)*

ADDITIONAL FINDINGS	COMMENTS
None.	Each of these drugs causes a diffuse reticulonodular pattern initially. With bleomycin or methotrexate, the pattern progresses to patchy acinar consolidation. (*See* page 607.)
Occasionally spontaneous pneumothorax, pleural effusion, and cor pulmonale; rarely segmental atelectasis.	This disease is felt by some to represent a stage of diffuse fibrosing alveolitis. (*See* page 655.)
Chylous pleural effusion and pneumothorax common. Sclerotic (and sometimes lytic) lesions in bone.	The basis pattern is coarse reticulonodular in type and may progress to a typical "honeycomb" appearance. (*See* page 660.)
Diffuse interstitial fibrosis usually associated with multiple bullae. Scoliosis and mediastinal neurofibromas.	Fibrosis is widespread, with some basal predominance, whereas bullae are predominantly upper zonal. (*See* page 659.)
None.	Possesses morphologic features exceedingly difficult to distinguish from pulmonary lymphoma. (*See* page 656.)
None.	The roentgenographic pattern is pathognomonic. Superimposition of millions of microliths can cause an almost uniformly white appearance to the lower lungs, often with obliteration of mediastinal and diaphragmatic contours. (*See* page 667.)
Those of the underlying disease for which oxygen therapy is administered.	Infants in respiratory distress who are placed on oxygen for long periods of time develop a "spongy" lung with fibrosis, atelectasis, and focal areas of emphysema. This may represent the late stage of hyaline membrane disease or the effects of long-term oxygen inhalation. Has also been described in adults. (*See* page 597.)
None.	Pattern may be reticulonodular or miliary. (*See* page 667.)

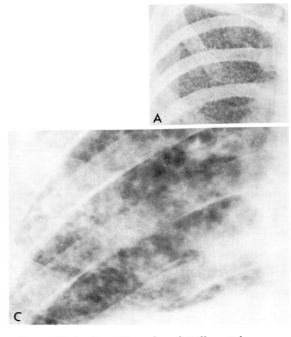

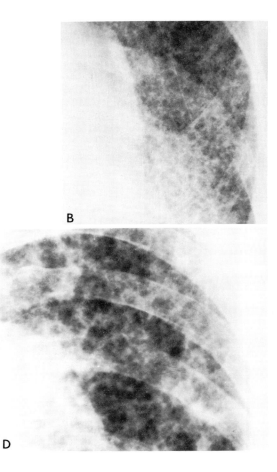

Figure 19–6. Four Examples of Diffuse Pulmonary Disease with a Predominantly Nodular, Reticular, or Reticulonodular Pattern. A, The micronodular pattern of miliary tuberculosis. B, A medium reticular pattern caused by diffuse interstitial pulmonary fibrosis of rheumatoid origin. C, A coarse reticulonodular pattern caused by diffuse interstitial pulmonary fibrosis of unknown etiology. D, The honeycomb pattern of chronic histiocytosis X.

DECISION TREE 19-6A

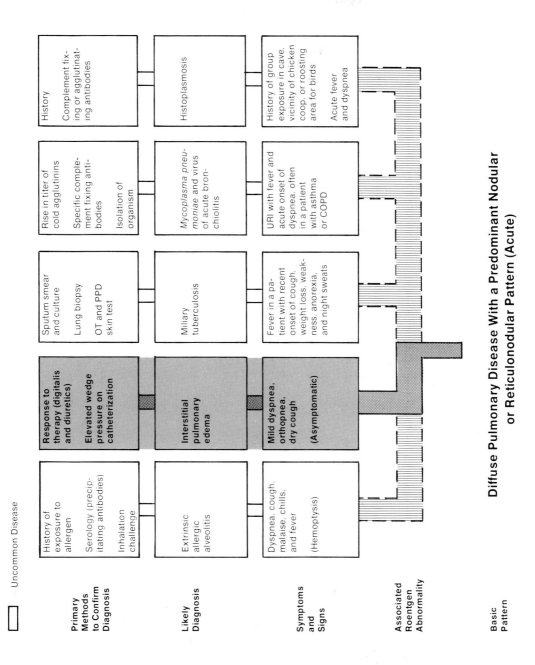

Diffuse Pulmonary Disease With a Predominant Nodular or Reticulonodular Pattern (Acute)

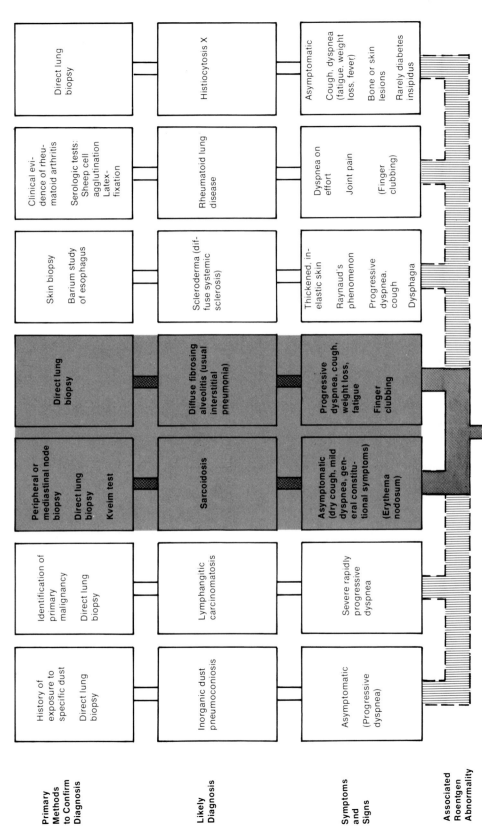

DECISION TREE 19-6B

■ = Common Disease

□ = Uncommon Disease

Primary Methods to Confirm Diagnosis

History of exposure to specific dust / Direct lung biopsy | Identification of primary malignancy / Direct lung biopsy | **Peripheral or mediastinal node biopsy / Direct lung biopsy / Kveim test** | **Direct lung biopsy** | Skin biopsy / Barium study of esophagus | Clinical evidence of rheumatoid arthritis / Serologic tests: Sheep cell agglutination / Latex-fixation | Direct lung biopsy

Likely Diagnosis

Inorganic dust pneumoconiosis | Lymphangitic carcinomatosis | **Sarcoidosis** | **Diffuse fibrosing alveolitis (usual interstitial pneumonia)** | Scleroderma (diffuse systemic sclerosis) | Rheumatoid lung disease | Histiocytosis X

Symptoms and Signs

Asymptomatic (Progressive dyspnea) | Severe rapidly progressive dyspnea | **Asymptomatic (dry cough, mild dyspnea, general constitutional symptoms) (Erythema nodosum)** | **Progressive dyspnea, cough, weight loss, fatigue / Finger clubbing** | Thickened, inelastic skin / Raynaud's phenomenon / Progressive dyspnea, cough / Dysphagia | Dyspnea on effort / Joint pain / (Finger clubbing) | Asymptomatic / Cough, dyspnea (fatigue, weight loss, fever) / Bone or skin lesions / Rarely diabetes insipidus

Associated Roentgen Abnormality

Basic Pattern

Diffuse Pulmonary Disease With a Predominant Nodular or Reticulonodular Pattern (Chronic)

TABLE 19–7

DIFFUSE PULMONARY DISEASE WITH A MIXED ACINAR AND RETICULONODULAR PATTERN

The pattern created by combined air-space consolidation and interstitial disease is best exemplified by pulmonary edema secondary to pulmonary venous hypertension. The roentgenographic manifestations of interstitial involvement consist in increased size and loss of definition of lung markings due to the presence of edema fluid within the bronchovascular sheath; air-space consolidation is manifested by discrete and confluent "fluffy" opacities characteristic of acinar-filling processes.

Another example of the mixed pattern is that produced by generalized bronchioloalveolar carcinoma: nodular and acinar components reflect the replacement of air spaces by malignant cells, and the linear or reticular component is due to the extension of carcinoma along the bronchovascular bundles, chiefly within lymphatics (lymphangitic carcinoma).

TABLE 19–7. *(Continued)*

	ETIOLOGY	ANATOMIC DISTRIBUTION	VOLUME OF THORAX
INFECTIOUS	Cytomegalovirus (cytomegalic inclusion disease)	Generalized, uniform.	Usually unaffected.
	Pneumocystis carini	"Butterfly" or diffuse distribution.	Unaffected.
	Mycoplasma pneumoniae and many viruses	Generalized, uniform.	Unaffected or slightly decreased.
	Strongyloides stercoralis	Generalized.	Unaffected.
IMMUNOLOGIC	Idiopathic pulmonary hemosiderosis Goodpasture's syndrome	Usually widespread but may be more prominent in the perihilar areas and the mid- and lower lung zones.	Usually unaffected.
	Alveolar hypersensitivity diseases (extrinsic allergic alveolitis)	Generalized.	Unaffected.
NEOPLASTIC	Bronchiolo-alveolar carcinoma	Generalized.	Unaffected.
CARDIOVASCULAR	Pulmonary edema	Usually generalized.	May be reduced.
IDIOPATHIC	Drug-induced pulmonary disease Bleomycin	Generalized.	Unaffected.

TABLE 19–7. *(Continued)*

ADDITIONAL FINDINGS	COMMENTS
None.	Combined interstitial and air-space disease with production of mixed reticulonodular and acinar patterns. (*See* page 335.)
None.	Dissemination probably by inhalation. Pattern is combined reticulonodular and acinar. Sometimes occurs in combination with cytomegalovirus infection. (*See* page 341.)
None.	Diffuse reticular pattern early, with superimposition of patchy air-space consolidation. (*See* page 325.)
None.	Represents overwhelming infestation, often in a compromised host. (*See* page 343.)
Rarely hilar lymph-node enlargement. Coalescence of lesions may permit visualization of an air bronchogram.	The mixed pattern is caused by a combination of patchy air-space consolidation from hemorrhage and the presence of hemosiderin and fibrous tissue in the interstitium. It may clear completely or may leave a residuum of reticulation due to irreversible interstitial fibrosis. (*See* page 360.)
Vary somewhat, depending on specific disease entity, chiefly regarding hilar and mediastinal lymph-node enlargement.	The majority of these diseases produce a relatively pure "interstitial" pattern which is either nodular or reticulonodular. However, in some cases acinar shadows representing air-space involvement are superimposed on the reticular pattern during the acute stage of the disease. (*See* page 389.)
Prominent linear opacities extending along the bronchovascular bundles toward the hila usually represent lymphatic permeation. Pleural effusion in 8 to 10 per cent. Mediastinal lymph-node enlargement uncommon.	The mixed pattern consists of acinar, nodular, and reticulonodular components. (*See* page 423.)
Cardiomegaly common but not invariable.	Combined interstitial and air-space edema. (*See* page 497.)
None.	This antineoplastic agent causes pulmonary disease in 2.6 to 10 per cent of patients. Begins with a reticular pattern and progresses to acinar consolidation. (*See* page 608.)

Table continued on following page

TABLE 19–7. *(Continued)*

	ETIOLOGY	ANATOMIC DISTRIBUTION	VOLUME OF THORAX
	Methotrexate	Generalized.	Unaffected.
IDIOPATHIC *(Cont.)*	Sarcoidosis	Generalized.	Unaffected.
	Desquamative interstitial pneumonitis (DIP)	Generalized but with lower zone predominance.	Progressive loss of lung volume common.

TABLE 19-7. *(Continued)*

ADDITIONAL FINDINGS	COMMENTS
None.	Incidence of pulmonary disease complicating use of this antileukemic agent is high (41 per cent in one series). Pulmonary manifestations usually clear on drug withdrawal. Initially the pattern is reticular, progressing to patchy acinar consolidation. (*See* page 609.)
Hilar and mediastinal lymph-node enlargement may coexist.	A mixed acinar and reticulonodular pattern is more common than a predominantly acinar pattern alone. (*See* page 644.)
Hilar and mediastinal lymph-node enlargement uncommon.	Early changes have been described as "ground-glass" opacification of both lungs. (*See* page 655.)

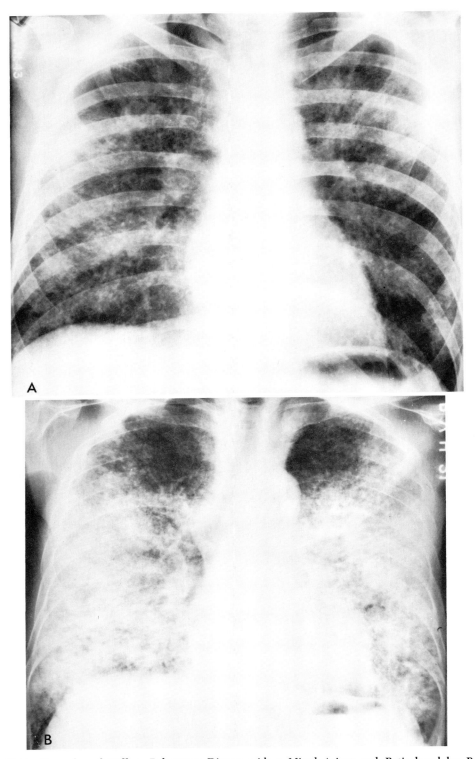

Figure 19–7. Examples of Diffuse Pulmonary Disease with a Mixed Acinar and Reticulonodular Pattern. *A,* *Pneumocystis carinii* pneumonia; the basic pattern is reticulonodular, indicating diffuse disease of the interstitium but superimposed upon this pattern in the upper lung zones are confluent acinar shadows representing air-space consolidation. *B,* Generalized bronchioloalveolar carcinoma; in the mid- and lower lung zones, acinar shadows are largely confluent, whereas in the upper zones the pattern is predominantly reticulonodular as a result of lymphangitic permeation of the neoplasm.

DECISION TREE 19-7

☐ Common Disease
☐ Uncommon Disease

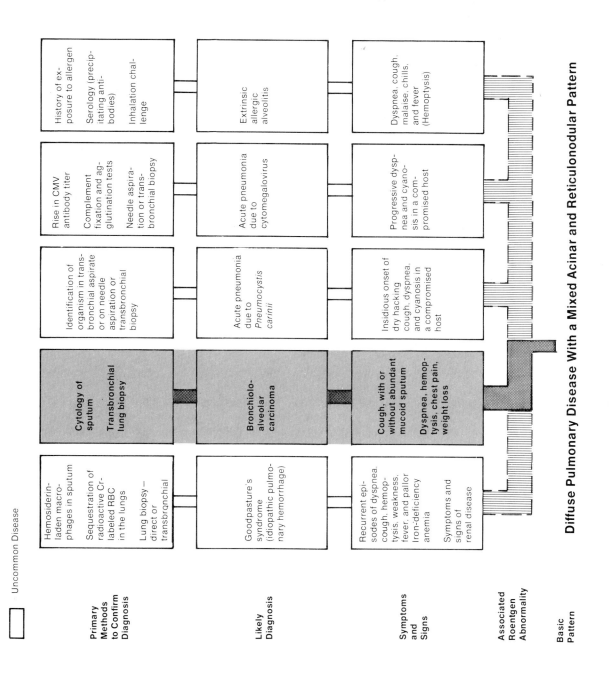

Diffuse Pulmonary Disease With a Mixed Acinar and Reticulonodular Pattern

Primary Methods to Confirm Diagnosis

- Hemosiderin-laden macrophages in sputum; Sequestration of radioactive Cr-labeled RBC in the lungs; Lung biopsy—direct or transbronchial
- **Cytology of sputum; Transbronchial lung biopsy**
- Identification of organism in transbronchial aspirate or on needle aspiration or transbronchial biopsy
- Rise in CMV antibody titer; Complement fixation and agglutination tests; Needle aspiration or transbronchial biopsy
- History of exposure to allergen; Serology (precipitating antibodies); Inhalation challenge

Likely Diagnosis

- Goodpasture's syndrome (idiopathic pulmonary hemorrhage)
- **Bronchiolo-alveolar carcinoma**
- Acute pneumonia due to *Pneumocystis carinii*
- Acute pneumonia due to cytomegalovirus
- Extrinsic allergic alveolitis

Symptoms and Signs

- Recurrent episodes of dyspnea, cough, hemoptysis, weakness, fever, and pallor; Iron-deficiency anemia; Symptoms and signs of renal disease
- **Cough, with or without abundant mucoid sputum; Dyspnea, hemoptysis, chest pain, weight loss**
- Insidious onset of dry hacking cough, dyspnea, and cyanosis in a compromised host
- Progressive dyspnea and cyanosis in a compromised host
- Dyspnea, cough, malaise, chills, and fever (Hemoptysis)

Associated Roentgen Abnormality

Basic Pattern

Table continued on following page

TABLE 19–8

**PLEURAL EFFUSION AS THE SOLE ROENTGENOGRAPHIC
ABNORMALITY IN THE THORAX**

This title is self-explanatory. Effusion may be unilateral or bilateral. It must be emphasized that the lack of association with other abnormalities in the chest implies the absence of other *roentgenologically demonstrable* abnormality. Obviously, disease may be present but be roentgenographically invisible; for example, pulmonary involvement in rheumatoid disease may have no definite roentgenographic mani-

	ETIOLOGY	CHARACTER OF THE FLUID
	Bacteria *Mycobacterium tuberculosis*	Serous exudate. Predominantly lymphocytic reaction; erythrocytes may be present but seldom in great numbers. Blood glucose levels below 25 mg/100 ml highly suggestive (N.B.: differentiate from effusions of rheumatoid disease).
INFECTIOUS	**Viruses** All viruses and Mycoplasma	Serous exudate.
	Extrathoracic infection Pancreatitis	Usually serous exudate but may be serosanguinous. Pleural fluid amylase higher than serum amylase.
	Subphrenic abscess	Serous exudate.
	Systemic lupus erythematosus	Serous exudate.
IMMUNOLOGIC	Rheumatoid disease	Serous exudate; tends to be turbid and greenish-yellow. Predominance of lymphocytes. Glucose concentration characteristically low, with failure to rise on I.V. glucose infusion (failure of glucose-transport mechanism).

festations, although a considerable degree of pulmonary interstitial fibrosis may be apparent histologically. Conversely, diseases in which pulmonary abnormality is obscured by an effusion (*e.g.*, lobar collapse due to an obstructing endobronchial cancer) are *not* included in this table, since the presence of underlying pulmonary disease would be clearly demonstrable roentgenographically after thoracentesis.

CRITERIA FOR PRESUMPTIVE DIAGNOSIS	CRITERIA FOR POSITIVE DIAGNOSIS	COMMENTS
Combination of positive tuberculin reaction and predominantly lymphocytic pleural fluid.	Positive pleural biopsy. Culture of tubercle bacilli from pleural fluid.	A negative tuberculin test may be found in early cases. Strong tendency to subsequent development of active pulmonary tuberculosis if effusion not treated. Effusions rarely bilateral. A manifestation of primary tuberculosis more common in the adult (approximately 40 per cent) than in children (10 per cent). (*See* page 675.)
None.	Elevated agglutinin titer to offending organism.	May be bilateral. (*See* page 677.)
Clinical picture of acute abdomen.	Elevated level of pleural fluid amylase.	May occur in acute, chronic, or relapsing pancreatitis. Majority of effusions left-sided. (*See* page 683.)
Elevation and fixation of hemidiaphragm.	Gas and fluid in subphrenic space.	More commonly associated with basal pulmonary disease ("plate" atelectasis or pneumonitis). (*See* page 683.)
Clinical findings of typical rash, renal disease, heart murmur, and so forth.	Positive antinuclear antibodies or L.E.-cell test in association with characteristic clinical findings.	Occurs as isolated abnormality in slightly more than 10 per cent of cases. Effusion usually small, but may be moderate or even massive; bilateral in about 50 per cent. Usually clears without residua. Often associated with pericardial effusion. (*See* page 678.)
Clinical or roentgenologic changes of rheumatoid arthritis. High titer of rheumatoid factor in serum highly suggestive but not conclusive.	Biopsy of pleura showing typical rheumatoid granulation tissue.	Almost exclusively in men. Usually unilateral, on right slightly more often than on left. May antedate signs and symptoms of rheumatoid arthritis, but usually follows. Effusion often persists for several months. (*See* page 678.)

Table continued on following page

TABLE 19–8. *(Continued)*

	ETIOLOGY	CHARACTER OF THE FLUID
	Neoplasms arising within thorax Lymphoma	Usually serosanguinous exudate; may be chylous or chyliform.
NEOPLASTIC	**Neoplasms arising outside the thorax** Metastatic carcinoma	Serous exudate; varies in blood content from none to grossly hemorrhagic. Glucose content greater than 80 mg/100 ml is common but not diagnostic.
	Ovarian neoplasms (Meigs-Salmon syndrome)	Usually serous exudate; occasionally serosanguinous.
	Carcinoma of the pancreas	Serous exudate.
	Retroperitoneal lymphoma	Serous exudate.
THROMBOEMBOLIC	Pulmonary embolism	Almost invariably serosanguinous.
INHALATIONAL	Asbestosis	Sterile, serous, or blood-tinged exudate.
TRAUMATIC	Closed-chest trauma	Blood (hemothorax).
		Chyle (chylothorax).

TABLE 19–8. *(Continued)*

CRITERIA FOR PRESUMPTIVE DIAGNOSIS	CRITERIA FOR POSITIVE DIAGNOSIS	COMMENTS
Peripheral lymph-node enlargement, hepatosplenomegaly, and so forth.	Finding of typical cells in pleural fluid or biopsy of remote lymph node. White cell count in leukemia.	This broad heading includes leukemia as well as Hodgkin's disease and non-Hodgkin's lymphoma. Approximately 30 per cent of cases have pleural effusion, but seldom without associated pulmonary or mediastinal node involvement. (*See* page 680.)
Identification of remote primary neoplasm.	Finding of characteristic tissue on needle biopsy or malignant cells in pleural fluid.	Most commonly from breast; also from pancreas, stomach, ovary, kidney. (*See* page 680.)
Pleural fluid negative for malignant cells; pelvic mass.	Presence of ovarian neoplasm with ascites; disappearance of effusion following oophorectomy.	Ovarian neoplasm may be fibroma, thecoma, cystadenoma, adenocarcinoma, granulosa-cell tumor; occasionally fibromyoma of uterus. (*See* page 683.)
Pleural fluid negative for malignant cells; clinical signs of intra-abdominal neoplasia.	Disappearance of fluid following removal of primary.	Effusion may occur without direct involvement of thorax by primary; probably related to transport of fluid into thorax via diaphragmatic lymphatics.
Pleural fluid negative for malignant cells; clinical signs of intra-abdominal neoplasia.	Disappearance of fluid following treatment of primary.	
History of sudden onset of pleural pain with or without peripheral thrombophlebitis. Rarely may observe relative diminution of peripheral vasculature roentgenologically.	Lung scan or pulmonary angiogram or both.	Frequency of effusion as sole manifestation of pulmonary embolism not precisely known, but probably very uncommon. (*See* page 681.)
History of asbestos exposure.	Only following exclusion of other diagnostic possibilities, particularly tuberculosis and mesothelioma.	Diagnosis should be made with caution. Effusions frequently recurrent, usually bilateral, and often associated with chest pain. (*See* page 679.)
History.	Thoracentesis and history.	May originate from chest wall, diaphragm, mediastinum, or lung. (*See* page 682.)
History. Time lag between trauma and development of effusion.	Thoracentesis; lymphangiography.	Side of chylothorax depends on site of thoracic duct rupture. (*See* page 684.)

Table continued on following page

TABLE 19-8. *(Continued)*

	ETIOLOGY	CHARACTER OF THE FLUID
TRAUMATIC *(Cont.)*		Contains ingested food (esophageal rupture).
	Following abdominal surgery	Serous exudate.
	Nephrotic syndrome and other causes of diminished plasma osmotic pressure	Transudate.
	Acute glomerulo-nephritis	Transudate (?).
	Myxedema	Serous exudate.
	Cirrhosis with ascites	Transudate.
	Hydronephrosis	Serous exudate.
INCIDENTAL CAUSES	Uremic pleuritis	Serous exudate. Sometimes fibrinous.
	Dialysis	Serous exudate, sometimes sanguineous as a result of anticoagulation.
	Lymphedema	High protein content.
	Familial recurring polyserositis	Serofibrinous exudate.

TABLE 19–8. *(Continued)*

CRITERIA FOR PRESUMPTIVE DIAGNOSIS	CRITERIA FOR POSITIVE DIAGNOSIS	COMMENTS
History.	Thoracentesis; esophagogram.	Almost always left-sided. Generally due to surgical or endoscopic procedure. (*See* page 623.)
History of recent abdominal surgery.	Unnecessary. Almost always self-limited.	Usually requires lateral decubitus roentgenograms for identification. Present in 49 per cent of patients in one series. (*See* page 683.)
General edema.	Thoracentesis; biochemical assay of serum and urine.	Effusion commonly infrapulmonary. (*See* page 683.)
Usual findings of acute glomerulonephritis.	——	(*See* page 684.)
Studies of thyroid activity.	——	Effusion occurs more often in pericardium. (*See* page 684.)
Demonstration of cirrhosis and ascites (N.B.: exclude carcinoma of liver).	——	Ascitic fluid enters pleural space via diaphragmatic lymphatics (as in Meigs-Salmon syndrome). (*See* page 684.)
Demonstration of hydronephrosis.	Disappearance of effusion following removal of urinary obstruction.	Mechanism not clear; possibly related to transport of fluid via diaphragmatic lymphatics.
Clinical findings of uremia.	——	May not be possible to distinguish from effusion associated with dialysis. (*See* page 684.)
History of peritoneal or hemodialysis.	——	May not be possible to distinguish from effusion associated with uremia itself.
Associated clinical findings of lymphedema elsewhere.	——	Results from hypoplasia of the lymphatic system. May be associated with Milroy's disease.
Combination of symptoms and signs in specific racial groups.	——	Heredofamilial; limited to Armenians, Arabs, and Jews. Episodic acute attacks of abdominal and chest pain. Most episodes of pleurisy associated with arthritis and arthralgia.

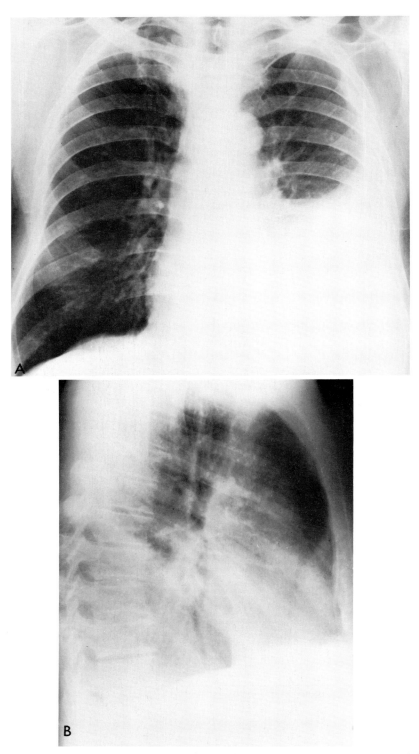

Figure 19–8. Pleural Effusion in Rheumatoid Pleuropulmonary Disease. Posteroanterior (*A*) and lateral (*B*) roentgenograms reveal the typical appearance of a moderate accumulation of fluid in the left pleural space. Following thoracentesis, the lungs were regarded as normal roentgenologically, although subsequent examination of the lungs at necropsy established the presence of extensive changes compatible with rheumatoid disease.

DECISION TREE 19-8

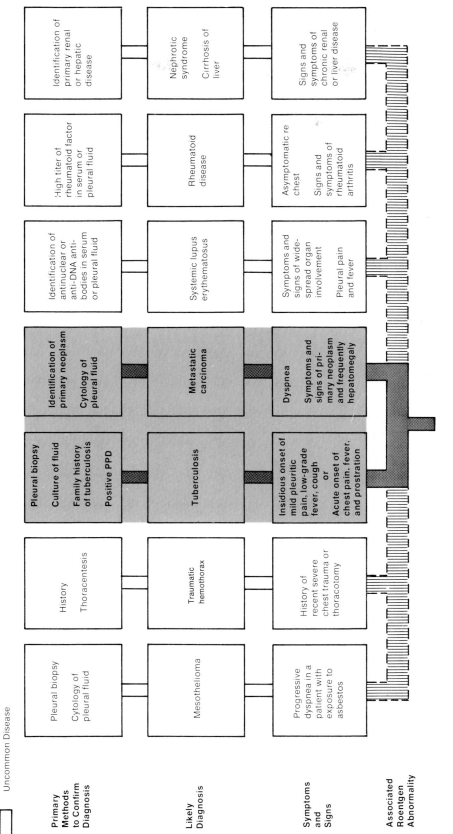

Pleural Effusion Unassociated With Other Roentgenographic Evidence of Disease in the Thorax

Common Disease

Uncommon Disease

Primary Methods to Confirm Diagnosis

Likely Diagnosis

Symptoms and Signs

Associated Roentgen Abnormality

Basic Pattern

TABLE 19–9

HILAR AND MEDIASTINAL LYMPH-NODE ENLARGEMENT

This table includes all conditions producing lymph-node enlargement within the thorax, either alone or in combination with other roentgenographic abnormalities. It is to be noted that a number of diseases are included in which node enlargement is a common manifestation in

	ETIOLOGY	SYMMETRY	NODE GROUPS INVOLVED
	Bacteria		
	Mycobacterium tuberculosis (primary)	Unilateral in 80 per cent of cases.	Approximately 60 per cent hilar and 40 per cent combined hilar and paratracheal.
	Francisella tularensis	Unilateral.	Hilar.
	Bordetella pertussis	Unilateral.	Hilar.
	Bacillus anthracis	Symmetric.	All.
	Yersinia pestis (the plague)	Symmetric.	Hilar and paratracheal.
	Mycoplasma and Viruses		
	Mycoplasma pneumoniae	Unilateral or bilateral.	Hilar.
INFECTIOUS	Rubeola	Bilateral.	Hilar.
	ECHO virus pneumonia	Bilateral.	Hilar.
	Varicella pneumonia	Bilateral.	Hilar.
	Psittacosis (ornithosis)	Unilateral or bilateral.	Hilar.
	Epstein-Barr mononucleosis	Bilateral symmetric.	Predominantly hilar.
	Fungi		
	Histoplasma capsulatum	May be unilateral or bilateral.	Hilar, mediastinal, or intrapulmonary.

TABLE 19–9 — HILAR AND MEDIASTINAL LYMPH-NODE ENLARGEMENT / **825**

infants and children but uncommon in adults; sinze we have excluded much reference to pediatric diseases of the chest in the text, their inclusion here is a compromise to space limitation.

ADDITIONAL FINDINGS	COMMENTS
Almost always associated with ipsilateral parenchymal disease.	Rarely the presentation may be bilateral, symmetric hilar-node enlargement as sole manifestation. (*See* page 290.)
Oval areas of parenchymal consolidation; pleural effusion common.	Ipsilateral hilar-node enlargement in 25 to 50 per cent of pneumonic tularemia. (*See* page 283.)
Ipsilateral segmental pneumonia.	Pneumonia is the result of secondary infection in some cases. (*See* page 283.)
Occasionally patchy nonsegmental opacities throughout lungs due to pulmonary hemorrhage; pleural effusion is common.	Node enlargement due to hemorrhage and edema; extension of inflammatory reaction into adjacent mediastinal tissues may obscure typical nodal configuration. (*See* page 272.)
———	Rarely, roentgenographic changes may be restricted to node enlargement, without associated pulmonary manifestations. (*See* page 284.)
Always with segmental inhomogeneous or homogeneous pneumonia.	Lymph-node enlargement is rare in adults but common in children. (*See* page 325.)
Diffuse interstitial pattern throughout the lungs.	This pattern results from infection with rubeola virus itself and not from secondary infection. (*See* page 331.)
Accompanied by increase in bronchovascular markings.	Lymph-node enlargement rare in adults and pneumonia extremely rare in infants. (*See* page 333.)
Diffuse air-space pneumonia may mask hilar node enlargement.	(*See* page 334.)
Parenchymal involvement may be homogeneous consolidation or a diffuse reticular pattern.	Hilar node enlargement has not been reported as sole manifestation of the disease. (*See* page 337.)
Splenomegaly.	Rarely associated with roentgenographic changes in the lungs. (*See* page 337.)
Enlarged nodes may obstruct airways through extrinsic pressure, resulting in pneumonitis.	Node enlargement is usually associated with parenchymal disease but may occur without, particularly in children. (*See* page 302.)

Table continued on following page

TABLE 19–9. *(Continued)*

	ETIOLOGY	SYMMETRY	NODE GROUPS INVOLVED
INFECTIOUS *(Cont.)*	*Coccidioides immitis*	Unilateral or bilateral.	Hilar or paratracheal or both.
	Sporotrichum schenkii	Unilateral.	Hilar.
	Parasites Tropical eosinophilia	Bilateral.	Hilar.
IMMUNOLOGIC	Extrinsic allergic alveolitis	Symmetric.	Bronchopulmonary.
NEOPLASTIC	Bronchogenic carcinoma	Unilateral almost invariably.	Hilar nodes almost invariably; paratracheal and posterior mediastinal nodes in some cases.
	Hodgkin's disease	Typically bilateral but asymmetric; unilateral node enlargement is very unusual.	Paratracheal and bifurcation group involved as often or more often than bronchopulmonary group. Involvement of anterior mediastinal and retrosternal nodes frequent.
	Non-Hodgkin's lymphoma	Bilateral but asymmetric.	Similar to Hodgkin's disease.
	Leukemia	Usually symmetric.	Mediastinal and bronchopulmonary.
	Metastatic lymphangitic carcinoma	Unilateral or bilateral.	Hilar or mediastinal or both.
	Bronchiolar carcinoma	Unilateral or bilateral.	Hilar or mediastinal or both.
	Broncho-pulmonary amyloidosis	Symmetric.	Hilar and mediastinal.
	Heavy-chain disease	Symmetric.	Mediastinal.

TABLE 19–9 — HILAR AND MEDIASTINAL LYMPH-NODE ENLARGEMENT / **827**

TABLE 19-9. *(Continued)*

ADDITIONAL FINDINGS	COMMENTS
Node enlargement may occur with or without associated parenchymal disease.	Involvement of paratracheal lymph nodes should raise suspicion of imminent dissemination. (*See* page 307.)
Associated with parenchymal disease in some cases.	A rare form of mycotic infection. (*See* page 321.)
A widespread micronodular pattern throughout the lungs.	Diffuse parenchymal disease is usually not accompanied by node enlargement. (*See* page 344.)
Diffuse reticulonodular (sometimes acinar) pattern invariably associated.	Hilar node enlargement fairly common in mushroom-worker's lung but rare in other varieties. (*See* page 389.)
Involvement of the bifurcation or posterior mediastinal groups of nodes may displace the barium-filled esophagus.	Enlargement of mediastinal lymph nodes other than bronchopulmonary may be the sole abnormality roentgenographically and almost always indicates spread from an undifferentiated carcinoma. (*See* page 410.)
Pulmonary involvement occurs in less than 30 per cent of patients and is almost invariably associated with mediastinal node enlargement. Pleural effusion in approximately 30 per cent of cases, usually in association with other intrathoracic manifestations. The sternum may be destroyed by direct extension from retrosternal nodes.	Intrathoracic involvement occurs in 90 per cent of patients at some stage of the disease, most commonly in the form of mediastinal lymph-node enlargement; the latter is seen on the initial chest roentgenogram of approximately 50 per cent of patients. (*See* page 430.)
Sometimes associated with pleuropulmonary involvement.	The most common intrathoracic manifestation of the disease; however, histiocytic lymphoma tends to be manifested by parenchymal consolidation without associated node enlargement. (*See* page 436.)
Both pleural effusion and parenchymal involvement may be associated.	The most common roentgenographic manifestation of leukemia within the thorax (25 per cent of patients). A much more common manifestation of lymphocytic than of myelocytic leukemia. (*See* page 440.)
Usually associated with a diffuse reticular or reticulonodular pattern throughout the lungs, predominantly basal in distribution.	Septal (Kerley B) lines are frequently present. (*See* page 445.)
Node enlargement may occur in association with either local or diffuse pulmonary disease.	A rare finding in this neoplasm. (*See* page 423.)
Enlarged nodes may be densely calcified. Sometimes associated with diffuse pulmonary involvement.	One of the plasma cell dyscrasias. (*See* page 443.)
Lung involvement rare. Hepatosplenomegaly.	One of the plasma cell dyscrasias. (*See* page 442.)

Table continued on following page

TABLE 19–9. *(Continued)*

	ETIOLOGY	SYMMETRY	NODE GROUPS INVOLVED
NEOPLASTIC *(Cont.)*	Immunoblastic lymphadenopathy	Bilateral but asymmetric.	Similar to Hodgkin's disease.
INHALATIONAL	Silicosis	Symmetric.	Predominantly bronchopulmonary.
	Chronic berylliosis	Symmetric.	Bronchopulmonary.
IDIOPATHIC	Sarcoidosis	Almost invariably symmetric, unilateral node enlargement occurring in 1 to 3 per cent of cases only. The outer borders of the enlarged hila are usually lobulated.	Paratracheal, tracheobronchial, and bronchopulmonary groups. Paratracheal enlargement seldom if ever occurs without concomitant enlargement of hilar nodes.
	Histiocytosis-X (eosinophilic granuloma)	Symmetric.	Hilar and mediastinal.
	Idiopathic pulmonary hemosiderosis	Symmetric.	Hilar.
AIRWAYS	Cystic fibrosis	Unilateral or bilateral.	Hilar.

TABLE 19–9—HILAR AND MEDIASTINAL LYMPH-NODE ENLARGEMENT / **829**

TABLE 19–9. *(Continued)*

ADDITIONAL FINDINGS	COMMENTS
The lungs are occasionally affected in a pattern similar to Hodgkin's disease.	A hyperimmune disorder, most probably of B lymphocytes. Lymph-node enlargement predominates and is identical to that of Hodgkin's disease. (*See* page 439.)
Diffuse nodular or reticulonodular disease throughout both lungs. Pleural thickening in late stages. "Eggshell calcification" of lymph nodes occurs in approximately 5 per cent of cases and may also be observed in lymph nodes in the anterior and posterior mediastinum, the thoracic wall, and occasionally the retroperitoneal and intraperitoneal nodes.	Enlargement of bronchopulmonary nodes may occur without roentgenographic evidence of pulmonary disease, although this is a rare presenting picture. (*See* page 480.)
Diffuse micronodular pattern invariably associated.	Hilar node enlargement occurs in a minority of cases. (*See* page 596.)
75 to 90 per cent of patients with sarcoidosis show mediastinal and hilar lymph-node enlargement and approximately 50 per cent of these will show diffuse parenchymal disease as well.	75 per cent of patients with hilar lymph-node enlargement show complete resolution of the enlarged nodes. Symmetric appearance, lack of involvement of retrosternal nodes, and diminution of lymph-node size with onset of diffuse lung disease aid in differentiating sarcoidosis from lymphoma and tuberculosis. (*See* page 643.)
Early diffuse micronodular pattern which may become coarse in later stages.	Intrathoracic lymph-node enlargement is rarely a manifestation of this disease. (*See* page 664.)
Diffuse alveolar and interstitial disease.	Predominantly in acute stage. (*See* page 361.)
Diffuse increase in markings with hyperinflation and areas of atelectasis and bronchiectasis.	Hilar node enlargement is an uncommon finding in this disease. (*See* page 562.)

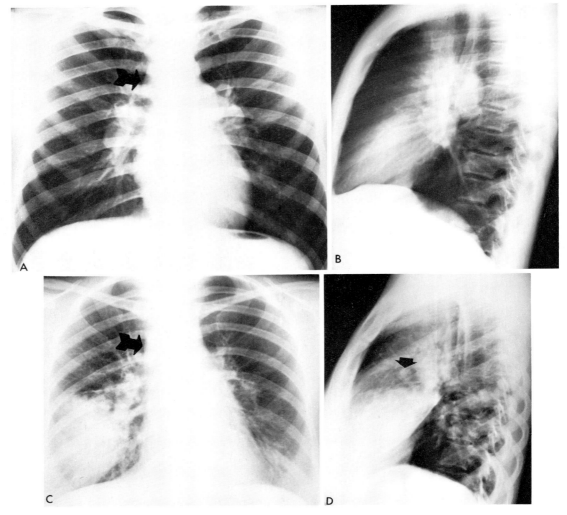

Figure 19–9. Hilar and Mediastinal Lymph Node Enlargement, with and without Roentgenographic Disease. The posteroanterior and lateral roentgenograms illustrated in *A* and *B* reveal marked enlargement of both hila by nodular opacities typical of enlarged lymph nodes. Bilateral paratracheal and tracheobronchial lymph node enlargement is also present (the azygos lymph node is indicated by an *arrow*). Proved sarcoidosis. *C* and *D* are similar roentgenograms from a patient with Hodgkin's disease in which there is evidence of b lateral paratracheal lymph node enlargement; note particularly the enlarged azygos node in the right tracheobronchial angle *(arrow in C)*. In addition, there is almost complete consolidation of the right middle lobe and a small, well-defined nodule in the right upper lobe *(arrow in D)*.

DECISION TREE 19–9A

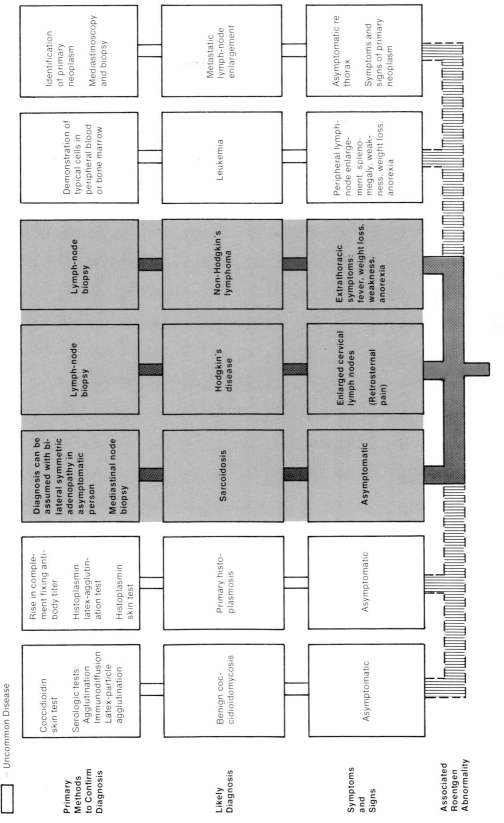

Hilar and Mediastinal Lymph-Node Enlargement, Unassociated With Other Roentgenographic Evidence of Disease

DECISION TREE 19-9B

Legend:
- ▓ = Common Disease
- ☐ = Uncommon Disease

Primary Methods to Confirm Diagnosis

- Rise in complement fixing antibody titer; Histoplasmin latex-agglutination test; Histoplasmin skin test
- PPD skin test; Sputum smear and culture
- Identification of primary malignancy; Lung biopsy
- Bronchoscopy and biopsy
- Lymph-node biopsy
- Diagnosis virtually certain with bilateral hilar node enlargement in asymptomatic person; Mediastinoscopy and node biopsy; Bronchoscopic lung biopsy
- History of exposure to specific dust; Direct lung biopsy
- Coccidioidin skin test; Serologic tests: Agglutination, Immunodiffusion, Latex-particle agglutination

Likely Diagnosis

- Primary histoplasmosis
- Primary tuberculosis
- Lymphangitic carcinomatosis
- Primary bronchogenic carcinoma
- Hodgkin's disease
- Sarcoidosis
- Silicosis
- Benign coccidioidomycosis

Symptoms and Signs

- Asymptomatic or mild respiratory symptoms—fever, cough with mucopurulent sputum (Erythema nodosum)
- Asymptomatic (fever, cough, anorexia. weight loss, chest pain) (Erythema nodosum)
- Severe and progressive dyspnea
- Fever, chest pain, cough (Hemoptysis)
- Enlarged peripheral (cervical) lymph nodes; Cough and dyspnea (Pleural or retrosternal pain)
- Asymptomatic (Erythema nodosum)
- Asymptomatic (Progressive dyspnea)
- Asymptomatic (Flulike symptoms—fever, cough, myalgia)

Associated Roentgen Abnormality

Basic Pattern

Hilar and Mediastinal Lymph-Node Enlargement Associated With Other Roentgenographic Evidence of Disease

GLOSSARY OF WORDS AND TERMS IN CHEST ROENTGENOLOGY

"Then you should say what you mean," the March Hare went on.

"I do," Alice hastily replied; "at least—at least, I mean what I say—that's the same thing, you know."

"Not the same thing a bit!" said the Hatter. "Why, you might just as well say that 'I see what I eat' is the same thing as 'I eat what I see!'"

This well-known excerpt from Lewis Carroll's *Alice's Adventures in Wonderland* points out a problem that confronts many physicians in today's constantly expanding scientific literature—the use of words and terms that mean different things to different people. The frequency with which imprecise or frankly erroneous words are employed to describe roentgenographic images (for example) is astonishing; common usage has created a jargon that has led to confusion if not to actual communication breakdown. In 1975, a joint committee of the American College of Chest Physicians and the American Thoracic Society published a glossary of pulmonary terms and symbols* pertinent to the medical and physiologic aspects of chest disease, but it omitted words that specifically related to chest roentgenology. The Fleischner Society formed a Committee on Nomenclature several years ago under the chairmanship of Dr. Wm. Tuddenham to draw up a glossary of roentgenologic words and terms that it was hoped would topple the "tower of Babel." This task is nearing completion and with the permission of the Fleischner Society we list herewith a number of words and terms selected from its glossary (as prepared by the Committee) that we hope our readers will refer to and use. The precise definition of some words has been altered slightly to coincide with usage in this book.

---

*Pulmonary Terms and Symbols; A report of the ACCP-ATS Joint Committee on Pulmonary Nomenclature. Chest, 67:583, 1975.

WORD OR TERM	COMMENTS
abscess *n.* 1. (pathol.) An inflammatory mass within lung parenchyma, the central portion of which has undergone purulent liquefaction necrosis. There may or may not be communication with the bronchial tree. 2. (radiol.) A mass within lung parenchyma that can present in one of two ways: (a) it has communicated with the bronchial tree and thus represents a cavity (*q.v.*); or (b) it has not communicated with the bronchial tree and thus can be considered to represent an abscess in the morphologic sense only by inference. *Qualifiers* may be employed to indicate clinical course (*e.g.*, acute, chronic); etiology (*e.g.*, bacterial, fungal); or anatomic site (*e.g.*, lung, mediastinum).	Should be used only with reference to masses of presumed infectious etiology. The word is not synonymous with cavity (*q.v.*).
acinar pattern *n.* (radiol.) A collection of round or elliptical, ill-defined, discrete or partly confluent opacities in the lung, each	An inferred conclusion usually used as a descriptor. An acceptable term, pre-

WORD OR TERM	COMMENTS

measuring 4 to 8 mm in diameter and together producing an extended, inhomogeneous shadow.

Synonyms: Rosette pattern; acino-nodose pattern (used specifically with reference to endobronchial spread of tuberculosis); alveolar pattern.

ferred to cited synonyms (especially "alveolar pattern," which is an inaccurate descriptor).

acinar shadow *n.* (radiol.) A round or slightly elliptical pulmonary opacity 4 to 8 mm in diameter presumed to represent an anatomic acinus rendered opaque by consolidation. Usually employed in the presence of many such opacities (*see* acinar pattern).

An inferred conclusion sometimes applicable as a roentgenologic descriptor.

acinus *n.* (anat.) The portion of lung parenchyma distal to the terminal bronchiole and consisting of respiratory bronchioles, alveolar ducts, alveolar sacs, and alveoli (*see* acinar shadow, acinar pattern).

A specific feature of pulmonary anatomy.

aeration *n.* (physiol./radiol.) 1. The state of containing air. 2. The state or process of being filled or inflated with air. *Qualifiers:* overaeration (preferred) or hyperaeration; underaeration (preferred) or hypoaeration.

Synonym: Inflation.

An acceptable term with reference to the inspiratory phase of respiration. Inflation is preferred in sense 2.

air bronchiologram *n.* (radiol.) The equivalent of air bronchogram but in airways assumed to be bronchioles because of their peripheral location and diameter.

An acceptable term. Note that because alveoli cannot be seen roentgenographically, the term "air alveologram" is inaccurate and its use is to be condemned.

air bronchogram *n.* (radiol.) The roentgenographic shadow of an air-containing bronchus peripheral to the hilum and surrounded by airless lung (whether by virtue of absorption of air, replacement of air, or both), a finding generally regarded as evidence of the patency of the more proximal airway. Hence, any bandlike tapering and/or branching lucency within opacified lung corresponding in size and distribution to a bronchus or bronchi and presumed to represent an air-containing segment of the bronchial tree.

A specific feature of roentgenologic anatomy whose identity is often inferred. A useful and recommended term.

air-fluid level *n.* (radiol.) A local collection of gas and liquid that, when traversed by a horizontal x-ray beam, creates a shadow characterized by a sharp horizontal interface between gas density above and liquid density below.

A useful roentgenologic descriptor. Since with rare exception (*e.g.*, fat-fluid level) the upper of the two absorbant media is "air" (gas), it is sufficient to describe such an appearance as a "fluid level."

air space *n.* (*adj.* air-space) (anat./radiol.) The gas-containing portion of lung parenchyma, including the acini and excluding the interstitium and purely conductive portions of the lung.

Synonyms: Acinar consolidation, alveolar consolidation (when used as an adjective in relation to air-space consolidation).

An inferred conclusion usually used as a roentgenologic descriptor. An acceptable term whose use as an adjective is also appropriate.

air-trapping *n.* (pathophysiol./radiol.) The retention of excess gas in all or part of the lung at any stage of expiration.

A specific roentgenologic sign to be employed only if excess air retention is demonstrated by a dynamic study, *e.g.*, inspiration-expiration roentgenography or fluoroscopy. *Not* to be used with reference to overinflation of the lung at full inspiration (total lung capacity).

airway *n., adj.* (anat./radiol.) A collective term for the air-conducting passages from the larynx to and including the respiratory bronchioles.

Synonyms: Conducting airway; trancheobronchial tree.

A useful anatomic term. May be used as an adjective in relation to disease or abnormality. Note that the respiratory bronchioles are both conducting and gas-exchanging airways and thus constitute the transitory zone.

Word or Term	**Comments**

alveolarization *n.* (radiol.) The opacification of groups of alveoli by a contrast medium.

A misnomer whose use is to be deplored. Excessive filling of peripheral lung structure by contrast media usually employed for bronchography may opacify respiratory bronchioles but not alveoli. Thus, the correct term is "bronchiolar filling or opacification."

anterior junction line *n.* (radiol.) A vertically oriented linear or curvilinear opacity approximately 1 to 2 mm wide, commonly projected on the tracheal air shadow. It is produced by the shadows of the right and left pleurae in intimate contact between the aerated lungs anterior to the great vessels (and sometimes the heart); hence, it never extends above the suprasternal notch (*cf.* posterior junction line).

Synonyms: Anterior mediastinal septum, line, or stripe.

A specific feature of roentgenologic anatomy; to be preferred to cited synonyms.

aortopulmonary window *n.* 1. (anat.) A mediastinal space bounded anteriorly by the posterior surface of the ascending aorta; posteriorly by the anterior surface of the descending aorta; superiorly by the inferior surface of the aortic arch; inferiorly by the superior surface of the left pulmonary artery; medially by the left side of the trachea, left main bronchus, and esophagus; and laterally by the left lung. Within it are situated fat, the ductus ligament, the left recurrent laryngeal nerve, and lymph nodes. 2. (radiol.) A zone of relative lucency in the mediastinal shadow that is seen to best advantage in the left anterior oblique or lateral projection and that corresponds to the anatomic space defined above. On a posteroanterior roentgenogram of the chest, the lateral margin of the space constitutes the aortopulmonary window interface.

Synonym: Aortic-pulmonic window.

A specific feature of roentgenologic anatomy.

atelectasis *n.* (pathophysiol./radiol.) Less than normal inflation of all or a portion of the lung with corresponding diminution in volume. *Qualifiers* may be employed to indicate severity (mild, moderate, severe), mechanism (resorption, relaxation, cicatrization, adhesive), or distribution (*e.g.*, lobar, platelike (*q.v.*), discoid).

Synonyms: Collapse, loss of volume, anectasis.

Generally this term is preferable to "collapse" in describing loss of volume. The word "collapse" connotes total atelectasis in which lung tissue has been reduced to its smallest volume. Anectasis is usually used in reference to failure of lung expansion in the newborn.

azygoesophageal recess *n.* 1. (anat.) A space or recess in the right side of the mediastinum into which the medial edge of the right lower lobe (crista pulmonis) extends. It is limited superiorly by the arch of the azygos vein, inferiorly by the diaphragm, posteriorly by the azygos vein in front of the vertebral column, and medially by the esophagus and its adjacent structures. (The exact relationship between the medial edge of the lung and the mediastinal structures is variable.) 2. (radiol.) In a frontal chest roentgenogram, a vertically oriented interface between air in the right lower lobe and the adjacent mediastinum that represents the medial limit of the anatomic azygoesophageal recess.

Synonyms: Infra-azygos recess; right pleuroesophageal line or stripe; right paraesophageal line or stripe.

A specific feature of roentgenologic anatomy. The use of the term "recess" to identify an interface is inappropriate; thus, anygoesophageal recess interface is preferred.

bat's-wing distribution *n.* (radiol.) A spatial arrangement of roentgenographic opacities in a frontal roentgenogram that bears a vague resemblance to the shape of a bat in flight; said of coalescent, ill-defined opacities that are approximately bilaterally symmetrical and that are confined to the medulla of the lungs (*q.v.*).

Synonym: Butterfly distribution.

A roentgenologic descriptor of limited usefulness.

WORD OR TERM	COMMENTS
bleb *n.* 1. (pathol.) A gas-containing space within or contiguous to the visceral pleura of the lung. 2. (radiol.) A local, thin-walled lucency contiguous with the pleura, usually at the lung apex. *Synonyms:* Type I bulla (pathol.); bulla; a form of pulmonary air cyst (radiol.)	An inferred conclusion seldom justifiable by roentgenogram alone. Bulla or air cyst is preferred.
bronchiole *n.* (anat./radiol.) An airway that contains no cartilage in its wall. A bronchiole may be purely conducting (up to and including the terminal bronchiole) or transitory (the respiratory bronchioles that carry out both conduction and gas exchange).	A specific feature of pulmonary anatomy.
bronchocele *n.* *See* mucoid impaction.	
bronchus *n.* (anat./radiol.) A conducting airway distal to the tracheal bifurcation that contains cartilage in its wall	A specific feature of pulmonary anatomy.
bulla *n.*, *pl.* -lae. 1. (pathol.) A sharply demarcated region of emphysema; a gas-containing space that may contain nothing but gas or may contain overdistended and ruptured alveolar septa and blood vessels. 2. (radiol.) Sharply demarcated hyperlucent area of avascularity within the lung, measuring 1 cm or more in diameter and possessing a wall less than 1 mm in thickness. *Qualifiers:* small, medium, large.	The preferred term to describe all thin-walled air-containing spaces in the lung with the exception of pneumatocele (*q.v.*).
butterfly distribution *n.* (radiol.) *See* bat's-wing distribution.	To be distinguished from the use of this term in general medicine to describe the distribution of certain cutaneous lesions.
calcification *n.* 1. (pathophysiol.) (a) The process by which one or more deposits of calcium salts are formed within lung tissue or within a pulmonary lesion. (b) Such a deposit of calcium salts. 2. (radiol.) A calcific opacity within the lung that may be organized (*e.g.*, concentric lamination), but which does not display the trabecular organization of true bone. *Qualifiers:* "eggshell," "popcorn," target, laminated, flocculent, nodular, etc.	An explicit conclusion; may be used as a descriptor. To be distinguished from ossification (*q.v.*).
carina *n.* (anat./radiol.) The keel-shaped ridge that separates the right and left main bronchi at the tracheal bifurcation.	A specific feature of pulmonary anatomy.
carinal angle *n.* (anat./radiol.) The angle formed by the right and left main bronchi at the tracheal bifurcation. *Synonyms:* Bifurcation angle; angle of tracheal bifurcation.	A definitive anatomic and roentgenologic measurement.
cavity *n.* 1. (pathol.) A mass within lung parenchyma, the central portion of which has undergone liquefaction necrosis and has been expelled via the bronchial tree, leaving a gas-containing space, with or without associated fluid. 2. (radiol.) A gas-containing space within the lung surrounded by a wall whose thickness is greater than 1 mm and usually irregular in contour.	A useful descriptor without etiologic connotation. The word must not be used interchangeably with abscess (*q.v.*), which may exist without bronchial communication and therefore without cavitation.
circumscribed *adj.* (radiol.) Possessing a complete or nearly complete visible border.	An acceptable descriptor.
clot *n.* (pathol.) A semisolidified mass of blood elements.	*Cf.* thrombus.
coalescence *n.* (radiol.) The joining together of a number of opacities into a single opacity; confluence (*q.v.*).	An acceptable descriptor.
coin lesion *n.* (radiol.) A sharply defined, circular opacity within the lung suggestive of the appearance of a coin and usually representing a spherical or nodular lesion. *Synonyms:* Pulmonary nodule, pulmonary mass.	A roentgenologic descriptor, the use of which is to be condemned. The term "coin" may be descriptive of the shadow, but certainly not of the lesion producing it.

WORD OR TERM	COMMENTS
collapse *n.* (radiol.) A state in which lung tissue has undergone complete atelectasis.	The term is acceptable when employed strictly as defined, but "atelectasis" is preferred, since the degree of loss of lung volume can be qualified by mild, moderate, or severe.
collateral ventilation *n.* (physiol./radiol.) The process by which gas passes from one lung unit (acinus, lobule, segment, or lobe) to a contiguous unit via alveolar pores (pores of Kohn), canals of Lambert, or direct airway anastomoses. *Synonym:* Collateral air drift.	An inferred conclusion usually based on fairly reliable signs. A useful term. The channels of peripheral airway communication also function as a mechanism for transmission of liquid from one unit to another (*e.g.,* in acute airspace pneumonia).
confluence *n.* (radiol.) The nature of opacities that are contiguous with or adjacent to one another. *Antonym:* Discrete (*q.v.*)	A useful descriptor; confluence is to be distinguished from coalescence (*q.v.*), which is the act of becoming confluent.
consolidation *n.* 1. (pathophysiol.) The process by which air in the lung is replaced by the products of disease, rendering the lung solid (as in pneumonia). 2. (radiol.) An essentially homogeneous opacity in the lung characterized by little or no loss of volume, by effacement of pulmonary blood vessels, and sometimes by the presence of an air bronchogram (*q.v.*).	An inferred conclusion, applicable only in an appropriate clinical setting when the opacity can with reasonable certainty be attributed to replacement of alveolar air by exudate, transudate, or tissue. Not to be used with reference to all homogeneous opacities.
corona radiata *n.* (radiol.) A circumferential pattern of fine linear spicules, approximately 5 mm long, extending outward from the margin of a solitary pulmonary nodule through a zone of relative lucency.	A sign of limited usefulness in the differentiation of benign and malignant nodules.
cor pulmonale *n.* 1. (pathol./clin.) Right ventricular hypertrophy and/or dilatation occurring as a result of an abnormality of lung structure or function. 2. (radiol.) The combination of pulmonary arterial hypertension and chronic lung disease, with or without evidence of enlargement of right heart chambers. *Qualifiers:* acute, chronic.	An inferred roentgenologic conclusion based on usually reliable signs. An acceptable descriptor. Despite the pathologic definition, roentgenologic evidence of cardiomegaly need not be present.
cortex *n.* (radiol.) The peripheral 2 to 3 cm of lung parenchyma adjacent to the visceral pleura, either over the convexity of the thorax or in the interlobar fissures. (*See* medulla and hilum.)	The peripheral part of an arbitrary subdivision of the lung into three zones from the hilum to the visceral pleura. Of limited usefulness.
CT number *n.* (radiol./physics) In computed tomography, a quantitative numerical statement of the relative attenuation of the x-ray beam at a specified point; loosely, the relative attenuation of a specified tissue absorber, usually expressed in Hounsfield units (HU).	
cyst *n.* 1. (pathol.) A circumscribed space whose contents may be liquid or gaseous and whose wall is generally thin and well defined and composed of a variety of cellular elements. 2. (radiol.) A gas-containing space of any size possessing a thin wall. *Qualifiers:* foregut (bronchogenic, esophageal duplication); postinfectious.	This term is entirely nonspecific and should not possess inferred conclusion as to etiology. It is the preferred term to describe any thin-walled gas-containing space in the lung possessing a wall thickness greater than 1 mm.
defined *adj.* (radiol.) The character of the border of a shadow. *Qualifiers:* well, sharply, poorly, distinctly.	An acceptable descriptor.
demarcated *adj.* (radiol.) Distinct from adjacent structures. *Qualifiers:* well, sharply, poorly.	An acceptable descriptor. (*Cf.* defined.)
dense *adj.* (radiol.) Possessing density (*q.v.*). Usually used in describing or comparing roentgenographic shadows with respect to their light transmission.	A recommended term in the context defined. Should not be used in referring to the opacity of an absorber of x-radiation. (*See* opaque, opacity.)

WORD OR TERM	COMMENTS

density *n.*   1. (physics) The mass of a substance per unit volume. 2. (photometry/radiol.) The opacity of a roentgenographic shadow to visible light; film blackening. 3. (radiol.) The shadow of an absorber more opaque to x-rays than its surround; an opacity or radiopacity. 4. The degree of opacity of an absorber to x-rays, usually expressed in term of the nature of the absorber (*e.g.*, bone, water, or fat density).

In sense 2, the term refers to a fundamental characteristic of the roentgenogram, and its use is recommended. In senses 3 and 4, it refers to the character of the absorber and has an exactly opposite connotation with respect to film blackening. Because of this potential confusion, the term should *never* be used to mean an "opacity" or "radiopacity."

diffuse *adj.*   1. (pathophysiol.) Widely distributed through an organ or type of tissue. 2. (radiol.) Widespread and continuous (said of shadows and by inference of the states or processes producing them).

Synonyms: Disseminated, generalized, systemic, widespread.

A useful and acceptable term. In the context of chest radiology, "diffuse" connotes widespread, anatomically continuous but not necessarily complete involvement of the lung or other thoracic structure or tissue; "disseminated" connotes widespread but anatomically discontinuous involvement; and "generalized" connotes complete or nearly complete involvement, whereas "systemic" connotes involvement of a thoracic structure or tissue as part of a process involving the entire body.

discrete *adj.*   (radiol.) Separate, individually distinct; hence, with respect to opacities, usually circumscribed.

Antonyms: Confluent, coalescent.

An acceptable descriptor.

disseminated *adj.*   1. (pathophysiol.) Widely but discontinuously distributed through an organ or type of tissue. 2. (radiol.) Widespread but anatomically discontinuous (said of shadows and by inference of the states or processes producing them).

Synonyms: Diffuse (*q.v.*), generalized, systemic.

A useful and acceptable term.

doubling time *n.*   (radiol.) The time span over which a pulmonary nodule or mass doubles in volume (increases its diameter by a factor of 1.25).

An acceptable term. The concept should be used with caution as a criterion for distinguishing benign from malignant nodules.

embolus *n.*   1. (pathol.) A clot or mass of foreign material that has been carried by the bloodstream to occlude partly or completely the lumen of a blood vessel. 2. (radiol.) (a) A lucent defect or obstruction within an opacified blood vessel presumed to represent an embolus in the pathologic sense. (b) An acutely dilated pulmonary artery presumed to represent the presence of blood clot or other embolic material. *Qualifiers:* acute, chronic; air, fat, amniotic fluid, parasitic, neoplastic, tissue, foreign material (*e.g.*, iodized oil, mercury, talc); septic, therapeutic, paradoxical.

In sense 2(a), an inferred conclusion based on reliable evidence (arteriography); in sense 2(b), based on highly suggestive evidence (conventional roentgenography) in the appropriate clinical setting. A useful descriptor, particularly in arteriography.

emphysema *n.*   1. (pathol.) (a) A morbid condition of the lung characterized by abnormally expanded air spaces distal to the terminal bronchiole, with or without destruction of the air-space walls (per Ciba Conference, 1959). (b) As above, but "with destruction of the walls of involved air spaces" specified (per World Health Organization, 1961, and American Thoracic Society, 1962). 2. (radiol.) Overinflation of all or a portion of one or both lungs, with or without associated oligemia (*q.v.*), presumed to represent morphologic emphysema.

In radiology, an inferred conclusion based on usually reliable signs (if the disease is moderate or advanced). Applicable only in an appropriate clinical setting and, in the sense of the ATS definition, not applicable to spasmodic asthma or compensatory overinflation.

fibrocalcific *adj.*   (radiol.) Of or pertaining to sharply defined, linear, and/or nodular opacities containing calcification(s) (*q.v.*), usually occurring in the upper lobes and presumed to represent old granulomatous lesions.

A widely used and acceptable roentgenologic descriptor.

WORD OR TERM	COMMENTS
fibronodular *adj.* (radiol.) Of or pertaining to sharply defined, approximately circular opacities occurring singly or in clusters, usually in the upper lobes, and associated with linear opacities and distortion (retraction) of adjacent structures. A finding usually presumed to represent old granulomatous disease.	An inferred conclusion usually employed as a roentgenologic descriptor. Its use is not recommended.
fibrosis *n.* 1. (pathol.) (a) Cellular fibrous tissue or dense acellular collagenous tissue. (b) The process of proliferation of fibroblasts leading to the formation of fibrous or collagenous tissue. 2. (radiol.) Any opacity presumed to represent fibrous or collagenous tissue; applicable to linear, nodular, or stellate opacities that are sharply defined, that are associated with evidence of loss of volume in the affected portion of the lung and/or with deformity of adjacent structures, and that show no change over a period of months or years. Also applicable with caution to a diffuse pattern of opacity if there is evidence of progressive loss of lung volume or if the pattern of opacity is unchanged over time.	In radiology, an inferred conclusion often used as a descriptor. An acceptable term if used in strict accordance with the criteria cited.
fissure *n.* 1. (anat.) The infolding of visceral pleura that separates one lobe or a portion of a lobe from another. 2. (radiol.) A linear opacity normally 1 mm or less in width that corresponds in position and extent to the anatomic separation of pulmonary lobes or portions of lobes. *Qualifiers:* minor, major, horizontal, oblique, accessory, anomalous, azygos, inferior accessory. *Synonym:* Interlobar septum.	A specific feature of anatomy.
Fleischner's line(s) *n.* (radiol.) A straight, curved, or irregular linear opacity that is visible in multiple projections; is usually situated in the lower half of the lung; is usually approximately horizontal, but may be oriented in any direction; and may or may not appear to extend to the pleural surface. Such lines vary markedly in length and width; their exact pathologic significance is unknown.	An acceptable term. However, the term "linear opacity," properly qualified with respect to location, dimensions, and orientation, is preferred. There are no synonyms ("platelike," "discoid," and "platter" atelectasis should *not* be employed as synonyms; in the absence of clear histologic evidence of the significance of Fleischner's lines, the inferred identification of such lines with a form of atelectasis is unwarranted).
fluffy *adj.* (radiol.) In describing opacities: Ill-defined, lacking clear-cut margins; resembling down or fluff. *Synonyms:* Shaggy, poorly defined.	An imprecise descriptor of limited usefulness.
ground-glass pattern *n.* (radiol.) Any extended, finely granular pattern of pulmonary opacity within which normal anatomic details are partly obscured. Term derived from a fancied resemblance to etched or abraded glass. *Synonym:* Granular pattern.	A nonspecific roentgenologic descriptor of limited usefulness; the synonym is preferred.
hernia *n.* (clin./morphol./radiol.) The protrusion of all or part of an organ or tissue through an abnormal opening.	An inferred conclusion to be used only within the precise terms of the definition. Thus, in the thorax the word is appropriate in relation to the diaphragm but should not be used with reference to pulmonary overinflation and mediastinal displacement.
hilum *n, pl.* -la. 1. (anat.) A depression or pit in that part of an organ where the vessels and nerves enter. 2. (radiol.) The composite shadow at the root of each lung composed of bronchi, pulmonary arteries and veins, lymph nodes, nerves, bronchial vessels, and associated areolar tissue. *Synonyms:* Lung root; hilus (hili).	A specific element of pulmonary anatomy. Hilum (hila) is preferred to hilus (hili).

WORD OR TERM	COMMENTS

homogeneous *adj.*   (radiol.) Of uniform opacity or texture throughout.

A useful roentgenologic descriptor. Inhomogeneous is the preferred antonym.

Antonyms: Inhomogeneous, nonhomogeneous, heterogeneous.

honeycomb pattern *n.*   1. (pathol.) A multitude of irregular cystic spaces in pulmonary tissue that are generally lined with bronchiolar epithelium and have markedly thickened walls composed of dense fibrous tissue, with or without associated chronic inflammation. 2. (radiol.) A number of closely approximated ring shadows representing air spaces 5 to 10 mm in diameter with walls 2 to 3 mm thick that resemble a true honeycomb; a finding whose occurrence implies "end-stage" lung.

It is recommended that the term be used strictly in accordance with the dimensional limits cited, in which case it possesses specific connotation.

hyperemia *n.*   1. (pathol./physiol.) An excess of blood in a part of the body; engorgement. 2. (radiol.) Increased blood flow.

Synonym: Pleonemia (*q.v.*).

While semantically correct, this word has come through common usage to mean the increased blood flow that is part of the inflammatory response. We recommend that it be used as a descriptor only in arteriography. The synonym is preferred when indicating increased blood flow to the lungs.

hypertension *n.*   (clin./radiol.) Elevation above normal levels of systolic and/or diastolic pressure within the systemic or pulmonary vascular bed. Generally accepted empirical levels of pressure for systemic arterial hypertension are 140 systolic, 90 diastolic; systemic venous hypertension, 12 mm Hg; pulmonary arterial hypertension, 30 mm Hg systolic, 15 diastolic; pulmonary venous hypertension, 12 mm Hg.

Synonym: High blood pressure.

With the exception of systemic arterial hypertension, roentgenologic assessment of hypertension in each of the four vascular compartments constitutes an inferred conclusion, although based on usually reliable signs.

infarct *n.*   (Literally, a portion of tissue stuffed with extravasated blood or serum.) 1. (pathol.) A zone of ischemic necrosis surrounded by hyperemic lung resulting from occlusion of the region's feeding vessel, usually by an embolus. 2. (radiol.) A pulmonary opacity that, by virtue of its temporal development and in the appropriate clinical setting, is considered to result from thromboembolic occlusion of a feeding vessel. The opacity is commonly but not exclusively hump-shaped and pleural based when viewed in profile and poorly defined and round when viewed *en face*.

An inferred roentgenologic conclusion acceptable in the proper clinical setting and with appropriate signs. Subsequent events may establish that the opacity was the result of either hemorrhage or tissue necrosis. The word should not be used in the absence of an opacity (*e.g.*, with oligemia).

infiltrate *n.*   1. (pathophysiol.) Any substance or type of cell that occurs within or spreads through the interstices (interstitium and/or alveoli) of the lung, which is foreign to the lung or which accumulates in greater than normal quantity within it. 2. (radiol.) (a) An ill-defined opacity in the lung that neither destroys nor displaces the gross morphology of the lung and is presumed to represent an infiltrate in the pathophysiologic sense. (b) Any ill-defined opacity in the lung.

An inferred and often unwarranted conclusion used as a descriptor. The term is almost invariably used in sense 2(b) in which it serves no useful purpose, and, lacking a specific connotation, is so variably used as to cause great confusion. The term's use as a descriptor is to be condemned. The preferred word is "opacity," properly qualified with respect to location, dimensions, and definition.

inflation *n.*   (physiol./radiol.) The state or process of being expanded or filled with gas; used specifically with reference to the expansion of the lungs with air. *Qualifiers:* overinflation (preferred) or hyperinflation; underinflation (preferred) or hypoinflation.

Synonyms: Aeration, inhalation, inspiration.

"Inflation" connotes expansion with gas or air. "Aeration" connotes the admission of air, exposure to air. "Inhalation" refers specifically to the act of drawing air into the lungs in the process of breathing (as opposed to exhalation); "inspiration," with reference to breathing, is similar in connotation. The word "inflation" is the preferred term, since it avoids the confusion that surrounds the meaning of aeration as a result of common misusage.

WORD OR TERM	COMMENTS

interface *n.* (radiol.) The common boundary between the shadows of two juxtaposed structures or tissues of different texture or opacity (*e.g.*, lung and heart).

Synonyms: Edge, border.

A useful roentgenologic descriptor.

interstitium *n.* (anat./radiol.) A continuum of loose connective tissue throughout the lung consisting of three subdivisions: (a) broncho-arterial (axial), surrounding the broncho-arterial bundles from the hila to the point at which bronchiolar walls become intimately related to lung parenchyma; (b) parenchymal (acinar), situated between alveolar and capillary basement membranes; and (c) subpleural, situated between the pleura and lung parenchyma and continuous with the interlobular septa and perivenous interstitial space that extends from the lung periphery to the hila.

Synonym: Interstitial space.

A useful anatomic term. The interstitium of the lung is not normally visible roentgenographically and only becomes visible when disease (*e.g.*, edema) increases its volume and attenuation.

Kerley line *n.* (radiol.) A linear opacity, which, depending on its location, extent, and orientation, may be further classified as follows: Kerley A line—an essentially straight linear opacity 2 to 6 cm in length and 1 to 3 mm in width, usually situated in an upper lung zone, that points toward the hilum centrally and is directed toward but does not extend to the pleural surface peripherally. Kerley B line—a straight linear opacity 1.5 to 2 cm in length and 1 to 2 mm in width, usually situated at the lung base, and oriented at right angles to the pleural surface with which it is usually in contact. Kerley C lines—a group of branching, linear opacities producing the appearance of a fine net, situated at the lung base and representing Kerley B lines seen *en face*.

Synonym: Septal line(s).

A specific feature of pathologic/roentgenologic anatomy. Except when it is essential to distinguish A, B, and C lines, the term "septal line" is preferred. "Lymphatic line" is anatomically inaccurate and should never be used.

line *n.* (radiol.) A longitudinal opacity no greater than 2 mm in width (*cf.* stripe).

A useful word appropriately employed in the description of roentgenographic shadows within the mediastinum (*e.g.*, anterior junction line) or lung (interlobar fissures).

linear opacity *n.* (radiol.) A shadow resembling a line; hence, any elongated opacity of approximately uniform width.

Synonyms: Line, line shadow, linear shadow, band shadow.

A generic roentgenologic descriptor of great usefulness. "Band shadow" and "line shadow" have been employed by some to identify elongated shadows more than 2 mm wide and less than 2 mm wide, respectively; "linear opacity," qualified by a statement of specific dimensions, is the preferred term. The length, width, anatomic location, and orientation of such a shadow should be specified.

lobe *n.* (anat./radiol.) One of the principal divisions of the lungs (usually three on the right, two on the left), each of which is enveloped by the visceral pleura except at the hilum and in areas of developmental deficiency where fissures are incomplete. The lobes are separated in whole or in part by pleural fissures.

A specific feature of pulmonary anatomy.

lobule *n.* (anat./radiol.) A unit of lung structure. A subdivision of lung parenchyma that is of two types: (a) primary, arising from the last respiratory bronchiole and consisting of a series of alveolar ducts, atria, alveolar sacs, and alveoli, together with their accompanying blood vessels and nerves; (b) secondary, composed of a variable number of acini (usually 3 to 5) and bounded in most cases by connective tissue septa.

Acinus is the preferred anatomic/physiologic unit of lung structure. Since a primary lobule is not visible roentgenographically, the use of the term has been largely abandoned. When unmodified, the word "lobule" refers to a secondary lobule. A secondary pulmonary lobule occasionally becomes visible when it is either selectively

WORD OR TERM	COMMENTS

consolidated or its surrounding connective tissue septa become visible from a process such as edema.

lucency *n.* (radiol.) The shadow of an absorber that attenuates the primary x-ray beam less effectively than do surrounding absorbers. Hence, in a roentgenogram, any circumscribed area that appears more nearly black (of greater photometric density) than its surround. Usually applied to local shadows of air density whose attenuation is less than that of surrounding lung (*e.g.*, a bulla) or of fat density when surrounded by a more effective absorber such as muscle.

Synonyms: Radiolucency, translucency, transradiancy.

This term, employed by analogy with "opacity," is acceptable in American usage, although it is etymologically indefensible. In British usage, "transradiancy" is preferred.

lymphadenopathy *n.* (clin./pathol./radiol.) Any abnormality of lymph nodes; by common usage usually restricted to enlargement of lymph nodes.

Synonym: Lymph node enlargement.

Since "adeno-" specifically relates to a glandular structure and since lymph nodes are not glands, the term is a misnomer and its use is to be condemned in favor of its synonym.

marking(s) *n.* (radiol.) A descriptor variously used with reference to the shadows produced by a combination of normal pulmonary structures (blood vessels, bronchi, etc.). Usually used in the plural and following "lung" or "bronchovascular."

Synonym: Linear opacity.

When used alone, a vague descriptor of little value and not recommended. With proper qualification, the term is acceptable.

mass *n.* (radiol.) Any pulmonary or pleural lesion represented in a roentgenogram by a discrete opacity greater than 30 mm in diameter (without regard to contour, border characteristics, or homogeneity), but explicitly shown or presumed to be extended in all three dimensions.

Synonym: Tumor (q.v.).

A useful and recommended descriptor. Should always be qualified with respect to size, location, contour, definition, homogeneity, opacity, and number. Its use as a qualifier of "lesion" is to be deplored.

medulla *n.* (radiol.) That portion of the lung situated between the hilum and cortex (*q.v.*).

A term and concept of limited usefulness.

miliary pattern *n.* (radiol.) A collection of tiny discrete opacities in the lungs, each measuring 2 mm or less in diameter, and generally uniform in size and widespread in distribution.

Synonym: Micronodular pattern.

An acceptable descriptor without etiologic connotation.

mucoid impaction *n.* (radiol.) A broad I-, Y-, or V-shaped roentgenographic opacity caused by the presence within a proximal airway (lobar, segmental, or subsegmental bronchus) of thick, tenacious mucus, usually associated with airway dilatation. The shape of the opacity depends upon the branching pattern of airway involved.

Synonym: Bronchocele.

An inferred conclusion based on usually reliable signs. A useful descriptor preferred to its synonym.

Mueller maneuver *n.* (physiol.) Inspiration against a closed glottis, usually but not necessarily from a position of residual volume.

A useful technique for producing transient decrease in intrathoracic pressure.

nodular pattern *n.* (radiol.) A collection of innumerable, small discrete opacities ranging in diameter from 2 to 10 mm, generally uniform in size and widespread in distribution, and without marginal spiculation (*cf.* reticulonodular pattern).

An acceptable roentgenologic descriptor without specific pathologic or etiologic implications. The size of the nodules should be specified, either as a range or as an average.

nodule *n.* (radiol.) Any pulmonary or pleural lesion represented in a roentgenogram by a sharply defined, discrete, approximately circular opacity 2 to 30 mm in diameter (*cf.* mass).

Synonym: Coin lesion (*q.v.*).

A useful and recommended descriptor to be used in preference to its synonym, which is a colloquial abomination. Should always be qualified with respect to size, location, border characteristics, number, and opacity.

WORD OR TERM	COMMENT

oligemia *n.*   1. (pathol./physiol.) Reduced blood flow to the lungs or a portion thereof. 2. (radiol.) General or local decrease in the apparent width of visible pulmonary vessels, suggesting less than normal blood flow. *Qualifiers:* acute, chronic; local, general.

Synonym: Reduced blood flow.

> An inferred conclusion usually used as descriptor and appropriately based on reliable signs. An acceptable term.

opacity *n.*   (radiol.) The shadow of an absorber that attenuates the x-ray beam more effectively than do surrounding absorbers. Hence, in a roentgenogram, any circumscribed area that appears more nearly white (of lesser photometric density) than its surround. Usually applied to the shadows of nonspecific pulmonary collections of fluid, tissue, etc., whose attenuation exceeds that of the surrounding aerated lung.

Synonym: Radiopacity (*cf.* density).

> An essential and recommended roentgenologic descriptor. In the context of roentgenologic reporting, "radiopaque" is acceptable but seems redundant; however, it is preferred in British usage. "Density" (*q.v.*) should *never* be used in this context.

opaque *adj.*   (radiol.) Impervious to x-rays.

Synonym: Radiopaque.

> Opaque and radiopaque are both acceptable terms, although the former is preferred (*see* opacity).

ossification *n.*   (radiol.) Calcific opacities within the lung that represent trabecular bone; applicable to calcific opacities that either display morphologic characteristics of trabecular bone (trabeculation and a defined cortex) or occur in association with a lesion known histologically to produce trabecular bone within lung (*e.g.*, mitral stenosis).

Synonyms: Ossific nodulation, ossific nodule(s).

> A useful roentgenologic term, although usually an inferred conclusion. To be distinguished from "calcification" (*q.v.*).

paraspinal line *n.*   (radiol.) A vertically oriented interface usually seen in a frontal chest roentgenogram to the left (rarely to the right) of the thoracic vertebral column. It extends from the aortic arch to the diaphragm and represents contact between aerated lower lobe and adjacent mediastinal tissues. The anatomic interface is situated posterior to the descending aorta and is seen between the left lateral margin of the aorta and the spine.

Synonyms: Left paraspinal pleural reflection; left paraspinal interface.

> A specific feature of roentgenologic anatomy. Either of the synonyms cited is preferred inasmuch as the shadow represents an interface, not a line.

parenchyma *n.*   1. (anat.) The gas-exchanging portion of the lung consisting of the alveoli and their capillaries, estimated to comprise approximately 90 per cent of total lung volume. 2. (radiol.) All lung tissue exclusive of visible pulmonary vessels and airways.

> A useful anatomic concept and an acceptable roentgenologic descriptor.

perfusion *n.*   (physiol./radiol.) The passage of blood into and out of the lung.

Synonym: Pulmonary blood flow.

> A useful and recommended term.

phantom tumor *n.*   (radiol.) A shadow produced by a local collection of fluid in one of the interlobar fissures (most often the minor fissure), usually possessing an elliptical configuration in one roentgenographic projection and a rounded configuration in the other, thus resembling a tumor. It is commonly caused by cardiac decompensation and usually disappears with appropriate therapy.

Synonyms: Vanishing tumor, pseudotumor.

> An explicit diagnostic conclusion from serial roentgenograms but only an inferred conclusion from a single examination. An acceptable descriptor.

platelike atelectasis *n.*   (radiol.) A linear or planar opacity presumed to represent diminished volume in a portion of the lung; usually situated in lower lung zones.

Synonyms: Platter, linear, or discoid atelectasis.

> An inferred conclusion usually not subject to proof and often unwarranted. Its use as a descriptor is not recommended. "Linear opacity" is preferred.

pleonemia *n.*   (pathol./physiol./radiol.) Increased blood flow to the lungs or a portion thereof, manifested roentgenologically by a general or local increase in the width of visible pulmonary vessels.

Synonyms: Increased blood flow, hyperemia.

> An inferred conclusion often used as a descriptor and based on usually reliable signs. An acceptable term preferable to hyperemia (*q.v.*).

WORD OR TERM	COMMENTS

pneumatocele *n.* (pathol./radiol.) A thin-walled, gas-filled space within the lung usually occurring in association with acute pneumonia (most commonly of staphylococcal etiology) and almost invariably transient.

An inferred conclusion. An acceptable descriptor if used in accordance with the precise definition.

pneumomediastinum *n.* (pathol./radiol.) A state characterized by the presence of gas in mediastinal tissues outside the esophagus, tracheobronchial tree, or pericardium. *Qualifiers:* spontaneous, traumatic, diagnostic.

Synonym: Mediastinal emphysema.

An appropriate descriptor based on roentgenologic signs alone; preferred to its synonym.

pneumonia *n.* (pathol./radiol.) Infection of the air spaces and/or interstitium of the lung. *Qualifiers* may be employed to indicate temporal course (acute, chronic), predominant anatomic involvement (air-space or lobar, interstitial, bronchial), or etiology (bacterial, viral, fungal).

Synonym: Pneumonitis.

An inferred conclusion, based on usually reliable signs. Generally preferred to its synonym, although the latter is sometimes used to designate infection caused by viruses or Mycoplasma pneumoniae.

pneumothorax *n.* (pathol./radiol.) A state characterized by the presence of gas within the pleural space. *Qualifiers:* spontaneous, traumatic, diagnostic, tension (*q.v.*).

A diagnostic conclusion appropriately based on roentgenologic evidence alone.

popcorn calcification *n.* (radiol.) A cluster of sharply defined, irregularly lobulated, calcific opacities, usually within a pulmonary nodule, suggesting the appearance of popcorn.

An acceptable descriptor.

posterior junction line *n.* (radiol.) A vertically oriented, linear or curvilinear opacity approximately 2 mm wide, commonly projected on the tracheal air shadow, and usually slightly concave to the right. It is produced by the shadows of the right and left pleurae in intimate contact between the aerated lungs. It represents the plane of contact between the lungs posterior to the trachea and esophagus and anterior to the spine; hence, in contrast to the anterior junction line, it may project both above and below the suprasternal notch.

Synonyms: Posterior mediastinal septum; posterior mediastinal line; supra-aortic posterior junction line or stripe; mesentery of the esophagus.

A specific feature of roentgenologic anatomy; to be preferred to cited synonyms.

posterior tracheal stripe *n.* (radiol.) A vertically oriented linear opacity ranging in width from 2 to 5 mm, extending from the thoracic inlet to the bifurcation of the trachea, and visible only on lateral roentgenograms of the chest. It is situated between the air shadow of the trachea and the right lung and is formed by the posterior tracheal wall and contiguous mediastinal interstitial tissue.

Synonym: Posterior tracheal band.

A specific feature of radiologic anatomy; to be preferred to its synonym.

primary complex *n.* 1. (pathol.) The combination of a focus of pneumonia due to a primary infection (*e.g.*, tuberculosis or histoplasmosis) with granulomas in the draining hilar or mediastinal lymph nodes. 2. (radiol.) (a) One or more irregular opacities of variable extent and location assumed to represent consolidation of lung parenchyma, associated with enlargement of hilar or mediastinal lymph nodes, an appearance presumed to represent active infection. (b) One or more small, sharply defined parenchymal opacities (often calcified) associated with calcification of hilar or mediastinal lymph nodes, an appearance usually regarded as evidence of an inactive process.

A useful inferred conclusion. "Primary complex" is to be preferred to "Ranke complex," which is acceptable but rarely used. "Ghon complex" represents an inappropriate use of the eponym and is unacceptable (Ghon described the pulmonary abnormality alone, which thus becomes a Ghon focus or Ghon lesion).

profusion *n.* (radiol.) The number of small opacities per unit area or zone of lung. In the ILO classification of radiographs of the pneumoconioses, the qualifiers 0 through 3 subdivide the profusion into 4 categories. The profusion categories may be further subdivided by employing a 12-point scale.

A useful word to describe the number of opacities in any diffuse disease, including the pneumoconioses.

WORD OR TERM	COMMENTS

pseudocavity *n.* (radiol.) A state in which a pulmonary nodule or mass possesses a central portion that is more lucent than its periphery (thus suggesting cavitation) but in which subsequent computed tomography or pathologic examination reveals only the presence of necrotic tissue high in lipid content, with no true cavity.

An inferred conclusion sometimes used as a descriptor. The term is without etiologic connotation.

Synonym: Simulated cavity.

pulmonary edema *n.* 1. (pathophysiol.) The accumulation of liquid in the interstitial compartment of the lung with or without associated alveolar filling. Specifically, the accumulation of water, protein, and solutes (transudate), usually due to one or a combination of the following: (a) increased pressure in the microvascular bed, (b) increased microvascular permeability, or (c) impaired lymphatic drainage. Also, the accumulation of water, protein, solutes, and inflammatory cells (exudate) in response to inflammation of any type (*e.g.*, infection, allergy, trauma, or circulating toxins). 2. (radiol.) A pattern of opacity (usually bilaterally symmetrical) believed to represent interstitial thickening or alveolar filling when associated findings and/or history suggest one of the processes enumerated above. *Qualifiers:* interstitial, air-space, alveolar.

An inferred conclusion often employed as a descriptor, based on usually reliable signs. A useful and acceptable term when used in an appropriate clinical setting. The synonyms are colloquialisms to be avoided.

Synonyms: Wet, boggy, or moist lung.

respiratory failure *n.* (physiol.) A state characterized by an arterial P_{O_2} below 60 mm Hg or an arterial P_{CO_2} above 49 mm Hg, at rest at sea level, resulting from impaired respiratory function.

A useful term that should be restricted to clinical and physiologic usage. It is preferred to its synonym.

Synonym: Pulmonary insufficiency.

reticular pattern *n.* (radiol.) A collection of innumerable small linear opacities that together produce an appearance resembling a net. *Qualifiers:* fine, medium, coarse.

A recommended descriptor that usually indicates predominant abnormality of the pulmonary interstitium. The synonym should be restricted to the roentgenographic characterization of pneumoconiosis.

Synonym: Small irregular opacities (in the ILO classification of radiographs of the pneumoconioses).

reticulonodular pattern *n.* (radiol.) A collection of innumerable small, linear, and nodular opacities that together produce a composite appearance resembling a net with small superimposed nodules. In common usage, the reticular and nodular elements are dimensionally of similar magnitude. *Qualifiers:* fine, medium, coarse.

An acceptable roentgenologic descriptor that usually indicates predominant abnormality of the pulmonary interstitium.

right tracheal stripe *n.* (radiol.) A vertically oriented linear opacity approximately 2 to 3 mm wide extending from the thoracic inlet to the right tracheobronchial angle. It is situated between the air shadow of the trachea and the right lung and is formed by the right tracheal wall and contiguous mediastinal interstitial tissue and pleura.

A specific feature of radiologic anatomy; to be preferred to the cited synonym since the opacity is caused chiefly by the tracheal wall itself.

Synonym: Right paratracheal stripe or band.

segment *n.* (anat./radiol.) One of the principal anatomic subdivisions of the pulmonary lobes served by a major branch of a lobar bronchus. *Qualifier:* bronchopulmonary.

A useful anatomic and roentgenologic descriptor.

septal line(s) *n.* (radiol.) Usually used in the plural, a generic term for linear opacities of varied distribution produced when the interstitium between pulmonary lobules is thickened (*e.g.*, by fluid, dust deposition, cellular material).

A specific feature of roentgenologic pathology, sometimes inferred. A recommended term. "Kerley line" is acceptable, particularly when seeking to identify a particular type of septal line (*e.g.*, Kerley B line).

Synonym: Kerley line (*q.v.*).

shadow *n.* (radiol.) In clinical roentgenography, any perceptible discontinuity in film blackening (or fluoroscopic image or CRT display) attributed to the attenuation of the x-ray beam by a

A useful and recommended descriptor to be employed only when more specific identification is not possible.

WORD OR TERM	COMMENTS

specific anatomic absorber or lesion on or within the body of the patient; an opacity or lucency. The word should always be qualified as precisely as possible with respect to size, contour, location, opacity, lucency, and so on.

silhouette sign *n.* (radiol.) The effacement of an anatomic soft tissue border within the thorax by a process of equal or similar density in contiguous lung or pleura (*e.g.*, consolidation of adjacent lung or accumulation of fluid in the contiguous pleural space).

Useful in detecting and localizing an opacity along the axis of the x-ray beam. Although the physical basis underlying the production of this sign is contentious, the term is a widely accepted and useful descriptor. Despite the fact that the definition implies *loss* of silhouette, the term has acquired such common popularity that its continued use is recommended.

small irregular opacities *n.* (radiol.) A collection of innumerable small linear opacities that together produce an appearance resembling a net. In the ILO/1980 classification of radiographs of the pneumoconioses, the qualifiers s, t, and u subdivide the dimensions of the opacities into three diameter ranges—up to 1.5 mm, 1.5 to 3 mm, and 3 to 10 mm, respectively.

Synonym: Reticular pattern (*q.v.*).

A term to be employed specifically to describe roentgenographic manifestations of the pneumoconioses; the synonym is preferred for nonpneumoconiotic disease.

small rounded opacities *n.* (radiol.) A collection of innumerable pulmonary nodules ranging in diameter from bare visibility up to 10 mm, usually widespread in distribution. In the ILO/1980 classification of radiographs of the pneumoconioses, the qualifiers p, q, and r subdivide the dimensions of the opacities into three diameter ranges—up to 1.5 mm, 1.5 to 3 mm, and 3 to 10 mm, respectively.

Synonym: Nodular pattern (*q.v.*).

A term to be employed specifically to describe roentgenographic manifestations of the pneumoconioses; the synonym is preferred for nonpneumoconiotic disease.

stripe *n.* (radiol.) A longitudinal composite opacity measuring 2 to 5 mm in width (*cf.* line).

An acceptable descriptor when limited to anatomic structures within the mediastinum (*e.g.*, right tracheal stripe).

subsegment *n.* (anat./radiol.) A unit of pulmonary tissue supplied by a bronchus of lesser order than a segmental bonchus.

A useful anatomic and roentgenologic descriptor.

tension *adj.* 1. (physiol./clin.) When used with reference to pneumo- or hydrothorax, a state characterized by cardiorespiratory functional impairment. 2. (radiol.) The accumulation of gas or fluid in a pleural space in an amount sufficient to cause airlessness of the ipsilateral lung, marked depression of the ipsilateral hemidiaphragm, and displacement of the mediastinum to the opposite side.

An inferred conclusion to be used only in the presence of clinical cardiorespiratory embarrassment. In fact, "tension" in relation to pneumothorax exists only during the expiratory phase of the respiratory cycle, since pleural pressure on inspiration is usually subatmospheric. The word should not be employed as in the term "tension cyst," which does not satisfy the criteria cited.

thromboembolism *n.* (pathol./clin./radiol.) Partial or complete occlusion of the lumen of a blood vessel by a clot originating from a thrombus (*q.v.*).

An inferred conclusion sometimes based on reliable signs (in conventional roentgenography) or a diagnostic conclusion based on roentgenologic evidence alone (in angiography).

thrombosis *n.* (pathol./radiol.) The state or process of thrombus formation within a blood vessel or heart chamber.

Cf. clot.

thrombus *n.* (pathol./radiol.) A mass of semisolidified blood, composed chiefly of platelets and fibrin with entrapped cellular elements, at the site of its formation in a blood vessel or heart chamber.

A useful descriptor to be employed only in the precise sense of the definition. (*Cf.* embolus.)

WORD OR TERM	COMMENTS

tramline shadow *n.* (radiol.) Parallel or slightly convergent linear opacities that suggest the planar projection of tubular structures and that correspond in location and orientation to elements of the bronchial tree. They are generally assumed to represent thickened bronchial walls.

Synonyms: Thickened bronchial wall, tubular shadow (*q.v.*).

A roentgenologic descriptor which is not recommended in deference to either of the synonyms. Such shadows are of possible pathologic significance only when they occur outside the limits of the hilar shadows where bronchial walls may be seen normally.

tubular shadow *n.* (radiol.) 1. Paired, parallel, or slightly convergent linear opacities presumed to represent the walls of a tubular structure seen *en face* (*e.g.*, a bronchus). 2. An approximately circular opacity presumed to represent the wall of a tubular structure seen end-on.

Synonyms: Tramline shadow (*q.v.*), thickened bronchial wall.

Acceptable if the anatomic nature of a shadow is obscure; otherwise the more precise "thickened bronchial wall" is to be preferred.

tumor *n.* 1. (general) A swelling or morbid enlargement. 2. (pathol./radiol.) Literally, a mass (*q.v.*), not differentiated as to its neoplastic or non-neoplastic nature.

Synonym: Mass.

A useful descriptor, although "mass" is preferred. The use of the word as a synonym for neoplasm is to be condemned.

Valsalva maneuver *n.* (physiol.) Forced expiration against a closed glottis, usually but not necessarily from a position of total lung capacity.

A useful technique to produce transient increase in intrathoracic pressure.

vasoconstriction *n.* (physiol.) Narrowing of muscular blood vessels (mainly arterioles) by contraction of their muscle layer. 2. (radiol.) Local or general reduction in the caliber of visible pulmonary vessels (oligemia [*q.v.*]), presumed to result from decreased flow occasioned by contraction of muscular pulmonary arteries. *Qualifiers:* hypoxic, reflex.

An inferred conclusion based on usually reliable signs. The word is not synonymous with oligemia; although the latter is a *sign* of vasoconstriction, it may also occur when vessel narrowing is organic (as in emphysema) rather than functional and potentially reversible.

vasodilation *n.* (radiol.) The local or general increase in the width of visible pulmonary vessels resulting from increased pulmonary blood flow.

Synonym: Vasodilatation.

An inferred conclusion based on usually reliable signs.

ventilation *n.* (physiol./radiol.) The movement of air into and out of the lungs; inspiration and expiration. *Qualifiers:* hyperventilation (preferred), or overventilation; hypoventilation (preferred), or underventilation.

The term always implies a biphasic dynamic process of admission and expulsion; hence, it cannot be assessed from a single static image (*see* inflation).

INDEX

Page numbers in *italics* indicate illustrations; page numbers followed by t indicate tables.